Physiotherapy for Respiratory and Cardiac Problems

To our families and to our teachers

For Churchill Livingstone:

Editorial Director, Health Professions: Mary Law
Project Development Manager: Katrina Mather
Design Direction: Judith Wright

Physiotherapy for Respiratory and Cardiac Problems

Adults and Paediatrics

Edited by

Jennifer A Pryor MBA MSc FNZSP MCSP
Research Fellow, Physiotherapy, Royal Brompton & Harefield NHS Trust, London, UK

S Ammani Prasad MCSP
Research Physiotherapist, Cystic Fibrosis Unit, Great Ormond Street Hospital for Children NHS Trust, London, UK

THIRD EDITION

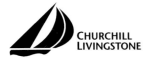
CHURCHILL
LIVINGSTONE

EDINBURGH LONDON NEW YORK OXFORD PHILADELPHIA ST LOUIS SYDNEY TORONTO 2002

CHURCHILL LIVINGSTONE
An imprint of Elsevier Science Limited

First edition 1993
Second edition 1998
Third edition 2002
Reprinted 2002

ISBN 0 443 07075 X

British Library Cataloguing in Publication Data
A catalogue record for this book is available from the British Library

Library of Congress Cataloging in Publication Data
A catalog record for this book is available from the Library of
Congress

Note
Medical knowledge is constantly changing. As new information
becomes available, changes in treatment, procedures, equipment and
the use of drugs become necessary. The author, contributors and the
publishers have taken care to ensure that the information given in this
text is accurate and up to date. However, readers are strongly advised
to confirm that the information, especially with regard to drug usage,
complies with the latest legislation and standards of practice.

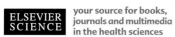 your source for books,
journals and multimedia
in the health sciences
www.elsevierhealth.com

The
publisher's
policy is to use
**paper manufactured
from sustainable forests**

Printed in China

Contents

Contributors

Ian Balfour-Lynn BSc MD MBBS MRCP FRCS (Ed)
FRCPCH DHMSA
Consultant in Paediatric Respiratory Medicine,
Royal Brompton & Harefield NHS Trust,
London, UK

Anne Ballinger MD FRCP
Senior Lecturer, Digestive Diseases Research
Centre, St Bartholomew's and Royal London
School of Medicine and Dentistry, London, UK

Stephen J Barton RGN RMN BSc (Hons)
Senior Nurse, Royal Brompton & Harefield
NHS Trust, London, UK

Jenny Bell BA MPhil PhD
Project Director, British Association for Cardiac
Rehabilitation, British Cardiac Society, London,
UK

Delva Bethune MHSc DipPT DipOT RPT
Formerly Associate Professor, Queen's
University, School of Rehabilitation Therapy,
Faculty of Health Sciences, Division of Physical
Therapy; Downtown Physiotherapy Clinic and
Health Centre, Kingston, Ontario, Canada

Catherine E Bray BAppSci
Director, Cardiorespiratory Therapy Services,
Therapy Services, Darlinghurst, Australia

Mandy Bryon BA MSc PhD
Consultant Clinical Psychologist, Department of
Psychological Medicine, Great Ormond Street
Hospital for Children NHS Trust, London, UK

Wendy Burford RGN BTTA
Clinical Nurse Specialist, Lung Cancer, University
of London College Hospitals, London, UK

Conor D Collins BSc MB MRCPI FRCR
Consultant Radiologist, St Vincent's Hospital,
Dublin, Ireland

Susan J Copley MD MRCP FRCR
Consultant Radiologist, The Hammersmith
Hospitals NHS Trust, London, UK

Elizabeth Dean PhD PT
Professor, School of Rehabilitation Sciences,
University of British Columbia, Vancouver,
British Columbia, Canada

Mary E Dodd FCSP
Specialist Physiotherapy Clinician, Bradbury
Cystic Fibrosis Unit, Wythenshawe Hospital,
Manchester, UK

Elizabeth R Ellis Grad Dip Phty PhD MHL
Senior Lecturer, School of Physiotherapy,
Faculty of Health Sciences, Lidcombe, Australia

Stephanie Enright MCSP MSc MPhil PhD
Senior Lecturer, Department of Physiotherapy,
University of Salford, Salford, UK

Rachel Garrod PhD MSc PG Cert Ed HE Grad Dip Phys
MCS
Senior Lecturer in Physiotherapy, School of
Physiotherapy, St George's Hospital Medical
School, London, UK

Christopher D George FRCS FRCR
Consultant Radiologist, Department of
Radiology, Epsom and St Helier NHS Trust,
Surrey, UK

Isky Gordon FRCR FRCP
Professor in Paediatric Radiology, Great
Ormond Street Hospital for Children NHS
Trust, London, UK

David M Hansell FRCP FRCR MD
Professor of Thoracic Imaging, Royal Brompton
& Harefield NHS Trust, London, UK

Kathryn Harris Grad Dip Phys, MCSP, SRP
Respiratory Clinical Specialist Physiotherapist,
The Duke of Cornwall Spinal Treatment Centre,
Salisbury District Hospital, Salisbury, UK

Amanda Heinl-Green Grad Dip Phys MCSP
Physiotherapist, Research Fellow, Department of
Gene Therapy, National Heart & Lung Institute,
Imperial College of Science, Technology and
Medicine, London, UK

Amanda Howarth B Med Sci (Hons) MSc RGN
Clinical Nurse Specialist, Pain Clinic, Royal
Hallamshire Hospital, Sheffield, UK

Ian Hudson MD FRCP
Consultant Cardiologist, Leicester General
Hospital, Gwendolen Road, Leicester, UK

Diana M Innocenti FCSP
Formerly Head of Physiotherapy, Guy's
Hospital, London, UK

Sue Jenkins Grad Dip Phys PhD
Associate Professor in Cardiopulmonary
Science, School of Physiotherapy, Curtin
University of Technology, Shenton Park,
Physiotherapy Department, Sir Charles
Gairdner Hospital Nedlands, Western Australia

Mandy Jones PhD MSc Grad Dip Phys
Research Fellow, Respiratory Medicine, Royal
Brompton & Harefield NHS Trust, London,
UK

Fiona Lough MCSP MPhil
Cardiac Rehabilitation Coordinator, Medical
Sciences, Addenbrookes NHS Trust, Cambridge,
UK

Eleanor Main PhD BA MCSP
Lecturer in Children's Physiotherapy Research
Institute of Child Health, London, UK

Sally Middleton MSc (Med) BApplSci (Phty)
Clinical Research Assistant, David Reed
Laboratory, University of Sydney, Sydney,
Australia

Peter G Middleton MBBS (Hons) BSc (Med) PhD
FRACP
Senior Staff Specialist & Head, Cystic Fibrosis
Unit, Department of Respiratory Medicine,
Westmead Hospital, Westmead, Australia

Stephen Patchett MD FRCPI
Consultant Physician/Gastroenterologist,
Beaumont Hospital, Dublin, Ireland

Amanda J Piper BAppSci (Phty) Med PhD
Senior Physiotherapist, Respiratory Failure
Service, Sleep Disorders Unit, Royal Prince
Alfred Hospital, Camperdown, New South
Wales, Australia

Helen M Potter BAppSci (Phty) Grad Dip Manip
Therapy MSc
Manipulative Physiotherapist, In Touch
Physiotherapy, West Perth, Australia

S Ammani Prasad MCSP
Research Physiotherapist, Cystic Fibrosis Unit,
Great Ormond Street Hospital for Children NHS
Trust, London, UK

Jennifer A Pryor MBA MSc FNZSP MCSP
Research Fellow, Physiotherapy, Royal
Brompton & Harefield NHS Trust, London, UK

Sarah C Ridley MCSP
Superintendent Physiotherapist, Physiotherapy
Department, Western General Hospital,
Edinburgh, UK

Julius Sim BA MSc (Soc) PhD MCSP
Professor, Department of Physiotherapy Studies,
University of Keele, Staffordshire, UK

Sally J Singh PhD BA MCSP
Lecturer and Cardiopulmonary Rehabilitation
Coordinator, Department of Respiratory
Medicine, The Glenfield Hospital, Leicester, UK

Linda Tagg GradDipPhys MCSP SRP
Chartered Physiotherapist, Back to Work,
Basingstoke, UK

Robert C Tasker MA MB MD FRCP
Consultant Paediatric Intensivist, Department of
Paediatrics, Addenbrookes Hospital,
Cambridge, UK

Ann Taylor PhD MSc BA MCSP DipTP
Lecturer, Physiotherapy Division, Guy's, King's
and St Thomas' School of Biomedical Sciences,
King's College London, London, UK

Beatrice Tucker BAppSci(Phty) PGradDip Phty MSc
Lecturer, School of Physiotherapy, Curtin
University of Technology, Shenton Park,
Western Australia

John S Turner MBChB MMed MD (UCT) FCP(SA) FCCP
Physician/Critical Care Specialist, Cape Town,
South Africa

Trudy Ward MSc Grad Dip Phys
Therapy Manager, The Duke of Cornwall Spinal
Treatment Centre, Salisbury District Hospital,
Salisbury, UK

A Kevin Webb FRCP
Professor of Respiratory Medicine, Clinical
Director Bradbury Cystic Fibrosis Unit,
Wythenshawe Hospital, Manchester, UK

Barbara A Webber FCSP DSc (Hon)
Formerly Head of Physiotherapy, Royal
Brompton Hospital, London, UK

Jadwiga Wedzicha MA MD FRCP
Professor of Respiratory Medicine,
St Bartholomew's and Royal London School of
Medicine and Dentistry, London, UK

Fran H Woodard MCSP SRP
Head of Therapy Services, Clinical and
Diagnostic Services Directorate, St Mary's NHS
Trust, London, UK

Preface to third edition

This third edition has a much greater emphasis on paediatrics. We have a number of new authors, for both the adult and paediatric sections, who are internationally recognized in their field. We are most grateful to all the authors who have contributed so much of their time both in writing and in updating their sections. It is owing to the multiauthor, multidisciplinary and international characteristics of this book that such a wealth of knowledge can be contained within one text.

A textbook is neither a meta-analysis nor a systematic review of each and every topic covered. Papers on particular topics will be published both during and after publication of this book. When pursuing a subject in detail it is important that the reader also searches the literature but it is hoped that this text will provide a basis for further review and research.

We wish to acknowledge the tremendous help from the many people who have advised and supported us during this project including Guy Thorpe Beeston, Barbara Webber, Margaret Hodson, Robert Dinwiddie, Mary Dodd, Colin Wallis, Peter Pryor and the Medical Illustration Departments at the Institute of Child Health and the Royal Marsden Hospital NHS Trust, particularly Nicholas Geddes, Milena Potucek and Paul Hyett. Our thanks also to our colleagues in the Cystic Fibrosis Departments of the Royal Brompton & Harefield NHS Trust and Great Ormond Street Hospital for Children NHS Trust.

London 2002 J.A.P.
S.A.P.

Preface to second edition

During the last five years the term 'evidence-based medicine' has had an increasing profile in medicine and 'purchasers' of physiotherapy services are asking for outcomes and evidence that physiotherapy is of benefit in specific patients with specific problems.

We cannot answer all these questions but the database of clinical trials is growing. In assessing the evidence it is important to remember the definition of Sackett et al (1996): 'Evidence-based medicine involves integrating individual clinical expertise and the best external evidence available from systematic research'.

In this book we have referenced statements where possible, but there are still many areas of practice which are anecdotal. We must not lose the skills and techniques in these areas if there are indications of patient benefit.

The second edition includes separate and new chapters on surgery and intensive care, and new chapters on non-invasive ventilation and pulmonary rehabilitation. Other chapters have been expanded with sections written by physiotherapy specialists in the field – manual therapy and acupuncture. All the chapters have been updated and new references included.

No text can meet every reader's need but we hope that the material here will lead the reader on to other sources and contacts and, by open exchange of information and ideas, we should be able to take the profession forward to benefit our patients.

London 1997   J.A.P.
                                                        B.A.W.

Preface to first edition

This book is intended for physiotherapy students, new graduates and postgraduate physiotherapists with an interest in patients with respiratory and cardiac problems.

Assessment of the patient should reveal the patient's problems. If some or all of these problems can be influenced by physical means, physiotherapy is indicated. Physiotherapy is also indicated when potential problems have been identified and preventative measures should be taken. The role of the physiotherapist as an educator in both the prevention and treatment of problems is another important aspect.

Diagnoses will continue to provide useful medical categories, but treatment can become prescriptive and inappropriate or ineffective if given in response to a diagnosis alone. The pathology behind the problem provides the key as to whether it is a physiotherapy problem or a medical problem.

It is by accurate assessment of the patient that short- and long-term patient goals can be identified and agreed, and an effective treatment plan outlined. Continuous reassessment of the patient and the treatment outcomes will identify the need for continuation or modification of treatment.

This book begins with assessment of the patient and the interpretation of medical investigations. This is followed by a section on mechanical support and cardiopulmonary resuscitation.

An important part of our role is communication, counselling and health education. The skills available to the cardiorespiratory physiotherapist are many and varied. Practical skills have been outlined and referenced where possible. All skills are not yet supported by rigorous clinical studies, but it is important that we continue to use them if outcome measures support their place in clinical practice. In the future measurement tools could validate their use. Research should be an integral part of the practice of physiotherapy.

Patients' problems and their management are outlined in the context of differing pathologies. One pathological process may present as several patient problems. Pneumothorax, for example, appears under the problems of both pain and breathlessness. The characteristic problems of some patient groups and diagnostic categories are then discussed detailing the pathology, medical management, physiotherapy and evaluation of treatment.

This book should be read in conjunction with specialized texts on anatomy, physiology and pathology. Further reading is indicated within each chapter. Throughout the text, for simplicity, the patient is referred to as he/him and the physiotherapist as she/her, but it is not intended to imply that all patients are male or that all physiotherapists are female.

It is hoped that the problem-orientated approach to physiotherapy practice will facilitate the learning process for the physiotherapist and improve the quality of the care we provide.

London 1993   B.A.W.
                                               J.A.P.

Acknowledgement

We wish to express our debt to Barbara Webber, who, as co-editor and author of the first and second editions of this book, has made a significant contribution to the foundation of the third edition.

Assessment, investigations, skills, techniques and management

SECTION CONTENTS

1

Assessment and investigation of patients' problems

Sally Middleton   *Peter G Middleton*

INTRODUCTION

The aim of assessment is to define the patient's problems accurately. It is based on both a subjective and an objective assessment of the patient. Without an accurate assessment it is impossible to develop an appropriate plan of treatment. Equally, a sound theoretical knowledge is required to develop an appropriate treatment plan for those problems which may be improved by physiotherapy. Once treatment has commenced it is important to assess its effectiveness regularly in relation to both the problems and goals.

The system of patient management used in this book is based on the problem-oriented medical system (POMS) first described by Weed in 1968. This system has three components:

- problem-oriented medical records (POMR)
- audit
- educational programme.

The POMR is now widely used as the method of recording the assessment, management and progress of a patient. It is divided into five sections, as shown in Figure 1.1, and summarized below:

- *Database.* Here personal details, medical history, relevant social history, results of investigations and tests, together with the physiotherapist's assessment of the patient are recorded.
- *Problem list.* This is a concise list of the patient's problems, compiled after the assessment is complete. Problems are not always

3

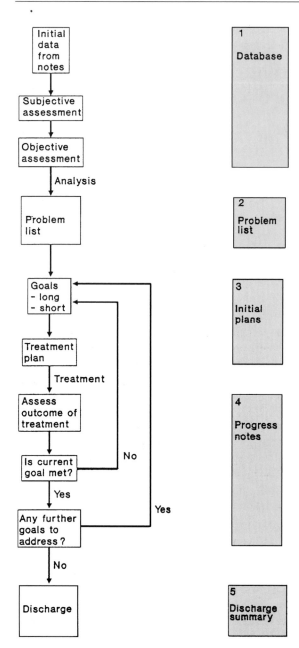

Figure 1.1   The process of problem-oriented medical records.

- *Initial plan and goals.* A treatment plan is formulated to address the physiotherapy-related problems, with consideration given to the patient's other problems. Long- and short-term goals are then formulated. Long-term goals are what the patient and the physiotherapist want to finally achieve and should relate to the problems. Short-term goals are the stages by which the long-term goals should be achieved.
- *Progress notes.* These are written to document the patient's progress, especially highlighting any changes. The notes are written in the 'subjective, objective, analysis, plan' (SOAP) format for each problem and provide an up-to-date summary of the patient's progress.
- *Discharge summary.* This is written when the patient is discharged from treatment or transferred to another institution. It includes presenting problems, treatment given, outcomes of treatment, together with any home programme or follow-up instructions.

DATABASE

The database contains a concise summary of the relevant information about the patient taken from the medical notes, together with the subjective and objective assessment made by the physiotherapist. The format may differ from hospital to hospital but will contain the same information.

The first part contains the patient's personal details, including name, date of birth, address, hospital number and referring doctor. It may also contain the diagnosis and reason for referral. The second part summarizes the history from the medical notes and the physiotherapy assessment. This is often divided into several sections.

- *History of presenting condition (HPC)* summarizes the patient's current problems, including relevant information from the medical notes.
- *Previous medical history (PMH)* summarizes the entire list of medical and surgical problems that the patient has had in the past. It may be written in disease-specific groupings or as a chronological account.

written in order of priority. The list includes problems both amenable to physiotherapy and problems that must be taken into consideration during treatment. The resolution of problems and the appearance of new ones are noted appropriately.

- *Drug history (DH)* is a list of the patient's current medications (including dosage) taken from the medication charts. Drug allergies should also be noted.
- *Family history (FH)* includes a list of any major diseases suffered by members of the immediate family.
- *Social history (SH)* provides a picture of the patient's social situation. It is important to specifically question the patient about the level of support available at home and to gain an idea of the patient's expected contribution to household duties. The layout of the patient's home should also be ascertained, with particular emphasis on stairs. Occupation and hobbies, both past and present, give further information about the patient's lifestyle. Finally, history of smoking and alcohol use should be noted.
- *Patient examination* includes all information collected in the physiotherapist's subjective and objective assessment of the patient.
- *Test results* contain any significant findings as they become available. These may include arterial blood gases, spirometry, blood tests, sputum analysis, chest radiographs, computed tomography (CT) and any other relevant tests (e.g. hepatitis B positive).

Subjective assessment

Subjective assessment is based on an interview with the patient. It should generally start with open-ended questions *What is the main problem? What troubles you most?* allowing the patient to discuss the problems that are most important to him at that time. Indeed, by asking such questions, previously unmentioned problems may surface. As the interview progresses, questioning may become more focused on those important features that need clarification. There are five main symptoms of respiratory disease:

- breathlessness (dyspnoea)
- cough
- sputum and haemoptysis
- wheeze
- chest pain.

With each of these symptoms, enquiries should be made concerning:

- *duration* – both the absolute time since first recognition of the symptom (months, years) and the duration of the present symptoms (days, weeks)
- *severity* – in absolute terms and relative to the recent and distant past
- *pattern* – seasonal or daily variations
- *associated factors* – including precipitants, relieving factors and associated symptoms, if any.

Breathlessness

Breathlessness is the subjective awareness of an increased work of breathing. It is the predominant symptom of both cardiac and respiratory disease. It also occurs in anaemia where the oxygen-carrying capacity of the blood is reduced, in neuromuscular disorders where the respiratory muscles are affected, and in metabolic disorders where there is a change in the acid–base equilibrium (see pp. 77 and 137) or metabolic rate (e.g. hyperthyroid disorders). Breathlessness is also found in hyperventilation syndrome where it is due to psychological factors (e.g. anxiety).

The pathophysiological mechanisms causing breathlessness are still the subject of intensive investigation. Many factors are involved, including respiratory muscle length–tension relationships, respiratory muscle fatigue, stimulation of pulmonary stretch receptors and alterations in central respiratory drive.

The duration and severity of breathlessness are most easily assessed through enquiries about the level of functioning in the recent and distant past. For example, a patient may say that 3 years ago he could walk up five flights of stairs without stopping but now cannot even manage one flight. Some patients may deny breathlessness as they have (unconsciously) decreased their activity levels so that they do not get breathless. They may only acknowledge breathlessness when it interferes with important activities, e.g. bathing. The physiotherapist should always relate breathlessness to the level of function that the patient can achieve.

Comparison of the severity of breathlessness between patients is difficult because of differences in perception and expectations. To overcome these difficulties, numerous gradings have been proposed. The New York Heart Association grading (1964), shown in Box 1.1, was developed for patients with cardiac disease but is also applicable to respiratory patients. The Borg Rating of Perceived Exertion Scale (Tables 15.1 and 15.2 on p. 500) is another scale that is frequently used for both respiratory and cardiac patients. No scale is universal and it is important that all staff within one institution use the same scale.

Breathlessness is usually worse during exercise and better with rest. The one exception is hyperventilation syndrome where breathlessness may improve with exercise. Two patterns of breathlessness have been given specific names.

- *Orthopnoea* is breathlessness when lying flat.
- *Paroxysmal nocturnal dyspnoea (PND)* is breathlessness that wakes the patient at night.

In the cardiac patient, lying flat increases venous return from the legs so that blood pools in the lungs, causing breathlessness. A similar pattern, may be described in patients with severe asthma but here the breathlessness is caused by nocturnal bronchoconstriction.

Further insight into a patient's breathlessness may be gained by enquiring about precipitating and relieving factors. Breathlessness associated with exposure to allergens and relieved by bronchodilators is typically found in asthma.

Box 1.1 The New York Heart Association classification of breathlessness

Class I	No symptoms with ordinary activity, breathlessness only occurring with severe exertion, e.g. running up hills, fast bicycling, cross-country skiing
Class II	Symptoms with ordinary activity, e.g. walking up stairs, making beds, carrying large amounts of shopping
Class III	Symptoms with mild exertion, e.g. bathing, showering, dressing
Class IV	Symptoms at rest

Cough

Coughing is a protective reflex which rids the airways of secretions or foreign bodies. Any stimulation of receptors located in the pharynx, larynx, trachea or bronchi may induce cough. Cough is a difficult symptom to clarify as most people cough normally every day, yet a repetitive persistent cough is both troublesome and distressing. Smokers may discount their early morning cough as being 'normal' when in fact it signifies chronic bronchitis.

Important features concerning cough are its effectiveness and whether it is productive or dry. The severity of cough may range from an occasional disturbance to a continual trouble. A loud, barking cough, which is often termed 'bovine', may signify laryngeal or tracheal disease. Recurrent coughing after eating or drinking is an important symptom of aspiration. A chronic productive cough every day is a fundamental feature of chronic bronchitis and bronchiectasis. Interstitial lung disease is characterized by a persistent, dry cough. Nocturnal cough is an important symptom of asthma in children and young adults, but in older patients it is more commonly due to cardiac failure. Drugs, especially beta-blockers and some other antihypertensive agents, can cause a chronic cough. Chronic cough may cause fractured ribs (cough fractures) and hernias. Stress incontinence is a common complication of chronic cough, especially in women. As this subject is often embarrassing to the patient, specific questioning may be required (see p. 8).

Postoperatively, the strength and effectiveness of cough is important for the physiotherapist to assess.

Sputum

In a normal adult, up to 100 ml of tracheobronchial secretions are produced daily and cleared subconsciously. Sputum is the excess tracheobronchial secretions cleared from the airways by coughing or huffing. It may contain mucus, cellular debris, microorganisms, blood and foreign particles. Questioning should

Table 1.1   Sputum analysis

	Description	Causes
Saliva	Clear watery fluid	
Mucoid	Opalescent or white	Chronic bronchitis without infection, asthma
Mucopurulent	Slightly discoloured, but not frank pus	Bronchiectasis, cystic fibrosis, pneumonia

Purulent	Thick, viscous:
	  Yellow
	  Dark green/brown
	  Rusty
	  Redcurrant jelly
		
		Haemophilus
		Pseudomonas
		Pneumococcus, mycoplasma
		Klebsiella

Frothy	Pink or white	Pulmonary oedema
Haemoptysis	Ranging from blood specks to frank blood, old blood (dark brown)	Infection (tuberculosis, bronchiectasis), infarction, carcinoma, vasculitis, trauma, also coagulation disorders, cardiac disease
Black	Black specks in mucoid secretions	Smoke inhalation (fires, tobacco, heroin), coal dust

determine the colour, consistency and quantity of sputum produced each day. This may clarify the diagnosis and the severity of disease (Table 1.1).

A number of grading systems for mucoid–mucopurulent–purulent sputum have been proposed. For example, Miller (1963) suggested:

M1   mucoid with no suspicion of pus
M2   predominantly mucoid, suspicion of pus
P1   1/3 purulent, 2/3 mucoid
P2   2/3 purulent, 1/3 mucoid
P3   >2/3 purulent.

However, in clinical practice sputum is often classified as mucoid, mucopurulent or purulent, together with an estimation of the volume (1 teaspoon, 1 egg cup, 1/2 cup, 1 cup). Odour emanating from sputum signifies infection. In general, particularly offensive odours suggest infection with anaerobic organisms (e.g. aspiration pneumonia, lung abscess).

In patients with allergic bronchopulmonary aspergillosis (ABPA), asthma and occasionally bronchiectasis, sputum 'casts' may be expectorated. Classically these take the shape of the bronchial tree.

Haemoptysis is the presence of blood in the sputum. It may range from slight streaking of the sputum to frank blood. Frank haemoptysis can be life threatening, requiring bronchial artery embolization or surgery. Isolated haemoptysis may be the first sign of bronchogenic carcinoma, even when the chest radiograph is normal.

Patients with chronic infective lung disease often suffer from recurrent haemoptyses.

Wheeze

Wheeze is a whistling or musical sound produced by turbulent airflow through narrowed airways. These sounds are generally noted by patients when audible at the mouth. Stridor, the sound of an upper airway obstruction, is often mistakenly called 'wheeze' by patients. Heart failure may also cause wheezing in those patients with significant mucosal oedema. Wheezing is discussed in more detail later in this chapter.

Chest pain

Chest pain in respiratory patients usually originates from musculoskeletal, pleural or tracheal inflammation, as the lung parenchyma and small airways contain no pain fibres.

● *Pleuritic chest pain* is caused by inflammation of the parietal pleura and is usually described as a severe, sharp, stabbing pain which is worse on inspiration. It is not reproduced by palpation.
● *Tracheitis* generally causes a constant burning pain in the centre of the chest, aggravated by breathing.
● *Musculoskeletal (chest wall) pain* may originate from the muscles, bones, joints or nerves of the

thoracic cage. It is usually well localized and exacerbated by chest and/or arm movement. Palpation will usually reproduce the pain.

- *Angina pectoris* is a major symptom of cardiac disease. Myocardial ischaemia characteristically causes a dull central retrosternal gripping or band-like sensation which may radiate to the arm, neck or jaw.
- *Pericarditis* may cause pain similar to angina or pleurisy.

A differential diagnosis of chest pain is given in Table 1.2.

Incontinence

Incontinence is a problem which is often aggravated by chronic cough (Orr et al 2001, Thakar & Stanton 2000). Coughing and huffing increase intra-abdominal pressure which may precipitate urine leakage. Fear of this may influence compli-

Table 1.2 Syndromes of chest pain

Condition	Description	Causes
Pulmonary		
Pleurisy	Sharp, stabbing, rapid onset, limits inspiration, well localized, often 'catches' at a certain lung volume, not tender on palpation	Pleural infection or inflammation of the pleura, trauma (haemothorax), malignancy
Pulmonary embolus	Usually has pleuritic pain, with or without severe central pain	Pulmonary infarction
Pneumothorax	Severe central chest discomfort, with or without pleuritic component, severity depends on extent of mediastinal shift	Trauma, spontaneous, lung diseases (e.g. cystic fibrosis, AIDS)
Tumours	May mimic any form of chest pain, depending on site and structures involved	Primary or secondary carcinoma, mesothelioma
Musculoskeletal		
Rib fracture	Localized point tenderness, often sudden onset, increases with inspiration	Trauma, tumour, cough fractures (e.g. in chronic lung diseases, osteoporosis)
Muscular	Superficial, increases on inspiration and some body movements, with or without palpable muscle spasm	Trauma, unaccustomed exercise (excessive coughing during exacerbations of lung disease), accessory muscles may be affected
Costochondritis (Tietze's syndrome)	Localized to one or more costochondral joints, with or without generalized, non-specific chest pain	Viral infection
Neuralgia	Pain or paraesthesia in a dermatomal distribution	Thoracic spine dysfunction, tumour, trauma, herpes zoster (shingles)
Cardiac		
Ischaemic heart disease (angina or infarct)	Dull, central, retrosternal discomfort like a weight or band with or without radiation to the jaw and/or either arm, may be associated with palpitations, nausea or vomiting	Myocardial ischaemia, onset at rest is more suggestive of infarction
Pericarditis	Often retrosternal, exacerbated by respiration, may mimic cardiac ischaemia or pleurisy, often relieved by sitting	Infection, inflammation, trauma, tumour
Mediastinum		
Dissecting aortic aneurysm	Sudden onset, severe, poorly localized central chest pain	Trauma, atherosclerosis, Marfan's syndrome
Oesophageal	Retrosternal burning discomfort, but can mimic all other pains, worse lying flat or bending forward	Oesophageal reflux, trauma, tumour
Mediastinal shift	Severe, poorly localized central discomfort	Pneumothorax, rapid drainage of a large pleural effusion

ance with physiotherapy. Thus identification and treatment of incontinence is important. Questions may need to be specific to elicit this symptom: *'When you cough, do you find that you leak some urine?'*, *'Does this interfere with your physiotherapy?'*

Other symptoms

Of the other symptoms a patient may report, a number have particular importance.

- *Fever (pyrexia)* is one of the common features of infection but low-grade fevers can also occur with malignancy and connective tissue disorders. Equally, infection may occur without fever, especially in immunosuppressed (e.g. chemotherapy) patients or those on corticosteroids. High fevers occurring at night, with associated sweating (night sweats), may be the first indicator of pulmonary tuberculosis.
- *Headache* is an uncommon feature of respiratory disease. Morning headaches in patients with severe respiratory failure may signify nocturnal carbon dioxide retention. Early morning arterial blood gases or nocturnal transcutaneous carbon dioxide monitoring are required for confirmation.
- *Peripheral oedema* in the respiratory patient suggests right heart failure which may be due to cor pulmonale (right ventricular failure secondary to hypoxic pulmonary vasoconstriction). Peripheral oedema may also occur in patients taking high-dose corticosteroids, as a result of salt and water retention.

Functional ability

It is important to assess the patient as a whole, enquiring about his daily activities. If the patient is employed, what does his job *actually* entail? For example, a surveyor may sit behind a desk all day or he may be climbing 25-storey buildings. The home situation should also be documented, in particular the number of stairs to the front door and within the house. With whom does the patient live? What roles does the patient perform in the home (shopping, housework, cooking)?

Finally, questions concerning activities and recreation often reveal areas where significant improvements in quality of life can be made.

Quality of life

Assessment of quality of life (QOL) is becoming increasingly important to measure the impact of disability on the patient and of response to treatment. QOL scales measure the effect of an illness and its management upon a patient as perceived by the patient. Often there is little correlation between physiological measures (e.g. lung function) and QOL. A number of both generic (for example, SF-36; Ware & Sherbourne 1992) and disease-specific QOL scales are available which allow data to be gathered principally by self-report questionnaires or interview. QOL scales available for assessment of patients with respiratory or cardiovascular disease are reviewed elsewhere (Juniper et al 1999, Kinney et al 1996, Mahler 2000, Pashkow et al 1995). The choice of a QOL measure requires an evaluation of QOL scales with respect to their reliability, validity, responsiveness and appropriateness (Aaronson 1989).

Disease awareness

During the interview it is important to ascertain the patient's knowledge of his disease and treatment. The level of compliance with treatment, often difficult to assess initially, may become evident as rapport develops. These issues will influence the goals of treatment.

Objective assessment

Objective assessment is based on examination of the patient, together with the use of tests such as spirometry, arterial blood gases and chest radiographs. Although a full examination of the patient should be available from the medical notes, it is worthwhile making a thorough examination at all times as the patient's condition may have changed since the last examination and the physiotherapist may need greater detail of certain aspects than is available from the notes. A good examination will provide an objective base-line for the future measurement of the patient's progress. By developing a standard method of examination, the findings are quickly assimilated and the physiotherapist remains confident that nothing has been omitted. This chapter refers mainly to assessment of the adult patient although much of the information is also relevant to the paediatric population. Specific details for the assessment of infants and children and normal values can be found in the relevant paediatric sections (Chapters 3, 9 and 13).

General observation

Examination starts by observing the patient from the end of the bed. Is the patient short of breath, sitting on the edge of the bed, distressed? Is he obviously cyanosed? Is he on supplemental oxygen? If so, how much? What is his speech pattern – long fluent paragraphs without dis-cernible pauses for breath, quick sentences, just a few words or is he too breathless to speak? When he moves around or undresses, does he become distressed? With a little practice, these observations should become second nature and can be noted whilst introducing yourself to the patient.

In the intensive care patient there are a number of further features to be observed. The level of ventilatory support must be ascertained. This includes both the mode of ventilation (e.g. sup-plemental oxygen, continuous positive airway pressure, intermittent positive pressure ventil-ation) and the route of ventilation (mask, endo-tracheal tube, tracheostomy). The level of cardiovascular support should also be noted, including drugs to control blood pressure and cardiac output, pacemakers and other mechanical devices. The patient's level of consciousness should also be noted. Any patient with a decreased level of consciousness is at risk of aspiration and retention of pulmonary secretions. In those patients who are not pharmacologically sedated, the level of consciousness is often meas-ured using the Glasgow Coma Scale (Box 1.2). This gives the patient a score (from 3 to 15) based on his best motor, verbal and eye responses.

Box 1.2 The Glasgow Coma Scale		
Eye opening	Spontaneous	4
	To speech	3
	To pain	2
	None	1
Best verbal response	Oriented	5
	Confused speech	4
	Inappropriate words	3
	Incomprehensible sounds	2
	None	1
Best motor response	Obeys commands	6
	Localizes to pain	5
	Withdraws (generalized)	4
	Flexion	3
	Extension	2
	No response	1

Maximum total score is 15; minimum total score is 3.

The patient's chart should then be examined for recordings of temperature, pulse, blood pres-sure and respiratory rate. These measurements are usually performed by the nursing staff imme-diately on admission of the patient and regularly thereafter.

Body temperature. Body temperature can be measured in a number of ways. Oral temper-atures are the most convenient method in adults but should not be performed for at least 15 minutes after smoking or consuming hot or cold food or drink. Aural, axillary and rectal temper-ature may also be measured.

Body temperature is maintained within the range 36.5–37.5°C. It is lowest in the early morning and highest in the afternoon.

Fever (pyrexia) is the elevation of the body temperature above 37.5°C and is associated with an increased metabolic rate. For every 0.6°C (1°F) rise in body temperature, there is an approxi-mately 10% increase in oxygen consumption and carbon dioxide production. This places extra demand on the cardiorespiratory system which causes a compensatory increase in heart rate and respiratory rate.

Heart rate. Heart rate is most accurately meas-ured by auscultation at the cardiac apex. The pulse rate is measured by palpating a peripheral artery (radial, femoral or carotid). In most situ-ations, the heart rate and pulse rate are identical;

a difference between the two is called the 'pulse deficit'. This indicates that some heart beats have not caused sufficient blood flow to reach the periphery and is commonly found in atrial fibrillation and some other arrhythmias. The normal adult heart rate is 60–100 beats per minute.

Tachycardia in adults is defined as a heart rate greater than 100 beats/min at rest. It is found with anxiety, exercise, fever, anaemia and hypoxia. It is also common in patients with cardiac disorders. Medications such as bronchodilators and some cardiac drugs may also increase heart rate.

Bradycardia is defined as a heart rate less than 60 beats/min in adults. It may be a normal finding in athletes and may also be caused by some cardiac drugs (especially beta-blockers).

Blood pressure (BP). With every contraction of the heart (systole) the arterial pressure increases, with the peak called the 'systolic' pressure. During the relaxation phase of the heart (diastole), the arterial pressure drops, with the minimum called the 'diastolic' pressure. Blood pressure is usually measured non-invasively by placing a sphygmomanometer cuff around the upper arm and listening over the brachial artery with a stethoscope. The cuff width should be approximately one-half to two-thirds of the length of the upper arm, otherwise readings may be inaccurate. Cuff inflation to above systolic pressure collapses the artery, blocking flow. With release of the air, the cuff pressure gradually falls to a point just below systolic. At this point, the peak pressure within the artery is greater than the pressure outside the artery, so flow recommences. This turbulent flow is audible through the stethoscope. As the cuff is further deflated the noise continues. When the cuff pressure drops to just below diastolic, the pressure within the artery is greater than that of the cuff throughout the cardiac cycle, so turbulence abates and the noise ceases.

Blood pressure is recorded as systolic/diastolic pressure. Normal adult blood pressure is between 95/60 and 140/90 mmHg.

Hypertension is defined as a blood pressure of greater than 145/95 mmHg, usually due to changes in vascular tone and/or aortic valve disease.

Hypotension is defined as a blood pressure of less than 90/60 mmHg. It is often a normal finding during sleep. Daytime hypotension may be due to heart failure, blood loss or decreased vascular tone.

Postural hypotension is a drop in blood pressure of more than 5 mmHg between lying and sitting or standing and may be due to decreased circulating blood volume or loss of vascular tone.

Pulsus paradoxus is the exaggeration of the drop in blood pressure that occurs with inspiration. Normally, during inspiration the negative intrathoracic pressure reduces venous return and decreases cardiac output slightly. Exaggeration of this normal response where blood pressure drops by more than 10 mmHg is seen in situations where the intrathoracic pressure swings are greater, as occurs in severe airway obstruction.

Respiratory rate. Respiratory rate should be measured with the patient seated comfortably. The normal adult respiratory rate is approximately 12–16 breaths/min.

Tachypnoea is defined as a respiratory rate greater than 20 breaths/min and can be seen in any form of lung disease. It may also occur with metabolic acidosis and anxiety.

Bradypnoea is defined as a respiratory rate of less than 10 breaths/min. It is an uncommon finding and is usually due to central nervous system depression by narcotics or trauma.

Body weight. Weight is often recorded on the observation chart. Respiratory function can be compromised by both obesity and severe malnourishment. As ideal body weight has a large normal range, the body mass index (BMI) has been proposed as an alternative. This is calculated by dividing the weight in kilograms by the square of the height in metres (kg/m^2); the normal range is 20–25 kg/m^2. Patients with values below 20 are underweight, those with values of 25–30 are overweight and those with values over 30 are classified as obese.

Malnourished patients often exhibit depression of their immune system with increased risk of infection. They also have weaker respiratory muscles which are more likely to fatigue. Obesity causes an increase in residual volume (RV) and a decrease in functional residual capacity (FRC)

(Rubinstein et al 1990). Thus tidal breathing occurs close to closing volumes. This is particularly important postoperatively, where the obese are more prone to subsegmental lung collapse.

An accurate daily weight gives a good estimate of fluid volume changes, as any change in weight of more than 250 g/day is usually due to fluid accumulation or loss. Daily weights are commonly used in intensive care, renal and cardiac patients to assess fluid balance.

Other measures. In the intensive care patient there is a plethora of monitoring that can be performed. As well as the parameters listed above, measures of central venous pressure (CVP), pulmonary artery pressure (PAP) and intracranial pressure (ICP) will need to be reviewed as part of the physiotherapy assessment. Some intensive care units now record this information on bedside computer terminals. Further details of intensive care monitoring can be found in Chapters 4 and 9.

Apparatus. The presence of lines and tubes should be noted. Venous lines provide constant direct access to the bloodstream and vary widely in site, complexity and function. The simplest cannula in a small peripheral vein, usually in the forearm, is called a 'drip'. It is used for the administration of intravenous (IV) fluids and most IV drugs. At the other end of the spectrum are the multilumen lines placed in the subclavian, internal jugular or femoral veins, ending in the venae cavae close to the heart. These central lines allow simultaneous administration of multiple drugs and can be used for central venous pressure monitoring. Central lines can be potentially dangerous, as disconnection of the line can quickly suck air into the central veins, causing an air embolus which may be fatal.

Some patients, especially those in intensive care, may have an arterial line for continuous recording of blood pressure and for repeated sampling of arterial blood. These lines are usually inserted in the radial or brachial artery. If accidentally disconnected, rapid blood loss will occur.

After cardiac surgery, most patients have cardiac pacing wires which exit through the skin overlying the heart. In most cases these wires are not required and are removed routinely before discharge. In the event of clinically significant cardiac arrhythmias, these wires are connected to a pacing box that electrically stimulates the heart. In medical patients, pacemaker wires are introduced through one of the central veins and rest in the apex of the right ventricle. Care must be taken with all pacing wires as dislodgement may be life threatening.

Intercostal drains are placed between two ribs into the pleural space to remove air, fluid or pus which has accumulated. They are also used routinely after cardiothoracic surgery. In general, the tube is attached to a bottle partially filled with sterile water, called an 'underwater seal drain'. The bottle should be positioned at least 0.5 metre below the patient's chest (usually on the floor). Bubbling indicates that air is entering the tube from the pleural space at that time. Frequent observations must be made of the fluid level within the tube which should oscillate or 'swing' with every breath. If the fluid does not swing, the tube is not patent and requires medical attention. In certain situations the bottle may be connected to continuous suction which will dampen the fluid 'swing'. Those patients who are producing large volumes of fluid or pus may be connected to a double bottle system, where the first bottle acts as a reservoir to collect the fluid and the second provides the underwater seal. More recently, fully enclosed disposable plastic systems have been devised. Any patient with a chest drain should have a pair of large forceps available at all times to clamp the tube if any connection becomes loosened.

Postoperatively, drains may be placed at any operation site (e.g. abdomen) to prevent the collection of fluid or blood. These are generally connected to sterile bags. Nasogastric tubes are placed for two reasons: soft, fine-bore tubes are used to facilitate feeding, whilst firm, wider-bore tubes allow aspiration of gastric contents.

The hands. Significant findings can be identified by observing and examining the hands. A fine tremor will often be seen in association with high-dose bronchodilators. Warm and sweaty hands with an irregular flapping tremor may be due to acute carbon dioxide retention.

Weakness and wasting of the small muscles in the hands may be an early sign of an upper lobe tumour involving the brachial plexus (Pancoast's tumour). Examination of the fingers may show nicotine staining from smoking.

Clubbing is the term used to describe the changes in the fingers and toes as shown in Figure 1.2. The first sign of clubbing is the loss of the angle between the nail bed and the nail itself. Later, the finger pad becomes enlarged. The nail bed may also become 'spongy', but this is a difficult sign to elicit. A summary of the diseases associated with clubbing is given in Box 1.3. The exact cause of clubbing is unknown. It is interesting to note that clubbing in cystic fibrosis patients disappears after heart and lung or lung transplant.

The eyes. The eyes should be examined for pallor (anaemia), plethora (high haemoglobin) or jaundice (yellow colour due to liver or blood disturbances). Drooping of one eyelid with enlargement of that pupil suggests Horner's syndrome where there is a disturbance in the sympathetic nerve supply to that side of the head (sometimes seen in cancer of the lung).

Box 1.3	Causes of clubbing
Lung disease	Infective (bronchiectasis, lung abscess, empyema) Fibrotic Malignant (bronchogenic cancer, mesothelioma)
Cardiac disease	Congenital cyanotic heart disease Bacterial endocarditis
Other	Familial Cirrhosis Gastrointestinal disease (Crohn's disease, ulcerative colitis, coeliac disease)

Cyanosis. This is a bluish discolouration of the skin and mucous membranes. Central cyanosis, seen on examination of the tongue and mouth, is caused by hypoxaemia where there is an increase in the amount of haemoglobin not bound to oxygen. The degree of blueness is related to the quantity of unbound haemoglobin. Thus a greater degree of hypoxia is necessary to produce cyanosis in an anaemic patient (low haemoglobin), whilst a patient with polycythaemia (increased haemoglobin) may appear cyanosed with only a small drop in oxygen levels. Peripheral cyanosis, affecting the toes, fingers and earlobes, may also be due to poor peripheral circulation, especially in cold weather.

Jugular venous pressure. On the side of the neck the jugular venous pressure (JVP) is seen as a flickering impulse in the jugular vein. It is normally seen at the base of the neck when the patient is lying back at 45°. The JVP is usually measured in relation to the sternal angle as this point is relatively fixed in relation to the right atrium. A normal JVP at the base of the neck corresponds to a vertical height approximately 3–4 cm above the sternal angle. The JVP is generally expressed as the vertical height (in centimetres) above normal. The JVP provides a quick assessment of the volume of blood in the great vessels entering the heart. Most commonly it is elevated in right heart failure. This may occur in patients with chronic lung disease complicated by cor pulmonale. In contrast, dehydrated patients may only have a visible JVP when lying flat.

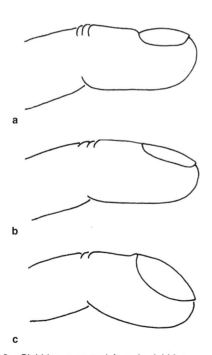

Figure 1.2   Clubbing: **a** normal; **b** early clubbing; **c** advanced clubbing.

Peripheral oedema. This is an important sign of cardiac failure, but may also be found in patients with a low albumin level, impaired venous or lymphatic function or those on high-dose steroids. When mild, it may only affect the ankles; with increasing severity it may progress up the body. In bedbound patients, it is important to check the sacrum.

Observation of the chest

When examining the chest it is important to remember the surface landmarks of the thoracic contents (Fig. 1.3). Some important points are:

- The oblique fissure, dividing the upper and middle lobes from the lower lobes, runs underneath a line drawn from the spinous process of T2 around the chest to the sixth costochondral junction anteriorly.
- The horizontal fissure on the right, dividing the upper lobe from the middle lobe, runs from the fourth intercostal space at the right sternal edge horizontally to the midaxillary line, where it joins the oblique fissure.
- The diaphragm sits at approximately the sixth rib anteriorly, the eighth rib in the midaxillary line and the 10th rib posteriorly.
- The trachea bifurcates just below the level of the manubriosternal junction.
- The apical segment of both upper lobes extends 2.5 cm above the clavicles.

Chest shape. The chest should be symmetrical, with the ribs, in adults, descending at approximately 45° from the spine. The transverse diameter should be greater than the anteroposterior (AP) diameter. The thoracic spine should have a slight kyphosis. Important common abnormalities include:

- *kyphosis*, where the normal flexion of the thoracic spine is increased
- *kyphoscoliosis*, which comprises both lateral curvature of the spine with vertebral rotation

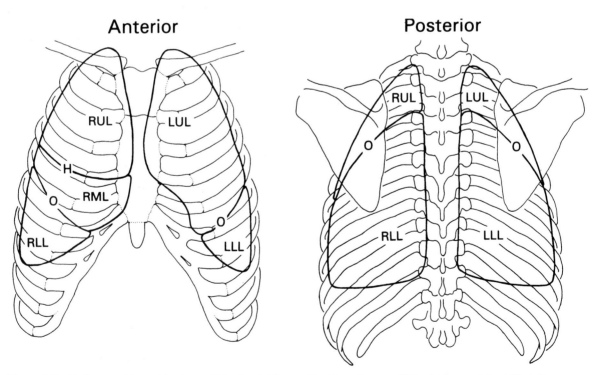

Figure 1.3 Surface markings of the lungs: H, horizontal fissure; O, oblique fissures; RUL, right upper lobe; LUL, left upper lobe; RML, right middle lobe; LLL, left lower lobe; RLL, right lower lobe.

(scoliosis) and an element of kyphosis. This causes a restrictive lung defect which, when severe, may cause respiratory failure

- *pectus excavatum*, or 'funnel' chest, is where part of the sternum is depressed inwards. This rarely causes significant changes in lung function but may be corrected surgically for cosmetic reasons
- *pectus carinatum*, or 'pigeon' chest, is where the sternum protrudes anteriorly. This may be present in children with severe asthma and rarely causes significant lung function abnormalities
- *hyperinflation*, where the ribs lose their normal 45° angle with the thoracic spine and become almost horizontal. The anteroposterior diameter of the chest increases to almost equal the transverse diameter. This is commonly seen in severe emphysema.

Breathing pattern. Observation of the breathing pattern gives further information concerning the type and severity of respiratory disease.

Normal breathing should be regular with a rate of 12–16 breaths/min, as mentioned previously. Inspiration is active and expiration passive. The approximate ratio of inspiratory to expiratory time (I : E ratio) is 1 : 1.5 to 1 : 2.

Prolonged expiration may be seen in patients with obstructive lung disease, where expiratory airflow is severely limited by dynamic closure of the smaller airways. In severe obstruction the I : E ratio may increase to 1 : 3 or 1 : 4.

Pursed-lip breathing is often seen in patients with severe airways disease. By opposing the lips during expiration the airway pressure inside the chest is maintained, preventing the floppy airways from collapsing. Thus overall airflow is increased.

Apnoea is the absence of breathing for more than 15 seconds.

Hypopnoea is diminished breathing with inadequate ventilation. It may be seen during sleep in patients with lung disease.

Kussmaul's respiration is rapid, deep breathing with a high minute ventilation. It is usually seen in patients with metabolic acidosis.

Cheyne–Stokes respiration refers to irregular breathing with cycles consisting of a few relatively deep breaths, progressively shallower breaths (sometimes to the point of apnoea) and then slowly increasing depth of breaths. This is usually associated with heart failure, severe neurological disturbances or drugs (e.g. narcotics).

Ataxic breathing consists of haphazard, uncoordinated deep and shallow breaths. This may be found in patients with cerebellar disease.

Apneustic breathing is characterized by prolonged inspiration and is usually the result of brain damage.

Chest movement. During normal inspiration, there are symmetrical increases in the anteroposterior, transverse and vertical diameters of the chest. The increase in vertical diameter is achieved by contraction of the diaphragm, causing the abdominal contents to descend. Sternal and rib movements are responsible for the increases in anteroposterior and transverse diameters of the chest. These movements can be divided into two components (Fig. 1.4). When elevated, the anterior ends of the ribs move forward and upwards with anterior movement of the sternum. This increase in anteroposterior diameter is likened to the movement of an old-fashioned 'pump handle'. At the same time, rotation of the ribs causes an

Pump handle

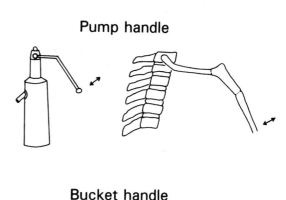

Bucket handle

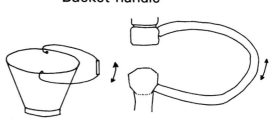

Figure 1.4 Chest wall movement.

increase in the transverse diameter, likened to the movement of a 'bucket handle'.

During normal quiet breathing, the diaphragm is the main inspiratory muscle increasing the vertical diameter. There is also an increase in the lower thoracic transverse diameter due to external intercostal muscle contraction. Expiration is passive, caused by the elastic recoil of the lung and chest wall. When breathing is increased, all the accessory inspiratory muscles (sternomastoid, scalenes, trapezii) contract to increase the anteroposterior and transverse diameters and the diaphragm activity increases, thus further increasing the vertical dimensions. Expiration may become active with contraction of the abdominal and internal intercostal muscles.

Intercostal indrawing occurs where the skin between the ribs is drawn inwards during inspiration. It may be seen in patients with severe inspiratory airflow resistance. Larger negative pressures during inspiration suck the soft tissues inwards. This is an important sign of respiratory distress in children, but is less often seen in adults.

Palpation of the chest

Trachea. Firstly, the trachea is palpated to assess its position in relation to the sternal notch. Tracheal deviation indicates underlying mediastinal shift. The trachea may be pulled towards a collapsed or fibrosed upper lobe or pushed away from a pneumothorax or large pleural effusion.

Chest expansion. This can be assessed by observation but palpation is more accurate. The patient is instructed to expire slowly to residual volume. At residual volume the examiner's hands are placed spanning the posterolateral segments of both bases, with the thumbs touching in the midline posteriorly, as shown in Figure 1.5. In obese patients, it helps if the skin of the anterior chest wall is slightly retracted by the fingertips. The patient is then instructed to inspire slowly and the movement of both thumbs is observed. Both sides should move equally, with 3–5 cm being the normal displacement.

A similar technique may be used anteriorly, again to measure basal movements. Measurement of apical movement is more difficult. By placing

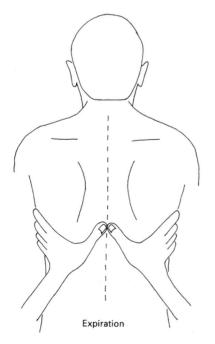
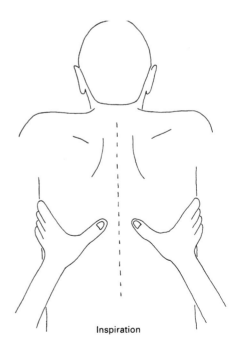

Expiration

Inspiration

Figure 1.5 Palpation of thoracic expansion.

the hand over the upper chest anteriorly, a qualitative comparison of the two sides can be made. In all cases, diminished movement is abnormal.

Paradoxical breathing is where some or all of the chest wall moves inwards on inspiration and outwards on expiration. It can involve anything from a localized area to the entire chest wall. Localized paradox occurs when the integrity of the chest wall is disrupted. Fractures of multiple ribs with two or more breaks in each rib will result in the central section losing the support usually provided by the rest of the thoracic cage. Thus, during inspiration, this loose segment (often called a 'flail segment') is drawn inwards as the rest of the chest wall moves out. In expiration the reverse occurs.

Paradoxical movement of one hemithorax may be remarkably difficult to observe. It may be caused by unilateral diaphragm paralysis. Paradox of the entire chest wall occurs in bilateral diaphragm weakness or paralysis. It is most apparent when the patient is supine.

Paradoxical movement of the lower chest can occur in patients with severe chronic airflow limitation who are extremely hyperinflated. As the dome of the diaphragm cannot descend any further, diaphragm contraction during inspiration pulls the lower ribs inwards. This is called 'Hoover's sign'.

Surgical emphysema. Air in the subcutaneous tissues of the chest, neck or face should also be noted. On palpation there is a characteristic crackling in the skin. This occurs when a pneumomediastinum (air in the mediastinum) has tracked outwards. A chest radiograph must be performed immediately, as a pneumomediastinum may be associated with a pneumothorax.

Vocal fremitus. Vocal fremitus is the measure of speech vibrations transmitted through the chest wall to the examiner's hands. It is measured by asking the patient to repeatedly say '99', whilst the examiner's hands are placed flat on both sides of the chest. The hands are moved from apices to bases, anteriorly and posteriorly, comparing the vibration felt. Vocal fremitus is increased when the lung underneath is relatively solid (consolidated), as this transmits sound better. As sound transmission is decreased through any interface between lung and air or fluid, vocal fremitus is decreased in patients with a pneumothorax or a pleural effusion.

Percussion

Percussion of the chest provides further information that can help in the assessment and localization of lung disease. It is performed by placing the left hand firmly on the chest wall so that the fingers have good contact with the skin. The middle finger of the left hand is struck over the distal interphalangeal joint with the middle finger of the right hand. The right wrist should be relaxed so that the weight of the entire right hand is transmitted through the middle finger. Both sides of the chest from top to bottom should be percussed alternately, paying particular attention to the comparison between sides.

Resonance is generated by the chest wall vibrating over the underlying tissues. Normal resonance is heard over aerated lung, whilst consolidated lung sounds dull, and a pleural effusion sounds 'stony dull'. Increased resonance is heard when the chest wall is free to vibrate over an air-filled space, such as a pneumothorax or bulla. In situations where the chest wall is unable to move freely, as may occur in obese patients, the percussion note may sound dull even if the underlying lung is normal.

Auscultation

Chest auscultation is the process of listening to and interpreting the sounds produced within the thorax. A stethoscope simplifies auscultation and facilitates localization of any abnormalities. It consists of a diaphragm and bell connected by tubing to two earpieces. The diaphragm is generally used for listening to breath sounds, whilst the bell is best for the very low frequencies generated by the heart (especially the third and fourth heart sounds). The diaphragm and bell must be intact for a sound to be heard properly and the tubing relatively short to minimize absorption of the sound. The earpieces, made of plastic or rubber, should fit snugly within the ears, pointing slightly forward in order to maximize sound transmission into the auditory canal.

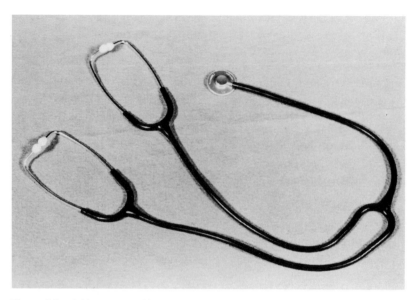

Figure 1.6 A Littmann teaching stethoscope.

A teaching stethoscope (Fig. 1.6) is a useful tool to allow both the experienced and inexperienced physiotherapist to hear the same sounds simultaneously (Ellis 1985). More recently, a number of electronic stethoscopes have been produced, allowing teacher and students to listen together.

Chest auscultation should ideally be performed in a quiet room, with the chest exposed. The patient is instructed to take deep breaths through an open mouth, as turbulence within the nose can interfere with the breath sounds. There is a wide variation in the intensity of breath sounds depending on chest wall thickness. The terms used are described below.

Breath sounds. *Normal breath sounds* are generated by turbulent airflow in the trachea and large airways. These sounds, which can be heard directly over the trachea, comprise high, medium and low frequencies. The higher frequencies are attenuated by normal lung tissue so that breath sounds heard over the periphery are softer and lower pitched. Originally it was thought that the higher-pitched sounds were generated by the bronchi (bronchial breath sounds) and the lower ones by airflow into the alveoli (vesicular breath sounds). It is now known that normal breath sounds (previously called 'vesicular') simply represent filtering of the 'bronchial' breath sounds generated in the large airways. Although technically incorrect, normal breath sounds are still sometimes referred to as 'vesicular' or 'bronchovesicular'. Normal breath sounds are heard all over the chest wall throughout inspiration and for a short period during expiration.

Bronchial breath sounds are the normal tracheal and large airway sounds, transmitted through airless lung which does not attenuate the higher frequencies. Thus, the sounds heard over an area of consolidated lung are similar to those heard over the trachea itself. Bronchial breath sounds are loud and high pitched, with a harsh quality. They are heard equally throughout inspiration and expiration, with a short pause between the two. Thus in all three respects, bronchial breath sounds differ from normal breath sounds which are faint, lower pitched and absent during the latter half of expiration.

If the bronchus supplying an area of consolidated lung is obstructed (e.g. carcinoma, large sputum plug) bronchial breath sounds may not be heard as the obstruction blocks sound transmission.

Diminished sounds occur when there is a reduction in the initial generation of the sound or an increase in sound attenuation. As the breath sounds are generated by flow-related turbulence, reduced flow causes less sound. Thus patients who will not (e.g. due to pain) or cannot (e.g. due to muscle weakness) breathe deeply will have globally diminished breath sounds. Similarly, diminished breath sounds are heard in some patients with emphysema where the combination of parenchymal destruction and hyperinflation cause greater attenuation of the normal breath sounds.

Locally diminished breath sounds may represent obstruction of a bronchus by tumour or large sputum plugs. Localized accumulation of air or fluid in the pleural space will block sound transmission so that breath sounds are absent.

Added sounds. *Wheezes*, previously called 'rhonchi', are musical tones produced by airflow vibrating a narrowed or compressed airway. A fixed, monophonic wheeze is caused by a single obstructed airway, while polyphonic wheezes are due to widespread disease. Any cause of narrowing, for example, bronchospasm, mucosal oedema, sputum or foreign bodies, may cause wheezes. As the airways are normally compressed during expiration, wheezes are first heard at this time. When airway narrowing is more severe, wheezes may also be heard during inspiration. The pitch of the wheeze is directly related to the degree of narrowing, with high-pitched wheezes indicating near-total obstruction. However, the volume of the wheeze may be misleading as the moderate asthmatic may have loud wheezes while the very severe asthmatic may have a 'quiet chest' because he is not generating sufficient airflow to cause wheezes.

Low-pitched, localized wheezes are caused by sputum retention and can change or clear after coughing.

Crackles, previously called 'crepitations' or 'rales', are clicking sounds heard during inspiration. They are caused by the opening of previously closed alveoli and small airways during inspiration. Crackles are described as 'early' or 'late', 'fine' or 'coarse', and 'localized' or 'widespread'. Coarse, early inspiratory crackles occur when bronchioles open (often heard in bronchiectasis and bronchitis), whilst fine, late inspiratory crackles occur when alveoli and respiratory bronchioles open (often heard in pulmonary oedema and pulmonary fibrosis). When severe, the late inspiratory crackles of pulmonary oedema and pulmonary fibrosis may become coarser and commence earlier in inspiration.

Localized crackles may occur in dependent alveoli which are gradually closed by compression from the lung above. This early feature of subsegmental lung collapse resolves when the patient breathes deeply or coughs. The crackles of pulmonary oedema are also more marked basally, but only clear transiently after coughing. The differentiation between subsegmental lung collapse and pulmonary oedema may be difficult and sometimes auscultation will not clarify the situation. Elevation of the JVP and peripheral oedema suggest pulmonary oedema, whereas ineffective cough, recent anaesthesia and pyrexia suggest sputum retention which could lead to subsegmental lung collapse (Table 1.3). Postoperative and intensive care patients may have a combination of both pulmonary oedema and sputum retention.

Table 1.3   Differentiation between pulmonary oedema and sputum retention

Chest sign	Pulmonary oedema	Sputum retention
Auscultation	Fine crackles, especially at bases, with or without wheezes	Scattered or localized crackles, with or without wheezes, may move with coughing
Sputum	Frothy white or pink	Thicker, more viscid, any colour
Other signs	Elevated JVP Peripheral oedema Increased weight, positive fluid balance History of previous cardiac disease	Pyrexia History of intercurrent chest disease, recent anaesthetic, aspiration, respiratory muscle weakness

Pleural rub is the creaking or rubbing sound which occurs with each breath when the pleural surfaces are roughened by inflammation, infection or neoplasm. Normally the visceral and parietal pleura slide silently. Pleural rubs range from being localized and soft to being loud and generalized, sometimes even palpable. In certain instances, they may be difficult to differentiate from crackles. An important distinguishing feature is that pleural rubs are heard equally during inspiration and expiration, with the sounds often recurring in reverse order during expiration.

Vocal resonance. Vocal resonance is the transmission of voice through the airways and lung tissue to the chest wall where it is heard through a stethoscope. It is usually tested by instructing the patient to say '99' repeatedly (like vocal fremitus which is felt with the hands). As mentioned previously, normal lung attenuates the higher frequencies so that the lower frequencies dominate. Thus, speech normally becomes a low-pitched mumble. Consolidated lung transmits all sounds better, especially the high frequencies, so the transmitted sound is louder and higher pitched. In this situation speech can actually be understood. Whispered speech lacks the lower frequencies and is normally not transmitted to the chest wall. However, over areas of consolidation the whisper is clearly heard and intelligible – this is called 'whispering pectoriloquy'.

As with auscultation of breath sounds, vocal resonance is decreased when the transmission of sound through the lung or from the lung to chest wall is impeded. This occurs with emphysema, pneumothorax, pleural thickening or pleural effusion.

A summary of the chest examination in selected chest problems is given in Table 1.4.

Heart sounds. The normal heart sounds represent the closure of the four heart valves. The first heart sound is caused by closure of the mitral and tricuspid valves, while the second heart sound is due to closure of the aortic and pulmonary valves. A third heart sound indicates cardiac failure in adults but may be normal in children. It is attributed to vibration of the ventricular walls caused by rapid filling in early diastole. The fourth heart sound is caused by vibration of the ventricular walls in late diastole as the atria contract. It may be heard in heart failure, hypertension and aortic valve disease.

A murmur is the sound generated by turbulent flow through a valve. The murmur of valvular incompetence is caused by back flow across the valve, whilst stenotic valves generate murmurs by turbulent forward flow.

Sputum

At the end of the respiratory examination, it is often worthwhile instructing the patient to huff to a low lung volume to assess the presence of retained secretions. Any sputum produced should be examined for colour, consistency and quantity as previously described.

Physiotherapy techniques

In those patients who have previously been taught physiotherapy, it is important to ascertain which techniques are used, how well they are performed and their effectiveness. For example, patients who use huffing to clear retained secretions should

Table 1.4 Summary of chest examination in selected chest problems

Disease	Breath sounds	PN	VF	VR
Consolidation:				
With open airway	Bronchial	Dull	↑	↑
With blocked airway	↓	Dull	↓	↓
Pneumothorax	↓ or absent	Hyperresonant	↓ or absent	↓ or absent
Pleural effusion	↓ or absent	Stony dull	↓ or absent	↓ or absent

PN, percussion note; VF, vocal fremitus; VR, vocal resonance; ↑, increased; ↓, decreased have its effectiveness assessed. Suboptimal techniques need to be identified and their correction incorporated in the treatment plan.

Exercise capacity

For a complete assessment of the respiratory system, exercise capacity should also be measured. Depending on the situation, this may vary from a full exercise test for measuring maximum oxygen uptake to a simple assessment of breathlessness during normal activities. An exercise test provides the best measure of functional limitation, which may differ from that suggested by a patient's lung function. Two of the most common methods used to assess patients with respiratory disease are the 6-minute walking test (Butland et al 1982) and the shuttle walking tests (Bradley et al 1999, Revill et al 1999, Singh et al 1992).

Test results

The final stage of assessment of a respiratory or cardiac patient involves the use of tests, in particular spirometry, arterial blood gases and chest radiography. The following is a brief summary of the application of these tests. A full discussion is given in Chapters 2 and 3.

Spirometry

The forced expiratory volume in 1 second (FEV_1), the forced vital capacity (FVC) and peak expiratory flow (PEF) are important measures of ventilatory function. Normal values, based on population studies, depend on age, height, sex and race. Weight is not an important determinant of lung function, except in the markedly obese or malnourished.

Although often expressed as absolute values, lung function should always be compared with the predicted values and with the previous recordings for that patient. For example, a 21-year-old, 6-foot-tall male asthmatic changing his spirometry (FEV_1/FVC) from 4.0/5.0 litres to 1.5/3.0 litres should cause concern, while a normal 81-year-old, 5-foot female may never manage to blow more than 1.3/1.8 litres!

Arterial blood gases

Arterial blood gases (ABGs) provide an accurate measure of oxygen uptake and carbon dioxide removal by the respiratory system as a whole. The arterial blood is usually sampled from the radial artery at the wrist. Rarely, arterialized capillary samples may be taken from the earlobe. Arterial blood gases are best used as a measure of steady-state gas exchange; thus it is imperative that the patient is resting quietly with a constant inspired oxygen level (FiO_2) and mode of ventilation for at least 30 minutes prior to sampling. When analysing the results, consideration must be given to all these factors.

Normal values for arterial blood gases are:

pH	7.35–7.45
PaO_2	10.7–13.3 kPa (80–100 mmHg)
$PaCO_2$	4.7–6.0 kPa (35–45 mmHg)
HCO_3^-	22–26 mmol/l
Base excess	–2 to +2

Chest radiographs

Chest radiographs are an important aid to physical examination as they provide a clear picture of the extent and severity of disease at that time. In some instances, chest radiographs may show more extensive disease than expected, whilst in others they may underestimate the pathology present. Comparison with previous radiographs provides an excellent measure of improvement or deterioration over time and an objective assessment of the response to treatment. However, the chest radiograph may sometimes lag 1–2 days behind the clinical findings.

Electrocardiograph and echocardiograms

The electrocardiograph (ECG) and echocardiogram provide important information regarding cardiac electrical and mechanical function. An understanding of these is essential as abnormalities may alter the treatment plan. More detailed information about their measurement and implications is covered in Chapter 3.

PROBLEM LIST

The second part of POMR is the problem list (see Fig. 1.1). The information in the database, together with the subjective and objective assessment, are then analysed as a whole and integrated with the physiotherapist's knowledge of disease processes.

The problem list is then compiled. It consists of a simple, functional and specific list of the patient's problems at that time, not always listed in order of priority. Each problem is numbered and dated at the time of assessment. The problem list should not only include those problems amenable to physiotherapy (e.g. breathlessness on exertion), but should also include other problems for consideration when designing and implementing a treatment plan (e.g. anaemia). The problem list should not be a list of signs and symptoms, as this would provide the wrong emphasis for treatment. In the past, disease-based treatment tended to result in standardized treatment, ignoring the patient's individual problems. This meant that all chronic airflow limitation patients were given treatment for impaired airway clearance. All intubated patients also received standard treatment, irrespective of the presence or absence of excess secretions and the patient's ability to clear them. The best system is one that is individualized to each patient.

Once problems are resolved they should be signed off and dated. Any subsequent problems are added and dated appropriately.

INITIAL PLANS

For each of the physiotherapy problems listed, long- and short-term goals are formulated. These should be Specific, Measurable, Achievable, Realistic and Timed (SMART). Prioritizing the problem list and developing the goals for each problem should be performed, where possible, in consultation with the patient. The importance of involving the patient cannot be overstressed, as cooperation is fundamental to nearly all physiotherapy treatment. The patient assessment will have identified important factors which must be considered when developing a plan and goals.

Such factors may include coexisting conditions or disease (e.g. diabetes mellitus) or other factors such as age, motivation, cultural or social factors.

Long-term goals are generally directed at returning the patient to his maximum functional capacity. Specifically, goals may be simplified to functions that are important to the patient, e.g. to be able to walk home from the shops carrying one bag of shopping. When setting goals for an inpatient, consideration must be given to discharge. If the home situation includes two flights of stairs to the bedroom then the goal of exercise ability should reflect this. If physiotherapy is to be continued at home after discharge, one of the goals must be to teach the patient or a relative how to perform the treatment effectively.

Short-term goals are the steps taken to achieve the long-term goals. In general, these are small, simple activities that are more easily achieved. All goals, both short- and long-term, should state expected outcomes and time frames. The goals, especially the short-term goals, should be reviewed regularly as some patients may improve faster than others. If goals are not met within the agreed time frame, then revision is necessary. The time frame may have been too short, the goal inappropriate or other problems need attention before this goal can be met.

The treatment plan includes the specifics of treatment, together with its frequency and equipment requirements. Patient education must not be omitted from the treatment plan as it is an important component of physiotherapy.

A summary, as a reminder of the key points of assessment, is given in Box 1.4.

PROGRESS NOTES

These are written on a daily basis using the 'subjective, objective, analysis, plan' (SOAP) format.

- **Subjective** – what the patient, doctors or nurses report.
- **Objective** – any change in physical examination or test, e.g. auscultation, chest radiograph.
- **Analysis** – the physiotherapist's professional opinion of the subjective and objective findings.

Box 1.4   Key points of assessment

Database
- Medical records

Subjective assessment
- Breathlessness, cough, sputum, wheeze, chest pain
- Duration, severity, pattern, associations
- Functional ability, disease awareness

Objective assessment
- General observation from end of bed
- Chest – observation, palpation, percussion, auscultation
- Sputum
- Physiotherapy techniques, exercise capacity

Test results
- Spirometry
- Arterial blood gases
- Chest radiographs

Problem list → Treatment plan

- **P**lan – including changes in treatment and any further action.

Entries are made for each physiotherapy problem, signed and dated. If there have been no changes, nothing further needs to be written.

Progress notes may also include a graph or flow chart. Graphs are particularly useful in displaying the change in a parameter over time, for example an asthmatic's peak expiratory flow rates. Flow chart displays are useful if multiple factors are changing over a period of time, as may occur in the intensive care patient.

Outcomes

The short- and long-term goals provide a basis for evaluating the effectiveness of treatment for each problem. One of the best indicators of outcome is the change in objective findings after treatment. Although changes that occur immediately after a single treatment are related to physiotherapy intervention alone, changes over longer periods of time reflect treatment by the entire health team. Chest auscultation before and after a treatment may provide a simple indication of the effectiveness of that treatment. Similarly, the chest radiograph can demonstrate the effectiveness of physiotherapy treatment by showing diminution in the area of collapsed/consolidated lung. On a long-term basis, changes in lung function or exercise tolerance provide the most valuable measures of treatment outcome. If there are discrepancies between the actual and expected outcomes then the plan (P) should document the changes to the goals and/or treatment, as required.

The selection and use of appropriate outcome measures is fundamental to the evaluation of any therapy. Demonstrating the effects of physiotherapy intervention, using instruments which have high reliability and validity is increasingly being required by healthcare providers and physiotherapists themselves. Other parties which may require outcome data include the patient, caregivers, community and patient support groups.

To standardize the measurement of outcomes the World Health Organization (WHO) has developed a scale of functioning and disability, the International Classification of Functioning, Disability and Health (ICIDH-2) (WHO 2001). This scale focuses on human functioning at the level of the body, the whole person and the person within the social/environmental context. It classifies functioning of the affected body part and the whole person in terms of impairment to bodily function and structure, limitation of activity and restriction on participation. It is designed to measure the effectiveness of an intervention using a patient-focused measure rather than the more traditional medical focus. For example, a patient with bronchiectasis who has had three admissions to hospital for chest infections over the last year is taught the active cycle of breathing techniques (ACBT) to assist sputum clearance. Over the next 12 months the outcome measure important to the patient is the ability to maintain a full-time job, whilst the outcome measure important to the area health service is the cost saving achieved by a reduction in hospital admissions. Thus when selecting an outcome measure it is important to take into account for whom the data is needed.

DISCHARGE SUMMARY

Upon discharge or transfer elsewhere, a summary should be written of the patient's initial problems, treatment and outcomes. Instruction for home programmes and any other relevant information should also be included. Discharge summaries are helpful to other physiotherapists who may treat the patient in the future. The summary should always contain adequate information for future audit and studies of patient care.

AUDIT

'Audit' refers to the systematic and critical analysis of the quality of care. There are three main forms of audit: structure, process and outcome.

1. *Structural audit* examines the organization of resources within a certain area. This may address the availability of human and/or equipment resources, e.g. a hospital's requirements for TENS machines, batteries and electrodes.
2. *Process audit* investigates the system of delivery of care, e.g. studying the methods of patient referral.
3. *Outcome audit* is the most clinically based audit. It examines the results of physiotherapy care, e.g. assessing whether the goals of treatment have been met within the stated time frames.

The audit process is cyclical. First, a standard of care is defined. The actual practice is then audited in comparison with the agreed standard. Discrepancies provoke further discussion. Changes are then made to eliminate these discrepancies. After an appropriate length of time the cycle begins again.

EDUCATIONAL PROGRAMME

By using a structured system of problem-oriented medical records and audit, the problem-oriented medical system allows identification of areas where goals are not being met within an appropriate time frame. Audit may also reveal situations where the agreed standards are not met. In both instances staff education programmes will improve patient care.

CONCLUSION

Accurate assessment should reveal the exact nature of the patient's problems and delineate those that are amenable to physiotherapy. Only then can the best treatment be chosen for that patient. Subsequent reassessment is essential to ensure that treatment is specific, effective and efficient. This process ensures high-quality patient care.

REFERENCES

Aaronson NK 1989 Quality of life assessment in clinical trials: methodological issues. Controlled Clinical Trials 10: 195S–208S

Bradley J, Howard J, Wallace E, Elborn S 1999 Validity of a modified shuttle test in adult cystic fibrosis. Thorax 54: 437–439

Butland RJA, Pang J, Gross ER, Woodcock AA, Geddes DM 1982 Two-, six-, and 12-minute walking tests in respiratory disease. British Medical Journal 284: 1607–1608

Ellis E 1985 Making a teaching stethoscope. Australian Journal of Physiotherapy 31: 244

Juniper EF, Guyatt GH, Cox FM, Ferrie PJ, King DR 1999 Development and validation of the mini asthma quality of life questionnaire. European Respiratory Journal 14(1): 32–38

Kinney MR, Burfitt SN, Stullenbarger E, Rees B, DeBott MR 1996 Quality of life in cardiac patient research: a meta-analysis. Nursing Research 45(3): 173–180

Mahler DA 2000 How should health-related quality of life be assessed in patients with COPD? Chest 117(2) (Suppl): 54S-57S

Miller DL 1963 A study of techniques for the examination of sputum in a field survey of chronic bronchitis. American Review of Respiratory Disease 88: 473–483

Orr A, McVean RJ, Webb AK et al 2001 Urinary incontinence in women with cystic fibrosis is a marginalised and undertreated problem: questionnaire survey. British Medical Journal 322: 1521

Pashkow P, Ades PA, Emery CF et al 1995 Outcome measurement in cardiac and pulmonary rehabilitation. Journal of Cardiopulmonary Rehabilitation 15(6): 394–405

Revill SM, Morgan MDL, Singh SJ, Williams J, Hardman AE 1999 The endurance shuttle walk: a new field test for the assessment of endurance capacity in chronic obstructive pulmonary disease. Thorax 54: 213–222

Rubinstein I, Zamel N, DuBarry L, Hoffstein V 1990 Airflow limitation in morbidly obese, nonsmoking men. Annals of Internal Medicine 112(11): 828–832

Singh SJ, Morgan MDL, Scott S, Walters D, Hardman AE 1992 The development of the shuttle walking test of disability in patients with chronic airways obstruction. Thorax 47(12): 1019–1024

Thakar R, Stanton S 2000 Management of urinary incontinence in women. British Medical Journal 321: 1326–1331

Ware JE, Sherbourne CD 1992 The MOS-short-form health survey (SF-36). Medical Care 30: 473–483

Weed LL 1968 Medical records that guide and teach. New England Journal of Medicine 278: 593–600, 652–657

World Health Organization 2001 International Classification of Functioning, Disability and Health. In press. Final draft available at www.who.int/icidh

2

Thoracic imaging

Adults

*Susan J Copley   Connor D Collins
David M Hansell*

Paediatrics[1]

Christopher D George   Isky Gordon

ADULTS

CHEST RADIOGRAPHY AND OTHER TECHNIQUES

Different types of chest radiograph

Chest radiography has been used as the main radiological investigation of the chest since the discovery of X-rays by Röentgen in 1895 and chest radiographs comprise 25–40% of all radiological investigations. Chest radiographs are indicated in almost any condition in which a pulmonary abnormality is suspected.

The majority of chest radiographs are obtained in the main radiology department. The radiograph is obtained with the patient standing erect. Patients who are immobile or too ill to come to the main department have a chest radiograph performed using a mobile machine (portable film); the resulting radiograph differs from a departmental film in terms of projection, positioning, exposure and film used and is therefore not strictly comparable with a conventional posteroanterior (PA) film. Other types of chest radiograph are the lateral, lordotic, apical and decubitus views; these are generally taken in the main department.

Departmental films are referred to as 'posteroanterior' (or PA) chest radiographs and describe

---

[1] Reproduced with permission of Nelson Thornes Ltd from Paediatric Respiratory Care, ISBN 0 1425 5000 8 first published 1995.

the direction in which the X-ray beam traverses the patient. The patient is positioned with his anterior chest wall against the film cassette and his back to the X-ray tube. The arms are abducted to rotate the scapulae away from the posterior chest and the radiograph is taken during full inspiration. The tube is centred at the spinous process of the fourth thoracic vertebra. For portable films taken in an anteroposterior (AP) projection, the patient's back is against the film cassette and the X-ray tube is positioned at a variable distance from the patient. As the heart is placed anteriorly within the chest it is further from the cassette and is therefore magnified in an AP radiograph. The degree of magnification depends on the distance between the patient and the X-ray tube.

For a lateral radiograph the patient is turned 90° and the side of interest placed against the film cassette. The arms are extended forwards and the radiograph is again taken in full inspiration.

Lateral decubitus views are sometimes useful for the demonstration of small pleural effusions. For this projection the patient lies horizontally with the side in question placed downwards. The film cassette is positioned at the back of the patient and the X-ray beam is horizontal centred at the midsternum. This provides a sensitive means of detecting small quantities of pleural fluid (50–100 ml) that cannot be identified on a frontal chest radiograph. However, ultrasonography is increasingly being used as a reliable means of confirming the presence of small pleural effusions.

Lordotic films are sometimes used to confirm middle lobe collapse and for demonstrating a questionable apical opacity otherwise obscured by the clavicle and ribs. For this AP projection, the patient arches back so that the shoulders are touching the cassette with the centring point remaining the same. Linear tomography is another technique designed to reveal lesions otherwise hidden by the skeleton by blurring out everything overlying and underlying the lesion in question. This is achieved by having the X-ray tube and film cassette move at the same time but in opposite directions. These two techniques are less frequently used with the advent of computed tomography (CT).

Factors influencing the quality of a chest radiograph

The quality and thus diagnostic usefulness of a chest radiograph depend critically on the conditions under which it is obtained. Of particular importance are the radiographic exposure, the projection, the orientation of the patient relative to the film cassette, the X-ray tube to film distance, the depth of inspiration of the patient and the type of film–screen combination used.

The ideal chest radiograph provides an image of structures within the chest whilst exposing the patient to the lowest possible dose of radiation. Most radiology departments have a policy of obtaining either high kilovoltage (kVp) or low kilovoltage chest radiographs. Radiographs performed at high kilovoltage (e.g. 140 kVp) have much to recommend them. Even at total lung capacity with the patient erect, nearly a third of the lungs is partially obscured by the mediastinal structures, diaphragm and ribs. With the low-kilovoltage technique (80 kVp or less) these areas are often poorly visualized. This problem is partially overcome by using films exposed at high kVp. The normal vessel markings and subtle differences in soft tissue densities are better demonstrated and a further advantage is the better penetration of the mediastinum which improves visualization of the trachea and main bronchi. The disadvantage of high-kilovoltage radiographs is the relatively poor demonstration of calcified structures so that rib fractures and calcified pulmonary nodules or pleural plaques are less conspicuous.

During exposure the X-ray beam is modified according to the structures through which it passes. The photons that have passed through the patient carry information which then must be converted into a visual form. Some of the photons emerging from the patient are aligned in a virtually parallel direction and other photons are scattered. These scattered photons degrade the final image but can be absorbed by using lead strips embedded in an aluminium sheet positioned in front of the cassette. This device is known as a grid. Photons that are travelling in parallel pass through the grid to form the image on the film.

The sensitivity of film to direct X-ray exposure is very low and if film were used alone as the image receptor, this would result in a prohibitively large X-ray dose to the patient. Intensifying screens made of phosphorescent material are positioned on the inside of the cassettes and they convert the incident X-ray photons into visible light which is recorded by the adjacent film. These phosphor screens are composed of either calcium tungstate or a rare-earth containing compound. Rare-earth phosphors emit more light in response to X-ray photons and therefore less radiation is necessary to produce the image. Similarly, improvements in the quality of X-ray film have also occurred over the years. Standard film emulsions tend to lack detail in the relatively under- or overexposed areas of the radiograph and newer emulsions have been developed so that detail is similar in all areas of the chest radiograph. The choice of film–screen combination has a crucial influence on the quality and 'look' of the radiograph produced. Further variations may result from film-processing problems.

Over the years much effort has been expended on producing radiographs that are less affected by technical factors so that accurate comparisons can be made on serial radiographs of the same patient. Newer devices designed to accurately expose the various parts of the chest using automatic exposure devices are now being installed. One of these, the advanced multiple beam equalization radiography (AMBER) system, produces chest radiographs which greatly improve the demonstration of mediastinal abnormalities and pulmonary nodules which would otherwise be obscured by the overlying heart or diaphragm by continuously modulating X-ray output in response to transmitted radiation (Fig. 2.1).

In the intensive care setting, portable chest radiographs are often taken in less than ideal conditions. Multiple tubes, lines and dressings in conjunction with an immobile, supine patient and the use of a mobile low-kilovoltage machine often result in suboptimal radiographs. One approach to this is the development of phosphor plate technology which is ultimately expected to replace conventional film–screen radiography. The phosphor plate is placed inside a conventional cassette and stores some of the energy of the incident X-ray photons as a latent image (the image produced on

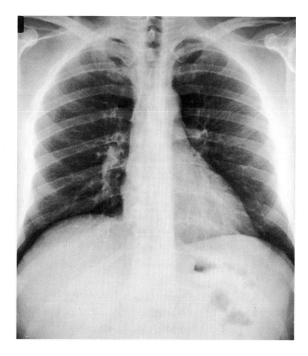

Figure 2.1   A normal AMBER chest radiograph (PA). This technique provides better detail of the lung parenchyma than conventional radiography.

a film or phosphor plate prior to development). The plate is scanned with a laser beam and the light emitted from the 'excited' latent image is detected by a photomultiplier or solid state image receptors. Thereafter this signal is processed in digital form. This digital image may be viewed either on a television monitor or on film (on which it has been laser printed). The great advantage of this system is that it can retrieve an image of diagnostic quality from a suboptimal exposure. Similar gross over- or underexposure would result in a non-diagnostic conventional radiograph. Manipulation of the digital image, particularly 'edge enhancement', aids the detection of linear structures such as the edge of a pneumothorax or central venous catheters (Fig. 2.2).

Other techniques

Fluoroscopy

The patient is positioned, either standing or lying, in a screening unit allowing 'real-time' visualization of the area in question on a television

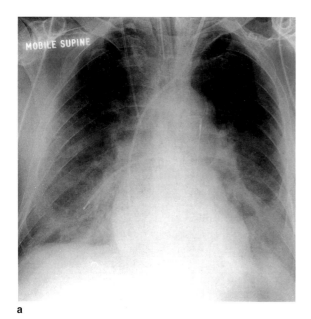

a

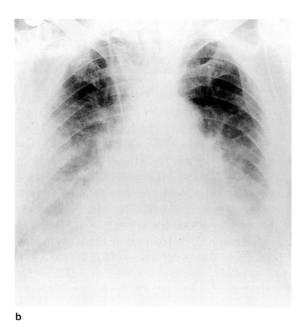

b

Figure 2.2 The same AP digital chest radiograph of a patient on the intensive care unit imaged on different settings. This technique has the advantage that the image can be made darker (**a**) or lighter (**b**) after it has been taken to allow better visualization of lines and tubes or lung parenchyma. Note the patient's endotracheal tube, right internal jugular central line, pulmonary artery catheter and intraaortic balloon pump.

monitor. The patient can be turned in any direction and this technique can help to distinguish pulmonary from extrapulmonary opacities. One of the main uses of fluoroscopy is to 'screen' the diaphragm to demonstrate paralysis or abnormal movement. It is also useful in needle placement during biopsy of lung masses.

Ultrasonography

High-frequency sound waves do not traverse air and the use of this technique is therefore limited in the chest. It is mainly used for cardiac imaging (echocardiography) and has become an essential technique in the investigation of patients with valvular and ventricular function problems. Outside the heart, ultrasonography is very useful in distinguishing between fluid above the diaphragm (pleural effusion; Fig. 2.3), fluid below the diaphragm (subphrenic) and pleural thickening. Chest radiography often cannot differentiate between pleural fluid and thickening with any certainty. Ultrasound can also be used to guide the placement of a percutaneous drain into a pleural effusion.

Computed tomography

Computed tomography (CT) scanning depends on the same basic physical principle as conventional radiography, namely the absorption of X-rays by tissues of different densities. The basic components of a CT machine are a table on which the patient lies and a gantry through which the table slides. An X-ray tube and a series of detectors are housed within the gantry. The X-ray tube and detectors rotate around the patient. A computer is used to reconstruct the signals received by the detectors into an image. The images acquired are transverse (axial) cross-sections of the patient. In orienting the patient's right and left sides, it is the convention to view all CT images as if from the patient's feet.

Because of the cross-sectional nature of CT it can accurately localize lesions seen on only one view on plain chest radiographs. The superior contrast resolution of CT allows superb demonstration of mediastinal anatomy (e.g. lymph

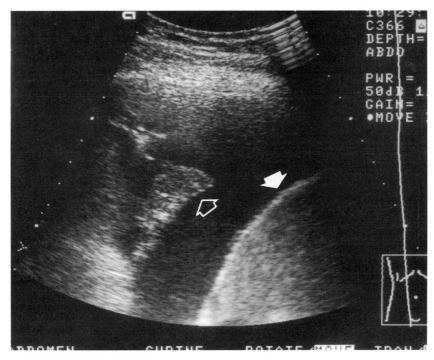

Figure 2.3 Ultrasound of lower right hemithorax/upper abdomen demonstrating a right basal effusion with fluid interposed between collapsed right lower lobe (open arrow) and diaphragm (closed arrow).

nodes and vessels) (Fig. 2.4) as well as calcification within a pulmonary nodule. Highly detailed thin sections of the lung parenchyma can also be obtained, allowing the complex morphology of many interstitial lung diseases to be more accurately defined. The disadvantages of CT are its relatively high cost and increased radiation exposure to the patient compared with chest radiography.

A relatively recent development has been the introduction of helical (spiral) CT scanning. Whereas conventional CT scanning involves alternating table movement through the gantry with exposure, helical CT involves simultaneous table movement and X-ray exposure. The technique allows faster scan times and advantages are the elimination of respiratory artefacts, minimization of motion artefacts and production of overlapping images without additional radiation exposure. Helical (spiral) CT is so named because the X-ray can be thought of as tracing a helix or spiral curve on the patient's surface.

Common indications for CT of the chest.

1. CT scanning is used to further evaluate hilar or mediastinal masses seen or suspected on a chest radiograph.
2. Within the lungs it can be used to further define the nature of a mass or cavitating lesion not clearly seen on the plain film.
3. In patients with normal chest radiographs but abnormal pulmonary function tests, thin high-resolution CT sections of the lung may provide the first radiological evidence of parenchymal disease. This type of scanning is also very useful for assessing patients with suspected bronchiectasis.
4. CT is useful in patients with neoplasms, in assessing both their operability and their response to treatment.
5. Detection of pulmonary embolism (spiral CT).
6. For guiding the percutaneous needle biopsy of lung lesions, mediastinal masses or chest wall abnormalities.

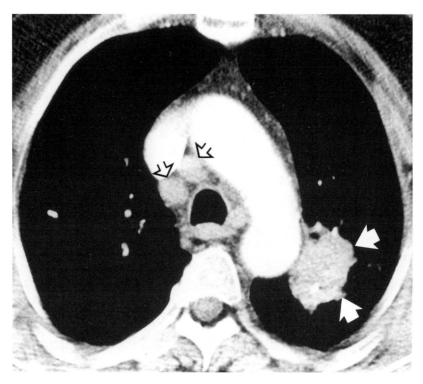

Figure 2.4 Computed tomography (CT) image post intravenous contrast showing a lung tumour adjacent to the arch of the aorta (closed arrows). Lymph nodes are seen anterior to the trachea (open arrows) which were not visible on chest radiography.

Magnetic resonance imaging

The physical principles of magnetic resonance imaging (MRI) are more complex and very different from those of CT scanning. The equipment consists of a sliding table on which the patient lies within the bore of a large magnet. A combination of the intense magnetic field and a series of radiofrequency waves produces an alteration in the alignment of protons (mostly in water) resulting in the emission of different signals which are detected and subsequently analysed for their intensity and position by a computer. The major advantages of MRI are that images may be obtained in any plane without the use of ionizing radiation. The disadvantages are its inability to produce detailed images of the lung, cost and reduced acceptability to patients because of the claustrophobic bore of the magnet. There are also important contraindications such as permanent cardiac pacemaker devices. Its application to chest imaging is limited at present but the technique is good for imaging chest wall lesions (Fig. 2.5), the great vessels and the heart.

Interventional procedures

Percutaneous needle biopsy

Percutaneous needle biopsy of a pulmonary or mediastinal mass, to provide a histological specimen, is usually performed in patients in whom a bronchoscopic biopsy has failed or a thoracotomy is inappropriate. Different types of needle are used and the complication rate (pneumothorax and haemoptysis) bears some relation to the site of the lesion, the size of the needle and the number of attempts to obtain tissue. Contraindications to the procedure include any patient with poor respiratory reserve unable to withstand a pneumothorax, pulmonary arterial hypertension and a previous contralateral pneumonectomy.

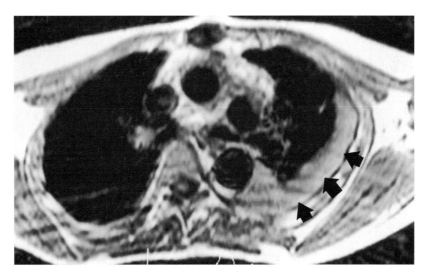

Figure 2.5   Magnetic resonance image (MRI) of the thorax. There is a left-sided pleural effusion (arrows).

Pulmonary and bronchial arteriography, superior vena cavography

Pulmonary arteriography. This is usually undertaken in the investigation of suspected pulmonary arteriovenous malformations and, less commonly since the development of helical (spiral) CT, pulmonary embolism. It requires puncture of either the femoral vein in the groin or the antecubital vein in the elbow and the guiding of a catheter through the right side of the heart under fluoroscopy. The tip of the catheter is positioned in the main pulmonary artery or selectively placed in a smaller pulmonary artery. Contrast is then injected. Arteriography remains the most specific method of identifying pulmonary emboli; these are shown as filling defects which cause non-filling of branches of the arterial tree. It is also the best and most appropriate technique for the demonstration of pulmonary arteriovenous malformations. These can be treated at the time of the arteriogram by the injection of occlusive materials (embolization).

Bronchial arteriography. Demonstration of the bronchial arteries requires catheterization of the femoral artery and passage of a catheter into the midthoracic aorta from where the bronchial arteries are selectively catheterized. The major indication for this procedure is recurrent or life-threatening haemoptysis in patients with a chronic inflammatory disease, usually bronchiectasis. Accurate placement of the catheter not only allows demonstration of the bleeding vessel but also allows embolization to be performed simultaneously.

Superior vena cavography. This is performed for the evaluation of superior vena caval (SVC) obstruction and the investigation of anatomical variants. More recently, patients with SVC compression due to tumour have been palliated by the insertion of an expandable metallic mesh wire stent at the site of the SVC narrowing, thus restoring flow and relieving symptoms.

THE NORMAL CHEST

Anatomy

On the normal posteroanterior radiograph (Fig. 2.6) the following structures can be identified:

- outline of the mediastinum and heart
- the hila
- pulmonary vessels and main bronchi
- diaphragm
- soft tissues and bones of the thoracic cage.

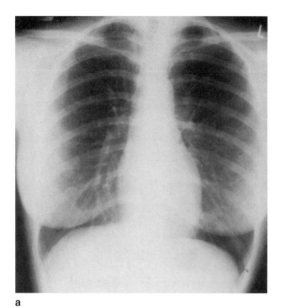

a

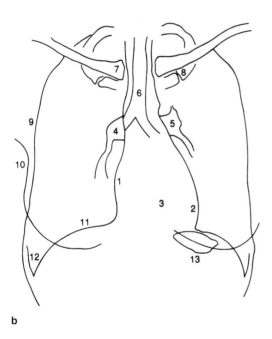

b

Figure 2.6 a Normal PA chest radiograph. **b** Normal structures visible on a PA chest radiograph: 1 right atrium; 2 left ventricle; 3 right ventricle; 4 right pulmonary artery; 5 left pulmonary artery; 6 air within trachea; 7 clavicle; 8 first rib; 9 lateral border of hemithorax; 10 breast shadow; 11 right hemidiaphragm; 12 costophrenic angle; 13 gastric air bubble.

The heart and mediastinum

The mediastinum consists of the organs and soft tissues in the central part of the chest. These comprise the trachea, aortic arch and great vessels, superior vena cava and oesophagus. In children the thymus gland is a prominent component. On the two-dimensional chest radiograph these structures are superimposed and cannot be clearly distinguished from each other. The mediastinum is conventionally divided into superior, anterior, middle and posterior compartments. Whilst the boundaries of the latter three are arbitrary, it is usual to divide the mediastinum into equal thirds. The superior mediastinum is that portion lying above the aortic arch and below the root of the neck.

The mediastinal border on the right is formed superiorly by the right brachiocephalic vein and superior vena cava. The mediastinal shadow to the left of the trachea above the aortic arch comprises the left carotid and left subclavian arteries together with the left brachiocephalic and jugular veins. On a correctly exposed chest radiograph, air in the trachea can be seen throughout its length as it descends downwards, deviating slightly to the right above the carina (where the trachea divides into the right and left main bronchi) due to displacement by the aortic arch.

The heart lies eccentrically in the chest, with one-third of the cardiac shadow to the right of the spine and two-thirds to the left. The density of the cardiac shadow on the left and right of the spine should be identical. The right cardiac border on a chest radiograph is formed by the right atrium. The left cardiac border is composed of the apex of the left ventricle and superiorly the left atrial appendage. The outline of the right ventricle, which is superimposed on the left ventricle, cannot be identified on a frontal radiograph. The maximum transverse diameter of the heart should be less than half the maximum transverse diameter of the thorax, as measured from the inside border of the ribs (the so-called 'cardiothoracic ratio').

The hila

Hilar shadows are a complex summation of the pulmonary arteries and veins with minor contributions from other components (the main bronchi and lymph nodes). In general, the hila are of equal density and are approximately the same size. Adjacent to the left hilum, the main pulmonary artery forms a localized bulge just above the left atrial appendage and just below the aortic arch. The area between the aortic arch and the main pulmonary artery is known as the 'aortopulmonary window'.

The superior pulmonary veins run vertically and converge on the upper and midhilum on both sides. It is not possible to distinguish arteries from veins in the outer two-thirds of the lungs. The inferior pulmonary veins run obliquely in a near-horizontal plane below the lower lobe arteries to enter the left atrium beneath the carina. The hilar point is where the superior pulmonary vein on each side crosses the basal artery. This is more easily assessed on the right than on the left. Using this as an index point, the left hilum is normally 0.5–1.5 cm higher than the right one.

Abnormalities of the hilar shadows in the form of increased density or abnormal configuration are usually the result of lymph node or pulmonary artery enlargement. The detection of subtle hilar abnormalities is difficult and requires experience and knowledge of the many outlines that the hila may assume in normal individuals.

Fissures, vessels and segmental bronchi within the lungs

Each lung is divided into lobes surrounded by visceral pleura. There are two lobes on the left (the upper and lower, separated by the major (oblique) fissure) and three on the right (the upper, middle and lower lobes which are separated by the major (oblique) and minor (horizontal or transverse) fissures). In the majority of normal subjects some or all of the minor fissure is seen on a frontal radiograph. The major fissures are only identifiable on the lateral projection. Each lobe of the lung contains a number of segments which have their own segmental bronchi. The walls of the segmental bronchi are invisible on the chest radiograph, except when seen end-on as ring shadows measuring up to 7 mm in diameter.

The pulmonary blood vessels are responsible for the branching and linear structures within the lungs. The diameter of the blood vessels beyond the hilum varies with the position of the patient and with haemodynamic factors. In the erect position there is a gradual increase in the diameter of the vessels, travelling from apex to base. This increase in size is seen in both the arteries and veins and is abolished if the patient lies supine.

The diaphragm

The interface between the lung and diaphragm should be sharp and, in general, the diaphragm is dome shaped with its highest point medial to the midclavicular line. The margin of the right hemidiaphragm at its highest point lies between the anterior ends of the fifth and seventh ribs. The right hemidiaphragm is usually higher than the left by up to 2 cm in the erect position. Laterally, the diaphragm dips downwards, forming a sharp angle with the chest wall known as the 'costophrenic angle'. Filling in or blunting of these angles reflects pleural disease, either fluid or thickening.

Thoracic cage

On a high kilovoltage chest radiograph it should be possible to identify the edges of the vertebral bodies of the dorsal spine through the heart shadow. However, a high kilovoltage radiograph may 'burn out' the ribs, particularly the posterior portions. Because of this the chest radiograph may be an insensitive means of demonstrating rib abnormalities, particularly fractures.

Common anatomical variants

The trachea lies centrally, but in the elderly may deviate markedly to the right in its lower portion due to unfolding and dilatation of the aortic arch. A small ovoid soft tissue shadow just above the origin of the right main bronchus represents the azygos vein. This may be enlarged as a result of posture (supine position) or haemodynamic factors. It may be indistinguishable from an azygos lymph node.

Occasionally, extra fissures are seen in the lungs. The most common of these is the azygos lobe fissure; this is seen as a fine white line running obliquely from the apex of the right lung to the azygos vein. Other accessory fissures are the superior and inferior accessory fissures, both of which are in the right lower lobe.

The surfaces of the two lungs abut each other anteriorly and posteriorly and give rise to two white lines projected over the vertebral column, known as the 'anterior and posterior junction lines' respectively. Both of these may be seen overlying the trachea – the anterior line extending from the clavicles to the left main bronchus and the posterior line lying more medially and extending above the clavicles. The azygo-oesophageal recess line is a curved line projected over the vertebral column and extending from the azygos vein to the diaphragm. It represents the interface between the right lung and right oesophageal wall.

A small 'nipple' may occasionally be seen projecting laterally from the aortic knuckle due to the left superior intercostal vein. The term 'paraspinal line' refers to the line that parallels the left and right margin of the thoracic spine. The left is thicker than the right because of the adjacent aorta.

The lateral view

It is conventional to read the lateral film (Fig. 2.7) with the heart to the viewer's left and the dorsal spine to the right, irrespective of whether the film is labelled 'right' or 'left'. The chamber of the heart that touches the sternum is the right ventricle. Behind and above the heart lies lung, the density of which should be the same both behind the heart and behind the sternum. As the eye travels down the spine, the vertebral column should appear increasingly transradiant or 'dark' (Fig. 2.7a); the loss of this phenomenon suggests the presence of disease in the posterobasal segments of the lower lobes. In the middle of the lateral film lie the hilar structures with the main pulmonary artery anteriorly. The aortic arch should be easily identified but only a variable proportion of the great vessels is visible depend-

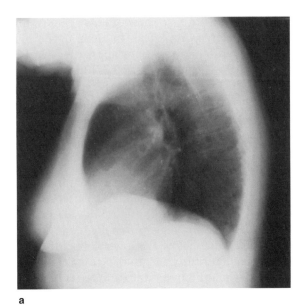

a

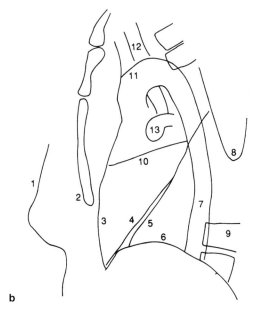

b

Figure 2.7 a Normal lateral chest radiograph. **b** Normal structures visible on a lateral chest radiograph: 1 breast shadow; 2 sternum; 3 position of right ventricle; 4 right oblique fissure; 5 left oblique fissure; 6 hemidiaphragm; 7 descending aorta; 8 inferior angle of scapula; 9 dorsal vertebrae; 10 horizontal fissure; 11 aortic arch; 12 trachea; 13 pulmonary artery.

ing on the degree of aortic unfolding. The brachiocephalic artery is most frequently identified arising anterior to the tracheal air column. The left and right brachiocephalic veins form an extrapleural bulge behind the upper sternum in about a third of individuals.

The course of the trachea is straight with a slight posterior angulation but no visible indentation from adjacent vessels. The carina is not seen on the lateral view. The posterior wall of the trachea is always visible and is known as the 'posterior tracheal stripe'.

The oblique fissures are seen as fine diagonal lines running from the upper dorsal spine to the diaphragm anteriorly. The left is more vertically oriented and is visible just behind the right. The minor fissure extends forwards horizontally from the mid-right oblique fissure. Care must be taken not to confuse rib margins with fissure lines. As the fissures undulate, two distinct fissure lines may be generated by a single fissure. The fissures should be of no more than hairline width.

The scapulae are invariably seen in the lateral view and since they are incompletely visualized, lines formed by the edge of the scapula can easily be confused with intrathoracic structures. The arms are held outstretched in front of the patient on a lateral view and these give rise to soft tissue shadows projected over the anterior and superior mediastinum. A band-like opacity simulating pleural disease is often seen along the lower half of the anterior chest wall immediately behind the sternum. The left lung does not contact the most anterior portion of the left thoracic cavity at these levels because the heart occupies the space. This band-like opacity is known as the 'retrosternal line'.

Useful points in interpreting a chest radiograph

Documentary information. The name of the patient and the time and date on which the radiograph was taken, particularly in relation to other films in a series, should all be noted. Often the film is annotated with the patient's date of birth. Of particular importance is the presence of the side markers ('right' or 'left'). The radiograph should also be marked 'AP' if the anteroposterior projection was used; departmental posteroanterior (PA) films are generally not marked as such.

Radiographic projection. A judgement as to whether a radiograph is AP or PA can be made from the following evidence.

1. The position of the label (this varies from department to department and is open to error).
2. The relationship of the scapulae to the lung margins (in the PA projection the scapulae are projected clear of the lungs and in AP projection they overlie the lungs).
3. The appearance of the vertebral bodies in the cervicodorsal region. The vertebral endplates are seen more clearly in the AP projection and the laminae are more clearly seen in the PA projection.

Supine versus prone position. It is important to know whether a chest radiograph was taken in the erect or supine position. In the supine position, blood flow is more evenly distributed throughout the lungs, making the upper zone vessels equal in size to those in the lower zones. This has implications in assessing the chest radiograph of a patient suspected of being in cardiac failure. In addition, fluid is distributed throughout the dependent part of the pleural space and any air–fluid levels that might be present on an erect film are impossible to detect. The position and contours of the heart, mediastinum and diaphragm are also different compared with an erect film. In the absence of any indication on the radiograph, one clue is the position of the gastric air bubble: if it is just under the left hemidiaphragm it is in the fundus and the patient is erect, whereas in the supine position air collects in the antrum of the stomach which lies centrally or slightly to the right of the vertebral column, well below the diaphragm.

Patient rotation. The patient may be rotated around one of three axes. Axial rotation is the most common cause of unilateral transradiancy (one lung appearing darker than the other). It also distorts the mediastinal outline. The degree of rotation can be assessed by relating the medial ends of the clavicles to the spinous process of the vertebral body at the same level – they should be equidistant from the spinous processes.

Rotation about the horizontal coronal axis results in a more kyphotic or lordotic projection than normal. The main pulmonary artery and subclavian vessels may appear unduly prominent. Rotation around the horizontal sagittal axis usually leads to obvious tilt of the chest in relation to the edge of the radiograph which is assumed to be upright.

Physical attributes of the patient, such as a kyphoscoliosis or a depressed sternum (pectus excavatum), may also distort the appearance of the thoracic cage and its contents.

State of inspiration or expiration. The degree of inspiration is an important consideration for the correct interpretation of a chest radiograph. A poor inspiratory effort does not necessarily imply lack of patient cooperation and may as often be related to a pathological process. At full inspiration the midpoint of the right hemidiaphragm lies between the anterior end of ribs 5–7. A shallow inspiration affects the contour of the heart and mediastinum and may mimic the appearances of pulmonary congestion because the upper zone vessels will have the same diameter as the lower zone vessels.

Films taken deliberately with the patient in full expiration are invaluable in the investigation of air trapping. They are mandatory in any patient suspected of having inhaled a foreign body with consequent obstruction of a lobar bronchus. An expiratory film is also useful in accentuating a small pneumothorax.

Review areas. Several areas are difficult to assess on a frontal radiograph and should be scrutinized carefully. These review areas are:

- apices
- behind the heart
- hilar regions
- bones
- lung periphery just inside the chest wall.

Detection and description of radiographic abnormalities should then be undertaken and a differential diagnosis listed based on the abnormalities detected. With experience, the structured search gives way to the rapid identification of abnormalities and a search for confirmatory radiological signs and associated abnormalities.

COMMON RADIOLOGICAL SIGNS
Consolidation

'Consolidation' is the term used to describe lung in which the air-filled spaces are replaced by the products of disease, e.g. water, pus or blood. The two most important radiological signs of consolidation are (a) an air bronchogram and (b) the silhouette sign. The causes of widespread consolidation may be divided into four categories (Box 2.1).

An air bronchogram is present when the airways contain air and appear as radiolucent (black) branching structures against a now white background of airless lung. The silhouette sign is present when the border of a structure is lost because the normally air-filled lung outlining the border is replaced by radio-opaque fluid or tissue. Recognition of this sign can help localize the affected area of abnormality within the chest. Thus, loss of a clear right heart border is due to right middle lobe consolidation or collapse.

Localized areas of consolidation are usually due to infection. In some cases the borders of the consolidation are clearly demarcated. This usually corresponds to a fissure and the consolidation is confined to one lobe (lobar pneumonia) (Fig. 2.8). If consolidation is slow to clear with treatment, it may be secondary to partial obstruc-

Box 2.1 Causes of widespread pulmonary consolidation	
Fluid transudation	Pulmonary oedema due to cardiac failure, renal failure, hepatic failure
Exudation	Infection, e.g. lobar pneumonia and bronchopneumonia, tuberculosis Acute respiratory distress syndrome (ARDS) Pulmonary haemorrhage due to contusion Pulmonary eosinophilia
Inhalation	Gastric contents Toxic fumes Oxygen toxicity
Infiltration	Lymphoma Alveolar cell carcinoma

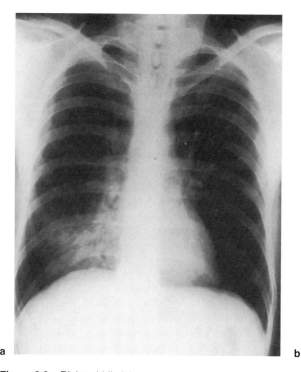
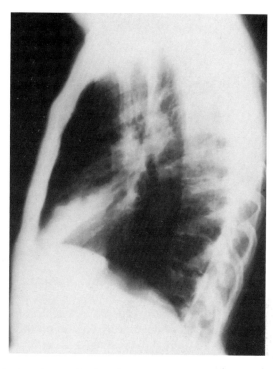

a   b

Figure 2.8   Right middle lobe consolidation. **a** The right heart border is not seen clearly owing to adjacent consolidation. Note that the right hemidiaphragm is clearly visible as far as the vertebral column. **b** The lateral view confirms the presence of consolidation in the right middle lobe with the posterior aspect well demarcated by the oblique fissure.

tion of a lobar bronchus, such as carcinoma of the bronchus. Consolidation may also be widespread and affect both lungs (Figs 2.9, 2.10).

Collapse (atelectasis)

'Collapse' (atelectasis) is the radiological term used when there is loss of aeration and, therefore, expansion in part or all of a lung. Collapse of a lobe or an entire lung is most frequently due to an endobronchial tumour, an inhaled foreign body or a mucus plug.

Although collapse is most often thought of as occurring at a lobar level, focal areas of pulmonary collapse at a subsegmental level occur very commonly in postoperative patients. There

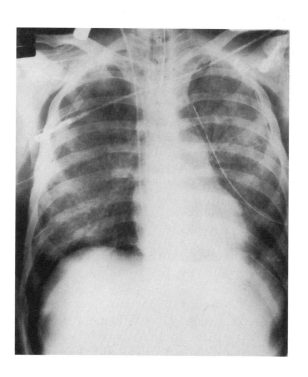

Figure 2.9   Widespread airspace consolidation in a patient with acute respiratory distress syndrome (ARDS). There are multiple chest drains for bilateral pneumothoraces.

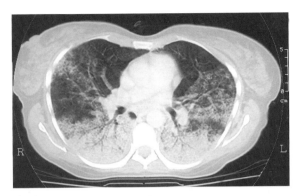

Figure 2. 10 Diffuse consolidation within apical segments of both lower lobes. Note prominent bilateral air bronchograms within consolidated lung. Infection due to *Pneumocystis carinii* and cytomegalovirus in an immunocompromised patient.

Box 2.2 Signs associated with a collapsed lobe

- Increased density of the collapsed lobe
- Shift of fissures
- Silhouette sign
- Hilar shift and distortion
- Crowding of vessels and airways
- Mediastinal shift
- Crowding of the ribs
- Elevation of hemidiaphragm

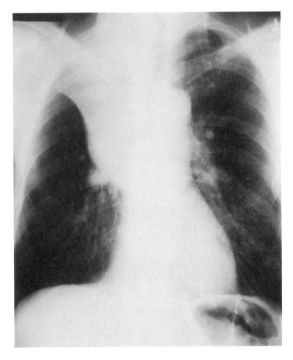

Figure 2.11 Right upper lobe collapse. There is increased density medial to the elevated horizontal fissure. The cause was a large central tumour obstructing the right upper lobe bronchus.

---

are many signs of lobar collapse but it is important to realize that not all these signs occur together. In addition, some non-specific signs may be present which indirectly point to the diagnosis and alert the observer to look for the more specific signs.

The most reliable and frequently present finding in lobar collapse is shift of the fissures, which invariably occurs to some extent. If air stays in the collapsed lobe, the contained blood vessels remain visible and appear crowded. If there is marked volume loss the density of the collapsed and airless lobe increases. The hila may show two types of change consisting either of gross displacement upwards or downwards or of rearrangement of individual hilar components (i.e. vessels and airways) leading to changes in shape and prominence. Elevation of the hemidiaphragm, reflecting volume loss, is most marked in collapse of a lower lobe. 'Peaking' of the mid-portion of the hemidiaphragm occurs in upper lobe collapse due to displacement of the oblique fissure. The signs associated with collapse are listed in Box 2.2.

Collapse of individual lobes

Right upper lobe

On the PA radiograph there is elevation of the transverse fissure and the right hilum. If the collapse is complete the non-aerated lobe is seen as an increased density alongside the superior mediastinum adjacent to the trachea (Fig. 2.11). On the lateral view the minor fissure moves upwards and the major fissure moves forwards. The retrosternal area becomes progressively more opaque and the anterior margin of the ascending aorta becomes effaced.

Right middle lobe

On the PA radiograph the lateral part of the minor fissure moves down and there is blurring of the normally sharp right heart border. This may be a subtle abnormality which is easily overlooked. On the lateral view the minor fissure moves downwards and the lower half of the major fissure moves forwards, giving rise to a triangular shadow visible behind the lower sternum (Fig. 2.12).

Right lower lobe

On the PA view there is an increase in density overlying the medial portion of the right hemidiaphragm and the right hilum is displaced inferiorly. The right heart border usually remains sharply defined since this is in contact with the aerated right middle lobe. On the lateral view the oblique fissure moves backwards and with increasing collapse, there is loss of definition of the right hemidiaphragm as well as increased density overlying the lower dorsal vertebrae.

Right lower lobe collapse is a mirror image of left lower lobe collapse (Fig. 2.13).

Left upper lobe

The main finding on the PA radiograph is of a veil-like increase in density, without a sharp margin, spreading outwards and upwards from the left hilum which is elevated. The aortic knuckle, left hilum and left heart border may have ill-defined outlines. As volume loss increases, the collapsed lobe moves closer to the midline and the lung apex may become lucent due to hyperinflation of the apical segment of the left lower lobe. A sharp border may also return to the aortic arch. On the lateral view the oblique fissure moves upwards and forwards, remaining relatively straight and roughly parallel to the anterior chest wall (Fig. 2.14). On the PA projection, collapse (or consolidation) of the

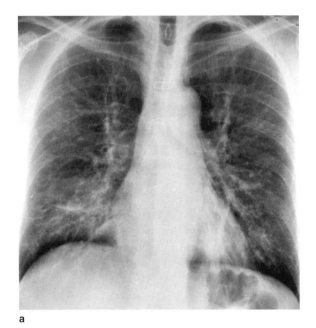

a

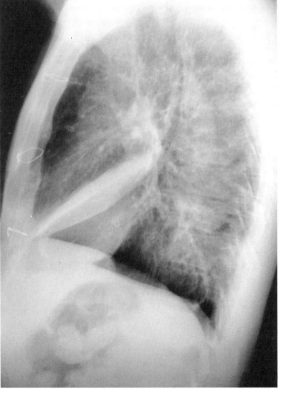

b

Figure 2.12 Right middle lobe collapse in a patient post-thoracotomy. **a** Loss of the right heart border may be subtle on the frontal film (note the patient also has some left lower lobe consolidation). **b** The lateral view shows the typical triangular opacity overlying the cardiac shadow.

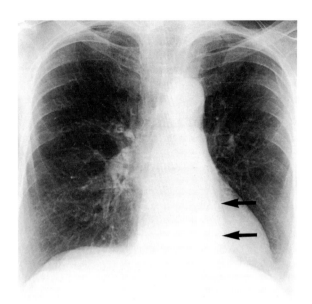

Figure 2.13 Left lower lobe collapse. A PA radiograph shows loss of the outline of the medial portion of the left hemidiaphragm and a triangular density behind the left side of the heart (arrows). There is also volume loss of the left hemithorax and the mediastinum is deviated to the left, allowing increased visibility of the thoracic spine.

lingular segment of the left upper lobe should be suspected when the left cardiac border is ill defined.

Left lower lobe

This is most commonly seen in patients following cardiac surgery and a thoracotomy due to the retention of secretions in the left lower lobe bronchus. On the PA view there is a triangular density behind the heart with loss of the medial portion of the left hemidiaphragm (Fig. 2.13); if the PA radiograph is underexposed, it may be impossible to see this triangular opacity. On the lateral view there is backwards displacement of the oblique fissure and with increasing collapse there is increased density over the lower dorsal vertebrae.

Pneumothorax

When air is introduced into the pleural space, the resulting pneumothorax can be recognized radio-

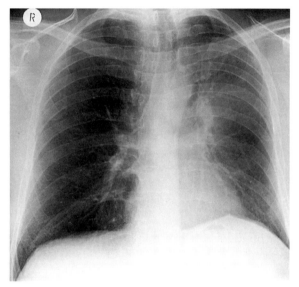

a

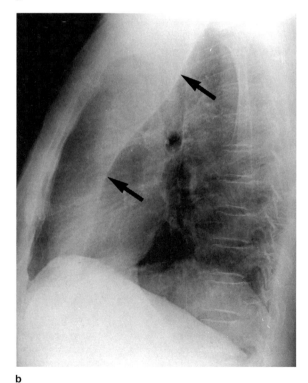

b

Figure 2.14 Left upper lobe collapse. **a** There is a veil-like density of the left hemithorax which obscures the outline of the aortic knuckle and left heart border superiorly. There is also volume loss on the left (the trachea is deviated to the left and the left hemidiaphragm is raised with 'peaking' centrally). **b** The lateral radiograph shows increased density anterior to the oblique fissure (arrows).

graphically. There are numerous causes of a pneumothorax but the most common include penetrating injuries (e.g. stab wound, placement of a subclavian line) and breaches of the visceral pleura (e.g. spontaneous rupture of a subpleural bulla or mechanical ventilation with high pressures). The cardinal radiographic sign is the visceral pleural edge: lateral to this edge no vascular shadows are visible and medial to it the collapsed lung is of higher density than the contralateral lung (Fig. 2.15). It is important to remember that in the supine position, the air of a small pneumothorax will collect anteriorly in the pleural space; thus on a portable supine chest radiograph, the pneumothorax will be visible as an area of relative translucency without a visceral pleural edge necessarily being identifiable.

If air enters the pleural space during inspiration but cannot leave on expiration (usually because of a check-valve effect of the torn flap of the visceral pleura), pressure increases rapidly and this results in a life-threatening tension pneumothorax. This can be recognized by a shift of the mediastinum to the opposite side (Fig. 2.16).

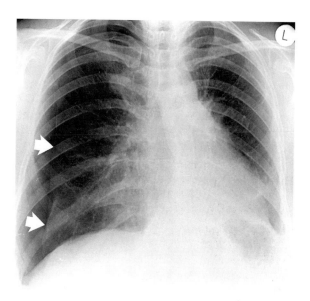

Figure 2.16 Tension pneumothorax post thoracoscopic biopsy of a right upper zone lung nodule. The pneumothorax in Fig. 2.15 involves more of the hemithorax but this pneumothorax is causing deviation of the mediastinum to the opposite side and is potentially life threatening unless treated promptly. The visceral pleural edge is visible (arrows).

The opaque hemithorax

If one-half of a chest is completely opaque (a white-out) it is due either to collapse of a lung or a large pleural effusion. If there is a shift of the mediastinum to the affected side it implies that volume loss in the lung (i.e. collapse) on that side must have occurred. Where there is no shift of the mediastinum or it is shifted slightly to the side of the white-out, this is usually due to constricting pleural disease (including pleural tumour). A pleural effusion which is large enough to cause complete opacification of a hemithorax will displace the mediastinum away from the side of the white-out. Whilst penetrated PA and lateral films may help, it is sometimes surprisingly difficult to differentiate between the causes of an opaque hemithorax. Ultrasound and computed tomography allow the distinction to be made with confidence and the latter may give further information about the underlying disease.

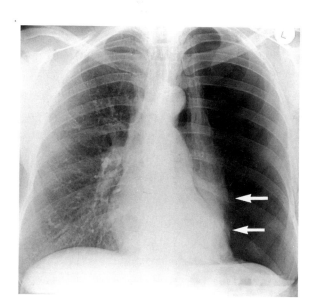

Figure 2.15 Spontaneous pneumothorax. There is a large left-sided pneumothorax with loss of vascular markings lateral to the edge of the collapsed lung. The visceral pleural edge is visible (arrows).

Decreased density of a hemithorax

The conditions outlined so far have all focused on increased density of the lungs on plain radiographs. However, there are a number of causes where one lung appears less dense than the other side. When a chest radiograph demonstrates greater radiolucency of one lung compared with the other, it is necessary first to determine whether this appearance is due to a pulmonary abnormality; the radiograph should be checked for patient rotation and for soft tissue asymmetry, e.g. a mastectomy.

The pulmonary vessels are a helpful pointer to abnormalities causing a true decrease in density. In compensatory hyperinflation they are splayed apart. A search should also be made for a collapsed lobe. The vessels are considerably diminished or truncated in emphysema. Further radiological examination should include an expiration film if a pneumothorax is suspected. This will also demonstrate air trapping that occurs with bronchial obstruction. Computed tomography may also be useful in elucidating the cause of a hyperlucent lung. The lungs can be seen on computed tomography without the problem of overlying tissues and any decrease in density is more readily apparent.

Elevation of the diaphragm

The right or left dome of the diaphragm may be elevated because it is paralysed, pushed up or pulled up. However, there are a number of circumstances in which the diaphragm appears to be elevated without actually being so.

The radiographic evaluation of an apparently elevated diaphragm should begin with an assessment of the plain film, in particular evidence of prior surgery. Old radiographs are essential to determine whether the diaphragmatic elevation is of long standing. A decubitus film is particularly useful in ruling out a suspected subpulmonary effusion; in this instance the pleural effusion is confined to the space between the lung base and the superior surface of the diaphragm. The radiograph will show what appears to be an elevated hemidiaphragm. Ultrasound will assist in determining if fluid is present above and/or below the diaphragm.

If the hemidiaphragm is paralysed, fluoroscopic examination is useful as it may demonstrate paradoxical movement on vigorous sniffing (instead of the diaphragm moving down, it moves up). An important proviso is that a few normal individuals show this paradoxical movement of the diaphragm on sniffing. In congenital eventration part or all of the hemidiaphragm muscle is made up of a thin layer of fibrous tissue and it may be difficult to distinguish from paralysis even on fluoroscopy.

Pleural disease

Because the chest radiograph is a two-dimensional image, abnormalities of the pleura and chest wall are often difficult to assess. Gross pleural abnormalities are usually obvious on a chest radiograph (Fig. 2.17), but even when there is extensive pleural pathology it may be difficult to distinguish between pleural fluid, pleural thickening (e.g.

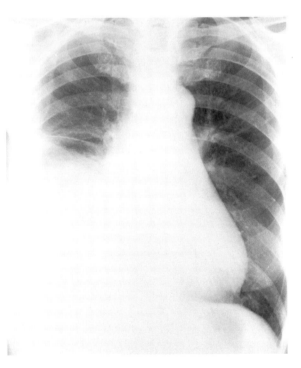

Figure 2.17 Pleural effusion. The right lower and mid zones are opaque due to a large right-sided pleural effusion.

secondary to a previous inflammatory process) and a neoplasm of the pleura. In such cases a lateral decubitus film or ultrasound scan is useful in identifying the presence of fluid. Computed tomography can readily identify the encasing and constricting nature of a mesothelioma.

The pulmonary mass

Most pulmonary nodules or masses are discovered by plain chest radiography. It is important to obtain previous films if at all possible. If the mass was present on the previous films and has not changed over a number of years, it can be assumed that the lesion is benign and no further action needs to be taken. However, if the nodule was not previously present or has increased in size, further investigation is warranted.

Computed tomography (see Fig. 2.4) will detect or exclude the presence of other lesions within the lungs. The presence of calcification within the nodule, although often thought to be an indicator of benignity, will not exclude malignancy with complete certainty. In addition, computed tomography can be used to determine the presence of hilar or mediastinal lymph node enlargement as well as direct invasion of the adjacent mediastinum or chest wall. In patients in whom surgical resection of the pulmonary mass is not indicated, a cytological or histological specimen by percutaneous needle biopsy may be taken. This is usually reserved for small peripheral lesions that are not accessible by bronchoscopy. It can be performed under computed tomography guidance or fluoroscopy but complications include pneumothorax or pulmonary haemorrhage (see other interventional techniques).

Pulmonary nodules

A large number of conditions are characterized by multiple pulmonary nodules (Fig. 2.18). Combining the clinical information with an accurate description of the size and distribution of the nodules narrows down the list of differential diagnoses.

Metastatic deposits are by far the most common cause of multiple pulmonary nodules of varying

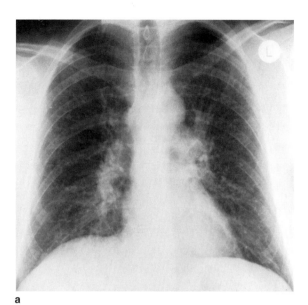

a

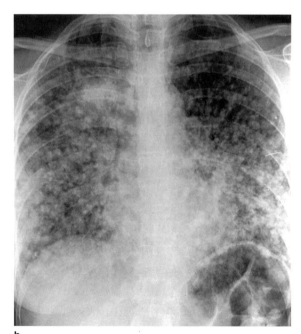

b

Figure 2.18 Multiple pulmonary nodules. **a** Pulmonary sarcoidosis. These pulmonary nodules are small (2–3 mm) and subtle and there is bilateral hilar lymphadenopathy. **b** Multiple pulmonary metastases. These nodules are more well defined, larger (most 0.5–1 cm in diameter) and are so numerous that they have coalesced in the right upper zone.

sizes in adult patients in the United Kingdom (Fig. 2.18) but this is not the case worldwide. In some parts of the USA, histoplasmosis is endemic and multiple lesions due to this condition may be more common than those due to malignancy. Making this important distinction may be difficult and biopsy of one lesion may be the only reliable means of distinguishing a benign from a malignant cause for the multiple nodules.

Nodules are described as 'miliary' when they are less than 5 mm in diameter and are so numerous that they cannot be counted. The crucial diagnosis to consider, even if the patient is not particularly unwell, is miliary tuberculosis, since this life-threatening disease can be readily treated. If the patient is asymptomatic the differential diagnosis is more likely to lie between sarcoidosis, metastatic disease or a coal worker's pneumoconiosis. As ever, previous radiographs showing the rate of growth of the nodules may give valuable clues to the likely nature of the disease.

Cavitating pulmonary lesions

The radiological definition of cavitation is a lucency representing air within a mass or an area of consolidation. The cavity may or may not contain a fluid level and is surrounded by a wall of variable thickness (Fig. 2.19).

The two most likely diagnoses in an adult presenting with a cavitating pulmonary lesion on a chest radiograph are a cancer or a lung abscess. In children, infection is the most common cause. Cavitation secondary to necrosis is well recognized in a variety of bacterial pneumonias, particularly those associated with tuberculosis, *Staphylococcus aureus*, anaerobes and *Klebsiella*. Diagnosis is usually by plain chest radiograph in the first instance but computed tomography is also useful for localizing the abscess and sometimes to enable percutaneous aspiration to be undertaken. It also allows assessment of the relationship of the abscess to adjacent airways so that appropriate postural drainage can be planned.

In all age groups it is important to consider tuberculosis, especially if the cavitating lesions are in the lung apices. Linear or computed tomography may be necessary if the presence of cavitation is questionable; in addition, computed

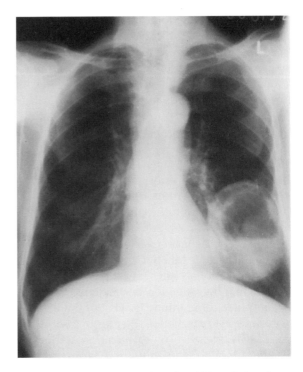

Figure 2.19 Lung abscess: there is a thick-walled cavity containing a fluid level in the left lower lobe.

tomography may show other features which help to narrow the differential diagnosis (e.g. pulmonary calcifications in tuberculosis, mediastinal lymph node enlargement in metastatic disease). In general, radiology alone cannot distinguish one cause of a cavitating mass from another.

SPECIFIC CONDITIONS

The postoperative and critically ill patient

In the context of intensive care medicine, the portable radiograph is one of the main means of monitoring critically ill patients. However, it is a far from perfect technique as the degree of inspiration is usually poor and may vary widely on serial radiographs. In addition, evaluation of cardiac size and the lung bases is, at best, difficult. This is often compounded by the rapidly changing haemodynamic state of the patient.

To some extent the advent of phosphor plate radiography has enabled more accurate assessments to be made because variations in exposure are not such a problem. Decubitus radiographs can be useful to evaluate the dependent side for fluid and the non-dependent side for small but clinically important pneumothoraces. For convenience it is useful to consider the various disease processes in the categories described below.

Support and monitoring apparatus

Careful radiographic monitoring of the position of various tubes and catheters used in the postoperative and critically ill patient is essential to decrease complications. Before evaluating the heart and lungs it is good practice to check each of these lines for proper positioning. The ideally placed central venous line ends in the superior vena cava (see Fig. 2.2). Catheters terminating in the right atrium or ventricle may cause arrhythmias or perforation. Swan–Ganz catheters used to monitor pulmonary capillary wedge pressure are ideally sited in a main or lobar pulmonary artery (see Fig. 2.2). Drugs inadvertently injected directly into the wedged catheter may cause lobar pulmonary oedema or necrosis. Both catheters (central venous pressure line and Swan–Ganz) are inserted percutaneously and therefore share certain complications. The most frequent is a pneumothorax due to puncture of the lung at the time of subclavian vein insertion. If the catheter is inserted into the mediastinum or perforates a vein or artery, there may be dramatic widening of the superior mediastinum due to haematoma. If the catheter enters the pleural space, infused fluid rapidly fills the pleural space. Catheter perforation of the right atrium or ventricle may lead to cardiac tamponade which may result in progressive enlargement of the heart shadow on serial radiographs.

The intra-aortic balloon pump is usually inserted via the femoral artery and is used in patients with intractable heart failure or in weaning the patient from cardiopulmonary bypass. On the frontal radiograph the tip of the catheter should be seen lying just inferior to the aortic arch (see Fig. 2.2).

A cardiac pacemaker wire is usually inserted via the external jugular, the cephalic or femoral vein and passed under fluoroscopic control into the apex of the right ventricle. Kinks or coils of wire are undesirable and the wire should be examined carefully along its entire length.

The tip of a correctly positioned endotracheal tube (see Fig. 2.2) lies in the midtrachea, approximately 5–7 cm above the carina. This distance is needed to ensure that it does not descend into the right main stem bronchus with flexion of the head and neck or ascend into the pharynx when the head and neck are extended. If the endotracheal tube is inadvertently passed into the right main stem bronchus (the more vertical of the two main bronchi), the left lung may collapse with a shift of the mediastinum to the left and hyperinflation of the right lung. If the endotracheal tube is positioned just below the vocal cords, the tube may retract into the pharynx, airway protection is lost and aspiration may occur. If the tube remains high in the trachea, inflation of the cuff may cause vocal cord damage. Delayed complications include focal tracheal necrosis leading ultimately to a localized stricture. It is worth noting that, even with correct positioning and cuff inflation, an endotracheal tube is not an absolute guarantee against aspiration of stomach contents into the airways.

Tracheostomy for long-term support has its own complications. A correctly placed tracheostomy tube should be parallel to the long axis of the trachea, approximately one-half to two-thirds the diameter of the trachea and end at least 5 cm from the carina. Marked subcutaneous or mediastinal emphysema may be due to tracheal injury or a large leak around the stoma. After prolonged intubation some tracheal scarring is inevitable. Symptomatic tracheal stenosis or collapse of a short length of the trachea is less common now owing to use of low-pressure occlusion cuffs on endotracheal tubes. When positive end expiratory pressure (PEEP) is added, the patient's tidal volume and functional residual capacity increase. This is reflected in the radiograph as increased lung aeration. PEEP may open up areas of collapse and cause radiographic clearing. However, this may be spurious as any densities present will be less obvious owing to the increased lung volume. Similarly, when the patient is weaned off PEEP, the lung volume drops and the lungs may appear to be dramatically worse. Pulmonary barotrauma (air leakage due to elevated pressure) complicates approximately 10% of patients on positive pressure ventilation. If air continues to leak due to continued ventilation, a tension pneumothorax may develop. The chest radiograph is often the first indicator of this potentially fatal complication.

Collapse

Following laparotomy, at least half of all patients develop some postoperative pulmonary collapse. Volume loss is most often attributed to hypoventilation and retained secretions and it is most frequent in patients with chronic bronchitis, emphysema, obesity, prolonged anaesthesia or unusually heavy analgesia. The most common radiographic manifestation is of linear densities which appear in the lower lung zones soon after surgery. Patchy, segmental or complete lobar consolidation is less common. When due to hypoventilation or large airway secretions, marked volume loss rather than dense consolidation is the usual appearance. Careful attention should be paid to unilateral elevation of the diaphragm and shifts of the minor fissure or hilar vessels. When collapse is due to multiple peripheral mucus plugs, the radiographic picture may be of pulmonary consolidation rather than volume loss. Areas of collapse tend to change rapidly and often clear with suction or physiotherapy. Postoperative collapse is not usually an infectious process but if not treated promptly, areas of collapse will usually become secondarily infected.

Aspiration pneumonia

Another postoperative complication is the aspiration of gastric contents. A depressed state of consciousness and the presence of a nasogastric tube which disables the protective oesophagogastric sphincter are the most frequent predisposing factors. An endotracheal or tracheostomy tube does not always protect the patient from aspiration. The radiographic appearance of patchy, often bilateral, consolidation appears any time within the first 24 hours of aspiration and then progresses rapidly. In an uncomplicated case there is usually evidence of stability or regression by 72 hours, with complete clearing within 1–2 weeks. The infiltrates are usually patchy and diffuse and are most often seen at the lung bases, more commonly on the right. Complications include progression to acute respiratory distress syndrome (ARDS). Any worsening of the radiograph on the third day or thereafter should suggest the diagnosis of secondary infection.

Acute respiratory distress syndrome

Acute respiratory distress syndrome (ARDS) consists of progressive respiratory insufficiency following a major bodily insult and can be due to a large number of factors. Over the years it has been known as 'shock lung', 'stiff lung syndrome' and 'adult hyaline membrane disease'.

At the pathophysiological level there is increased permeability of the pulmonary capillaries and the formation of platelet and fibrin microemboli. This results in alveolar oedema and haemorrhage which can affect the entire lung. After several days, hyaline membranes form within the distal air spaces. As a general rule, symptoms occur on the second day after insult or injury, but the radiograph remains normal during the initial hours of clinical distress. Interstitial oedema is the first radiographic abnormality, which may be of a faint, hazy ground-glass appearance (Fig. 2.20), and this is followed rapidly by patchy air-space oedema. By 36–72 hours after insult, diffuse global air-space consolidation is evident. It is the timing of the radiographic changes relative to the insult and the onset of symptoms, rather than the radiological appearance alone, that suggest the diagnosis of ARDS.

Pneumonia

Pulmonary infection may occur several days after surgery. Pneumonia may complicate col-

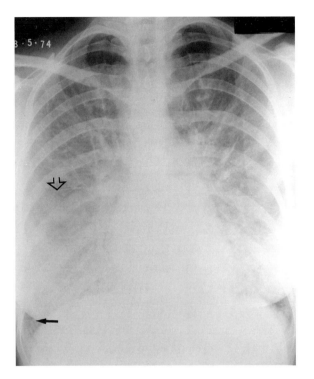

Figure 2.20 Pulmonary oedema due to mitral valve disease. There is increased opacity or 'haziness' throughout the lungs. There is fluid within the horizontal fissure (open arrow) and septal lines (closed arrow) corresponding with fluid in the interstitium of the lung.

lapse but may result from aspiration or inhalation of infected secretions from the pharynx.

The features of consolidation have already been covered but the critically ill or postoperative patient may not show typical appearances of consolidation. Numerous factors, such as prior antibiotic therapy and coexistent heart or lung disease, may alter the radiographic features. The radiographic appearance may vary from a few ill-defined or discrete opacities to a pattern of coalescence and widespread patchy consolidation. Cavity or pneumatocele (a thin-walled air-filled space) formation is not infrequent.

Extrapulmonary air

The diagnosis of a pneumothorax is made by the identification of the thin line of the visceral pleura. Free air may also be found in the pulmonary interstitium, the mediastinum, the pericardial space and the subcutaneous tissues. In the intensive care setting, extrapulmonary air is most often due to barotrauma from mechanical ventilation or secondary to surgery or other iatrogenic procedures. Pulmonary interstitial emphysema is difficult to recognize radiographically and is invariably due to ventilator-induced barotrauma. Unlike air bronchograms, the interstitial air is seen as black lines and streaks radiating from the hila; they do not branch or taper towards the periphery. Interstitial emphysema usually culminates in a pneumomediastinum and this is shown on a frontal radiograph as a radiolucent band against the mediastinum bordered by the reflected mediastinal pleura. Air may outline specific structures such as the aortic arch, the descending aorta or the thymus.

Cardiac failure

The radiographic diagnosis of early left ventricular failure is largely dependent on changes in the calibre of the pulmonary vessels in the erect patient. As the left atrial pressure rises, blood is shunted to the upper zones. This is the first and most important radiographic sign of elevated left ventricular pressure but it is important to remember that, because of redistribution of blood flow in the supine position, a supine radiograph does not allow this criterion to be used.

Interstitial pulmonary oedema then follows; this is manifested by blurring of the vessel margins, a perihilar haze and a vague increased density over the lower zones. When fluid fills and distends the interlobular septa, Kerley B lines (septal lines) may be visible (see Fig. 2.20). These are best visualized in the costophrenic angles as thin white lines arising from the lateral pleural surface. As the left ventricular pressure continues to rise, multiple small, ill-defined opacities occur in the lower half of the lungs. These represent alveoli filling with fluid. Alveolar oedema may also appear as poorly defined bilateral 'butterfly' perihilar opacification. Increasing cardiac size usually accompanies cardiac failure but, if it occurs following acute myocardial infarction or an acute arrhythmia, cardiac failure may be present without an increase in cardiac size. Bilateral pleural effusions often accompany cardiac failure.

Pulmonary embolism

The postoperative or critically ill patient has numerous risk factors for the development of deep venous thrombosis and thus pulmonary embolism. In this group, where respiratory distress is often multifactorial, the diagnosis of pulmonary embolism is extremely difficult.

Conventional radiographic findings are non-specific and include elevation of the diaphragm, collapse or segmental consolidation. A small pleural effusion may appear during the first 2 days following the embolus. It is important to recognize that a normal chest radiograph does not exclude a major pulmonary embolus; indeed, a normal radiograph in a patient with acute respiratory distress is suggestive of the diagnosis. A radionuclide perfusion scan is of use because if it is normal a pulmonary embolus can be excluded; however, this is not a practical test for a patient in an intensive care unit and the decision to treat with anticoagulants is often made clinically.

The success of helical CT in the diagnosis of pulmonary embolism relates to its rapid scan time, volumetric data acquisition and high degree of vascular enhancement.

Kyphoscoliosis

Kyphoscoliosis makes assessment of the chest radiograph difficult and it is useful to reduce the distortion of thoracic contents due to the kyphoscoliosis by obtaining an oblique radiograph, positioning the patient in such a way that the spine appears at its straightest. Severe kyphoscoliosis may cause pulmonary arterial hypertension and cor pulmonale. Some congenital chest anomalies such as pulmonary agenesis (absence of a lung) and neurofibromatosis are associated with dorsal spine abnormalities. Because of the problems associated with getting a true posteroanterior and lateral view, computed tomography scanning is often the most satisfactory method of visualizing the lungs.

Bronchiectasis

Bronchiectasis is a chronic condition characterized by local, irreversible dilatation of the bronchi, usually associated with inflammation. On a chest radiograph (Fig. 2.21a) the findings include:

- the bronchial wall visible either as single thin lines or as parallel 'tram-lines'
- ring and curvilinear opacities which represent thickened airway walls seen end on. These tend to range in size from 8 to 20 mm, have thin (hairline) walls and may contain air–fluid levels
- dilated airways filled with secretions giving rise to broad-band shadows some 5–10 mm wide and several centimetres long (seen end on, these dilated fluid-filled airways produce rounded or oval nodular opacities)
- overinflation throughout both lungs (particularly in cystic fibrosis)
- volume loss where bronchiectasis is localized (this may give rise to crowding of bronchi or collapse due to mucus plugging that can be severe and result in complete collapse of a lobe)
- less specific signs including consolidation, scarring and pleural thickening.

The definitive diagnosis of bronchiectasis used to be made by bronchography (injection of contrast into the bronchial airway), but this is an invasive and unpleasant procedure and a viable alternative is high-resolution computed tomography (Fig. 2.21b). With this technique, thin slices are taken throughout both lungs and the findings are similar to those on the plain film (thickened bronchial walls, bronchial dilatation, ring opacities containing air–fluid levels). Comparing the diameter of the bronchial wall with the adjacent vessel is helpful, as both should be approximately the same size. Computed tomography may also be helpful in determining the optimum position for postural drainage. Upper lobe predominance is present in early cystic fibrosis and after tubercle infection and allergic bronchopulmonary aspergillosis. The remaining causes of bronchiectasis (e.g. post childhood infection) affect predominantly the middle and lower lobes.

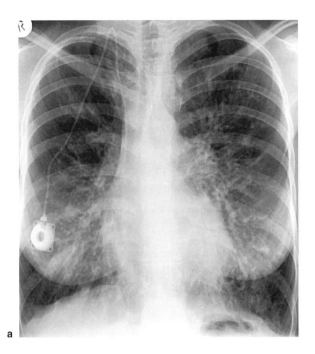

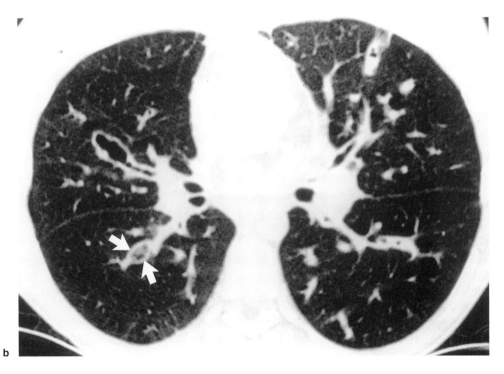

Figure 2.21 Cystic fibrosis. **a** The lungs are overinflated on the PA chest radiograph and there is widespread increased shadowing due to bronchial wall thickening and peribronchial consolidation. Note the prominent central pulmonary artery (pulmonary arterial hypertension may be a complication) and the catheter for long-term intravenous antibiotics. **b** A thin-section CT image of the same patient shows the dilated, bronchiectatic airways, some of which are plugged with mucus (arrows).

Chronic airflow limitation

This comprises three conditions which are present simultaneously in a given patient to a greater or lesser degree: chronic bronchitis, asthma and emphysema. The first is diagnosed by the patient's history and, strictly speaking, does not have any characteristic radiological features. In asthma the chest radiograph is normal in the majority of patients between attacks, but as many as 40% reveal evidence of hyperinflation during an acute severe episode. In asthmatic children with recurrent infection, bronchial wall thickening occurs. Collapse of a lobe or an entire lung because of mucus plugging is another feature and may be recurrent, affecting different lobes. Complications include pneumomediastinum which arises secondarily to pulmonary interstitial emphysema and pneumothorax due to rupture of a subpleural bulla. Expiratory radiographs may aid detection of a pneumothorax as well as demonstrating any air trapping secondary to bronchial occlusion.

Emphysema is a condition characterized by an increase in air spaces beyond the terminal bronchiole owing to destruction of alveolar walls. Whilst it is strictly a pathological diagnosis, certain radiographic appearances are characteristic in more advanced cases. These include overinflation of the lungs, an alteration in the appearance of the pulmonary vessels and the presence of bullae. Overinflation results in flattening of the diaphragmatic dome (Fig. 2.22) resulting in an apparently small heart and a decreased cardiothoracic ratio. On the lateral chest radiograph the large retrosternal translucency caused by the hyperinflated lungs is particularly striking (Fig. 2.22b). The pulmonary vessels are abnormal: the smooth gradation in size of vessels from the hilum outwards is lost, with the hilar vessels being larger than normal and tapering abruptly, so-called 'pruning' of the vessels. However, the lungs are usually unevenly involved and this is mirrored by the uneven distribution of pulmonary vessels. When emphysema is predominantly basal in distribution, there is prominent upper lobe blood diversion which should not be mistaken

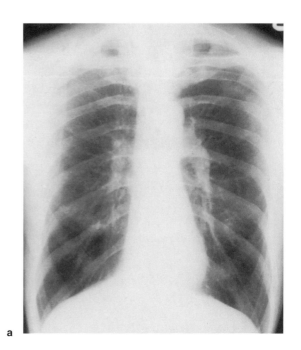

a

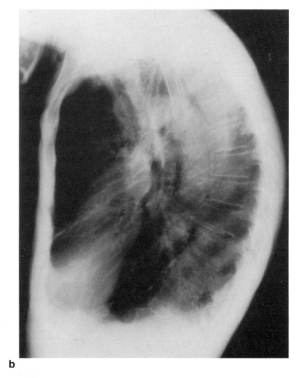

b

Figure 2.22 Emphysema. **a** Both lungs are hyperinflated. There is dilatation of the proximal pulmonary arteries with pruning of the peripheral vasculature. **b** The retrosternal and retrocardiac areas are strikingly transradiant.

for evidence of left heart failure. Bullae are recognized by their translucency, their hairline walls and a distortion of adjacent pulmonary vessels. They vary greatly in size and are occasionally big enough to occupy an entire hemithorax. When large they are an important cause of respiratory distress. Complications of bullae formation are infection and haemorrhage, which are usually manifested as the presence of an air–fluid level. Pneumothorax is another complication and occasionally may be difficult to distinguish from a large bulla.

PAEDIATRICS

INTRODUCTION

Despite the advent of new imaging modalities, such as ultrasound, computed tomography (CT), magnetic resonance imaging (MRI) and ventilation/perfusion lung scans ($\dot{V}/\dot{Q}$ scan), the plain chest radiograph remains the mainstay of paediatric chest imaging. In most circumstances the clinical history and examination will be augmented by a chest radiograph before a working diagnosis is made and treatment or further investigations planned.

This section aims to provide a concise and practical introduction to imaging the paediatric chest, emphasizing the importance of the plain chest radiograph but also indicating where other modalities provide additional information or allow the same information to be acquired with less use of ionizing radiation. The first part provides an overview of imaging modalities currently available, the second reviews important radiological signs commonly seen in paediatric chest radiographs and the final part discusses common paediatric chest problems and their radiological signs.

The text has not been referenced extensively but a number of selected general references suitable for further reading are given at the end of the section.

MODALITIES IN PAEDIATRIC CHEST IMAGING

Plain chest radiographs and fluoroscopy

Chest radiographs may be taken in the erect posteroanterior (PA) or anteroposterior (AP) position or in the supine AP position. In some circumstances, such as on the neonatal unit (NNU) where patient handling is minimized, all films are obtained in the supine AP projection. Up to the age of 3 any of the projections may be used depending on the policy of the department. Over the age of 3 most units obtain erect PA films. It is important that within any given unit techniques are standardized and films clearly labelled as the appearances of some radiological signs, particularly those of pleural fluid and pneumothorax, are profoundly different in the erect and supine positions. These changes will be discussed in greater detail below. Frontal chest radiographs should be obtained in inspiration, using a short exposure time and with attention to technical factors so as to minimize the radiation exposure to the patient and attendants.

The lateral chest radiograph necessitates a significantly higher exposure than the frontal and is not required routinely. It is usually obtained during the follow-up of patients with cystic fibrosis or malignant disease likely to metastasize to the chest and in the assessment of recurrent chest infections. A lateral view may also be performed to clarify an abnormality seen on the frontal projection.

Coned, AP plain radiographs using a high kV technique and filtration to give an optimal exposure are used to demonstrate the anatomy and calibre of the major airways.

One of the disadvantages of conventional radiographs is that it is difficult to adequately demonstrate all soft tissue and bony structures using the same exposure factors. Two major recent developments have attempted to overcome these disadvantages. The first is digital chest radiography in which a phosphor plate is used for the exposure. The plate is then scanned with a laser beam which reads the information and stores it in digital form. The information can then be reconstructed as the 'chest X-ray' on a computer screen and manipulated to allow optimal visualization of areas of interest. Hard copies of the images can be printed on a laser imager. The advantages of this technique in paediatric radiology are the uniformity of image that can be maintained from day to day, the facility for image manipulation and a reduction in radiation dose.

The second technique, scanning equalization radiography (SER), uses a beam of X-rays which scans the patient. The exposure is continuously changing according to the tissues within the beam at any given time. This results in a more even exposure and a more uniform image.

Fluoroscopy remains a useful technique for assessing diaphragmatic movements and for detecting changes in airway calibre during respiration in conditions like tracheomalacia.

Bronchography and tomography

Since CT and MRI have become widely available conventional tomography is no longer used and bronchography is only rarely undertaken to demonstrate focal bronchial narrowing.

Ultrasound

Ultrasound is useful for examining the pleural space for fluid (Fig. 2.23). Effusions and empyemas can be located, measured and drained under ultrasound control. Because the ultrasound beam is strongly reflected by aerated lung, ultrasound is less useful for assessing lung lesions unless they are peripheral, lie against the chest wall and consist of either solid or fluid. The movement and integrity of the hemidiaphragms can be assessed using ultrasound. The disadvantage is that each hemidiaphragm can only be assessed independently and not in relationship to each other. This is important in mild hemidiaphragm paresis. Cardiac ultrasound is an extremely accurate non-invasive way of assessing congenital heart disease.

Computed tomography and magnetic resonance imaging

In many ways these techniques are complementary and will be discussed together. Both techniques require the patient to remain still for the duration of the scan and this is particularly important in MRI. Neonates and young infants may be examined if asleep after a feed but older infants and children usually require sedation or general anaesthesia.

CT uses a narrow beam of X-rays to image the patient in 'slices'. The thickness of the slice may be varied from 1.5 mm to 1 cm and slices may be taken with or without gaps between them depending on the region being examined and the likely pathology. Assessment of the mediastinum and of vascular structures is facilitated by using intravascular contrast medium.

High-resolution computed tomography (HRCT) uses a thin slice thickness and special software to demonstrate the lung parenchyma. HRCT is used in the diagnosis of diffuse parenchymal disease and bronchiectasis.

In MRI the patient lies within a strong magnetic field and is exposed to pulses of radiofrequency energy. This energy is absorbed by protons within the body. When the radiofrequency pulses are stopped the protons return to their normal state but as they do so they release energy, the magnetic resonance signal, which can be detected by coils placed around the body. Magnetic resonance signals are different for different tissues and may be altered by disease. Intravascular contrast medium for MRI is available.

CT has better spatial resolution and can detect fine calcification which affords it an advantage in evaluating mediastinal masses and lymphadenopathy. Bone structure and in particular cortical changes are best imaged on CT. Currently lung pathology is best evaluated on CT, using HRCT if necessary. Vascular structures are well demonstrated on CT if intravascular contrast is used and ultrafast CT scanners, which enable the entire chest to be scanned in a matter of seconds, facilitate the investigation of congenital vascular and cardiac abnormalities.

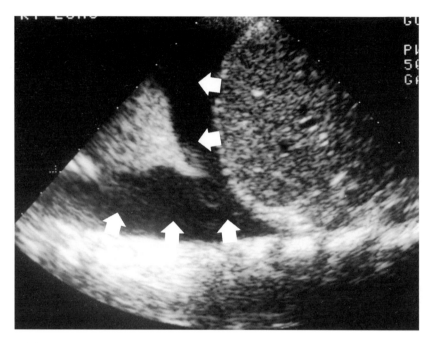

Figure 2.23   Sagittal ultrasound of a large pleural effusion which is poorly echogenic and appears black (white arrows). The patient's back is seen to the bottom and the liver lies to the right of the image. The effusion surrounds the partly collapsed, triangular lower lobe.

MRI of the chest is complicated by cardiac and respiratory movements. These effects can be minimized by only taking images at the same point in each cardiac and respiratory cycle, a technique known as gating. MRI has three major advantages over CT: its superior soft tissue contrast, its ability to acquire images in any plane and the fact that it does not use ionizing radiation. Sagittal and coronal images are of immense value in assessing the extent of a mediastinal mass and in deciding whether a paraspinal mass extends into the spinal canal.

One of the most exciting branches of MRI is magnetic resonance angiography (MRA) which allows blood vessels and the heart to be imaged without the need for artery puncture or the injection of any contrast media.

Angiography and cardiac catheterization

Cardiac ultrasound and the advent of MRA have reduced the indications for conventional angio-graphy and cardiac catheterization to assess congenital anomalies of the aorta and pulmonary vessels and congenital arteriovenous malformations.

Barium studies

These studies have a limited but very important role in the assessment of chest problems, specifically the barium swallow to evaluate extrinsic oesophageal compression by aberrant vessels or masses and the swallow/meal to assess intrinsic abnormalities such as incoordinated swallowing, abnormal oesophageal peristalsis or gastro-oesophageal reflux which can cause aspiration. If a tracheo-oesophageal fistula is suspected a tube oesophagram must be performed in the prone position.

There is no reliable technique for the positive diagnosis of aspiration; this includes the barium swallow/meal as well as the isotope milk scan. Recurrent aspiration may be inferred when there is severe gastro-oesophageal reflux.

Radionuclide studies

Radionuclide studies provide quantifiable functional information which complements the anatomical information provided by other imaging modalities. The ventilation/perfusion scan ($\dot{V}/\dot{Q}$ scan) uses krypton ([81mKr]) gas for ventilation and technetium ([99mTc]) labelled macroaggregates for perfusion. The $\dot{V}/\dot{Q}$ scan is the only method which will provide information on regional lung function. The radiation burden from the $\dot{V}$ scan is less than one-fifth of a chest radiograph while the $\dot{Q}$ scan has a dose equal to less than 60 seconds of fluoroscopy.

Most ventilatory disturbances result in a corresponding reduction in perfusion whereas if the pulmonary artery to a region is occluded (pulmonary embolus, sequestrated segment or pulmonary artery disease) that region remains ventilated. Occasionally other radionuclide studies such as bone scans or milk scans are indicated in the assessment of chest pathology.

BASIC SIGNS ON THE PLAIN CHEST RADIOGRAPH

Consolidation

Replacement of air in the very distal airways and alveoli by fluid or solid is called consolidation. The cardinal signs of consolidation are an area of increased opacity which may have an irregular shape, irregular margins, a non-segmental distribution and contains an air bronchogram (Fig. 2.24). The volume of the affected lung remains unchanged and consequently there are no signs of loss of volume. If an area of consolidation abuts the mediastinum, heart or diaphragm their clear silhouette, which is dependent upon the sharp radiological contrast between normally aerated lung (black) and solid structures (white), is lost (Fig. 2.24). Similarly the presence of air bronchograms within an area of consolidation can be explained by the sharp contrast between air in the medium and large bronchi (black) and the surrounding non-aerated and 'solid' lung (white) (Figs 2.24, 2.25).

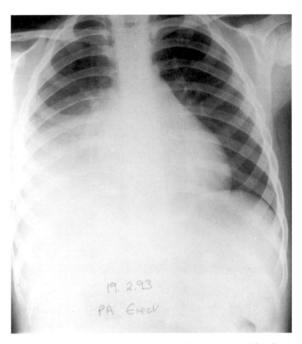

Figure 2.24   Right lower lobe consolidation caused by the bacterium *Strep. pneumoniae*. There is increased opacity in the right lower and mid zones, loss of the clear outline of the right hemidiaphragm and a proximal air bronchogram.

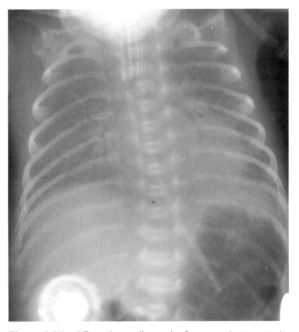

Figure 2.25   AP supine radiograph of a premature neonate with respiratory distress syndrome (RDS). The lungs show generalized opacity due to consolidation and a prominent air bronchogram.

A variant of infective consolidation frequently seen in infants and children is the 'round pneumonia'. This may mimic a mass lesion radiologically since it has well-defined borders but the clinical picture points to an infective aetiology. While infection is the most common cause of consolidation, it is also caused by any pathological process in which the alveoli are filled by fluid or solid. The most common causes of consolidation are listed in Box 2.3.

Collapse

Collapse means loss of lung volume and this may affect a lung, lobe or segment. This is manifest on the radiograph by shift of the normal fissures and crowding of airways in the collapsed lung (Figs 2.26, 2.27). If the volume loss is large there may also be mediastinal shift towards the affected side, elevation of the ipsilateral hemidiaphragm, ipsilateral rib crowding and alteration in hilar position. The collapsed lobe may or may not cause increased radio-opacity and there may be compensatory hyperinflation of unaffected lobes. If the collapsed lobe abuts on part of the diaphragm or cardiomediastinal silhouette the clear outline of these may be lost on the radiograph, as in consolidation (Figs 2.26, 2.27). Collapse is most often due to obstruction of a large airway by foreign body, mucus plug, tumour or extrinsic

compression. Less commonly it occurs secondary to poor ventilation.

Pleural fluid

The radiological appearance of pleural fluid is largely determined by the position of the patient. In the erect position the fluid collects at the bases and initially causes blunting of the costophrenic angles. Larger effusions cause a homogeneous opacity with a concave upper border higher laterally than medially – the meniscus. Very large effusions may cause mediastinal shift to the opposite side.

In the supine position, often used for neonatal and infant radiographs, an effusion causes reduced transradiancy (whiter hemithorax) of the affected side and may collect around the apex of the lung. In larger effusions a peripheral band of soft tissue density appears between the chest wall and the lung; on the right this band has a characteristic step at the position of the horizontal fissure (Figs 2.23, 2.28). Pleural fluid may collect and loculate within fissures or between the inferior surface of the lung and the diaphragm, the 'subpulmonic' effusion.

Pneumothorax

In the erect position pleural air collects at the apex, causing increased apical transradiancy (darker apex) and absent lung markings beyond a visible lung edge. In the supine position air collects initially in the anteroinferior chest, causing quite different and often subtle signs. These include small slivers of air at the apex, around the heart and between the lung and the diaphragm. Where free air as opposed to aerated lung abuts part of the cardiomediastinal or diaphragmatic silhouette, the clarity of that border is especially sharp, this being the opposite of the effect seen in consolidation (see above). A large pneumothorax in neonates and infants when supine may collect anteriorly and cause an increased ipsilateral transradiancy (darker hemithorax) and increased sharpness of the cardiomediastinal silhouette (Fig. 2.29).

A tension pneumothorax occurs when a pleural tear acts as a one-way flap valve, allow-

Box 2.3	Common causes of consolidation
Pulmonary oedema	Cardiogenic Non-cardiogenic Respiratory distress syndrome Aspiration
Pulmonary exudate	Infection
Blood	Traumatic contusion Infarction Aspiration
Other rare causes	Alveolar proteinosis Alveolar microlithiasis Lymphoma Sarcoidosis

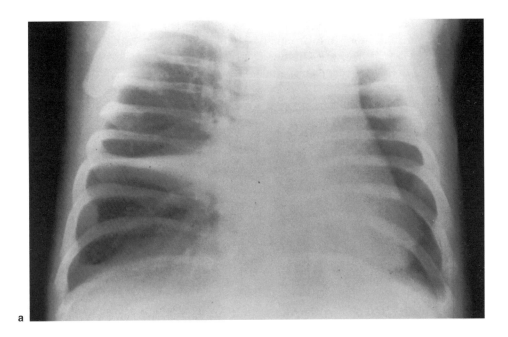

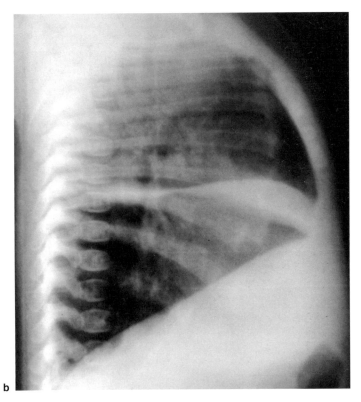

Figure 2.26   **a** AP radiograph taken in a lordotic projection to show the band-like opacity of middle lobe collapse. Part of the right heart silhouette is lost where the collapsed lobe abuts the heart. **b** Lateral radiograph showing the collapsed middle lobe and displaced fissures. In addition, the lungs show generalized overinflation with some flattening of the diaphragm.

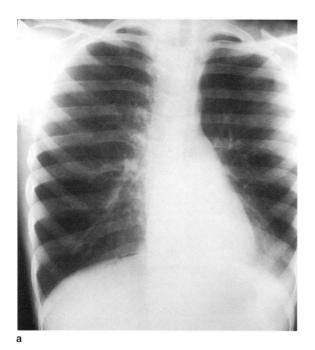

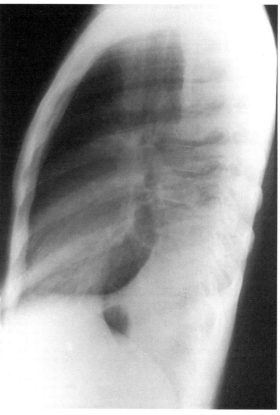

Figure 2.27 **a** Frontal radiograph of a patient with asthma and a left lower lobe collapse caused by a mucus plug. Generalized overinflation, increased opacity in the left cardiac region and loss of clarity of the outline of the medial left hemidiaphragm. **b** The lateral radiograph shows the collapsed left lower lobe as a wedge-shaped opacity in the lower chest posteriorly.

ing air into the pleural space but preventing egress. The pressure within the hemithorax rises and may remain positive for much of the respiratory cycle, causing mediastinal shift to the contralateral side and flattening, or even eversion, of the ipsilateral hemidiaphragm (Fig. 2.30).

COMMON PAEDIATRIC CHEST PROBLEMS

Congenital abnormalities of the chest

Congenital diaphragmatic hernia

Large congenital diaphragmatic hernias frequently present as neonatal respiratory distress although many are now diagnosed antenatally on routine antenatal ultrasound examination. Many are associated with other congenital anomalies. Most hernias are left sided, situated posteriorly and large. Abdominal organs are sited in the chest and appear on the radiograph as a cystic/solid mass. The mediastinum is shifted to the contralateral side and one or both lungs may be hypoplastic (Fig. 2.31). When large, the condition carries a high mortality.

Hiatus hernia

A sliding hiatus hernia exists when the lower oesophageal sphincter and part of the stomach are situated in the thorax, above the diaphragm. This condition is usually associated with incompetence

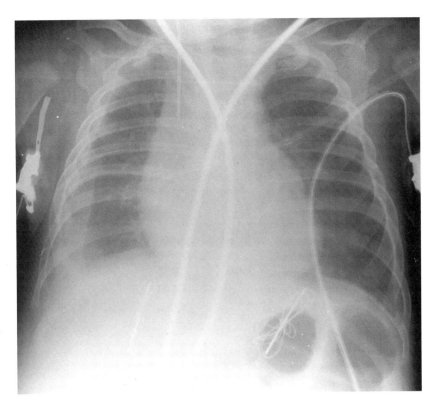

Figure 2.28 Supine radiograph showing a pleural effusion. There is reduced transradiancy on the right and a peripheral band of soft tissue density paralleling the chest wall with a 'step' at the position of the horizontal fissure.

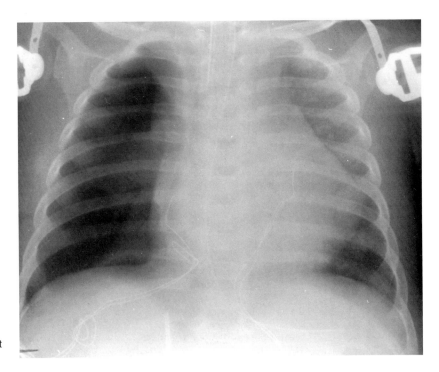

Figure 2.29 Supine radiograph showing a postoperative right pneumothorax. There is increased transradiancy of the right hemithorax. The right heart border is very clearly defined and the right lung edge is visible.

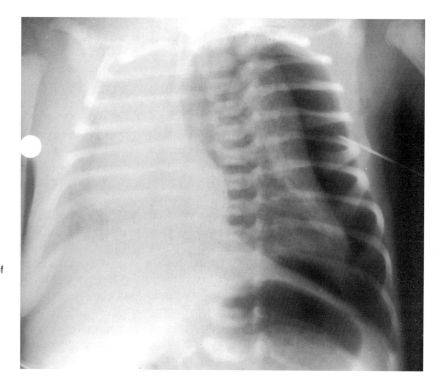

Figure 2.30 Supine radiograph of a patient with RDS. There is a left tension pneumothorax causing flattening of the hemidiaphragm and mediastinal shift to the right. The pneumothorax is seen surrounding a consolidated left lung. A needle drain has been inserted.

of the sphincter and may result in feeding problems, gastro-oesophageal reflux and aspiration.

Congenital lobar emphysema

A focal abnormality of a lobar bronchus leads to a ball valve effect, causing air trapping and overinflation of the affected lobe. The left upper, right middle and right upper lobes are most frequently affected. Initial radiographs in the first few hours of life may show an opaque mass in the region of the affected lobe. As fluid clears the appearances are those of an overinflated lobe with compression of normal surrounding lung and mediastinal shift to the contralateral side (Fig. 2.32). Treatment is surgical excision of the affected lobe if the neonate is in respiratory distress; if found in the older infant, conservative management is advocated.

Cystic adenomatoid malformation

This condition, caused by a disorganized and usually cystic mass of pulmonary tissue, can

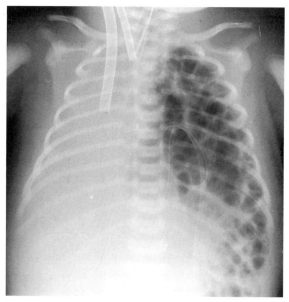

Figure 2.31 A large left diaphragmatic hernia. The left hemithorax contains the stomach (nasogastric tube) and loops of small bowel. The mediastinum is shifted to the right. The right lung is airless and opaque because the patient is on an extracorporeal membrane oxygenator (ECMO).

mimic both congenital diaphragmatic hernia and congenital lobar emphysema. The hamartomatous mass can affect any lobe, although the middle lobe is rarely affected, and in one-fifth of cases more than one lobe is affected. The radiograph shows a well-defined cystic mass which may be large, compress adjacent lung and cause mediastinal shift.

Neonatal chest problems

Respiratory distress syndrome (RDS)

Immature surfactant production in premature infants, infants of diabetic mothers and infants who experience perinatal asphyxia fails to reduce the alveolar surface tension sufficiently to prevent alveolar collapse. This is the most common cause of respiratory distress in premature neonates and causes tachypnoea, cyanosis, expiratory grunting and chest wall retraction. The radiograph shows bilateral symmetrical hypo-aeration, small volume lungs, ground-glass granularity of the pulmonary parenchyma and well-defined air bronchograms extending from the hilum into the peripheral lung (see Fig. 2.25).

These neonates frequently require intermittent positive pressure ventilation which may give rise to specific complications of pulmonary interstitial emphysema (PIE) (Fig. 2.33), pneumothorax (Figs 2.30, 2.33), pneumomediastinum and bronchopulmonary dysplasia (BPD) (Fig. 2.34).

Pulmonary interstitial emphysema is caused by gas leaking from overdistended alveoli and tracking along bronchovascular sheaths. The radiographic appearance is that of a branching pattern of gas with associated bubbles affecting all or part of the lung (Fig. 2.33).

Bronchopulmonary dysplasia is seen exclusively in infants who have been on positive pressure ventilation, usually for RDS. The combination of high pressure trauma and oxygen toxicity results in lung damage. The lung passes through a number of radiological stages during the evolution of BPD, Initially there is an RDS pattern which progresses to almost complete opacification and then to a coarse pattern of linear opacities and cystic lucencies (Fig. 2.34). The lack of adequate oxygenation in RDS may result in failure of the ductus arteriosus to close. The consequent left-to-right shunt may progress to frank plethora and heart failure.

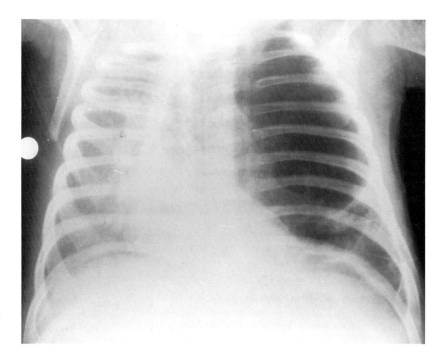

Figure 2.32 Congenital lobar emphysema of the left upper lobe. The lower lobe is compressed and the mediastinum is shifted to the right.

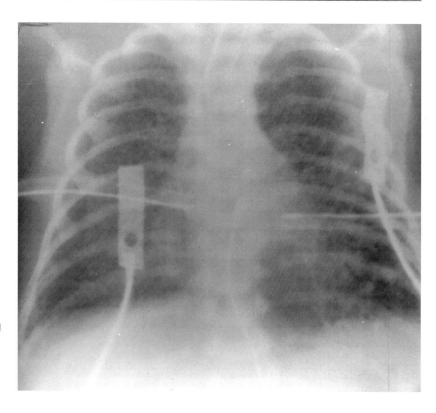

Figure 2.33 Pulmonary interstitial emphysema (PIE) complicating RDS. There is a branching pattern of gas with associated small bubbles. Bilateral chest drains and persistent right pneumothorax.

Meconium aspiration syndrome

This is the most common cause of respiratory distress in full or post-term neonates. The aspirated meconium causes a chemical pneumonitis and bronchial obstruction. The radiographic picture is of bilateral diffuse patchy collapse with other areas of overinflation (Fig. 2.35). Spontaneous pneumothorax, pneumomediastinum and small effusions are common but air bronchograms are rare.

Respiratory tract infections

Viral infections

Viral infections generally affect the bronchi and peribronchial tissues and this is reflected in the radiological signs: symmetrical parahilar, peribronchial streaky shadowing radiating for a variable distance into the lung periphery, hilar lymphadenopathy, occasionally reticulonodular shadowing, segmental/lobar collapse and generalized overinflation secondary to narrowing of the bronchi (Fig. 2.36). Effusions are rare. Organisms commonly encountered are the respiratory syncytial virus (RSV), influenza and parainfluenza viruses, adenovirus and rhinovirus.

Bacterial and mycoplasma infections

In the neonatal period the most common organisms are non-haemolytic streptococci, *Staphylococcus aureus* and *Escherichia coli*. Lobar consolidation is rare and more often the following signs are seen: radiating perihilar streakiness, coarse patchy parenchymal infiltrates, nodular or reticulonodular shadowing, or diffuse hazy shadowing, most often basal. One important pattern to recognize is the diffuse bilateral granularity of group B haemolytic streptococcal pneumonia which so closely mimics RDS.

In infants bacterial infection is more often seen as lobar or patchy consolidations (see Fig. 2.24). The organisms are most commonly *Haemophilus influenzae, Streptococcus pneumoniae,*

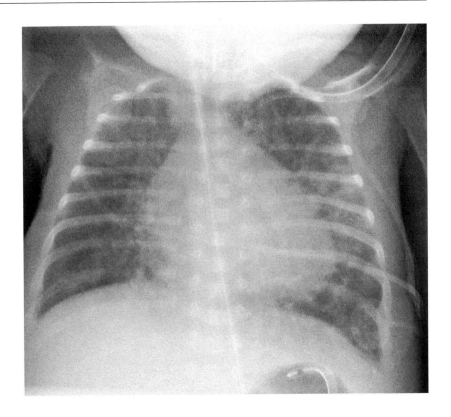

Figure 2.34 Bronchopulmonary dysplasia. A coarse pattern of linear opacities and cystic lucencies.

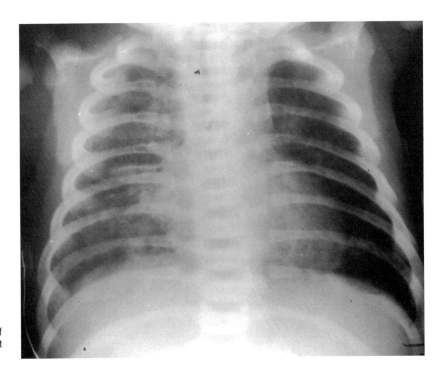

Figure 2.35 Meconium aspiration syndrome. Areas of patchy collapse with other areas of overinflation. The right lung is most affected.

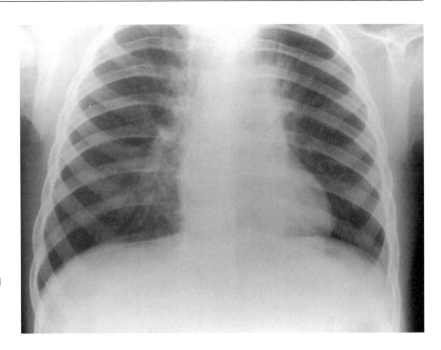

Figure 2.36 Viral pneumonia caused by the respiratory syncytial virus (RSV). There is symmetrical parahilar, peribronchial streaky shadowing and mild hilar lymphadenopathy.

Staphylococcus aureus and *Mycoplasma pneumoniae*. Pleural effusions, empyemas, abscesses and pneumatoceles are well-recognized complications. The 'round pneumonia' is an area of infective consolidation which transiently has a rounded configuration and mimics a mass lesion. *Mycoplasma pneumoniae* infection can mimic the radiographic appearances of both bacterial and viral pneumonia. However, one pattern that is highly specific is unilobar reticulonodular infiltration, especially if associated with hilar lymphadenopathy and/or a small pleural effusion.

Tuberculosis

Tuberculosis acquired in infancy is usually manifest by unilateral hilar or paratracheal lymphadenopathy and occasionally the primary or Ghon focus is seen as an area of consolidation in the periphery of the ipsilateral lung (Fig. 2.37). Collapse is seen, usually due to compression of a bronchus by lymph nodes. Bronchopneu-monic spread, with widespread areas of consolidation, occurs if either an infected node discharges into a bronchus or when host resistance is very low, facilitating spread through the airways. Miliary tuberculosis, with multiple small nodules, is caused by the haematogenous spread that occurs when an infected node discharges into the bloodstream. Cavitation is unusual in children.

Airway obstruction

Asthma

The radiological features are rarely seen before the age of 3. In chronic asthma there is generalized overinflation of the lungs with parahilar, peribronchial infiltrates but hilar lymphadenopathy is rare. Plugs of viscid mucus obstruct the airways and cause recurrent segmental or lobar collapse (see Fig. 2.27). Pneumomediastinum is a common complication but rarely requires specific treatment; pneumothorax is seen less frequently.

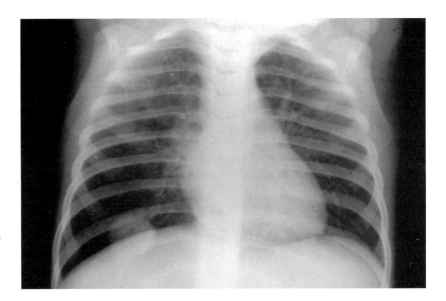

Figure 2.37 Primary tuberculous infection. Unilateral right hilar lymphadenopathy and an area of consolidation (Ghon focus) in the ipsilateral lower zone.

Obstruction by foreign bodies

Aspirated foreign bodies most commonly lodge in the major bronchi and act like a ball valve, causing a distal obstructive emphysema (Fig. 2.38). Radiographs are taken in inspiration and expiration to demonstrate the air trapping. Less commonly, the lung distal to the obstruction collapses and may become infected.

Cystic fibrosis

This autosomal recessive condition causes excessively thick and viscid mucus. In the neonatal period bowel obstruction due to meconium ileus may draw attention to the condition. In the chest the earliest signs are very similar to those of viral bronchiolitis: overinflation, focal collapse and parahilar, peribronchial infiltrates (Fig. 2.39). Recurrent infections lead to bronchiectasis, fib-

rosis and generalized overinflation with segmental areas of collapse. Bronchial collaterals are recruited and when these become large, haemoptysis may be a problem.

Acknowledgements

CDG and IG are most grateful to Dr BJ Loveday at the Royal Surrey County Hospital, Guildford, and Dr DB Reiff at St George's Hospital, London, for allowing us to use their radiographs as illustrations. We wish to thank Mrs Hazel Cook, Mrs Mary Shoesmith and Mrs Susan Ranson of the Department of Diagnostic Radiology and the Royal Surrey County Hospital, Guildford, and the Department of Medical Illustration at the Hospital for Sick Children, Great Ormond Street, for their help in preparing the illustrations.

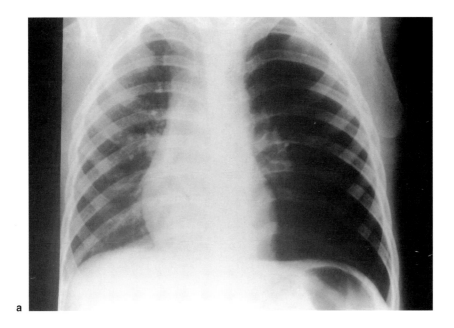

a

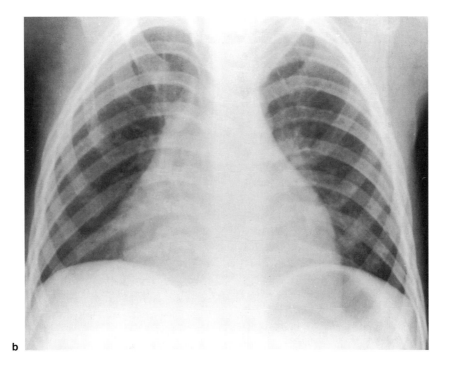

b

Figure 2.38 **a** Aspirated foreign body lodged in the left main stem bronchus. Marked air trapping in the affected lung causing overinflation, increased transradiancy and mediastinal shift. **b** Same patient after bronchoscopic removal of the obstruction.

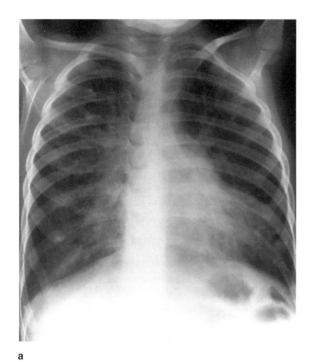

Figure 2.39 Cystic fibrosis: overinflation, focal collapse and parahilar, peribronchial infiltrates.

a

FURTHER READING: THORACIC IMAGING

Armstrong P, Wilson AW, Dee P, Hansell DM 2000 Imaging of diseases of the chest, 3rd edn. Mosby-Year Book, St Louis

De Bruyn R 1993 Paediatric chest. In: Cosgrove D, Meire H, Dewbury K (eds) Clinical ultrasound: abdominal and general ultrasound, vol. 2. Churchill Livingstone, London, pp. 983–988

Edelman RL, Warach S 1993 Magnetic resonance imaging (part 1). New England Journal of Medicine 328: 708–716

Edelman RL, Warach S 1993 Magnetic resonance imaging (part 2). New England Journal of Medicine 328: 785–791

Goodman LR 1999 Felson's principles of chest roentgenology, 2nd edn. WB Saunders, Philadelphia

Goodman LR, Putman CE 1991 Intensive care radiology: imaging of the critically ill, 3rd edn. WB Saunders, Philadelphia

Gordon I, Helms P, Fazio F 1981 Clinical applications of radionuclide lung scanning. British Journal of Radiology 54: 576–585

Gordon I, Matthew DJ, Dinwiddie R 1987 Respiratory system. In: Gordon I (ed.) Diagnostic imaging in paediatrics. Chapman and Hall, London, pp 27–57.

Grainger RG, Allison DJ 2000 Diagnostic radiology. An Anglo-American textbook of imaging, 4th edn. Churchill Livingstone, Edinburgh

Hayden CK, Swischuk LE (eds) 1992 Pediatric ultrsonography, 2nd edn. Williams and Wilkins, Baltimore.

Heitzmann ER 1988 The mediastinum: radiologic correlations with anatomy and pathology, 2nd edn. Springer-Verlag, Berlin

Keats TE 1996 Atlas of normal roentgen variants that may simulate disease, 6th edn. Mosby-Year Book, St Louis

Lipscombe DJ, Flower CDR, Hadfield JW 1981 Ultrasound of the pleura: an assessment of its clinical value. Clinical Radiology 32: 289–290.

Newman B. 1993 The pediatric chest. Radiology Clinics of North America 31: 453–719

Piepsz A, Gordon I, Hahn K 1991 Paediatric nuclear medicine. European Journal of Nuclear Medicine 18: 41–66.

Swischuk LE 1989 Imaging of the newborn, infant and young child, 3rd edn. Williams and Wilkins, Baltimore

Weinberger E, Brewer DK 1992 Pediatric body imaging. In: Moss AA, Gamsu G, Genant HK (eds) Computed tomography of the body with magnetic resonance imaging, 3rd edn. WB Saunders, Philadelphia, pp 1267–1296

Reed JC 1997 Chest radiology: plain film patterns and differential diagnosis, 4th edn. Mosby-Year Book, St Louis

Simon G 1975 The anterior view chest radiograph – criteria for normality derived from a basic analysis of the shadows. Clinical Radiology 26: 429–437

Vix VA, Klatte EC 1970 The lateral chest radiograph in the diagnosis of hilar and mediastinal masses. Radiology 96: 307–316

Webb RW, Müller NL, Naidich DP 1996 High-resolution CT of the lung, 2nd edn. Lippincott-Raven, Philadelphia

3

Cardiopulmonary function testing

Adults
Sally J Singh   Ian Hudson

The electrocardiogram (ECG) and cardiac arrest[1]
Anne Ballinger   Stephen Patchett

Paediatrics
Ian Balfour-Lynn

ADULTS

ASSESSMENT OF PULMONARY FUNCTION

Introduction

In health the human cardiorespiratory system has enormous reserve capacity to cope with the demands of exercise or illness. We are not normally aware of breathlessness or fatigue as a feature of resting activity. Furthermore, unless we harbour athletic ambitions, we are unlikely to explore the boundaries of our physiological limitations and assure ourselves that spare capacity would be present if it ever became necessary. The measurement of physiological capacity in health is, therefore, a matter of relevance only to the curious or the serious competitor who wishes to improve his or her performance. In patients with heart or lung disease the erosion of physiological reserve eventually imposes limitations upon the activities of daily life. Under these circumstances the measurement

---

[1] Reproduced from Ballinger & Patchett 1999 Saunders Pocket Essentials of Clinical Medicine 2e, WB Saunders, with permission.

of cardiopulmonary function allows the accurate assessment of disability and of the effect of therapeutic intervention. This chapter examines the scientific basis of clinical measurement and its relevance to physiotherapy.

It is reasonable and conventional to consider the function of the cardiovascular system in three compartments. First the lungs themselves, second the effectiveness of the integrated activity of gas exchange and acid–base balance, and finally the capacity of the circulatory system to deliver.

Lung function

The apparently simple function of the lung is to deliver oxygen to the gas-exchanging surface and exhaust carbon dioxide to the atmosphere. To achieve this, air is drawn by conductive flow into the alveoli and presented to the gas-exchanging surface where diffusion effects the process of exchange. The carriage of air through the airways depends on the patency of the tubes as well as on the consistency of the lung and the power of the respiratory muscles. These aspects of pulmonary function are commonly measured in lung function laboratories.

General principles of measurement

Lung function measurements are made to describe the lung for diagnostic purposes and subsequently in monitoring change. Accuracy and consistency are therefore very important and conventions exist for the procedures of measurement and expression of results. In general, a measurement will only be accepted after multiple attempts have been scrutinized and expressed under standard conditions. These are usually body temperature and atmospheric pressure (BTPS). To guarantee accuracy, laboratory practice should include regular physical and biological calibration of the equipment. Standards for good laboratory conduct have been described (British Thoracic Society/Association of Respiratory Technologists and Physiologists 1994). In health there are several factors which influence the magnitude of lung function. These include height, sex and age and to a lesser degree weight and ethnic origin (Anthonisen 1986, Cotes 1993). As a result, assessment of normality can only be made by comparison with reference values. The latter are obtained from the study of large numbers of normal people from the relevant population (European Community for Coal and Steel 1983). Once obtained, results can be expressed as percentage predicted or, more correctly, by comparison with the 95% confidence interval for that value.

Airway function

For the purposes of measurement the lung has only one portal of entry and exit, i.e. through the mouth, and airway function is assessed by quantification of gas flow or volume. The calibre of the airways reduces through their generations and the major resistance to gas flow is normally in the upper airway. The larger airways are supported by cartilage, while the smaller airways are held patent by the radial traction of the surrounding lung so that their calibre increases with the volume of the lung. The diameter of these airways is also controlled by neural tone which is predominantly parasympathetic.

The disruption of airway function can occur through physical or rigid obstruction to a large airway by, for example, a tracheal tumour. It may also occur because of more widespread disease in asthma, when large numbers of smaller airways are affected by episodic alteration of their calibre by smooth muscle contraction, mucosal oedema and intraluminal secretions. In chronic bronchitis, obstruction occurs by mucosal thickening and mucous secretion but in emphysema the mechanism is different. Though seldom occurring in isolation from other forms of airway obstruction, the result of parenchymal emphysema is to weaken the elastic structure which maintains radial traction on the airways and allows them to close too early in expiration.

Tests of airway function measure airway calibre and are now well established in clinical practice. Most tests of airway patency examine expiratory function. There are three common methods:

- spirometry (FEV$_1$ and FVC)
- flow–volume curves
- peak expiratory flow (PEF)

Production of the spirogram from a maximal forced expiration following a full inspiration is reliable and provides the forced expiratory volume in 1 second (FEV$_1$) and the forced vital capacity (FVC) (Fig. 3.1). The measurement is usually made using a spirometer which measures volume or is derived from a flow signal

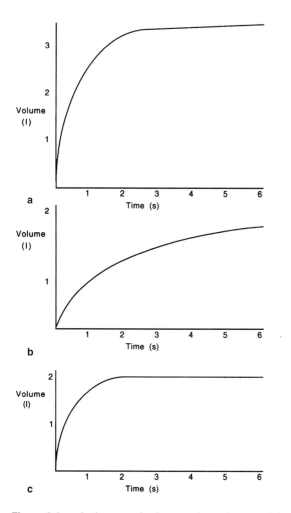

Figure 3.1 **a** In the normal spirogram the major part of the vital capacity (FVC) is expelled in 1 s (FEV$_1$). **b** In patients with airway obstruction the FEV$_1$ is reduced to a greater degree than the FVC. This pattern is known as 'obstructive'. **c** When the lungs are small and empty quickly the pattern is known as 'restrictive'.

obtained from a pneumotachograph or turbine. Most commonly, the FEV$_1$ and FVC are measured during the same manoeuvre, but a greater vital capacity may be obtained in patients with airway disease if it is performed slowly. Reduction in FEV$_1$ with relative preservation of FVC or vital capacity (VC) is known as an 'obstructive' pattern, which indicates and grades airway obstruction: FEV$_1$/FVC < 75% is graded as mild, <60% as moderate and < 40% as severe impairment (American Thoracic Society 1986). Simultaneous reduction in both FEV$_1$ and FVC with an increase in the FEV$_1$/FVC ratio is called a 'restrictive' defect and is usually associated with a reduction in lung volume. Abnormal values are defined as those recognized to be outside the normal range of two standard deviations for sex, height and age. This usually requires a reduction of about 15% from predicted values. Thus simple spirometry can detect and quantify airway obstruction, but gives no indication of the cause.

Measurement of the flow–volume curve is now commonplace and can provide information about the nature of airway obstruction. In this test, the gas flow from a full maximum expiration is plotted against the expired volume as the lung empties (Fig. 3.2). The flow of gas from the lung reaches a peak expiratory flow (PEF) after about 100 milliseconds and then declines linearly as the lung empties. If the measurement is continued into the subsequent full inspiration, a flow–volume 'loop' is produced and inspiratory flow rates can be measured. The shape of the expiratory and inspiratory portions are different, since in expiration the active expulsion is assisted by the elastic recoil of the lung while inspiratory flow rates are a reflection of airway calibre and inspiratory muscle strength only. Something of the nature of the airway obstruction can be learnt from consideration of the actual and relative values of PEF, peak inspiratory flow (PIF) and the values of expiratory flow at 50% and 75% vital capacity (MEF$_{50}$ and MEF$_{75}$). Simple inspection of the loop is often sufficient to distinguish between rigid upper airway obstruction, intraluminal obstruction in chronic bronchitis and asthma, and the 'pressure-dependent' collapse

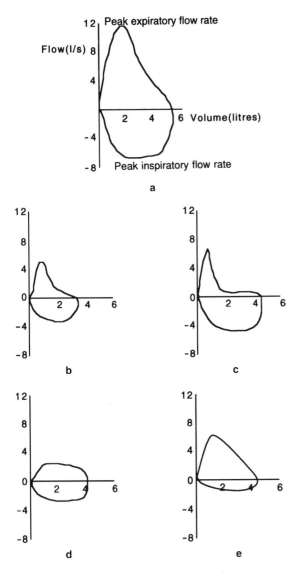

Figure 3.2 **a** The normal flow–volume loop has a characteristic shape. **b** Airway obstruction from asthma or chronic bronchitis appears as a concave expiratory limb and reduced inspiratory flows. **c** In emphysema the expiratory flows are suddenly attenuated but the inspiratory flows are relatively well preserved. **d** A rigid obstruction to a major airway can produce an oval loop. **e** Inspiratory flows are reduced in diaphragm weakness or extrathoracic tracheal obstruction.

seen in pure emphysema with relative preservation of inspiratory flow rates.

The PEF is one component of the flow–volume manoeuvre which has become increasingly popular. This has been encouraged by the avail-

ability of simple devices for its measurement. Provided that the patient does not have weak respiratory muscles and has made a maximum effort, the PEF will reflect airway calibre. The absolute values obtained are not particularly helpful unless they are extremely low but the easily repeated measurements can be used to obtain valuable insight into the mechanisms of variable airway obstruction in asthma. There is a normal diurnal variation in airway calibre of about 50 ml/min which is exaggerated in patients with poorly controlled asthma (Benson 1983). Wider variation will be seen approaching or recovering from an attack and following exposure to trigger factors.

The real value of the PEF lies in its repeatability and its portability. The issue of meters to patients with asthma allows domiciliary and occupational investigation of asthma. It also provides a tool for patients to use to monitor their asthma objectively as part of a self-management plan. In past years, the PEF chart has been used during hospital admissions to record the progress and predict the discharge of patients with airway disease. Although this is valuable in asthma where the airway obstruction is variable, it can show no change at all in patients with chronic airflow limitation in spite of a clinical improvement. In this case the twice-weekly measurement of FEV_1 and FVC is more likely to mirror progress than will the slavish recording of the PEF chart (Gibson 1995).

Changes in spirometry are poorly related to clinical improvements after bronchodilator therapy in COPD. O'Donnell et al (1999) have suggested that an increase in inspiratory capacity (a reflection of resting lung hyperinflation) may reflect improvements in exercise endurance capacity and dyspnoea more accurately than FEV_1 or FVC measures. Airway responsiveness is a measure of the degree of airway narrowing to specific and non-specific stimuli. Histamine and methacholine are the most widely used non-specific stimuli in challenge tests. Using the tidal breathing method (Juniper et al 1994), doubling concentrations of methacholine (0.03 to 16 mg/ml) are nebulized via a Wright nebulizer. Airway hyperresponsiveness is defined as a >20% fall in FEV_1 with a concentration of <8 mg/ml ($PC_{20}FEV_1 < 8$ mg/ml).

Most asthmatics have a combination of eosinophilic airway, airway responsiveness and variable airflow obstruction to the extent that many definitions of asthma now include these three features. There is evidence that directing treatment at improving airway responsiveness reduces mild exacerbations of asthma. Elevated exhaled nitric oxide concentration due to increased inducible nitric oxide synthetase (INOS) expression and activity in the bronchial epithelium is a feature of untreated asthma (Kharitonov et al 1994). The relationship between NO and asthma severity or response to treatment is unclear (Sont et al 1999).

The physical properties of the lung

The two lungs contain millions of alveoli within a fibroelastic matrix. They do not have a very rigid structure and are held in contact with the rib cage by surface tension forces at the apposition of the two pleural surfaces. The resting volume of the lung (the functional residual capacity (FRC)) is thus determined by the outward spring of the rib cage and the inward elastic recoil of the lung matrix. Expansion and contraction of the lung therefore involves the controlled stretching or relaxation of the lung by the respiratory muscles away from FRC. The position of FRC can be influenced if the lung is stiffer than usual (as in interstitial disease) or if it is more compliant (as when damaged by emphysema). The measurement of the lung's volume can therefore give some insight into these conditions.

For obvious reasons direct measures of lung volume cannot be made. The most familiar method is helium dilution, which involves rebreathing through a closed circuit a mixture of gases containing a known concentration of helium which is not absorbed into the circulation. The measurement of the final concentration of helium is used to calculate the gas dilution, or the 'accessible' volume, of the lung. An alternative method uses the Boyle's law principle: gas in the chest is compressed and the change in pressure is used to calculate the volume of gas within the chest. This method requires a large airtight box or plethysmograph. In both methods the

actual volume that is estimated is the FRC and total lung capacity (TLC) and residual volume (RV) are obtained from an additional spirometric trace. A further method involves the calculation of the total volume of the lung from the dimensions of a chest radiograph. This volume includes the total volume of gas, tissue and blood. Since the techniques do measure different aspects of volume, consistency in sequential measurements is important. In normal lungs the results are very similar, but where there is airway obstruction the values may be disparate. Such disparity can be used to advantage, e.g. in calculating the degree of trapped gas as the difference between the plethysmographic and helium dilution lung volumes.

The chest wall and the respiratory muscles

To maintain their shape the lungs depend on the support of the rib cage and the patency of the airways and alveoli. The expansion of the rib cage by the respiratory muscles is responsible for the tidal flow of gas into and out of the lungs. Over the past few years there has been increasing awareness of the importance of dysfunction of the respiratory muscles and the bony rib cage in contributing to respiratory failure. Such conditions include myopathies and polio as well as skeletal malformations such as scoliosis which decrease rib cage compliance and reduce the effectiveness of the musculature.

The respiratory muscles include the diaphragm as the major muscle of inspiration and the intercostal muscles and scalenes. The latter, together with the sternomastoids, are known as the 'accessory muscles', but actually have a stabilizing role in tidal breathing. The combination of the respiratory muscles and the bony rib cage is called the 'chest wall' and conceptually is considered as the organ which inflates the lungs. Weakness of the respiratory muscles will eventually lead to ventilatory failure which may first become apparent during the night as an exaggeration of the normal nocturnal hypoventilation (Shneerson 1988).

The function of the respiratory muscles is difficult to study directly since the muscles have complex origins and insertions. Furthermore, their product, which is the pressure generated within the thoracic cavity, depends on the coordinated action of many muscles, the individual functions of which may be difficult to distinguish in life. It is possible to make some assessment of both the strength and endurance of the muscles and also to separate the diaphragm from the other muscles. The simple strength that the inspiratory and expiratory muscles can generate as pressure is easy to measure. The maximum inspiratory pressure ($P_i$max) and expiratory pressure ($P_e$max) are easy to measure with a manometer or electronic gauge. The normal values of approximately -100 cmH$_2$O and $+120$ cmH$_2$O (Black & Hyatt 1971) are well in excess of that needed to inflate the lungs (5–10 cmH$_2$O) and therefore provide a sensitive measure of developing muscle weakness. These measurements do have a learning requirement and are not suitable for monitoring of patients with rapidly developing muscle weakness, such as in Guillain–Barré syndrome. Under these circumstances the sequential measurement of the vital capacity is much more reliable, since a failure to maintain it will predict ventilatory failure.

The strength of the diaphragm can be separated from the other muscles by measuring the pressure gradient across it. This is achieved by using balloons attached to pressure transducers to estimate the pressure in the oesophagus and the stomach. The gradient across the diaphragm during a maximum inspiration or sniff is an indirect measure of the strength of the diaphragm. Normal values for sniff pressures have now been published (Uldry & Fitting 1995). If required, a value free of volition can be obtained by electrical stimulation of the phrenic nerve in the neck or even by magnetic stimulation of the cerebral cortex.

Fortunately, measurements of separate diaphragm strength are seldom required in clinical practice. A simple guide to diaphragm function can be obtained by observation of the change in vital capacity with posture. When supine, the vital capacity normally falls by 8–10%, but when diaphragm weakness is present it may fall by more than 30%. The measurement of the supine vital capacity is therefore a good screening test of diaphragm function (Green & Laroche 1990). More recently

the measurement of sniff pressures at the mouth or nose has become recognized as a reflection of pure diaphragmatic activity.

Gas exchange and oxygen delivery

The requirements of the average cell for oxygen are quite modest and a mitochondrion may need a PO_2 of as little as 1 kPa (7.5 mmHg) to function effectively. At sea level the atmospheric PO_2 is 20 kPa (150 mmHg) (FiO$_2$ = 0.21) and in the process of delivering oxygen to the cell, there is a loss along this gradient. The first step is the dilution of inspired air with expired air within the alveolus. Each tidal breath (V_T) contains a portion of gas which will remain within the airways and not come into contact with the alveoli. This is known as the 'dead-space ventilation' (V_D) and must be achieved before any effective alveolar ventilation ($\dot{V}_A$) can take place:

$$V_T = V_D + \dot{V}_A$$

Alveolar gas therefore contains a mixture of fresh gas and some expired CO$_2$ and the alveolar PO_2 is reduced to about 16 kPa (120 mmHg) before gas exchange begins.

At the alveolar level, gas exchange involves the transfer across the alveolar–capillary membrane of oxygen molecules to the blood and the reverse transfer of carbon dioxide. This is achieved by simple diffusion, which is amplified in the case of oxygen by the affinity of haemoglobin. It normally takes mixed venous blood about 300 milliseconds (ms) to traverse a capillary and complete equilibrium usually occurs in about 100 ms. This aspect of oxygen transfer from the lung to the blood can be tested using carbon monoxide. Carbon monoxide has a very strong affinity for haemoglobin, follows the same path into the blood and can be measured easily. This principle forms the basis of the carbon monoxide transfer test which measures the amount of carbon monoxide which can be transferred to the blood in the course of a single breath (TLCO). This gives a rough indication of the gas-transferring ability of the lung as a whole and is reduced in conditions like fibrosing alveolitis, emphysema and pneumonectomy where the quality or quantity of the gas-exchanging surface is reduced. If the total TLCO is corrected for lung volume then the subsequent value is known as the 'coefficient of gas transfer' (KCO) and describes the gas-exchanging quality of the lung that is available for ventilation. For example, a very large normal man and a small child should have different TLCOs but their KCO values should be identical.

The carbon monoxide transfer test can give some information about the ability of the lung to transfer gas, but there is not a direct relationship between the TLCO and arterial oxygenation. The lung contains millions of alveolar capillary units and adequate oxygenation depends on the coordinated, satisfactory function of the whole unit. The pulmonary causes of arterial hypoxaemia have four major origins:

- hypoventilation
- interference with pulmonary diffusion
- ventilation/perfusion imbalance
- true shunt.

Hypoventilation is fairly easy to recognize because the fall in arterial PO_2 is associated with a rise in arterial PCO_2. This occurs in ventilatory failure associated with airway obstruction, chest wall disease and drug intoxication. Interference with pulmonary diffusion is quite rare because the process is very efficient. However, the system may be stretched at altitude or in the presence of disease such as fibrosing alveolitis. Even in this disease the hypoxia is related to increased pulmonary capillary transit time rather than to diffusion failure. The most common contribution to hypoxaemia in many diseases is ventilation/perfusion $(\dot{V}/\dot{Q})$ imbalance. Since effective lung function depends on the coordination of equivalent ventilation and perfusion to all units, it is not surprising that failure of the local matching mechanisms can cause trouble. The most extreme example would be a pulmonary embolus where ventilation continues in an area with no circulation. In other conditions such as asthma, the patchy distribution of airway obstruction will have similar but less dramatic effects. Some blood passes through the lung without coming into contact with the gas-exchanging surface. Normally this is a very small quantity (<5%), but effective shunts can be considerable in pneumonia and other conditions where the alveoli are blocked by inflammatory exudate although the circulation continues through the ineffective portion of the lung. This results in extreme hypoxia which cannot easily be corrected by additional oxygen.

Oxygen carriage and arterial blood gases

Oxygen and carbon dioxide are carried in the blood in different ways. Oxygen is immediately bound to haemoglobin and released in the tissues under conditions of low oxygen tension or acidosis. Very little oxygen is carried in solution in the blood under conditions of normal pressure, although this can be increased in a hyperbaric chamber. By contrast, carbon dioxide is carried in the blood entirely in solution, mostly as bicarbonate. The difference between the two forms of carriage of the metabolic gases is fundamental to the interpretation of the measurement of arterial blood gases. The individual cell requires oxygen to survive, but the carriage of oxygen in the blood will have no effect on the body other than the delivery. By contrast, the chemistry involved in the carriage of carbon dioxide controls the short-term acid–base state of the body. When considering blood gas measurements, it is best to examine these functions separately.

The normal atmospheric PO_2 is approximately 20 kPa (150 mmHg) falling to 16 kPa (120 mmHg) within the alveolus. The arterial PO_2 (PaO_2) is usually about 14 kPa (105 mmHg) in a healthy subject. Although we are used to these values they are only true at sea level and really only have relevance because the partial pressure is easy to measure. What matters to the individual cell is the quantity of oxygen that it receives, not the partial pressure. Oxygen delivery to the tissues depends on other factors which include the amount of haemoglobin, the degree of saturation of haemoglobin with oxygen and the rate at which oxygenated blood is delivered to the tissues. Assuming that the haemoglobin and the cardiac output are normal, then the measurement of oxygen saturation of haemoglobin is more relevant to oxygen delivery than is the PaO_2. The PaO_2 is related to oxygen saturation in a complex manner determined by the properties of haemoglobin and known as the 'oxygen dissociation curve' (Fig. 3.3). This relationship demonstrates that, under most conditions, once PaO_2 reaches 8 kPa (60 mmHg), haemoglobin is fully saturated and cannot carry more oxygen. Thus an arterial PO_2 above that value is only an insurance measure.

The availability of pulse oximeters has made the non-invasive measurement of oxygen saturation (SpO_2) commonplace. Pulse oximeters work by transcutaneous examination of the colour spectrum of haemoglobin which changes with its degree of saturation. These instruments are reasonably accurate over the top range of saturation, but become unreliable below about 50% (Tremper & Barker 1989). The measurement of SpO_2 is an extremely valuable tool for monitoring patients' safety. There are, however, some important aspects of interpretation of its use which may be potentially hazardous. Oximetry provides information about oxygen saturation and this will relate to ventilation only if the inspired oxygen level is normal. Monitoring oxygen saturation will not detect underventilation and a rising $PaCO_2$. In patients who are breathing additional oxygen, a false sense of security can be given by a normal SpO_2 even though the $PaCO_2$ is rising. Furthermore, accurate recording of SaO_2 requires a good peripheral circulation which may often be compromised in patients who are hypovolaemic.

The assessment of acid–base status requires the measurement of arterial blood gas tensions. The average blood gas analyser measures PO_2, PCO_2 and pH. It subsequently calculates from the Henderson–Hasselbalch equation the values of bicarbonate, standard bicarbonate and base excess. The appreciation of the acid–base state requires examination of $PaCO_2$ and pH. Abnormalities are usually described in terms of their generation (Fig. 3.4). For example, a respiratory acidosis resulting from underventilation will display a low pH and an elevated $PaCO_2$. If this has been present for any length of time the serum bicarbonate will have become elevated and acid is excreted by the kidneys to compensate. In cases of nocturnal hypoventilation the daytime PaO_2 may be normal, but the elevation of the base excess gives a clue to the ventilatory history. If an alkalosis (high pH) is associated with a low $PaCO_2$, then this could be due to voluntary hyperventilation and is termed a 'respiratory alkalosis'. The build-up of acid products in diabetes or renal failure will result in a low pH and bicarbonate together with a low

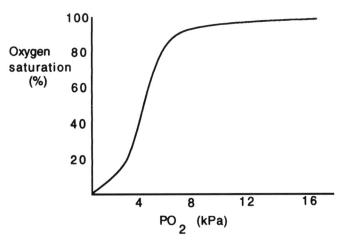

Figure 3.3 The oxygen dissociation curve relates oxygen saturation to ambient PO_2. In lung disease it is important to recognize that oxygen delivery is assured if PaO_2 is in excess of 8 kPa.

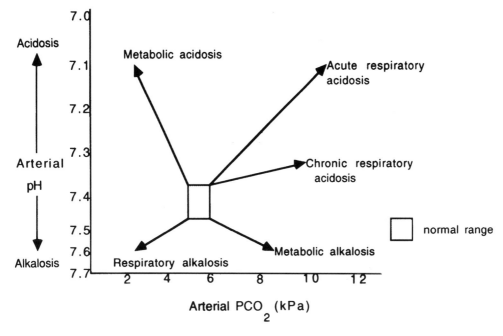

Figure 3.4   Acid–base relationships.

$PaCO_2$ in an attempt to compensate for a metabolic acidosis. Finally, the loss of acid from the stomach in prolonged vomiting can produce a metabolic alkalosis which is characterized by high pH, high bicarbonate and normal $PaCO_2$. These sketches of blood gas disturbance are superficial interpretations, but they provide a useful framework for clinical management under most circumstances.

Respiratory failure

Respiratory failure is defined as inadequate oxygen delivery. As we have seen, this can be due to a variety of circumstances and may or may not be accompanied by a disturbance of the CO_2 level. The critical PaO_2 level is approximately 8 kPa (60 mmHg), since a lower pressure than this will prejudice oxygen saturation and delivery. Therefore, respiratory failure is defined by convention as PaO_2 <7.3 kPa (54.8 mmHg). If the $PaCO_2$ is elevated above 6.5 kPa (48.8 mmHg), this is termed 'ventilatory failure' and is associated with chronic airflow limitation or other forms of hypoventilation.

The understanding of respiratory failure has changed in recent years with the recognition that it is seldom due to a single malfunction of the respiratory system. For example, the rise in $PaCO_2$ and hyperinflation associated with worsening airway obstruction may adversely affect the respiratory muscles and introduce a chest wall contribution to failure. Conversely, the loss of lung volume associated with muscle weakness may lead to atelectasis and decreased pulmonary compliance, which will in turn put a greater load on the lung. Understanding of the complexities of chronic respiratory failure has helped to improve the outlook for some groups of patients, e.g. those with ventilatory failure due to chest wall disease or obstructive sleep apnoea. In these conditions there are abnormalities of breathing during sleep, which may result in nocturnal hypoventilation or transient apnoea, that produce periods of oxygen desaturation which may spill over to the daytime. Recognition of this by oximetry and other more detailed somnography may result in effective treatment by nocturnal nasal intermittent positive pressure ventilation or continuous positive airway pressure (CPAP) (see Ch. 10). By extension these techniques may also have a role in the acute management of selected patients with COPD who have diminished respiratory drive (Wedzicha 1996).

Oxygen prescription

The prescription of oxygen for patients with COPD is well defined for long-term (more than 15 hours/day) use. An indication for long-term oxygen therapy (LTOT) is a PaO_2 less than 7.3 kPa, when breathing room air during a period of clinical stability. Clinical stability is defined as the absence of exacerbation of COPD and of peripheral oedema for the last 4 weeks. Ambulatory oxygen should be provided to those individuals who are on LTOT, need to be mobile and to leave the house. Patients without chronic hypoxaemia and LTOT should be considered for ambulatory oxygen if they have demonstrable desaturation on exercise. It is suggested that the level of desaturation should be at least 4%, to a saturation below 90%, on a standard exercise test whilst breathing room air. An improvement of at least 10% in distance and/or breathlessness score on repeat testing with supplemental oxygen warrants the prescription of an ambulatory system. The prescription of short-burst oxygen is less well defined. There is no evidence to support firm recommendation and further research is required to establish its role. A recent report by the Royal College of Physicians (1999) describes in some detail the prescription of domiciliary oxygen in the British National Health Service.

Posture and thoracic surgery

A knowledge of the effect of posture and thoracic surgery on pulmonary function is obviously very important to the physiotherapist. The circumstances of treatment make this knowledge of practical benefit. Lung function measurements are usually made sitting or standing, but the major postural effect occurs due to gravity in the supine position. There is a small fall in VC (8%) and a reduction in FRC while lying down which results from repositioning of the diaphragm and pooling of blood in the chest. This change can be used to advantage to identify patients with covert diaphragm weakness where the VC may drop by more than 30%. Gravity also produces a change in the distribution of ventilation and perfusion within the lungs. In the supine posture ventilation and perfusion are preferentially directed to the dependent zones (Kaneko et al 1966). This is important in adults if the lung disease is unilateral since oxygenation will be better if the good lung is dependent.

Physiotherapists are often involved in the assessment of patients for cardiothoracic surgery and their subsequent management. Some thoracic surgery, such as lung volume reduction surgery, bullectomy or decortication, improves lung function but most procedures impair the lung. The mechanisms of impairment include the anaesthetic, the thoracotomy and pulmonary resection. Following anaesthesia there is an immediate loss of FRC and subsequently VC which reaches a trough of about 40% at 24 hours and may take up to 2 weeks to recover (Jenkins et al 1988). This immediate loss of volume is associated with a widened gradient across the lung (A–aDO$_2$) and potential hypoxia which is worsened by obesity, age and smoking. Thoracotomy itself, without pulmonary surgery, will reduce the VC by approximately 10%, which recovers over a period of 3 months. There are no strong arguments for the benefit of median sternotomy over thoracotomy as far as recovery of long-term lung function is concerned. In the short term the physiotherapist should be cautious during treatment as gas exchange will be impaired if the patient is lying on the thoracotomy side.

The surgical removal of lung tissue does not necessarily have the predictable effects on function that might be imagined. Following pneumonectomy the functional state of the patient is remarkably stable and in the long term the VC and total lung capacity (TLC) become slightly larger than expected for one lung. The TLCO eventually settles to 80% predicted and the KCO may be high since the whole pulmonary blood flow now travels through one lung. The changes after lobectomy are surprisingly different. The long-term effects may be small but in the post-operative phase the disruption may be unexpectedly large. The contusion of lung adjacent to the lobectomy sets up $\dot{V}/\dot{Q}$ disturbances which may in the short term be as significant as removal of the whole lung.

The physiological assessment of patients for thoracic surgery is not straightforward. There is no single test which allows a distinction to be made between success and failure. It is important to consider the nature of the operation and the preoperative function as well as general health, weight and smoking habit. If there is any doubt about the suitability of a candidate from his spirometry, full lung function and oxygen saturation at rest then some assessment of exercise capacity is advisable (British Thoracic Society and Society of Cardiothoracic Surgeons 2001).

Lung volume reduction surgery

There has been a recent resurgence of interest in this technique, which can potentially make a dramatic improvement to the function of patients with more diffuse pulmonary emphysema. The technique is a development of bullectomy which removes approximately 30% of the substance of the lung which results in deflation of the chest wall. Surprisingly this operation can produce improvements in FEV_1 and elastic recoil pressure while reducing hyperinflation. There appear to be promising results in selected patients with more heterogeneous emphysema who have marked symptomatic hyperinflation (Criner et al 1999, Geddes et al 2000). Selection of patients for this procedure has yet to be well defined but preliminary data suggest that exercise capacity as measured by a SWT distance > 150 m (Geddes et al 2000), or a 6 MWD > 200 m and a resting $PaCO_2$ < 45 mmHg (Szekely et al 1997) were associated with a successful surgical outcome.

The effect of growth and ageing on lung function

The respiratory system reaches its peak in the third decade of life. Development of the lung continues from birth until the end of adolescence and starts to deteriorate after the age of 25 years. Fortunately, in the absence of disease there is sufficient reserve capacity to see out old age without discomfort!

The actual measurement of pulmonary function in childhood is problematic because of the obvious lack of cooperation. It is possible to measure lung volume and partial flow–volume curves in infancy by using an adapted plethysmograph. This is possible in the sedated child by producing a pneumatic 'hug' as an alternative to active expiration. In older children it is difficult to obtain cooperation for measurements until they are about 8 years old. After this age lung function can be measured easily, but there are difficulties in interpretation and production of reference values (see paediatric section of this chapter). The inconsistency of the timing of puberty and rapid growth spurts make comparisons difficult, but normal ranges have been produced for these age groups (Polgar & Promadhat 1971).

The most obvious differences between children and adults lie in the development of airway function. The airways develop faster than the alveoli, which may not reach maturity until about the seventh year. As the lung matrix develops, the airway walls remain strong and relatively patent. As a result expiratory flow rates, although lower than in adulthood, are relatively high. For example, the FEV_1/FVC ratio may be greater than 90% and the expiratory flow–volume curve may have a flat or convex appearance. In addition to airway patency there are also developments in the behaviour of the chest wall with growth. In childhood the musculoskeletal structures are immature and flexible. Rib cage distortion is often seen in childhood during illness, but disappears with growth and muscularization. The combination of airway patency and plasticity of the chest wall allows an interesting experiment. In childhood the residual volume (RV) is not determined by airway closure but by the strength of the expiratory muscles. Thus if children or young adults are hugged at the end of a forced expiration more air can be expelled. After the age of 25 years, RV is determined by premature airway closure and the lungs cannot be emptied further.

Life after 25 years is all downhill for the respiratory system. As with general ageing, the tissues become less elastic and the lung elastic recoil diminishes. TLC tends to remain static but RV rises as the FEV_1 and FVC fall with age. Arterial PO_2 and A–aDO_2 worsen but do not reach critically low values. Exercise capacity, as judged by oxygen consumption, shows a decline with age but it can be retarded by regular activity. As general levels of activity reduce with age, these effects are not usually important, but smoking or disease may accelerate the changes.

Interpretation of lung function tests

Once a baseline has been established, changes in function can be used to assess progress with natural history or treatment. Although there may be some investigations, which are specific to various diseases, it is seldom possible to rely on a single investigation for the purpose. The usual description of disease requires the combination of spirometry, lung volume and gas transfer measurement. The addition of bronchodilator response, a flow–volume loop and blood gases would provide further information, while additional specific tests are requested as indicated. The additional tests may include an exercise study or respiratory muscle function test to examine the relevant aspect. Interpretation of the tests involves the comparison of the values to the reference population and a description of the pattern of abnormality; if present. A helpful report will also give some guidance on the accuracy of the clinical diagnosis and suggest confirmatory investigations if the diagnosis is unclear. Some examples of clinical cases and the patterns of abnormal lung function are given in Table 3.1.

The measurement of disability and exercise testing

Static lung function tests can describe the physical properties of the lungs, but do not always reflect the performance of the cardiopulmonary system in action. The relationship between disability and spirometry is poor. To assess disability it must be

Table 3.1 Conclusions from pulmonary function tests are best derived from the examination of several measurements. **a** A 66-year-old man with chronic airflow limitation. There is an increase in lung volumes or hyperinflation of TLC and RV. The spirometry is obstructive but there is good bronchodilator reversibility, especially in the vital capacity. TLCO is slightly reduced but not as low as would be found in severe emphysema. The picture is one of smoking-related airflow obstruction, with the potential for some improvement. **b** A 49-year-old man with cryptogenic fibrosing alveolitis. There is a 'restrictive' defect with loss of lung volumes. Spirometry is not restrictive because of coexisting smoking-related airway obstruction. After treatment with prednisolone (10 March 1992) all values improved. **c** A 40-year-old woman with severe muscle weakness. There is a 'restrictive' picture, but the KCO is elevated because gas exchange is relatively normal. Respiratory muscle strength is reduced.

a	Predicted	Observed	Post-bronchodilator
FEV_1 (l)	2.86	1.15	1.30
FVC (l)	4.11	2.80	3.55
FEV_1/FVC (%)	70.00	41.00	37.00
TLC (l)	6.98	7.47	
RV (l)	2.54	4.24	
TLCO (mmol/min/kPa)	8.80	6.72	
KCO (mmol/min/kPa/l)	1.33	1.06	
VA (l)		6.33	

b	Predicted	23 April 1991	10 March 1992
FEV_1 (l)	3.75	1.70	2.45
FVC (l)	4.94	2.40	3.30
FEV_1/FVC (%)	75.00	71.00	74.00
TLC (l)	7.59	4.34	5.55
RV (l)	2.41	1.67	2.10
TLCO (mmol/min/kPa)	10.95	5.82	7.36
KCO (mmol/min/kPa/l)	1.57	1.38	1.77
VA (l)		4.06	4.20

c	Predicted	Observed
FEV_1 (l)	2.27	0.8
FVC (l)	2.83	1.10
FEV_1/FVC (%)	77.00	73.00
TLC (l)	4.25	1.89
RV (l)	1.22	0.85
TLCO (mmol/min/kPa)	7.49	3.84
KCO (mmol/min/kPa/l)	1.79	2.44
VA (l)	4.15	1.58
$P_e$max (cmH_2O)	59–127	50.00
$P_i$max (cmH_2O)	29–117	40.00

measured by an exercise test or inferred from questioning. Exercise tests are valuable in making an objective assessment of disability and in observing the physiological response to exercise in order to assist diagnosis. Tests of exercise performance can either be performed in a complex manner in the laboratory or simply by observation of walking achievement down a hospital corridor. The former generally examines the detailed physiological response while walking tests can give a useful and reproducible assessment of disability. A further value of exercise testing is to use the stimulus to provoke bronchoconstriction where exercise-induced asthma is suspected. In this use the exercise should be performed in an environment as close as possible to that which produces the symptoms.

Questionnaires

Most people do not ordinarily stress the lungs to their physiological limit. Furthermore, patients with exercise limitation adopt a restricted lifestyle which may hide their disability. Sometimes simple questions can identify the disruption of normal activity. An overall picture of disability can be judged by application of a detailed questionnaire designed to cover either general features of disability or those which relate to specific examples. There are several disease-specific questionnaires available for chronic lung disease. The Chronic Respiratory Questionnaire (CRQ) and St George's Respiratory Questionnaire have been validated for patients with COPD and asthma (Guyatt et al 1987, Jones 1991). These questionnaires are quite good at distinguishing change after an intervention but not so good at comparisons between patients. This is particularly true of the CRQ which uses individualized questions to obtain sensitivity. The Breathing Problems Questionnaire (BPQ) is another self-administered, disease-specific instrument which can provide a good comparative description of disability (Hyland et al 1994). More recent developments include the shortened BPQ developed specifically for rehabilitation (Hyland et al 1998) and the AQ-20 (Hajiro et al 1999). The Medical Research Council (MRC) dyspnoea scale has been shown to

relate reasonably well to shuttle walk test performance (Bestall et al 1999) and may give a quick and simple yet reasonably accurate measure of function in a clinical setting.

Laboratory estimation of exercise capacity

Observation of the physiological response to exercise in the laboratory is the gold standard measurement of disability. This is usually performed during a progressive maximal test which is completed when the subject is unable to continue on either a treadmill or a cycle ergometer. The latter provides a stable platform and more accurate assessment of workload, while the walking action on the treadmill will be more familiar to most patients. In health a greater $\dot{V}O_2$ is achieved on the treadmill, but this is not necessarily the case in severe COPD where the cycle may be a greater exercise stimulus (Mathur et al 1995).

While the exercise is progressing the basic physiological response is observed by measuring ventilation, heart rate and oxygen uptake and carbon dioxide production. Other measurements such as oxygen saturation or cardiac output can be made if necessary. The test is conducted in such a fashion as to obtain a symptom-limited duration of about 10 minutes with the increments of workload increased every minute by about 50 watts (W) for healthy subjects (10 W or less for patients with COPD). During this period the heart rate will rise linearly with workload. Ventilation also rises linearly until about 60% of maximum workload when it increases disproportionately. Oxygen uptake ($\dot{V}O_2$) will also rise linearly until the same point above which the rate of uptake slows and eventually reaches a plateau at the maximum oxygen uptake ($\dot{V}O_2$max) (Fig. 3.5). The $\dot{V}O_2$max is determined in health by the cardiovascular delivery of oxygen to the muscles and is a crude estimate of capacity and cardiopulmonary fitness. The point of inflection of pulmonary ventilation on the V_E versus $\dot{V}O_2$ slope is known as the 'anaerobic threshold'. It is usually measured by the gas exchange method ($\dot{V}O_2$ v $\dot{V}CO_2$ plot) or lactate accumulation. In patients with lung disease the limits to maximal

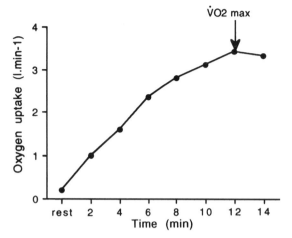

Figure 3.5   The relationship between work and oxygen uptake during progressive exercise.

exercise may be different. For example, maximal performance may be limited by low muscle mass, ventilation, respiratory muscle impairment and gas exchange. For this reason patients with COPD do not demonstrate a true $\dot{V}O_2$max because performance is terminated prematurely by the ventilatory limit imposed by airway obstruction. Fatigue from limb muscle weakness may also be a significant factor in these patients.

The value of exercise testing in lung disease lies in the measurement of the degree of functional impairment by assessment of the maximal workload and $\dot{V}O_2$max in comparison with reference values. If a patient fails to achieve his or her predicted performance the mode of failure can help to identify the mechanism. For example, in patients with lung disease the early rise of $\dot{V}_E$ may be characteristically in excess of expectations but reach a premature limit imposed by the physical constraints of damaged lungs. Concurrently the heart rate response may be attenuated, in contrast to patients with cardiac disease where the test may have to be terminated because of early attainment of maximum predicted heart rate or chest pain. It is always important to determine why the subject stops at the end of a test.

The value of exercise testing

- Differential diagnosis of dyspnoea
- Objective assessment of disability
- Assessment of therapeutic intervention
- Identification of exercise-induced asthma
- Prescription of an exercise training programme

Muscle function (biopsies)

It is now becoming clearer that peripheral muscle dysfunction makes an important contribution to disability in patients with chronic respiratory disease (American Thoracic Society 1999). There is increasing evidence of reduced size and strength of muscles of the lower limb compared to healthy controls (Gosselink et al 1996, 1998). Others have shown an altered metabolic response to exercise (Maltais et al 1996). The sampling of peripheral muscle in healthy individuals is commonplace both at rest and during exercise. To date only sampling at rest has been fully described in COPD patients (Maltais et al 1996). This technique, whilst not applicable to all respiratory centres, may provide useful information for future therapies (Steiner & Morgan 2001).

Field exercise tests

Laboratory tests of performance are the most accurate but are not always available and require expensive equipment. As an alternative, several field tests have been developed which can measure performance and their results relate quite well to laboratory estimates. There are two main categories of field test – those which are unpaced and those where the speed of activity is imposed.

One of the first unpaced tests was the 12-minute running test which was developed to assess the fitness of military personnel. This concept was adapted to the needs of the respiratory patient by downgrading the activity to a walk along a hospital corridor. Later, a reduction of the time to 6 minutes appeared to have no disadvantages. The 12- and 6-minute walks have become familiar forms of assessment for respiratory patients (Butland et al 1982, McGavin et al 1976). The test procedure is extremely simple, with a course marked out along the corridor and the patient given the simple instruction to cover as much ground as possible in the time permitted. These tests have proven value but also have some limitations. There is quite a large learning effect and the reproducibility only becomes acceptable after two or more attempts (Knox et al 1988, Mungall & Hainsworth 1979). In addition, no two patients will attack the test in the same way and the relative stresses may not allow direct comparison. Lastly, the lack of pace constraint makes the test performance vulnerable to mood and encouragement. Nevertheless, these simple tests require no equipment and, within their limitations, provide valuable information about general exercise capacity and major therapeutic changes.

The second type of field exercise test imposes a pace on the patient which reduces the effect of motivation and encouragement. An endurance walking test instructs the patient to walk at a constant fast pace for an unlimited distance and measures the time and distance travelled. Another form of constrained exercise is the step test where the subject steps up and down a couple of steps in time to a metronome signal. Inability to continue, signals the end of the test and could be due to fatigue or breathlessness. This test has the capacity for incremental progression by increasing the pacing rate, but is a rather unnatural form of exercise.

An attempt to combine the comprehensive nature of incremental laboratory tests and the flexibility of the 6-minute walk has been made in the shuttle walk test. This is an adaptation of the 20 m shuttle running test where a subject runs between two cones 20 m apart with the pace determined by a series of audio signals (Léger & Lambert 1982). At intervals the pace increases until the subject can continue no longer. For patients with lung disease the shuttle distance is reduced to 10 m and the pace increments altered to provide a comfortable start and reasonable range (Singh et al 1992) (Fig. 3.6). Under these

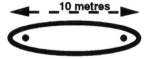

Level	Shuttles /level	Speed (mph)
1	3	1.12
2	4	1.50
3	5	1.88
4	6	2.26
5	7	2.64
6	8	3.02
7	9	3.40
8	10	3.78
9	11	4.16
10	12	4.54
11	13	4.92
12	14	5.30

a

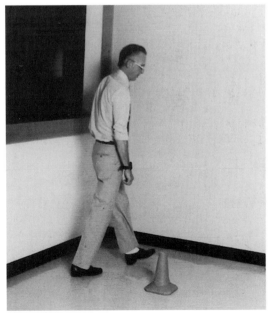

b

Figure 3.6   **a** The shuttle walk test involves the perambulation of an oval 10 m course. The walking speeds are increased every minute and thereby increase the number of shuttles per level. **b** The subject turns around the cone in the shuttle walk in time with an audio signal. This subject is wearing a heart rate telemeter on his wrist.

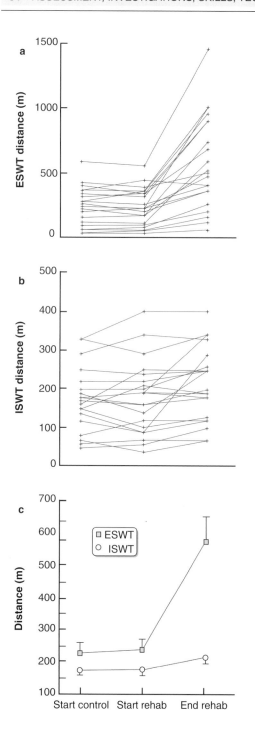

circumstances the test provides a similar physiological stimulus to an incremental treadmill test and can be combined with measurements of heart rate and breathlessness to obtain almost as much information as provided by the laboratory standard. The standard shuttle walking test has been applied successfully in defining disability in patients with chronic respiratory disease and more recently in chronic heart failure (Keell et al 1998).

A modification of the shuttle walking test has been described by Bradley et al (1999). This modified test allows the subject to run when required and includes an additional two levels. It has been validated in patients with cystic fibrosis, who were previously unchallenged by the standard test.

The endurance shuttle walking test (Revill et al 1999) complements the incremental test; patients are required to walk around an identical course for as long as possible at a constant speed (after a short warm-up) and the test result is recorded as time.

These functional walking tests are very useful in the context of pulmonary rehabilitation where mass laboratory testing is impractical; they provide a baseline measure of disability and have been shown to be sensitive to change (Griffiths et al 2000). Rehabilitation provokes significant changes in both incremental and endurance performance (Revill et al 1999). The magnitude of change reported was far greater for the endurance shuttle walking test than the incremental, reflecting the mode of training employed in this study (Fig. 3.7).

ASSESSMENT OF CARDIAC FUNCTION

Introduction

The heart is a more straightforward organ compared to the lungs and assessment of cardiac function can be made employing a variety of reliable and reproducible techniques. It is, however, a less forgiving organ and minor abnormalities of the coronary arteries or cardiac muscle function may have dramatic consequences.

Figure 3.7 Changes observed in the endurance shuttle walking test (ESWT) (a), incremental shuttle walking test (ISWT) (b) and the mean (SE) distances for both tests after a short course of rehabilitation (c). (Reproduced with permission from Revill et al 1999.)

The heart is composed of specialized muscle cells (myocytes) which together act as a coordinated pump to eject blood through the two major vascular circuits: the systemic vasculature and the pulmonary vasculature. Within the myocardium are electrical pathways which are responsible for the coordinated and rhythmical contraction of the heart, starting with the atria and followed by the ventricles. Within the four cardiac chambers are the heart valves which prevent the ejection of blood in the wrong direction. On the surface of the heart are the coronary arteries, which supply the myocardium with blood. Apart from congenital defects in the structure of the heart, disease processes can affect any of these components.

The symptomatic response to disease or malfunction depends very much on the individual structures affected. Angina pectoris and myocardial infarction are caused by disturbances of myocardial blood supply and usually result in the development of retrosternal chest tightness, heaviness and pain. Distinction between the two conditions can be difficult. Stable angina pectoris is more usually characterized by pain and/or dyspnoea on effort, whereas unstable angina and myocardial infarction tend to be more severe and may occur at any time, including at rest.

When left ventricular function is impaired, such as with myocardial cell death following myocardial infarction, symptoms may include breathlessness. When severe enough to cause pulmonary oedema, severe breathlessness at rest associated with sweating and severe distress may ensue. If both ventricles are damaged or impaired (congestive cardiac failure) or if there is right ventricular dysfunction in isolation, in addition to breathlessness, significant peripheral oedema or ascites may be present along with elevation in the neck veins.

Rhythm disturbances of the heart (arrhythmias) can manifest in a variety of ways. The presentation depends partly on the rhythm concerned and partly on whether there is underlying cardiac disease. Atrial fibrillation is a rhythm characterized by an irregularly irregular pulse and can produce symptoms of fatigue and breathlessness in the absence of a cardiac abnormality, but is much more likely to produce symptoms if myocardial function is already impaired. It may also be characterized by an inappropriately fast pulse with a rapid increase in rate associated with exertion. This makes assessment of function more difficult in patients with this arrhythmia. Severe slowing of the heart (bradycardia) or acceleration (tachycardia) may present with dizziness or syncope.

The chest radiograph

The simple chest radiograph can provide valuable information about the presence of heart failure and is probably the most useful clinical tool for monitoring its progress. Enlargement of the heart can be measured if the radiograph is taken in the posteroanterior (PA) projection and the cardiothoracic ratio (CTR) documented. This is the width of the cardiac border divided by the width of the thorax and should be less than 0.5. Enlargement of the heart represents either increased muscle bulk or, more commonly, dilatation of the ventricular cavities. Pulmonary venous pooling will fill the upper lobe vessels followed by the engorgement of the interlobular lymphatics which become visible as horizontal lines at the costophrenic angles (Kerley B lines). If the pulmonary venous pressure rises above 25 mmHg there is the risk of interstitial oedema. This is first visible as loss of definition of the hilum, but subsequently may produce widespread shadowing (bat's wing appearance). If congestive cardiac failure is present the picture may be complicated by pleural effusions.

The electrocardiograph (ECG)

The ECG or electrocardiograph records the electrical activity of the heart (Fig. 3.8). Normally the ECG employs 12 different leads which record the activity over various aspects of the heart so that areas of abnormality can be anatomically located. For instance, if there are signs consistent with abnormality over the anterior leads (V2 to V6), then it is probable that there is a problem with the anterior wall of the heart which is composed predominantly of the left ventricle. Similarly, changes confined to the inferior leads (II, III and

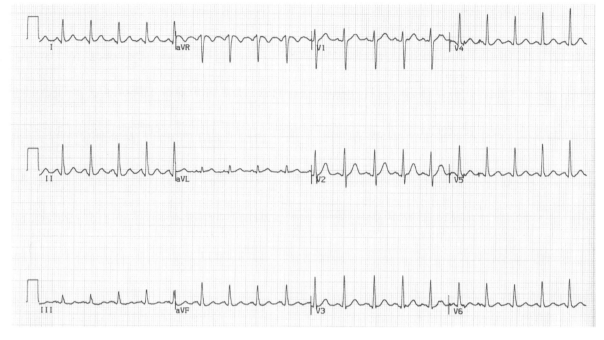

Figure 3.8   Normal 12-lead ECG.

aVF) suggest a problem with the inferior surface of the heart which consists of both right and left ventricles.

The ECG is a well-established cardiological investigation and can provide a whole variety of information. First, it allows the reliable identification of the underlying cardiac rhythm. Normal rhythm is regular and is called sinus rhythm. Abnormal rhythms (arrhythmias) such as atrial flutter may also be regular but the ECG will allow ready identification. For intermittent arrhythmias a 24- or 48-hour ECG recording may be helpful. For patients with persistent symptoms of cardiac arrhythmia but in whom no abnormality can be recorded, other techniques are available. Devices can be loaned to patients for several days which allow them to record their episodes and transmit them to a local centre via the telephone for analysis (cardiac memo recorders). For patients in whom more serious arrhythmias are suspected, devices can be implanted under the skin and activated by means of an external magnet (Reveal© device).

This will automatically store the ECG for a pre-determined period. This allows patients to store the event even following recovery from attacks that may have induced syncope. The device can then be interrogated via an external analyser and any abnormality of rhythm documented.

Some cardiac conditions produce characteristic abnormalities of the ECG waveform. For example, myocardial infarction tends to produce elevation in the ST segment of the waveform.

In addition to helping diagnose the condition, the ECG also gives the clinician an indication of the territory involved and the potential consequences of the episode (Figs. 3.9, 3.10). Often the presence of a previous myocardial infarction can also be determined. Episodes of ischaemia such as angina also tend to produce classic appearances on the ECG such as ST depression or T-wave inversion. These appearances are looked for during exercise testing (see below). However, a normal ECG does not exclude angina, especially if the patient was not symptomatic during the recording.

The presence of heart failure cannot be determined from the ECG but it can be said that a completely normal ECG makes the diagnosis of heart failure very unlikely.

Exercise testing

The exercise ECG is the first-line investigation in the assessment of patients with known or suspected ischaemic heart disease. In this investigation the 12-lead ECG is recorded during a progressive exercise test. This is usually by means of a treadmill, but cycle and step tests have been used for patients who cannot use a treadmill. A popular treadmill protocol is the Bruce protocol in which the difficulty increases in 3-minute stages. Stage 1 is at 1.7 mph on an incline of 10%, stage 2 is at 2.5 mph and 12%, stage 3 is at 3.4 mph and 14% and stage 4 is at 4.2 mph on an incline of 16%. This is a difficult protocol, especially for elderly patients or individuals of short stature. Other gentler protocols are available: Sheffield, modified Bruce, Balke, Naughton, etc. (see Table 3.2).

The normal response to exercise is a steady increase in heart rate. This is accompanied by a gradual rise in systolic blood pressure and a small (if any) rise in diastolic pressure. A lack of rise or a fall in the systolic pressure raises the possibility of multivessel coronary disease or left ventricular dysfunction.

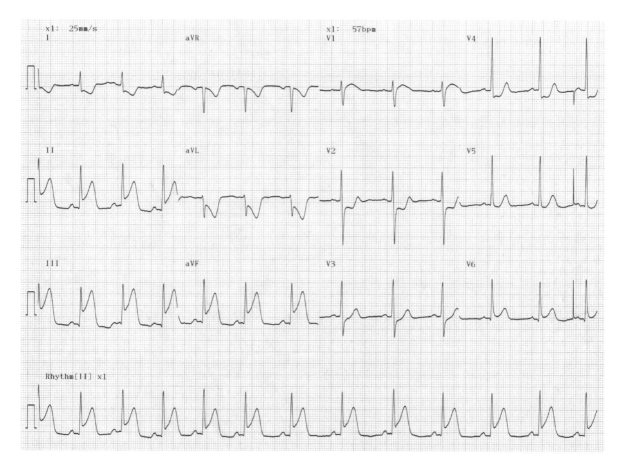

Figure 3.9 Inferior myocardial infarction. There is elevation in the ST segment of the ECG in leads II, III and aVF which look at the inferior surface of the heart.

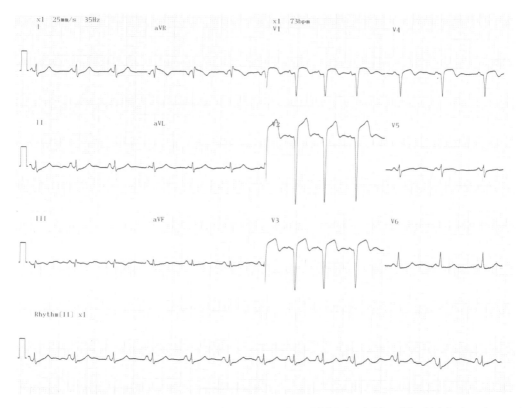

Figure 3.10 Anterior myocardial infarction. There is ST elevation of the ECG in leads V1 to V4 which look at the anterior surface of the heart.

The exercise ECG is deliberately provocative compared to those used to assess respiratory function. The aim is to place demands on the heart and achieve an adequate level of work accompanied by a rise in heart rate. In general, achievement of 85% or greater of the target heart rate provides an adequate level of stress for diagnostic purposes. Target heart rate can be calculated by the equation:

$$220 - \text{the patient's age.}$$

The main indication for exercise testing is for the assessment of myocardial ischaemia and coronary artery disease, in particular the diagno-

Table 3.2 Examples of exercise testing protocols

	Bruce		Sheffield or Mod. Bruce		Northwick Park		Mod. Sheffield	
	Speed mph	Incline %	Speed mph	Incline %	Speed mph	Incline %	Speed mph	Incline %
Stage 1	1·7	10	1·7	0	2·0	0	1·7	0
Stage 2	2·5	12	1·7	5	3·0	4	1·7	5
Stage 3	3·4	14	1·7	10	3·0	8	1·7	10
Stage 4	4·2	16	2·5	12	3·0	12	2·5	10
Stage 5	5·0	18	3·4	14	3·0	16	2·5	12
Stage 6	5·5	20	4·2	16	3·0	20	3·4	12
Stage 7	–	–	5·0	18	4·5	20	–	–
Stage 8	–	–	5·5	20	–	–	–	–

sis of chest pain, assessment of ischaemic risk, prognosis and residual ischaemia following myocardial infarction, evaluation of medical or surgical therapy, evaluation of cardiac function and exercise capacity and detection of exercise-induced arrhythmias.

False positive tests can occur, as can false-negative tests, but overall the exercise test is an extremely useful guide to the presence or absence of ischaemic heart disease and a good predictor of prognosis. Patients who cannot exceed 3 minutes of the Bruce protocol and who have ECG changes consistent with ischaemia (Fig. 3.11) have a mortality at 1 year in excess of 5%, whereas those who exceed 9 minutes (with no ECG changes) have a mortality of less than 1%. Similarly, patients who exercise for less than 3 minutes have a 3.5 fold greater risk of dying than patients who exercise for more than 6 minutes.

Electrophysiological studies

For patients with more complex cardiac arrhythmias, more invasive ECG assessment is possible. Electrophysiological studies involve the positioning of a number of electrodes within the cardiac chambers (usually via the femoral artery and/or vein) under radiological guidance. Intracardiac recordings of electrical activity can then be made. The appearance of the ECG is very different from that obtained by the standard 12-lead ECG. The procedure allows for the more accurate assessment and diagnosis of arrhythmias and particularly allows identification of extra cardiac circuits (so-called 'accessory pathways') which may predispose the individual to inappropriately fast rhythms. Ultimately this may allow therapeutic procedures to be offered whereby these extra circuits can be destroyed (radiofrequency ablation).

Radioisotope studies

A variety of radioisotope investigations are available in the assessment of cardiac function. Overall myocardial function can be accurately measured using isotope studies – for example, multigated acquisition (MUGA) scans – so that a reliable assessment of the ejection fraction can be made. The ejection fraction is the amount of blood ejected by the heart in each cycle and in normal individuals is in excess of 50%. In

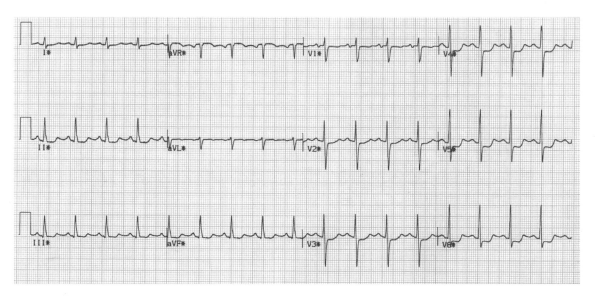

Figure 3.11   Example of a positive stress test with ST segment depression (consistent with ischaemia) in leads V4 to V6 during stage 2 of the Bruce protocol.

patients with left ventricular dysfunction, the ejection fraction may be anywhere between 10% and 45%. Obviously the lower the ejection fraction, the more severe the problem. The MUGA scan also allows for separate measurement of right ventricular function.

Radioisotope studies can also be used to assess myocardial perfusion (Fig. 3.12). This is particularly useful if the exercise ECG test fails to give an adequate assessment or answer.

Pre-existing ECG abnormalities (such as left bundle branch block) do not allow for identification of the development of ischaemia. In some there may be a suspicion that the test was a false negative and the isotope study is more sensitive and specific for the identification of ischaemia.

Radioisotope studies also give the opportunity to assess patients who cannot walk on the treadmill, as the heart can be stressed pharmacologically using agents such as dobutamine or adenosine. Scanning patients before and after stress (be it exercise or pharmacological) allows a comparison to be made between images. Gamma cameras are employed to detect uptake of the isotope by the myocardium and areas of underperfusion can be seen. The test also allows for the identification of areas of fixed ischaemia which do not improve with rest. These often suggest the presence of scar tissue which would not benefit

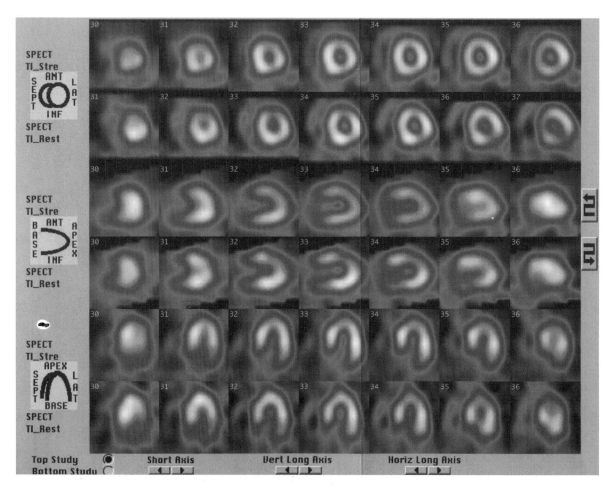

Figure 3.12 Images obtained following a stress radioisotope study comparing images taken during rest (rows 2, 4 and 6) and stress (rows 1, 3 and 5). The brighter the image, the better the blood supply to that region. This is a normal scan with no evidence of ischaemia.

from a revascularization procedure (such as bypass surgery or angioplasty). Another potential use is to assess the physiological significance of coronary artery stenoses detected by angiography (see later) and allow the clinician to determine whether revascularization is required.

Echocardiography

Ultrasound examination of the heart has become an invaluable asset to cardiac investigation and has superseded many invasive techniques. Standard transthoracic echocardiography provides an ultrasound image of the structure of the heart, while Doppler studies allow the assessment of flow patterns and pressure gradients within the chambers.

M-mode echocardiography involves a one-dimensional view of structures in the path of the ultrasound beam. This technique allows for the assessment of movement and the quantification of chamber size and a rough estimate of cardiac function. Two-dimensional echocardiography produces more anatomically pleasing images which allow the direct visualization of the myocardium, heart valves and associated structures (Fig. 3.13). Doppler echocardiography records direction and velocity of blood flow within the heart and great vessels. Superimposing colour flow Doppler on two-dimensional images

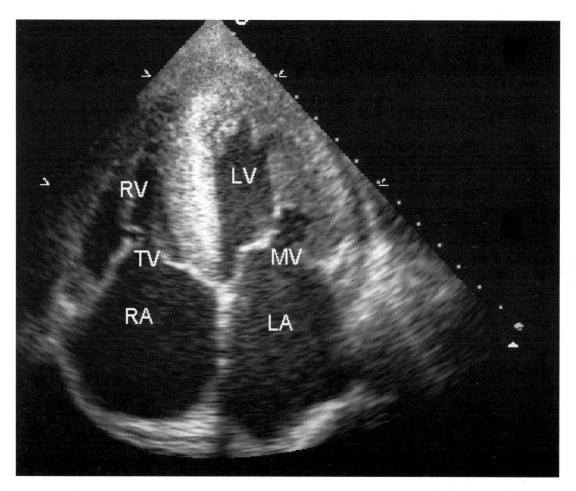

Figure 3.13 A two-dimensional echocardiography image showing all four cardiac chambers, the right atrium (RA), right ventricle (RV), the left atrium (LA) and the left ventricle (LV). The mitral (MV) and tricuspid (TV) valves are clearly seen.

produces clear images of flow across structures and illustrates the presence or absence of abnormal flow such as valve regurgitation and turbulence.

Transoesophageal echocardiography is a technique which utilizes all the features of transthoracic echocardiography, but involves the passage of an ultrasound transducer mounted on an endoscope into the oesophagus. Extremely clear images of the heart and great vessels can be obtained because the oesophagus is in such close proximity to the relevant structures and there is little air or tissue interface. It is useful when transthoracic images are inconclusive because of poor image quality or when more detailed assessment is desirable (such as in mitral valve morphology or the diagnosis of endocarditis).

Stress echocardiography is a technique which involves the visualization of myocardial performance during infusion of various pharmacological stressing agents such as dobutamine. This allows the determination of ventricular performance and can give an indication of areas of underperfusion and of irreversible left ventricular damage.

Contrast echocardiography involves the injection of microbubbles that appear as clouds of echoes on the ultrasound image. This helps accurate determination of the outline of the myocardium, particularly when measuring movement of the ventricle. Precise areas of impaired movement can be visualized.

Cardiac catheterization

Cardiac catheterization allows the accurate assessment of coronary artery anatomy. The procedure involves the insertion of catheters into the arterial circulation (usually via the femoral artery) and the selective intubation of each of the coronary arteries. The presence of narrowings (stenoses) or blockages can be determined by the injection of dye to outline the vessels (Fig. 3.14). Images are acquired in various planes because of the three-dimensional nature of the heart. In addition, the procedure allows for a variety of other assessments to be made.

Continuous pressure monitoring gives the opportunity to measure pressures within the cardiac chambers, particularly the left ventricle during left heart catheterization. Elevation in the left ventricular end-diastolic pressure over 12 mmHg (the pressure trough immediately before ventricular contraction) suggests left ventricular dysfunction. Withdrawal of the catheter across the aortic valve also allows pressure gradients across the valve to be determined and the severity of any stenosis to be made.

Quantification of coronary stenoses is made visually and with the aid of computer programs. Other methods include the passage of tiny ultrasound probes mounted over flexible guidewires into the arteries themselves. This technique is called intravascular ultrasound (IVUS) and images of the inside of the coronary arteries and arterial wall are obtained. Recently the development of guidewires with pressure sensors has allowed the pressure within the arteries to be measured before and after a stenosis and an assessment of the severity of any given stenosis made.

Right heart catheterization (access being gained via the femoral vein) can measure pressures in the right heart chambers (right atrium and ventricle) and also the pulmonary arteries. Wedging of catheters or employing balloon-tipped catheters in the pulmonary arterial tree also enables the measurement of wedge pressure, which is an indirect measurement of left atrial pressure. Once left atrial pressure rises above 20 mmHg, pulmonary oedema can ensue and therefore wedge pressure allows further assessment of left ventricular function.

A variety of other parameters can be assessed by the sampling of blood in various chambers and vessels which ultimately can allow very accurate measurements of cardiac output, intracardiac shunts and vascular resistance.

The major drawback of cardiac catheterization is the invasive nature of the procedure and the potential risks.

Magnetic resonance imaging (MRI)

Magnetic resonance imaging (MRI) is a rapidly developing non-invasive technique for cardiac

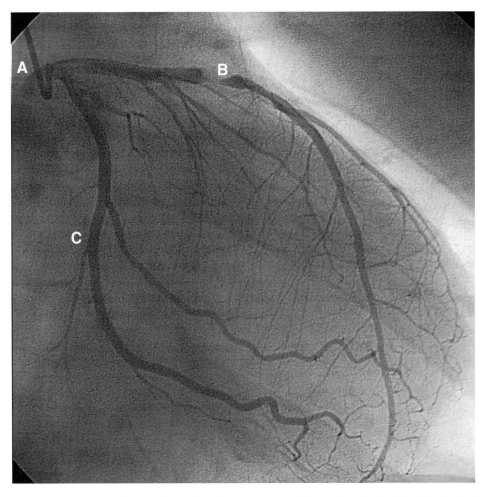

Figure 3.14 Example of cardiac catheterization of the left coronary artery. The catheter is illustrated (A) situated in the origin of the left coronary artery. A severe stenosis (narrowing) of the left anterior descending branch is seen (B). The circumflex branch (C) is relatively healthy.

investigation. Previously, cardiac motion from patient respiration and the cyclic motion of the heart hampered imaging with this modality. However, the advent of ultrafast imaging sequences has enabled MRI to become the gold standard for evaluation of cardiac anatomy and function. The high resolution of MRI and the ability to image in any plane allows three-dimensional measurement of ejection fraction without need for geometrical assumptions. Studies have shown excellent intra- and inter-observer variability and so small changes in function over time can be estimated reliably. No ionizing radi-

ation is required and so longitudinal (serial) patient studies are safe.

First pass contrast enhanced imaging can be used to evaluate myocardial perfusion. Both qualitative and quantitative parameters of myocardial blood flow can be obtained, although the latter is largely research based. Pharmacological stress protocols can be applied in a manner analogous to echocardiography and radioisotope studies so that regional abnormalities in function and/or perfusion can be assessed at rest and during stress.

Not all patients are suitable for magnetic resonance. Contraindications include patients with permanent pacing systems, metallic implants and severe claustrophobia. As scanners with cardiac specifications and trained personnel become more widely available in the workplace, MRI is likely to become a cardiac investigation of increasing usefulness.

THE ELECTROCARDIOGRAM

The electrocardiogram (ECG) is a recording from the body surface of the electrical activity of the heart. The standard ECG has 12 leads.

- Chest leads, V1–V6, which look at the heart in a *horizontal plane* (Fig. 3.15).
- Limb leads, which look at the heart in a *vertical plane* (Fig. 3.16). Limb leads are unipolar (AVR, AVL and AVF) or bipolar (I, II, III).

The ECG machine is arranged so that when a depolarization wave spreads towards a lead the needle moves upwards, and when it spreads away from the lead the needle moves downwards.

ECG WAVEFORM AND DEFINITIONS
(Fig. 3.17)

The *heart rate*. At normal paper speed (25 mm/s in the UK) each 'big square' is 0.2 s. The heart rate (if the rhythm is regular) is calculated by counting the number of big squares between consecutive R waves and dividing into 300.

The *P wave* is the first deflection and is caused by atrial depolarization. When abnormal it may be:

- broad and notched (> 0.12 s) in left atrial enlargement ('P mitrale', e.g. mitral stenosis)
- tall and peaked (> 2.5 mm) in right atrial enlargement ('P pulmonale', e.g. pulmonary hypertension)
- replaced by flutter or fibrillation waves (p. 98)
- absent in sinoatrial block (p. 97).

The QRS *complex* represents ventricular depolarization.

- A negative (downward) deflection preceding an R wave is called a Q wave. Normal Q waves are small and narrow; deep wide Q waves (except in AVR and V1) indicate myocardial infarction.
- A deflection upwards is called an R wave whether or not it is preceded by a Q wave.
- A negative deflection following an R wave is termed an S wave.

Ventricular depolarization starts in the septum and spreads from left to right (Fig. 3.18). Subsequently the main free walls of the ventricles are depolarized. Thus, in the right ventri-

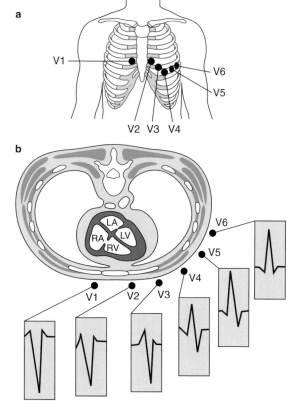

Figure 3.15 **a** The V leads are attached to the chest wall overlying the intercostal spaces as shown: V4 in the midclavicular line, V5 in the anterior axillary line, V6 in the midaxillary line. **b** Leads V1 and V2 look at the right ventricle, V3 and V4 at the interventricular septum, and V5 and V6 at the left ventricle. The normal QRS complex in each lead is shown.

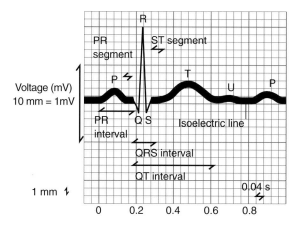

a The bipolar leads   **b** The augmented
bipolar leads

Figure 3.16 Lead I is derived from electrodes on the right arm (negative pole) and left arm (positive pole), lead II is derived from electrodes on the right arm (negative pole) and left leg (positive pole), and lead III from electrodes on the left arm (negative pole) and left leg (positive pole).

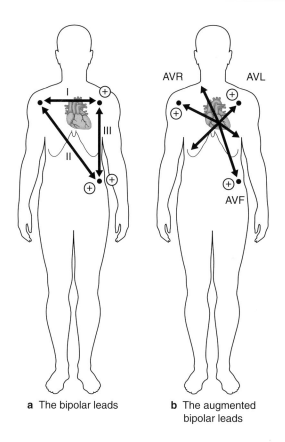

Voltage (mV)
10 mm = 1mV

Figure 3.17 The waves and elaboration of the normal ECG Modified from Goldman (1976).

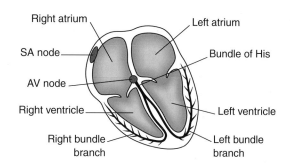

Figure 3.18 In normal circumstances only the specialized conducting tissues of the heart undergo spontaneous depolarization (automaticity) which initiates an action potential. The sinus node discharges more rapidly than the other cells and is the normal pacemaker of the heart. The impulse generated by the sinus node spreads first through the atria, producing atrial systole, and then through the atrioventricular node to the His–Purkinje system, producing ventricular systole.

cular leads (V1 and V2) the first deflection is upwards (R wave) as the septal depolarization wave spreads towards those leads. The second deflection is downwards (S wave) as the bigger left ventricle (in which depolarization is spreading away) outweighs the effect of the right ventricle (see Fig. 3.15). The opposite pattern is seen in the left ventricular leads (V5 and V6), with an initial downwards deflection (small Q wave reflecting septal depolarization) followed by a large R wave caused by left ventricular depolarization.

In left ventricular hypertrophy, the increased bulk of the left ventricular myocardium increases the voltage-induced depolarization of the free wall of the left ventricle. This gives rise to tall R waves (> 25 mm) in the left ventricular leads (V5, V6) and/or deep S waves (> 30 mm) in the right ventricular leads (V1, V2). The sum of the R wave in the left ventricular leads and the S wave in the right ventricular leads exceeds 40 mm. In addition to these changes there may also be ST segment depression and T wave flattening or inversion in the left ventricular leads.

Right ventricular hypertrophy (e.g. in pulmonary hypertension) causes tall R waves in the right ventricular leads.

The QRS duration reflects the time that excitation takes to spread through the ventricle. A wide QRS complex (> 0.10 s) occurs if conduction is delayed, e.g. with right or left bundle branch block, or if conduction is through abnormal pathways, e.g. ventricular ectopic.

T waves result from ventricular repolarization. In general the direction of the T wave is the same as that of the QRS complex. Inverted T waves occur in many conditions and, although usually abnormal, they are a non-specific finding.

The *PR interval* is measured from the start of the P wave to the start of the QRS complex. It is the time taken for excitation to pass from the sinus node, through the atrium, atrioventricular node and His–Purkinje system to the ventricle. A prolonged PR interval (> 0.22 s) indicates heart block (p. 97).

The *ST segment* is the period between the end of the QRS complex and the start of the T wave. ST elevation (> 1 mm above the isoelectric line) occurs in the early stages of myocardial infarction and with acute pericarditis. ST segment depression (> 0.5 mm below the isoelectric line) indicates myocardial ischaemia.

CARDIAC ARRHYTHMIAS

An abnormality of the cardiac rhythm is called a cardiac arrhythmia. Such a disturbance may cause sudden death, syncope, dizziness, palpitations or no symptoms at all. Paroxysmal arrhythmias may not be detected on a single ECG recording. Twenty-four hour ambulatory ECG monitoring (continuous recording for 24 hours) and event recorders (a portable device activated by the patient to record the ECG when symptoms occur) are outpatient investigations often used to detect arrhythmias causing intermittent symptoms.

There are two main types of arrhythmia.

- *Bradycardia*, where the heart rate is slow (< 60 beats/min). The slower the heart rate the more probable that the arrhythmia will be symptomatic.
- *Tachycardia*, where the heart rate is fast (> 100 beats/min). Tachycardias are more likely to be symptomatic when the arrhyth-

mia is fast and sustained. They are subdivided into *supraventricular tachycardias*, which arise from the atrium or the atrioventricular junction, and *ventricular tachycardias*, which arise from the ventricles.

Sinus rhythms

Sinus arrhythmia. Fluctuations of autonomic tone result in phasic changes in the sinus discharge rate. Thus, during inspiration parasympathetic tone falls and the heart rate quickens and on expiration the heart rate falls. This variation is normal, particularly in children and young adults.

Sinus bradycardia. Sinus bradycardia is normal during sleep and in well-trained athletes. During the acute phase of a myocardial infarction it often reflects ischaemia of the sinus node. Other causes include hypothermia, hypothyroidism, cholestatic jaundice, raised intracranial pressure and drug therapy with beta-blockers, digitalis and other antiarrhythmic drugs. Patients with symptomatic bradycardia are treated with a permanent cardiac pacemaker. Intravenous atropine (600 mg IV) is used in the acute situation.

Sinus tachycardia. Sinus tachycardia is a physiological response during exercise and excitement. It may also occur with fever, anaemia, cardiac failure, thyrotoxicosis and drugs (e.g. catecholamines and atropine). Treatment is aimed at correction of the underlying cause. If necessary, beta-blockers may be used to slow the sinus rate but not in uncontrolled heart failure.

Pathological bradycardias

There are two main forms of severe bradycardia: sinus node disease and atrioventricular block.

Sinus node disease (sick sinus syndrome). Most cases of chronic sinus node disease are the result of idiopathic fibrosis occurring in elderly people. Bradycardia is caused by intermittent failure of sinus node depolarization or failure of the sinus impulse to propagate through the perinodal tissue to the atria. This is seen on the ECG as a long pause between consecutive P waves (>2 s). The slow heart rate predisposes to ectopic pacemaker activity and tachyarrhythmias are common (tachy–brady syndrome).

Insertion of a permanent pacemaker is only indicated in symptomatic patients to prevent dizzy spells and blackouts. Antiarrhythmic drugs are used to treat tachycardias. Thromboembolism is common in sick sinus syndrome and patients should be anticoagulated unless there is a contra-indication.

Atrioventricular block. There are three forms: first-degree heart block, second-degree (partial block) and third-degree (complete) block. The common causes are ischaemic heart disease, cardiomyopathy and, particularly in elderly people, fibrosis of the conducting tissue.

- *First-degree atrioventricular (AV) block* is the result of delayed atrioventricular conduction and reflected by a prolonged PR interval on the ECG. No change in heart rate occurs and treatment is unnecessary.
- *Second-degree (partial AV) block* occurs when some atrial impulses fail to reach the ventricles. Asymptomatic patients require no treatment other than careful follow-up, because there may be progression to complete heart block. Symptomatic patients are treated with insertion of a permanent pacemaker. There are three forms (Fig. 3.19).
  - Mobitz type 1 block (Wenckebach's phenomenon), in which the PR interval gradually increases, culminating in a dropped beat
  - Mobitz type II block occurs when a dropped QRS complex is not preceded by progressive PR prolongation.
  - a 2:1 or 3:1 block occurs when every second or third P wave conducts to the ventricles. A 4:1 or 5:1 block can also occur.
- *Third-degree (complete) AV block.* There is no association between atrial and ventricular activity and ventricular contractions are maintained by a spontaneous escape rhythm (usually about 40/min) from an automatic centre below the site of the block. The ECG shows regular P waves and QRS complexes which occur independently of one another. The usual symptoms are dizziness and black-

outs (Stokes–Adams attacks). If the ventricular rate is very slow, cardiac failure may occur. Insertion of a permanent pacemaker is always required for sustained complete heart block. In the acute situation, e.g. myocardial infarction, recovery may be expected and intravenous atropine or a temporary pacemaker may be all that is necessary.

Intraventricular conduction disturbances. The intraventricular conduction system consists of the His bundle, the right and left bundle branches and the anterosuperior and postero-inferior divisions of the left bundle branch block. Complete block of a bundle branch is associated with a wider QRS complex (0.12 s or more). The shape of the QRS depends on whether the right or the left bundle is blocked.

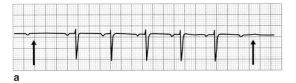

a

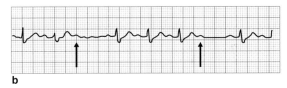

b

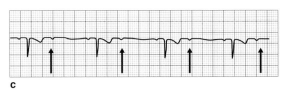

c

Figure 3.19   Three varieties of second-degree atrioventricular (AV) block. **a** Wenckebach (Mobitz-type I) AV block. The PR interval gradually prolongs until the P wave does not conduct to the ventricles (arrows). **b** Mobitz-type II AV block. The P waves that do not conduct to the ventricles (arrows) are not preceded by gradual PR interval prolongation. **c** Two P waves to each QRS complex. The PR interval prior to the dropped P wave is always the same. It is not possible to define this type of AV block as type I or type II Mobitz block and it is therefore a third variety of second-degree AV block (arrows show P waves).

Pathological tachycardias

The mechanisms responsible for most tachy-arrhythmias are abnormal automaticity and re-entry mechanisms.

Arrhythmias arise if there is enhanced automaticity of the normal conducting tissue or automaticity is acquired by damaged cells of the atria or ventricles; this causes ectopic beats and, if sustained, tachyarrhythmias.

Re-entry may occur if there are two separate pathways for impulse conduction (Fig. 3.20).

Atrial tachyarrhythmias. Ectopic beats, tachycardia, flutter and fibrillation may all arise from the atrial myocardium. They share common aetiologies, which are listed in Table 3.3.

Table 3.3   Causes of atrial arrhythmias

Ischaemic heart disease
Rheumatic heart disease
Thyrotoxicosis
Cardiomyopathy
Lone atrial fibrillation (i.e. no cause discovered)
Wolff–Parkinson–White syndrome
Pneumonia
Atrial septal defect
Carcinoma of the bronchus
Pericarditis
Pulmonary embolus
Acute and chronic alcohol abuse
Cardiac surgery

Atrial ectopic beats. These are caused by premature discharge of an ectopic atrial focus. On the ECG this produces an early and abnormal P wave, usually followed by a normal QRS complex. Treatment is not usually required unless they cause troublesome palpitations or are responsible for provoking more significant arrhythmias.

Atrial flutter. Atrial flutter is almost always associated with organic disease of the heart. The atrial rate is usually about 300 beats/min. The AV node usually conducts every second flutter beat, giving a ventricular rate of 150 beats/min. The ECG (Fig. 3.21a) characteristically shows 'sawtooth' flutter waves (F waves), which are most clearly seen when AV conduction is transiently impaired by carotid sinus massage or drugs. Treatment of an acute paroxysm is electrical cardioversion. Prophylaxis is achieved with class Ia, Ic or III drugs (Table 3.4). Rate control of a chronic arrhythmia is with AV nodal blocking drugs, e.g. digoxin.

Atrial fibrillation (AF). This is a common arrhythmia, occurring in between 5% and 10% of patients over 65 years of age. It also occurs, particularly in a paroxysmal form, in younger patients. Atrial activity is chaotic and mechanically ineffective. The AV node conducts a proportion of the atrial impulses to produce an irregular ventricular response. There are no clear P waves

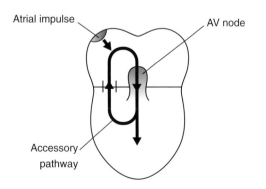

Figure 3.20   A re-entry circuit. The impulse is conducted normally through the AV node and initiates ventricular depolarization. In certain circumstances the accessory pathway is able to transmit the impulse retrogradely back into the atria, thus completing a circuit and initiating a self-sustaining re-entry tachycardia.

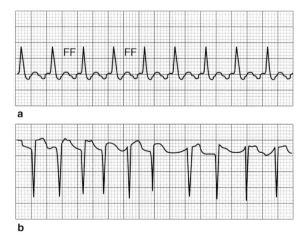

Figure 3.21   a Atrial flutter. The flutter waves are marked with an F, only half of which are transmitted to the ventricles. **b** Atrial fibrillation. There are no P waves and the ventricular response is fast and irregular.

Table 3.4 Vaughan Williams classification of antiarrhythmic drug therapy

Class	Mechanism of action	Individual drugs
Ia		Quinidine, procainamide, disopyramide
Ib	Membrane-stabilizing action	Lidocaine (lignocaine), mexiletine
Ic		Flecainide, propafenone
II	Beta-adrenergic blockers	Metoprolol, atenolol, propranolol
III	Increases refractory period of conducting system	Amiodarone, sotalol, bretylium
IV	Calcium channel blocking agents	Verapamil, diltiazem

Adenosine and digoxin are other antiarrhythmic drugs which do not fit into this classification.
These drugs all have proarrhythmic side effects (among others) and should be used with caution.
All except amiodarone are negatively inotropic and may exacerbate heart failure.

on the ECG (Fig. 3.21b), only a fine oscillation of the baseline (so-called fibrillation or f waves).

When AF arises in an apparently normal heart it is sometimes possible to convert to sinus rhythm, either electrically (by cardioversion) or chemically (with class Ia, Ic or III drugs). When AF is caused by an acute precipitating event, such as alcohol toxicity, chest infection or thyrotoxicosis, the underlying cause should be treated initially. Chronic AF occurring in a diseased heart will usually not respond to cardioversion and treatment is by control of the ventricular rate, usually with digoxin. Atrial fibrillation is associated with an increased risk of thromboembolism and antigcoagulation should be given for at least 3 weeks before (with the exception of those who require emergency cardioversion) and 4 weeks after cardioversion. Most patients with chronic AF should also be anticoagulated (INR 2.0–3.0). The exception is young patients with lone AF who are not diabetic or hypertensive. This group has a low incidence of thromboembolism and is treated with aspirin alone.

Junctional tachycardia. Junctional tachycardias are paroxysmal in nature and usually occur in the absence of structural heart disease. They are re-entrant arrhythmias caused by an abnormal pathway in the AV node or by an accessory pathway (bundle of Kent), as in the Wolff–Parkinson–White syndrome (Fig. 3.22). The usual history is of a sudden onset of fast (140–280/min) regular palpitations. On the ECG the P waves may be seen very close to the QRS complex or not seen at all. The QRS complex is usually of normal shape because, as with other

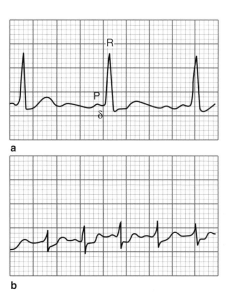

Figure 3.22 **a** An ECG showing Wolff–Parkinson–White syndrome. During sinus rhythm electrical impulses are conducted quickly through the abnormal pathway, resulting in a short PR interval and a slurred proximal limb of the QRS complex (δ wave). **b** A trace demonstrating the paroxysmal tachycardia which may result from this syndrome.

supraventricular arrhythmias, the ventricles are activated in the normal way, down the bundle of His. Occasionally the QRS complex is wide, because of a rate-related bundle branch block, and it may be difficult to distinguish from ventricular tachycardia.

Termination of an attack

● Manoeuvres that increase vagal stimulation of the sinus node: carotid sinus massage, ocular pressure or the Valsalva manoeuvre.

- Drug treatment: adenosine is a very short-acting AV nodal blocking drug given as a 3 mg bolus dose intravenously. It will terminate most junctional tachycardias. If there is no response after 1–2 minutes a further bolus of 6 mg is given. A third bolus of 12 mg may be given if there is still no response. Transient side effects include complete heart block, hypotension, nausea and bronchospasm. Asthma and second- or third-degree AV block are contraindications to adenosine. An alternative treatment is intravenous verapamil 10 mg IV over 5–10 minutes (contraindicated if the QRS complex is wide and therefore differentiation from ventricular tachycardia difficult).
- Rapid atrial pacing or DC cardioversion is used if adenosine fails.

Prophylaxis

- Radiofrequency ablation of the accessory pathway via a cardiac catheter.
- Flecainide, disopyramide, amiodarone and beta-blockers are the drugs most commonly used.

Ventricular arrhythmias

Ventricular ectopic beats (extrasystoles, premature beats). Ventricular ectopic beats may be asymptomatic or patients may complain of extra beats, missed beats or heavy beats. The ectopic electrical activity is not conducted to the ventricles through the normal conducting tissue and thus the QRS complex on the ECG is widened, with a bizarre configuration (Fig. 3.23). In normal individuals ectopic beats are of no significance, but treatment is sometimes given for symptoms. In patients with heart disease they are associated with an increased risk of sudden death. A recent meta-analysis of published trials suggests that prophylaxis with amiodarone may reduce mortality by preventing arrhythmias and sudden death.

Ventricular tachycardia Ventricular tachycardia and ventricular fibrillation are usually associated with underlying heart disease, e.g. ischaemia, cardiomyopathy and hypertensive heart disease. Ventricular tachycardia is defined as three or more consecutive ventricular beats occurring at a rate of 120/min or more. The ECG shows a rapid ventricular rhythm with broad abnormal QRS complexes which can sometimes be confused with a broad complex junctional tachycardia. Ventricular tachycardia may produce severe hypotension, when urgent DC cardioversion is necessary. If there is no haemodynamic compromise, treatment is usually with intravenous lidocaine (50–100 mg IV over 5 minutes followed by an intravenous infusion of 2–4 mg/min). Prophylaxis is usually with mexiletine, disopyramide, flecainide or amiodarone. Patients who are refractory to all medical treatment may need an implantable defibrillator (a small device implanted behind the rectus abdominis and connected to the heart; it recognizes ventricular tachycardia or ventricular fibrillation and automatically delivers a defibrillation shock to the heart).

Ventricular fibrillation. This is a very rapid and irregular ventricular activation (see Fig. 3.23) with no mechanical effect and hence no cardiac output. Ventricular fibrillation rarely reverts spontaneously and management is immediate cardioversion.

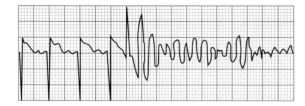

Figure 3.23 A rhythm strip demonstrating four beats of sinus rhythm followed by a ventricular ectopic beat that initiates ventricular fibrillation. The ST segment is elevated owing to acute myocardial infarction.

PAEDIATRICS

MEASUREMENT OF LUNG FUNCTION

History and examination

Taking a history is still the starting place when assessing a child's lung function. Questions need to reflect the child's age, and must take into account symptoms at rest, and when the child is running around playing, or taking part in school games or sport. For example, can a baby drink a full bottle of milk or does he become breathless and start spluttering? Does a boy keep up during a game of football or is he always put in goal? Can a schoolgirl carry her books up several flights of stairs to lessons or does she have to rest at each floor? Questions are easier to answer if they relate to normal activities and information is then obtained about how the child functions in everyday life. When discussing noisy breathing, it is well to remember that many parents do not understand what is meant by terms such as wheezing (Cane et al 2000) and an ability to demonstrate these sounds is helpful.

Physical examination is critical although it will only give information about the child at rest. Nevertheless, inspection will soon reveal whether the patient is in respiratory distress with, for example, tachypnoea and/or dyspnoea. The normal respiratory rate is dependent on age and decreases exponentially with body weight in children under 3 years (Gagliardi et al 1997) (Table 3.5). Note should also be taken of whether accessory muscles are being used and if the child has intercostal or subcostal recession. It is also important to determine whether the child can speak sentences without becoming breathless. Cyanosis, if present, ought to be fairly obvious. When reviewing a child with cystic fibrosis (CF) or bronchiectasis, it is important to inspect the sputum (colour, consistency).

Palpation is good for assessing chest expansion and placing the hands on the chest will indicate, by a feeling of vibration, whether the chest

is full of sputum – a method used by many parents of children with CF. Percussion is most useful for determining the presence of a pleural effusion (parapneumonic or empyema) indicated by dullness. Before auscultating with a stethoscope, it is worth simply listening to the child's breathing for wheeze (an expiratory sound), stridor (an inspiratory sound) or upper respiratory tract secretions heard in the throat (harsh expiratory and inspiratory sounds that are transmitted throughout the chest). The presence of a cough and its nature (dry, moist, productive, spasmodic) should be listened for. A forceful huff may also reveal abnormal sounds not obvious with quiet breathing. Finally, listening with the stethoscope may indicate abnormal sounds that can then be located to a particular area or lobe. It is always worth asking the patient to cough before listening again, as often some of the added sounds will have disappeared.

Dynamic lung function

In clinical practice, lung function tests mainly help with the management of a child with respiratory disease, for example in assessing severity, time trends, response to treatment and sometimes prognosis (Silverman & Stocks 1999). Although the tests may confirm that there is a respiratory problem, they rarely produce a specific diagnosis. To an extent, asthma is an exception, since demonstration of obstructive lung disease that responds to a bronchodilator or worsens with exercise is an important diagnostic aid.

Peak expiratory flow rate (PEFR)

This provides information on large airway function and normal values relate to the height of the child (Godfrey et al 1970). A child over 5–6 years ought to be able to use a peak flow meter after appropriate training and practise but the test is very effort dependent and easy to fake. After a maximal inhalation, the child needs to blow with a short hard blast, which is different from the full expiratory manoeuvre required in spirometry (see below). For this reason, PEFR must be ascertained separately using a peak flow meter rather

Table 3.5 Respiratory rate by age (adapted from Hooker et al 1992)

Age (years)	Respiratory rate (per minute) mean ± 2 SD	
1	30	18–42
2	29	19–39
4	26	16–36
8	23	13–33
12	21	13–29
16	20	12–28

than using the value calculated by a spirometer. It is most often used in management of asthmatic children and cheap peak flow meters are available on prescription for home use. It may be valuable when assessing a new therapy but regular use with a peak flow diary is of limited value due to the poor compliance with such a regimen (Redline et al 1996). Many children simply make up the results and fill in the diary the day before their clinic appointment. However, knowledge of a child's personal best and usual PEFR can help with asthma management, as a gradual drop in PEFR tends to precede an exacerbation and may sometimes occur before symptoms are recognized. Self-management plans can include guidance on when to take bronchodilators, start oral corticosteroids or seek medical help. Poor control is also indicated by an increase in day-to-day variability of PEFR measurements.

Spirometry

Spirometry, which can be performed in a clinic or at the bedside, is the most valuable and reproducible lung function test used in children. Most 6-year-olds can perform the technique reliably, with some 5-year-olds managing it as well. Normal values are available which take into account the child's gender and height (Polgar & Weng 1979, Rosenthal et al 1993a). Results are usually expressed as a 'percent predicted' but it is better to use standard deviation (SD) scores, even though these are more difficult for parents to understand. Generally, FEV_1 (forced expiratory volume at 1 second) and FVC (forced vital capacity) >80% of the predicted mean are considered normal, while a cut-off of 60% is used for $MEF_{25-75\%}$ (maximal expiratory flow at 25–75% vital capacity), as these correspond roughly to values that lie within 2 SD of the mean (Pattishall 1990). FEV_1 values of 60–79% are considered to represent mild, 40–59% moderate and <40% severe dysfunction, particularly when related to CF lung disease. Puberty has a dramatic effect on lung function in that both before and after there is a linear increase of lung function with height, while during puberty the relationship is more

complex (Rosenthal et al 1993a). Pubertal correction factors exist but in practice are rarely used.

Spirometry is effort dependent and it is important to watch the child's technique; the flow–volume and volume–time curves will also indicate whether a proper effort was made. The child inhales maximally then exhales as hard as possible and for as long as possible. Expiratory flow–volume loops are obtained along with data such as FVC and FEV_1. Flow rates at smaller lung volumes, e.g. maximal expiratory flow at 25% vital capacity ($MEF_{25\%}$), or mean flows across the mid-portion can also be obtained ($MEF_{25-75\%}$). Although these give more sensitive information about flow in the small airways, the measurements are less reliable due to their greater variability. It is best to view trends over time and FVC and FEV_1 are the two measurements most often followed. The shape of the flow–volume loop can indicate the presence of airway obstruction (a scooped-out concave appearance) and is particularly useful in children when assessing for the possible diagnosis of asthma.

The ratio of FEV_1 to FVC, used in adult practice to differentiate restrictive from obstructive disease, is less important in children where this differentiation is usually more obvious. However, children have relatively higher flows for their size than adults so the FEV_1/FVC ratio tends to be higher at around 90% (compared to 75–85% in adults). Inspiratory flow–volume curves can also be obtained and may be useful when considering extrathoracic obstruction, e.g. from a vascular ring. Infection control is important when using spirometers, particularly in a CF clinic.

Bronchodilator responsiveness

Evidence of airway reversibility is useful for both the diagnosis of asthma and its further management. Bronchodilators should ideally be withheld for 4 hours before assessing reversibility and long-acting beta-2 agonists are withheld that morning. Baseline FEV_1 should be measured, followed by the administration of a short-acting bronchodilator. In an effort to demonstrate reversibility, a large dose should be used, such as 1000 µg (10 puffs) of salbutamol via a metered dose inhaler with a spacer device or 5 mg via a nebulizer. FEV_1 should then be measured 15 minutes later. Bronchodilator reversibility is commonly expressed as a calculated increase in FEV_1 >15% of the baseline value but this is now felt not to be the best statistical method. In adults, change in FEV_1 should be expressed in absolute terms with an increase of >190 ml indicating reversibility (Editorial 1992). However, in children it has been suggested that an absolute increase >9% of the predicted value (e.g. from 60% predicted to > 69%) is the most appropriate way of defining reversibility (Waalkens et al 1993). In some children with genuine asthma, it may not be possible to document reversibility because they have near normal lung function at the time of testing. In children with CF, the variability of spirometric testing is greater than in normal children, so a larger response is needed to be confident that bronchodilator responsiveness is present (Cooper et al 1990, Nickerson et al 1980).

Bronchial challenge

Tests of bronchial hyperreactivity (BHR) involve challenging the airway with cold air or pharmacological agents such as methacholine or histamine. Although commonly performed in adults, in children bronchial challenge tends to be reserved for research protocols and clinical studies. The principal outcome is PC_{20}, which is the dose of bronchoconstricting agent that produces a 20% fall in FEV_1 sustained for 3 minutes. Using methacholine and histamine produces similar results and may be more sensitive than an exercise test at diagnosing non-specific BHR. These challenges do not produce a late-phase response. Spirometry is performed at baseline (and the test should not proceed if FEV_1 is <70% predicted), then the subject inhales the agent (diluted in 3 ml 0.9% saline) via a nebulizer. The starting dose is 0.03 mg/ml and it is doubled each time to a maximum of 16 mg/ml. After 2 minutes of nebulization with a mouthpiece, spirometry is performed 30 seconds and then 90 seconds after the finish. If the second measure is above the first, the subject proceeds to the next challenge dose, with a 4-minute interval between

nebulizations. If it is less, then spirometry is repeated at 1-minute intervals until FEV_1 starts to rise. Once FEV_1 has fallen by 20% or more from baseline, no more inhalations are given. The dose that produced the fall is recorded as the PC_{20} and a bronchodilator is given. Spirometry is repeated 15–20 minutes later to ensure lung function has been restored to pretest levels and to inform about bronchodilator responsiveness.

Static lung volume measurements

Plethysmography to measure static absolute lung volumes has been discussed in the adult section. Data on total lung capacity (TLC), residual volume (RV) and functional residual capacity (FRC) can be obtained in children usually over the age of 5 years although some of the younger ones are not keen on getting inside the box. Normative data have been published for UK children aged 4–19 years and male puberty leads to a profound change in lung function, mostly related to size of the thoracic cage, an effect not observed in girls (Rosenthal et al 1993b). The use of these techniques, however, tends to be limited to tertiary care; for example, during annual review in children with CF or as part of investigations for difficult refractory asthma. Useful information is gained on gas trapping but their use, as an aid to differentiating obstructive from restrictive disease, is less applicable in paediatric practice.

Resistance and compliance

Measurements of airway resistance and conductance can also be performed but they are quite variable. Their greatest use in children is to help in the assessment of difficult asthma as they are non-volitional, unlike spirometry which is easy to fake. Compliance measurements are rarely done in children as they involve swallowing an oesophageal balloon.

Diffusing capacity of the lungs

Diffusing capacity or transfer factor (TLCO) estimates the transfer of oxygen from the alveolar gas to the red blood cells. A correction is used to take into account the patient's size (KCO). Children need to be able to hold their breath for 10 seconds (this is usually possible over the age of 5 years) and need a minimum vital capacity of 800 ml, although rebreathing techniques can be used in smaller children. The test is not often used in children but in practice it has its greatest role in assessment of interstitial lung disease or sarcoidosis. Normal data have been published for UK children aged 4–19 years (Rosenthal et al 1993b).

Preschool children

Measurement of lung function in this age group is problematic due to lack of coordination and cooperation. This is unfortunate, as it is in this age group that diagnosis of conditions such as asthma is most difficult and where objective information from lung function testing would be useful.

Infant lung function

Techniques have been developed to measure certain aspects of lung function in infants from birth to age 18–24 months, by which time the infants are usually too big. Due to methodological difficulties, lack of standardization and limited reference data, these techniques still largely remain a research tool rather than of great use to the clinician. The infants are usually sedated with oral medication such as triclofos or chloral hydrate for the procedure, although some newborns (usually under 4 weeks) may be tested whilst sleeping naturally. Several techniques are available; for example, whole-body plethysmography measures lung volumes such as functional residual capacity (FRC) or thoracic gas volume (TGV), simultaneously with airway resistance. Unlike in adults, well babies frequently have evidence of gas trapping (Kraemer 1993). Total respiratory resistance can also be measured by a method called the forced oscillation technique. A different method, called rapid thoracoabdominal compression (RTC), produces partial expiratory flow–volume curves. The sleeping child breathes quietly until a jacket, placed around the chest, is suddenly inflated (squeeze technique). This produces a sharp expiration resulting in a recorded flow–volume curve and a measurement of maximal flow at FRC ($\dot{V}$maxFRC). In a variation, called raised volume RTC, the chest is passively inflated prior to the squeeze. This gives $FEV_{0.4}$, which is similar to the information provided by the FEV_1 in an older child. Normal data are available although ideally each infant lung function laboratory will have generated its own data.

Standards for infant respiratory function testing have been produced jointly by the European Respiratory Society and American Thoracic Society and published as a series of six articles (Stocks & Gerritsen 2000, 2001).

Resistance measured by the interruptor technique (R_{int})

R_{int} is a method, recently applied to young children, whereby airways resistance and bronchodilator responsiveness can be measured in children as young as 2–3 years (Bridge et al 1999). The child, wearing a nose-clip, breathes quietly (tidal breathing) into the mask. Then, in response to a trigger during expiration, at the peak of a tidal flow, a shutter closes off airflow automatically for 100 milliseconds (ms). This gives a measure for airways resistance, which can then be repeated after administration of a bronchodilator or even a bronchial challenge. Normal data are becoming available and this technique may find a place in clinical practice, particularly as this is an ambulatory test that can be carried out anywhere. It has been shown recently that R_{int} could differentiate children aged 2–5 years with a history of wheezing from those with recurrent cough and those with no history of respiratory symptoms (McKenzie et al 2000).

Oxygen and carbon dioxide monitoring

Pulse oximetry

Pulse oximetry measures arterial oxygen saturation (SaO_2) in a non-invasive way that avoids the need for painful arterial blood sampling. It is thus immensely useful, but its shortcomings must be recognized (Gaskin & Thomas 1995), particularly the lack of accuracy at SaO_2 <70% (Schnapp & Cohen 1990). With children, it is important that the correct sized probe is used otherwise poor contact with the skin may result in an inaccurate reading. Finger clubbing does not seem to cause problems with finger probes.

Particular caution must be used when a pulse oximeter is the only measure of oxygenation available in a sick premature baby where too much oxygen is positively harmful. Due to the shape of the oxyhaemoglobin dissociation curve (oxygen saturation vs partial pressure of oxygen; see Fig. 3.3), pulse oximetry is unreliable at diagnosing hyperoxia due to the flat part of the curve. This means, for example, that although a SaO_2 >97% might at first sight be fine, the PaO_2 may be so high as to cause toxicity (Table 3.6). Furthermore, the shape and variability of the oxyhaemoglobin dissociation curve in critically ill children mean that a given SaO_2 is compatible with a range of arterial oxygen tensions (Clark et al 1992). In these situations, direct measurement of the PaO_2 is more appropriate. An alternative non-invasive method is transcutaneous PaO_2 monitoring, although this tends to be restricted to use in neonatal units (Clark et al 1992). Particular care must be taken in the newborn not to overheat the skin and the electrode needs changing every 3–4 hours.

Overnight SaO_2 monitoring is also an important technique; for example, when assessing whether a child with CF requires nocturnal oxygen during a chest exacerbation or when evaluating a child with difficult asthma. It is important that a continuous paper recording is

Table 3.6 Arterial PO_2 with corresponding SaO_2 from oxyhaemoglobin dissociation curve

Arterial PO_2 (kPa)	O_2 saturation (%)
13	97
9	93
8	89
6	80
5	75
4	57

produced that can be analysed the next morning, although these need to be looked at manually rather than simply relying on the computer-generated data summaries. These summaries inevitably include periods when movement artefact produces a falsely low reading that gets included in the summary data. This form of monitoring has been used in certain circumstances as a screening procedure for deciding on the need for full polysomnography in suspected cases of obstructive sleep apnoea (OSA), although a negative oximetry result will not necessarily rule out the diagnosis (Brouillette et al 2000). However, although it is true that a normal overnight SaO_2 is encouraging, significant hypercarbia can sometimes accompany normal oxygen levels so caution must be exercised. In addition, arousal may be so rapid in some children with OSA that there is not enough time for hypoxaemia to develop and the diagnosis can be missed with oximetry alone.

Domiciliary pulse oximetry is useful for children receiving home oxygen, particularly for infants with chronic lung disease. It has been recommended that oxygen therapy should be considered in infants with baseline SaO_2 <93% and that levels be maintained $\geqslant$95% (Poets 1998).

Non-invasive CO_2 monitoring

As mentioned above, measurement of SaO_2 alone gives only half the picture. This is particularly true in children with neuromuscular disease and occasionally so in cases of OSA. Ideally, continuous CO_2 levels should be measured to detect alveolar hypoventilation. This is usually done using a transcutaneous monitor with an electrode that can be left on the skin for up to 8 hours. These measurements correlate reasonably well with the arterial PCO_2 although the response time is too slow to pick up changes secondary to brief apnoeas or hypopnoeas (Clark et al 1992). If a transcutaneous monitor is not available, then a compromise is to measure a capillary PCO_2 immediately the child awakes. Another method for continuous CO_2 monitoring is measurement of airway end-tidal CO_2, but usually this can only be accurately carried out on an intubated patient as ambient air dilutes the measurements if used with mask ventilation (Clark et al 1992). Furthermore a mask would have to be so tightly fitting that it may be too uncomfortable to be used during a sleep study.

Capillary blood gases

Measurement of 'capillary gases', i.e. pH, PO2, PCO2, bicarbonate and base excess is very useful, especially in infancy, an age at which arterial sampling is difficult. Up to 12 months, blood is obtained by a heel prick and in older children a finger prick is used. Although the capillary PO2 is unrepresentative of arterial levels (normally reading only about 4–5 kPa), the rest of the measurements give a reasonable guide to the child's respiratory status. It is important that the child's heel is warmed to ensure sufficient blood flow and after a heel prick with a sterile lancet, 150 microlitres (μl) of free-flowing blood is collected into a heparinized capillary tube. It is important that air bubbles are not sucked up into the capillary tube, otherwise the sample is spoiled, and the blood should be put into the blood gas analyser promptly.

Arterial blood gases

For a complete picture of blood gas analysis, an arterial blood sample is required. In practice, this tends to be routinely available only in neonatal and paediatric intensive care units, where an indwelling arterial or umbilical catheter has been placed. A single arterial stab is painful and difficult in a child who understandably will not cooperate. This means that the resultant analysis may not be valid, as a screaming child will have a reduced $PaCO_2$ and possibly an altered PaO_2.

EXERCISE TESTING

Exercise testing has become an important tool in the evaluation and treatment of many paediatric disorders, although its value is often overlooked. Exercise stresses many aspects of normal physiology (including ventilation and gas exchange,

cardiovascular, neuromuscular and thermoregulatory functions), hence exercise testing may reveal symptoms or physiological abnormalities that are not apparent at rest.

Physiological response to exercise in children

The cardiovascular response of children to exercise is broadly similar to that of adults but there are important age-related differences, which have been reviewed (Braden & Carroll 1999). Oxygen consumption ($\dot{V}O_2$) can increase up to 10-fold from rest to maximal exercise in children compared to 10–15-fold in healthy adults. Maximal $\dot{V}O_2$ ($\dot{V}O_2max$) increases with age until puberty after which the rate of increase accelerates in adolescent boys and levels off in girls. However, if $\dot{V}O_2max$ is related to body mass or weight, it changes little during childhood in boys and actually decreases a little in girls. Maximal cardiac output increases with increasing body size, mainly due to the increase in ventricular size and stroke volume.

The maximal heart rate is fairly stable through childhood then begins to decline in the late teens towards adult values, whereas resting heart rate progressively decreases throughout childhood. A commonly used formula for predicting the maximal expected heart rate in children is 220 – age (in years) ± 10 beats per minute (Nixon & Orenstein 1988). Gender differences are present throughout childhood but are more marked after puberty; for example, boys have a greater $\dot{V}O_{2max}$ and maximal cardiac output, whereas girls have higher heart rate values. The effect of training on cardiovascular responses to exercise is small in prepubertal children but after puberty, increases brought about by training are similar to those found in adults.

Rationale behind exercise testing

There are more paediatric than adult disorders in which exercise testing is clinically relevant (Tomassoni 1996a). Guidelines have been produced by the American College of Cardiology and American Heart Association to make recommendations on the appropriate use of exercise testing in the diagnosis or treatment of patients with known or suspected cardiovascular disease, which includes a section on children (Gibbons et al 1997). Use of exercise testing can be broadly categorized as follows.

Diagnostic tool

Exercise testing may help identify abnormal cardiovascular, respiratory or metabolic responses to exercise; for example, cardiac arrhythmias, hypertension, hypoxaemia or hypoglycaemia (Nixon & Orenstein 1988). The test may amplify pathophysiological changes and trigger changes not seen at rest. Sometimes testing can help make a specific diagnosis, particularly when the symptoms appear only with exertion, in which case the exercise acts as a provocation test. The classic examples are exercise-induced bronchospasm and exercise-induced cardiac arrhythmias. Exercise testing may also be useful for differentiating non-specific symptoms, such as chest pain which may be due to asthma or cardiac ischaemia, or breathlessness which may be due to asthma or poor fitness levels. Sometimes a test may identify a deficiency in a specific component of fitness; for example, it may differentiate a problem of muscle endurance and strength from aerobic capacity (Tomassoni 1996a).

Determine severity and functional effects of known disease

Exercise testing may provide information about the effect of the disease on a child's ability to tolerate exercise, giving useful information on how well the child can function in everyday life. This information is often only partially obtainable from standard lung function testing performed with the child essentially at rest. Day-to-day functioning is critical to a child's quality of life. Regular exercise testing can also help chart disease progression. This may be useful as part of the annual review of children with CF or for children affected by neuromuscular disorders such as Duchenne muscular dystrophy. It can also help

determine the severity of cardiac dysrhythmias. Finally, in some circumstances, it may be possible to estimate prognosis from exercise ability; for example, cycle ergometry in CF (Nixon et al 1992), or 6-minute walking test in severe left ventricular dysfunction (Bittner et al 1993).

Outcome measure for therapeutic interventions

Exercise testing may help in deciding the appropriateness of a particular therapeutic intervention; for example, the use of certain drugs in the management of exercise-induced bronchospasm. Another example would be its use as one of the criteria for deciding whether listing for heart-lung transplant is appropriate. Having established a baseline, repeat testing can then be used as a measure of the effectiveness of a particular intervention. This may be particularly useful in assessing the functional success of surgical correction of a congenital heart lesion.

Aid to improving fitness in (health and) disease

Many children and their parents are anxious about allowing the child to exercise if the child has an underlying cardiac or respiratory disorder. Exercise testing, conducted with the reassurance of the supervising staff, in the protective environment of the laboratory can be used to provide evidence that it is safe for the child to exercise. Children can then be encouraged to adopt an active lifestyle to increase their exercise tolerance and improve their level of fitness. In addition, testing can then provide the basis for prescribing individualized exercise conditioning programmes – something not often undertaken in the United Kingdom for children. Periodic exercise testing can then monitor changes in fitness.

Outcome measure in clinical trials

Exercise tests are a useful outcome measure for clinical trials (Ramsey & Boat 1994). If the test is simple and portable it may have a place in phase III multicentre trials (Pike et al 2001).

Types of tests available and their application in children

There are many types of exercise tests available and choosing the appropriate test depends on the question being asked and the aspect of exercise tolerance that needs elucidating (Orenstein 1998). It is important that children understand what is expected of them and that they enjoy the test otherwise they certainly will not make much of an effort. Tests may be categorized as either maximal or submaximal and their relative merits have recently been reviewed (Noonan & Dean 2000).

Maximal tests – cycle ergometry and the treadmill

Progressive maximal tests, in which workload on a cycle ergometer or treadmill is increased until subjects reach their maximal level of tolerance, with on-line analysis of inspired and expired gases have already been described in the adult section. They are usually considered the gold standard for adults, with oxygen uptake as the principal outcome measure. Children can also perform these tests (once over the age of about 6 years) although a degree of coordination is required (Fig. 3.24). The cycle ergometer is familiar as most children ride bicycles; however, some children find it easier to run than pedal so prefer the treadmill. Some children also find it difficult to maintain a constant pedalling rate. For smaller children, the speed of the treadmill must be adjusted to account for their shorter strides. A treadmill does take up more space and requires a bigger exercise laboratory. A more detailed evaluation of different maximal exercise protocols suitable for children can be found in the review by Nixon & Orenstein (1988).

One of the main problems with peak or maximal exercise tests in children is that they do not represent their normal daily activities (Cooper 1995). Children tend to engage in very short bursts of high-intensity physical activity interspersed with variable periods of low and moderate intensity (Bailey et al 1995). Children do not tend to perform sustained heavy exercise, which is the format of most maximal tests. Furthermore, they are highly effort dependent and healthy control children can be strongly encouraged, even cajoled, to make a maximal effort. In contrast, children who have an underlying cardiorespiratory disorder will not be pushed so hard, making comparison with normal values less valid (Cooper 1995). Other problems with these types of tests is that they are time consuming and require a high level of expertise with expensive equipment (including a mass spectrometer). Furthermore, they are physiologically stressful and there may be concerns over taking unnecessary risks in children with moderate to severe cardiorespiratory compromise.

Normal reference ranges and ventilatory variables for children undergoing cycle ergometry

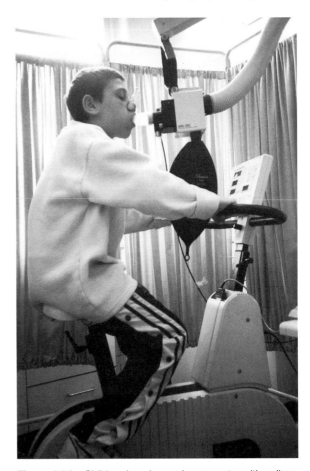

Figure 3.24 Child undergoing cycle ergometry with online respiratory gas analysis.

have recently been published (Rosenthal & Bush 2000).

Wingate anaerobic test (WanT)

Whilst some children's daily activities are predominantly aerobic, most activities rely on both aerobic and anaerobic energy (Boas et al 1996). The intensity and duration of the activity, as well as the child's level of fitness, determine the relative contribution of these energy sources; for example, high-intensity exercise of short duration is principally anaerobic in nature. As discussed above, this form of exercise is typical of children, hence the relevance of this form of exercise testing in paediatric practice. Anaerobic capacity is determined by the muscle's ability to produce energy quickly from anaerobic sources and to test this, the subject performs a 30-second all-out sprint at the highest tolerable workload on a cycle ergometer. This is designed to test anaerobic performance only and the indices of performance are peak power and mean power. A version also exists using arm cranking that has been used in children with neuromuscular disorders (Bar-Or 1996). Studies in children and adolescents with CF have shown that anaerobic exercise capacity is reduced and this mainly reflects decreased nutritional status, with pulmonary function playing a smaller role (Boas et al 1996, Cabrera et al 1993). Children with asthma have also been found to have a reduced anaerobic capacity (Counil et al 1997) and have been compared to children with CF and normal children (Boas et al 1999).

Walking tests

Self-paced walking tests were initially developed for adults with COPD (see adult section) and the techniques have been reviewed by Noonan & Dean (2000). The distance covered in a given period of time (usually 6 or 12 minutes) provides an estimate of functional capacity and is predictive of morbidity and mortality (Nixon et al 1996); the other outcome used is change in SaO_2 measured on a pulse oximeter. The 6-minute test has been validated by comparison with cycle ergometry in children with severe cardiorespiratory disease being assessed for heart-lung transplantation (Nixon et al 1996). It was reported that the distance walked correlated with $\dot{V}O_{2peak}$ and physical work capacity and the minimum SaO_2 was also significantly correlated, although 11/17 children had a greater fall in SaO_2 on the walk compared to the more energetic bike. It was felt that the submaximal walking test might better assess changes in SaO_2 that occur with the normal day-to-day activities carried out by these children. The 6-minute walk has been further validated in children with mild and moderate CF lung disease, being compared with cycle ergometry (Gulmans et al 1996) and the 3-minute step test (Balfour-Lynn et al 1998). Finally, there has been a shortened version (2 minutes) that has been used in CF children who demonstrated an improved distance after treatment of their chest exacerbations (Upton et al 1988).

Walking tests are cheap, easy to learn and can be used in an ambulatory setting by children as young as 5 years. However, they require adequate space and are effort dependent so that the patient's attitude and motivation are major factors in determining the distance walked.

Three-minute step test

The 3-minute step test was developed for use in children over 6 years as a means of assessing submaximal exercise tolerance by a simple quick method (Balfour-Lynn et al 1998). Adapted from an adult cardiac test used since the 1920s, it consists of stepping up and down a commercially available aerobic step for 3 minutes (Fig. 3.25). The following protocol is used:

- Subjects step up and down a single 15 cm (6 inch) aerobic step.
- Stepping rate is 30 steps per minute. A metronome set at 120 regulates the rate.
- Test duration is 3 minutes and a stopwatch is used.
- Subjects are shown how to change the lead leg whilst stepping (i.e. the leg placed on the step first) so that one leg does not get overtired (muscle fatigue).

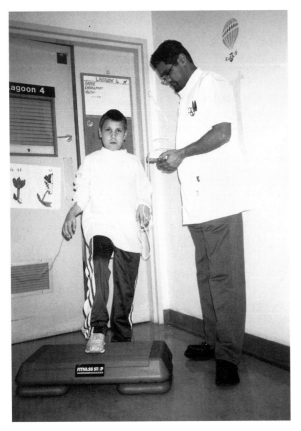

Figure 3.25 Child performing the 3-minute step test.

- It is best for children to practise the test first with sufficient resting time before the test begins.
- Comfortable shoes should be worn (not high heels, preferably trainers) and ideally there should be a cushioned mat on the floor to lessen impact on knee joints.
- A pulse oximeter is used with the probe attached to the patient's finger and the lead taped to the forearm to ensure minimal trace interference during stepping.
- Standard encouragement at 1 and 2 minutes is given. This should state how far into the test the patient is and that they are doing well.

Outcome measures used are:

- Baseline and lowest oxygen saturation (SaO_2) during the test. This may occur at any time within the 3 minutes. A fall in SaO_2 over 4% should be considered abnormal.
- Baseline and highest pulse rate during the test. This usually occurs towards the end of the test.
- Breathlessness determined at the start and end of the test using a subjective score (10 cm visual analogue) and the objective 15-count breathlessness score (Prasad et al 2000).

The patients are told that they can stop the test at any time if they feel unable to continue for any reason. The investigator should stop the test if the SaO_2 falls below 75%, the patient is unduly breathless or is struggling to keep pace and rhythm. If patients stop stepping within 3 minutes, the reason why they felt unable to continue should be recorded as well as the time they stopped.

The step test has been compared with the 6-minute walk in 54 CF children; the step produced significantly greater changes in heart rate and breathlessness than the walk, with a comparable fall in SaO_2 (Balfour-Lynn et al 1998). A fall in SaO_2 >4% was felt to be clinically significant and could not always have been predicted from the baseline FEV_1. The test was found to be simple to learn, quick to perform and required little space or expense. Importantly, motivation is excluded as a possible variable and although patients can stop if they wish, in practice this rarely happens. The ambulatory nature of the test means it has even been used in outdoors high-altitude exercise testing of children with CF (Dinwiddie et al 1999). The step test has also been studied in children with severe CF lung disease being assessed for heart-lung transplantation (Aurora et al 2001). In this patient group it produced a greater fall in SaO_2 and rise in heart rate than the 6-minute walk and although it may have a role in transplant assessment, further work is needed.

The step test has also been used to assess the effects of intravenous antibiotics on exercise tolerance in 36 children with CF and all exercise outcomes were shown to improve (Pike et al 2001). It was found that it complemented spirometry and simple SaO_2 monitoring and, importantly, it was demonstrated that the step test was sensitive to changes after a therapeutic intervention. A modified incremental version of the original test has also been used in the evaluation of breathlessness in both normal children and children with CF. In this test the stepping rate rises at 2-minute intervals using rates of 20/min, 30/min then 40/min and although incremental, this test remains submaximal (Prasad et al 2000). It was used to study means of measuring breathlessness in both normal children and children with CF.

A criticism of the step test is that the workload varies with each subject (Orenstein 1998). This is because the work performed in the test is a product of the stepping height and rate (both fixed) as well as the subject's weight and height (particularly leg length). In order to keep the amount of work constant between subjects, the height or rate could be adjusted to account for differences in patient size. However, in practice this is neither feasible nor important in the context of the way the test is used, although the pubertal growth spurt might affect interpretation of longitudinal results from annual testing through puberty.

Shuttle tests

There are various forms of the shuttle test (reviewed by Noonan & Dean 2000). The original 20-metre shuttle running test is well described but was felt to be too strenuous for many patients. This resulted in the development of a 10-metre, 12-level shuttle walking test that was studied in adults with COPD (Singh et al 1992). However, in some patient groups the test was felt to be too easy for patients with less severe disability and often failed to elicit a maximal response. Hence the development of the modified shuttle test, in which three additional levels have been added and the subject is allowed to run (15 levels with the distance between the cones remaining at 10 m) (Bradley et al 1999). The 20-metre shuttle running test has been used in normal children and is often used in schools during sports and games. In a study of 15–16-year-old schoolboys, it provoked exercise-induced bronchospasm in 8/73 children, six of whom were not previously known to be asthmatic (Freeman et al 1990). It has potential for use as a diagnostic test and physical education teachers should be aware of its possible adverse effects. It has also been used to study the effects of

training on a group of asthmatic children aged 12–17 years, when, compared to standard cycle ergometry, it had sufficient validity to register training effects (Ahmaidi et al 1993). To date, there are no publications in which the more recent modifications to the shuttle test have been studied in children with cardiorespiratory disease.

Tests of muscle strength

Various tests exist to measure muscle strength, such as lifting simple weights or measuring isometric muscle force using a dynamometer or myometer. Peripheral muscle force is impaired in children with CF, even in the absence of reduced pulmonary or nutritional status (De Meer et al 1999). It is also possible to measure inspiratory muscle strength non-invasively and in children with CF, it has been found to be impaired, again, even in those with good nutritional status (Hayot et al 1997).

Outcome measures

O_2 consumption ($\dot{V}O_2$)

$\dot{V}O_2$ is the principal outcome measure from maximal exercise testing such as cycle ergometry or a treadmill test and it is the single measure most commonly used to represent overall aerobic fitness in children (Nixon & Orenstein 1988). $\dot{V}O_2$ increases rapidly at the start of dynamic exercise and after the second minute at each level of intensity, it usually reaches a plateau (Washington et al 1994). During progressively increasing exercise, $\dot{V}O_2$ increases linearly with increases in work level. Maximum $\dot{V}O_2$ ($\dot{V}O_2$max) is the highest amount of oxygen that a given individual can consume while performing dynamic exercise, whereas peak $\dot{V}O_2$ ($\dot{V}O_2$peak) is the maximal $\dot{V}O_2$ observed during a specific exercise test (Washington et al 1994).

A true $\dot{V}O_2$max is attained when the $\dot{V}O_2$ plateaus off despite an increase in exercise intensity, i.e. the child has the same $\dot{V}O_2$ for two successive workloads. However, this is observed in less than a third of children and adolescents (unlike adults) (Cooper 1995), so $\dot{V}O_2$max cannot be precisely determined in many paediatric studies. Part of the reason for this is that the test is effort dependent so many children feel tired and stop before the true $\dot{V}O_2$max is reached. Instead, $\dot{V}O_2$peak is often used as the endpoint, whereby the $\dot{V}O_2$ is measured at the point of exhaustion when the child will go no further; sometimes this is referred to as the symptom-limited $\dot{V}O_2$ (Nixon & Orenstein 1988). Typical values in healthy children are 40–50 ml O_2/kg body weight/minute, whilst children with cardiorespiratory disease may have values as low as 10 ml/kg/min (Nixon & Orenstein 1988). The intraindividual day-to-day variation in $\dot{V}O_2$max is around 4–6% in fit subjects, although this figure is higher in those with pulmonary disease (Noonan & Dean 2000).

In children, it has been suggested that the data collected during the submaximal phases, rather than from the final single data point at peak or maximal power, should be utilized more than is currently the case (Cooper 1995). An alternative method of analysis is the concept of the oxygen uptake efficiency slope (OUES), which is derived from a logarithmic curve fitting model for $\dot{V}O_2$ and minute ventilation (Baba et al 1999). It has been well validated in children and the OUES correlates strongly with $\dot{V}O_2$max. A further advantage is that it is not affected by exercise intensity so that data are obtained even if the child is unwilling or unable to complete the test to maximal intensity.

As well as O_2, the CO_2 is measured in the inspired and expired gas collected during formal maximal testing. This gives the full picture of ventilation and pulmonary gas exchange. In addition to $\dot{V}O_2$, CO_2 output ($\dot{V}CO_2$), minute ventilation ($\dot{V}_E$), respiratory gas exchange ratio ($\dot{V}CO_2/\dot{V}O_2$), and the oxygen ventilatory equivalent ($\dot{V}_E/\dot{V}O_2$) can be calculated. With the addition of flow measurements (by turbine or pneumotachograph) the average respiratory rate and tidal volume can also be measured.

Ventilatory anaerobic threshold

When performing maximal exercise tests, the last half of the test is usually performed at work rates that are above the subject's lactate or anaerobic threshold. This is the point when the oxygen demand of the exercising muscle exceeds the oxygen supply and anaerobic metabolism is required to enable the subject to continue further exercise (reviewed by Washington 1999). At this point, there is an abrupt rise in blood lactate levels that follows the rise of lactate in muscle cells, termed the onset of blood lactate accumulation (OBLA). However, routine venepuncture is impractical and undesirable in children (particularly when for research purposes). During the process of buffering the blood lactate levels, there is an increased production of bicarbonate, which leads to a rise in $PaCO_2$, and this in turn results in reflex hyperventilation. The onset of this hyperventilation is known as the ventilatory anaerobic threshold (VAT) and it can be seen as the point of inflexion on the minute ventilation/$\dot{V}O_2$ curve; it is usually expressed as a percent of the $\dot{V}O_2$max or total exercise time (Washington et al 1994).

Measurement of the anaerobic threshold is one of the better ways of determining aerobic fitness, as the fitter the person, the higher the $\dot{V}O_2$ before the blood lactate starts to rise; this has been validated in children as young as 6 years old (Hebestreit et al 2000). The VAT is probably most useful in children who are unable to exercise to maximum levels to attain $\dot{V}O_2$max. Those with congenital heart disease limiting exercise will have a rise in lactate at an extremely low $\dot{V}O_2$, although patients with significant pulmonary disease or any type of airway obstruction may not attain a true VAT (Washington 1999). VAT decreases with age and is higher in boys; typical values are around 66% of $\dot{V}O_2$max.

Oxygen saturation (SaO_2)

Online respiratory gas analysis as described above requires expensive equipment and a high level of expertise to interpret. Probably the most useful measure of gas exchange that is readily available and accessible is the SaO_2 determined by pulse oximetry; and desaturation <90% during exercise is an abnormal response in children. In practice, even dramatic falls in SaO_2 have no untoward results and most children gain preexercise levels within 5 minutes and all by 15 minutes (Henke & Orenstein 1984). The recovery time to preexercise levels may also be a useful outcome measure.

It is particularly important that movement artefact is eliminated during exercise otherwise measurements are invalid. In our experience, a flexi-probe taped to the index finger with the lead strapped to the forearm overcomes this problem (Balfour-Lynn et al 1998). Generally, using a finger is now preferred to having the probe clipped to an earlobe (Gaskin & Thomas 1995). Ideally, traces are also recorded on to a computer program alongside the numbers, for later review; this allows elimination of false reading due to low-quality signals. The type of test may also affect the frequency of movement artefact; for example, fewer occur during the step test compared to the walking test, as the children's arms can be kept relatively still whilst stepping whereas they tend to swing their arms when walking (Balfour-Lynn et al 1998). In addition, the oximeter and its lead are kept stationary during the step test rather than being wheeled or carried up and down a corridor.

There are also potential problems with the oximeters themselves during exercise and these have been reviewed by Gaskin & Thomas (1995). Different oximeters have varying degrees of accuracy under exercise conditions. In general, they are more accurate in the higher saturation ranges but tend to overestimate in the lower ranges (SaO_2 < 90%), which has been demonstrated in CF during cycle ergometry (Orenstein et al 1993). While this means they may be reliable when used with healthy subjects, drops in SaO_2 may be underestimated in patients with cardio-respiratory problems. Measurement of heart rate is also limited at higher ranges and an underestimation may be seen with heavy exercise (Gaskin & Thomas 1995).

Cardiovascular response

Measurement of heart rate is mandatory for all exercise testing and is usually done by a pulse oximeter or cardiorater with electrodes attached to the chest; potential problems of using the former method have been discussed. During dynamic exercise, the heart rate increases in a linear fashion with the rate of work and increases up to three-fold from resting can be seen (Braden & Carroll 1999). Variables that affect heart rate during exercise include the type of exercise, body position during testing, gender, state of health and fitness of the subject and environmental conditions (temperature, humidity, altitude) (Washington et al 1994). Young children compensate for their relatively small heart size (with lower stroke volume) by an increased heart rate for a given amount of work, so they attain higher maximal heart rates than adults do. In pulmonary disease, the patients may not attain the expected maximal heart rate, as their exercise is ventilation limited. Resting heart rate is also a useful measure in children with lung disease and was shown to be significantly reduced after treatment of a chest exacerbation in children with CF (Pike et al 2001). Presumably this is due to a reduction in the high metabolic rate and increased work of breathing associated with a chest infection. In addition, a high resting age-adjusted heart rate is associated with a poorer prognosis in children with CF (Aurora et al 2000).

Other cardiovascular outcomes tend to be reserved for testing children with known or suspected cardiac disease (reviewed by Washington et al 1994). Electrocardiographic changes are one of the main outcome measures used, particularly for patients suspected of having myocardial ischaemia, e.g. aortic stenosis, and ST segment changes may indicate mismatch of myocardial oxygen demand and supply. Onset of dysrhythmias is also looked for carefully. More complex measurements, such as cardiac output and stroke volume, can also be tested and cardiac output usually rises 3–5-fold during maximal exercise. As well as the state of health, the type of exercise is a variable and treadmill testing generally results in a higher maximal cardiac output than does cycle ergometry. Finally, blood pressure changes may be monitored, although the response to exercise can be complex. In children, this is done by indirect methods using a cuff, even though motion artefact and noise can make the measurement difficult, as direct arterial measurements are painful and invasive. Systolic blood pressure increases with progressive workloads and maximal systolic blood pressure rarely exceeds 200 mmHg in children although there is no evidence of danger if it reaches 250 mmHg. A lack of increase or a decrease in systolic blood pressure has been thought to be an ominous sign of severe cardiac dysfunction, but in fact an exertional drop in blood pressure may occur in normal subjects (Washington et al 1994). Data on diastolic blood pressure changes are less certain due to the technical difficulties often encountered when measuring it in exercising children (Braden & Carroll 1999).

Lung function

The normal response to exercise is transient bronchodilation mediated by release of endogenous catecholamines (Cypcar & Lemanske 1994). The airway calibre usually returns to normal by the end of the exercise period and can be monitored by regular peak flow or FEV_1 measures. The main use of this form of testing is in the investigation of possible exercise-induced bronchospasm (see later section on Asthma). The response of children with CF is variable and not always predictable from baseline spirometry (Balfour-Lynn et al 1998).

Work

Maximal work capacity is the highest workload achievable on a progressive test and is influenced by age, body size and gender – older and larger children have a greater work capacity, as do boys (Nixon & Orenstein 1988). Obviously children with higher levels of aerobic fitness also can do more work. Estimates of the amount of exercise performed are made using the following definitions (Washington et al 1994).

- *Work* is force expressed by distance irrelevant of time.
- *Power* is the rate of performing work.
- *Maximal power output* is the highest rate of work achieved during the test.
- *Endurance time* is the total test time until exhaustion on a continuous graded test.

- *Physical working capacity-170* (PWC-170) is the highest rate of submaximal work on a cycle ergometer corresponding to a heart rate of 170 bpm.
- *Total work* is the total amount of work performed until exhaustion or another predetermined endpoint.

Units of work on a cycle ergometer are joules, whilst power is joules/second (= 1 watt). On a treadmill, work is expressed as kilopond*metre and power as kilopond*metre/min. PWC-170 is invalid in cases of congenital heart disease where inherent control of heart rate is part of the abnormality.

Distance

This is relevant in walking and shuttle tests and although one of the main outcomes in this form of testing (see above), it is very dependent on the subject's motivation (Guyatt et al 1984). This is particularly true of walking tests where the subjects determine their own pace. In severe lung disease, the distance covered has been shown to correlate with survival in adults (Kadikar et al 1997). Although this is true in CF children being assessed for transplantation, the minimum SaO_2 during the walking test has been shown to be a stronger predictor (Aurora et al 2000).

Symptoms

Breathlessness. It is normal for breathlessness to increase alongside the increase in O_2 uptake and CO_2 output, which accompanies exercise. The significance of breathlessness is related to the intensity of the exercise that produces the symptoms. Clearly a child who is breathless at rest has a greater problem than one that is only breathless during intense exercise. This makes the measurement of breathlessness an important outcome of exercise testing as long as it can be quantified reliably.

The usual means of assessing the subjective elements of breathlessness are the modified Borg scale of perceived breathlessness (Table 3.7) and standard visual analogue scores (Fig. 3.26)

Table 3.7 Modified Borg scale of perceived breathlessness. The original Borg scale of perceived exertion (Borg 1982) has been modified for measurement of breathlessness (Burdon et al 1982). It has 12 points, 10 of which have accompanying verbal descriptors

0	Nothing at all
0.5	Very very slight (just noticeable)
1	Very slight
2	Slight
3	Moderate
4	Somewhat severe
5	Severe
6	
7	Very severe
8	
9	Very very severe (almost maximal)
10	Maximal

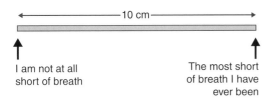

Figure 3.26 Visual analogue score. 10 cm horizontal line with two anchor points at each extreme (zero and 10 cm). The subject puts a mark through the line where they think their breathlessness fits on this scale, which is then measured (in cm) from the zero point.

(Prasad et al 2000). Generally, similar scores are obtained by these two methods despite them being quite different (Wilson & Jones 1989). It is interesting that they give such similar scores, as there is an in-built bias to score under 5 with the Borg scale since 5 represents 'severe' breathlessness, which is usually as high as patients wish to score themselves. In practice, use of the Borg scale is a problem for many children due to difficulty understanding some of the terminology (such as moderate or maximal). It is likely that many children simply use the number ratings 1 to 10 and ignore the accompanying descriptors, so that in the end the Borg scale is often used in a similar way to the visual analogue score. A theoretical advantage of the latter is that it is a continuous variable, which is supposed to be easier to use than scoring with discrete

numbers. However, one problem with the visual analogue score is that the anchor points ('I am not at all short of breath' or 'The most short of breath I have ever been') are specific to the individual, making comparisons of scores between different people less reliable. A score of 5 for one child may be very different to what another child considers 5 to represent. They often score themselves in the middle of the line as halfway represents an average day for them – 'I am as breathless as I usually feel after exercise', which of course may be very different for different individuals.

These problems with the Borg and visual analogue scores highlight the difficulties of measuring a subjective feeling or symptom. However, they do not invalidate their use, as it is important to know how breathless the child feels or thinks they feel, since this is the symptom that is causing them concern. Another problem is that just as in quantifying pain, what the patient says they are experiencing is not always in keeping with their appearance to others (parents and medical attendants).

In addition to subjective measures, an objective score has been validated in children, called the 15-count breathlessness score (Prasad et al 2000). This score is determined by asking the child to take a deep breath and count out loud to 15 (taking about 8 seconds to do so). The number of breaths required to reach 15 (including the initial breath) is the score, hence 1 is the minimum score. Most children score 1 at rest and when performing light exercise, many will still score 1, especially if they are healthy. For this reason, the 15-count score is best used in those prone to breathlessness or in healthy subjects undergoing intense exercise. It has shown that this score can differentiate degrees of breathlessness induced by exercise of varying intensity and also discriminate between healthy children and children with CF in terms of their exercise-induced breathlessness. It is simple to learn and easy to demonstrate and can be used by anyone old enough to count fluently to 15 in any language.

It is important to control certain variables when using the 15-count score (Prasad et al 2000). The speed of counting is important, as a subject counting quicker is likely to take fewer breaths (and hence obtain a lower score) than someone counting more slowly. A consistent speed of counting is particularly critical if a subject is repeating scores after exercise or a therapeutic intervention. In practice, it is easy to count at the correct speed and it has been found to be quite consistent. A metronome is not recommended as it can confuse children who take extra breaths since they can become out of synchrony with the metronome's beat. Another important variable to control is how deep a breath the subject takes at the start of the count, as a low starting lung volume will make it harder to reach 15 without taking further breaths. Subjects are told to take a deep breath, which is essentially to vital capacity, and although obviously it cannot be measured, it is not difficult to see whether the child has breathed in fully.

The 15-count score is designed to give a more objective and reproducible measure of breathlessness than the subjective modified Borg and visual analogue scores. However, it will not take into account the child's perception of their breathlessness, nor the intensity of the 'unpleasantness' of the breathlessness, something only the patient can know, and is therefore best used together with one of the subjective scores.

Fatigue. Fatigue has been defined as a gradual decline in force-generating capacity and using this physiological definition, it can be quantified formally (Fulco et al 1995). Another method is the fatigue index, which can be applied to high-intensity short-term exercise, using the definition of work performed during last five repetitions divided by the work performed during first five repetitions × 100 (Pincivero et al 2001). However, in practical terms, it is simply a feeling of tiredness, which is more difficult to quantify. Like breathlessness, it is somewhat subjective and motivation plays a large part in its perception. It can be a generalized body fatigue or localized leg muscle fatigue and levels of fitness tend to determine its onset. There are measures such as the Fatigue Severity Scale and the Fatigue Scale but these are best applied to everyday fatigue. For measuring exercise-induced fatigue, a visual analogue score can be used.

Chest pain. Non-specific chest pain is a fairly common symptom, particularly in adolescents, and exercise testing may offer reassurance to the child and family. Often no specific diagnosis is made but exercise testing can certainly indicate whether the pain is due to chest tightness from exercise-induced bronchospasm. The use of an ECG monitor can also exclude pain from cardiac ischaemia (e.g. aortic stenosis). Ratings of pain measurement exist but are not relevant here, as the exercise test should be terminated if chest pain occurs.

When to stop an exercise test

In general, the test can be stopped when the diagnosis is made or a predetermined endpoint is reached. Certain signs and symptoms should make the investigator halt the test.

- Subject feels unable to continue for *any* reason
- Chest pain, muscle cramps, headache, dizziness, syncope, light-headedness
- Excessive breathlessness or fatigue
- Significant desaturation, usually SaO_2 <75%
- ST segment depression or elevation greater than 3 mm
- Significant arrhythmia precipitated or aggravated by the exercise:
  - premature ventricular contractions with increasing frequency
  - supraventricular tachycardia
  - ventricular tachycardia
  - atrioventricular conduction block
- Blood pressure signs:
  - progressive decrease in systolic blood pressure by >10 mmHg
  - failure to increase with increased workload
  - hypertension (systolic > 250 mmHg, diastolic > 120 mmHg)

Disease-specific testing

Asthma

Exercise-induced asthma (EIA) or bronchospasm (EIB) usually results in a variable combination of wheeze, cough, breathlessness and chest pain or tightness which come on within 5–10 minutes of starting exercise. After the normal transient bronchodilation, asthmatic children experience progressive bronchoconstriction, which is usually at its worst 5–10 minutes after stopping the exercise (when symptoms are also usually at their worst). Symptoms have usually gone within 15–30 minutes of stopping and lung function is back to normal within 30–60 minutes (Cypcar & Lemanske 1994). The response is of course variable, with some patients able to continue the exercise with spontaneous resolution of their symptoms, giving them a 'second wind'. Rarely, a late response can be elicited with symptoms reported 4–12 hours after exercise (Nixon 1996). The severity of the response is determined by exercise intensity, climate (worst in cold dry air) and baseline airway reactivity and function. Some sports are more likely to cause problems, e.g. long-distance running, cycling, soccer, rugby and cross-country skiing, whilst less provoking sports include swimming, tennis and gymnastics. Between 40% and 95% of asthmatic patients experience a degree of EIA (Nixon 1996). The proposed mechanisms and management of EIA have been reviewed by Cypcar & Lemanske (1994).

Exercise testing therefore has an important role in evaluation of asthmatic children, particularly those who only develop symptoms with exercise or in whom standard treatment is not helping these exercise-induced symptoms. Often it is unnecessary though, since a known asthmatic with symptoms provoked by exercise should simply be treated for EIA without necessarily performing an expensive time-consuming test first.

At its most basic, a test can consist of measuring peak flow rates in clinic, then getting the child to run up and down the stairs and repeating the peak flow. Although somewhat crude, this method has been used in paediatric clinics in hospitals without comprehensive exercise-testing facilities. A screening test known as the free running exercise challenge has also been used for identifying asthma, in which children simply run as hard as possible around a gymnasium for 6 minutes. However, testing on reproducibility in 8–10-year-olds has now suggested it is not a suitable screening tool (Powell et al 1996).

There are various regimens for formally testing known or suspected asthmatic children. The Royal Brompton Hospital regimen involves the child running on a treadmill to elicit a heart rate 85% of age-predicted maximum, which in practice is usually up to 8 minutes of exercise. The speed and angle of the treadmill are adjusted to ensure adequate rise in heart rate. Peak flow is measured at baseline, then every 2 minutes until completion of exercise. Measurements then continue every 1 minute for 5 minutes (to ensure an early dip is not missed) then every 5 minutes for 30 minutes. A bronchodilator is then given to demonstrate reversibility using standard methods of testing bronchodilator responsiveness that have been described above. SaO_2 and heart rate are monitored throughout the procedure.

Asthmatic children are usually unfit and sometimes overweight. This owes more to psychological adjustment (including self-image and self-esteem) than measures of lung function (except in the rare cases of very severe disease). Prescription of exercise programmes may help the situation but only if the children are sufficiently motivated. Studies on the effects of training on frequency and severity of asthma have given inconsistent results (Nixon 1996). Supervised exercise testing may reassure the children and their parents that they can actually perform exercise without adverse effects, particularly if bronchodilators are taken 15–20 minutes before the start. Asthmatic children should realize that there are Olympic gold medallists and other famous sportsmen and women with asthma (Voy 1986).

Cystic fibrosis

In the 30 years since Godfrey & Mearns (1971) showed that exercise was limited by pulmonary mechanics in children with CF, these children have been subjected to all forms of exercise testing and there is now a wealth of publications in this area (Orenstein 1998). The importance lies in the fact that patients with CF suffer progressively impaired exercise tolerance, which can have a serious impact on quality of life. Furthermore, their exercise ability cannot always be predicted from their lung function or SaO_2 measured at rest. Maximal exercise testing has even been shown to predict mortality in this disease, with those with higher aerobic fitness having a three-fold increase in 8-year survival compared to those with lower fitness, even after controlling for lung function and nutritional status (Nixon et al 1992).

For these reasons, it is a recommended standard of care set by the United Kingdom Cystic Fibrosis Trust to perform exercise testing yearly to assess disease progression (Cystic Fibrosis Trust 2001). Exactly what form this testing should take is not clear but for logistical reasons it is likely to be one of the less complex and time-consuming submaximal tests such as the 6-minute walk, 3-minute step test or shuttle (once the latter has been evaluated in children). Exercise testing can be a useful guide to improvement in clinical status after a therapeutic intervention; for example, a course of intravenous antibiotics (Cerny et al 1982, Pike et al 2001). Finally, exercise testing may also be a useful outcome measure for clinical studies (Ramsey & Boat 1994).

In CF, generally, there is a direct correlation between lung function and exercise tolerance (Orenstein et al 1981). Patients with the worst FEV_1 at rest have the lowest exercise tolerance and aerobic fitness measured by $\dot{V}O_2$peak (Nixon 1996). However, there is such wide variability in exercise capacity and $\dot{V}O_2$peak for a given FEV_1 that it is not possible to predict results for an individual patient. The effect of CF on exercise physiology has been reviewed by Nixon (1996). To compensate for airways obstruction and increased dead space, patients often breathe with large minute ventilation ($\dot{V}_E$) to meet the demands of exercise. In healthy subjects, some ventilatory reserve remains at peak exercise, with minute ventilation remaining less than two-thirds of their maximum voluntary ventilation (MVV). In patients with CF, it is not unusual for $\dot{V}_E$ to reach or even exceed MVV at peak exercise; hence exercise is restricted by a

mechanical ventilatory limitation. Other limiting factors include breathlessness, muscle fatigue, nutritional status and psychological parameters. In those with severe disease, ventilation-perfusion mismatching results in O_2 desaturation and even CO_2 retention but significant desaturation is unusual in those with an FEV > 50% predicted (Henke & Orenstein 1981). Anaerobic performance is also limited in CF, principally due to nutritional factors (muscle mass) (Boas et al 1996).

Cardiovascular responses to exercise are normal in CF patients with mild disease. Those with moderate to severe disease may not attain expected peak heart rates and cardiac output, since non-cardiac factors, such as those already discussed, limit their ability to exercise before their cardiovascular systems are maximally stressed.

Measurement of exercise tolerance is an important part of heart-lung transplant assessment in children with CF, particularly since it may predict life expectancy and provide information about the patient's quality of life. Walking tests are often used, either the 12-minute (Whitehead et al 1991) or 6-minute (Kadikar et al 1997), and it has recently been shown that the step test may have a role to play (Aurora et al 2001).

Most but not all studies have shown that aerobic fitness can be improved by exercise training in patients with CF (Nixon 1996) and increased aerobic fitness is associated with an improved quality of life (Orenstein et al 1989). Benefit was more likely when the exercise programmes were supervised, included activities such as running or swimming, lasted for at least 8 weeks and patient adherence was good. Unfortunately, although ventilatory muscle endurance and strength have been shown to improve, the effect on actual lung function is less consistent. One of the main problems, however, is that improvements tend to be lost within weeks of finishing the exercise programmes. In addition, a recent study showed that even though a training programme led to significant improvements in perceptions of self-worth and physical appearance, the children did not wish to carry on with the programme (cycling 20 minutes a day for 5 days a week) (Gulmans et al 1999). Given all the other time-consuming burdens of CF therapy, perhaps that is not too surprising. In fact, adolescents with CF seem to engage in physical activity as much as their healthy peers (admittedly self-reporting), but this activity declines after the age of 17 years (Britto et al 2000). Exercise has been shown to aid airway clearance (Zach et al 1982) but generally it is not recommended as a substitute for the usual physiotherapy techniques. In practice, however, it is difficult to persuade those children who play regular sport and are fit to carry out regular chest physiotherapy.

Congenital heart disease

Exercise testing is an important part of evaluation of children with cardiac disease and the American Heart Association has produced comprehensive guidelines for paediatric testing (Washington et al 1994). In addition, they suggest when testing should be avoided:

● Severe pulmonary vascular disease
● Poorly compensated congestive heart failure
● Recent myocardial infarction
● Active rheumatic fever with carditis
● Acute myocarditis or pericarditis
● Severe aortic stenosis
● Severe mitral stenosis
● Unstable arrhythmia
● Marfan syndrome with suspected aortic dissection
● Uncontrolled severe hypertension
● Hypertrophic cardiomyopathy with history of syncope

Exercise testing is rarely diagnostic in congenital heart disease but has its greatest value in evaluating severity. In particular, it may reveal abnormalities that are not present at rest. Tomassoni (1996b) has outlined common reasons for using exercise testing in evaluation of cardiovascular disease:

● Objective assessment of exercise-induced symptoms, e.g. chest pain, palpitations, dizziness or syncope. In particular,

dysrhythmias or ischaemia can be determined.
● Evaluation of cardiac arrhythmia to see whether exercise has an effect.
● Establishment of severity of obstructive heart disease such as aortic stenosis or coarctation of the aorta. The onset of exercise-induced ischaemia can be determined.
● Determination of exercise tolerance and production of recommendations on what exercise it is safe for the child to take part in.
● Evaluation of responses to medical therapy or cardiac pacing.

For further details of specific congenital heart lesions and the role of exercise testing see Tomassoni (1996b) or the special review edition of *Pediatric Cardiology* 1999 (volume 20, part 1) edited by WB Strong.

Musculoskeletal disorders

Neuromuscular disease. The areas of testing most relevant to children with neuromuscular disease (NMD) relate to muscle function rather than cardiorespiratory function; for example, muscle strength and endurance, peak mechanical power and effect on O_2 status of physical movement. Due to the obvious limitations imposed by muscle weakness, children with neuromuscular disease have markedly reduced exercise tolerance but maximal aerobic power is seldom the limiting factor (Bar-Or 1996). At the advanced stage of diseases such as Duchenne muscular dystrophy, the heart muscles are also affected, further limiting the severely weakened movement ability. It is important to test several muscle groups as, depending on the condition, certain muscles are affected more than others. For more severe conditions, the arm-cranking version of the Wingate Anaerobic Test may be the only test that the patients can perform, as they are too weak to walk or cycle. Children with conditions such as spastic cerebral palsy may have reasonable muscle strength but the difficulties of incoordination make testing difficult. In addition, the inefficiency of movement means that for a given task, $\dot{V}O_2$ is much higher in these children (Nixon & Orenstein 1988).

Rationale for testing children with NMD is as follows (Bar-Or 1996):

- Monitoring progression of the disease, e.g. the rate of decline in thigh muscle strength can be useful in patients with Duchenne or Becker's muscular dystrophy.
- Measuring effect of treatment, e.g. improvement in movement seen after a child with cerebral palsy has had a procedure such as surgical release of hip adductors or lengthening of Achilles tendons.
- Assessing functional effect of exercise, e.g. a child with severe scoliosis who has ventilatory limitation may have a normal SaO_2 at rest but desaturate during exercise.
- Monitoring levels of fitness during training programmes or rehabilitation.

Scoliosis. Children with a marked scoliosis have a deformed thoracic cage that leads to a restrictive lung disorder, often accompanied by ventilation-perfusion mismatch. They may be able to perform spirometry and arm span is substituted for height to calculate predicted values. If a scoliosis is secondary to neuromuscular disease, then they will have the additional burden of severe muscle weakness, which may make even spirometry impossible. With severe scoliosis, exertional dyspnoea and reduced exercise tolerance are common (Nixon & Orenstein 1988).

Chronic lung disease (bronchopulmonary dysplasia)

Advances in neonatal care of prematurely born babies has led to better survival figures. Unfortunately this survival may be at the cost of damage to the developing lungs, resulting in an infant with chronic lung disease who is oxygen dependent, often for many years. There have been many studies on such children that have found abnormalities in lung function and exercise tolerance (reviewed by Pianosi & Fisk 2000). A recent study on 8–9-year-olds who had required mechanical ventilation for hyaline membrane disease found that, on average, $\dot{V}O_{2peak}$ was within the normal range although on the low side (Pianosi & Fisk 2000). They did not appear to have a significant cardiopulmonary limitation to exercise but they exhibited certain adaptations in their responses. They tended to increase their respiratory rate rather than their tidal volume, i.e. they breathed faster rather than deeper, resulting in a lower end-tidal PCO_2. The reason for this difference in regulation of breathing is not clear.

Obesity

Obesity is becoming a serious problem amongst an ever-increasing number of children due to poor eating habits and a sedentary lifestyle, with approximately one in five children and adolescents in the USA being classified as obese (Owens & Gutin 1999). Exercise is said to be a cornerstone of treating paediatric obesity along with dietary and behaviour modification but unfortunately research on the benefits gained by training has not been conclusive (Epstein et al 1996). Apart from simply weighing the child, exercise testing may be a useful way of monitoring progress and the response of the obese child to exercise has recently been reviewed by Owens & Gutin (1999), who conclude that the physiological changes are similar to those of non-obese children. It is particularly important to be sensitive and instil confidence in these children at the time of testing.

REFERENCES

Ahmaidi SB, Varray AL, Savy-Pacaux AM, Prefaut CG 1993 Cardiorespiratory fitness evaluation by the shuttle test in asthmatic subjects during aerobic training. Chest 103: 1135–1141

American College of Sports Medicine 2000 Guidelines for exercise testing and prescription, 6th edn. Lea and Febiger, Philadelphia

American Thoracic Society 1986 Evaluation of impairment/disability secondary to respiratory disorders. American Review of Respiratory Disease 133: 1205–1209

American Thoracic Society 1996 Lung volume reduction surgery. American Journal of Respiratory and Critical Care Medicine 154: 1151–1152

American Thoracic Society 1999 Skeletal muscle dysfunction in chronic obstructive pulmonary disease. A statement of the American Thoracic Society and European Respiratory Society. American Journal of Respiratory Critical Care Medicine 159: s1–40

Anthonisen NR 1986 Tests of mechanical function. In: Fishman AP (ed) Handbook of respiratory physiology: the respiratory system III. American Physiological Society, Bethesda

Aurora P, Wade A, Whitmore P, Whitehead B 2000 A model for predicting life expectancy of children with cystic fibrosis. European Respiratory Journal 16: 1056–1060

Aurora P, Prasad SA, Balfour-Lynn IM, Slade G, Whitehead B, Dinwiddie R 2001 Exercise tolerance in children with cystic fibrosis undergoing lung transplantation assessment. European Respiratory Journal 18: 293–297

Baba R, Nagashima M, Nagano Y, Ikoma M, Nihibata K 1999 Role of the oxygen uptake efficiency slope in evaluating exercise tolerance. Archives of Disease in Childhood 81: 73–75

Bailey RC, Olson J, Pepper SL, Porszasz J, Barstow TJ, Cooper DM 1995 The level and tempo of children's physical activities: an observational study. Medicine and Science in Sports and Exercise 27: 1033–1041

Balfour-Lynn IM, Prasad SA, Laverty A, Whitehead BF, Dinwiddie R 1998 A step in the right direction: assessing exercise tolerance in cystic fibrosis. Pediatric Pulmonology 25: 278–284

Bar-Or O 1996 Role of exercise in the assessment and management of neuromuscular disease in children. Medicine and Science in Sports and Exercise 28: 421–427

Benson MK 1983 Diseases of the airways. In: Weatherall DJ, Ledingham JGG, Warrel DA (eds) Oxford textbook of medicine, vol 2. Oxford University Press, Oxford, pp 15.60–15.70

Bestall JC, Paul EA, Garrod R, Garnham R, Jones PW, Wedzicha JA 1999 Usefulness of the MRC dyspnoea scale as a measure of disability in patients with chronic obstructive pulmonary disease. Thorax 54 (7): 581–586

Bittner V, Weiner DH, Yusuf S et al, for the SOLVD Investigators 1993 Prediction of mortality and morbidity with a 6-minute walk test in patients with left ventricular dysfunction. Journal of the American Medical Association 270: 1702–1707

Black LF, Hyatt RE 1971 Maximal static respiratory pressures in generalised neuromuscular disease. American Review of Respiratory Disease 103: 641–650

Boas SR, Joswiak ML, Nixon PA, Fulton JA, Orenstein DM 1996 Factors limiting anaerobic performance in adolescent males with cystic fibrosis. Medicine and Science in Sports and Exercise 28: 291–298

Boas SR, Danduran MJ, McColley SA 1999 Energy metabolism during anaerobic exercise in children with cystic fibrosis and asthma. Medicine and Science in Sports and Exercise 31: 1242–1249

Borg GAV 1982 Psychophysical bases of perceived exertion. Medicine and Science in Sports and Exercise 14: 377–381

Braden DS, Carroll JF 1999 Normative cardiovascular responses to exercise in children. Pediatric Cardiology 20: 4–10

Bradley J, Howard J, Wallace E, Elborn S 1999 Validity of a modified shuttle test in adult cystic fibrosis. Thorax 54: 437–439

Bridge PD, Ranganathan S, McKenzie SA 1999 Measurement of airway resistance using the interrupter technique in preschool children in the ambulatory setting. European Respiratory Journal 13: 792–796

British Thoracic Society/Association of Respiratory Technologists and Physiologists 1994 Guidelines for the measurement of respiratory function. Respiratory Medicine 88: 165–194

British Thoracic Society and Society of Cardiothoracic Surgeons of Great Britain and Ireland Working Party 2001 Guidelines on the selection of patients with lung cancer for surgery. Thorax; 56: 89–108

Britto MT, Garrett JM, Konrad TR, Majure JM, Leigh MW 2000 Comparison of physical activity in adolescents with cystic fibrosis versus age-matched controls. Pediatric Pulmonology 30: 86–91

Brouillette RT, Morielli A, Leimanis A, Waters KA, Luciano R, Ducharme FM 2000 Nocturnal pulse oximetry as an abbreviated testing modality for pediatric obstructive sleep apnea. Pediatrics 105: 405–412

Burdon GW, Juniper EF, Killian KJ, Hargreave FE, Campbell EJM 1982 The perception of breathlessness in asthma. American Review of Respiratory Diseases 126: 825–828

Butland RJA, Pang J, Gross ER et al 1982 Two-, six-, and 12-minute walking tests in respiratory disease. British Medical Journal 284: 1607–1608

Cabrera ME, Lough MD, Doershuk CF, De Rivera GA 1993 Anaerobic performance assessed by the Wingate test in patients with cystic fibrosis. Pediatric Exercise Science 5: 78–87

Cane RS, Ranganathan SC, McKenzie SA 2000 What do parents of wheezy children understand by 'wheeze'? Archives of Disease in Childhood 82: 327–332

Castile RG 1998 Pulmonary function testing in children. In: Chernick V, Boat TF (eds) Kendig's disorders of the respiratory tract in children. WB Saunders, Philadelphia, pp 196–214

Cerny FJ, Cropp GJA, Bye MR 1982 Hospital therapy improves exercise tolerance and lung function in cystic fibrosis. American Journal of Disease in Childhood 138: 261–265

Clark JS, Votteri B, Aragiano RL et al 1992 Noninvasive assessment of blood gases. American Review of Respiratory Disease 145: 220–232

Cooper DM 1995 Rethinking exercise testing in children: a challenge. American Journal of Respiratory and Critical Care Medicine 152: 1154–1157

Cooper DM, Springer C 1998 Pulmonary function assessment in the laboratory during exercise. In: Chernick V, Boat TF (eds) Kendig's disorders of the respiratory tract in children. WB Saunders, Philadelphia, pp 214–237

Cooper PJ, Robertson CF, Hudson IL, Phelan PD 1990 Variability of pulmonary function tests in cystic fibrosis. Pediatric Pulmonology 8: 16–22

Cotes JE 1993 Lung function: assessment and application in medicine, 5th edn. Blackwell Science, Oxford

Counil FP, Varray A, Karila C, Hayot M, Voisin M, Prefaut C 1997 Wingate test performance in children with asthma:

aerobic or anaerobic limitation? Medicine and Science in Sports and Exercise 29: 430–435

Criner GJ, Cordova FC, Furukawa S et al 1999 Prospective randomised controlled trial comparing bilateral lung volume reduction surgery to pulmonary rehabilitation in severe chronic obstructive pulmonary disease. American Journal of Respiratory and Critical Care Medicine 160: 2018–2027

Cypcar D, Lemanske Jr RF 1994 Asthma and exercise. Clinics in Chest Medicine 15: 351–368

Cystic Fibrosis Trust 2001 Standards for the clinical care of children and adults with cystic fibrosis in the UK 2001. Cystic Fibrosis Trust, Bromley

De Meer K, Gulmans VAM, Van Der Laag J 1999 Peripheral muscle weakness and exercise capacity in children with cystic fibrosis. American Journal of Respiratory and Critical Care Medicine 159: 748–754

Dinwiddie R, Madge S, Prasad SA, Balfour-Lynn IM 1999 Oxygen therapy for cystic fibrosis. Journal of the Royal Society of Medicine 92(suppl 37): 19–22

Editorial 1992 Reversibility of airflow obstruction: FEV1 vs peak flow. Lancet 340: 85–86

Epstein LH, Coleman KJ, Myers MD 1996 Exercise in treating obesity in children and adolescents. Medicine and Science in Sports and Exercise 28: 428–435

ERS Task Force 1997 Clinical testing with reference to lung diseases: indications, standardisation and interpretation strategies. European Respiratory Journal 10: 2662–2689

European Community for Coal and Steel 1983 Standardized lung function testing. Bulletin Europeén de Physiopathologie Respiratoire 19 (suppl 5): 1–95

Freeman W, Weir DC, Sapiano SB, Whitehead JE, Burge PS, Cayton RM 1990 The twenty-metre shuttle-running test: a combined test for maximal oxygen uptake and exercise-induced asthma? Respiratory Medicine 84: 31–35

Fulco CS, Lewis SF, Frykman PN et al 1995 Quantitation of progressive muscle fatigue during dynamic leg exercise in humans. Journal of Applied Physiology 79: 2154–2162

Gagliardi L, Rusconi F and the Working Party on Respiratory Rate 1997 Respiratory rate and body mass in the first three years of life. Archives of Disease in Childhood 76: 151–154

Gaskin L, Thomas J 1995 Pulse oximetry and exercise. Physiotherapy 81: 254–261

Geddes D, Davies M, Koyama H et al 2000 Effect of lung volume reduction surgery in patients with severe emphysema. New England Journal of Medicine 343: 239–245

Gibson GJ 1996 Clinical tests of respiratory function, 2nd edn. Chapman and Hall, London

Gibson GJ 1995 Respiratory function tests. In: Brewis RAL, Corrin B, Geddes DM, Gibson GJ (eds) Respiratory medicine, 2nd edn. WB Saunders, London, pp 229–243

Gibbons RJ, Balady GJ, Beasley JW et al 1997 ACC/AHA guidelines for exercise testing: executive summary. Circulation 96: 345–354

Godfrey S, Mearns M 1971 Pulmonary function and response to exercise in cystic fibrosis. Archives of Disease in Childhood 46: 144–151

Godfrey S, Kamburoff PL, Nairn JR 1970 Spirometry, lung volumes and airway resistance in normal children aged 5 to 18 years. British Journal of Diseases of the Chest 64: 15–24

Gosselink R, Troosters T, Decramer M 1996 Peripheral muscle weakness contributes to exercise limitation in COPD. American Journal of Respiratory and Critical Care Medicine 153: 976–980

Gosselink R, Decramer M 1998 Peripheral skeletal muscle and exercise performance in patients with chronic obstructive pulmonary disease. Monaldi Archives for Chest Disease 1998;53: 419–23

Green M, Laroche CM 1990 Respiratory muscle weakness. In: Brewis RAL, Corrin B, Geddes DM, Gibson GJ (eds) Respiratory Medicine. WB Saunders, London, pp 1373–1387

Griffiths TL, Burr ML, Campbell IA et al 2000 Results at 1 year of outpatient multi-disciplinary pulmonary rehabilitation: a randomised controlled trial. Lancet 335: 362–368

Gulmans VAM, Van Veldhoven NHMJ, De Meer K, Helders PJM 1996 The six-minute walking test in children with cystic fibrosis: reliability and validity. Pediatric Pulmonology 22: 85–89

Gulmans VAM, De Meer K, Brackel HJL, Faber JAJ, Berger R, Helders PJM 1999 Outpatient exercise training in children with cystic fibrosis: physiological effects, perceived competence and acceptability. Pediatric Pulmonology 28: 39–46

Guyatt GH, Berman LB, Townsend M et al 1987 A measure of the quality of life for clinical trials in chronic lung disease. Thorax 42: 773–778

Guyatt GH, Pugsley SO, Sullivan MJ et al 1984 Effect of encouragement on walking test performance. Thorax 39: 818–822

Hajiro T, Nishimura K, Jones PW, Tsukino M, Ikeda A, Koyama H, Izimi T 1999 A novel, short, and simple questionnaire to measure health related quality of life in patients with chronic obstructive pulmonary disease. American Journal of Respiratory and Critical Care Medicine 159: 1874–1878

Hayot M, Guillaumont S, Ramonatxo M, Voisin M, Préfaut C 1997 Determinants of the tension-time index of inspiratory muscles in children with cystic fibrosis. Pediatric Pulmonology 23: 336–343

Hebestreit H, Staschen B, Hebestreit A 2000 Ventilatory threshold: a useful method to determine aerobic fitness in children? Medicine and Science in Sports and Exercise 32: 1964–1969

Henke KG, Orenstein DM 1984 Oxygen saturation during exercise in cystic fibrosis. American Review of Respiratory Disease 129: 708–711

Hooker EA, Danzl DF, Brueggmeyer M, Harper E 1992 Respiratory rates in pediatric emergency patients. Journal of Emergency Medicine 10: 407–410

Hyatt RE, Scanlon PD, Nakamura M 1997 Interpretation of pulmonary function tests. A practical guide. Lippincott-Raven, Philadelphia

Hyland ME, Bott J, Singh SJ, Kenyon CAP 1994 Domains, constructs and the development of the breathing problems questionnaire. Quality of Life Research 3: 245–256

Hyland ME, Singh SJ, Sodergren SC, Morgan MD 1998 Development of a shortened vesion of the Breathing Problems Questionnaire suitable for use in a pulmonary rehabilitation clinic: a purpose specific, disease specific questionnaire. Quality of Life Research 7: 227–233

Jenkins SC, Soutar SA, Moxham J 1988 The effects of posture on lung volumes in normal subjects and in patients pre- and post-coronary artery surgery. Physiotherapy 74: 492–496

Jones PW 1991 Quality of life measurement for patients with disease of the airway. Thorax 46: 676–682

Juniper EF, Cockcroft DW, Hargreave FE 1994 Histamine and methacholine inhalation tests: a laboratory tidal breathing protocol, 2nd edn. Astra Draco AB, Lund, Sweden

Kadikar A, Maurer J, Kesten S 1997 The six-minute walk test: a guide to assessment for lung transplantation. Journal of Heart and Lung Transplantation 16: 313–319

Kaneko KM, Milic-Emili J, Dolovich MB et al 1966 Regional distribution of ventilation and perfusion as a function of body position. Journal of Applied Physiology 21: 767–777

Keell SD, Chambers JS, Francis DP, Edwards DF, Stables RH 1998 Shuttle walk test to assess chronic heart failure (letter). Lancet 352: 705

Kharitonov SA, Yates D, Robins RA et al 1994 Increased nitric oxide in exhaled air of asthmatic patients. Lancet 343: 133–135

Knox AJ, Morrison JFJ, Muers MF 1988 Reproducibility of walking test results in chronic obstructive airways disease. Thorax 43: 388–392

Kraemer R 1993 Assessment of functional abnormalities in infants and children with lung disease. Agents and Actions (suppl) 40: 41–55

Léger LA, Lambert J 1982 A multi-stage 20-m shuttle run test to predict VO_2 max. European Journal of Applied Physiology 49: 1–12

McKenzie SA, Bridge PD, Healy MJR 2000 Airway resistance and atopy in preschool children with wheeze and cough. European Respiratory Journal 15: 833–838

McGavin CR, Gupta SP, McHardy GJR 1976 Twelve-minute walking test for assessing disability in chronic bronchitis. British Medical Journal 1: 822–823

Maltais F, Simard AA, Simard C et al 1996 Oxidative capacity of the skeletal muscle and lactic acid kinetics during exercise in normal subjects and in patients with COPD. American Journal of Respiratory and Critical Care Medicine 153: 288–293

Mathur RS, Revill SM, Vara DD et al 1995 Comparison of peak oxygen consumption during cycle and treadmill exercise in severe chronic airflow obstruction. Thorax 50: 829–833

Morgan MDL 2001 Enhancing performance in chronic obstructive pulmonary disease. Thorax 56:73–77

Mungall IPF, Hainsworth R 1979 Assessment of respiratory function in patients with chronic obstructive airways disease. Thorax 34: 254–258

Nickerson BG, Lemen RJ, Gerdes CB, Wegmann MJ, Robertson G 1980 Within-subject variability and per cent change for significance of spirometry in normal subjects and patients with cystic fibrosis. American Review of Respiratory Disease 122: 859–866

Nixon PA 1996 Role of exercise in the evaluation and management of pulmonary disease in children and youth. Medicine and Science in Sports and Exercise 28: 414–420

Nixon PA, Orenstein DM 1988 Exercise testing in children. Pediatric Pulmonology 5: 107–122

Nixon PA, Orenstein DM, Kelsey SF, Doershuk CF 1992 The prognostic value of exercise testing in patients with cystic fibrosis. New England Journal of Medicine 327: 1785–1788

Nixon PA, Joswiak ML, Fricker FJ 1996 A six-minute walk test for assessing exercise tolerance in severely ill children. Journal of Pediatrics 129: 362–366

Noonan V, Dean E 2000 Submaximal exercise testing: clinical application and interpretation. Physical Therapy 80: 782–807

Nunn JF 1987 Applied respiratory physiology, 3rd edn. Butterworths, London

O'Donnell DE, Lam M, Webb KA 1999 Spirometric correlates of improvement in exercise perfromance after anticholinergic therapy in chronic obstructive pulmonary disease. American Journal of Respiratory and Critical Care Medicine 160: 542–549

Orenstein DM 1998 Exercise testing in cystic fibrosis. Pediatric Pulmonology 25: 223–225

Orenstein DM, Franklin BA, Doershuk CF, Hellerstein HK, Germann KJ, Horowitz JG, Stern RC 1981 Exercise conditioning and cardiopulmonary fitness in cystic fibrosis. The effect of a three-month supervised running program. Chest 80: 392–398

Orenstein DM, Nixon PA, Ross EA, Kaplan RM 1989 The quality of well-being in cystic fibrosis. Chest 95: 344–347

Orenstein DM, Curtis SE, Nixon PA, Hartigan ER 1993 Accuracy of three pulse oximeters during exercise and hypoxemia in patients with cystic fibrosis. Chest 104: 1187–1190

Owens S, Gutin B 1999 Exercise testing of the child with obesity. Pediatric Cardiology 20: 79–83

Pattishall EN 1990 Pulmonary function testing references values and interpretations in pediatric training programs. Pediatrics 85: 768–773

Pianosi PT, Fisk M 2000 Cardiopulmonary exercise performance in prematurely born children. Pediatric Research 47: 653–658

Pike SE, Prasad SA, Balfour-Lynn IM 2001 Effect of intravenous antibiotics on exercise tolerance (3-minute step test) in cystic fibrosis. Pediatric Pulmonology 32: 38–43

Pincivero DM, Gear WS, Sterner RL 2001 Assessment of the reliability of high-intensity quadriceps femoris muscle fatigue. Medicine and Science in Sports and Exercise 33: 334–338

Poets CF 1998 When do infants need additional inspired oxygen? A review of the current literature. Pediatric Pulmonology 26: 424–428

Polgar G, Promadhat V 1971 Pulmonary function testing in children: techniques and standards. WB Saunders, Philadelphia

Polgar G, Weng TR 1979 The functional development of the respiratory system from the period of gestation to adulthood. American Review of Respiratory Disease 120: 625–695

Powell CVE, White RD, Primhak RA 1996 Longitudinal study of free running exercise challenge: reproducibility. Archives of Disease in Childhood 74: 108–114

Prasad SA, Randall SD, Balfour-Lynn IM 2000 Fifteen-count breathlessness score: an objective measure for children. Pediatric Pulmonology 30: 56–62

Ramsey BW, Boat TF 1994 Outcome measures for clinical trials in cystic fibrosis. Summary of a Cystic Fibrosis Foundation Consensus Conference. Journal of Pediatrics 124: 177–192

Redline S, Wright EC, Kattan M, Kercsmar C, Weiss K 1996 Short-term compliance with peak-flow monitoring: results from a study of inner city children with asthma. Pediatric Pulmonology 21: 203–210

Revill SM, Morgan MDL, Singh SJ, Williams J, Hardman AE 1999 The endurance shuttle walk: a new field test for the assessment of endurance capacity in chronic obstructive pulmonary disease. Thorax 54: 213–222

Roca J, Whipp BJ 1997 Clinical exercise testing. European Respiratory Monograph. 2: 6 West JB 1990 Respiratory physiology, 4th edn. Williams and Wilkins, Baltimore

Rosenthal M, Bush A 2000 Ventilatory variables in normal children during rest and exercise. European Respiratory Journal 16: 1075–1083

Rosenthal M, Bain SH, Cramer D, Helms P, Denison D, Bush A, Warner JO 1993a Lung function in white children aged 4 to 19 years: I – spirometry. Thorax 48: 794–802

Rosenthal M, Cramer D, Bain SH, Denison D, Bush A, Warner JO 1993b Lung function in white children aged 4 to 19 years: II – single breath analysis and plethysmography. Thorax 48: 803–808

Royal College of Physicians 1999 Domiciliary oxygen therapy services. Clinical guidelines and advice for prescription. Royal College of Physicians, London

Schnapp LM, Cohen NH 1990 Pulse oximetry. Uses and abuses. Chest 98: 1244–1249

Schramm CM, Grunstein MM 1998. Pulmonary function tests in infants. In: Chernick V, Boat TF (eds) Kendig's disorders of the respiratory tract in children. WB Saunders, Philadelphia, pp 175–196

Shneerson J 1988 Disorders of ventilation. Blackwell Science, Oxford, pp 78–85

Silverman M, Stocks J 1999 Pediatric pulmonary function. In: Hughes JMB, Pride NB (eds) Lung function tests. Physiological principles and clinical applications. WB Saunders, London, pp 163–183

Singh SJ, Morgan MDL, Scott S et al 1992. The development of the shuttle walking test of disability in patients with chronic obstructive airways obstruction. Thorax 47: 1019–1024

Sont JK, Willems LN, Bel EH, Van Krieken HJ, Vandenbroucke JP, Sterk PJ 1999 Clinical control and histopathologic outcome of asthma when using airway responsiveness as an additional guide to long-term treatment. American Journal of Respiratory and Critical Care Medicine 159: 1043–1051

Steiner MC, Morgan MDL. Enhancing performance in chronic obstructive pulmonary disease. Thorax ;56: 73–77

Stocks J, Gerritsen J (eds) 2000 & 2001 Standards for infant respiratory function testing: ERJ / ATS Task Force. European Respiratory Journal Series number 1, 16: 731–740; Series number 2, 16: 741–748; Series number 3, 16: 1016–1022; Series number 4, 16: 1180–1192; Series number 5, 17: 141–148; Series number 6, 17: 302–312

Stocks J, Sly PD, Tepper RS, Morgan WJ 1996 Infant respiratory function testing. John Wiley, New York

Szekely LA, Oelberg DA, Wright C et al 1997 Pre-operative predictors of operative morbidity and mortality in COPD patients undergoing bilateral lung volume reduction surgery. Chest 111: 550–558

Tremper KK, Barker S 1989 Pulse oximetry. Anesthesiology 70: 98––108

Tomassoni TL 1996a Introduction: the role of exercise in the diagnosis and management of chronic disease in children and youth. Medicine and Science in Sports and Exercise 28: 403–405

Tomassoni TL 1996b Role of exercise in the management of cardiovascular disease in children and youth. Medicine and Science in Sports and Exercise 28: 406–413

Uldry C, Filling JW 1995 Maximal values of sniff nasal inspiratory pressures in healthy subjects. Thorax 50: 371–375

Upton CJ, Tyrrell JC, Hiller EJ 1988 Two minute walking distance in cystic fibrosis. Archives of Disease in Childhood 63: 1444–1448

Voy RO 1986 The U.S. Olympic Committee experience with exercise-induced bronchospasm, 1984. Medicine and Science in Sports and Exercise 18: 328–330

Waalkens HJ, Merkus PJFM, Van Essen-Zandvliet EE et al 1993 Assessment of bronchodilator response in children with asthma. European Respiratory Journal 6: 645–651

Washington RL 1999 Cardiorespiratory testing: anaerobic threshold/respiratory threshold. Pediatric Cardiology 20: 12–15

Washington RL, Bricker JT, Alpert BS et al 1994 Guidelines for exercise testing in the pediatric age group. Circulation 90: 2166–2179

Wedzicha J A 1996 Domiciliary ventilation in chronic obstructive pulmonary disease: where are we? Thorax 51: 455–457

West JB 1992 Pulmonary pathophysiology, 4th edn. Williams and Wilkins, Baltimore

Whitehead B, Helms P, Goodwin M et al 1991 Heart-lung transplantation for cystic fibrosis. I: Assessment. Archives of Disease in Childhood 66: 1018–1021

Wilson RC, Jones PW 1989 A comparison of the visual analogue scale and modified Borg scale for the measurement of dyspnoea during exercise. Clinical Science 76: 277–282

Zach M, Oberwaldner B, Hausler F 1982 Cystic fibrosis: physical exercise versus chest physiotherapy. Archives of Disease in Childhood 57: 587–589

FURTHER READING

American College of Sports Medicine 2000 Guidelines for exercise testing and prescription, 6th edn. Lea and Febiger, Philadelphia

Braunwald E 2001 Heart disease: a textbook of cardiovascular medicine, 5th edn. WB Saunders, Philadelphia

British Thoracic Society/Association of Respiratory Technologists and Physiologists 1994 Guidelines for the measurement of respiratory function. Respiratory Medicine 88: 165–194

Castile RG 1998 Pulmonary function testing in children. In: Chernick V, Boat TF (eds) Kendig's disorders of the respiratory tract in children. WB Saunders, Philadelphia, pp 196–214

Cooper DM, Springer C 1998 Pulmonary function assessment in the laboratory during exercise. In: Chernick V, Boat TF (eds) Kendig's disorders of the respiratory tract in children. WB Saunders, Philadelphia, pp 214–237

Cotes JE 1993 Lung function: assessment and application in medicine, 5th edn. Blackwell Science, Oxford

ERS Task Force 1997 Clinical testing with reference to lung diseases: indications, standardisation and interpretation strategies. European Respiratory Journal 10: 2662–2689

Houghton AR, Gray D 1997 Making sense of the ECG. Edward Arnold, London

Hyatt RE, Scanlon PD, Nakamura M 1997 Interpretation of pulmonary function tests. A practical guide. Lippincott-Raven, Philadelphia

Jones NL 1988 Clinical exercise testing, 3rd edn. WB Saunders, Philadelphia

Julian DG, Cowan JC, McLenachan JM 1998 Cardiology, 7th edn. WB Saunders, Philadelphia

Nunn JF 1987 Applied respiratory physiology, 3rd edn. Butterworths, London

Roca J, Whipp BJ 1997 Clinical exercise testing. European Respiratory Monograph. 2: 6 West JB 1990 Respiratory physiology, 4th edn. Williams and Wilkins, Baltimore

Schramm CM, Grunstein MM 1998. Pulmonary function tests in infants. In: Chernick V, Boat TF (eds) Kendig's disorders of the respiratory tract in children. WB Saunders, Philadelphia, pp 175–196

Stocks J, Sly PD, Tepper RS, Morgan WJ 1996 Infant respiratory function testing. John Wiley, New York

Sutton P 1999 Measurements in cardiology. Parthenon, London

West JB 1992 Pulmonary pathophysiology, 4th edn. Williams and Wilkins, Baltimore

4

Monitoring and interpreting medical investigations

John S Turner

MONITORING

Introduction

There has been an explosion of computer and video technology in recent years and patient monitoring has directly benefited from this. The ability to detect and rapidly react to changes in physiology is now possible and this has become the essence of modern intensive care.

The ideal monitoring system is not yet a reality (although several major manufacturers would deny this) but it is coming closer all the time. This system would need to be accurate, precise and reliable. It would be sensitive to small changes in the parameters it monitors, yet able to distinguish and eliminate artefacts. It would be non-invasive for the sake of safety. It would function on a real-time rather than an intermittent basis. It would have a memory for previous data and would be able to show trends. Its memory module would be moveable to allow it to capture data in the ward, in transport and in another environment such as an operating theatre. It would also almost certainly be extremely expensive!

Conventional observations

Back to reality. Nursing observations have for many years included the taking of the patient's temperature, pulse, respiratory rate and blood pressure. These are performed manually and carefully charted at intervals varying from quarter-hourly to 6-hourly to daily, being performed more frequently in high-care areas. These practices are quite adequate for general ward situations where patients are not critically ill and are even useful in intensive care units (ICUs), both for making physical contact with the patient and for checking the invasively monitored observations.

The major limitation of intermittently performed observations is that they may only establish the presence of an abnormality some time after it has developed. Thus the ability to react immediately to the development of an abnormality is lost. More frequently performed observations are obviously superior in this regard, but real-time continuous monitoring is the ultimate goal of monitoring.

Non-invasive monitoring

Non-invasive monitoring of a variety of parameters is now routinely practised in many areas, especially ICUs and operating theatres. Commonly monitored parameters include temperature, heart rate, blood pressure and oxygen saturation. Respiratory rate may be measured by some monitoring systems and in certain circumstances end-tidal CO_2 and transcutaneous PO_2 and PCO_2 monitoring may be performed. These may all be displayed on a single monitor screen. Technical problems and artefacts can occur with the display of any of these parameters, so the patient's clinical status must be checked before acting on a monitor display abnormality.

Temperature

Temperature is continuously monitored by means of an oesophageal or rectal probe. This determines core temperature, which is usually at least 1°C higher than axillary temperature and may be more in shock. Problems are rarely encountered with this method. The oesophageal temperature may be lower if the gases for respiratory support are unwarmed and the rectal probe may occasionally fall out without being noticed, leading to an erroneously low temperature being displayed. A rectum full of faeces may also lead to a lower temperature being recorded.

Heart rate

Heart rate is measured from the electrocardiogram (ECG) trace. Artefacts are common. Interference (usually from patient movement or a warming blanket) may confuse the monitor into showing the presence of a tachycardia or arrhythmia, while small complexes may be interpreted as asystole. Physiotherapy may also cause movement artefacts. On the ECG trace, large T waves (and occasionally P waves or a pacemaker spike) may be interpreted as QRS complexes, leading to the displayed heart rate being double the actual rate. Detached or dried-out electrodes will lead to asystole being displayed. Sinus tachycardia, sinus bradycardia and atrial fibrillation are described below.

Respiratory rate

Respiratory rate may be measured by making use of the changing impedance across the chest wall as it moves with respiration. In systems which offer this parameter, the sensors are built into the ECG leads. The heart rate and other movements of the chest can cause overreading of respiratory rate, while electrodes placed too far apart may not give a reading at all.

Appropriate physiotherapy treatment (e.g. for lobar lung collapse) may reduce a rapid respiratory rate, but it must be emphasized that an already tachypnoeic patient should not be allowed to become exhausted during treatment as he may rapidly decompensate. This may even necessitate emergency intubation. Close contact with the medical and nursing staff should therefore be maintained in such cases.

Blood pressure

Blood pressure is monitored with a pressure cuff around the upper arm. An oscillometric method is used to measure blood pressure, with automatic cuff inflation and deflation. The accuracy of such systems is generally good, but the cuff needs to be applied correctly and be of the appropriate size for the arm. The system also needs to be calibrated correctly against a mercury column.

Non-invasive blood pressure monitoring is performed intermittently but the interval between readings may be as short as one minute.

Physiotherapy treatment may cause a patient to become hypertensive, especially if the treatment causes pain or anxiety. The hypotensive patient may occasionally become more unstable and here the risks and benefits of treatment need to be carefully balanced.

Oxygen saturation

Oxygen saturation (Clark et al 1992) is continuously measured by a pulse oximeter with a probe on a finger or earlobe. There are two methods: the functional method, which measures the difference between oxyhaemoglobin and deoxyhaemoglobin, and the fractional method which measures all types of haemoglobin over a wide spectrum of light absorption. The former method may record erroneously high saturations if there is a high concentration of carboxyhaemoglobin (the combination of carbon monoxide and haemoglobin) in the blood, while the latter method will be inaccurate if a light-emitting diode (LED) or ultraviolet light (including sunlight) is close to the probe. Saturations are generally accurate between 100% and 80%, but may be inaccurate at lower levels. The saturation trace must be observed to correspond with the heart rate; if this is not so the reading may be erroneous. Low saturations with either method may be due to poor peripheral perfusion, painted or nicotine-stained fingernails, pierced ears, intravenous contrast medium or injected dyes. New software now allows better readings on cold and moving patients.

Hypoxaemia has been shown to occur both during and after chest physiotherapy; awareness and careful monitoring are therefore important. A patient on a ventilator and on high inspired oxygen concentrations or positive end-expiratory pressure may become dangerously hypoxaemic during tracheal suctioning. Strategies to limit this risk include preoxygenation, the use of a sealed suction port (as used for fibreoptic bronchoscopy) and the use of closed suctioning units.

End-tidal CO_2

End-tidal CO_2 (ETCO$_2$) may be measured on an intubated patient. The method works by the principle of absorption of infrared light. A probe from the monitor is inserted into the ventilator circuit close to the end of the endotracheal tube. ETCO$_2$ correlates well with PCO_2 in normal lungs, but less well in diseased lungs (Clark et al 1992). It is used widely in anaesthesia and for the ventilation of head-injured patients, but its use in other contexts is less well defined.

In paediatric (especially neonatal) patients, transcutaneous PO_2 and PCO_2 measurements are practised in many centres. The transcutaneous electrode is fixed to the skin which it heats and makes permeable to gas transport. Local hyperaemia arterializes the capillary blood. Good correlation between transcutaneous and arterial measurements has been shown. However, transcutaneous measurements have been shown to be sensitive but not specific indicators of blood gas status as they may be influenced not only by the partial pressure of the gas but also by a reduction in cardiac output or local blood flow. They have not gained acceptance in adult critical care practice.

Invasive monitoring

This requires the use of an invasive catheter, which is inserted into an artery, a central vein, the pulmonary artery or, in some neurosurgical centres, the extradural space (for intracranial pressure (ICP) monitoring). The catheter is connected to a transducer which is in turn connected to a pressure monitor (Fig. 4.1). The monitor displays pressure waveforms and values on a real-time basis (Fig. 4.2). We have become accustomed to seeing these displays (often in a variety of bright colours) and usually blindly accept that each component of the system is working correctly and accurately; this is unhappily not always the case and we may be lulled into a false and dangerous sense of security. Inaccuracies may (and commonly do) occur from any one (or a combination) of the following.

● The catheter may be incorrectly positioned.

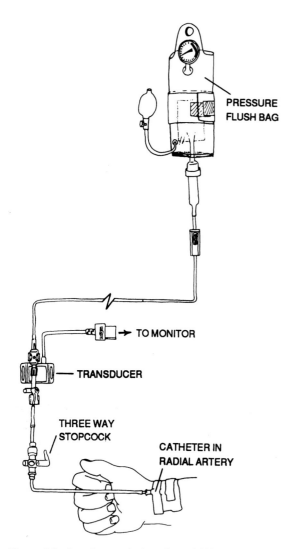

Figure 4.1   Invasive monitoring of arterial blood pressure.

- The catheter may be partially blocked or kinked.
- The connecting tubing may be partially blocked or kinked or it may allow too much resonance in the system, leading to exaggerated pressure waveforms (underdamping).
- The transducer may be faulty or incompatible with the other equipment.
- The monitor may be incorrectly calibrated.
- The pressure bag (which pressurizes the system for flushing and to prevent back flow) may not be properly inflated.

All these aspects of invasive pressure monitoring need to be checked regularly, especially if the readings do not correlate with the clinical appearance of the patient. In many cases, potentially harmful treatment has been instituted on the basis of totally incorrect information.

Common invasively monitored parameters include arterial blood pressure and central venous pressure (CVP). *Arterial cannulation* allows continuous monitoring of blood pressure as well as easy access for blood gas analysis. The radial artery on the non-dominant side is the most common site of insertion; other sites include brachial, dorsalis pedis and femoral arteries. The femoral artery is especially useful in states of shock, when peripheral pulses may be impalpable. The catheter is usually inserted percutaneously but may be introduced by surgical cut-down. Complications of arterial cannulation are uncommon and include infection and, rarely, thrombosis. Disconnection of the catheter from the line can easily occur with movement of the patient; vigorous bleeding will follow and exsanguination is a real risk. These lines should always therefore remain visible and care should be taken when moving the patient. Should disconnection occur, reconnection should be quickly performed; should displacement occur, firm pressure should be applied to the bleeding site.

CVP measurement involves placement of a catheter into a central vein (generally the superior vena cava), usually via the subclavian or internal jugular vein. The basilic, external jugular and femoral veins may also be used for access; the advantage of these sites is that there is no risk of pneumothorax and that bleeding is easier to control. Disadvantages of these routes include difficulty with accurate placement and a higher incidence of thrombosis. The CVP represents the state of filling of the vasculature and heart, more specifically the right side of the heart. If correctly interpreted, it can yield valuable diagnostic information and guide fluid therapy. The complications associated with all central venous catheters are not insubstantial: they include vascular erosion, air embolism, bleeding, thrombosis and infection. Again, disconnection can occur with movement. Bleeding will occur if the end of the

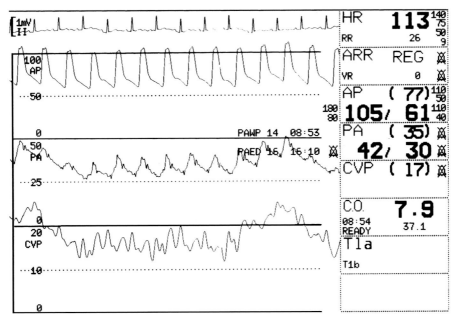

Figure 4.2   Display of pressure wave forms and ECG trace on monitor screen: HR, heart rate; ARR, arrhythmia monitoring; REG, regular; AP, arterial pressure; PA, pulmonary artery pressure; CVP, central venous pressure; CO, cardiac output.

catheter is below the level of the heart, while air may be sucked into the system and air embolism may result if the end of the catheter is above that level. Air embolism is a very serious event and can result in immediate collapse and death.

With a *pulmonary artery catheter*, pulmonary capillary wedge pressure (PCWP) may be monitored and cardiac output (CO) may be measured by means of the thermodilution technique. Systemic vascular resistance (SVR), pulmonary vascular resistance (PVR), oxygen delivery and oxygen consumption may also be calculated.

The pulmonary artery catheter is inserted via a central vein through the right side of the heart into the pulmonary artery. At its tip it has a balloon which is inflated when the catheter is in the heart and this allows the catheter to be carried through the heart chambers by the flow of blood (Fig. 4.3). When the inflated balloon occludes the pulmonary artery, the catheter no longer measures pulmonary artery pressure but PCWP. By a series of extrapolations, left atrial pressure and, therefore, left ventricular preload can be gauged (Fig. 4.4). This gives valuable information over and above CVP mea-

surement when the left and right sides of the heart are not functioning equally. The left heart alone may fail in anterior myocardial infarction and the right heart alone may fail in pulmonary embolism, cor pulmonale, pericardial constriction and right ventricular infarction. In all these settings, measurement of CVP alone may give totally misleading information about left ventricular filling. The interpretation of the PCWP is not always straightforward and has many pitfalls for the unwary (Raper & Sibbald 1986).

Measurement of cardiac output is an integral part of pulmonary artery catheterization. The resultant calculations of SVR, oxygen delivery and oxygen consumption give an enormous amount of information about the state of the heart and circulation. Manipulation of these variables by vasoactive drugs is useful in a variety of disease states, including sepsis, pulmonary oedema, adult respiratory distress syndrome and cardiogenic shock.

The use of pulmonary artery catheterization has been questioned (Connors et al 1996) and randomized controlled trials are in progress.

Left atrial pressure may be measured directly by means of a catheter inserted into the left atrium at the time of cardiac surgery. The catheter is brought out through the chest wall and monitoring takes place in the conventional way. All the above mentioned complications may occur; in addition, displacement may occasionally result in pericardial tamponade.

Intracranial pressure monitoring may be performed in patients with head injuries, brain surgery, intracranial and subarachnoid haemorrhage and cerebral oedema from other causes. However, the frequency of use of this technique depends on the enthusiasm of individual units. Such monitoring may give an indication of a rise in ICP before it becomes clinically evident, thus allowing therapeutic manoeuvres (hyperventilation, mannitol, surgery) to be initiated before cerebral damage occurs. The importance of ICP

measurement is that it provides an estimate of cerebral perfusion pressure (cerebral perfusion pressure = mean arterial pressure – ICP) which in turn relates to cerebral blood flow (CBF). Raised ICP causes reduced CBF which leads to tissue hypoxia and acidosis, raised PCO_2, cerebral vasodilatation and oedema, all of which cause a further rise in ICP.

ICP may be measured by means of an extradural or subarachnoid bolt, an intraventricular catheter (inserted through the skull into the lateral ventricle) or an epidural catheter. The former methods are the most widely used (Fig. 4.5). The intraventricular catheter has the additional advantage of being able to drain cerebrospinal fluid, thereby relieving raised ICP. More recently, a fibreoptic catheter is being used. It may be placed in any of the above spaces and is generally more robust and reliable. All these methods

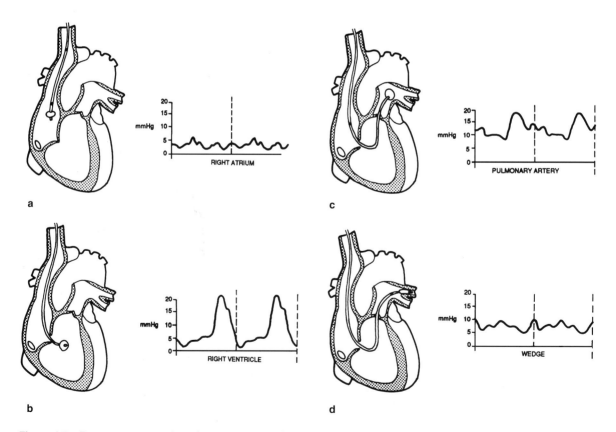

Figure 4.3 Pressure traces as the pulmonary artery catheter passes through the right side of the heart. **a** Right atrium. **b** Right ventricle. **c** Pulmonary artery. **d** Pulmonary capillary wedge pressure.

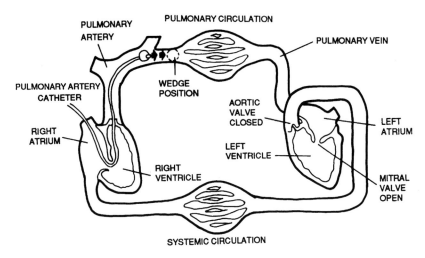

Figure 4.4   In diastole, with the mitral valve open, pulmonary capillary wedge pressure corresponds to left atrial pressure.

are invasive and the potential complications are not insignificant, the most serious being infection.

ECG monitoring

The more common arrhythmias are discussed below together with examples of ECG traces (Fig. 4.6). For further details on ECG monitoring refer to Chapter 3. Physiotherapy procedures may both cause arrhythmias (Hammon et al 1992) and worsen those already present. Great awareness and care are needed, especially in those patients at risk of developing arrhythmias.

1. *Sinus bradycardia* is a sinus rhythm below 60 beats/min. The common causes are drugs (e.g. beta-blockers) and hypoxaemia; bradycardia may be a warning sign that the latter is occurring and, as such, should be taken very seriously. Vagal stimuli from tracheal suctioning may also be implicated. Care with suctioning and generous preoxygenation may be necessary; occasionally it is reassuring to have atropine drawn up and ready to inject.
2. *Sinus tachycardia* is a sinus rhythm above 100 beats/min. Pain and anxiety are common causes, but occasionally it may be precipitated by haemodynamic instability or respiratory distress. Procedures should be carefully explained

to the patient and adequate analgesia should be given before physiotherapy begins.
3. *Atrial fibrillation* is a common arrhythmia in critically ill patients, especially after cardiac or thoracic surgery. It is a totally irregular rhythm that may reach a ventricular rate of up to 200 beats/min and cause haemodynamic instability. It may be paroxysmal. The cause is usually multifactorial, but common precipitating factors include hypokalaemia, hypoxaemia, dehydration or overhydration, ischaemic heart disease and cardiac surgery.

Patients at risk of developing arrhythmias often have ischaemic heart disease or a history of arrhythmias. However, critically ill patients may suddenly develop a rhythm disturbance, the cause of which is usually multifactorial. A patient may have recently had an arrhythmia (often of short duration) so it is vital to check the charts and to communicate with the doctors and nurses looking after the patient.

Most good monitoring systems today have memory capacity and can display past values on a minute-to-minute basis. Trends can be graphically displayed and analysed. A printer link may allow ECG or pressure traces to be printed and retained. Already in use in some centres are

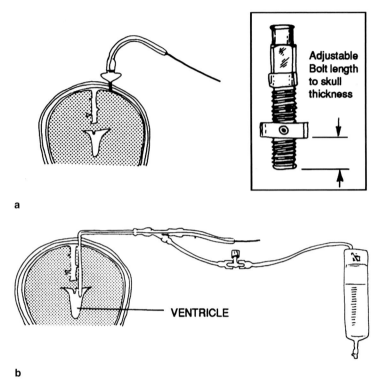

Adjustable
Bolt length
to skull
thickness

a

VENTRICLE

b

Figure 4.5 Intracerebral pressure monitoring. **a** Extradural or subarachnoid bolt. **b** Intraventricular catheter with cerebrospinal fluid drainage bag.

systems that utilize a specialized software package which enables the rapid recording, storage, display and reporting of a wide range of clinical data. Data are either downloaded directly from the patient monitors or entered manually. Hard copies of relevant data are produced using a printer. This system totally replaces nursing charts and is an extremely attractive option in terms of labour saving, accuracy, convenience and immediacy.

INTERPRETING MEDICAL INVESTIGATIONS

A number of blood and microbiological tests are regularly performed on patients in hospital, leading to an enormous amount of data which need to be responsibly interpreted (even when it is sometimes irresponsibly requested!). It is clearly vital to know the normal values for these tests, which abnormalities are important and which are not, and how to respond to any abnormalities which need treatment. The more commonly performed haematological, biochemical and microbiological tests are discussed with these issues in mind. Normal values depend on the test technique, the units in which the result is given and the local reference values.

Haematology

Full blood count

This is usually performed in an automated blood analyser which produces a printout of results. Included in most analysers are the following (the abbreviations given are commonly used).

Haemoglobin (Hb). Haemoglobin is the red oxygen-carrying pigment in red blood cells (RBCs). Its primary function is the transport

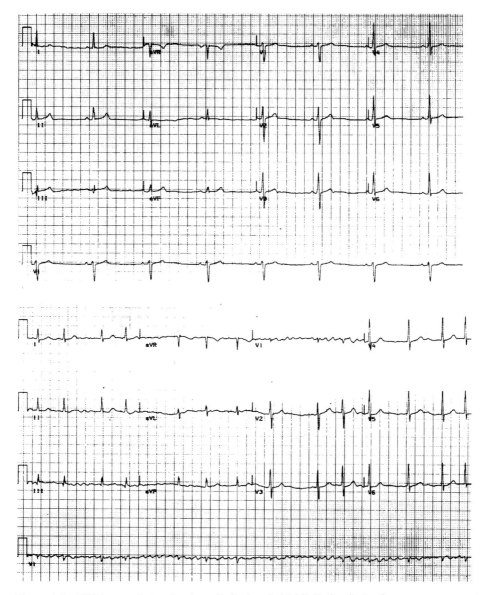

Figure 4.6 ECG traces of sinus bradycardia (top) and atrial fibrillation (bottom).

of oxygen. Hb is easy to measure (it can be measured in the ward with a Spencer haemoglobinometer) and is an indirect measure of the number of RBCs in the circulation and, therefore, of the total red cell mass. In states of dehydration or overhydration Hb may be falsely raised or lowered.

A reduced red cell mass is referred to as 'anaemia', while an increased red cell mass is known as 'polycythaemia' or 'erythrocytosis'. There are many causes of anaemia, but those most commonly seen are acute or chronic blood loss, iron deficiency and chronic illness or inflammation. Polycythaemia may be primary (from a disorder of the bone marrow) or secondary (due to chronic hypoxaemic lung disease or cyanotic heart disease, renal carcinoma, cerebellar haemangioblastoma or uterine fibroids).

Mean corpuscular volume (MCV). This is a measure of the size of the RBCs. A low MCV (small RBCs) is referred to as 'microcytosis': the most common cause is iron deficiency. A high MCV is referred to as 'macrocytosis' and is most often caused by vitamin B_{12} or folate deficiency. The MCV is useful in narrowing down the differential diagnosis of anaemia and other blood disorders.

Mean corpuscular haemoglobin (MCH). This is calculated by dividing the Hb by the total red cell count. It reflects the amount of Hb in the RBCs.

White cell count (WCC). The white blood cells, or leucocytes, perform a variety of functions in the body. Their major role is to defend the body against infection and their interaction in achieving this goal is remarkable. The neutrophils (the predominant type of leucocyte) perform the immediate response to infection by phagocytosing offending organisms. Lymphocytes are involved in the production of antibodies and play a pivotal role in both cell-mediated and humoral immunity. A certain subset of lymphocytes, known as CD4 cells, are destroyed by the human immunodeficiency virus (HIV). A CD4 count of less than 200 indicates particular susceptibility to opportunistic infections. The monocyte–macrophage cell line is also involved in immunity, primarily by processing antigens and presenting them to immunocompetent lymphocytes. They also have an important phagocytosing and scavenging function and incidentally play a role in the regulation of haematopoiesis.

The functions of eosinophils and basophils are poorly understood, but eosinophils seem to be important in the defence against parasitic infections and in allergic disorders.

Platelet count (Plt). Platelets circulate in the bloodstream as tiny discs less than half the size of RBCs and are an essential component in blood clotting. They are part of the first-line reaction to a breach in the vascular endothelium. A reduction in the platelet count is known as 'thrombocytopenia' while an increase is called 'thrombocytosis'. There are many causes for thrombocytopenia, but the common ones seen in critically ill patients include sepsis, disseminated intravascular coagulopathy, drug-

related causes, and consumption by dialysis machines or other extracorporeal circuits.

Differential count

This looks primarily at the white cells in the blood, but at the same time the morphology of the red blood cells and the platelets may be commented upon. A drop of blood is smeared smoothly across a glass slide; this is then stained and examined under a microscope. The different cells are counted in a high-power field and the numbers are given as a percentage. Absolute numbers of cells will thus depend upon the total white cell count. The differential count may be useful in diagnosis of specific infections or infiltrations, allergic or parasitic disorders and assessing immune status.

Clotting profile

This is generally performed in a patient who is either bleeding or at high risk of developing a bleeding problem. Indices measured include prothrombin time, partial thromboplastin time (PTT), platelets, fibrinogen and fibrin degradation products (FDPs). There is a wide variety of bleeding disorders with an even wider variety of causes; patients may be at risk for spontaneous haemorrhage or haemorrhage caused by minor trauma (and this may include physiotherapy procedures).

Prothrombin time and partial thromboplastin time measure the integrity of different limbs of the clotting cascade. The prothrombin time is now usually given as the ratio of measured time over control time, with international standardization of the reagents used: it is thus referred to as the 'international normalized ratio' (INR).

In acutely ill patients, there are two commonly found disorders of coagulation. First, a dilutional coagulopathy may occur from massive blood transfusions without the addition of clotting factors. The INR and PTT are prolonged and platelets and fibrinogen are reduced. Second, disseminated intravascular coagulopathy (DIC) may be caused by a wide variety of precipitating events, including sepsis, trauma and incompatible blood transfusions (Bick 1988). Clotting factors are consumed by inappropriate intravascular coagulation and there is thus a deficiency of them, which leads to bleeding. Again, INR and PTT are prolonged, platelets and fibrinogen are low (they may be extremely low) and FDPs are present in large amounts, representing the fibrinolysis (clot breakdown) that is taking place intravascularly.

Patients with a DIC or thrombocytopenia (especially when the platelet count is less than 20) may be at risk of pulmonary haemorrhage. Great care should be taken during suctioning and physiotherapy and the potential benefits should be weighed against this risk.

Biochemistry

Arterial blood gases

These not only give an indication of oxygenation and carbon dioxide clearance, but also of acid–base status. Most automated blood gas machines measure only pH, PO_2 and PCO_2 and extrapolate from these values the bicarbonate and oxygen saturation. These extrapolations are accurate under most circumstances, but oxygen saturation may be fallacious in the presence of carboxyhaemoglobin. Hypoxaemia (PaO_2 of less than 8 kPa or 60 mmHg at sea level) and hypercarbia ($PaCO_2$ of more than 6 kPa or 45 mmHg) are easy to recognize and their causes are not discussed here. The metabolic and respiratory causes of acidosis and alkalosis are a little more complex and may cause confusion.

In simple terms, in acidosis the pH is always low (normal pH is 7.36–7.44) and in alkalosis the pH is always high (remember that pH is an inverse and logarithmic expression of hydrogen ion concentration). Metabolic causes of acidosis and alkalosis involve a primary change of the bicarbonate concentration and respiratory causes involve a change of $PaCO_2$. The different disorders are discussed further below, a systematic approach to blood gases follows and some rather simplistic examples are given in Table 4.1.

Metabolic acidosis. This is probably the most serious acid–base disorder. It may be caused by either an excess of acid (lactate, ketoacids, metabolites or poisons) or a loss of bicarbonate by the small intestine or the kidneys. Lactate accumulates in states of inadequate oxygen delivery to the tissues; this is usually seen in shock of any cause. Ketoacids accumulate in diabetic ketoacidosis which is always associated with a raised blood glucose. Both lactate and ketoacids may be measured in the laboratory. In renal failure, tubular dysfunction reduces bicarbonate generation; in addition, there are unmeasured acidic anions in the blood and glomerular dysfunction leads to a reduction in the amount of sodium available for exchange with hydrogen ions. Poisons or drugs in overdose may be acidic, e.g. ethylene glycol and aspirin.

Compensation for the acidosis occurs by hyperventilation with a resultant fall in $PaCO_2$. This accounts for the deep sighing respiration (Kussmaul breathing) often seen in metabolic acidosis.

Treatment of metabolic acidosis is controversial. For many years bicarbonate was the mainstay of treatment, but evidence is now accumulating that its effects are mainly cosmetic and

Table 4.1 Examples of acid–base disturbances and the compensatory mechanisms

Disorder	pH	$PaCO_2$	Bicarbonate	Compensation
Metabolic acidosis	7.2	5	18	CO_2
Compensation	7.4	3	18	
Respiratory acidosis	7.2	8	26	Bicarbonate
Compensation	7.4	8	36	
Metabolic alkalosis	7.5	5	34	CO_2
Compensation	7.4	7	34	
Respiratory alkalosis	7.5	3	26	Bicarbonate
Compensation	7.4	3	20	

may be harmful (Cooper et al 1990). These include shifting the oxygen dissociation curve, thereby inhibiting the release of oxygen, causing hypernatraemia and hyperosmolarity and provoking an intracellular acidosis (Ritter et al 1990). It would seem that treatment of the cause of the acidosis should be the primary objective.

Respiratory acidosis. The primary problem is a raised $PaCO_2$. This is the result of alveolar hypoventilation, the cause of which may be inadequate minute volume (as in a weak or tired patient) or increased dead space (as in severe chronic obstructive airways disease). Often these occur in combination. Compensation occurs by an increase in plasma bicarbonate; this is done mainly by the kidneys, which increase bicarbonate reabsorption in the tubules.

The plasma bicarbonate level may be useful in differentiating acute from chronic respiratory acidosis. In the acute state bicarbonate is normal, while in the chronic state it is raised owing to the aforementioned compensatory mechanisms. This distinction may have important clinical consequences, for example in differentiating severe asthma from chronic lung disease.

Metabolic alkalosis. This may be caused by an excess of bicarbonate (always iatrogenic) or a loss of acid (either from the stomach or the kidneys). Acid may be lost from the stomach in cases of upper gastrointestinal tract obstruction or ileus; litres of fluid may be lost daily. The most common cause of acid loss by the kidneys is hypokalaemia. Here there is an inadequate amount of potassium ions available for exchange with sodium ions; hydrogen ions are sacrificed in their place.

Respiratory alkalosis. Here the primary problem is a low $PaCO_2$, which is always a result of hyperventilation. This may occur in a spontaneously breathing person who is anxious, in pain or has a respiratory disorder (causes include asthma, pneumonia, pulmonary embolus and adult respiratory distress syndrome). Rarely, neurological disorders (affecting the respiratory centre) will cause hyperventilation. It may also be seen in a mechanically ventilated patient who is being given too large a minute volume or who is tachypnoeic for any of the reasons mentioned above.

A systematic approach to blood gases follows. First look at the PaO_2. Determine whether it is normal or whether the patient is hypoxaemic. The PaO_2 is relatively independent of the other variables. Next look at the pH. Establish acidosis, alkalosis or normal. If abnormal, check if the problem relates to the $PaCO_2$ or the bicarbonate. It is sometimes said to be confusing as to which of these is the problem and which is the compensatory effect. It really is very easy. The one that correlates with the pH (i.e. acidosis, low bicarbonate) has to be the cause; the other is therefore the compensation (see examples in Table 4.1).

Electrolytes

Sodium and potassium are often measured as part of an automated biochemistry run, although many ICUs will have a separate electrolyte analyser that works on the principle of ion-selective electrodes. These analysers may be more accurate for potassium measurements than for sodium. Their advantage is obviously their immediacy.

Hyponatraemia has a variety of causes, but is more commonly caused by relative excess of water than deficiency of sodium. This is often iatrogenic, following excessive administration of hypotonic fluids. Another common cause is the syndrome of inappropriate antidiuretic hormone (ADH) secretion, in which ADH is secreted despite hypotonicity of the serum. The result is water retention and, thereby, hyponatraemia. The causes of this syndrome are numerous and include malignancies, pulmonary disorders and disturbances of central nervous system function. The treatment of hyponatraemia has been well described (Adrogue & Madias 2000).

Hypernatraemia is most often caused by water depletion. A true sodium excess is uncommon and is always iatrogenic. Both hyponatraemia and hypernatraemia may cause neurological signs ranging from confusion to coma.

Hypokalaemia, on the other hand, is potentially far more dangerous. It may predispose to cardiac arrhythmias, especially if combined with hypoxaemia. Hyperkalaemia may predispose to ventricular tachycardia and fibrillation. Physiotherapy treatment may have to be postponed until these abnormalities have been corrected.

Glucose

This needs to be regularly monitored in diabetics and in all critically ill patients. Blood glucose can easily be measured in the ward by means of reagent strips. A very high blood glucose level is almost always caused by diabetes mellitus or an intravenous infusion of high glucose content, while a slightly raised value may be caused by stress. The causes of a low blood glucose include starvation, liver failure (failure to produce glucose), insulin therapy or an insulin-secreting tumour.

Renal function tests

These include urea and creatinine. Urea is formed mainly from protein breakdown and creatinine mainly from muscle breakdown; there are obligatory amounts of both of these that need to be handled by the kidneys daily. If formation increases or excretion decreases, serum levels will rise. Renal failure causes both urea and creatinine to rise, though often at different rates. In hypovolaemic or low cardiac output states, urea rises more than creatinine, whilst in rhabdomyolysis (breakdown of skeletal muscle) creatinine rises faster than urea.

Liver function tests

Very few so-called 'liver function tests' actually measure liver function. Instead they simply represent the result of liver damage: raised enzymes reflect damage to cells and raised bilirubin may reflect a variety of abnormalities, not all of which actually occur in the liver.

Enzymes such as lactate dehydrogenase (LDH) and aspartate aminotransferase (AST) are not specific to liver tissue and even when they are produced by damaged liver cells, give little clue to the underlying pathology. Gamma glutamyl transferase (GGT) and alanine aminotransferase (ALT) are found in few other tissues, but again do not reflect causation. Alkaline phosphatase (ALP) is also not specific to liver cells, but that fraction which comes from the liver is concentrated in bile ducts and, as such, gives a clue to biliary disease or obstruction.

Bilirubin is a pigment that is produced from the breakdown of haem (from the haemoglobin in red blood cells). The liver takes up circulating bilirubin, conjugates it and excretes it in bile via the biliary tract. The clinical manifestation of a raised plasma bilirubin level is jaundice. In most hepatic disorders, both the conjugated and unconjugated fractions of bilirubin are raised. However, a predominantly unconjugated hyperbilirubinaemia (raised levels of unconjugated bilirubin in the blood) is often due to massive breakdown of red blood cells as in haemolysis or haematoma. Conjugated hyperbilirubinaemia is commonly seen in hepatitis or biliary tract obstruction; in the latter the classic clinical triad of dark urine, pale stools and pruritus is seen.

In critical illness, two distinct syndromes of liver dysfunction have been described (Hawker 1991). These are ischaemic hepatitis, occurring early and characterized by a massive rise in AST and ALT with only a slight rise in bilirubin, and ICU jaundice, which develops later, is part of the syndrome of multiple organ failure and is characterized by a progressive rise in bilirubin with only a slight enzyme rise.

Tests that reflect the synthetic capacity of the liver are more useful in determining actual liver function. Protein synthesis is one of the major functions of the liver; these proteins include clotting factors, albumin and globulins. Thus, measuring the INR (see above) and serum albumin can give a good idea of the synthetic function of the liver, provided there are no other reasons for these tests to be abnormal.

Cardiac enzymes

Enzymes are released by all damaged muscle cells. Cardiac enzyme estimations are therefore performed to confirm myocardial damage, usually caused by a myocardial infarct but occasionally caused by chest trauma. There is a characteristic pattern of enzyme rise, with creatine kinase (CK) rising first, followed by AST and then

LDH. For more specificity, isoenzymes (specific fractions of the enzymes) of CK and LDH may be measured. CK is also present in skeletal muscle, so the myocardial fraction (MB fraction) is measured to exclude skeletal muscle damage (from surgery, trauma or intramuscular injections) as a source. More recently, the enzymes specific to cardiac tissue have been used together. These include troponin T and I, CK-MB and myoglobin.

Electrical cardioversion has been said to cause CK (and specifically the MB fraction) to rise. This may be important in determining whether a patient has had a myocardial infarct. The evidence is that measurable myocardial damage rarely follows cardioversion and that when CK-MB is raised, the elevation is small.

Microbiology

Introduction

Infection control is becoming more and more important as more nasty and often antibiotic-resistant organisms are seen in hospitals, especially in ICUs. The importance of hand washing between going from one patient to another cannot be overemphasized. This is the simplest and still the most effective method of preventing cross-infection. Organisms such as methicillin-resistant *Staphylococcus aureus* (MRSA) and more recently vancomycin-resistant *enterococcus* (VRE) are becoming major problems in hospitals and have even caused closure of specialized units. In ICUs, Gram-negative organisms such as *pseudomonas* and *acinetobacter* have become particular problems, becoming impossible to eradicate.

Blood cultures

These are usually taken when the patient is pyrexial, in an attempt to isolate microorganisms which may be present in the bloodstream. The blood is drawn (usually from a forearm vein) in strictly aseptic conditions, placed in a special culture medium, incubated at 37°C and then cultured in the laboratory. A positive result is almost always of serious consequence, although contaminants may occur, usually from poor aseptic technique. A positive blood culture does not identify the site of sepsis, although the type of organism cultured may give a clue. The source of the sepsis needs to be found and dealt with in its own right.

Sputum/tracheal aspirate

Sputum is produced when a non-intubated patient coughs up pulmonary secretions, while a tracheal aspirate is a suctioned specimen from an endotracheal tube or tracheostomy. There is always a risk that a sputum specimen may contain mainly saliva and that it may be contaminated by oral organisms. Tracheal aspirates, on the other hand, represent the microflora of the lower airways and are much less likely to be contaminated, although after prolonged mechanical ventilation the tracheobronchial tree is often colonized by oral organisms. Physiotherapists are often requested to obtain these specimens, upon which future treatment may be based, and great care should be taken to get adequate and representative samples.

Newer methods of obtaining uncontaminated specimens which accurately reflect the microbiology of a specific lung segment include protected specimen brushing with quantitative colony counts and bronchoalveolar lavage (Chastre et al 1995).

A sputum or tracheal aspirate specimen is stained with Gram's stain, examined under a microscope and cultured. Antibiotic sensitivities are performed on a positive culture. One must be aware that the presence of organisms on tracheal aspirate may not be indicative of pulmonary infection, but may simply represent colonization. To make the diagnosis of pulmonary infection (and, therefore, to start antibiotics) one needs to have most of the following criteria: purulent secretions, white blood cells on Gram's stain of tracheal aspirate, organisms on culture of tracheal aspirate, fever, raised white blood cell count, infiltrates on the chest radiograph and a reduction in PaO_2.

Community-acquired pneumonia has been well studied in many countries and the organisms accounting for most cases have been established.

Streptococcus pneumoniae is the commonest organism by far, followed by *Mycoplasma pneumoniae* (in epidemics) and influenza virus. The logical antibiotic management of community-acquired pneumonia is regularly revised.

Diagnosis of pneumonia in a patient already on a ventilator is often much more difficult, although some of the newer diagnostic methods mentioned above are useful (Meduri 1995). Clinical judgement may still be necessary to differentiate colonization from infection.

Swabs and specimens from other sites

These may be taken from superficial wounds or from deep sites. Positive superficial cultures may represent skin colonization, so it is important to look for local (redness, pus) and systemic (pyrexia, raised white blood cell count) evidence of sepsis before starting antibiotic therapy. Local therapy with frequent cleaning and dressings is

usually all that is required for superficial sepsis. Specimens obtained from needle aspiration or during operative procedures (i.e. from the abdominal cavity or chest) are not likely to represent colonization and such infections cannot be treated topically – surgical drainage and antibiotic therapy are needed.

Urine

Urine specimens may be contaminated with perineal flora, so they are either taken by a midstream urine collection with strict attention to aseptic technique or from a urinary catheter. The urine is spun down in a centrifuge and then stained, examined and cultured in the same way as sputum. Although patients with long-term indwelling urinary catheters may develop bacterial bladder colonization with no clinicalconsequence, in other patients urinary tract infections may be a considerable source of morbidity.

REFERENCES

Adrogue HJ, Madias NE 2000 Hyponatremia. New England Journal of Medicine 342: 1581–1589

Bick RL 1988 Disseminated intravascular coagulation and related syndromes: a clinical review. Seminars in Thrombosis and Haemostasis 14: 299–338

Chastre J, Fagon JY, Bornet-Lesco M et al 1995 Evaluation of bronchoscopic techniques for the diagnosis of nosocomial pneumonia. American Journal of Respiratory and Critical Care Medicine 152: 231–240

Clark JS, Votteri B, Ariagno RL et al 1992 State of the art. Noninvasive assessment of blood gases. American Review of Respiratory Disease 145: 220–232

Connors AF, Speroff T, Dawson NV et al 1996 The effectiveness of right heart catheterisation in the initial care of critically ill patients. Journal of the American Medical Association 276: 889–897

Cooper DJ, Walley KR, Wiggs BR, Russell JA 1990 Bicarbonate does not improve haemodynamics in critically ill patients who have lactic acidosis. Annals of Internal Medicine 112: 492–498

Hammon WE, Connors AF, McCaffree DR 1992 Cardiac arrhythmias during postural drainage and chest percussion of critically ill patients. Chest 102: 1836–1841

Hawker F 1991 Liver dysfunction in critical illness. Anaesthesia and Intensive Care 19: 165–181

Meduri GU 1995 Diagnosis and differential diagnosis of ventilator-associated pneumonia. Clinics in Chest Medicine 16: 61–94

Raper R, Sibbald WJ 1986 Misled by the wedge? The Swan–Ganz catheter and left ventricular preload. Chest 89: 427–434

Ritter JM, Doktor HS, Benjamin N 1990 Paradoxical effect of bicarbonate on cytoplasmic pH. Lancet 335: 1243–1246

5

Effects of positioning and mobilization

Elizabeth Dean

INTRODUCTION

The purpose of this chapter is to provide a framework for clinical decision making in the management of patients with cardiopulmonary dysfunction with special emphasis on positioning and mobilization. 'Cardiopulmonary dysfunction' refers to impairment of one or more steps in the oxygen transport pathway. First, the oxygen transport pathway and the factors that contribute to impairment of oxygen transport are described. Second, three clinically significant effects of positioning and mobilization are distinguished:

- to improve oxygen transport in acute cardiopulmonary dysfunction
- to improve oxygen transport in the post-acute and chronic stages of cardiopulmonary dysfunction
- to prevent the negative effects of restricted mobility, particularly those that adversely affect oxygen transport.

In addition, the physiological and scientific rationale for use of positioning and mobilization for each of the above effects is described. Conceptualizing cardiopulmonary dysfunction as impairment of the steps in the oxygen transport pathway and exploiting positioning and mobilization as primary interventions in remediating this impairment will maximize physiotherapy efficacy. Emphasis is placed on impairment of oxygen transport given that such impairment in large part determines disability and handicap (Verbrugge & Lette 1993), as defined by the World Health Organization (1980), secondary to cardiopulmonary dysfunction.

The following terms (Ross & Dean 1989) have been adopted in this chapter.

1. *Positioning* refers to the application of body positioning to optimize oxygen transport, primarily by manipulating the effect of gravity on cardiopulmonary and cardiovascular function.
2. *Mobilization and exercise* refer to the application of progressive exercise to elicit acute cardiopulmonary and cardiovascular responses to enhance oxygen transport. In the context of cardiopulmonary physiotherapy, 'mobilization' refers to low-intensity exercise for typically acutely ill patients or those with severely compromised functional work capacity.
3. *Optimizing oxygen transport* is the goal of positioning and mobilization. The 'adaptation' or 'training-sensitive' zone defines the upper and lower limits of the various indices of oxygen transport needed to elicit the optimal adaptation of the steps in the oxygen transport pathway. This zone is based on an analysis of the factors that contribute to cardiopulmonary dysfunction and thus is specific for each patient.

CONCEPTUAL FRAMEWORK FOR CLINICAL DECISION MAKING

The oxygen transport pathway

Optimal cardiopulmonary function and gas exchange reflect the optimal matching of oxygen demand and supply (Dantzker 1983, Weber et al 1983). Oxygen delivery and oxygen consumption based on demand are essential components of the oxygen transport system. Figure 5.1 shows the components of oxygen delivery ($\dot{D}O_2$), namely arterial oxygen content and cardiac output (CO) and the components of oxygen consumption ($\dot{V}O_2$), namely the arteriovenous oxygen content difference and CO. In health, $\dot{D}O_2$ is approximately fourfold greater than $\dot{V}O_2$ at rest so there is considerable oxygen reserve that is drawn upon during times of increased metabolic demand such as exercise, stress, illness and repair. Because of the large reserve, $\dot{V}O_2$ is thought to be normally supply independent. This reserve capacity, however, becomes compro-

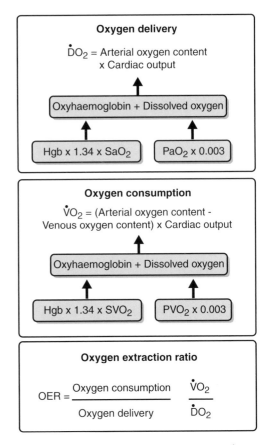

Figure 5.1 The components of oxygen delivery ($\dot{D}O_2$) and oxygen consumption ($\dot{V}O_2$).

mised secondary to acute and chronic pathological conditions. In critically ill patients in whom DO_2 is severely compromised, $\dot{V}O_2$ may be supply dependent until DO_2 reaches a critical threshold, i.e. the level at which metabolic demands are met (Phang & Russell 1993). Below this critical threshold, patients are increasingly dependent on anaerobic metabolism reflected by increased minute ventilation, respiratory exchange ratio and serum lactate levels.

The efficiency with which oxygen is transported from the atmosphere along the steps of the oxygen transport pathway to the tissues determines the efficiency of oxygen transport overall (Fig. 5.2). The steps in the oxygen transport pathway include ventilation of the alveoli, diffusion of oxygen across the alveolar capillary membrane, perfusion

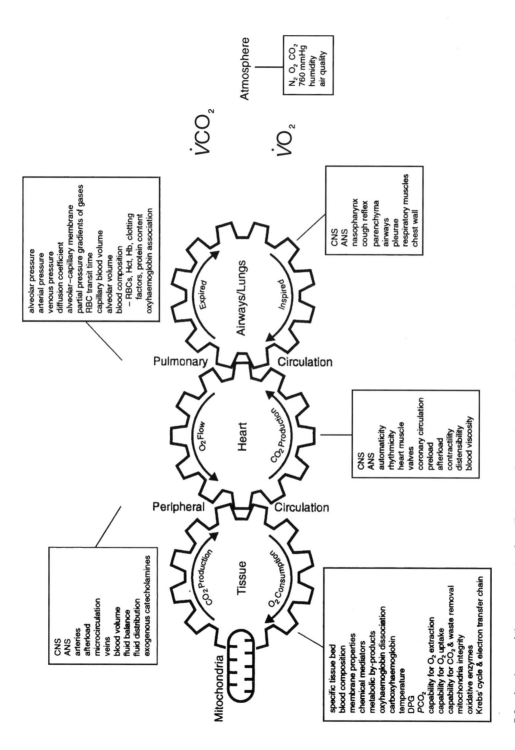

Figure 5.2 A scheme of the components of ventilatory–cardiovascular–metabolic coupling underlying oxygen transport modified from Wasserman et al (1987). CNS, central nervous system; ANS, autonomic nervous system; DPG, diphosphoglycerate; RBC, red blood cell; Hct, haematocrit; Hb, haemoglobin.

of the lungs, biochemical reaction of oxygen with the blood, affinity of oxygen with haemoglobin, cardiac output, integrity of the peripheral circulation and oxygen extraction at the tissue level (Johnson 1973, Wassermann et al 1987). At rest, the demand for oxygen reflects basal metabolic requirements. Metabolic demand changes normally in response to gravitational (positional), exercise and psychological stressors. When one or more steps in the oxygen transport pathway is impaired secondary to cardiopulmonary dysfunction, oxygen demand at rest and in response to stressors can be increased significantly. Impairment of one step in the pathway may be compensated by other steps, thereby maintaining normal gas exchange and arterial oxygenation. With severe impairment involving several steps, arterial oxygenation may be reduced, the work of the heart and lungs increased, tissue oxygenation impaired and, in the most extreme situation, multiorgan system failure may ensue.

While the oxygen transport pathway ensures that an adequate supply of oxygen meets the demands of the working tissues, the carbon dioxide pathway ensures that carbon dioxide, a primary byproduct of metabolism, is eliminated. This pathway is basically the reverse of the oxygen transport pathway in that carbon dioxide is transported from the tissues via the circulation to the lungs for elimination. Carbon dioxide is a highly diffusible gas and is readily eliminated from the body. However, carbon dioxide retention is a hallmark of diseases in which the ventilatory muscle pump is operating inefficiently or the normal elastic recoil of the lung parenchyma is lost.

Factors contributing to cardiopulmonary dysfunction

Cardiopulmonary dysfunction, in which oxygen transport is threatened or impaired, results from four principal factors: the underlying disease pathophysiology, bedrest/recumbency and restricted mobility, extrinsic factors imposed by the patient's medical care and intrinsic factors relating to the patient (Box 5.1) (Dean 1993a, Dean & Ross 1992a). An analysis of

---

Box 5.1 Factors contributing to cardiopulmonary dysfunction, i.e. factors that compromise or threaten oxygen transport (adapted from Dean 1993a, Dean & Ross 1992a and Ross & Dean 1992)

- **Cardiopulmonary pathophysiology**
  Acute
  Chronic – primary
         – secondary
  Acute and chronic

- **Bedrest/recumbency and restricted mobility**

- **Extrinsic factors**
  Reduced arousal
  Surgical procedures
  Incisions
  Dressings and bindings
  Casts/splinting devices/traction
  Invasive lines/catheters
  Monitoring equipment
  Medications
  Intubation
  Mechanical ventilation
  Suctioning
  Pain
  Anxiety
  Hospital admission

- **Intrinsic factors**
  Age
  Gender
  Ethnicity
  Congenital abnormalities
  Smoking history
  Occupation
  Air quality
  Obesity
  Nutritional deficits
  Deformity
  Fluid and electrolyte balance
  Conditioning level
  Impaired immunity
  Anaemia/polycythaemia
  Thyroid abnormalities
  Multisystem complications
  Previous medical and surgical history

---

those factors that contribute to cardiopulmonary dysfunction provides the basis for assessment and prescribing the parameters of positioning and mobilization to enhance oxygen transport for a given patient. The treatment is directed at the specific underlying contributing factors. In some cases, e.g. low haemoglobin, the underlying impairment of oxygen transport cannot be affected directly by physical intervention. However, mobilization and exercise can improve aerobic capacity in patients with anaemia, a factor not directly modifiable by non-invasive physiotherapy interventions, by increasing the efficiency of other steps in the oxygen transport pathway (Williams 1995). Further, even though some factors are not directly modifiable by non-invasive physio–therapy interventions, they influence treatment outcome and thus need to be considered when planning, modifying and progressing treatment.

Multisystem organ dysfunction and failure may lead to or result from cardiopulmonary dys-function; thus they are associated with significant mortality and morbidity. In these conditions, multiple factors impair multiple steps in the oxygen transport pathway so identifying which steps are affected and amenable to physiotherapy interventions is central to optimal treatment outcome (Dean & Frownfelter 1996).

THERAPEUTIC EFFECTS OF POSITIONING AND MOBILIZATION

To improve oxygen transport in acute cardiopulmonary dysfunction

Positioning and mobilization have profound acute effects on cardiovascular and cardiopulmonary function and hence on oxygen transport (Table 5.1). These effects translate into improved gas exchange overall: reduction in the fraction of inspired oxygen, pharmacological and ventilatory support (Burns & Jones 1975, Dean 1985, Svanberg 1957). Such effects need to be exploited in the management of acute cardiopulmonary dysfunc-tion with the use of positioning and mobilization as *primary* treatment interventions to enhance oxygen transport and as between-treatment inter-ventions (Dean & Ross 1992b, Ross & Dean 1992). The physiotherapist's role is to prescribe these

Table 5.1   Acute effects of upright positioning and mobilization on oxygen transport (adapted from Dean & Ross (1992a) and Imle & Klemic (1989))

Systemic response	Stimulus	
	Positioning (supine to upright)	Mobilization
Cardiopulmonary	↑ Total lung capacity ↑ Tidal volume ↑ Vital capacity ↑ Functioning residual capacity ↑ Residual volume ↑ Expiratory reserve volume ↑ Forced expiratory volumes ↑ Forced expiratory flows ↑ Lung compliance ↓ Airway resistance ↓ Airway closure ↑ PaO_2 ↑ AP diameter of chest ↓ Lateral diameter of rib cage and abdomen Altered pulmonary blood flow distribution ↓ Work of breathing ↑ Diaphragmatic excursion ↑ Mobilization of secretions	↑ Alveolar ventilation ↑ Tidal volume ↑ Breathing frequency ↑ A–aO_2 gradient ↑ Pulmonary arteriovenous shunt ↑ $\dot{V}_A/\dot{Q}$ matching ↑ Distension and recruitment of lung units with low ventilation and low perfusion ↑ Mobilization of secretions ↑ Pulmonary lymphatic drainage ↑ Surfactant production and distribution
Cardiovascular	↑ Total blood volume ↓ Central blood volume ↓ Central venous pressure ↓ Pulmonary vascular congestion ↑ Lymphatic drainage ↓ Work of the heart	↑ Cardiac output ↑ Stroke volume and heart rate ↑ Oxygen binding in blood ↑ Oxygen dissociation and extraction at the tissue level

AP, anteroposterior; ↑, increases; ↓, decreases.

interventions judiciously to optimize gas exchange and oxygen transport overall. This role is distinct from *routine* positioning and mobilization often performed jointly by the physiotherapy and nursing staff. The aim of routine positioning and mobilization is primarily to reduce the adverse effects of restricted mobility including pulmonary complications, bedsores and contractures.

To simulate the normal 'physiologic' body position, the primary goal of physiotherapy is to get the patient upright and moving. Mobilization and exercise are the most physiologic and potent interventions to optimize oxygen transport and aerobic capacity and so need to be exploited with every patient. Body positioning, however, is discussed in this chapter first because a patient cannot be in a position uninfluenced by gravity. Furthermore, a patient's oxygen transport status reflects the body position assumed regardless of whether the position is part of a treatment regimen, a routine positioning regimen or assumed randomly by the patient.

Positioning

Physiological and scientific rationale. The distributions of ventilation ($\dot{V}_A$), perfusion ($\dot{Q}$) and ventilation and perfusion matching in the lungs are primarily influenced by gravity and therefore body position (Clauss et al 1968, West 1962, 1977). The intrapleural pressure becomes less negative down the upright lung. Thus, the apices have a greater initial volume and reduced compliance than do the bases. Because the bases are more compliant in this position, they exhibit greater volume changes during ventilation. In addition to these gravity-dependent interregional differences in lung volume, ventilation is influenced by intraregional differences which are dependent on regional mechanical differences in the compliance of the lung parenchyma and the resistance to airflow in the airways. Perfusion increases down the upright lung such that the $\dot{V}_A/\dot{Q}$ ratio in the apices is disproportionately high compared with that in the bases. Ventilation and perfusion matching is optimal in the mid-lung region. Manipulating body position, however, alters both interregional and intraregional determinants of ventilation and perfusion and their matching. When choosing specific positions to enhance arterial oxygenation for a given patient, one needs to consider the underlying pathophysiology impairing cardiopulmonary function, the effects of bed rest/recumbency and restricted mobility, extrinsic factors related to the patient's care and intrinsic factors related to the patient.

Although the negative effects of the supine position have been well documented for several decades (Dean & Ross 1992b, Dripps & Waters 1941), supine or recumbent positions are frequently assumed by patients in hospital. These positions are non-physiologic and are associated with significant reductions in lung volumes and flow rates and increased work of breathing (Craig et al 1971, Hsu & Hickey 1976). The decrease in functional residual capacity (FRC) contributes to closure of the dependent airways and reduced arterial oxygenation (Ray et al 1974). This effect is accentuated in older persons (Leblanc et al 1970), patients with cardiopulmonary disease (Fowler 1949), patients with abdominal pathology, smokers and obese individuals.

The haemodynamic consequences of the supine position are also remarkable. The gravity-dependent increase in central blood volume may precipitate vascular congestion, reduced compliance and pulmonary oedema (Blomqvist & Stone 1983, Sjostrand 1951). The commensurate increase in stroke volume increases the work of the heart (Levine & Lown 1952). Within 6 hours, a compensatory diuresis can lead to a loss of circulating blood volume and orthostatic intolerance, i.e. haemodynamic intolerance to the upright position. Bed rest reconditioning has been attributed to this reduction in blood volume and the impairment of the volume-regulating mechanisms rather than physical deconditioning per se (Hahn-Winslow 1985). Thus, the upright position is essential to maximize lung volumes and flow rates and this position is the only means of optimizing fluid shifts such that the circulating blood volume and the volume-regulating mechanisms are maintained. The upright position coupled with movement is necessary to promote normal fluid regulation and balance (Lamb et al 1964).

The upright position is a potent stimulus to the sympathetic nervous system. This is an important effect clinically which offsets impaired blood volume and pressure-regulating mechanisms secondary to recumbency (Hahn-Winslow 1985). Stimulation of the sympathetic nervous system has been reported to augment the effects of potent sympathomimetic pharmacological agents such that the dosages of these drugs can be reduced (Warren et al 1983). The reduction or elimination of sympathomimetic drugs is an important outcome of non-invasive physiotherapy interventions.

Side-to-side positioning is frequently used in the clinical setting. If applied in response to assessment rather than routinely (Chuley et al 1982), the benefits derived from such positioning can be enhanced. Adult patients with unilateral lung disease may derive greater benefit when the affected lung is uppermost (Remolina et al 1981). Markedly improved gas exchange without deleterious haemodynamic effects has been reported for patients with severe hypoxaemia secondary to pneumonia (Dreyfuss et al 1992). Arterial oxygen tension is increased secondary to improved ventilation of the unaffected lung when this lung is dependent. Patients with uniformly distributed bilateral lung disease may derive greater benefit when the right lung is lowermost (Zack et al 1974). In this case, arterial oxygen tension is increased secondary to improved ventilation of the right lung, which may reflect the increased size of the right lung compared with the left and that, in this position, the heart and adjacent lung tissue are subjected to less compression. Improved gas exchange through non-invasive interventions can reduce or eliminate the need for supplemental oxygen which are primary treatment outcomes. Although various studies have shown beneficial effects of side lying, positioning should be based on multiple considerations including the distribution of disease if optimal results are to be obtained.

The prone position has long been known to have considerable physiological justification in patients with cardiopulmonary compromise (Douglas et al 1977), even those who are critically ill with acute respiratory failure (Bittner et al 1996,

Chatte et al 1997, Mure et al 1997) and patients with trauma-induced adult respiratory distress syndrome (Friedrich et al 1996). The beneficial effects of the prone position on arterial oxygenation may reflect improved lung compliance secondary to stabilization of the anterior chest wall, tidal ventilation, diaphragmatic excursion, FRC and reduced airway closure (Dean 1985, Pelosi et al 1998). In a dog model of acute lung injury, however, improved PaO_2 in prone has been attributed to a reduced shunt fraction (Albert et al 1987). A variant of the prone position, prone abdomen free, has shown additional benefits over prone abdomen restricted. In the prone abdomen-free position, the patient is positioned such that the movement of the abdomen is unencumbered by the bed. This can be achieved either by raising the patient's body in relation to the bed so that the abdomen falls free or by using a bed with a hole cut out at the level of the abdomen. Despite compelling evidence to support the prone position, it may be poorly tolerated in some patients or may be contraindicated in haemodynamically unstable patients. In these situations, intermediate positions approximating prone may produce many of the beneficial effects and minimize any potential hazard.

Positioning for drainage of pulmonary secretions may be indicated in some patients (Kirilloff et al 1985). Historically, these positions have been based on the anatomical arrangement of the bronchopulmonary segments to facilitate drainage of a particular segment. The bronchiole to the segment of interest is positioned perpendicular to facilitate drainage with the use of gravity. The efficacy of postural drainage compared with deep breathing and coughing induced with mobilization/exercise and repositioning of the patient has not been established. However, the fact that mobilization impacts on more steps in the oxygen transport pathway including the airways, to effect secretion clearance, supports the exploitation of mobilization coupled with deep breathing manoeuvres and coughing as a *primary* treatment intervention.

Physiotherapists need to consider two aspects of body positioning when the goal is to optimize oxygen transport. One is to select and apply specific body positions based on the patient's presentation, laboratory test results and radiographic imaging. The other is to elicit physiologic 'stir-up' (Dean 1996a, Dripps & Waters 1941). The purpose is to effect the normal gravitational stress on cardiopulmonary and cardiovascular function that is experienced in health. This is best simulated if patients are changed from one extreme position to another, e.g. supine to prone or upright, rather than from half to full side lying which is associated with a lesser 'stir-up' effect. Haemodynamically unstable patients, however, require greater monitoring during extreme position changes and may not tolerate some position changes well. Thus, based on assessment and patient response, frequent extreme position changes may be preferable to minimal shifts in body position in order to optimize cardiovascular, pulmonary and haemodynamic function.

Assessment and treatment planning. Body positioning, i.e. the specific positions selected, the duration of time spent in each position and the frequency with which the position is assumed, is based on a consideration of the factors that contribute to cardiopulmonary dysfunction, and treatment response. Understanding of the physi-

ology of cardiopulmonary and cardiovascular function and the effects of disease highlights certain positions that are theoretically ideal. However, these positions need to be modified or may be contraindicated for a given patient, based on other considerations (see Box 5.1). For example, if extreme positional changes are contraindicated, small degrees of positional rotation performed frequently can have significant benefit on gas exchange and arterial oxygenation. A three-quarters prone position may produce favourable results when the full prone position is contraindicated or is not feasible. This modification may simulate the prone abdomen-free position which has been shown to augment the effect of the traditional prone abdomen-restricted position (Douglas et al 1977). Furthermore, a three-quarters prone position may be particularly beneficial in patients with obese or swollen abdomens who may not tolerate other variations of the prone position. With attention to the patient's condition, invasive lines and leads and appropriate monitoring, a patient can be aggressively positioned (Fig. 5.3).

The time which a patient spends in a position and the frequency with which that position is assumed over a period of time are based on the

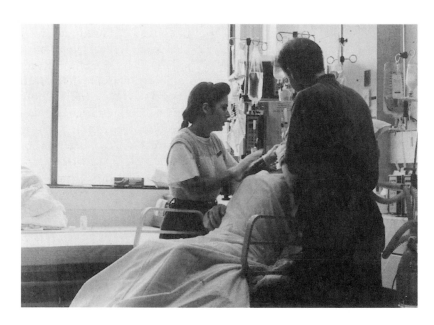

Figure 5.3 Positioning a critically ill patient may require several people and continual monitoring of the patient's response. Even though a position (particularly an upright position) may only be tolerated for a short period of time, the physiological benefits are considerable.

indications for the position and treatment outcome. Objective measures of the various steps that are compromised in the oxygen transport pathway as well as indices of oxygen transport overall are used in making these decisions. Subjective evaluation based on clinical judgement also has a role. A specific position can be justified, provided there is objective and subjective evidence of improvement. Signs and symptoms of deterioration need to be monitored so that deleterious positions can be avoided and deterioration secondary to excessive time in any one position can be detected. Prolonged duration in any single position will inevitably lead to compromise of the function of dependent lung zones and impaired gas exchange.

The ratio of treatment to between-treatment time is low. Typically, between-treatment time consists of some combination of positioning and mobilization. Positioning and mobilizing patients between treatments may be incorporated as an extension of treatment. Patients require monitoring and observation during these periods, as well as treatments. Between-treatment time may incorporate the use of maximally restful positions that do not compromise oxygen transport. Lastly, patients are positioned and mobilized between treatments to prevent the negative effects of restricted mobility and recumbency.

Special consideration (e.g. with respect to specific positioning and the use of supports) needs to be given to positioning patients who are comatose or paralysed because their joints and muscles are relatively unprotected and prone to trauma. Positions need to be selected that avoid injury to unprotected head, neck and limbs.

Progression. Progression of positioning involves new positions or modification of previous positions and modification of the duration spent in each position and the frequency with which each position is assumed over a period of time. These clinical decisions are based on the factors that contribute to cardiopulmonary dysfunction and objective and subjective indices of change in the patient's cardiopulmonary status. With improvement in cardiopulmonary status, the patient spends more time in erect positions and is mobilized more frequently and independently.

Mobilization

Physiological and scientific rationale. Compared with long-term exercise, the mechanisms underlying adaptation of the oxygen transport system to acute exercise, i.e. from session to session and day to day, are less well understood. However, although these mechanisms have yet to be elucidated, the responses to acute exercise are well documented. The acute response to mobilization/exercise reflects a commensurate increase in oxygen transport to provide oxygen to the working muscles and other organs. The increase is dependent on the intensity of the mobilization/exercise stimulus. The demand for oxygen and oxygen consumption ($\dot{V}O_2$) increases as exercise continues, with commensurate increases in minute ventilation ($\dot{V}_E$), i.e. the amount of air inhaled per minute, cardiac output and oxygen extraction at the tissue level. Relatively low intensities of mobilization can have a direct and profound effect on oxygen transport in patients with acute cardiopulmonary dysfunction (Dean & Ross 1992a, Dull & Dull 1983, Lewis 1980) and need to be instituted early after the initial pathological insult (Orlava 1959, Wenger 1982). The resulting exercise hyperpnoea, i.e. the increase in $\dot{V}_E$, is effected by an increase in tidal volume and breathing frequency. In addition, ventilation and perfusion matching is augmented by the distension and recruitment of lung zones with low ventilation and low perfusion. Spontaneous exercise-induced deep breaths are associated with improved flow rates and mobilization of pulmonary secretions (Wolff et al 1977). In clinical populations, these effects elicit spontaneous coughing. When mobilization is performed in the upright position, the anteroposterior diameter of the chest wall assumes a normal configuration compared with the recumbent position in which the anteroposterior diameter is reduced and the transverse diameter is increased. In addition, diaphragmatic excursion is favoured, flow rates augmented and coughing is mechanically facilitated. The work of breathing may be reduced with caudal displacement of the diaphragm and the work of the heart is minimized by the displacement of fluid away from the central circulation to the legs. Thus, despite increased metabolic demands of mobilization and exercise, the goal is to ensure that this increased demand is not wasteful and the demand can be met by the supply.

With respect to cardiovascular effects, acute mobilization/exercise increases CO by increasing stroke volume and heart rate. This is associated with increased blood pressure and increased coronary and peripheral muscle perfusion.

Passive movement of the limbs may stimulate deep breaths and heart function (West 1995). There is little scientific evidence, however, to support any additional benefit from various facilitation techniques (Bethune 1975). Thus, time allocated to the use of passive manoeuvres may compete with time for positioning and mobilization, i.e. interventions with demonstrated clinical efficacy. Although passive movements have a relatively small effect on cardiopulmonary function, they have several important benefits for neuromuscular and musculoskeletal function which support their use provided they do not replace active movement.

Assessment and treatment planning. For practical and ethical considerations, the mobilization plan for the patient with acute cardiopulmonary dysfunction cannot be based on a standardized exercise test, as is the case for patients with chronic conditions. However, response to a mobilization/exercise stimulus can be assessed during a mobilization challenge test, i.e. during the patient's routine activities such as turning or moving in bed, activities of daily living or responding to routine nursing and medical procedures (Dean 1996b). Comparable to prescribing exercise for the patient with chronic cardiopulmonary dysfunction, the parameters are specifically defined so that the stimulus is optimally therapeutic. The optimal stimulus is that which stresses the oxygen transport capacity of the patient and effects the greatest adaptation without deterioration or distress.

To promote adaptation of the steps in the oxygen transport pathway to the stimulation of acute mobilization, the stimulus is administered in a comparable manner to that in an exercise programme prescribed for chronic cardiopulmonary dysfunction. The components include a pre-exercise period, a warm-up period, a steady-state period, a cool-down period and a recovery period (Blair et al 1988). These components optimize the response to exercise by preparing the cardiopulmonary and cardiovascular systems for steady-state exercise and by permitting these systems to reestablish resting conditions following exercise. The cool-down period, in conjunction with the recovery period, ensures that exercise does not stop abruptly and allows for biochemical degradation and removal of the byproducts of metabolism. Mobilization consists of discrete warm-up, steady-state and cool-down periods; the components need to be identified, even in the patient with a very low functional capacity, i.e. a critically ill patient who may be only able to sit up over the edge of the bed. In such cases, preparing to sit up constitutes a warm-up period for the patient; the stimulus of sitting unsupported for several minutes while being aroused and encouraged to talk or be interactive non-verbally, if mechanically ventilated, constitutes a steady-state period; returning to bed constitutes the cool-down period. In the recovery period, observation of the patient continues to ensure that mobilization is tolerated well and that the indices of oxygen transport return to resting levels. This information is then used as the basis for mobilization in the next treatment.

Valid and reliable monitoring practices provide the basis for defining the parameters of mobilization, assessing the need for progression and defining the adaptation or training-sensitive zone. Monitoring is also essential given that subjecting patients to mobilization/exercise stimulation is inherently risky, particularly for patients with cardiopulmonary dysfunction. Indices of overall oxygen transport in addition to indices of the function of the individual steps in the oxygen transport pathway provide a detailed profile of the patient's cardiopulmonary status. In critical care settings, the physiotherapist has access to a wide range of measures to assess the adequacy of gas exchange. Minimally, in the general ward setting, measures of breathing frequency, arterial blood gases, arterial saturation, heart rate, blood pressure and clinical observation provide the basis for ongoing assessment, mobilization/exercise and progression. With appropriate attention to the patient's condition, invasive lines and leads and appropriate monitoring, a patient can be aggressively mobilized and ambulated (Fig. 5.4).

A fundamental requirement in defining the parameters for mobilization is that the patient's oxygen transport system is capable of increasing the oxygen supply to meet an increasing metabolic demand. If not, mobilization is absolutely contraindicated and the treatment of choice to optimize oxygen transport is body positioning. However, in the case of a patient being severely haemodynamically unstable, even the stress of positioning may be excessive. Thus, although critically ill patients may be treated aggressively, every patient has to be considered individually, otherwise the patient may deteriorate or be seriously endangered.

Progression. Progression and modification of the mobilization stimulus occur more rapidly in the management of the patient with acute cardiopulmonary dysfunction compared with the progression of the exercise stimulus for the patient with chronic illness. The status of acutely ill patients can vary considerably within minutes or hours. Whether the mobilization stimulus is increased or decreased in intensity depends on the patient's status and altered responses to mobilization. The mobilization stimulus is adjusted such that it remains optimal despite the patient's changing metabolic needs. Capitalizing on narrow windows of opportunity for therapeutic intervention must be exploited 24 hours a day with respect to the type of mobilization stimulus, its intensity, duration and frequency, particularly in the critically ill patient.

The 'immovable' patient. Given the well-documented negative effects of restricted mobility, the 'immovable' patient deserves special consideration. Although bed rest or activity restriction is ordered for patients frequently without reservation, the risks need to be weighed against the benefits. Restricted mobility coupled with recumbency constitutes a death knell for many severely compromised patients. Thus, an order for bed rest needs to be evaluated and challenged to ensure that this order is physiologically justified.

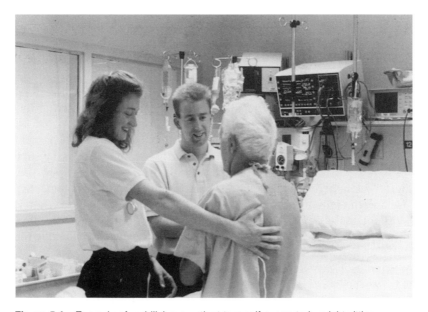

Figure 5.4 Example of mobilizing a patient to a self-supported upright sitting position. Mobilizing a critically ill patient needs to be a priority wherever possible. Short frequent sessions to the erect position (sitting or standing if possible) with continual monitoring of the patient's response should be the goal. As the patient progresses, sessions increase in intensity and duration and reduce in frequency.

Kinetic beds and chairs. Advances in furniture technology to facilitate positioning and mobilizing patients have lagged behind advances in clinical medicine, particularly in the critical care area. Conventional hospital beds are designed to be stationary and their widths and heights are often non-adjustable, making it difficult for the patient to get in and out of bed. Kinetic beds and chairs have become increasingly available over the past decade but they are not widely used clinically. These devices were originally designed to facilitate positioning and moving heavy and comatose patients. Some beds are designed to rotate on their long axis from side to side over several minutes. Other beds simulate a side-to-side movement with inflation and deflation of the two sides of an air-filled mattress. Although these beds have potential cardiopulmonary benefit (Glavis et al 1985, Kyle et al 1992), they do not replace active positioning and movement.

Mechanically adjustable bedside chairs constitute an important advance. These chairs adjust to a flat horizontal surface that can be matched to bed height and positioned beneath the patient lying on the bed. The device with the patient on top is then wheeled parallel to the bed where it can be adjusted back into a chair and thus the patient assumes a seated position. The degree of recline can be altered to meet the patient's needs and for comfort. This chair also facilitates returning the patient to bed. Comparable to these chairs are beds which can be converted into a chair while the patient is lying down. These avoid the negative effects of using tilt tables where the fluid shifts caudally are extreme and more risky by comparison.

The disadvantages of kinetic beds and chairs include the expense and the potential for overreliance on them. Without these devices, a heavy patient may require several people and several minutes to position in a chair which may be only tolerated for a few minutes. However, the cardiopulmonary benefits of the stimulation of preparing to be moved, the reflex attempts of the patient to assist and adjust to changing position, as well as actually sitting upright in a chair are not reproduced by bed positioning alone or by a kinetic bed. Research is needed to determine the indications and potential benefits of kinetic beds and chairs so that they can be used judiciously in the clinical setting as an integral therapeutic intervention.

To improve oxygen transport in post-acute and chronic cardiopulmonary dysfunction

In post-acute and chronic cardiopulmonary dysfunction, a primary consequence of impaired oxygen transport is reduced functional work capacity (Belman & Wasserman 1981, Wasserman & Whipp 1975). Work capacity can be improved with long-term exercise which improves the efficiency of the steps in the oxygen transport pathway and promotes compensation within the pathway as well as by other mechanisms. To optimize the patient's response, exercise can be carried out in judicious body positions in which oxygen transport is favoured.

Exercise is the treatment of choice for patients whose impaired oxygen transport has resulted from chronic cardiopulmonary dysfunction. Body positioning, however, may have some role in severe patients in optimizing oxygen transport at rest. Barach & Beck (1954), for example, reported that emphysematous patients were less breathless, had reduced accessory muscle activity and had a significant reduction in ventilation when positioned in a 16° head-down position. Some patients exhibited greater symptomatic improvement than in the upright position with supplemental oxygen. Classic relaxation positions, e.g. leaning forward with the forearms supported, can also be supported physiologically. Coupling such physiologically justifiable positions with mobilization/exercise will augment the benefits of exercise.

Physiological and scientific rationale. Although the physiological responses to long-term exercise in patients with chronic cardiopulmonary disease may differ from those in healthy persons, patients can significantly improve their functional work capacity (Table 5.2). In healthy persons, an improvement in aerobic capacity reflects improved efficiency of the steps in the oxygen transport pathway to adapt to increased oxygen demands imposed by exercise stress. This adaptation is effected by both central (cardiopulmonary) and peripheral (at the tissue level) changes (Dean & Ross 1992a, Wasserman & Whipp 1975). Such aerobic conditioning is characterized by a training-induced bradycardia secondary to an increased stroke volume and increased oxygen extraction capacity of the working muscle. These adaptation or training responses result in an increased maximal oxygen uptake and maximal voluntary ventilation and reduced submaximal V_E, cardiac output, heart rate, blood pressure and perceived exertion. Patients with chronic lung disease, however, are often unable to exercise at the intensity required to elicit an aerobic training response. Their functional work capacity is improved by other mechanisms, e.g. desensitization to breathlessness, improved motivation, improved biomechanical efficiency, increased ventilatory muscle strength and endurance or some combination (Belman & Wasserman 1981, Loke et al 1984). Patients with chronic heart disease, such as those with infarcted left ventricles, may be able to train aerobically; however, training adaptation primarily results from peripheral rather than central factors

(Bydgman & Wahren 1974, Hossack 1987, Ward et al 1987).

Planning an exercise programme. The exercise programme is based on the principle that oxygen delivery and uptake are enhanced in response to an exercise stimulus which is precisely defined for an individual in terms of the type of exercise, its intensity, duration, frequency and the course of the training programme. These parameters are based on an exercise test in conjunction with assessment findings. Exercise tests are performed on a cycle ergometer or treadmill or with a walk test. The general procedures and protocols are standardized to maximize the validity and reliability of the results (Dean et al 1989, Blair et al 1988). The principles of and guidelines for exercise testing and training patients with chronic lung and heart disease have been well documented (Dean 1993b). The training-sensitive zone is defined by objective and subjective measures of oxygen transport determined from the exercise test. The components of each exercise training session include baseline, warm-up, steady-state portion, cool-down and recovery period (Blair et al 1988, Dean 1993b). The cardiopulmonary and cardiovascular systems are gradually primed for sustaining a given level of exercise stress, whilst in addition the musculoskeletal system adapts correspondingly. Following the steady-state portion of the training session, the cool-down period permits a return to the resting physiological state. Cool-down and recovery periods are essential for the biochemical degradation and elimination of the metabolic byproducts of exercise.

Progression. Progression of the exercise programme is based on a repeated exercise test. This is indicated when the exercise prescription no longer elicits the desired physiological responses – specifically, when the steady-state work rate consistently elicits responses at the low end or below the lower limit of the training-sensitive zone for the given indices of oxygen transport. This reflects that maximal adaptation of the steps in the oxygen transport pathway to the given exercise stimulus has occurred. The degree of conditioning achieved is precisely matched to the demands of the exercise stimulus imposed.

Table 5.2 Chronic effects of mobilization/exercise on oxygen transport

Systemic response	Effect
Cardiopulmonary	↑ Capacity for gas exchange ↑ Cardiopulmonary efficiency ↓ Submaximal minute ventilation ↓ Work of breathing
Cardiovascular	Exercise-induced bradycardia ↑ Maximum $\dot{V}O_2$ ↓ Submaximal heart rate, blood pressure, myocardial oxygen demand, stroke volume, cardiac output ↓ Work of the heart ↓ Perceived exertion ↑ Plasma volume Cardiac hypertrophy ↑ Vascularity of the myocardium
Tissue level	↑ Vascularity of working muscle ↑ Myoglobin content and oxidative enzymes in muscle ↑ Oxygen extraction capacity

↑, increases; ↓, decreases.

To prevent the negative effects of restricted mobility

Although physiologically distinct, the effects of immobility are frequently confounded by the effects of recumbency in the hospitalized patient. Restricted mobility and the concomitant reduction in exercise stress affect virtually every organ system in the body with profound effects on the cardiovascular and neuromuscular systems. Recumbency and the elimination of the vertical gravitational stress exert their effects primarily on the cardiovascular and cardiopulmonary systems (Blomqvist & Stone 1983, Dock 1944, Harrison 1944). The most serious consequences of restricted mobility and recumbency are those resulting from the effects on the cardiopulmonary and cardiovascular systems and hence on oxygen transport. Although other consequences of restricted mobility, e.g. increased risk of infection, skin breakdown and deformity, may not constitute the same immediate threat to oxygen transport and tissue oxygenation, they can have significant implications with respect to morbidity and mortality (Rubin 1988). Thus, restricted mobility and recumbency need to be minimized and mobility and the upright position maximized to avert the negative consequences of restricted mobility, the risk of morbidity associated with these effects and the direct and indirect cardiopulmonary and cardiovascular effects. These negative consequences are preventable with frequent repositioning and mobilizing of the patient (Table 5.3). The prevention of these effects is a primary goal of positioning and mobilizing patients between treatments.

SUMMARY AND CONCLUSION

Cardiopulmonary dysfunction refers to impairment of one or more steps in the oxygen transport pathway which can impair oxygen transport overall. Thus, a conceptual framework for clinical problem solving in the management of patients with cardiopulmonary dysfunction, based on oxygen transport, can facilitate the identification of deficits and the directing of treatment to each specific deficit. Factors that can impair the transport of oxygen from the atmosphere to the tissues include cardiopulmonary pathology, bedrest, recumbency and restricted mobility, extrinsic factors related to the patient's medical care,

Table 5.3 Effects of positioning and mobilization that prevent the negative effects of restricted mobility and recumbency*

Systemic response	Effect
Cardiopulmonary	↑ Alveolar ventilation
	↓ Airway closure
	Alters the distributions of ventilation, perfusion and ventilation and perfusion matching
	Alters pulmonary blood volume
	Alters distending forces on uppermost lung fields
	↓ Secretion pooling
	Secretion mobilization and redistribution
	Alters chest wall configuration and pulmonary mechanics
	Varies work of breathing
Cardiovascular	Alters cardiac compression (positioning), wall tensions, filling pressures
	Alters preload, afterload and myocardial contraction
	Alters lymphatic drainage
	Varies work of the heart
	Promotes fluid shifts
	Stimulates pressure- and volume-regulating mechanisms of the circulation
	Stimulates vasomotor activity
	Maintains normal fluid balance and distribution
Tissue level	Alters hydrostatic pressure and tissue perfusion
	Maintains oxygen extraction capacity (mobilization)

*Some of the preventive effects of body positioning and mobilization are comparable; however, the magnitude of these effects in response to mobilization tends to be greater than with body positioning.

intrinsic factors related to the patient or a combination of these. Positioning and mobilization are two interventions that have potent and direct effects on several of the steps in the oxygen transport pathway. These interventions have a *primary* role in improving oxygen transport in acute and chronic cardiopulmonary dysfunction and in averting the negative effects of restricted mobility and recumbency, particularly those related to cardiopulmonary and cardiovascular function.

The principal goal of physiotherapy in the management of cardiopulmonary dysfunction is to optimize oxygen transport. A systematic approach to achieving this goal consists of:

1. Distinguishing the specific steps in the oxygen transport pathway which are impaired or threatened.
2. Establishing which factors contribute to this impairment
3. Distinguishing which factors are (a) amenable to positioning and mobilization and (b) not directly amenable to positioning and mobilization, as these factors will modify treatment
4. Specifying the parameters for positioning and mobilization so that they directly address the factors responsible for the cardiopulmonary

dysfunction wherever possible, i.e. to elicit the acute effects of these interventions to enhance oxygen transport or to elicit the long-term effects on oxygen transport, i.e. training responses and improved functional work capacity
5. Avoiding the multisystem consequences of restricted mobility and recumbency, particularly those that impair or threaten oxygen transport
6. Recognizing when positioning or mobilizing a patient needs to be modified to avoid a deleterious outcome.

Conceptualizing cardiopulmonary dysfunction as deficits in the steps in the oxygen transport pathway and identifying the factors responsible for each impaired step provides a systematic, evidence-based approach to clinical decision making in cardiopulmonary physiotherapy. Positioning and mobilization can then be specifically directed at the mechanisms underlying cardiopulmonary dysfunction wherever possible. Such an approach will maximize the efficacy of positioning and mobilizing patients with cardiopulmonary dysfunction and enhance the outcome of medical management overall.

REFERENCES

Albert RK, Leasa D, Sanderson M, Robertson HT, Hlastala MP 1987 The prone position improves arterial oxygenation and reduced shunt in oleic-acid-induced acute lung injury. American Review of Respiratory Diseases 138: 828–833

Barach AL, Beck GJ 1954 Ventilatory effect of head-down position in pulmonary emphysema. American Journal of Medicine 16: 55–60

Belman MJ, Wasserman K 1981 Exercise training and testing in patients with chronic obstructive pulmonary disease. Basics of Respiratory Disease 10: 1–6

Bethune DD 1975 Neurophysiological facilitation of respiration in the unconscious patient. Physiotherapy Canada 27: 241–245

Bittner E, Chendrasekhar A, Pillai S 1996 Changes in oxygenation and compliance as related to body position in acute lung injury. American Journal of Surgery 62: 1038–1041

Blair SN, Painter P, Pate RR et al 1988 Resource manual for guidelines for exercise testing and prescription. Lea and Febiger, Philadelphia

Blomqvist CG, Stone HL 1983 Cardiovascular adjustments to gravitational stress. In: Shepherd JT, Abboud FM (eds)

Handbook of physiology. Section 2: circulation, vol 2. American Physiological Society, Bethesda, pp 1025–1063

Burns JR, Jones FL 1975 Early ambulation of patients requiring ventilatory assistance. Chest 68: 608

Bydgman S, Wahren J 1974 Influence of body position on the anginal threshold during leg exercise. European Journal of Clinical Investigation 4: 201–206

Chatte G, Sab J-M, Dubois J-M 1997 Prone position in mechanically ventilated patients with severe acute respiratory failure. American Journal of Critical Care Medicine 155: 473–478

Chuley M, Brown J, Summer W 1982 Effect of postoperative immobilization after coronary artery bypass surgery. Critical Care Medicine 10: 176–178

Clauss RH, Scalabrini BY, Ray RF, Reed GE 1968 Effects of changing body position upon improved ventilation-perfusion relationships. Circulation 37(suppl 2): 214–217

Craig DB, Wahba WM, Don HF 1971 'Closing volume' and its relationship to gas exchange in seated and supine positions. Journal of Applied Physiology 31: 717–721

Dantzker DR 1983 The influence of cardiovascular function on gas exchange. Clinics in Chest Medicine 4: 149–159

Dean E 1985 Effect of body position on pulmonary function. Physical Therapy 65: 613–618

Dean E 1993a Bedrest and deconditioning. Neurology Report 17: 6–9

Dean E 1993b Advances in rehabilitation for older persons with cardiopulmonary dysfunction. In: Katz PR, Kane RL, Mezey MD (eds) Advances in long-term care. Springer-Verlag, New York, pp 1–71

Dean E 1996a Body positioning. In: Frownfelter D, Dean E (eds) Principles and practice of cardiopulmonary physical therapy, 3rd edn. Mosby, St Louis

Dean E 1996b Mobilization and exercise. In: Frownfelter D, Dean E (eds) Principles and practice of cardiopulmonary physical therapy, 3rd edn. Mosby, St Louis

Dean E, Frownfelter D 1996 Clinical case study guide to accompany principles and practice of cardiopulmonary physical therapy, 3rd edn. Mosby, St Louis

Dean E, Ross J 1992a Mobilization and exercise conditioning. In: Zadai C (ed) Pulmonary management in physical therapy. Churchill Livingstone, New York

Dean E, Ross J 1992b Discordance between cardiopulmonary physiology and physical therapy: toward a rational basis for practice. Chest 101: 1694–1698

Dean E, Ross J, Bartz J, Purves S 1989 Improving the validity of exercise testing: the effect of practice on performance. Archives of Physical Medicine and Rehabilitation 70: 599–604

Dock W 1944 The evil sequelae of complete bed rest. Journal of the American Medical Association 125: 1083–1085

Douglas WW, Rehder K, Froukje BM 1977 Improved oxygenation in patients with acute respiratory failure: the prone position. American Review of Respiratory Disease 115: 559–566

Dreyfuss D, Djedaini K, Lanore J-J, Mier L, Froidevaux R, Coste F 1992 A comparative study of the effects of almitrine bismesylate and lateral position during unilateral bacterial pneumonia with severe hypoxemia. American Review of Respiratory Disease 148: 295–299

Dripps RD, Waters RM 1941 Nursing care of surgical patients. I. The 'stir-up'. American Journal of Nursing 41: 530–534

Dull JL, Dull WL 1983 Are maximal inspiratory breathing exercises or incentive spirometry better than early mobilization after cardiopulmonary bypass? Physical Therapy 63: 655–659

Fowler WS 1949 Lung function studies. III. Uneven pulmonary ventilation in normal subjects and patients with pulmonary disease. Journal of Applied Physiology 2: 283–299

Fredrich P, Krafft P, Hochleuthner H 1996 The effects of long-term prone positioning in patients with trauma-induced adult respiratory distress syndrome. Anesthesia and Analgesia 83: 1206–1211

Glavis C, Sparacino P, Holzemer W, Skov P 1985 Effect of a rotating bed on mechanically ventilated critically ill patients. Paper presented at the Third Kinetic Therapy Seminar, San Antonio

Hahn-Winslow E 1985 Cardiovascular consequences of bed rest. Heart and Lung 14: 236–246

Harrison TR 1944 The abuse of rest as a therapeutic measure for patients with cardiovascular disease. JAMA 125: 1075–1078

Hossack KF 1987 Cardiovascular responses to dynamic exercise. In: Hanson P (ed) Exercise and the heart. WB Saunders, Philadelphia, pp 147–156

Hsu HO, Hickey RF 1976 Effect of posture on functional residual capacity postoperatively. Anesthesiology 44: 520–521

Imle PC, Klemic N 1989 Changes with immobility and methods of mobilization. In: Mackenzie CF (ed) Chest physiotherapy in the intensive care unit, 2nd edn. Williams and Wilkins, Baltimore, pp 188–214

Johnson RL 1973 The lung as an organ of oxygen transport. Basics of Respiratory Disease 2: 1–6

Kirilloff LH, Owens HR, Rogers RM, Mazzocco MC 1985 Does chest physical therapy work? Chest 88: 436–444

Kyle K, Jackiw A, Schroeder S et al 1992 Cardiopulmonary effects of kinetic bed therapy in mechanically ventilated patients. Paper presented at the American Thoracic Society Meeting, San Antonio

Lamb LE, Johnson RL, Stevens PM 1964 Cardiovascular deconditioning during chair rest. Aerospace Medicine 23: 646–649

Leblanc P, Ruff F, Milic-Emili J 1970 Effects of age and body position on airway closure in man. Journal of Applied Physiology 28: 448–451

Levine SA, Lown B 1952 'Armchair' treatment of acute coronary thrombosis. JAMA 148: 1365–1369

Lewis FR 1980 Management of atelectasis and pneumonia. Surgical Clinics of North America 60: 1391–1401

Loke J, Mahler DA, Man SFP 1984 Exercise improvement in chronic obstructive pulmonary disease. Clinics in Chest Medicine 5: 121–143

Mure M, Martling C-R, Lindahl SGE 1997 Dramatic effect on oxygenation in patients with severe acute lung insufficiency treated in the prone position. Critical Care Medicine 25: 1539–1544

Orlava OE 1959 Therapeutic physical culture in the complex treatment of pneumonia. Physical Therapy Review 39: 153–160

Pelosi P, Tubiolo D, Mascheroni D 1998 Effects of the prone position on respiratory mechanics and gas exchange during acute lung injury. American Journal of Critical Care Medicine 157: 387–393

Phang PT, Russell JA 1993. When does $\dot{V}O_2$ depend on $\dot{V}O_2$? Respiratory Care 38: 618–630

Ray JF, Yost L, Moallem S et al 1974 Immobility, hypoxemia and pulmonary arteriovenous shunting. Archives of Surgery 109: 537–541

Remolina C, Khan AV, Santiago TV, Edelman NH 1981 Positional hypoxemia in unilateral lung disease. New England Journal of Medicine 304: 523–525

Ross J, Dean E 1989 Integrating physiological principles into the comprehensive management of cardiopulmonary dysfunction. Physical Therapy 69: 255–259

Ross J, Dean E 1992 Body positioning. In: Zadai C (ed) Pulmonary management in physical therapy. Churchill Livingstone, New York

Rubin M 1988 The physiology of bed rest. American Journal of Nursing 88: 50–56

Sjostrand T 1951 Determination of changes in the intrathoracic blood volume in man. Acta Physiologica Scandinavica 22: 116–128

Svanberg L 1957 Influence of position on the lung volumes, ventilation and circulation in normals. Scandinavian Journal of Laboratory Investigation 25(suppl): 7–175

Verbrugge LM, Jette AM 1993 The disablement process. Social Sciences and Medicine 38: 1–14

Ward A, Malloy P, Rippe J 1987 Exercise prescription guidelines for normal and cardiac populations. Cardiology Clinics 5: 197–210

Warren JB, Turner C, Dalton N, Thomson A, Cochrane GM, Clark TJH 1983 The effect of posture on the sympathoadrenal response to theophylline infusion. British Journal of Clinical Pharmacology 16: 405–411

Wasserman K, Whipp BJ 1975 Exercise physiology in health and disease. American Review of Respiratory Disease 112: 219–249

Wasserman K, Hansen JE, Sue DY, Whipp BJ 1987 Principles of exercise testing and interpretation. Lea and Febiger, Philadelphia

Weber KT, Janicki JS, Shroff SG, Likoff MJ 1983 The cardiopulmonary unit: the body's gas transport system. Clinics in Chest Medicine 4: 101–110

Wenger NK 1982 Early ambulation: the physiologic basis revisited. Advances in Cardiology 31: 138–141

West JB 1962 Regional differences in gas exchange in the lung of erect man. Journal of Applied Physiology 17: 893–898

West JB 1977 Ventilation and perfusion relationships. American Review of Respiratory Disease 116: 919–943

West JB 1995 Respiratory physiology – the essentials. Williams and Wilkins, Baltimore

Williams C 1995 Haemoglobin – is more better? Nephrology Dialysis and Transplant 2 (suppl): 48–55

Wolff RK, Dolovich MB, Obminski G, Newhouse MT 1977 Effects of exercise and eucapnic hyperventilation on bronchial clearance in man. Journal of Applied Physiology 43: 46–50

World Health Organization 1980 International classification of impairments, disabilities and handicaps. A manual for classification relating to the consequences of disease. World Health Organization, Geneva

Zack MB, Pontoppidan H, Kazemi H 1974 The effect of lateral positions on gas exchange in pulmonary disease. American Review of Respiratory Disease 110: 49–55

FURTHER READING

American College of Sports Medicine 1991 Guidelines for exercise testing and prescription, 4th edn. Lea and Febiger, Philadelphia

Bates DV 1989 Normal pulmonary function. Respiratory function in disease, 3rd edn. WB Saunders, Toronto

Convertino VA 1987 Aerobic fitness, endurance training and orthostatic intolerance. Exercise and Sports Sciences Review 15: 223–259

Dantzker DR 1991 Cardiopulmonary critical care, 2nd edn. WB Saunders, Philadelphia

McArdle WD, Katch FI, Katch VL 1996 Exercise physiology. Energy, nutrition and human performance, 4th edn. Lea and Febiger, Philadelphia

Pollack ML, Wilmore JH 1990 Exercise in health and disease, 2nd edn. WB Saunders, Philadelphia

Reinhart K, Eyrich K (eds) 1989 Clinical aspects of oxygen transport and tissue oxygenation. Springer-Verlag, London

West JB 1990 Ventilation, blood flow and gas exchange, 5th edn. Blackwell Science, Oxford

West JB 1995 Respiratory physiology: the essentials, 5th edn. Williams and Wilkins, Baltimore

6

Physiotherapy techniques

Jennifer A Pryor   Barbara A Webber

Delva Bethune
(Neurophysiological facilitation of respiration)

Stephanie Enright
(Inspiratory muscle training)

Amanda Howarth
(Transcutaneous electrical stimulation)

Helen M. Potter
(Musculoskeletal dysfunction in respiratory disease)

Linda Tagg
(Acupuncture)

MUSCULOSKELETAL DYSFUNCTION IN RESPIRATORY DISEASE

The patient with chronic hyperinflation typically develops a barrel-shaped chest with an increase in the anteroposterior diameter of the chest, elevation of the first ribs and elevation or depression of the lateral shoulder girdle (Fig. 6.1). Tightness of pectoralis minor and levator scapulae together with weakness of serratus anterior and the middle and lower fibres of trapezius result in the scapulae being protracted, inferiorly rotated and anteriorly tilted. As the neck and head are drawn forwards by the sternocleidomastoids and the scalenes to balance the thoracic kyphosis, the mid-cervical region lordoses and the upper cervical spine may then hyperextend as the head tilts upward to maintain a vertical orientation of the face. Over time the long thoracic extensors and the deep upper cervical flexors lengthen and lose their endurance and stabilizing capacity and become less able to sustain the upright posture.

The stiff kyphotic thoracic spine and abnormal posture of the neck, shoulder girdle and first rib will limit the range of movement available in the cervical and thoracic spine and in the shoulder.

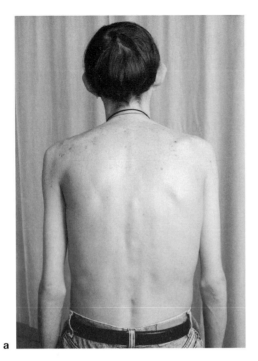
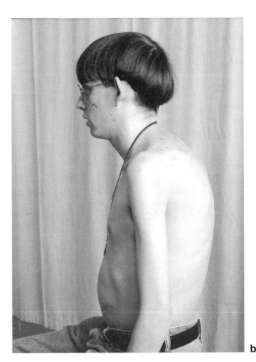

a   b

Figure 6.1 CJ, aged 16, cystic fibrosis. **a** Relaxed sitting posture (posterior view). *Note*: forward head position, tight suboccipital and mid-cervical extensors, tight upper and middle fibres of trapezius, asymmetry and abducted and protracted position of the scapulae, increased thoracic kyphosis, reduced upper lumbar lordosis, posterior rotation of pelvis. **b** Relaxed sitting posture (side view). *Note*: forward head position, increased sternocleidomastoid activity increased low cervical lordosis and thoracic kyphosis, abducted and protracted scapulae, anterior position of humerus in glenoid fossa, internal rotation of humerus, lax abdominal muscles.

Muscle fatigue related to the excess work of breathing may further accentuate poor posture in patients with moderate to severe chronic lung disease. Overactivity of the upper trapezius and levator scapulae muscles during shoulder flexion activities accentuates shortening of these muscle groups and a greater imbalance with the scapular stabilizers. In a study of 143 patients with cystic fibrosis, Henderson & Specter (1994) found 77% of females and 36% of males over 15 years of age had a kyphosis greater than 40° (the upper limit of normal). Both males and females with cystic fibrosis have also been found to have low bone mineral density (Bachrach et al 1994, Henderson & Madsen 1996).

Individuals with chronic respiratory disease may complain of acute or chronic cervical, thoracic or rib joint pain which may decrease their chest expansion as measured by a reduction in vital capacity (VC). Pain may restrict their ability to attain an upright posture and to use their muscles in a more efficient pattern. Loss of endurance of the deep cervical flexor muscles, associated with a forward head posture, has been linked to cervicogenic headache (Watson & Trott 1993). Tensioning of the neural tissues may also occur in some individuals (Butler 1991) associated with chronic overuse of the accessory muscles of respiration, elevated first rib and a depressed lateral shoulder girdle.

In patients who regularly swim or are involved in throwing sports, shoulder impingement problems may occur. Reduced range of thoracic extension will contribute to loss of the final 30° of shoulder flexion and abduction while tightness in anterior deltoid, teres major and latissimus dorsi muscles will decrease the range of external rotation and flexion available at the glenohumeral joint. Additionally, overstretching of infraspinatus and teres minor, associated with the internally rotated position of the humerus, may lead to poor stability of the humerus in the glenoid fossa. Figure 6.1 shows a very anterior position of the humerus in the glenoid cavity.

Subjective assessment

Initial assessment of a patient with respiratory disease or following surgery should include questioning regarding headache, neck, shoulder or thoracic pain and any upper limb pain or paraesthesia. The area of pain can be recorded on a body chart and the intensity quantified using an absolute visual analogue scale (AVAS) (Zusman 1986). The impact of any pain or movement restriction on activities of daily living may be assessed using a functional disability scale (e.g. Northwick Park Neck Pain questionnaire (Leak et al 1994) or the Modified Roland Morris questionnaire (Binkley et al 1996)). In the dyspnoeic patient, it may be helpful to quantify dyspnoea intensity using an AVAS or Borg scale prior to any postural correction or treatment.

Aggravating activities may involve either sustained end-range postures of the neck or thoracic spine, shoulder elevation or movements which require a reversal of the thoracic kyphosis. Pain may also be aggravated by coughing which loads the costotransverse joints. The behaviour of pain at night and in the morning will help clarify the degree of inflammation involved. Headache may be multifactorial in origin and may not be related to the musculoskeletal system.

Physical assessment

The musculoskeletal assessment should proceed in a systematic manner from evaluation of posture to assessment of joint mobility, muscle recruitment patterns, muscle length and strength and endurance. Any change in symptoms during assessment should be noted.

In the presence of chronic respiratory disease the physiotherapist should keep in mind the possibility of reduced bone density and fragile skin tissue as a result of long-term use of systemic steroids or increased age. Pain, dyspnoea and fatigue will need to be observed concur-

rently and the assessment adjusted as necessary. The presence of wound and drain sites in the postsurgical patient may require modified assessment positions. While the assessment is ideally performed in sitting, supine and prone, examination of dyspnoeic patients may need to be conducted in semi-supine, sitting or high side lying.

The resting posture of the cervical, thoracic and lumbar spine, the scapulae and arms should be observed posteriorly and laterally with the patient positioned in relaxed sitting. In particular, the degree of lumbar and thoracic kyphosis and the degree of mid- and upper cervical lordosis should be noted. The flexibility or permanence of any increase in these curves may be assessed by assisting the patient to roll the pelvis anteriorly (lumbosacral extension) and noting the automatic ability to reverse the lumbar and thoracic kyphosis. There should also be an automatic reduction in the mid-cervical lordosis and protracted position of the head (Fig. 6.2). If the slumped posture is severe and the thoracic extensors very weak, the patient may require passive assistance to reduce the thoracic kyphosis. Equally, the cervical spine and the head may need to be guided into a less protracted position to assess the reversibility of the resting posture. The ability of the patient to then maintain this corrected position will indicate the extent of loss of endurance of the postural muscles.

Total range of thoracic motion is dependent on the mobility of the apophyseal, costovertebral, costotransverse joints and ribs and the extensibility of the intercostal muscles and latissimus dorsi. Stiffness in the upper thoracic spine may be indicated by an inability to reverse the kyphosis during cervical extension and shoulder abduction. The major portion of thoracic rotation normally occurs in the middle thoracic spine (T6 to T8) (Gregersen & Lucas 1967) with lateral flexion occurring as a conjunct movement (Gregersen & Lucas 1967, White & Panjabi 1990). In the mid-thoracic region, a flattened or lordotic area usually indicates hypomobility (Boyling & Palastanga 1994). Normal thoracic rotation has a springy end-feel due to limitation by ligamentous tissue and joint capsules. During lateral flexion

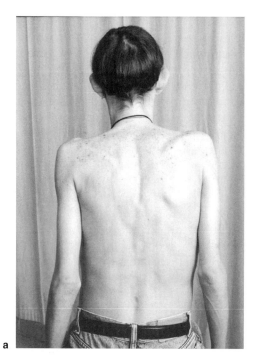 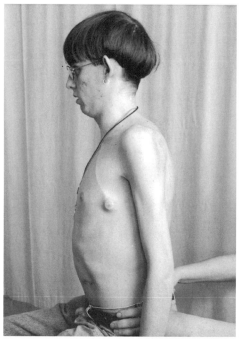

a   b

Figure 6.2 **a** Sitting posture (posterior view) following active assisted anterior rotation of pelvis. *Note*: decreased mid-cervical lordosis, improved position of scapulae, reduced thoracic kyphosis, neutral rotation of pelvis and improved lumbar lordosis.
b Sitting posture (side view) following active assisted anterior rotation of pelvis. *Note*: less forward head position, activation of deep cervical flexors, reduced sternocleidomastoid activity, improved scapulae and humeral position and thoracic kyphosis.

the ribs should flare and spread on the contra-lateral side and approximate on the ipsilateral side (Boyling & Palastanga 1994). Age changes at the costovertebral joints may restrict rib motion and lead to a harder end-feel (Nathan 1962).

During flexion the inferior facets of the apophyseal joint of the superior vertebra glide superoanteriorly on the facets of the inferior vertebra. In extension the reverse movement occurs. Although the initial limitation is from the anterior ligaments, the anterior annulus and the posterior longitudinal ligament, the normal end-feel is one of bony impingement as the inferior articular facets contact the lamina of the caudad vertebrae (White & Panjabi 1990). Gentle overpressure applied at end-range will assist determination of the quality of restriction. Overpressure should be used with caution, while manipulation of the thoracic spine is contraindicated.

The mobility of the upper and middle ribs may be assessed by palpating bilaterally anteriorly and posteriorly during a deep inspiration, while the lower ribs are assessed by palpating laterally.

The range of glenohumeral rotation will depend on tightness of the anterior and posterior shoulder muscles and position of the humerus. The range of bilateral shoulder flexion and abduction will in part be determined by the range of thoracic extension, particularly in the younger patient and in part by muscle length of latissimus dorsi and teres major. Any restriction in the range of thoracic lateral flexion and rota-tion will limit the range of unilateral shoulder elevation (Boyling & Palastanga 1994).

Abnormal patterns of muscle recruitment may be noted during shoulder elevation. The upper trapezius and levator scapulae muscles, sterno-cleidomastoid and the scalenes tend to be over-active and the deep upper cervical and scapular stabilizers underactive (Fig. 6.3). Abnormal scapulohumeral rhythm is usually most obvious as shoulder movement is initiated and towards

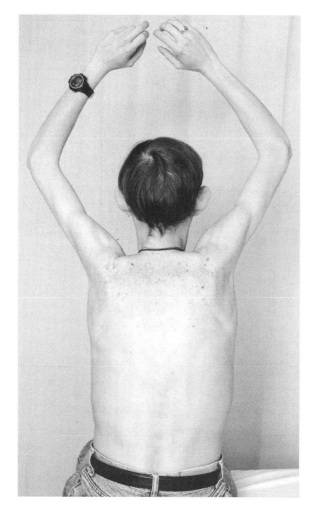

Figure 6.3 Shoulder abduction. *Note*: overactivity of upper trapezius, poor reversal of thoracic kyphosis, abducted, protracted and rotated scapulae, shortened teres major and latissimus dorsi and absence of lower trapezius activity.

the end of range. The excursion, strength and endurance of specific muscle groups identified as overactive or underactive need to be examined individually if a relationship to pain or dysfunction is found.

Neural tissue provocation tests (Butler 1991) and tests for reflexes, power and sensation should be performed if any arm pain or paraesthesia is reported. It is important to keep in mind that thoracic inlet/outlet complications may occur with altered posture.

Physiotherapy management

The patient's main problems need to be prioritized before treatment can be started. The time available, the severity of any musculoskeletal dysfunction and the chronicity need to be considered in the choice of technique. Joint restriction may be treated with passive mobilization techniques, active assisted exercises or active exercises. Posture may be improved by educating awareness of positioning and more efficient movement patterns using visual, auditory and sensory feedback.

Postural correction may change the patient's breathing pattern and intensity of dyspnoea; therefore these factors need to be monitored carefully during treatment. As the patient becomes familiar with the gentle effort required to activate the correct muscles, oxygen consumption may be reduced. Compliance with a home exercise programme will be improved if a direct link can be demonstrated between improvement in posture and relief of pain or shortness of breath.

Mobilization techniques

Physiotherapy management of joint restriction and pain may include passive mobilizations of cervical and thoracic apophyseal joints, the costotransverse, costochondral and sternochondral joints and the glenohumeral joint (Bray 1994, Vibekk 1991). The focus will usually be on improving the range and quality of thoracic extension and rotation and on increasing the mobility of the ribs. The patient's position during treatment will need to be carefully selected as many patients will not be able to lie prone or supine because of dyspnoea or pain. General techniques to the upper, mid or lower regions of the spine or localized techniques to a specific vertebral level or rib can be performed in sitting, forward lean sitting or in high side lying (Figs 6.4, 6.5).

In forward lean sitting with the head and arms supported on pillows, the rib cage will be free to move during mobilization techniques. Mobilization of the ribs may also be performed in side lying, with the upper arm elevated to stretch

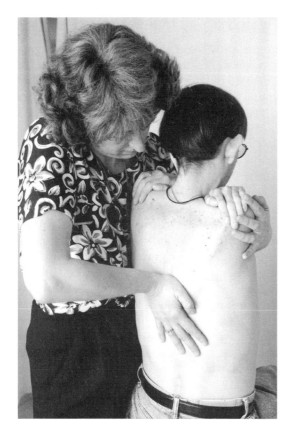

Figure 6.4 Mobilization of thoracic extension. Passive or active assisted, with fulcrum at T8.

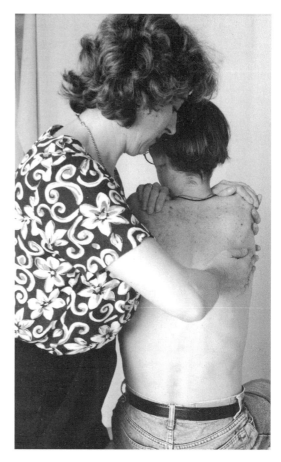

Figure 6.5 Mobilization of thoracic rotation. Passive or active assisted, with posteroanterior pressure on ribs 7 and 8.

the intercostal muscles or in sitting, using active shoulder abduction combined with lateral flexion. Bilateral arm flexion and spine extension may be combined with deep inspiration and expiration to improve rib mobility. In sitting, the patient may perform active extension or rotation while the therapist assists the movement to encourage an increase in range. Self-mobilizations can be performed over the back of a chair, in four-point kneel or leaning against a wall (Fig. 6.6). Home mobilization exercises will be necessary if the respiratory condition is chronic and the musculoskeletal dysfunction long-term.

For patients following sternotomy or thoracotomy, specific gentle passive mobilizations of the sternocostal joints or costotransverse joints may be required if localized painful limitation of shoulder or thoracic movement or pain on breathing is present. Bilateral arm movements are preferred in the early stage, initially avoiding abduction and external rotation. Following thoracotomy, patients may tend to immobilize the arm on the side of the incision and need to be encouraged to move within pain limits as early as possible to reduce the risk of frozen shoulder. The scapula may be taken through its range of protraction, retraction, elevation and depression while the patient is in side lying.

The long-term ventilated patient may also develop musculoskeletal problems. Routine passive mobilization of the shoulder through its full range of flexion, external rotation and abduction should be mandatory. Lateral flexion and extension of the thoracic spine can be performed via arm elevation when the patient is in side

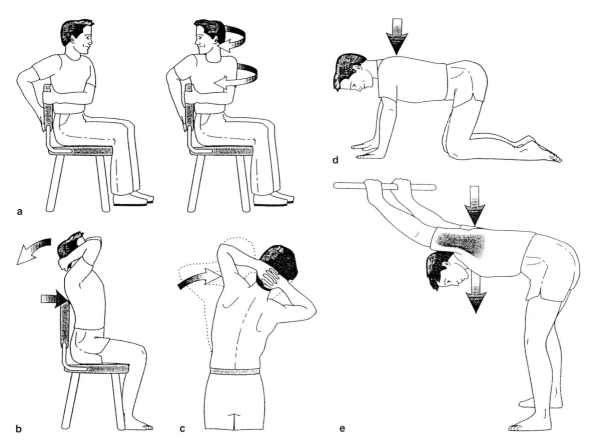

Figure 6.6 **a** Assisted active exercise for rotation of cervical and thoracic spine. **b** Active assisted exercise for thoracic spine extension. **c** Active exercise for thoracic spine lateral flexion and stretching of the intercostal muscles. **d** Active mobilization exercise for mid-thoracic extension. **e** Passive stretch of anterior shoulder muscles and mobilization of thoracic extension.

lying. Gentle passive rotation of the thoracic spine can also be performed in this position with the upper arm resting on the lateral chest wall.

Muscle-lengthening techniques

Stretching of tight muscle groups should precede or accompany endurance training of the lengthened muscle groups (Janda 1994). Stretching of the anterior deltoid and pectoralis major muscles using a proprioceptive neuromuscular facilitation hold–relax technique has been shown to increase VC and shoulder range of movement (Putt & Paratz 1996). Other muscles which may require stretching are: sternocleidomastoid, the scalenes, upper and middle fibres of trapezius, levator scapulae, pectoralis minor, teres major, latissimus dorsi, subscapularis and the suboccipital extensors (Table 6.1). Sustained stretches may be facilitated by conscious or reflex relaxation of the muscle during exhalation. Hold–relax techniques using the agonist or contract–relax techniques using the antagonist of the shortened muscle (White & Sahrmann 1994) may augment sustained stretches and myofascial release massage along the line of the muscle fibres. Where possible, patients should be taught to perform their own stretches and mobilizations as part of long-term maintenance.

Postural retraining

Postural correction utilizes motor learning with training of the holding ability of the postural

Table 6.1 Assessment of muscle length

Muscle	Observation if muscle tight	Length testing position
Pectoralis major	Internal rotation and anterior translation of the humerus	Horizontal extension and abduction to 140°
Pectoralis minor	Anterior and inferior position of coracoid process and elevation of ribs 3–5	Retraction and depression of scapula
Upper cervical extensors	Forward position of head on neck, increased upper cervical lordosis	Flexion of the head on the upper cervical spine
Upper trapezius	Elevation of scapula, palpable anterior border of trapezius (occiput to distal clavicle)	Cervical flexion with contralateral lateral flexion and ipsilateral rotation
Levator scapula	Increased muscle bulk anterior to upper trapezius and posterior to sternocleidomastoid from C2–4 to superior angle of scapula	Cervical flexion, contralateral lateral flexion and contralateral rotation keeping the medial superior scapula border depressed
Sternocleidomastoid	Forward position of head on neck, elevated 1st rib and prominence at the clavicular insertion of sternocleidomastoid	Upper cervical flexion with lower cervical extension
Anterior scalenes	Elevation of ribs 1–3, ipsilateral lateral flexion of head on neck	Exhalation with depression of ribs 1–3 and upper cervical flexion
Latissimus dorsi	Internal rotation of humerus	Elevation of shoulder in external rotation with posterior pelvic tilt
Teres major	Medial rotation of humerus, protracted and upward rotation of scapula	Flex shoulder while sustaining scapular retraction and depression
Diaphragm	Flexed thorax and localized lordosis at the thoraco-lumbar junction	Relaxed diaphragmatic breathing

stabilizers while avoiding substitution by the stronger prime movers (White & Sahrmann 1994). The principles of motor control require frequent repetition of the corrected movement or position. The initial focus should be on correcting any posterior pelvic rotation in sitting and on reducing the lumbar and thoracic kyphosis to bring the head back over the trunk. A small pillow or lumbar roll may then be used to maintain this position. If necessary, postural correction can be started in semi-supine or high side lying and then incorporated into maintenance of corrected posture during specific activities.

Taping

Reduction of the thoracic kyphosis may need to be assisted until the holding capacity of the thoracic extensors and lower fibres of trapezius has been improved. Strapping tape (over anti-allergy tape), applied with the patient in corrected sitting, may give proprioceptive feedback in the early stages of retraining. A long piece of tape starting anteriorly above the clavicle and crossing the mid-fibres of trapezius may inhibit overactivity of this muscle. The tape is then crossed over at the peak of the thoracic kyphosis and extended down to the lumbar spine. It should not be so firm that pain is produced or neural symptoms provoked. A horizontal tape to lift the lateral edge of the acromion and a tape around the inferior border of the scapula to facilitate serratus anterior action may all help.

Muscle retraining

Training of scapular retraction and depression using middle and lower fibres of trapezius is important to complement any gain in range of thoracic extension and to improve scapular stability (Fig. 6.7). The holding capacity of the deep upper cervical flexors and cervicothoracic extensors will need to be trained to reduce the degree of forward head posture and to assist relaxation of sternocleidomastoid and the scalene muscles (Table 6.2). The longus colli and rectus capitus

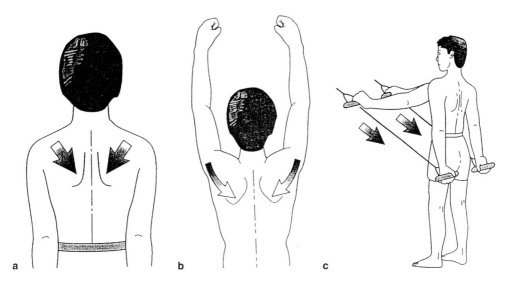

Figure 6.7   **a** Active scapulae retraction/depression (rhomboids, middle and lower trapezius). **b** Active scapulae retraction/depression in shoulder elevation. **c** Active scapulae retraction/depression in shoulder extension.

Table 6.2   Assessment of holding capacity of lengthened muscles

Muscle	Test position
Deep upper cervical flexors	Half supine, nodding of head on neck. Test holding ability
Middle and lower trapezius	With patient prone (or sitting if SOB), test holding ability by placing scapula in retraction and depression and asking patient to hold
Serratus anterior	Note ability to maintain scapula against chest wall during a partial push-up against a wall
Infraspinatus	Test strength of external rotation

anterior major may be trained initially in high sitting then progressed to supine if shortness of breath allows (Fig. 6.8). Alternatively, gentle nodding of the head on neck against slight resistance of the patient's thumb can be taught in sitting. Serratus anterior can be retrained to hold the scapula against the chest wall using a half push-up action against a wall (taking care that upper trapezius is not overactive).

Gym ball

A gym ball may be useful for encouraging a more upright sitting posture in younger patients. Prone positions over the ball may be used to stimulate the antigravity muscles. Side lying over the ball will assist with rib mobility and stretch-ing of the intercostal muscles if mobility and shortness of breath allow.

Neural tissue

The primary aim of treatment when neural tissue provocation tests reveal irritation or restriction is to mobilize the tight adjacent structures and improve posture while monitoring the effect on the neural system. If progress is inadequate, gentle mobilization (not stretching) of the neural tissues at the site of restriction may be required.

In summary, for patients with chronic respiratory disease it would seem logical to start postural education and a home mobilizing and strengthening programme as early as possible. For the more acute patient musculoskeletal techniques

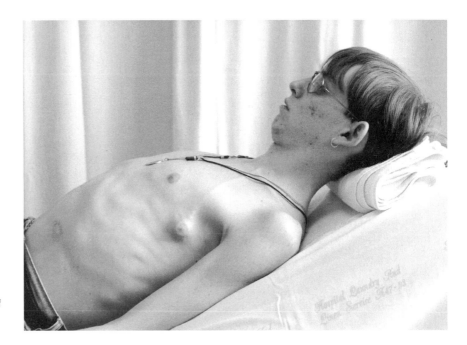

Fig 6. 8 Position for training activation of deep upper cervical flexors and lower trapezius and for stretching of upper cervical extensors and pectoralis minor and major.

could be integrated into the acute management. Research is required to evaluate whether the musculoskeletal complications described in this section can be prevented or minimized by an early intervention programme and whether treating the musculoskeletal system has a positive effect on respiratory function.

NEUROPHYSIOLOGICAL FACILITATION OF RESPIRATION

The respiration of mammals involves a ventilatory system in which the essential part, the lung, plays the role of exchange between the surrounding air and the blood. Even though this organ is richly supplied with nerves, it does not have an autonomous function. It can effectively fulfill its role only by the conjoint action of two elements, the rib cage and the diaphragm, which form the chamber enclosing it.

(Duron & Rose 1997)

Breathing is a complex behaviour. It is governed by a variety of regulating mechanisms under the control of large parts of the central nervous system. Ongoing research into the respiratory ventilatory system (rib cage and diaphragm) has dramatically altered traditional understanding of the respiratory muscles and their neural control.

The motor synergy of respiration includes the major and accessory respiratory muscles and motoneuron pools from the level of the fifth cranial nerve all the way down to the upper lumbar segments (Euler 1986).

Respiratory rhythmicity, as with other rhythmical repetitive motor actions (i.e. locomotion and mastication), is supported in the central nervous system by a central pattern generator (CPG). CPGs are neuronal networks capable of generating the characteristic rhythmic patterns in the complete absence of extrinsic reflexes and feedback loops (Atwood & McKay 1989, Euler 1986, Gordon 1991). However, in order to adapt the ventilatory system to prevailing and anticipated needs and to achieve coordination with the cardiovascular system, breathing is regulated by a multitude of reflexes, negative feedback circuits and feedforward mechanisms (Ainsworth 1997, Euler 1986, Koepchen et al 1986).

The purpose of this discussion is to assist the integration of evidence from recent biological research with clinical practice and to consider the implications of the newer models of respiratory neural control for clinical work. Much biological research now validates, in ways that previously were not possible, the empirical practices of earlier years. For example, research into the function of the abdominal muscles now supports empirical practices of the 1940s and 1950s when abdominal supports were used to assist persons with emphysema (Alvarez et al 1981, De Troyer 1997, Grassino 1974). The present models of the neural control of respiration, with their emphasis on the roles of spinal neurons and on the importance of afferent (sensory) input, provide further biological support for neurophysiological facilitation procedures, i.e. clinical use of selective afferent input in respiratory care.

Neurophysiological facilitation of respiration is the use of selective external proprioceptive and tactile stimuli that produce reflexive movement responses in the ventilatory apparatus to assist respiration. These procedures have been employed in physiotherapy chest care for the past 25 years. The responses they elicit appear to alter the rate and depth of breathing and can be demonstrated to occur in other mammals (dogs) as well as in humans (Bethune 1975, 1976). These procedures are particularly useful in the chest care of the

unconscious patient and of the conscious post-surgical patient who frequently find that the reflexive nature of the respiratory movements reduces the perception of pain (Bethune 1991, 1998).

Neural control

Research on ventilatory muscle control presently places considerable emphasis on spinal respiratory motoneurons and their controlling or modifying influence on central respiratory programmes. One of the newer theoretical models of the functional organization of the neural control of breathing identifies three major central nervous system levels: suprabulbar mechanisms, bulbar mechanisms and spinal motoneuron pools and integrating mechanisms (Euler 1986) (Fig. 6.9).

Based on a similar model, Miller et al (1997) discuss the many neural structures that can potentially modify the final output of the ventilatory muscles. Input from peripheral sensory

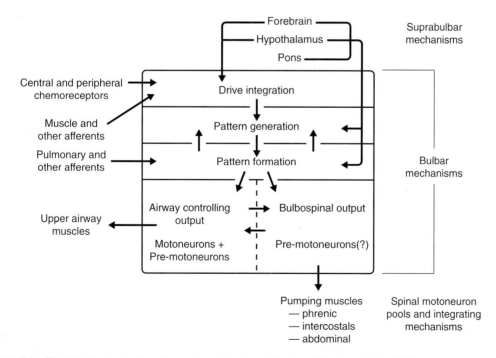

Figure 6.9   Functional organization of neural control of breathing (modified from Euler 1986).

structures (proprioceptive, cutaneous, vagal and chemoceptive) and from a variety of brain regions (cerebral cortex, pons, cerebellum and others) is all integrated in the premotor bulbo-spinal respiratory neurons. Adjustments to the respiratory control of these multifunctional muscles occurs to support their many non-respiratory behaviours during speech, swallowing, coughing, vomiting and so on. The motoneuron pools that drive these multifunctional ventilatory muscles are subjected to changes in their activity pattern due to their control by the neuronal networks recruited on the basis of the different incoming stimuli. The spinal respiratory motoneurons are the final common pathway. They detemine the output of the major respiratory muscles including their 'rhythmic breath-by-breath respiratory drive'. This discussion will be concerned with the actions of the ventilatory apparatus only during eupnic respiration (normal easy breathing).

Breathing in all mammalian species depends on a bilateral neuronal respiratory network within the lower brainstem which generates three neural phases: inspiration, post-inspiration and expiration. Inspiration involves augmenting activity in the inspiratory nerves and muscles. The post-inspiratory phase represents declining activity in the inspiratory nerves (early expiration). During late or active expiration the expiratory nerves and muscles exhibit augmenting activity which ends abruptly at the next inspiration. All phase activities are generated without the need for peripheral feedback. Although classical studies proposed a hierarchical organization of various 'centres' in the pons and medulla, recent studies have revealed that supra-medullary structures are not essential for the maintenance of respiratory rhythm. Respiratory neurons in the rostral pons, previously known as the 'pneumotaxic center' controlling respiratory rhythm, are not necessary for rhythm generation. These pontine neurons are now thought to stabilize the respiratory pattern, slow the rhythm and influence timing. Efferent axons from the medullary neurons project to the inspiratory neurons in the spinal cord (Atwood & MacKay 1989, Bianchi & Pasaro 1997, Richler et al 1997).

The origin of the respiratory rhythm remains unclear as precise knowledge of all possible interactions among neurons in the respiratory network is incomplete. 'Respiratory drive is regulated by information from sensory receptors within the airway, lungs and respiratory muscles, as well as central and peripheral chemoceptors' (Frazier et al 1997). Proprioceptive information arising from respiratory muscles may regulate the motor activity through long loop reflexes that include the medullary respiratory centres. Proprioceptive information through segmental and intersegmental loops at the spinal level may also influence the motor actiivity. Although complex spinal circuitry exists for modulating diaphragmatic activity through large and small phrenic afferents, proprioceptive regulation of phrenic motoneurons seems weak or absent. Afferent information from the lower intercostals and the abdominal muscles (T9–10) may facilitate phrenic motoneurons by a spinal reflex. Emerging evidence suggests that phrenic afferents are more involved in respiratory regulation during stressed breathing (Frazier et al 1997, Hilaire & Monteau 1997). There are apparent differences between the neural mechanisms controlling the diaphragm and those controlling the thoracic muscles. While phrenic motoneurons appear mainly under medullary control and seem insensitive to proprioception, thoracic respiratory neurons seem to receive respiratory drive mainly via a network of thoracic interneurons.

Respiratory muscles

The diaphragm

The diaphragm is the major inspiratory muscle in humans. Current understanding is that it does not expand the entire chest wall, as previously proposed. Actions of the diaphragm are being investigated with more attention being paid to the direction of the muscle fibres that compose it and the insertional and 'appositional' forces that are generated. The insertional forces are the result of muscular attachments. The appositional force is that pleural pressure that develops on the inner aspect of the lower ribs between the ribs and the diaphragm where the diaphragmatic fibres that are directed cranially, are in direct contact with the rib cage (De Troyer 1997).

Diaphragmatic muscle fibres originate from three major sites: the xiphisternal junction, the costal margin of the lower rib cage and the transverse processes of the lumbar vertebrae. All fibres insert into the central tendon. Thus, the orientation of these fibres differs. For example, midcostal diaphragmatic muscle fibres are perpendicular to midsternal and midcrural fibres. In humans, diaphragmatic muscle fibres have tendinous insertions within the muscle and do not traverse the full length of the muscle from origin to insertion, as in some smaller animals. Therefore, the mechanical action of these fibres is complex, depending on relationships imposed by the specific attachments and the loads imposed by the rib cage and abdominal wall.

Older literature raised the possibility that there might be motor innervation of some parts of the diaphragm from intercostal nerves. It is now clear that the only innervation is the phrenic nerve via the phrenic motoneurons originating in the third, fourth and fifth segments of the cervical cord in humans. Animal studies have demonstrated that the diaphragm is somatotopically innervated. In the cat C5 innervates the ventral portions of both costal and crural diaphragmatic fibres, while their dorsal portions are innervated by C6. Studies in other animals have produced similar data. The compartmentalization related to these innervation patterns and the further subcompartmentalization of motor unit territories within these areas 'provide the potential for differential control' of different regions of diaphragmatic muscle. The differences between the diaphragmatic fibres from the three sites of origin have prompted some investigators to suggest that the crural portion is a separate muscle, under separate neuromotor control (Sieck & Prakash 1997). The crural portion has no costal attachment. Crural fibres surrounding the oesophagus may be under separate neural control in order to act as a sphincter. Detailed histochemical studies have demonstrated other differences between fibres from the three originating sites. A recognized uniqueness of the diaphragm is that it has few muscle spindles. When they are present, they are found primarily in the crural portion (Agostoni & Sant' Ambrogio 1970, Sieck & Prakash 1997).

Studies of isolated diaphragmatic contractions, examined by electrical stimulation of the phrenic nerve in dogs, demonstrated that while the lower ribs moved cranially and the cross-sectional area of the lower rib cage increased, the upper ribs moved caudally and the cross-sectional area of the upper rib cage decreased. Similar studies, during phrenic nerve pacing, in human subjects with traumatic transection of the upper cord and during spontaneous breathing in subjects who, because of transection to the lower cord, use their diaphragm exclusively have yielded the same result. In seated humans (as in the dog) the diaphragm has both an expiratory action on the upper rib cage and an inspiratory action on the lower rib cage which increases in its transverse diameter.

It has been established that the inspiratory action of the diaphragm on the rib cage is due in part to the insertional force of its attachment to the lower ribs. During inspiration the muscle fibres of the diaphragm shorten and the dome descends relative to the costal insertions of the muscle. The descent of the dome, which remains relatively constant in size and shape during breathing, expands the thorax vertically, resulting in a fall in pleural pressure. The descent also displaces abdominal viscera caudally, increasing abdominal pressure which pushes the abdominal wall outwards. The diaphragmatic fibres inserting on the upper borders of the lower six ribs also apply a force on these ribs when they contract. This force equals the force exerted on the central tendon. If the abdominal viscera effectively oppose the diaphragmatic descent the lower ribs are lifted and rotated outwards.

The inspiratory force of the diaphragm is also related to its apposition to the rib cage. This is best explained in the words of De Troyer (1997).

The zone of apposition makes the lower rib cage, in effect part of the abdominal container and measurements in dogs have established that during breathing the changes in pressure in the pleural recess between the apposed diaphragm and the rib cage are almost equal to the changes in abdominal pressure. Pressure in the pleural recess rises, rather than falls during inspiration, thus indicating that the rise in abdominal pressure is truly transmitted through the apposed diaphragm to expand the lower rib cage.

The inspiratory efficiency of the insertional and appositional forces is largely dependent on the resistance the abdominal viscera provide to diaphragmatic descent. If the resistance of the abdominal contents was eliminated the zone of apposition would disappear during inspiration and the contracting diaphragmatic muscle would become oriented transversely at their attachments onto the ribs. In this case, the insertional force would have an expiratory action on the lower ribs. These studies reinforce the views of Goldman (1974) that 'abdominal muscle contraction, commonly associated only with an expiratory action, appears to have an important role in defending diaphragmatic length during inspiration'.

The intercostal muscles

The role of the intercostal muscles has been more difficult to establish. Conventional wisdom regards the external intercostals as inspiratory in function, elevating the ribs, and the internal intercostals as expiratory in function, depressing the ribs. This theory was based on geometric considerations proposed in 1848 (the Hamberger theory) and it has been challenged since 1867 when electrical stimulation of the intercostal muscles was done for the first time. These latter studies suggested that the external and internal intercostal muscles were synergistic in action. The Hamberger theory is regarded as being incomplete. Its theoretical model is planar but real ribs are curved. Therefore, the changes in length of the intercostal muscles (i.e. their mechanical advantage) vary with respect to the position of the muscle fibres along the rib. Also, the Hamberger theory assumed that all ribs rotate by equal amounts around parallel axes. The radii of curvature of the different ribs are different (Duron & Rose 1997).

Histological and electrophysiological studies have disclosed that the rib cage is non-homogeneous. It has motor components that vary with their location in the upper or lower thorax. In addition, each intercostal can be functionally different depending on its position in the same intercostal space (Gray 1973). It is now generally accepted that most of the external intercostal muscles do not participate in the ventilatory process during quiet breathing (De Troyer 1997, Duron & Rose 1997). Unlike the diaphragm, the intercostal muscles also have a postural function. Detailed studies of the respiratory and postural actions of the intercostal muscles have revealed functional differences from segment to segment and between external and internal intercostal muscles within the same segment. The major role of each intercostal muscle in postural activity and/or respiratory cycles is yet to be established. Nevertheless, Duron & Rose (1997) reviewed extensive studies in animal and human subjects and report rather precise distributions of inspiratory and expiratory activity. A summary of their findings follows.

1. In addition to the diaphragm, the inspiratory muscles active during normal breathing are the ventral intercartilaginous part of the intercostal muscles and the dorsal levator costae muscle.
2. The lateral part of the external and internal intercostal muscles of the upper rib spaces are synergistic muscles. They often have a postural type of activity. Their motoneurons may be activated by the central inspiratory drive; thus they may participate in respiration.
3. In the four lowest intercostal spaces the lateral parts of the external and internal intercostal muscles are also synergistic. The lateral part of the internal intercostal is active in expiration during quiet breathing. The lateral part of the external intercostal is also expiratory but only during dyspnoea, similar to abdominal expiratory action.
4. The lateral part of the intercostal muscles are antagonistic in the 5th–8th intercostal spaces. The external intercostals are inspiratory and the internal intercostals are expiratory.
5. In every intercostal space the dorsal part of the external (inspiratory) and the dorsal part of

the internal (expiratory) muscles are antagonistic during quiet breathing.
6. All intercostal muscles of the lateral part of the rib cage participate in posture. There appears to be a clear distinction between the dorsal and ventral part of each intercostal space from which phasic respiratory activities are always recorded and the lateral part of each intercostal space where tonic postural activities are observed.

The insertions of both the external and internal intercostal muscles suggest that their orientation would assist rotation of the thorax. Indeed, electromyographical (EMG) studies on normal human subjects have demonstrated that external intercostals on the right were activated when the torso was rotated to the left but silent when the torso was rotated to the right. On the other hand, the internal intercostals on the right were only active when the torso was rotated to the right. The abundance of muscle spindles and the preponderance of type 1 (slow) muscle fibres in intercostal muscles are consistent with postural activity. Eighty-five percent of external intercostal muscle fibres in dogs are type 1, a percentage that is higher than that of antigravity limb muscles.

Accessory muscles of inspiration

The scalene muscles in humans have traditionally been considered as accessory inspiratory muscles. However, EMG studies have established that scalene muscles invariably contract with the diaphragm and parasternal intercostals during inspiration. No clinical situation exists in which paralysis of all inspiratory muscles occurs without also affecting the scalene muscles, so it is impossible to accurately define the isolated action of these muscles on the human rib cage. Observations on quadriplegic patients have demonstrated that persistent inspiratory action in scalene muscles is observed in those subjects with a spinal transection at C7 or lower that preserves scalene innervation. In these situations the anteroposterior diameter of the rib cage remains constant or increases, as opposed to the inward

displacement of the upper rib cage when the level of transection interferes with scalene innervation (De Troyer 1997). Accessory muscles of the neck assist thoracic respiration by stabilizing the upper rib cage. This is a minor function in normal persons at rest. These muscles become more active during exercise and in the presence of diseases such as asthma and chronic obstructive pulmonary disease. Generally, neck and upper airway muscles have a higher proportion of fast muscle fibres, faster isometric contraction times and lower fatigue resistance than the diaphragm (Lunteren & Dick 1997).

Many other muscles can elevate the ribs when they contract and are therefore truly 'accessory' muscles of inspiration. These are muscles running between the head and the rib cage, shoulder girdle and rib cage, spine and shoulder girdle. Such muscles as the sternocleidomastoid, pectoralis minor, trapezius, serrati and erector spinae are primarily postural in function. They are active in respiration in healthy humans only during increased respiratory effort. Of these accessory muscles, only the sternocleidomastoids have been extensively studied. In patients with transection of the upper cord causing paralysis of the diaphragm, intercostals, scalene and abdominal muscles, the sternocleidomastoids (innervation cranial nerve 11) contract forcefully during unassisted inspiration, causing a large increase in the expansion of the upper rib cage but an inspiratory decrease in the transverse diameter of the lower rib cage (De Troyer 1997).

The abdominal muscles

The four muscles of the ventrolateral wall of the abdomen, the rectus abdominis, the external oblique, the internal oblique and the transversus abdominis, have significant respiratory function in humans. The fibres in each of these muscles assume a direction different from each other; consequently the mechanical action of an abdominal muscle contraction depends on fibre direction and the concurrent action of the other abdominal muscles. Added to this complexity is the fact that the force generated by the abdominal wall is applied to a load that is determined by viscous and non-linear elastic resistances. The capacity of the abdominal wall to function adequately varies markedly among individuals and correlates well with an individual's activity level, gender, corpulence and age.

Abdominal muscle fibres are similar to those of other skeletal muscle. Differences in fibre composition between them are minor. Generally speaking, type 1 (slow) muscle fibres predominate. Bishop (1997) reports that although details of the morphology of abdominal motor units are not known and information on the number and distribution of muscle proprioceptors (muscle spindles and tendon organs) in abdominal muscle is scarce, proprioceptive feedback is recognized as an important modulator of abdominal motoneuron excitability. Electrically evoked reflexes studied in cats under the conditions of bilateral rhizotomy of the lumbar segments or C6 spinal cord transection, demonstrated that both segmental feedback and supraspinal signals control abdominal motoneurons. Furthermore, studies on the phasic and tonic abdominal stretch reflexes suggest a special functional significance for the gamma-spindle loop. Normal individuals, when standing, develop tonic abdominal muscle activity unrelated to respiratory phases.

Many brain regions can modify abdominal motoneuron output via multliple descending pathways. Spinal abdominal motoneurons receive strong projections from the brainstem. However, brainstem and spinal abdominal motoneurons receive direct and indirect projections from the premotor cortex, the motor cortex, the cerebellum, the hypothalamus, the pons and many other regions of the brain. The voluntary control over the abdominal muscles via the motor cortex is very similar to control by the cortex over muscles of the limbs and digits.

The respiratory action of the abdominal muscles is first to contract and pull the abdominal wall inward and so increase abdominal pressure. This pressure causes the diaphragm to move upwards into the thoracic cavity which, in turn, results in an increase in pleural pressure and a decrease in lung volume. The abdominal muscles also displace the rib cage. By virtue of their insertions on the ribs, it would appear that the action of the abdominal

muscles is to pull the lower ribs caudally and thus deflate the rib cage in another expiratory action. However, experiments in dogs have shown that these muscles also have an inspiratory action. Because of the large zone where the diaphragm is directly apposed to the rib cage, the rise in abdominal pressure due to abdominal muscle contraction is transmitted to the lower rib cage. In addition, the rise in abdominal pressure forcing the diaphragm cranially and the consecutive increase in passive diaphragmatic tension also tend to raise the lower ribs and expand the lower rib cage (insertional force of the diaphragm). Regardless of their actions on the ribs, the abdominal muscles are primarily expiratory muscles through their actions on the diaphragm and the lung.

Neurophysiological facilitatory stimuli

The proprioceptive and tactile stimuli selected produce remarkably consistent reflexive responses in the ventilatory muscles. Inspiratory expansion of the ribs, increased epigastric excursion, visibly increased and often palpably increased tone in the abdominal muscles and change in the respiratory rate (usually slower) are among the responses observed. In the clinical setting these responses are often accompanied by involuntary coughing, changes in breath sounds on auscultation, rapid return of mechanical chest wall stability, less necessity for suctioning, a more normal respiratory pattern and retention of the improved breathing pattern for some time after the treatment period. In some unconscious patients there is an apparent increase in the level of consciousness (more reaction to other stimuli). These effects appear to be cumulative. Successive application of the stimuli elicit faster responses and longer retention of the altered pattern. The changes noted during treatment application are frequently dramatic. The responses are most pronounced in the most deeply unconscious. The facilitatory stimuli are:

- intercostal stretch
- vertebral pressure to the upper thoracic spine
- vertebral pressure to the lower thoracic spine

- anterior-stretch lift of the posterior basal area
- moderate manual pressure
- perioral pressure
- abdominal co-contraction.

The foregoing discussion of neural control models, with the emphasis that is now placed on the importance of afferent input and the role of spinal motoneurons, indicates that the majority of the responses to these stimuli are mediated by muscle stretch receptors via dorsal roots and intersegmental reflexes (Table 6.3).

Intercostal stretch (Fig. 6.10a)

Intercostal stretch is provided by applying pressure to the upper border of a rib in a direction that will widen the intercostal space above it. The pressure should be applied in a downward direction, not pushing inward into the patient. The application of the stretch is timed with an exhalation and the stretched position is then maintained as the patient continues to breathe in his usual manner. As the stretch is maintained a gradual increase in inspiratory movements in and around the area being stretched occurs. This may be done as a unilateral or bilateral procedure. It should not be performed on fractured or floating ribs. Care must be exercised around sensitive mammary tissue in females. When performed over areas of instability, as in the presence of paradoxical movement of the upper rib cage or over areas of decreased mobility, this procedure is effective in restoring normal breathing patterns. Epigastric excursions can be observed if intercostal stretch is performed over the lower ribs but above the floating ribs. This may represent the reflexive activation of the diaphragm by the intercostal afferents that innervate its margins.

Table 6.3 Neurophysiological facilitation for the chest

Procedure	Method	Observations	Suggested mechanism
Perioral stimulation	Pressure is applied to the patient's top lip by the therapist's finger – and maintained	<ul><li>Increased epigastric excursion</li><li>'Deep breathing'</li><li>Sighing</li><li>Mouth closure</li><li>Swallowing</li><li>'Snout phenomena'</li></ul>	Primitive reflex response related to sucking
Vertebral pressure – high	Manual pressure to thoracic vertebrae in region of T2–T5	<ul><li>Increased epigastric excursions</li><li>'Deep breathing'</li></ul>	Dorsal root-mediated intersegmental reflex
Vertebral pressure – low	Manual pressure to thoracic vertebrae in region of T7–T10	Increased respiratory movements of apical thorax	
Anterior stretch – lifting posterior basal area	<ul><li>Patient supine</li><li>Hands under lower ribs</li><li>Ribs lifted upward</li></ul>	<ul><li>Expansion posterior basal area</li><li>Increased epigastric movements</li></ul>	<ul><li>Dorsal root as above</li><li>Stretch receptors in intercostals, back muscles</li></ul>
Co-contraction – abdomen	<ul><li>Pressure laterally over lower ribs and pelvis</li><li>Alternate right and left sides</li></ul>	<ul><li>Increased epigastric movements</li><li>Increased muscle contraction (rectus abdominus)</li><li>Decreased girth in obese</li><li>Increased firmness to palpation</li><li>Depression of umbilicus</li></ul>	Stretch receptors in abdominal muscles ? intercostal to phrenic reflex
Intercostal stretch	Stretch on expiratory phase maintained	Increased movement of area being stretched	Intercostal stretch receptors
Moderate manual pressure	Moderate pressure open palm	Gradually increased excursion of area under contact	Cutaneous afferents

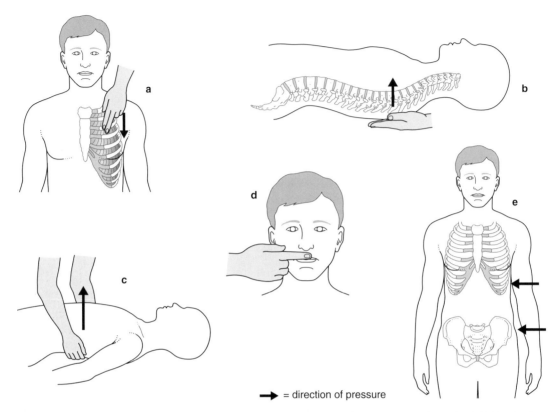

Figure 6.10 **a** Intercostal stretch: pressure down towards the next rib, not 'in' towards the patient's back. **b** Vertebral pressure (i) over T2, 3, 4, (ii) T9, 10, 11. **c** Lifting posterior basal area. **d** Perioral stimulation: moderate pressure on top lip (the airway should not be occluded). **e** Co-contraction of abdominal muscles: pressure over lower ribs and pelvic bone.

Vertebral pressure (Fig. 6.10b)

Firm pressure applied directly over the vertebrae of the upper and lower thoracic cage activates the dorsal intercostal muscles. Pressure should be applied with an open hand for comfort and must be firm enough to provide some (intrafusal) stretch. For this reason it is easier to apply when the patient is supine, as in the supine position it is not necessary to stabilize the body and one may also observe the patient's reactions. Afferent input that activates the dorsal intercostal muscles is consistent with the observations of Duron & Rose (1997) that in every intercostal space, the dorsal part of the external (inspiratory) and the dorsal part of the internal (expiratory) intercostal muscles are antagonistic during quiet breathing.

Firm presssure over the uppermost thoracic vertebrae results in increased epigastric excur-

sions in the presence of a relaxed abdominal wall. Pressure over the lower thoracic vertebrae results in increased inspiratory movements of the apical thorax. These responses correlate with the observations of Helen Coombs. In 1918 Coombs demonstrated that section of the thoracic roots diminished costal respiration. She stated:

If the spinal roots are cut in the thoracic region alone there is diminution of costal respiration although abdominal respiration remains unaltered and the rate is very little changed: if the cervical dorsal roots are also involved, independent costal respiration disappears ... .

In 1930, in research with kittens, Coombs & Pike found that:

when dorsal roots of spinal nerves are divided in the thoracic region, costal respiration in kittens from birth to ten days old almost ceases ... when dorsal roots of cervical nerves are sectioned, the thoracic nerves being intact, the movements of the diaphragm are much cut down and the respiratory rate is slower at no matter what age.

There is little to be found in the literature defining intersegmental respiratory reflexes. Sieck & Prakash (1997) noted that phrenic motoneurons do not receive a major excitatory input from muscle spindle afferents. However, they recognize that there are extrasegmental reflexes that affect phrenic motoneuron activation. Group I and II afferents from intercostal nerves have been shown to exert both inhibitory and facilitatory influences on phrenic nerve activity.

Anterior-stretch basal lift (Fig. 6.10c)

This procedure is performed by placing the hands under the ribs of the supine patient and lifting gently upwards. The lift is maintained and provides a maintained stretch and pressure posteriorly and an anterior stretch as well. This may be done bilaterally if the patient is small enough. If this is not possible or necessary, it is effective done unilaterally. As the lift is sustained, stretch is maintained and increasing movement of the ribs in a lateral and posterior direction can be seen and felt. Increased epigastric movements also often become obvious. The lift to the back places some stretch on the dorsal intercostal area and should also stretch the spaces between some of the mid-thoracic ribs (5–8). These are both areas where the intercostal muscles are considered to be antagonistic in action. The epigastric movements suggest that the diaphragm is being activated by intercostal afferents.

Maintained manual pressure

When firm contact of the open hand(s) is maintained over an area in which expansion is desired, gradual increasing excursion of the ribs under the contact will be felt. This is a useful procedure to obtain expansion in any situation where pain is present, for instance, when there are chest tubes or after cardiac surgery which

may have required splitting of the sternum. Manual contact over the posterior chest wall is also useful and comfortable for persons with chronic obstructive pulmonary disease. The inspiratory response is thought to be due to cutaneous tactile receptors. The contact should be firm so that it does not tickle.

In 1963 Sumi studied hair, tactile and pressure receptors in the cat amd reported thoracic cutaneous fields for both inspiratory and expiratory motoneurons. He proposed that since the excitatory skin fields for inspiratory motoneurons were more extensive than those for expiratory motoneurons, more inspiratory motoneurons could be excited by a single skin stimulus. Local cutaneous stimulation of the thoracic region would then tend to reflexly produce an inspiratory position of the rib cage. Duron & Bars (1986) also studied thoracic cutaneous stimulation in the cat. They directly electrically stimulated desheathed lateral cutaneous nerves in anaesthetized decerebrate cats and cats that were both decerebrate and spinal. Among their findings was widespread inhibition on both inspiratory and expiratory activity after stimulation of the cutaneous nerve. Their observations also suggested that responses from the upper and lower thoracic areas were different. They acknowledge that the roles of the different cutaneous afferent components need to be identified.

Perioral pressure (Fig. 6.10d)

Perioral stimulation is provided by applying firm maintained pressure to the patient's top lip, being careful not to occlude the nasal passage. (The use of surgical gloves is advised to avoid contamination.) The response to this stimulus is a brief (approximately 5 second) period of apnoea followed by increased epigastric excursions. The initial response may frequently be observed as a large maintained epigastric swell. Pressure is maintained for the length of time the therapist wishes the patient to breathe in the activated pattern. As the stimulus is maintained the epigastric excursions may increase so that movement is transmitted to the upper chest and the patient appears to be deep breathing. Respiratory rate is usually slower. The patient may sigh on initiation of the procedure or sometime after the response has become established.

The paucity of muscle spindles in the diaphragm determines that phrenic motoneurons which provide its motor activation do not receive any significant excitatory input from muscle spindle afferents and there are few, if any gamma motoneurons in the phrenic motor nucleus (Sieck & Prakash 1997). Information regarding afferent facilitation of phrenic motoneurons and/or other reflex interactions influencing their excitability is sparse. The responses that are observed on application of this stimulus correlate very well with the work of Peiper (1963).

When this perioral stimulus is applied to the unconscious patient, if the mouth is open, it will close. Swallowing is noted and sucking movements are often evident even in the presence of oral airways. Swallowing and sucking may not be evident initially, but may appear in the more deeply unconscious after repeated stimulation. Occasionally such a patient has been observed to push pursed lips forward in a 'mouth phenomenon' or 'lip phenomenon' or 'snout phenomenon'. These observations are similar to observations made by Peiper (1963) while studying the neurology of respiration and the neurology of food intake and the relationship between sucking, swallowing and breathing in infants. The 'mouth' or 'lip' or 'snout phenomenon' has been reported by Peiper and other investigators, as a reflex response to gentle tapping on the upper lip noted in young normal infants and in adults with severe cerebral disorders. Movement of the lips, sucking, swallowing and chewing motions have been reported on stroking the lips of comatose adults and are thought to be related to infantile rooting reflexes.

Peiper observed that three centrally directed rhythmic movements arise during an infant's food intake: sucking, breathing and swallowing. Earlier experiments on young animals had established that there was a sucking centre located bilaterally in the medulla. Peiper established the dominance of the sucking centre over respiration. Infants can breathe while they nurse, partly due to the high position of the larynx. The

initiation of sucking was observed to immediately disturb respiration. There was initial lowering of the diaphragm for 5 seconds or more before respirations began at a new rhythm led by the sucking centre. When the sucking movements ceased, the respiratory movements continued in the new pattern for a period (in this instance, faster rhythm). The similarity between the observations recorded by Peiper and those observed in response to the perioral stimulus suggests that these phenomena are related. The stimulus on the top lip is thought to imitate, in part, the pressure of the mother's breast against the lips of a nursing infant. The lack of recent recorded material would seem to indicate that the investigation into sucking centres per se has not been pursued much further. The related activity, swallowing, has been investigated, especially with respect to its interactions with respiration.

Swallowing is a complex behaviour. Although it is one of the most elaborate of motor functions in humans, swallowing is a primitive reflex with implications of a stereotyped and fixed behaviour (Jean et al 1997). In most mammals, including humans, all the muscles concerned with swallowing are striated. Similar to respiration, swallowing is considered an autonomic function, but is governed by the same neural principles as those serving some somatic functions, such as locomotion. Great differences among species are observed concerning swallowing during the respiratory cycle. Most of the significant data were obtained from sheep. The oropharynx serves both deglutition and respiration. Several muscles in the mouth, pharynx and larynx are active to ensure the patency of the upper airways and to regulate the airflow during the respiratory cycle. In humans, swallows occur mainly during expiration. When the swallowing rhythm is regular, one swallow occurs for every one or few breaths. A brief minor inspiration called a 'swallow breath' ('Schluckatmung' by pioneer investigators) occurs at the onset of swallowing. The functional significance of this brief inspiration is not known.

The central pattern generator (CPG) for swallowing is located in the medulla in two main groups of neurons in two regions that also contain respiratory neurons. The mechanisms that generate its rhythms are not understood. The factors regulating the functional interactions between swallowing and respiration have yet to be determined. Margaret Rood (1973) taught the use of perioral stimulation to reduce spastic muscle tone. She believed that it induced a parasympathetic bias (as opposed to a sympathetic bias) and that it promoted general relaxation. It was a prerequisite for her light, moving touch facilitation procedure to activate limb muscles. Her treatment focus and patient population probably accounts for Rood's lack of awareness of the respiratory responses to this stimulus.

Co-contraction of the abdomen (Fig. 6.10e)

Rood (1973) taught co-contraction of the abdomen as a procedure to facilitate respiration. Pressure is applied simultaneously over the patient's lower lateral ribs and over the ilium in a direction at right angles to the patient. Moderate force is applied and maintained. Rood believed that this procedure increased tone in the abdominal muscles and also activated the diaphragm. She proposed that the pressure directed across the abdomen produced intrafusal stretch, thus activating the muscle spindles (mainly in the rectus). She thought that the side contralateral to the pressure reacted first. As those muscles responded to the stretch and shortened, they would stretch the intrafusal fibres of the opposite muscles which in turn would activate their homonymous extrafusal muscles, which would contract, shorten and stretch the first set again and so the cycle would be repeated. A series of alternating contractions was thought to occur as long as the pressure was maintained. Co-contraction of the abdomen should be done bilaterally with pressure applied alternately and maintained for some seconds on either side. The maintained pressure is repeated as necessary to obtain and maintain the response for the desired period.

In practice, activation of the abdominal muscles does not always occur in the contralateral side first. There can be considerable variation in individual responses. Pre-existing muscle

tone, corpulence, postoperative status and the integrity of the abdominal wall are some of the influencing factors. Lax abdominal muscles (for any reason) appear to respond more slowly. If activation is slow it is often helpful to observe the umbilicus which may exhibit changes in its movement pattern, becoming more depressed on exhalations before changes in the muscles can be detected.

This is an effective procedure. As pressure is maintained, increasing abdominal tone can be both seen and palpated. In the presence of retained secretions abdominal co-contractions may produce coughing more readily than the other procedures. As ventilation increases with any procedure, coughing may occur. In obese patients abdominal co-contraction has frequently resulted in decreased abdominal girth.

Clinical application

In the clinical setting auscultation and standard chest assessment should be undertaken before, during and after treatment. Ventilatory movement patterns should be noted. Is chest expansion simultaneous and equal? Are there paradoxical movements or any areas of indrawing on inspiration? The therapist must be aware of the patterns of ventilation and how they are changing. Since the patient's response determines the duration of treatment, assessment is critical. The procedure of choice is continued until the desired treatment effect has been achieved, whether increased breath sounds, cough or stabilized respiratory pattern. Many patients raise secretions and cough. (Advice given to therapists was frequently 'co-contract and duck'.) Unconscious patients need assistance to get rid of their secretions, but suctioning may not be required as often or as deeply. Some unconscious patients appear to become less obtunded. Eyelids may flutter, eyes may open or there may be spontaneous movements. Sometimes, such a patient will initially turn the head away or push the therapist's hand away. These are positive signs as these patients are often thought to be unresponsive.

Responses to the facilitatory procedures are individual reactions and therefore every patient will not demonstrate the same level of responsiveness to each procedure. It is not necessary to do each procedure with every patient but it is imperative to observe the individual response and modify treatment accordingly. Treatment should not be continued in the presence of an undesirable response. A dramatic example of an undesirable response was seen in a decerebrate patient who was so hypertonic that abdominal co-contractions applied in the supine position began to elevate him into a sitting position. Such a response necessitates the use of other procedures. Conscious medical patients often appreciate the sense of relaxation and the lack of a sense of effort when facilitation procedures are used in their care. Many do their own perioral stimulation. Acute and chronic neurological conditions such as amyotrophic lateral sclerosis, Guillain–Barré, cerebral vascular accidents and others may also be treated with these procedures and derive benefit.

BREATHING CONTROL

Breathing techniques can be divided into normal breathing, known as 'breathing control', where minimal effort is expended and breathing exercises where either inspiration is emphasized, as in thoracic expansion exercises and inspiratory muscle training or expiration is emphasized, as in the huff of the forced expiration technique.

Breathing control is normal tidal breathing using the lower chest with relaxation of the upper chest and shoulders. This used to be known as 'diaphragmatic breathing', but this term is a misnomer as during normal tidal breathing there is activity not only in the diaphragm but also in the internal and external intercostal muscles, the abdominal and scalene muscles (Green & Moxham 1985).

To be taught breathing control, the patient should be in a comfortable well-supported position either sitting (Fig. 6.11) or in high side lying (Fig. 6.12). The patient is encouraged to relax his upper chest, shoulders and arms while using the lower chest. One hand, which may be either the patient's or the physiotherapist's or one hand of each, can be positioned lightly on the upper abdomen. As the patient breathes in, the hand should be felt to rise up and out; as the patient breathes out, the hand sinks down and in.

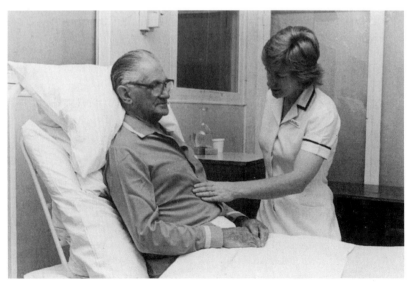

Figure 6.11   Breathing control in sitting.

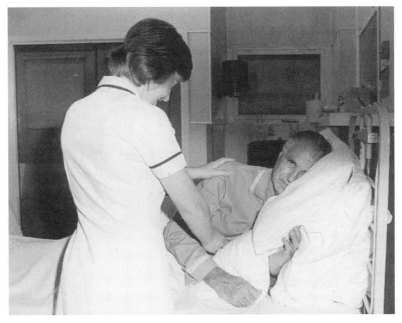

a

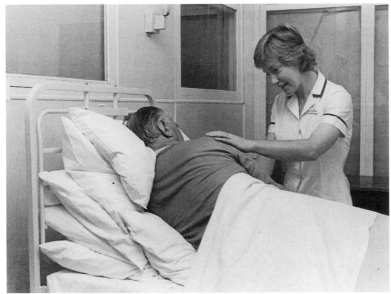

b

Figure 6.12 Breathing control in high side lying.

Inspiration is the active phase, expiration should be relaxed and passive and both inspiration and expiration should be barely audible. Inspiration through the nose allows the air to be warmed, humidified and filtered before it reaches the upper airways. If the nose is blocked, breathing through the mouth will reduce the resistance to the flow of air and will reduce the work of breathing. If the patient is very breathless, breathing through the mouth will reduce the anatomical dead space.

Some patients reflexly use pursed-lip breathing. Breathing through pursed lips has the effect of generating a small positive pressure during expiration which may to some extent reduce the collapse of unstable airways, for example in emphysema. This technique increases the work of breathing, particularly if it has become a forced noisy manoeuvre and many patients no longer need to use pursed-lip breathing when they have relearned breathing control (normal breathing), which minimizes the work of breathing.

There are positions which optimize the length tension status of the diaphragm (American Thoracic Society 1999, Dean 1985, O'Neill & McCarthy 1983, Sharp et al 1980). When the patient is sitting or standing leaning forward, the abdominal contents raise the anterior part of the diaphragm, probably facilitating its contraction during inspiration. A similar effect can be seen in the side lying and high side lying positions where the curvature of the dependent part of the diaphragm is increased. This effect, combined with relaxation of the head, neck and shoulders, promotes the pattern of breathing control.

Any breathless patient, for example those with emphysema, asthma, pulmonary fibrosis or lung cancer, will benefit from using breathing control in positions which encourage relaxation of the upper chest and shoulders and allow movement of the lower chest and abdomen. One of the most useful positions is high side lying (Fig. 6.12). For maximal relaxation of the head, neck and upper chest, the neck should be slightly flexed and the top pillow should be above the shoulder, supporting only the head and neck. Other useful positions are:

- relaxed sitting (Fig. 6.13)
- forward lean standing (Fig. 6.14)
- relaxed standing (Fig. 6.15)
- forward lean sitting (Fig. 6.16).

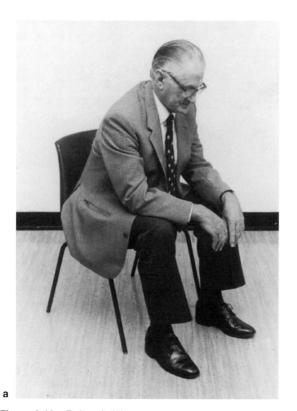

a

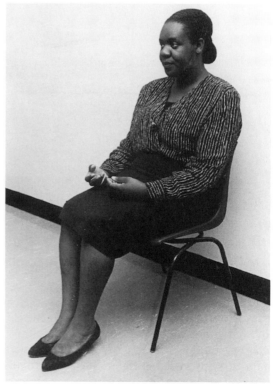

b

Figure 6.13 Relaxed sitting

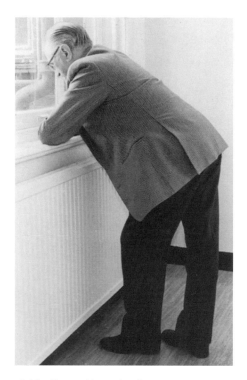

Figure 6.14 Forward lean standing.

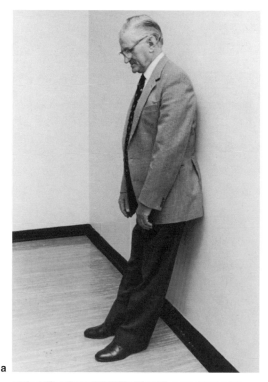

a

Breathless children may prefer a kneeling position (Fig. 6.17).

These positions discourage the tendency of breathless patients to push down or grip with their hands, which causes elevation of the shoulders and overuse of the accessory muscles of breathing. Figure 6.13b shows a position that is often preferred by patients who are overweight.

Breathing control is also used to improve exercise tolerance in breathless patients when walking up slopes, hills and stairs (Fig. 6.18). Breathless patients tend to hold their breath on exertion and rush, for example up a flight of stairs, arriving at the top extremely breathless and unable to speak. The simple technique of relaxing the arms and shoulders, reducing the walking speed a little and using the pattern of breathing *in* on climbing one step and breathing *out* on climbing the next step can lead to a marked reduction in breathlessness and the ability to converse on arrival at the top of the flight of stairs (Webber 1991). When this

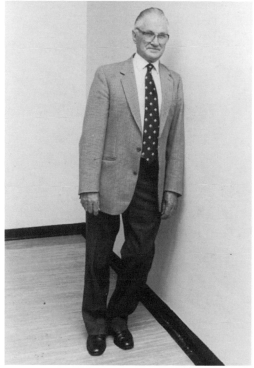

b

Figure 6.15 Relaxed standing.

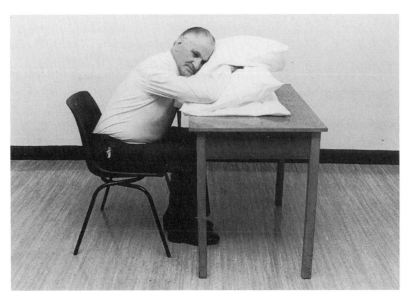

Figure 6.16 Forward lean sitting.

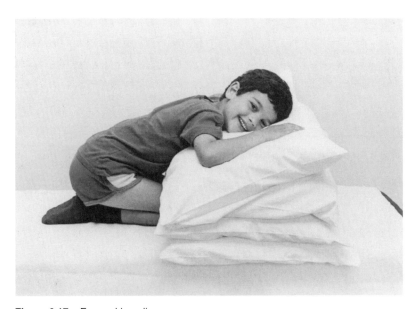

Figure 6.17 Forward kneeling.

technique has been mastered, some patients, on days when they are less breathless, may find breathing *in* for *one* step and *out* for *two* steps more comfortable.

The severely breathless patient may find the combination of breathing control with walking also helpful when walking on level ground. A respiratory walking frame (Fig. 6.19) with or without portable oxygen can be used to assist ambulation in the severely breathless patient.

Breathing control can also be used to control a bout or paroxysm of coughing.

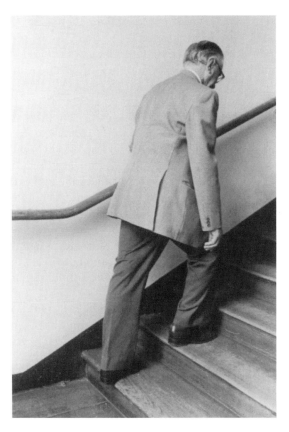

Figure 6.18   Breathing control while stair climbing.

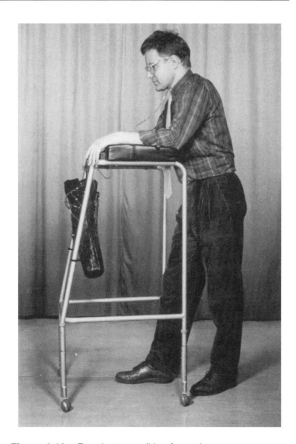

Figure 6.19   Respiratory walking frame in use.

INSPIRATORY MUSCLE TRAINING

During the last two decades, a plethora of studies have been performed examining the benefits of inspiratory muscle training (IMT), particularly in patients with chronic obstructive pulmonary disease (Asher et al 1982, Chen et al 1985, Dekhujzen et al 1991, Larson et al 1988). Despite this intensive investigation over this period, IMT has failed to become part of routine clinical practice. In part this has been due to the paucity of controlled clinical trials but, more importantly, it is due to the nature of the training adopted. In general, the trials were confounded by the nature of their training methodology in which the frequency, duration and intensity of training were less than that required to achieve a true training response (Smith et al 1992).

Training of the ventilatory muscles must follow the basic principles of training for any striated muscle with regard to the intensity and duration of the stimulus, the specificity of training and the reversibility of training. It is equally important to evaluate the outcome of training with appropriate criteria.

The principle of specificity of training states that the effects of training are very specific to the neural and muscular elements of overload. The overload principle states that overload must be applied to a muscle for a training response to occur. Overload may be applied by increasing the frequency or duration of training or the intensity of the loading or a combination of these factors. Overload may also include the concept of incremental loading. This involves decreasing the rest periods between muscle contractions (Komi & Hakkinen 1991), which has been shown to recruit a larger proportion of muscle fibres and, hence, a larger pool of fibres are trained for subsequent lower but potentially fatiguing loads (Reid & Samrai 1995, Reid et al 1994).

In humans, objective and quantitative data on the intensity of training required to improve inspiratory muscle function are lacking (Larson et al 1988). The load has to be high enough to induce training effects but in published data (Asher et al 1982, Dekhujzen et al 1991, Larson et al 1988, Leith & Bradley 1976) the training stimulus is extremely variable from one study to another. In 1991 Dekhuijzen and co-workers used a training load of 70% of maximum inspiratory pressure. They showed that in patients with a ventilatory limitation of exercise capacity, IMT had a positive effect on exercise performance that was greater than that of exercise training alone.

According to Pardy & Rochester (1992) one must ascertain that the inspiratory pressure per breath during training is set at a minimum of 50% and preferably at or above 70% of maximum inspiratory pressure (MIP). However, recommendations from the American College of Sports Medicine (1995) suggest that an optimal aerobic response can be achieved at training levels at or above 80% of maximum intensity. Indeed, studies which have employed high-intensity (85–95% $\dot{V}O_{2max}$) interval training have shown that oxidative capacity may be increased by 20–30% within the costal diaphragm in rats (Lawler et al 1993, Powers et al 1992). In support of these findings, more recent investigations in human subjects have identified low frequency fatigue in the diaphragm following repeated inspiratory manoeuvres to task failure in which the training intensity was set at 80% of MIP (Chatwin et al 2000).

In many previous investigations training methodologies have varied to include loads imposed on the respiratory muscles which can be characterized as flow, pressure and volume loads (McCool 1992). A flow load is imposed by any process that increases the level of ventilation needed to remain normocapnic. Flow loads may be imposed by increasing the level of ventilation either during exercise or through voluntary effort. In contrast to a flow load, a pressure load

occurs with any process that increases the transpulmonary pressure required to inspire. These loads can be experimentally imposed by inhaling from a rigid chamber or by breathing through an external resistance.

A volume load is a process that results in hyperinflation, thus decreasing the length of the inspiratory muscles as the subject approaches total lung capacity. This load may be imposed by reducing the time to exhale, thereby causing dynamic hyperinflation or by the application of continuous positive airways pressure. As with the techniques used in the assessment of the respiratory muscles, many training regimens have focused on repeated maximal inspiratory and expiratory efforts against a closed airway for strength training and isocapnoeic hyperpnoea, resistive and pressure loads for endurance training.

In many previous investigations, the volume at which training was performed has not been controlled. A potential problem with this is that patients tend to change their breathing strategy in order to tolerate the imposed load more easily. This may reduce the load on the inspiratory muscles below that which is necessary to induce training (Goldstein 1993). Smith et al (1992) included in their meta-analysis a criticism of the lack of control of imposed workloads during IMT, but the authors added the caveat that if workload was controlled and substantial pressures generated during training then improvements were possible.

A further important component to consider when training the inspiratory muscles is the control of the ratio of inspiratory time to expiratory time or the tension/time index. Bellemare & Grassino (1982) have described a tension/time index for the diaphragm (TTdi) which is derived from the comparison of work/rest ratios with a critical value of 0.15–0.2 (TTdi); a score of 1 would indicate continuous contraction at maximum force with no rest periods. Zocchi and co-workers (1993) applied the concept of TTdi to the inspiratory muscles, describing a critical value of 0.3 (TTdi) beyond which respiratory muscle fatigue would occur. If levels of IMT are fully fixed in compliance with the principles of overload, at a level that is consistent with a strength/endurance response, this would eventually lead to fatigue if the system were not unloaded by introducing periods of relative rest. These factors indicate that in addition to the fixation of pressure and flow during IMT, work/rest ratios should also be fixed to ensure that a true training load is applied.

Constant reassessment of maximal strength of contraction is also needed to allow changes in load which ensure that true overload is consistently applied throughout a training regimen (Komi & Hakkinen 1991). Studies which have incorporated an increase in the TTdi during repeated inspiratory manoeuvres to task failure at a training intensity of 80% of MIP have demonstrated an increase in exercise capacity in both moderately trained and highly trained subjects (Chatham et al 1999, Enright et al 2000) and in adult patients with cystic fibrosis (Enright et al, personal communication).

The frequency of training in IMT interventions has often been arbitrarily set at 30 minutes daily with some studies taking as little as 2–4 weeks (Chen et al 1985, Kim et al 1984, Nomori et al 1994). Neural adaptation is said to take place over the first 4 weeks of training (Fleck 1994) incorporating both learned response (Larson et al 1993) and increased frequency and improved coordination of neuromuscular firing (Epstein 1994). Improvements seen beyond this period are believed to be due to morphological adaptations, including increases in the oxidative capacity, the capillary bed of the muscle and muscle fibre hypertrophy (Komi & Hakkinen 1991). The optimal frequency of training is thought to be three times weekly, with maintenance achieved by continuing training at one or two times weekly (Fleck 1994). Thus, evidence from standard exercise training suggests that IMT interventions should take place three times weekly and continue beyond 4 weeks.

In conclusion, although there is much conflicting evidence in the literature which has cast doubt on the role of IMT in patients with respiratory muscle dysfunction, more recent data which have incorporated the appropriate physiological training principles during IMT look promising (Chatwin et al 2000). Thus with effective IMT regimens, exercise intolerance, dysp-

noea and hypercapnic ventilatory failure may be prevented or alleviated. These considerations are vital if IMT is to find a proven role in clinical practice (Goldstein 1993, Grassino 1989).

AIRWAY CLEARANCE TECHNIQUES

The term 'airway clearance techniques' is commonly used for the techniques described (alphabetically) in this section. For patients who need to use an airway clearance technique (ACT) in the long term, for example people with cystic fibrosis or bronchiectasis, a change of technique or the introduction of a device may improve adherence to treatment. There is as yet no evidence to support the use of any one airway clearance technique over and above any other (Prasad & Main 1998). Practice tends to be influenced by culture, patient preference and the experience of the physiotherapist. When a device is included in an airway clearance regimen meticulous cleaning and thorough drying of the equipment after use is essential to prevent the possibility of infection from the device.

Other techniques, for example intermittent positive pressure breathing and glossopharyngeal breathing, described later under 'Other techniques', may also assist in the clearance of secretions but have other additional effects.

It is important to introduce the concept of self-treatment at an early stage. Patients in hospital should be encouraged to take some responsibility for their treatment (Fig. 6.20). Surgical patients should continue their breathing exercises in between the treatment sessions with the physiotherapist. Medical patients can perhaps start by doing their own evening treatment. If the patient takes responsibility for his treatment before discharge home, both the patient and physiotherapist will have the confidence that treatment will be continued effectively. It is, however, important to negotiate rather than prescribe a physiotherapy home programme to increase compliance with treatment (Carr et al 1996). Programmes must be realistic and appropriate general physical activities should be encouraged.

Revision of techniques at intervals is necessary to assess the effectiveness of the treatment regimen and to correct and update techniques as

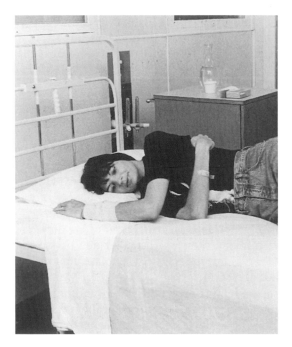

Figure 6.20 Self-treatment: thoracic expansion exercises.

necessary. Currie et al (1986) recognized the importance of reassessment in maintaining patient compliance.

Active cycle of breathing techniques

The active cycle of breathing techniques (ACBT) is used to mobilize and clear excess bronchial secretions. It has been shown to be effective in the clearance of bronchial secretions (Pryor et al 1979, Wilson et al 1995) and to improve lung function (Webber et al 1986), without increasing hypoxaemia (Pryor et al 1990) or airflow obstruction (Pryor & Webber 1979, Pryor et al 1994, Thompson & Thompson 1968).

The ACBT is a flexible method of treatment which can be adapted for use in any patient in whom there is a problem of excess bronchial secretions and can be used with or without an assistant. It is a cycle of breathing control, thoracic expansion exercises and the forced expiration technique (FET). The original studies on 'the forced expiration technique' (Hofmeyr et al 1986, Pryor et al 1979, Webber et al 1986) used this cycle of techniques, but people began to use

a regimen of huffing alone or other variations on the FET (Falk et al 1984, Reisman et al 1988) and the literature became confusing. In order to emphasize the use of thoracic expansion exercises and the periods of breathing control, in addition to the FET, the whole regimen was renamed the active cycle of breathing techniques (ACBT) (Webber 1990). The regimen did not change in practice and the early studies on the FET were controlled trials of the ACBT.

Thoracic expansion exercises

Thoracic expansion exercises are deep breathing exercises emphasizing inspiration. Inspiration is active and may be combined with a 3-second hold before the passive relaxed expiration. The postoperative manoeuvre of a 3-second hold at full inspiration has been said to decrease collapse of lung tissue (Ward et al 1966). This 'hold' is probably also of value in patients with medical chest conditions.

In the normal lung the resistance to airflow via the collateral ventilatory system is high, but with increasing lung volume and in the presence of lung pathology the resistance decreases, allowing air to flow via the collateral channels – the pores of Kohn, channels of Lambert and channels of Martin (Menkes & Traystman 1977) (Fig. 6.21). Air behind secretions may assist in mobilizing them.

The effectiveness of thoracic expansion exercises in re-expanding lung tissue and in mobilizing and clearing excess bronchial secretions can

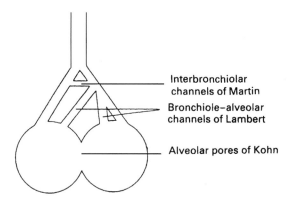

Figure 6.21 Collateral ventilation pathways.

Interbronchiolar
channels of Martin

Bronchiole–alveolar
channels of Lambert

Alveolar pores of Kohn

also be explained by the phenomenon of inter-dependence (Mead et al 1970). This is the effect of the expanding forces exerted between adjacent alveoli. At high lung volumes the expanding forces between alveoli are greater than at tidal volume and assist in re-expansion of lung tissue. Three or four expansion exercises are usually appropriate before pausing for a few seconds for a period of breathing control. Any more deep breaths could produce the effects of hyperventilation or could tire the patient.

Thoracic expansion exercises can be encouraged with proprioceptive stimulation by placing a hand, either the patient's or the physiotherapist's, over the part of the chest wall where movement of the chest is to be encouraged. There may be an initial increase in ventilation to this part of the lung (Tucker et al 1999) and there is an increase in chest wall movement.

Sometimes an additional increase in lung volume can be achieved by using a 'sniff' manoeuvre at the end of a deep inspiration. This manoeuvre may not be appropriate in patients who are hyperinflated, but for surgical patients who need further motivation to increase their lung volume it may be a useful technique.

Thoracic expansion exercises may be combined with chest shaking, vibrations and/or chest clapping. These techniques may further assist in the clearance of secretions.

The forced expiration technique (FET)

The forced expiration technique is a combination of one or two forced expirations (huffs) and periods of breathing control. Huffing to low lung volumes will move the more peripherally situated secretions and when secretions have reached the larger more proximal upper airways a huff or cough from a high lung volume can be used to clear them. 'Forced expiratory manoeuvres are probably the most effective part of chest physiotherapy' (van der Schans 1997).

With any forced expiratory manoeuvre there is dynamic compression and collapse of the airways downstream (towards the mouth) of the equal pressure point (West 1997). This is an important part of the clearance mechanism of

either a huff or a cough. As lung volume decreases during a forced expiratory manoeuvre, the equal pressure points move out and into the smaller, more peripheral airways. At lung volumes above functional residual capacity the equal pressure points are located in lobar or segmental bronchi (Macklem 1974). A series of coughs without intervening inspirations was advocated by Mead et al (1967) to clear bronchial secretions, but clinically a single continuous huff down to the same lung volume is as effective and less exhausting. Hasani et al (1994), comparing cough and the FET, concluded that both were equally effective in clearing lung secretions, but that the FET required less effort.

The mean transpulmonary pressure during voluntary coughing is greater than during a forced expiration. This results in greater compression and narrowing of the airways which limits airflow and reduces the efficiency of bronchial clearance (Langlands 1967). In 1989 Freitag et al demonstrated an oscillatory movement, 'hidden' vibrations, of the airway walls in addition to the squeezing action produced by the forced expiratory manoeuvre.

The viscosity of mucus is shear dependent (Lopez-Vidriero & Reid 1978) and the shear forces generated during a huff should reduce mucus viscosity. This, together with the high flow of a forced expiratory manoeuvre, would also be expected to aid mucus clearance and the expectoration of sputum.

When mobilizing and clearing peripheral secretions it is an unnecessary expenditure of energy to start the huff from a high lung volume. A huff from mid-lung volume is more efficient and probably more effective. To huff from mid-lung volume a medium-sized breath should be taken in and, with the mouth and glottis open, the air is squeezed out using the chest wall and abdominal muscles. It should be long enough to loosen secretions from the more peripherally situated airways and should not just be a clearing noise in the back of the throat. However, if the huff is continued for too long it may lead to unnecessary paroxysmal coughing. Too short a huff may be ineffective (Partridge et al 1989), but when the secretions have reached the upper airways, a shorter huff or a cough from a high lung volume is used to clear them.

The huff is a forced but not violent manoeuvre. To be maximally effective the length of the huff and force of contraction of the expiratory muscles should be altered to maximize airflow and to minimize airway collapse. A peak flow mouthpiece or similar piece of tubing, may improve the effectiveness of the huff as it helps to keep the glottis open. Some people find that huffing through a tube at a tissue or cotton wool ball is helpful in perfecting the technique. The huff can be introduced to children as blowing games (Thompson 1978) and from about the age of 2 years they are usually able to copy others huffing (Fig. 6.22).

An essential part of the forced expiration technique is the pause for breathing control after one or two huffs, which prevents any increase in airflow obstruction. The length of the pause will vary from patient to patient. In a patient with bronchospasm or unstable airways or in one who is debilitated and fatigues easily, longer pauses (perhaps 10–20 seconds) may be appropriate. In patients with no bronchospasm the periods of breathing control may be considerably shorter (perhaps two or three breaths or 5–10 seconds).

In the tetraplegic patient, clearance of secretions from the upper airways is difficult because maximum lung volume cannot be achieved and the equal pressure points will therefore never reach the largest airways (Morgan et al 1986). Secretions can be cleared from the smaller airways, but accumulate in the larger upper airways.

Application of the active cycle of breathing techniques

The cycle of breathing control, thoracic expansion exercises and the forced expiration technique are adapted for each patient (Fig. 6.23). Sometimes one set of thoracic expansion exercises will be followed by the forced expiration technique (Fig. 6.23a,b), but if secretions loosen slowly it may be more appropriate to use two sets of thoracic expansion exercises (Fig. 6.23c). The surgical patient will probably benefit from the 3-second hold with the thoracic expansion exercises (Fig. 6.24) and there is probably no indication, in the surgical patient, for the use of chest clapping. Wound support may be more suitable than chest compression during huffing and coughing (Fig. 6.25).

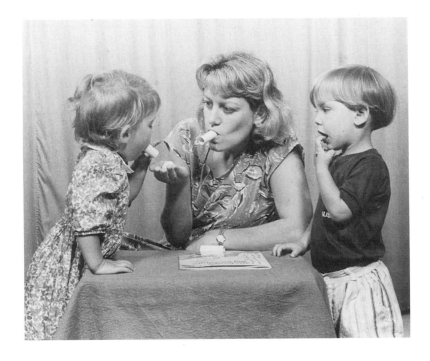

Figure 6.22 Huffing games.

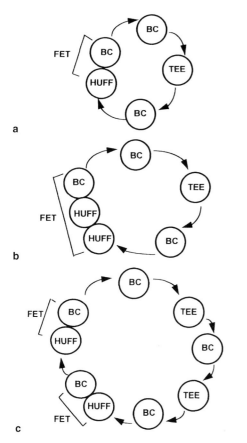

a

b

c

Figure 6.23   Examples to demonstrate the flexibility of the active cycle of breathing techniques: BC, breathing control; TEE, thoracic expansion exercises; FET, forced expiration technique.

In many patients the ACBT will effectively clear secretions in the sitting position, but in others gravity-assisted positions may be required. Cecins et al (1999) studied the effects of gravity (positions with and without a head-down tilt) in a group of patients with cystic fibrosis, bronchiectasis and immotile cilia syndrome, using the ACBT. There were no significant differences in lung function or in the weight of sputum expectorated during treatment. Most of the patients preferred the horizontal position and felt less breathless without a head-down tilt. Further work needs to be undertaken to determine whether the majority of patients in the study, who had cystic fibrosis, influenced the outcome or whether the results also reflect the effects in patients with bronchiectasis and immotile cilia syndrome.

For patients with a moderate amount of bronchial secretions, for example with bronchiectasis or cystic fibrosis, clinical experience suggests that a minimum of 10 minutes in any productive position is usually necessary. For patients with minimal secretions, for example some asthmatics, some chronic bronchitics or following surgery, less time is required. The 'endpoint' of a treatment session can be recognized either by the physiotherapist or the patient treating himself when an effective huff to low lung

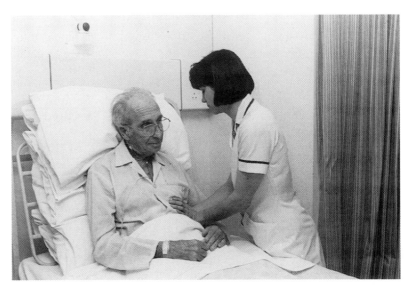

Figure 6.24   Thoracic expansion exercises.

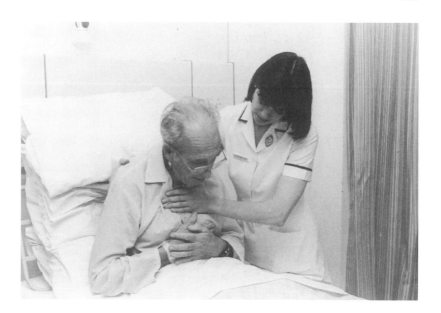

Figure 6.25 Huffing with wound support.

volume, in two consecutive cycles, has been dry sounding and non-productive. The sicker patient may not reach this end-point before tiring and should stop when fatigue is recognized.

Autogenic drainage

Autogenic drainage (AD) aims to maximize airflow within the airways to improve the clearance of mucus and ventilation (David 1991). Chevaillier developed this concept in Belgium in the late 1960s, but little was published until 1979 (Dab & Alexander 1979). Autogenic drainage utilizes gentle breathing at different lung volumes to loosen, mobilize and clear bronchial secretions.

Chevaillier originally described three phrases: 'unstick', 'collect' and 'evacuate' (Schöni 1989). The breathing technique is that of a slow breath in, keeping the upper airways (mouth and glottis) open while using breathing control. It is recommended that the breath be held for 2–4 seconds. This 'hold' facilitates more equal filling of lung segments, by allowing for the variation in time constants within different lung regions. Expiration is also performed keeping the upper airways open, as if sighing. The expiratory force is balanced so that the expiratory flow reaches the highest rate possible without causing airway

compression. Breathing out at a high velocity enhances shear forces. As mucus is mobilized it can be both heard and felt (by placing the hands on the chest). This cycle is repeated through the varying lung volumes.

Breathing at low lung volumes is said to mobilize peripheral mucus. This is the first or 'unstick' phase. It is followed by a period of breathing around the individual's tidal volume which is said to 'collect' mucus from the middle airways. Then, by breathing around high lung volumes, the 'evacuate' phase, expectoration of secretions from the central airways is promoted. When sufficient mucus has been collected in the large airways it may be cleared by coughing or huffing. Coughing before this point is discouraged (Chevaillier 1995, Chevaillier 2001 personal communication). Autogenic drainage is usually practised in the sitting (Fig. 6.26) or supine lying position.

AD has been altered in Germany (David 1991) and is not split into the three phases as the patients were found to be uncomfortable breathing at low lung volumes. This technique is known as modified autogenic drainage (M AD) (Kieselmann 1995). The patient breathes around tidal volume while breath holding for 2–3 seconds at the end of each inspiration. Coughing is used to clear mucus from the larynx (Kieselmann 1995).

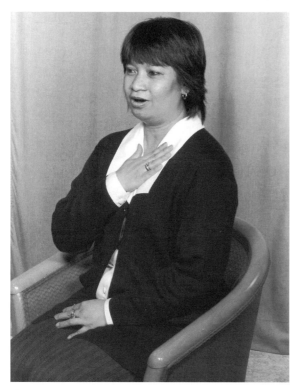

Figure 6.26   Autogenic drainage.

The flow–volume loop is frequently used to support the theory of an increase in airflow with the unforced expiratory manoeuvre of autogenic drainage (Schöni 1989). Airflow near functional residual capacity is low. It is only possible to move outside the flow–volume loop if pressure-dependent airway collapse exists, which is often the case as lung disease progresses. However, in patients without pressure-dependent airway collapse, this phenomenon may not exist. In a long-term study of patients with cystic fibrosis AD was compared with 'conventional' percussion and postural drainage. AD was found to be at least as effective as the conventional treatment and the patients had a marked preference for AD (Davidson et al 1992).

Oscillating positive expiratory pressure

These devices combine an oscillation of the air within the airways during expiration and a vari-able positive expiratory pressure. Two commonly used devices are described below.

Flutter®

The Flutter® is a small, portable device (Fig. 6.27). It is pipe shaped with a single opening at the mouthpiece and a series of small outlet holes at the top of the bowl. The bowl contains a high-density stainless steel ball enclosed in a small cone. During expiration the movement of the ball along the surface of the cone creates a positive expiratory pressure (PEP) and an oscillatory vibration of the air within the airways. In addition, intermittent airflow accelerations are produced by the same movements of the ball. The device is held horizontally and tilted slightly either downwards or upwards until a maximal oscillatory effect can be felt. It is usually used either sitting or in supine lying, but may be used in other positions provided an effective oscillation can be maintained. Sputum viscoelasticity has been shown to be reduced after the use of the Flutter (App et al 1998).

The Flutter is placed in the mouth and inspiration is either through the nose or through the mouth by breathing around the Flutter (it is not

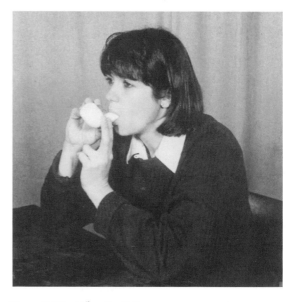

Figure 6.27   Using the flutter.

possible to breathe in through the Flutter). A slow breath in, only slightly deeper than normal, with a breath hold of 3–5 seconds is followed by a breath out, through the Flutter, at a slightly faster rate than normal. After 4–8 of these breaths, a deep breath with a 'hold' at full inspiration is followed by a forced expiration through the Flutter. This may precipitate expectoration and should be followed by a pause for breathing control following a huff or cough. In some parts of Europe this forced expiratory manoeuvre is not used as a part of the regimen.

Konstan et al (1994) compared three regimens: the Flutter, voluntary coughing and a regimen of postural drainage which included up to 10 positions. Each session lasted 15 minutes. The Flutter regimen was the most effective as measured by the weight of sputum expectorated. Homnick et al (1998) and Gondor et al (1999) have supported the findings of Konstan et al. Ambrosino et al (1995) showed the Flutter to be as effective as 'conventional physiotherapy'. This is important evidence but when the above studies were undertaken, other parts of the world were already using airway clearance regimens which

had been shown to be more effective than 'postural drainage'.

Originally the recommended technique for the Flutter was a gentle exhalation through the device. Treatment was continued for a period of 10 minutes. Secretions were expectorated by spontaneous coughing. It was this regimen that was shown by Pryor et al (1994) to be less effective than the ACBT. The inclusion of the forced expiratory manoeuvre in the regimen would be likely to increase the effectiveness of airway clearance and this was demonstrated, in the short term, by Pike et al (1999).

When autogenic drainage was compared with the Flutter it was concluded that both regimens were equally effective, but the Flutter was easier to teach (Lindemann 1992). A clinical trial was undertaken using the Flutter in patients following thoracotomy, but no advantage could be found in its inclusion (Chatham et al 1993).

RC-Cornet®

The R-C Cornet® (Fig. 6.28) consists of a curved, hard plastic outer tube, mouthpiece and flexible

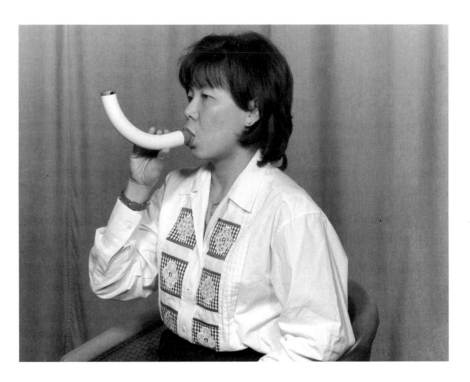

Figure 6.28 R-C Cornet.

latex-free inner tube (valve-hose). The Cornet is placed in the mouth and inspiration is either through the nose or through the mouth, by breathing around the Cornet (it is not possible to breathe in through the Cornet). During expiration through the Cornet, a positive expiratory pressure and an oscillatory vibration of the air within the airways are generated. The flow, pressure and frequency of the oscillations can be adjusted to suit the individual and it can be used in any position (e.g. sitting, side lying, head-down tilt) as it is independent of gravitional forces. Initially the individual breathes out through the Cornet at approximately his normal rate and depth, but these breaths may be interspersed with deeper ones. Huffing or coughing is used to clear secretions mobilized to the upper airways and is followed by breathing control. It is recommended that the Cornet be used for 10–15 minutes (Cegla 1999, personal communication). The Cornet has been shown to be as effective as the Flutter in airway clearance (Cegla et al 1997) and to decrease the cohesiveness and viscoelasticity of sputum from patients with bronchiectasis (Nakamura et al 1998).

Positive expiratory pressure

The positive expiratory pressure (PEP) mask was described by Falk et al (1984) who found an increase in sputum yield and an improvement in transcutaneous oxygen tension when compared with postural drainage, percussion and breathing exercises. It was suggested that the increase in sputum yield was produced by the effect of PEP on peripheral airways and collateral channels. Falk & Andersen (1991) suggest that with the PEP treatment the increase in lung volume may allow air to get behind secretions blocking small airways and assist in mobilizing them.

The PEP apparatus consists of a facemask and a one-way valve to which expiratory resistances can be attached. A manometer is inserted into the system between the valve and resistance to monitor the pressure which should be between 10 and 20 cmH$_2$O during mid-expiration (Falk & Andersen 1991).

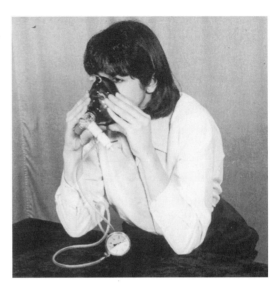

Figure 6.29   Using the PEP mask.

The patient sits leaning forward with his elbows supported on a table and holding the mask firmly over the nose and mouth (Fig. 6.29). A mouthpiece and nose clip can be used in place of the mask if this is preferred. The patient breathes at tidal volume with a slightly active expiration for approximately 6–10 breaths. The lung volume should be kept up by avoiding complete expiration. This is followed by the forced expiration technique to clear the secretions that have been mobilized. The duration and frequency of treatment are adapted to each individual, but treatment is usually performed for approximately 15 minutes, twice a day, in patients with stable chest disease and excess bronchial secretions (Falk & Andersen 1991). This should be adjusted according to the patient's signs and symptoms. In postoperative patients short periods of PEP used every hour as a prophylactic treatment have been described by Ricksten et al (1986).

The study by Falk et al (1984) in patients with cystic fibrosis compared an assisted 'conventional' postural drainage treatment with an unassisted PEP mask regimen and found that the PEP mask regimen was more effective and the one preferred by the patients. In order to reduce the variables studied, Hofmeyr et al (1986) compared the unassisted treatment of PEP combined with the forced expiration technique, with thoracic expansion exercises combined with the forced expiration technique (the active cycle of breathing techniques). In this study the ACBT was found to be advantageous in terms of the amount of sputum expectorated. van der Schans et al (1991) studied mucus clearance with PEP using a radio-aerosol technique in patients with cystic fibrosis. They showed that PEP temporarily increased lung volume, but did not lead to an improvement in mucus transport.

Lung function has been shown to improve with PEP in a long-term study (one year) when compared with postural drainage and percussion (McIlwaine et al 1997). McIlwaine et al (2001) also compared the use of PEP and the Flutter in the long term (one year). They concluded that PEP was more effective than the Flutter in maintaining pulmonary function.

High-pressure PEP is a modified form of PEP mask treatment described by Oberwaldner et al (1986) for the treatment of patients with cystic fibrosis. The mask is used during tidal volume breaths and also for a full forced expiratory manoeuvre. By applying a positive expiratory pressure during forced expiration, secretions may be mobilized more easily in patients with unstable airways. Assessment for the technique involves forced vital capacity manouevres with the mask attached to a spirometer (Oberwaldner et al 1986). The resultant expiratory flow volume curves are used to determine the appropriate resistor for the PEP mask. It is the resistance that allows the patient to expire to a volume greater than his usual forced vital capacity. The technique is only recommended where full lung function equipment is available for regular reassessment of the appropriate expiratory resistance for each individual. Meticulous care must be taken as an incorrect resistance may lead to a deterioration in lung function.

For treatment the patient sits upright holding the mask firmly against the face. Six to ten rhythmical breaths at tidal volume are followed by an inspiration to total lung capacity and then a forced expiratory manoeuvre against the resistance to low lung volume. The pressure generated during this manouevre ranges from 50–120 cmH$_2$O and usually results in the expectoration of sputum (Oberwaldner et al 1991).

Pfleger et al (1992) compared high-pressure PEP and autogenic drainage. More sputum was cleared with high-pressure PEP than with AD or with a combination of PEP and AD. Using this technique there is no evidence of any increase in pneumothorax (Zach & Oberwaldner 1992). The technique does require considerable effort and is perhaps less suitable for the patient who tires easily.

Mechanical percussion, vibration, oscillation and compression

A variety of mechanical devices are available to provide either percussion or oscillation to the chest wall, but the evidence for the use of these devices is inconclusive (Thomas et al 1995).

Mechanical percussors have been shown to increase intrathoracic pressure (Flower et al 1979), but Pryor et al (1981) could not demonstrate any increase in sputum clearance or improvement in lung function with mechanical percussion.

Goodwin (1994) undertook a review of mechanical percussion, vibration, high-frequency oscillation and chest wall compression in airway clearance. He concluded that mechanical vibration may increase mucociliary clearance and that high-frequency chest wall compression (Arens et al 1994, Hansen et al 1994) was more promising than oral high-frequency oscillation (George et al 1985, Pryor at al 1989, Van Hengstum et al 1990). Further work needs to be undertaken on the frequency of the vibration which may be patient dependent.

High-frequency chest wall oscillation (HFCWO) is the application of positive pressure air pulses to the chest wall, for example by means of an inflatable vest. The hypothesis is that an increase in cough clearability may be due to an increase in mucus/airflow interaction and/or a shearing mechanism leading to a decrease in the viscoelasticity of mucus (Tomkiewicz et al 1994).

Intrapulmonary percussive ventilation (IPV) is the delivery of a pulsatile flow of gas to the lungs during inspiration. The pulsatile flow results in an internal percussion. The subject's inspiratory effort initiates the flow of gas and the volume of gas released with each pulse and the pulsation frequency can be adjusted (Homnick et al 1995, Langenderfer 1998).

High-frequency chest compression may be considered a cost-effective alternative to chest physiotherapy (Hansen et al 1994). In other parts of the world where patients are already using independent airway clearance treatments it is unlikely that the expensive and cumbersome alternative of a mechanical device will be seriously considered.

Adjuncts to airway clearance techniques

Chest clapping

Chest clapping is performed using a cupped hand with a rhythmical flexion and extension action of the wrist. The technique is often done with two hands but, depending on the area of the chest, it may be more appropriate to use one hand. For the infant, chest clapping is performed using two or three fingers of one hand. Single-handed chest clapping is probably the technique of choice for self-chest clapping.

Chest clapping should never be uncomfortable and should be done over a layer of clothing to avoid sensory stimulation of the skin. It should not be necessary to use extra layers of clothing or towelling as the force of the chest clapping should be adapted to suit the individual.

Mechanical percussion has been shown to increase intrathoracic pressure (Flower et al 1979) and chest clapping may have a similar effect but this change in intrathoracic pressure has not been correlated with an increase in the clearance of bronchial secretions. Andersen (1987, personal communication) hypothesized that the air-filled alveoli would buffer increases in intrathoracic pressure and markedly reduce the mechanical effect of chest clapping.

Some studies (Campbell et al 1975, Wollmer et al 1985) have demonstrated an increase in airflow obstruction when chest clapping is included in the regimen, but other studies (Gallon 1991, Pryor & Webber 1979) have shown no increase in airflow obstruction with chest clapping.

In infants and small children not yet old enough to do voluntary breathing techniques and in patients with neuromuscular weakness or paralysis and the intellectually impaired, chest clapping is a useful technique to stimulate coughing probably by the mobilization of secretions.

Chest clapping has been shown to cause an increase in hypoxaemia (Falk et al 1984, McDonnell et al 1986), but when short periods of chest clapping (less than 30 seconds) have been combined with 3–4 thoracic expansion exercises no fall was seen in oxygen saturation (Pryor et al 1990).

In a group of clinically stable patients with cystic fibrosis no advantage was shown when self-chest clapping was used in addition to thoracic expansion exercises (Webber et al 1985), but this cannot be extrapolated to either all medical chest conditions or to acute chest problems. Single-handed chest clapping is advocated in self-treatment as it is difficult to coordinate two-handed clapping at the same time as using thoracic expansion exercises.

If a patient feels that self-chest clapping is beneficial, but the physiotherapist thinks it is tiring and may be causing hypoxaemia, the patient could be monitored using an oximeter. If oxygen desaturation of clinical significance occurs during the self-chest clapping the patient should be encouraged to omit the clapping but to continue with the thoracic expansion exercises. Patients studied by Carr et al (1995) felt that self-chest clapping was useful when they were clinically stable, but more particularly when they were unwell. The benefits of chest clapping remain uncertain, but if chest clapping is considered to be clinically beneficial for an individual it should be continued, provided there are no adverse effects.

There is probably no indication for chest clapping in postoperative patients and in patients following chest injury. Severe osteoporosis and frank haemoptysis are contraindications, although chest clapping is unlikely to increase bleeding when bronchial secretions are lightly streaked with blood.

Vigorous and rapid chest clapping may lead to breath holding and may induce bronchospasm in a patient with hyper-reactive airways. There is no evidence that alteration in the rate of chest clapping increases or decreases the mobilization of bronchial secretions. A rhythmical comfortable rate for both patient and physiotherapist is probably the most appropriate.

Chest shaking, vibrations and compression

The hands are placed on the chest wall and, during expiration, a vibratory action in the direction of the normal movement of the ribs is transmitted through the chest using body weight. This action augments the expiratory flow and may help to mobilize secretions. It is unknown whether airway closure will be increased if the vibratory action is continued into the expiratory reserve volume, but the techniques are frequently combined with thoracic expansion exercises which would counteract any resulting airway closure.

The vibratory action may be either a coarse movement (chest shaking) or a fine movement (chest vibrations). Little work has been done on the effects of either coarse or fine vibrations and physiotherapists have tended to adopt the techniques that they find the most helpful clinically.

In infants, vibrations are performed using two fingers in contact with the chest wall. Chest vibrations and shaking should never be uncomfortable and should be adapted to suit the individual patient. Some patients doing their own chest physiotherapy find self-chest vibrations helpful. One hand is placed on top of the other on the appropriate part of the chest wall and vibrations or shaking are carried out during expiration. With the hands in a similar position chest compression throughout expiration is often helpful to augment the forced expiratory manoeuvre of the huff. When in side lying self-compression can be given over the side of the chest with the upper arm and elbow and the hand of the other arm.

The physiotherapist or other carer may give compression during huffing or coughing. Some patients find this helpful, but others prefer to be unsupported. Postoperative patients usually find that supporting the wound facilitates both huffing and coughing. With fractured ribs and other chest injuries shaking of the chest wall would be inappropriate, but compressive support may assist the clearance of secretions.

In the paralysed patient the technique of rib springing may be used where compression of the chest wall is continued throughout expiration and overpressure is applied at the end of the breath out. By releasing the hands quickly inspiration is encouraged. This technique is inappropriate in the non-paralysed patient and may be harmful as compression against a reflexly splinted chest wall may produce rib fractures. Assisted coughing for the paralysed patient is described in Chapter 17.

In the drowsy, semicomatosed patient (for example, the chronic bronchitic in respiratory failure with sputum retention), chest compression similar to but less vigorous than rib springing may stimulate a deeper inspiration.

Chest shaking or chest vibrations can also be used during the expiratory phase of a manual hyperinflation treatment (Ch. 11, p. 368) to assist the clearance of secretions.

Care must be taken when using the techniques of chest shaking, vibrations and compression if there are signs of osteoporosis or metastatic deposits affecting the ribs or vertebral column.

Gravity-assisted positions

Gravity-assisted positions can be used to:

- assist the clearance of bronchial secretions
- improve ventilation and perfusion.

Clearance of bronchial secretions. Gravity can be used to assist the clearance of bronchial secretions (Hofmeyr et al 1986, Sutton et al 1983). Nelson (1934) described the use of positioning for draining secretions, based on the anatomy of the bronchial tree. The recognized positions (Thoracic Society 1950) (Fig. 6.30) are shown in Figures 6.31 to 6.41 and described in Table 6.4.

Some patients cannot tolerate the recognized positions and for others they may be contraindicated. Modified positions such as high side lying (Fig. 6.42) or side lying may be more appropriate. At school, college, work or when on holiday, positions such as side lying or sitting may be easier, more convenient and more likely to encourage patient compliance.

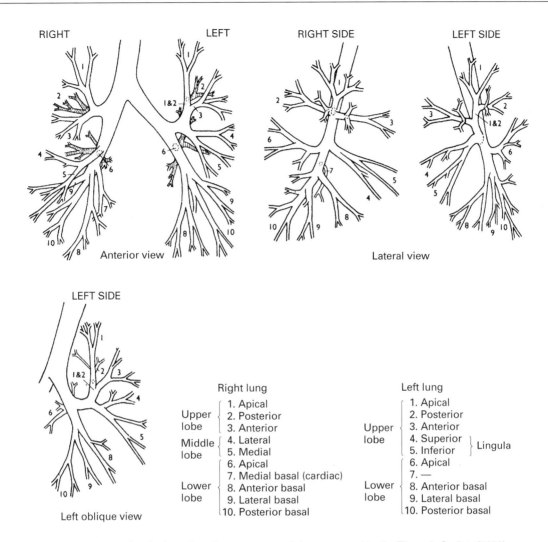

Figure 6.30 Diagram illustrating the bronchopulmonary nomenclature approved by the Thoracic Society (1950). (Reproduced by permission of the Editor of *Thorax.*)

Individual assessment will indicate whether gravity-assisted drainage positions are of clinical benefit. In some patients with very tenacious secretions gravity is unlikely to help and a comfortable position in which effective breathing techniques can be carried out is likely to be the most beneficial. In patients with cystic fibrosis the upper lobes are frequently the most severely afffected, although the cause is unknown (Tomashefski et al 1986) and positions other than sitting may only occasionally be indicated.

It is inappropriate to use the downward chest tilted positions immediately following meals and in the following conditions: cardiac failure, severe hypertension, cerebral oedema, aortic and cerebral aneurysms, severe haemoptysis, abdominal distension, gastro-oesophageal reflux and after recent surgery or trauma to the head or neck.

Ventilation/perfusion. In the adult, both ventilation and perfusion are preferentially distributed to the dependent parts of the lung (West

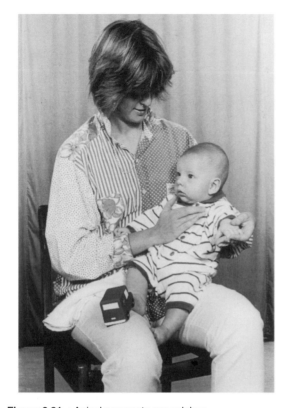

Figure 6.31 Apical segments upper lobes.

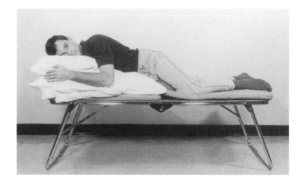

Figure 6.32 Posterior segment right upper lobe.

Figure 6.33 Posterior segment left upper lobe.

Table 6.4 Gravity-assisted drainage positions (numbers refer to Fig. 6.30 and patient position is shown in Figs 6.31 to 6.41)

	Lobe		Position	
Upper lobe	1	Apical bronchus	1	Sitting upright
	2	Posterior bronchus		
		(a) Right	2a	Lying on the left side horizontally turned 45° on to the face, resting against a pillow, with another supporting the head
		(b) Left	2b	Lying on the right side turned 45° on to the face, with three pillows arranged to lift the shoulders 30 cm from the horizontal
	3	Anterior bronchus	3	Lying supine with the knees flexed
Lingula	4	Superior bronchus	4 & 5	Lying supine with the body a quarter turned to the right maintained by a pillow under the left side from shoulder to hip. The chest is tilted downwards to an angle of 15°
	5	Inferior bronchus		
Middle lobe	4	Lateral bronchus	4 & 5	Lying supine with the body a quarter turned to the left maintained by a pillow under the right side from shoulder to hip. The chest is tilted downwards to an angle of 15°
	5	Medial bronchus		
Lower lobe	6	Apical bronchus	6	Lying prone with a pillow under the abdomen
	7	Medial basal (cardiac) bronchus	7	Lying on the right side with the chest tilted downwards to an angle of 20°
	8	Anterior basal bronchus	8	Lying supine with the knees flexed and the chest tilted downwards to an angle of 20°
	9	Lateral basal bronchus	9	Lying on the opposite side with the chest tilted downwards to an angle of 20°
	10	Posterior basal bronchus	10	Lying prone with a pillow under the hips and the chest tilted downwards to an angle of 20°

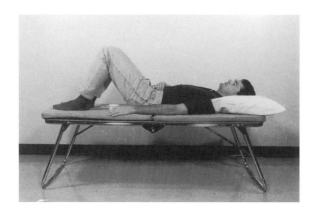

Figure 6.34 Anterior segments upper lobes.

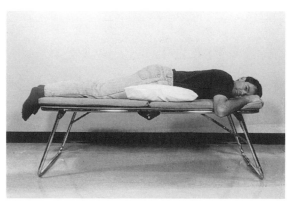

Figure 6.37 Apical segments lower lobes.

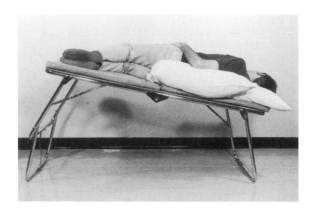

Figure 6.35 Lingula.

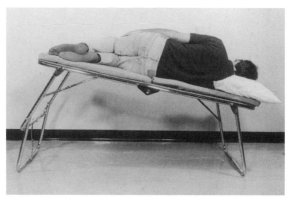

Figure 6.38 Right medial basal and left lateral basal segments lower lobes.

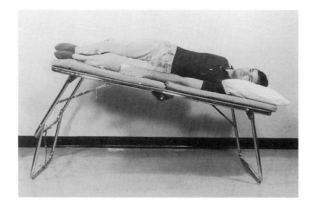

Figure 6.36 Right middle lobe.

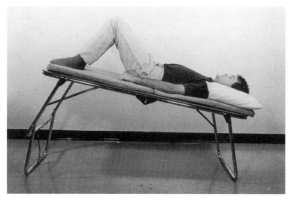

Figure 6.39 Anterior basal segments

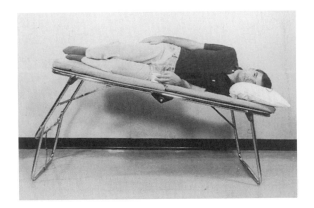

Figure 6.40 Lateral basal segment right lower lobe.

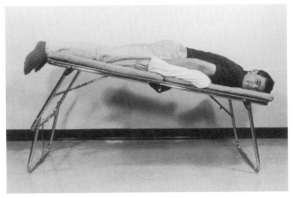

Figure 6.41 Posterior basal segments lower lobes.

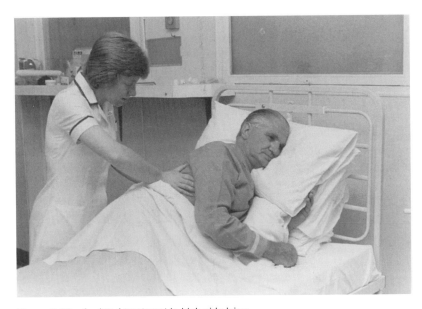

Figure 6.42 Assisted treatment in high side lying.

1997) whereas in children this differs (p. 428). In adults with unilateral lung disease gas exchange may be improved by using the side-lying position with the unaffected lung dependent (Zack et al 1974). Postoperatively the easiest method of increasing functional residual capacity (FRC) and preventing lung collapse is appropriate positioning and early ambulation (Jenkins et al 1988). Most patients can sit out of bed the day after surgery (Fig. 6.43a). If they cannot sit in a chair, they should be encouraged to either sit upright in bed or adopt a side-lying position, but they should not be in a slumped sitting position (Fig. 6.43b).

See also Chapter 5, Effects of positioning and mobilization.

Management of stress incontinence

Many patients with chronic cough and requiring airway clearance techniques suffer from stress incontinence which often causes embarrassment.

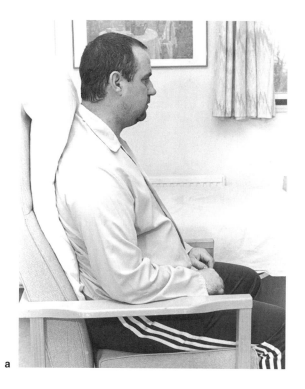

a

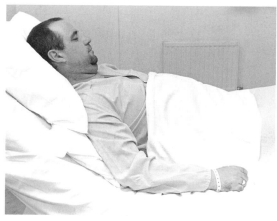

b

Figure 6.43 Positioning: **a** sitting upright; **b** slumped sitting.

The physiotherapist, during assessment (p. 8), should include questions to identify whether this is a problem. Instruction in pelvic floor exercises will probably be helpful but referral to an expert physiotherapist would ensure the best treatment programme and advice.

OTHER TECHNIQUES

Incentive spirometry

Incentive spirometers are mechanical devices introduced in an attempt to reduce postoperative pulmonary complications. The patient takes a slow deep breath in, with his lips sealed around the mouthpiece (Fig. 6.44), and is motivated by visual feedback, for example a ball rising to a preset marker. The patient aims to generate a predetermined flow or to achieve a preset volume and he is encouraged to hold his breath for 2–3 seconds at full inspiration. A short, sharp inspiration can activate the flow-generated incentive spirometry devices with little increase in tidal

volume, but with a volume-dependent device an increase in tidal volume must be achieved before the preset level can be reached.

The pattern of breathing while using an incentive spirometer is important. Expansion of the lower chest should be emphasized rather than the use of the accessory muscles of respiration which would encourage expansion of the upper chest.

Diaphragmatic movement (Chuter et al 1990) is thought to be an important factor in the prevention of postoperative pulmonary complications. Incentive spirometry has been shown to increase abdominal movement in normal subjects, but not in subjects following abdominal surgery (Chuter et al 1989). Postoperatively, an increase in diaphragmatic movement has been observed by encouraging an increase in lung volume while using the pattern of breathing control without the resistive loading of an incentive spirometer (Chuter et al 1990). This may help to reduce postoperative pulmonary complications by increasing ventilation to the dependent parts of the lungs.

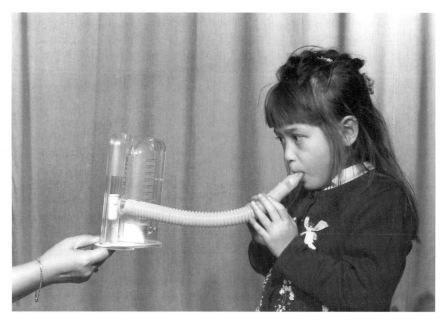

Figure 6.44 An incentive spirometer (Voldyne®, Sherwood Medical Company).

Incentive spirometry has been compared with intermittent positive pressure breathing (Oikkonen et al 1991), continuous positive airway pressure (Stock et al 1985) and chest physiotherapy (Gosselink et al 1997, Hall et al 1991) in patients following surgery. Few differences between the regimens have been reported.

There may be a place for the use of incentive spirometry in children and in some adolescents to provide motivation to increase lung volume following surgery, but the use of breathing control and thoracic expansion exercises with an inspiratory hold should be encouraged and, combined with ambulation, may be more effective in the prevention of postoperative pulmonary complications.

Glossopharyngeal breathing

Glossopharyngeal breathing (GPB) is a technique useful in patients with a reduced vital capacity resulting from respiratory muscle weakness or paralysis. Although its original use was in rehabilitation of patients with poliomyelitis, it can be invaluable when taught to tetraplegics (Alvarez et al 1981, Bach & Alba 1990) and in some neuro-muscular diseases (Bach 1995, Baydur et al 1990).

GPB was first described by Dail (1951) when patients with poliomyelitis were observed to be gulping air into their lungs. It was this gulping action that gave the technique the name 'frog breathing'. GPB is a form of positive pressure ventilation produced by the patient's voluntary muscles where boluses of air are forced into the lungs. Paralysed patients dependent on a mechanical ventilator are sometimes able to use GPB continuously, other than during sleep, to substitute for the mechanical ventilation. GPB is very useful in patients who are able to breathe spontaneously but whose power to cough and clear secretions is inadequate. The technique also enables these patients to shout to attract attention and to help to maintain or improve lung and chest wall compliance (Bach et al 1987, Dail et al 1955). For patients dependent on a ventilator, either non-invasively or via a tracheostomy, GPB can be life saving (Bach 1995) in an emergency if the ventilator becomes disconnected or if there should be a power failure and can increase the feeling of independence (Make et al 1998).

To breathe in, a series of pumping strokes is produced by action of the lips, tongue, soft palate, pharynx and larynx. Air is held in the chest by the larynx which acts as a valve as the mouth is opened for the next gulp. Expiration occurs by normal elastic recoil of the lungs and rib cage.

Before starting to teach GPB it may be helpful for the patient to inflate his chest using an intermittent positive pressure ventilator with a mouthpiece. After inflating the lungs, the mouthpiece is removed and he should try and hold all the air in the lungs with the mouth open, avoiding escape of air through the larynx or nose. A teaching video is available that may help both patient and physiotherapist when learning or teaching GPB (Webber & Higgens 1999).

The first and most important step in learning GPB is the enlargement of the mouth and throat cavity by depressing the tracheal and laryngeal cartilages. The tongue should remain flat with the tip touching the inside of the lower teeth. When correct, the uvula should be visible. The patient may find it helpful to watch the movement in a mirror and possibly by feeling the cartilages with his fingers. To emphasize this movement, practice should progress to holding the throat in this open position for about 5 seconds.

When this movement has been achieved two other stages are added to complete the cycle. The three stages are practised.

1. Enlarge the throat cavity to fill the mouth and pharynx with air by depressing the cartilages and tongue (Fig. 6.45a).
2. While maintaining this position the lips are closed, trapping the air (the jaw must not be closed) (Fig. 6.45b).
3. The floor of the mouth and cartilages are allowed to rise to their normal position while air is pumped through the larynx into the trachea (Fig. 6.45c).

This cycle should be practised slowly at first and then gradually speeded up until the movement flows.

The next stage is to take a maximum breath in and, while holding this breath, to add several glossopharyngeal gulps, to augment the vital capacity. When correct, the patient will feel his chest filling with air and the physiotherapist can test the 'GPB vital capacity' by putting a mouthpiece attached to the expiratory limb of a Wright's respirometer in the patient's mouth before he exhales.

The respirometer can be used to measure the volume per gulp; the patient will require less effort and reach his maximum capacity more quickly if he develops a large volume gulp. The volume per gulp is directly related to the amount of downward movement of the cartilages. A study by Kelleher & Parida (1957) reported a group of patients in whom the average volume per gulp varied from 25 to 120 ml and when teaching GPB an attempt should be made to achieve at least 80 ml per gulp.

If GPB were being used continuously as a substitute for normal tidal breathing, approximately 6–8 gulps would be taken before breathing out. When used for clearance of secretions, 10–25 gulps may be required to obtain a maximal vital capacity. Volumes of 2.5–3.0 litres can be achieved and the expiratory flow produced is sufficient to mobilize secretions (Make et al 1998).

GPB would normally be taught with the patient in a comfortable sitting position, but for patients with postural hypotension following spinal cord injury, a reclined position would be more appropriate at first. When mastered, GPB should be practised in positions useful for the patient to clear his bronchial secretions. After filling his chest to capacity he signals to the physiotherapist who compresses his chest as he lets the air out. The patient may have sufficient muscle power to apply compression himself or carers can be taught to give assistance.

GPB is learnt easily by some patients, but others need time and patience to acquire this skill. Although frequent self-practice can be very helpful in the learning stages it is recommended to ensure correct opening of the throat (stage 1) before encouraging the patient to practise on his own as bad habits are difficult to eradicate. It can be tiring to learn GPB and therefore short frequent sessions are most effective. Once learnt, it is not tiring to use the technique.

There are reasons why a person may fail to achieve GPB initially. The soft palate may not be

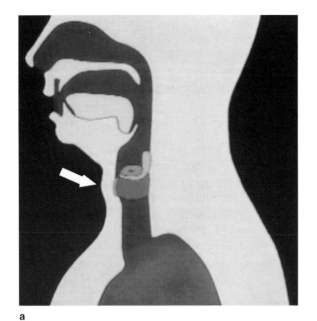

a

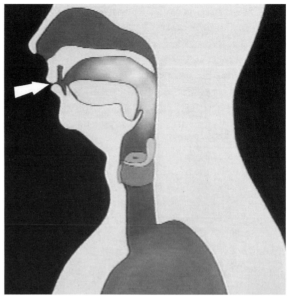

b

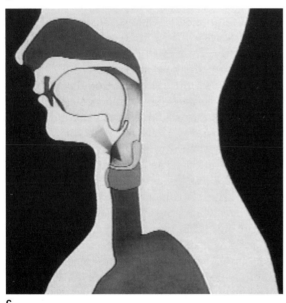

c

Figure 6.45 The stages of glossopharyngeal breathing (a,b,c).

closing so that air passes out through the nose instead of into the trachea. This can often be corrected by asking the patient to take several gulps while the nose is alternately pinched closed for two gulps and released for two gulps. When the nose is held closed the patient will feel pressure inside the mouth and throat and possibly in the ears. GPB should then be repeated without the nose being pinched and the patient should attempt to reproduce the same feeling of pressure with every gulp. Occasionally patients have very poor soft palate control and will need to wear a nose clip. Exercises to improve soft palate control may be helpful.

Another problem that may be found during the learning stages is weakness of the vocal cords. If the cords are unable to hold the air in the lungs, the vital capacity is decreased after attempting some gulps. This can be tested by asking the patient to take a very deep breath using intermittent positive pressure by mouthpiece and then, with the mouthpiece removed, he should say 'Ah, ah, ah ...' in short staccato bursts during expiration. If all the 'Ahs' run into a continuous sound, the cords are failing to shut off the flow of air under pressure. To strengthen the cords, the patient can start to take a volume of air just greater than his vital capacity and practise the 'Ah, ah' sounds. When this is achieved, the volume of air can be gradually increased and the expiration exercises repeated.

GPB is a valuable technique to consider when treating tetraplegics or patients with a neuromuscular disease with a vital capacity of less than 2 litres. Instruction can begin when the patient has reached a stable condition but it is inappropriate in the acute phase or during an acute chest infection. When successfully learnt, it is invaluable during a period of chest infection to assist in the clearance of secretions. With neuromuscular disease it is often easiest to teach GPB as a 'normal' part of treatment, before deterioration in respiratory muscle function has occurred.

It is possible to teach GPB to patients with an uncuffed tracheostomy tube, provided there is an effective seal round the tube to avoid air leaks and some form of plug to the tube. A one-way valve, for example a Passy-Muir valve, fitted between the tracheostomy tube and the ventilator tubing, acts as a plug preventing air escaping into the ventilator tubing, but allowing it to enter the lungs. If a ventilator dependent patient has a one-way valve in situ and can do GPB, it gives a great sense of security should a ventilator tube become kinked or disconnected. Before starting to learn GPB it is essential that patients who are entirely ventilator dependent learn to use intermittent positive pressure by mouthpiece. It gives them a reliable respiratory support during the learning stages. While increasing the period of time using GPB, it is important to ensure that normal blood gases are maintained. Patients usually take 6–8 gulps per breath, 10–12 times per minute, to provide a normal minute volume. When learning to build up their endurance they may have a sense of desperate need for air but by taking a larger number of gulps, perhaps 20 or 25, at high speed, this feeling can be relieved and the normal pattern can be resumed.

Weakness of the oropharyngeal muscles may make it impossible to do GPB. The technique is contraindicated in patients with pulmonary disease, for example tuberculosis and obstructive airways disease where the positive pressure could increase air trapping. It is also contraindicated in cardiac failure where the long inspiratory period with high intrathoracic pressure could decrease venous return, causing a fall in blood pressure.

Intermittent positive pressure breathing

Intermittent positive pressure breathing (IPPB) is the maintenance of a positive airway pressure throughout inspiration, with airway pressure returning to atmospheric pressure during expiration. The Bird Mark 7 ventilator (Fig. 6.46) is a pressure-cycled device convenient to use for providing IPPB as an adjunct to physiotherapy in the spontaneously breathing patient.

IPPB has been shown to augment tidal volume (Sukumalchantra et al 1965) and using an IPPB device in the completely relaxed subject, the work of breathing during inspiration approaches zero (Ayres et al 1963). These two effects support the use of IPPB to help in the clearance of bronchial secretions when more simple airway clearance techniques alone are not maximally effective, for example in the semicomatose patient with chronic bronchitis and sputum retention (Pavia et al 1988) or in a patient with neuromuscular disease and a chest infection. The reduction in the work of breathing can be used with effect in the acute severe exhausted asthmatic, but there is no evidence that the effect of bronchodilators delivered by IPPB is greater than from a nebulizer alone (Webber et al 1974).

An ideal IPPB device for use with physiotherapy should be portable and have simple controls. Other important features are as follows.

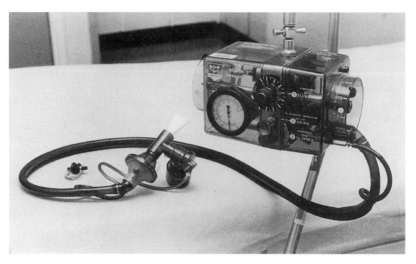

Figure 6.46 The Bird Mark 7 ventilator

Positive pressure. The range of pressures is likely to be from 0 to 35 cmH$_2$O.

Sensitivity. The patient should be able to 'trigger' the inspiratory phase with minimal effort. Fully automatic control is unpleasant for most patients and unnecessary for physiotherapy. A hand triggering device is useful to test the ventilator and nebulizer.

Flow control. With ventilators such as the Bird Mark 7 the inspiratory gas is delivered at a flow rate which can be preset by means of a control knob. Optimal distribution of gas to the more peripheral airways is achieved at relatively slow flow rates, but if the patient is very short of breath and has a fast respiratory rate, a slow inspiratory phase may be unacceptable. It is often useful to alter the flow control several times during a single treatment session, providing slow breaths during the periods attempting to mobilize peripheral secretions and a faster flow rate when a patient is recovering his breath after expectoration. The Bennett PR-1 and AP-5 (which are no longer available to purchase in the UK, but may be available within a hospital for use) do not require flow rate adjustment because automatic variable flow is provided with each breath. This feature is known as 'flow sensitivity' and means that the flow of the

inspired gas adapts to the resistance of the individual's airways.

Nebulizer. An efficient nebulizer in the circuit is necessary to humidify the driving gas and, when appropriate, to deliver bronchodilator drugs. The nebulizer in the Bird circuit is driven automatically with the inspiratory phase of the ventilator, but the Bennett has a separate control knob for the nebulizer.

Air-mix control. When driven by oxygen, air must be entrained by the apparatus to provide an air/oxygen mixture for the patient. Some Bird devices have a control which should be set to give a mixture, while others have no control but automatically entrain air. The use of 100% oxygen for a patient is very rare and when it is indicated, an IPPB device with an air-mix control will be needed. When air is not entrained through the apparatus the flow rate control must be regulated to provide an adequate flow to the patient.

When IPPB is driven by oxygen and the air-mix control is in use, the percentage of oxygen delivered to the patient is approximately 45% (Starke et al 1979). This percentage will be considerably higher than the controlled percentage delivered by an appropriate Venturi mask, for example to a patient with chronic bronchitis. This higher percentage is rarely dangerous during treatment because the patient's ventilation is assisted and the removal of secretions as a result of treatment is likely to lead subsequently to an improvement in arterial blood gas tensions (Gormezano & Branthwaite 1972).

It has been suggested that a few patients become more drowsy during or after IPPB as a result of the high percentage of oxygen received. Starke et al (1979) showed that increased drowsiness caused by hypercapnia occurred whether oxygen or air was the driving gas for IPPB and that the deterioration was dependent on inappropriate settings of the ventilator. The pressure and flow controls must be set to provide an adequate tidal volume, this being particularly important when treating patients with a rigid thoracic cage (Starke et al 1979).

Occasionally, IPPB may be powered by Entonox (p. 383) and in this case the air-mix control would need to be in the position to provide 100% of the driving gas with no additional air entrained.

Breathing circuit. To prevent cross-infection it is essential for each patient to have his own breathing circuit which consists of tubing, nebulizer, exhalation valve and a mouthpiece or mask. The majority of patients prefer to use a mouthpiece but a face mask is required when treating confused patients. A flange mouthpiece (Fig. 6.47) is useful for patients who have difficulty making an airtight seal around the mouthpiece.

The type of breathing circuit used will depend on the local means of sterilization. They can be autoclavable, non-disposable but non-autoclavable, or disposable.

Preparation of the apparatus

1. Normal saline solution or the drug to be nebulized (3–4 ml in total) is inserted into the nebulizer chamber.
2. The breathing circuit is connected to the IPPB ventilator and the ventilator connected to the driving gas source. It can be used from an oxygen or air cylinder if piped compressed gas is unavailable.
3. If there is an air-mix control, this should be in the position for entrainment of air.

4. If there is an automatic control (expiratory timer) this should be turned off to allow the patient to 'trigger' the machine at his desired rate.
5. The sensitivity, flow and pressure controls are set appropriately for the individual. With the Bird Mark 7 the sensitivity control is usually adjusted to a low number (5–7) where minimal inspiratory effort is required. The pressure and flow controls are adjusted to provide regular assisted ventilation without discomfort. A patient with a rigid rib cage will require a higher pressure setting to obtain an adequate tidal volume than someone with a more mobile rib cage.

When adjusting the settings for a new patient it may be easiest to start with a pressure at approximately 12 cmH$_2$O and the flow at about 10, then gradually increase the pressure and reduce the flow until the pattern of breathing is the most appropriate for the individual. Some IPPB devices do not have numbered markings, but after finding the most effective settings for a patient during one treatment, it is useful to note the positions of the controls in order to use these as a starting point at the next treatment. The controls to be set on the Bennett PR-1 are the nebulizer, sensitivity and pressure.

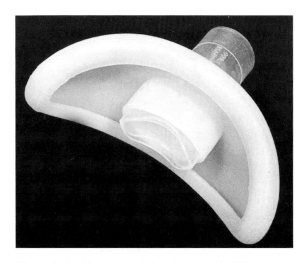

Figure 6.47 Flange mouthpiece for use with IPPB.

6. Before starting a treatment the hand triggering device is operated to check that there are no leaks in the breathing circuit and that the nebulizer is functioning well.

Treatment of the patient

The position in which IPPB is used depends on the indication for treatment. It may be used in side lying, high side lying or in the sitting position. The patient should be positioned comfortably and encouraged to relax the upper chest and shoulder girdle.

After the purpose of the IPPB treatment has been explained, the patient is asked to close his lips firmly around the mouthpiece and then to make a slight inspiratory effort which will trigger the device into inspiratory flow. He should then relax throughout inspiration, allowing his lungs to be inflated. When the preset pressure is reached at the mouth the ventilator cycles into expiration; the patient should remain relaxed and let the air out quietly.

If the patient attempts to assist inspiration there will be a delay in reaching the cycling pressure. A delay will also occur if there is a leak around the mouthpiece, at any of the circuit connections or from the patient's nose. A nose clip may be required until he becomes familiar with the technique.

The physiotherapist will find it useful to watch the manometer on the ventilator in order to detect any faults in the patient's technique. At the start of inspiration the needle should swing minimally to a negative pressure and then swing smoothly up to the positive pressure set, before cutting out into expiration and returning to zero. A larger negative swing at the beginning of inspiration shows that the patient is making an unnecessary effort in triggering the device. If the patient makes an active effort throughout inspiration the needle will rise very slowly to the inspiratory set pressure and if he attempts to start expiration before the preset pressure is reached, the needle will rise sharply above the set pressure and then cut out into expiration.

When IPPB is taught correctly the work of breathing is relieved, but if the patient is allowed to assist either inspiration or expiration there will be an increase in the work of breathing.

The patient should pause momentarily after expiration before the next inspiration, to avoid hyperventilation and possible dizziness. Occasionally children using IPPB tend to swallow air during treatment. It is important to observe the size of the abdomen before and during IPPB to recognize signs of abdominal distension and discontinue IPPB if this occurs.

When IPPB is used to relieve the work of breathing while delivering bronchodilator drugs, e.g. in the acute severe asthmatic patient, it is often helpful for the physiotherapist to hold the breathing circuit to allow the patient to relax his shoulders and arms as much as possible (Fig. 6.48).

A facemask for IPPB is used in the drowsy or confused patient and in those with facial weakness unable to make an airtight seal at the mouth. When using IPPB to assist in mobilizing secretions, the patient would be positioned to assist drainage of secretions, for example in side lying. The patient's jaw should be elevated and the mask held firmly over the face, ensuring an airtight fit. Chest shaking during the expiratory phase may be used to assist in mobilizing secretions. In a drowsy patient it may be necessary to stimulate coughing using nasotracheal suction (p. 214) if spontaneous coughing is not stimulated by IPPB and chest shaking.

In medical patients with retained secretions and poor respiratory reserve IPPB may be useful both to mobilize secretions and to relieve the effort of breathing following expectoration. The flow control on a Bird ventilator should be adjusted to give a slow but comfortable breath to mobilize secretions, but the patient's increased respiratory requirements following the exertion of expectoration necessitate increasing the flow and possibly reducing the pressure until he has returned to his normal breathing pattern.

IPPB may be used in patients with chest wall deformity, for example kyphoscoliosis, when they have difficulty clearing secretions during an infective episode. To achieve an adequate increase in ventilation in patients with a rigid rib cage, the pressure setting needs to be higher than for a more mobile rib cage.

Occasionally, in postoperative patients, IPPB is the adjunct of choice when the patient is unable to augment his tidal volume adequately during treatment. In these patients, in contrast to the relaxed technique normally used with IPPB, thoracic expansion may be actively encouraged during the inspiratory phase.

Bott et al (1992) have reviewed the literature on IPPB and concluded that it is an important adjunct to chest physiotherapy.

Contraindications for IPPB

- Pneumothorax.
- Large bullae.
- Lung abscess as the size of the air space may increase.
- Severe haemoptysis as treatment is inappropriate until the bleeding has lessened.
- Postoperative air leak unless the advantages of IPPB would outweigh the possibility of increasing the air leak during treatment.
- Bronchial tumour in the proximal airways. Air may flow past the tumour during inspiration and may be trapped on expiration as the airways narrow. There would be no

contraindication if the tumour were situated peripherally.

Manual hyperinflation

The technique of manual hyperinflation may be indicated to mobilize and assist clearance of excess bronchial secretions and to reinflate areas of lung collapse in the intubated patient. It is described in Chapter 11 (p. 368).

Airway suction

Airway suction is usually necessary to clear secretions from the intubated patient with an endotracheal tube, tracheostomy, minitracheostomy or the patient with an 'airway'. Brazier's review (1999) highlights the evidence for this technique. For intubated adults the technique is described in Chapter 11 (p. 369). For children including the non-intubated infant and small child, see Chapter 13 (p.434).

Suction is required occasionally in the *non-intubated adult* who has retained secretions. The vacuum pressure should be kept as low as possible and usually in the range 60–150 mmHg

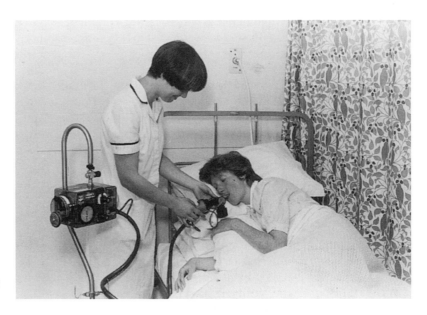

Figure 6.48 IPPB to reduce the work of breathing during inhalation of nebulized bronchodilator.

(8.0–20 kPa), but this will vary with the viscosity of the mucus. A built-in finger tip control or Y-connector is recommended to allow a more gradual build-up of suction pressure than is possible by the release of a kinked catheter tube.

Before any suction procedure it is important to give an explanation to the patient.

Nasotracheal suction is a means of stimulating a cough, but is an unpleasant procedure for the patient and should only be performed when absolutely necessary. The indication for suction is the inability to cough effectively and expectorate when secretions are retained. It may be necessary, for example, when an acute exacerbation of chronic bronchitis has led to carbon dioxide narcosis and respiratory failure, in neurological disorders, postoperative complications or laryngeal dysfunction. It is contraindicated when there is stridor or severe bronchospasm.

Airway suction causes damage to the tracheal epithelium and this can be minimized by the appropriate choice of catheter and technique (Brazier 1999). A flexible catheter of suitable size, usually 12 FG in adults, is lubricated with a water-soluble jelly and gently passed through the nasal passage so that it curves down into the pharynx. Occasionally a cough may be stimulated when the catheter reaches the pharynx and suction can then be applied, the secretions aspirated and the catheter withdrawn. More often, it is necessary to pass the catheter between the vocal cords and into the trachea to stimulate coughing. The catheter is less likely to enter the oesophagus if the patient's neck is extended and if he is able to cooperate, it is often helpful if he can put his tongue out. The catheter should be inserted during the inspiratory phase and if it passes into the trachea, will stimulate vigorous coughing.

Oxygen should always be available during the suction procedure and the patient observed for signs of hypoxia. If it has been difficult to insert the catheter and the patient looks cyanosed, instead of withdrawing the catheter from the trachea, suction should be stopped and oxygen administered until the patient's colour has improved. Suction can then be restarted.

Adults nursed in the sitting position can be suctioned in that position but comatose patients should be suctioned in side lying to avoid the possibility of aspiration if vomiting occurs.

Using the technique of nasotracheal suction it is important to be aware of the possibility of causing laryngeal spasm (Sykes et al 1976) or vagal nerve stimulation which may lead to cardiac arrhythmias (Jacob 1990). Provided that suction is carried out carefully and oxygen is always available, it is a valuable technique and may avoid the need for the more invasive treatments of bronchoscopy, endotracheal intubation or minitracheotomy. However, it should not be undertaken until every attempt to achieve effective coughing has failed.

Suction via the nose is contraindicated in patients with head injuries where there is a leak of cerebrospinal fluid into the nasal passages. *Oropharyngeal suction* through an airway would be an alternative method. An oropharyngeal airway is a plastic tube shaped to fit the curved palate. It is inserted with its tip directed towards the roof of the mouth and is then rotated so that the tip lies over the back of the tongue.

Although retention of secretions may be a problem in patients with respiratory muscle paralysis there is no benefit in using suction in an attempt to stimulate an effective cough. It is the lack of volume of air that prevents clearance of secretions in these patients and it is the combination of gravity-assisted drainage positions, chest compression and intermittent positive pressure breathing or glossopharyngeal breathing (p. 206) which should provide an effective means of clearance.

Portable suction units are available for domiciliary use and for patients in transit. They may be powered manually, by mains electricity or by battery, e.g. from a car cigarette lighter adapter.

Minitracheotomy

A minitracheotomy (Fig. 6.49) may be considered when a spontaneously breathing patient is retaining bronchial secretions. It has been used successfully in surgical and medical patients (Preston et al 1986). Nasotracheal suction may have been successful in clearing some secretions but is unpleasant and traumatic for the patient if it needs to be repeated frequently. A minitracheotomy is a means of clearing secretions more easily while avoiding the more invasive techniques of bronchoscopy, endotracheal intubation or tracheostomy (Ryan 1990). It would not provide an adequate airway for ventilation and it offers no airway protection.

A cannula with an internal diameter of 4 mm is inserted into the trachea through the cricothyroid membrane (Matthews & Hopkinson 1984). The procedure can be carried out under local anaesthesia and the minitracheotomy allows tracheal suction as often as necessary.

With the small tube in position the patient is able to breathe normally through the mouth and nose and the inspired air is humidified as it passes through the nasal passages. The patient can talk, eat and drink normally and the tube does not prevent him from coughing effectively.

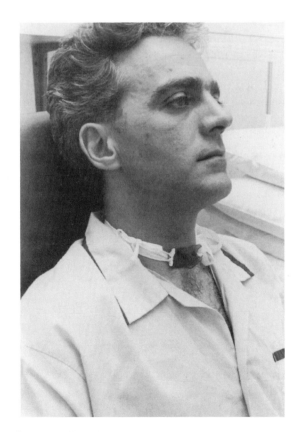

Fig 6.49   Minitracheotomy.

Oxygen can be administered by a facemask or nasal cannulae if required.

With a minitracheotomy a size 10 FG suction catheter is the maximum size that can be used. Size 8 FG is usually too narrow to clear secretions effectively. Normal saline solution (1–2 ml) is instilled via the minitracheotomy before suction to assist in maintaining patency of the tube. The catheter is gently inserted either until a cough is stimulated or the carina is reached and suction is applied when starting to withdraw it. There may be copious secretions which will take longer to clear using this small catheter, but the patient is able to breathe with the narrow tracheal tube in situ and the procedure should not be distressing.

As soon as the patient is capable of clearing his secretions effectively without becoming exhausted the minitracheotomy is removed and the small incision heals quickly.

The size of the minitracheotomy was designed for the adult trachea and is not recommended for children under the age of 12 years (Preston et al 1986).

INHALATION: DRUGS AND HUMIDIFICATION

As the knowledge base of inhalation therapy has increased it has become more complex and the advantages and disadvantages of the different systems and patient preferences need to be considered (Pedersen 1996). An understanding of the aerosol particle and its pattern of deposition within the airways is essential when considering the delivery of drugs by the inhaled route. A suspension of fine liquid or solid particles in air is known as an 'aerosol'. The pattern of deposition of aerosol particles within the bronchial tree depends on particle size, method of inhalation and on the degree of airflow obstruction (Newman et al 1986).

Large particles in the size range 5–10 μm deposit by impaction in the oropharynx and upper airways where the cross-sectional diameter of the airway is small and the airflow high. The total cross-section of the airway increases rapidly beyond the 10th generation of bronchi, airflow slows significantly and particles of 0.5–5 μm, known as the 'respirable particles', deposit in the small airways and alveoli by gravitational sedimentation. It is the particles of less than 2 µm that reach the alveoli. Gravitational sedimentation is time dependent and enhanced by breath holding. A more central patchy deposition is seen in patients with airflow obstruction (Clarke 1988).

The topical deposition of a drug by inhalation allows a smaller dose to be given than when other routes are used, the onset of action is often more rapid and with minimal systemic absorption the side effects are lessened.

Metered-dose inhaler (MDI) and dry powder inhalers

Numerous devices are available for the inhalation of drugs, ranging from the simple MDI or powder inhalers to breath-actuated inhalers and a variety of nebulizers. The physiotherapist should be aware of the range of possibilities to enable the patient to gain maximum benefit from the prescribed drugs. The choice of device will depend on the patient's age, coordination and dexterity, severity of the respiratory condition and patient preference.

Practice with placebo inhalers may be necessary to perfect the technique. Even if a patient has been using an inhalation device for a long time, it is always worth observing his technique as it may not be effective.

To gain maximum effect from an MDI it should first be shaken to ensure that the drug is evenly distributed in the propellant gases. The inhaler is held upright and the cap is removed. The patient breathes out gently but not fully and then, with the mouth around the mouthpiece of the inhaler, the device is pressed to release the drug as soon as inspiration has begun. The breath in should be slow and deep and inspiration should be held for 10 seconds if possible, before breathing out gently through the nose (Burge 1986, Clarke 1988). Effective technique is essential as it is known that only about 10% of the drug reaches the lungs (Clarke 1988).

Frequently, the prescribed dose will involve the inhalation of more than one 'puff'. It is recommended that puffs be taken one after the other. If the inhalation technique described above is used, the length of time between inhalations is likely to be 15–20 seconds which allows sufficient time to overcome the problem of cooling of the metering chamber as the gas evaporates. Compliance is improved when doses are taken one after the other (Burge 1986).

Large volume spacers (Fig. 6.50) can be used to improve the deposition of the drug in the lungs to approximately 15% (Clarke 1988) and to reduce the deposition in the oropharynx as the larger particles drop out in the spacer rather than the oropharynx. This helps to minimize any adverse effects.

Spacers may be cone or pear shaped, the shape of a 'puff' from an MDI. The patient is encouraged to take a slow deep breath with a hold, but if this is difficult tidal breathing can be used. Gleeson & Price (1988) showed that a bronchodilator was equally effective when a child breathed several times at tidal volume through a spacer when compared with a deep breath and inspiratory hold.

For patients with a poor inhaler technique, severely breathless or with candidiasis or dysphonia from inhaled steroids, a spacer may be appropriate (Clarke 1988). The addition of a piece of corrugated tubing (approximately 15 cm in length) attached to the mouthpiece of an MDI may act as a cheap and effective spacer. Oral candidiasis can be minimized by rinsing the mouth thoroughly following inhalation.

For people with poor coordination a breath-actuated inhaler may be considered (Newman et al 1991) or a dry powder device. The dry powder inhalers may also be breath-actuated, releasing the drugs on inspiration, but require a faster inspiratory flow rate than a pressurized (MDI) inhaler. The inspiratory flow required depends on the resistance within the device.

It is not only important that the patient can use the device effectively but also that the patient or parent can easily recall whether a dose of the drug has been taken and many devices incorporate a monitoring system.

For inhalation therapy to be effective in infants and children, the appropriate device for the age and ability of the child (p. 458) must be selected (British Thoracic Society et al 1997). It may be

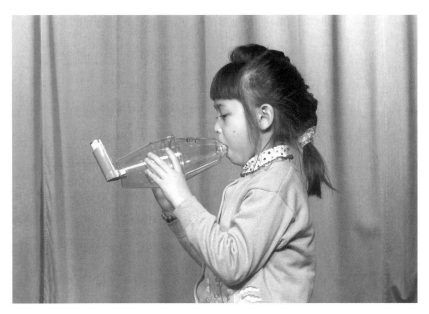

Figure 6.50   Spacer device (Volumatic®, Allen & Hanbury)

necessary to use a domiciliary nebulizer system in early childhood.

For each inhalation device the individual instructions should be carefully read and followed.

Nebulizers

A nebulizer may be used for the inhalation of drugs if a more simple method cannot produce the optimal effect or the drug cannot be administered by other means. A nebulizer converts a solution into aerosol particles (fine droplets) which are suspended in a stream of gas. The aim of nebulizer therapy (Nebuliser Project Group 1997) is to deliver a therapeutic dose of a prescribed drug as an aerosol in the form of respirable particles (particles <5 µm in diameter) in an acceptable period of time, approximately 5–10 minutes. There are two types of nebulizers – jet nebulizers and ultrasonic nebulizers.

Jet nebulizers

With the jet nebulizer a driving gas (electric air compressor or compressed air or oxygen from a hospital line or cylinder) is forced through a narrow orifice. The negative pressure created around the orifice draws the drug solution up the feed tube from the liquid reservoir and the jet of gas fragments the liquid into droplets. A screening baffle allows the smaller particles in the form of a mist to be available for inhalation by the patient and the larger particles to drop back into the reservoir to be recycled (Medic-Aid Ltd 1996).

A newer generation of jet nebulizer is the Adaptive Aerosol Delivery System™ (Nikander & Denyer 2000). The device assesses the individual patient's breathing pattern over three or four breaths and delivers the aerosol during the first half of inspiration. Almost no drug is lost during expiration, obviating the need for the use of filters or wide-bore tube systems.

Ultrasonic nebulizers

An aerosol can also be created by high-frequency (1–2 MHz) sound waves. An electric current applied to a piezo-electric crystal causes ultrasonic vibrations. The sound waves will travel through a liquid to the surface where they produce an aerosol. The particle size is influenced by the frequency of oscillation of the crystal. Ultrasonic nebulizers can produce a higher output than jet nebulizers. An advantage of ultrasonic nebulizers is that they operate quietly. A small volume of drug can be nebulized in a large volume ultrasonic nebulizer by the insertion of a drug chamber.

The majority of ultrasonic nebulizers are fan assisted, but a few models require the patient to breathe in actively to open a valve to the nebulizing chamber. Patients with very poor respiratory reserve and children, may find this additional effort difficult.

Nebulizer performance

The performance of a nebulizer can be measured by its *respirable output*. The respirable output is the mass of *respirable particles* (particles less than 5 μm in diameter) produced per minute, i.e.:

aerosol output (mg/min) × respirable fraction.

The *respirable fraction* is the percentage of respirable particles within the aerosol output. It is recommended that a nebulizer should provide a respirable fraction of at least 50% at its recommended driving gas flow (British Standards Institution 1994) and a number of nebulizers exceed this level.

The performance of an individual nebulizer has often been described by the mass median aerodynamic diameter (MMAD) of the particles. The MMAD indicates the range of size of particles leaving the nebulizer. Half of the aerosol mass from the nebulizer is of particles smaller than the MMAD and half of the aerosol mass is of particles larger than the MMAD. This is a less useful measurement of nebulizer performance as it is not related to the mass of drug.

It is important to consider an air compressor and nebulizer system as a unit. They should be matched to provide an acceptable output (Kendrick et al 1995).

Factors which affect individual nebulizer performance include the following (Nebuliser Project Group 1997).

Driving gas. Most jet nebulizers operate efficiently with a flow rate of 6–8 l/min. For patients in hospital it is often convenient to use the piped oxygen supply and in hypoxic patients without carbon dioxide retention, oxygen should be used. For patients retaining carbon dioxide who are dependent on their hypoxic drive to stimulate breathing, compressed air should be the driving gas (Gunawardena et al 1984). Occasionally it may be appropriate to increase the inspired oxygen concentration by entraining a low flow of oxygen.

Nebulizer chamber design. With a *'conventional'* nebulizer the output flow (from the nebulizer, towards the patient) is equal to the input flow (from the driving gas source) and nebulization is continuous. With a *'venturi'* nebulizer the output flow is greater than the input flow due to the presence of an open vent, but the output flow does not change with the patient's breathing pattern. With an *'active venturi'* nebulizer the output flow is breath assisted and is increased during inspiration. There is therefore less wastage of the drug during expiration.

When selecting a nebulizer the age of the patient must be considered. The inspiratory flow of an infant will probably be less than the output from a venturi nebulizer. The concentration of the aerosolized drug may be increased as there will be little or no air entrainment, but the total dose of the drug may be reduced (Collis et al 1990).

Consideration should also be given to the optimal particle size of the drug to be delivered. Inhaled pentamidine or antibiotics need to be delivered to the more peripheral airways (requiring a high percentage of particles of less than 2 μm), whereas bronchodilator drugs probably have their effect in the more central airways.

Residual volume. This is the volume of solution which remains in the nebulizer after nebulization has stopped. The Nebuliser Project Group of the BTS (1997) recommends that a fill volume of 2–2.5 ml may be adequate if the residual volume is less than 1 ml, but nebulizers with a higher residual volume will probably require a fill volume of 4 ml. The patient should be encouraged to tap the side of the nebulizer to allow as much as possible to be delivered (Everard et al 1994).

Fill volume. For effective nebulization it is important not to exceed the manufacturer's recommended fill volume.

Physical properties of drug solution or suspension. Most bronchodilator solutions when nebulized have a similar volume output to normal (0.9%) sodium chloride, but solutions with a higher viscosity or a high surface tension (e.g. carbenicillin) are slow to nebulize.

Breathing pattern of the patient. The optimal pattern of breathing has not yet been ascertained, but a recommended one is to intersperse one or two slow deep breaths with breathing at tidal volume. The deep breathing may increase peripheral deposition of the drug and the periods of breathing control will prevent hyperventilation. When inhaling from a nebulizer, the patient should be in a comfortable and well-supported position.

Drug delivery

A range of drugs often administered via a nebulizer include bronchodilators, corticosteroids, antibiotics, pentamidine, antifungals, local anaesthetics, rhDNase and surfactant. The nebulizer system used must be appropriate for the drug that has been prescribed. The evidence for drug device matching is outlined in the European Respiratory Society nebulizer guidelines: clinical aspects (2000). It is important to remember that the relative proportions of the airway and the anatomy and structure of the lung will alter during childhood. This will affect the deposition of inhaled drugs (Barry et al 2000).

Other points for consideration

- The dose of a prescribed nebulized bronchodilator may seem large compared with that from a pressurized aerosol, but only 10–20% of the initial dose is received by the patient and only 50% of this reaches the lungs. The drug which does not reach the patient is lost in the equipment and exhaled gas (Lewis & Fleming 1985).
- A facemask is necessary for the infant and child (Fig. 6.51), but as soon as the child will

cooperate a mouthpiece should be used to minimize deposition of the drug on the face and in the nasal passages (Wolfsdorf et al 1969). Other disadvantages of a mask are facial skin irritation from nebulized antibiotics and steroids and nebulized ipratropium bromide and salbutamol by mask have been associated with glaucoma in a group of adults with chronic airflow limitation (Shah et al 1992).

- For infants and children, parents should be given written instruction in addition to verbal instruction to improve adherence to treatment (Barry et al 2000).
- For nebulized antibiotics and pentamidine a one-way valve system is recommended (Wilson et al 2000). This can be achieved either with an effective filter on the exhalation port (Fig. 6.52) or wide-bore tubing to allow the exhaled gas to be vented out through a window (Fig. 6.53). This is to prevent small quantities of antibiotics remaining in the atmosphere which could lead to patients, family members and medical personnel in the vicinity receiving a subtherapeutic dose (Smaldone et al 1991) and environmental organisms becoming resistant to the antibiotic (Sanderson 1984). A nose clip is necessary if the patient is breathing partially through the nose.
- If inhaled antibiotics are prescribed for a pseudomonal infection in the upper respiratory tract, for example a patient with cystic fibrosis following lung transplantation, a nebulizer producing large particles is necessary (Webb et al 1996). A mask should be used and the patient encouraged to breathe through his nose.
- More than one antibiotic may be prescribed. A few antibiotics are compatible when mixed, but others must be inhaled separately. Either normal saline or sterile water is used to reconstitute a powdered antibiotic or to make a prescribed solution up to the necessary volume for nebulization. Information on the advisability of mixing drugs should be obtained from a pharmacist.
- Nebulized antibiotics may be isotonic, hypo- or hypertonic solutions and may cause airflow

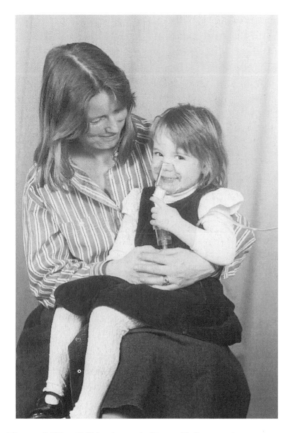

Figure 6.51 Child using nebulizer with facemask

obstruction (Cunningham et al 2001, Dodd et al 1997). The first dose of a nebulized anti-biotic should be monitored by recording the FEV_1 and FVC before, immediately after, 15 minutes after and, if evidence of airflow obstruction persists, 30 minutes after the inhalation (Maddison et al 1994). Individual patients respond differently and this response will vary with different drugs. Airflow obstruction can usually be controlled by the inhalation of a bronchodilator taken before physiotherapy for the clearance of secretions, preceding the inhalation of the antibiotic.

- Hypertonic saline (3–7%) may assist in the clearance of secretions (Eng et al 1996). It may cause an increase in airflow obstruction (Schoeffel et al 1981) and a test dose using spirometry is necessary.
- The mucolytic acetylcysteine should be used with caution. A reduction in sputum viscosity does not necessarily produce an increase in expectoration of sputum and bronchospasm may be induced. A test dose using spirometry is also necessary with this drug. Acetylcysteine is inactivated by oxygen and, if nebulized, the driving gas should be air (Reynolds 1996).

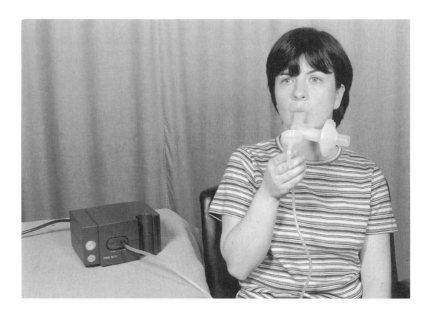

Figure 6.52 Inhalation of antibiotics using an active venturi nebulizer (LC STAR) and air compressor (PARI TurboBOY) (PARI Medical Ltd).

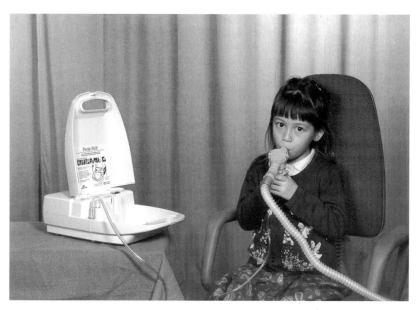

Figure 6.53   Inhalation of antibiotics using an active venturi nebulizer (Ventstream) and air compressor (Porta Neb) (Medic-Aid Ltd).

- Sputum induced by the inhalation of hypertonic saline by ultrasonic nebulizer (Pin et al 1992) is used for investigative procedures, as the proportion of viable cells obtained is higher than that found in spontaneous sputum (Bhowmik et al 1998).

Domiciliary nebulization

If there is an indication for domiciliary nebulization, careful instructions are essential, both verbal and written and equipment should be appropriately selected. Ideally, the air compressor should be portable, lightweight and quiet when in operation. Instructions in the care and cleaning of the equipment must be given in accordance with local infection control policies.

A spare jet nebulizer should be available and an inlet filter for the air compressor if necessary. The nebulizer must be washed and dried thoroughly after each treatment to reduce the possibility of bacterial infection (Hutchinson et al 1996) and to keep the jets clear. The transducer of an ultrasonic nebulizer should be cleaned regularly with acetic acid (white vinegar) to maintain its efficiency. An annual check of output and general and electrical safety should be undertaken and there should be provision for servicing as required (Dodd et al 1995).

Some patients may benefit from a compressor that can be used when travelling, either by using a 12 volt adaptor in a socket in the car, 'crocodile clips' fitted on to a battery or, more conveniently, a compact battery pack supplied with the compressor (Fig. 6.54). Those travelling to a country using a different voltage may require a transformer or a dual-voltage compressor. Some compressors incorporate a universal power pack which adapts to voltages throughout the world. An international travel plug adaptor is an accessory required for all who travel abroad. A foot pump may be useful to power a nebulizer where no electricity is available, but it requires considerable energy to operate. It is advisable to take a letter from a doctor explaining the need to travel with drugs and possibly syringes and needles, when travelling abroad.

Bronchodilator response studies

The value of bronchodilator response studies in the assessment of patients for nebulized bronchodilators is controversial (Goldman et al 1992, Mestitz et al 1989, O'Driscoll et al 1990). Short-term responses may not reflect a long-term response. A peak flow meter (Fig. 6.55) (Miller 2000) is often used to assess bronchodilator response. This will be suitable in a patient with asthma, but will not detect the more subtle response of a change in FVC which can occur in those with more irreversible airflow obstruction (Fig. 6.56). For these patients the response to a bronchodilator, detected by a change in FVC, may lead to an increase in exercise ability and improved quality of life.

The unnecessary use of nebulized broncho-dilators can restrict activities of daily living. A nebulizer and air compressor system should only be prescribed if a simple device used correctly is not as effective.

Objective measurements of bronchodilator response can be made by serial recordings of FEV_1 and FVC. Preceding the study, the drugs to be tested should be withheld for 4–6 hours, but all other drugs should be continued as prescribed.

Stable baseline readings, with correct technique, must first be obtained. The best result

of two or three attempts is taken, allowing a pause of at least 30 seconds between each attempt. Baseline readings are repeated at 5-minute intervals until the maximum pretreatment level is known. Some patients will continue to improve over several minutes, while others will soon reach a plateau or decrease their FEV_1 or FVC.

Having ensured a correct technique, the bronchodilator is inhaled and spirometry repeated at the appropriate time interval for the particular drug. After salbutamol (Ventolin) or terbutaline (Bricanyl), readings can be made at 15 and 30-minute intervals (Ruffin et al 1977), whereas with

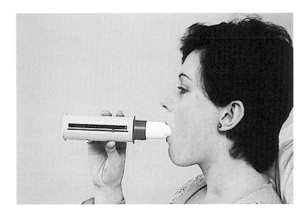

Figure 6.55 Peak flow meter (mini-Wright).

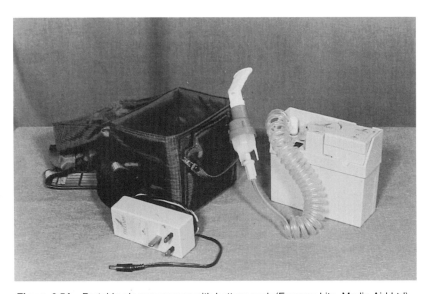

Figure 6.54 Portable air compressor with battery pack (Freeway Lite, Medic-Aid Ltd).

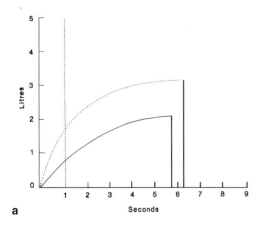

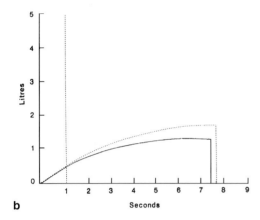

Figure 6.56 **a** Increase in FEV_1 and FVC. **b** increase in FVC only. Spirometry before bronchodilator ———; spirometry after bronchodilator ⋯⋯⋯ .

the slower acting ipratropium bromide (Atrovent), recordings are made 40 and 60 minutes from the time of inhalation (Loddenkemper 1975). In each case recordings should be continued until the maximum response is achieved; for example, if the response to salbutamol is greater at 30 minutes than at 15 minutes the spirometry is repeated at 10-minute intervals until a plateau or fall in FEV_1 or FVC is recorded. If time is limited, this outline can be modified, recordings being taken at the expected times of maximal improvement (30 minutes following Ventolin and Bricanyl and 60 minutes following Atrovent).

The same principle can be applied when comparing different methods of delivery of the same drug or when comparing the response to two different bronchodilators. If comparing the response

of a patient to Ventolin by an MDI (or other simple device) and a nebulized solution of Ventolin, measurements are made until maximum response is reached after inhalation by MDI and then the nebulized solution is given immediately. Any additional response is determined by the post-nebulizer recordings. If response to one method of delivery is determined on one occasion and to the other method on a separate occasion, the results are unlikely to be comparable because the baseline readings and other factors such as the time of testing and dose of steroid drugs may be different. Similarly, when comparing the response to two different drugs (for example, Ventolin and Atrovent) the second should be given as soon as maximum response has been achieved with the first (Webber 1988).

McGavin et al (1976) demonstrated that the inhalation of a bronchodilator preceding exercise can improve exercise tolerance, but the improvement does not correlate with changes in FEV_1 and FVC.

O'Driscoll et al (1990), in their study on home nebulizers, could not demonstrate a correlation between formal lung function testing and the domiciliary use of a nebulizer system. They recommended that patients who are referred for consideration of home nebulizer therapy be given the equipment to try under supervision for several weeks at home and that the patient's subjective assessment should be considered.

In assessing bronchodilator treatment Vora et al (1995) concluded that a quality of life measure and shuttle walking test appeared to be sensitive outcome measures. More recently, the St George's Respiratory Questionnaire (SRQ) has been shown to be a sensitive measurement tool (Jones 2000, personal communication).

An objective study which demonstrates to the patient a positive response to a simple inhalation device, with no further response to nebulized drugs, often relieves the patient who has felt that a compressor system would be necessary.

Many patients with asthma keep a diary card at home which will include recordings of peak expiratory flow before and after bronchodilator drugs. These will only be valid if the technique when using the meter is correct. Points to emphasize are:

- The patient should take a maximum breath in (in his haste to carry out the manoeuvre the patient may not take a full deep breath).
- Expiration should be short and sharp.
- Sufficient rests (at least 15 seconds) should be allowed between 'blows' to prevent any increase in airflow obstruction with the forced expiratory manoeuvre.
- The same position, sitting or standing, should be used for taking the readings.

Oxygen therapy

Oxygen therapy is indicated for many patients with hypoxaemia. The physiotherapist frequently treats patients requiring added inspired oxygen and may be involved with the setting up of oxygen therapy equipment. Oxygen is a drug and should be prescribed by a medical practitioner. The delivery device, flow rate/concentration and frequency/duration should be documented on the patient's drug chart (Dodd et al 2000, Thiagamoorthy et al 2000). It should be monitored using arterial blood gas analysis or oxygen saturation (SpO_2) recordings. When measuring SpO_2 recordings only, it must be remembered that an increase in PaO_2 may be associated with an increase in $PaCO_2$, but any rise in $PaCO_2$ will be difficult to detect. If a patient is on continuous oxygen therapy the mask should be removed only briefly for expectoration, eating and drinking and sometimes during these periods it may be appropriate to continue oxygen therapy using nasal cannulae.

Devices for administering oxygen therapy may be divided into fixed and variable performance devices (Hinds & Watson 1996). A *variable performance device* supplies a flow of oxygen which is less than the patient's minute volume. The inspired oxygen concentration (FiO_2) will vary with the rate and volume of breath and considerable variations between and within subjects have been demonstrated (Bazuaye et al 1992). Commonly used variable performance devices are the simple facemask (Fig. 6.57a) and nasal cannulae (Fig. 6.57b). Nasal cannulae are often preferred as the patient can eat, drink and speak more comfortably and often finds them less

claustrophobic than a mask. Although high flows of oxygen can be delivered via nasal cannulae, 1–4 l/min (approximately 24–36%) is the range for patient comfort. Higher flows, up to 6 l/min, tend to irritate and dry the nasal mucosa, but this can be alleviated by including a bubble-through humidifier in the circuit. However, humidification via narrow bore tubing is not an effective means of humidifying secretions (Campbell et al 1988) and to humidify secretions, a system using a specific concentration of oxygen should be used. Nasal cannulae should be used with caution with very breathless hypoxic patients as they are likely to be breathing through the mouth and not benefiting from the nasal oxygen.

When accurate delivery of oxygen is required, especially at low concentrations, a fixed performance device is essential because wide variations in inspired oxygen concentration have been shown to be produced by variable performance devices, even with the recommended flows (Jeffrey & Warren 1992).

A *fixed performance device* will deliver a known inspired oxygen concentration (FiO_2), by providing a sufficiently high flow of premixed gas that should exceed the patient's peak inspiratory flow rate. A venturi system allows a relatively low flow of oxygen to entrain a large volume of air and the mixed gas is conveyed to the facemask (Fig. 6.57c). With a 24% venturi mask the usual setting of 2 l/min flow of oxygen will entrain approximately 50 l/min of air, giving a total flow of approximately 52 l/min. An extremely breathless patient, with a greatly increased work of breathing and high peak inspiratory flow rate, may find this flow too low and then it is necessary to increase the flow to exceed the inspiratory flow of the patient (Hill et al 1984). The manufacturer should provide information for each mask (e.g. a 24% mask run at 3 l/min may augment the total flow to 78 l/min without changing the oxygen concentration). It is not possible to measure the critically ill patient's peak inspiratory flow, but by careful observation the physiotherapist will be able to tell if the total flow is sufficient. If gas can be felt flowing out through the holes and around the edges of the mask during inspiration, the flow will be exceeding the patient's requirements.

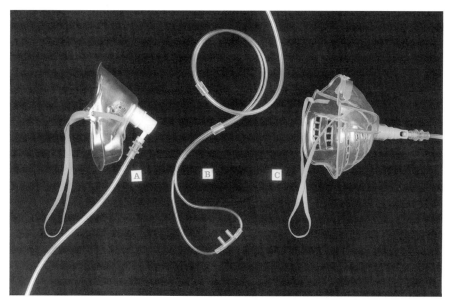

Figure 6.57   Oxygen delivery devices: **a** variable performance mask (Intersurgical); **b** nasal cannulae (Inrsurgical); **c** fixed performance venturi mask (Flexicare Medical).

For most patients using a venturi mask the entrained room air provides sufficient humidification, but occasionally additional humidification is indicated (p. 229). A bubble-through humidifier attached to the narrow bore tubing of a venturi mask is inappropriate as the flow of oxygen is likely to be reduced by the back pressure from the humidifier device and by condensation blocking the narrow bore tubing.

When high concentrations of oxygen, at high flows, are required a *high-flow variable FiO$_2$ generator* can be used. The gas flows along wide bore tubing from the generator across an appropriate heated humidifier to the facemask. It is essential to have an oxygen analyser in the circuit. Oxygen concentrations between 35% and 100% can be delivered at flows of up to 130 l/min. High-flow oxygen should be considered when patients requiring oxygen concentrations greater than or equal to 40% are not responding to a fixed performance device.

Nebulizers for the delivery of drugs in hospital are frequently powered by piped oxygen but in the patient dependent on his hypoxic drive to breathe, air should be used as the driving gas.

Occasionally in the severely hypoxic patient, who is also hypercapnic and dependent on a controlled 24% oxygen mask, the patient should not be deprived of this added oxygen while using a nebulizer. The level of oxygen entrained to maintain the baseline oxygen saturation can be monitored using an oximeter.

For most patients an *intermittent positive pressure breathing device* (IPPB) should be driven by compressed oxygen. Starke et al (1979) demonstrated that in hypercapnic patients oxygen can be used as the driving gas (p. 210). In hypoxic patients without hypercapnia, for example in acute asthma, oxygen is required and it is dangerous to use air alone as the driving gas for IPPB.

Long-term oxygen therapy (LTOT) has been shown to improve the length and quality of life in selected patients with severe chronic airflow limitation (Medical Research Council Working Party 1981, Nocturnal Oxygen Therapy Trial Group 1980). The expected gradual progression of pulmonary hypertension associated with this condition is slowed down by the use of long-term oxygen therapy. This benefit will not occur unless oxygen is used at a low flow for a minimum of 15 hours/day and should be prescribed only for carefully selected patients. Studies have been undertaken to evaluate the effects of LTOT and non-invasive ventilation (NIV) (Leach & Bateman 1994, Wedzicha 2000). Clinical guidelines for the prescribing of domiciliary oxygen have been established (Royal College of Physicians 1999).

An *oxygen concentrator* (Fig. 6.58) is a convenient and efficient means of providing long-term oxygen therapy in the home. Oxygen tubing can be fitted in areas of the home to allow for mobility, but a maximum length of 50 feet (15.25 metres) is recommended (DeVilbiss Oxygen Services 2000). A back-up oxygen cylinder is necessary for emergency use. Humidifiers are sometimes fitted to oxygen concentrators but care must be taken, as these are a potential source of infection (Pendleton et al 1991).

Small *oxygen cylinders* (e.g. PD 300) can be used for short trips outside the home. These may be transported on a lightweight trolley.

In an attempt to give patients who are dependent on oxygen greater mobility and the opportunity to participate in activities outside the home, an *inspiratory phased delivery system* or *oxygen by transtracheal catheter* may be considered (Shneerson 1992). A microcatheter inserted into the trachea will reduce the dead space and decrease the requirement for oxygen. Some patients find this more cosmetically acceptable than nasal cannulae, but there is the increased possibility of infection.

Liquid oxygen systems are used in some parts of the world. These are portable, lightweight, convenient and may improve compliance with treatment (Lock et al 1992, Wurtemberger & Hutter 2000).

The physiotherapist may be involved in *assessing* patients who may benefit from portable oxygen. Careful attention should be paid to the required flow rate and concentration. Repeated walking tests, for example the shuttle walking test, with the patient 'blind' to whether he is using oxygen or air during the walk, can be used as a means of assessment. The measurement of oxygen saturation using an oximeter may be included in the assessment.

Entonox

The inhalation of Entonox (50% nitrous oxide and 50% oxygen) has an analgesic effect which is easily and rapidly induced. See Chapter 12 (p. 383).

Heliox

A mixture of helium (79%) and oxygen (21%) is sometimes used on a temporary basis to relieve respiratory distress in patients with upper airways obstruction, for example a tumour causing partial obstruction of the trachea.

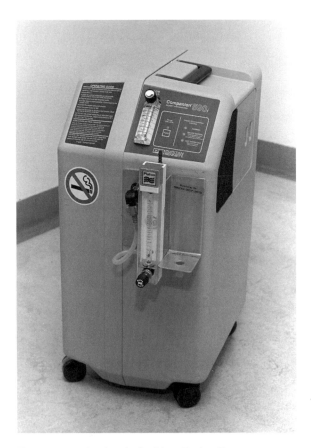

Figure 6.58 An electrically driven Puritan Bennett Companion® 590i oxygen concentrator.

Helium is lighter than the nitrogen in air and the mixture passes more easily through the narrowed airway, requiring less effort from the patient (Vater et al 1983). A side-effect of heliox is an alteration in the pitch of the voice, due to its effect on the vocal cords. This is only temporary, but should be explained to the patient before use of heliox to avoid unnecessary concern.

Humidification

A device to provide humidification of the airways may be considered if either the normal means of humidifying the airways or the mucociliary escalator is not functioning effectively.

The mucous membranes of the upper airways normally provide warmth and humidification of the inspired air. The temperature and humidity of the inspired air vary, but the gas in the alveoli is fully saturated with water vapour at body temperature. There is a temperature and humidity gradient from the nose to the point where the gas reaches 37°C and 100% relative humidity (Shelly et al 1988). This point is normally just below the carina in the adult, but varies depending on the temperature and water content of the inspired gas and the tidal volume. The upper airways act as a heat and moisture exchanger with the fully saturated expired gas giving up some heat and water to the mucosa (Chatburn 1987).

The epithelial lining of the airways, from the trachea to the respiratory bronchioles, contains ciliated cells which are responsible for moving mucus and particulate matter proximally to the level of the larynx. The optimal temperature for cilial activity is normal body temperature with reduced activity occurring below 20°C and above 40°C (Wanner 1977). The cilia beat within a watery fluid, the 'periciliary' or 'sol' layer. A mucus layer 'gel' covers the periciliary layer and interacts with the tips of the cilia.

The efficiency of mucus transport is dependent on correctly functioning cilia and the composition of the periciliary and mucus layers. If the periciliary layer becomes too shallow, as with dehydration, the cilia become enmeshed in the viscous mucus layer and cannot function effec-

tively. If the periciliary layer is too deep the tips of the cilia are not in contact with the mucus layer and propulsion of the mucus is inefficient.

The viscosity of mucus is increased during bacterial infection owing to an increase in the DNA content of the mucus (Wilson & Cole 1988). With hypersecretory disorders of, for example, bronchiectasis, cystic fibrosis and chronic airflow limitation, there is an increase in both quantity and viscosity of mucus secretions. Bacteria directly affect cilial beating and coordination, disrupt the epithelium, stimulate mucus secretion and alter periciliary fluid composition (Cole 1995). Humidification has been shown to enhance tracheobronchial clearance when used as an adjunct to physiotherapy in a group of patients with bronchiectasis (Conway et al 1992).

Clarke (1995) has suggested that the efficiency of cough increases with a decrease in viscosity of mucus and an increase in the periciliary layer of the airway. Conway (1992) hypothesizes that humidification by water or saline aerosol produces an increase in depth of the periciliary and mucus layers, thereby decreasing viscosity and enhancing the shearing of secretions by huffing or coughing.

Humidification may be indicated to assist clearance of secretions when the clearance mechanism is not optimally effective or when the normal heat and moisture exchange system of the upper airways is bypassed by an endotracheal or tracheostomy tube. Patients with a long-term tracheostomy may develop metaplasia of the tracheal epithelium. While adequate humidification of the inspired gas occurs normally, additional humidification may be required during an episode of respiratory infection (Oh 1990).

Methods of humidification

Systemic hydration

Adequate humidification may be obtained by increasing the oral or intravenous fluid intake of a patient. Breathless patients find drinking fluids an effort, but need encouragement to avoid dehydration. Patients should be reminded to maintain an adequate fluid intake as this may help to prevent secretions from becoming more tenacious. During periods of infection and fever a higher fluid intake is required.

Heated water bath humidifiers

Gas is blown over a reservoir of heated sterile water and absorbs water vapour which is then inhaled by the patient (Fig. 6.59). If the delivery tube is cold there is a temperature drop as the gas passes along the tube and condensation occurs. The humidifier should be positioned below the level of the patient's airway to avoid flooding of the airway by condensed water. Sealed (to prevent contamination) water traps should be included in the circuit to allow regular emptying without interrupting ventilation. A heated delivery tube eliminates the problem of condensation and allows the gas to be delivered at a desired temperature of 32–36° with a water content of 33–43 g/m^3 (Hinds & Watson 1996). Sterile water must be used in these devices. If saline is used, it is the water only which vaporizes and the sodium chloride crystallizes out.

Humidifiers can be used for the spontaneously breathing patient or can be incorporated into ventilator circuits including continuous positive airway pressure and non-invasive ventilation (see Fig. 10.5, p. 338). In some patients using 'high continuous flow CPAP systems', it may be necessary to use two humidifiers in series to increase the humidification (Harrison et al 1993).

Heat and moisture exchangers (HME)

A heat and moisture exchanger or the 'Swedish nose' is a lightweight disposable device and may be used in the intubated patient either mechanically ventilated or breathing spontaneously. In the spontaneously breathing patient it is important to be aware of the slight resistance that will increase the work of breathing. The humidifier acts in a similar way to the nasopharynx. The heat and moisture of the exhaled gas are retained either by condensation (condenser humidifier) or by absorption and returned in the inhaled gas as it passes through the device. A variety of hygro-

scopic materials and chemicals are used for absorption within heat and moisture exchangers.

Heat and moisture exchangers are inefficient if there is a large air leak around an uncuffed tracheostomy tube (Tilling & Hayes 1987) and do not provide adequate humidification for infants. If the secretions of a patient using a heat and moisture exchanger become tenacious, a more effective form of humidification will be required (Bransen et al 1993). The humidifier must be changed at least every 24 hours and immediately if it becomes soiled with secretions. In children with an increased work of breathing, the additional resistance from a heat and moisture exchanger may further compromise breathing.

Nebulizers

A nebulizer for humidification may be a jet or ultrasonic nebulizer (Fig. 6.60). Nebulizers produce an aerosol mist of droplets. Some jet nebulizers have a heater incorporated in the system. This increased temperature raises the rel-

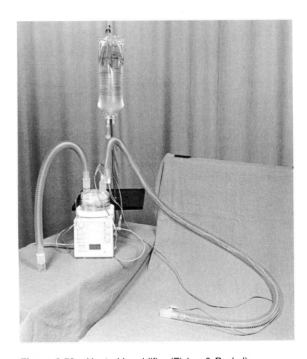

Figure 6.59 Heated humidifier (Fisher & Paykel).

ative humidity, is less irritative for patients with hyperreactive airways and is less likely to increase airflow obstruction than cold humidification. When a jet nebulizer is powered by oxygen the amount of air entrained by the nebulizer will be determined by the oxygen concentration required. If the concentration of oxygen is not important, consideration should be given to the optimal density of mist and flow produced by the specific device.

The mist particles delivered with a venturi closed (98% setting) appear more dense, but the total flow (approximately 10 l/min) will be insufficient to meet the patient's inspiratory requirement and additional room air will be entrained through the holes in a facemask or mouthpiece, effectively reducing the degree of humidification. A 35% setting on a venturi system will produce a flow of approximately 40 l/min. This would provide a higher degree of humidification as it would meet the inspiratory demand of the patient most of the time.

Many ultrasonic nebulizers do not have a heater, but the mist is at ambient temperature and warmer than that produced from a jet nebulizer powered from compressed piped gas. There is often an airflow control valve in addi-

tion to a control for the density of the mist. By regulating these two controls a density of mist can be obtained that the patient can inhale comfortably.

Sterile normal saline (0.9%) is an isotonic solution and probably the most acceptable to patients inhaling from a nebulizer. Sterile water can be used if saline is unavailable, but has been shown to cause bronchoconstriction in patients with hyperreactive airways (Schoeffel et al 1981).

Bubble-through humidifiers

A device containing cold water, through which the inspired gas is bubbled, is not an effective means of humidification. If connected to an oxygen mask with narrow bore tubing, it may alter the oxygen concentration as water condenses in the tubing. A bubble-through humidifier is often connected to nasal cannulae, but there are neither objective nor subjective benefits from this form of humidification (Campbell et al 1988).

Steam inhalations

Inhalation of steam may be useful in patients with postoperative sputum retention if they are

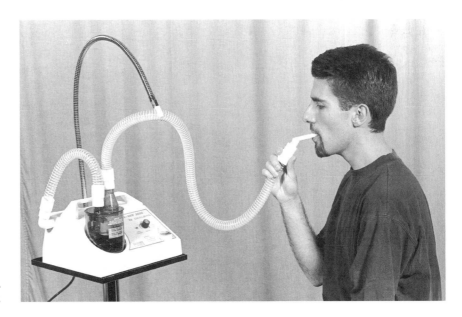

Figure 6.60 DeVilbiss Ultraneb 2000 ultrasonic nebulizer.

encouraged to breathe deeply. Precautions must be taken to avoid spilling the hot water.

Delivery to the patient

Patients with retained secretions postoperatively or those with excess viscous secretions due to a chronic bronchopulmonary infection may benefit from a period of 10–20 minutes' humidification before physiotherapy to assist the clearance of secretions. If the concentration of oxygen required by the patient is not critical, a *mouthpiece* with a hole for entrainment of additional air is simple and comfortable to use. Deep breathing interspersed with tidal volume breathing may encourage peripheral deposition of an aerosol, while avoiding hyperventilation.

If a patient requires an oxygen concentration of 28% or more, a *facemask* can be connected by wide-bore tubing to a nebulizer and the venturi of the nebulizer should be set to the appropriate concentration.

Patients requiring an inspired oxygen concentration of 24% will probably wear a venturi mask connected to the oxygen by narrow bore tubing. It is impossible to give high humidification through a narrow bore tube owing to condensation within the tubing. Effective humidification can be obtained by using a *humidity adaptor* which allows the air entrained by the mask to be humidified. It is a cuff fitted over the air-entraining holes of the mask and connected by wide bore humidity tubing to a humidifier powered by an air source. This can be piped compressed air, if it is available or an air cylinder or an electric air compressor capable of continuous use ('continuously rated') (Fig. 6.61). An ultrasonic nebulizer, set at a high flow, can be used and is quieter than a jet nebulizer system. A humidity adaptor can be used to give humidification to venturi masks delivering accurate higher concentrations of oxygen (e.g. 28% or 35%), but is unsatisfactory with a 60% venturi mask because the air-entraining holes are too small to entrain the humidity.

If a patient is breathing spontaneously through a tracheostomy, a *tracheostomy mask* may be attached to a humidifier or nebulizer via wide bore tubing. Alternatively a 'Swedish nose' or a 'laryngectomy-permanent tracheostomy protector' (tracheostomy 'bib') may be used.

Humidification through a *head box* (see Fig. 13.6 p.438) is often used in the treatment of spontaneously breathing infants. With the narrow airways of an infant the risk of mucus plugging is higher than in adults. Humidity to a head box may be either from a heated water bath humidifier or a heated nebulizer system.

Hazards of humidification

Inhalation of cold mist or water (a hypotonic solution) may cause bronchoconstriction in patients with hyperreactive airways (Schoeffel et al 1981). Heated humidification and normal saline solution are less likely to cause this problem. It may be appropriate to take peak flow or spirometry recordings before and immediately after the first treatment.

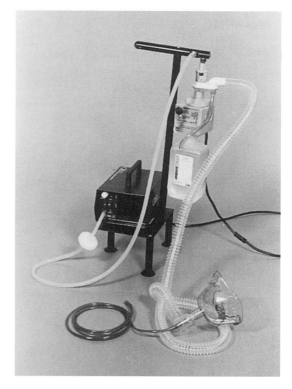

Figure 6.61 Heated humidification of 24% oxygen using a humidity adaptor (Vickers, Kendall, Medic-Aid).

Water reservoirs may become infected with *Pseudomonas* and other organisms, many of which multiply rapidly at 45°C. A particularly vulnerable site is the catheter mount of the ventilator circuit in the intubated patient. Some control of infection can be obtained by using an operating temperature of 60°C (Oh 1990). Regular disposal, disinfection or sterilization of all humidification equipment is essential to prevent infection and local infection control policies must be observed.

TRANSCUTANEOUS ELECTRICAL NERVE STIMULATION

Transcutaneous electrical nerve stimulation (TENS) is the application of electricity to relieve pain. It is not a new treatment; carvings from Egypt dating back to 2500BC illustrate the use of electric fish for the treatment of pain (Walsh 1997). TENS units deliver a small electrical current to the sensory cutaneous nerve endings through electrically conductive pads. The patients experience a buzzing, prickling, tingling sensation when the machine is switched on. TENS machines are battery powered, usually by a regular 9 volt battery. Rechargeable batteries can be used in most machines and are useful if the machine is going to be used for prolonged periods of time. The units are the size of a small personal stereo and easily fit into patients' bags and pockets or can be clipped onto a belt or waistband of clothes. The machines have controls to alter the intensity of the stimulus and should have the facility to change the mode. Machines should have the facility for a constant mode (also known as continuous or conventional), a burst mode (also known as acupuncture TENS) and a modulation mode. On the constant mode (high frequency/low intensity) a constant tingling sensation is felt, on burst mode (low frequency/high intensity) a pulsing sensation is felt and on modulation mode (variation of pulse duration and frequency in a cyclical pattern) an increase and decrease in the tingling sensation are felt. To accommodate these three modes the machine should have the facility to alter the pulse rate (frequency) and pulse width. The frequency of the pulse rate, that is measured in hertz (Hz), can be altered between 1 and 150 Hz per second and the width or duration of each pulse ranges from 10 to 120 microseconds (μs). Both of these settings should be altered according to the aetiology of pain a patient is experiencing and the mode that the machine is being used on (Table 6.5). TENS units either have one or two channels allowing the use of either two or four pads. The dual-channel machines are preferable to allow coverage of a larger area or treatment of two separate areas. Each pair of pads includes an anode (positive/red) and a cathode (negative/black). The electroconductive pads adhere to the skin and can be either self-adhesive or plain carbon rubber that requires electroconductive gel and tape to secure them. The self-adhesive pads are recommended if the machine is to be used over a long period of time, as they are much easier to use and therefore promote patient compliance.

Analgesic mechanism

It is thought that TENS relieves pain by several mechanisms. The main principle behind the effect of TENS is the gate control theory of pain (Melzack & Wall 1988). Electrical impulses are conducted more quickly than pain impulses and subsequently provide a competitive barrage of sensory input in the dorsal horns. This enhanced sensation inhibits the activity of the spinal cord pain neurons. The stimulus therefore closes the 'gate' by nociceptor inhibition (Walsh 1997). TENS may also close the gate in the thalamus where pain stimuli and normal sensation converge before distribution to the brain. Researchers hypothesize that TENS may stimulate the production of endorphins and encephalins, the body's own natural analgesics at spinal cord level, especially if used at low frequency when the patient will experience sharper and more intense pulses (Sjolund & Eriksson 1979).

Indications for TENS

TENS can be used for a variety of painful conditions and to assist in the undertaking of various procedures. It is, however, necessary to identify the cause of the pain so that the appropriate mode and settings can be chosen. The types of pain TENS is suitable for are listed below.

Neuropathic pains

- Peripheral neuropathy
- Trigeminal neuralgia
- Postherpetic neuralgia
- Rhizopathy
- Central pain
- Sympathetically mediated pain

Nociceptive pain

- Muscular pain
- Ischaemic pain, e.g. angina resultant from ischaemic heart disease (Jessurun et al 1998)
- Dermal pain
- Skeletal pain

TENS is probably not effective in the treatment of visceral pain and may not be effective in patients with active psychiatric disorders (Sjolund et al 1990). Once the mechanism of the pain has been identified then the mode, settings and electrode stimulation can be chosen as illustrated in Table 6.5.

The positioning of the electrodes can be crucial but little decisive evidence can be drawn from studies that specifically evaluate electrode positioning (Wheeler et al 1984, Wolf et al 1981). The therapist must therefore be prepared to use a degree of 'trial and error'. When using the constant or modulation mode the pads should be placed around the area of pain. With the burst mode it is necessary to place the pads in the dermatomal distribution of the pain in order to elicit a muscle twitch (Sjolund et al 1990, Walsh 1997). This twitch can initially be distressing and alarming for patients but with reassurance they usually become accustomed to it.

Time should be spent with the patient explaining, teaching and demonstrating the use of the machine and trying it out with them. An opportunity should be made available to review the use and efficacy of the machine either at an appointment or over the telephone. This allows for troubleshooting and is felt to increase patient compliance.

Contraindications

TENS machines should not be used with the following:

- pacemaker
- percutaneous CVP
- first trimester of pregnancy
- skin lesion around the area to be treated
- confusion.

There is some suggestion that TENS should not be used on patients with epilepsy but there is no evidence for this exclusion.

Table 6.5 TENS stimulation modes and settings (adapted from Lockwood 1986, Mannheimer & Lampe 1984, Sjolund et al 1990)

Mode	Conventional/modulation mode	Burst mode
Settings	Rate 50–100 Hz Width 200 μs	Rate 1–4 Hz Width 200 μs
Electrode positioning	Cathode proximal Anode distal	Cathode distal Anode proximal
Time	At least an hour 2–3 times a day. Can be used for longer provided that skin integrity is maintained	30–45 minutes 4–6 times a day
Types of pain	Skeletal pain Dermal pain Ischaemic pain Periosteal pain Neuropathy without sensory loss	Muscular pain Rhizopathic pain Neuropathy with sensory loss

Conclusion

TENS can be a very useful tool in facilitating the management of pain. If TENS is being used to allow procedures to be undertaken, e.g. breathing exercises and ambulation, enough time must be given to allow the machine to become effective. In the long-term use of TENS, its limitations must be recognized in that it will only work while the machine is in use and possibly for short periods of time afterwards.

ACUPUNCTURE

Acupuncture has been used successfully for many years. Its use in pain relief is well documented and backed up by scientific research (Anonymous 1981, Kosterlitz et al 1975, Sweet 1981). The stimulation of acupuncture points (acupoints) results in the release of certain chemicals including endorphins, enkephalins and serotonin, which can relieve both acute and chronic pain by working on the gating and descending pain inhibition mechanisms. Palpation of an acupoint stimulates the A-beta touch fibres, which close the gate to pain and also work via the descending inhibitory pain pathways. Insertion of a needle stimulates the A-delta fibres which work on the descending pathways to relieve pain (Bowsher 1990, Melzack & Wall 1988). Acupoints are usually more tender than the surrounding area and hence can be found by palpation on healthy subjects. If a point is active and in need of treatment, it will be much more tender than normal. Palpation is therefore the way of accurately locating the points that need stimulating. Sometimes, a point which is tender on palpation on initial assessment is no longer tender when treatment with a needle is instigated. This is probably because it has responded to treatment by the acupressure used during the assessment.

Acupuncture can be a very effective method of dealing with various pain syndromes linked with respiratory illnesses, but there is little evidence to explain how it works in the treatment of respiratory disease and its associated symptoms (Fung et al 1986, Jobst 1986). It is therefore necessary to look to some of the traditional Chinese medicine ideas to try and explain what is happening. Traditional theories revolve around the hypothesis that stimulation of acupoints balances the body's energy, 'chi', putting the body in an ideal state to allow healing to take place and for the body to become at ease (Veith 1949). When the chi energy, made up of yin and yang, is out of balance, the body is said to be at dis-ease. Interestingly, we do have some evidence that these energies exist. In 1983, Kenyon produced a piezo-electric pressure sensor which gave oscilloscope evidence of different energy patterns present in the meridian pulses in the radial artery.

There are many different acupuncture techniques available today and one way to obtain the most successful outcome from treatment is to use a combination of both body and ear acupuncture (auriculotherapy). Every structure and physiological function of the body is represented by an acupoint on the ear (Nogier 1981, Practical Ear Needling Therapy 1980). Stimulation of these has an effect on the corresponding area of the body. An electromagnetic balancing of the points is achieved, internal opiates are released and there can be an immediate reflex effect on, for example, relief of pain. Auriculotherapy (Fig. 6.62) is one of the safest and effective ways of dealing with symptoms and conditions more complicated than pain.

Safety is of prime importance in the use of acupuncture and training revolves around this. With an invasive procedure the risk of infection is ever present, especially in the ear. However, there are now many non-invasive options available for therapists who do not wish to needle, for patients in whom needling is contraindicated or for those who do not like the idea of needles. These methods include electrical, laser and magnetic stimulation together with acupressure (Baxter 1995, Kenyon 1983, 1988, Lawrence et al 1998). The patient can be taught to use acupressure at home to enhance and maintain the effect of treatment. Unpublished case studies have shown that non-invasive methods can be as effective as needling and in some cases more effective. With auriculother-

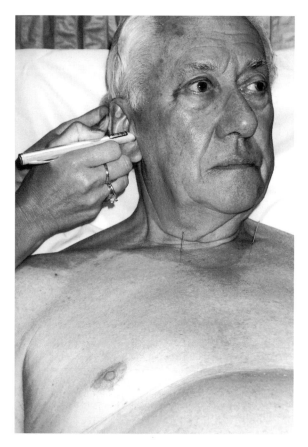

Figure 6.62 Lasers and magnetic ball therapy to the ear with body needles to help coughing and asthma.

apy, tiny gold-plated magnets can be placed over selected points. These stay on between treatments, creating both pressure and a magnetic field over the point, and prolong the effectiveness of treatment. The patient can press them and get immediate relief of symptoms, thus reducing the frequency and number of visits required.

Auriculotherapy and non-invasive body methods can be particularly useful for patients with respiratory problems, as in many of these patients needling and the use of certain body acupoints may be contraindicated. Certain drugs will reduce the effectiveness of body acupuncture, for example corticosteroids acting

as a partial opiate antagonist, but these same drugs do not reduce the effectiveness of auriculotherapy.

Following the stimulation of acupoints, the desired effect can be anything from immediate total relief to a delayed reduction in symptoms. With invasive acupuncture, the needles can be inserted and left to 'drain' for 20 minutes, manipulated by hand or a combination of these two methods can be used. If the patient does not respond to these initial techniques, an electroacupuncture machine can be connected to the needles by crocodile clips and an electrical stimulation applied via the needles. For osteoarthritic symptoms, chronic bronchitis and chronic asthma, heat can be applied to certain acupoints, both invasively and non-invasively, as a progression of treatment.

These techniques are contraindicated on pregnant women and people with pacemakers.

The following are some examples of particularly useful acupoints which may be used for certain respiratory symptoms. The points can be found by palpating for a tender spot and acupressure given using a circular massage over the point for about a minute.

CV 17   On the sternum roughly midway between the nipples.
This is used for shortness of breath and if used in conjunction with breathing exercises, works well by applying straight pressure to the point on exhalation.

P 6   In the centre of the anterior aspect of the forearm, three fingers' breadth from the anterior wrist crease. This is effective for stress reduction and the relief of nausea and vomiting (Stainton & Neff 1994).

Co 4   Adduct the thumb, find the high point of the interosseus muscle and press towards the second metacarpal. This is one of the most useful points in the body. It can be used for pain relief and stress reduction.

Stimulation of acupoints, whether by needle or non-invasive means, can act as a very effective complementary therapy to work alongside the conventional treatment of respiratory diseases and the concomitant symptoms, to enhance the outcome of treatment.

REFERENCES

Agostoni E, Sant'Ambrogio G 1970 The diaphragm. In: Campbell EJM, Agostoni E, Newsom Davies J (eds). The respiratory muscles, mechanics and neural control. Saunders, Philadelphia

Ainsworth D 1997 Respiratory muscle recruitment during exercise. In: Miller AD, Bianchi A, Bishop BP (eds) Neural control of the respiratory muscles. CRC Press, New York

Alvarez SE, Peterson M, Lunsford BR 1981 Respiratory treatment of the adult patient with spinal cord injury. Physical Therapy 61 (12): 1737–1745

Ambrosino N, Callegari G, Galloni C, Brega S, Pinna G 1995 Clinical evaluation of oscillating positive expiratory pressure for enhancing expectoration in diseases other than cystic fibrosis. Monaldi Archives of Chest Disease 50(4): 269–275

American College of Sports Medicine 1995 Guidelines for exercise testing and prescription, 5th edn.: Lea & Febiger, Philadelphia, p. 91

American Thoracic Society 1999 Dyspnea. Mechanisms, assessment and management: a consensus statement. American Journal of Respiratory and Critical Care Medicine 159: 321–340

Anonymous 1981 How does acupuncture work? (Editorial) British Medical Journal 283: 746–748

App EM, Kieselmann R, Reinhardt D, Lindemann H, Dasgupta B, King M, Brand P 1998 Sputum rheology changes in cystic fibrosis lung disease following two different types of physiotherapy. Flutter vs autogenic drainage. Chest 114: 171–177

Arens R, Gozal D, Omlin KJ, Vega J, Boyd KP, Keens TG, Woo MS 1994 Comparison of high frequency chest compression and conventional chest physiotherapy in hospitalized patients with cystic fibrosis. American Journal of Critical Care Medicine 150: 1154–1157

Asher MI, Pardy RL, Coates AL, Thomas E, Macklem PT 1982 The effects of inspiratory muscle training in patients with cystic fibrosis. American Review of Respiratory Disease 26: 855–859

Atwood HL, MacKay WA 1989 Essentials of neurophysiology. Decker, Toronto

Ayres SM, Kozam RL, Lukas DS 1963 The effects of intermittent positive pressure breathing on intrathoracic pressure, pulmonary mechanics and the work of breathing. American Review of Respiratory Disease 87: 370–379

Bach JR 1995 Respiratory muscle aids for the prevention of pulmonary morbidity and mortality. Seminars in Neurology 15 (1): 72–83

Bach JR, Alba AS 1990 Noninvasive options for ventilatory support of the traumatic high level quadriplegic patient. Chest 98 (3): 613–6 19

Bach JR, Alba AS, Bodofsky E, Curran FJ, Schultheiss M 1987 Glossopharyngeal breathing and noninvasive aids in the management of post-polio respiratory insufficiency. Birth Defects 23: 99–113

Bachrach LK, Loutit CW, Moss RB, Marcus R 1994 Osteopenia in adults with cystic fibrosis. American Journal of Medicine 96: 27–34

Barry PW, Fouroux B, Pedersen S, O'Callaghan C 2000 Nebulizers in childhood. European Respiratory Review 10 (76): 527–535

Baxter GD 1995 Therapeutic lasers theory and practice. Churchill Livingstone, Edinburgh

Baydur A, Gilgoff I, Prentice W et al 1990 Decline in respiratory function and experience with long-term assisted ventilation in advanced Duchenne's muscular dystrophy. Chest 97: 884–889

Bazuaye EA, Stone TN, Corris PA, Gibson GJ 1992 Variability of inspired oxygen concentration with nasal cannulas. Thorax 47: 609–611

Bellemare F, Grassino A. 1982 Effect of pressure and timing of contraction on human diaphragmatic fatigue. Journal of Applied Physiology 53: 1190–1195

Bethune D 1975 Neurophysiological facilitation of respiration in the unconscious adult patient. Physiotherapy Canada 27(5): 241–245

Bethune D 1976 Facilitation of respiration in unconscious adult patients. Respiratory Technology 12(4): 18–21

Bethune D 1991 Neurophysiological facilitation of respiration. In: Pryor JA (ed) Respiratory care. Churchill Livingstone, Edinburgh

Bethune D 1998 Neurophysiological facilitation of respiration. In: Pryor JA, Webber BA (eds) Physiotherapy for respiratory and cardiac problems, 2nd edn. Churchill Livingstone, Edinburgh

Bhowmik A, Seemungal TAR, Sapsford RJ et al 1998 Comparison of spontaneous and induced sputum for investigation of airway inflammation in chronic obstructive pulmonary disease. Thorax 53: 953–956

Bianchi AL, Pasaro R 1997 Organization of central respiratory neurons. In: Miller AD, Bianchi AL, Bishop BP (eds) Neural control of the respiratory muscles. CRC Press, New York

Binkley J, Soloman P, Finch E, Gill C, Moreland J 1996 Defining the minimal level of detectable change for the Roland–Morris questionnaire. Physical Therapy 76: 359–365

Bishop BP 1997 The abdominal muscles. In: Miller AD, Bianchi A, Bishop BP (eds) Neural control of the respiratory muscles. CRC Press, New York

Bott J, Keilty SEJ, Noone L 1992 Intermittent positive pressure breathing – a dying art? Physiotherapy 78: 656–660

Bowsher D 1990 Physiology and pathophysiology of pain. Journal of British Medical Acupuncture Society 7: 17–20

Boyling JD, Palastanga N 1994 In: Grieve GP (ed) Modern manual therapy of the vertebral column, 2nd edn. Churchill Livingstone, Edinburgh

Bransen RD, Davis K, Campbell RS, Johnson DJ, Porembka DT 1993 Humidification in the intensive care unit: prospective study of a new protocol utilizing heated humidification and a hygroscopic condenser humidifier. Chest 104: 1800–1805

Bray C 1994 Thoracic mobilisation in the management of respiratory and cardiac problems. In: The forgotten thoracic spine. Manipulative Physiotherapists Association of Australia Symposium, University of Sydney, Australia

Brazier D 1999 Endotracheal suction technique – putting research into practice. Journal of the Association of Chartered Physiotherapists in Respiratory Care 32: 13–17

British Standards Institution 1994 Specification for gas powered nebulisers for the delivery of drugs. BS7711 Part 3. British Standards Institution, London

British Thoracic Society, National Asthma Campaign, Royal College of Physicians of London et al 1997 The British guidelines on asthma management – 1995 review and position statement. Thorax 52 (suppl 1): S1–S21

Burge PS 1986 Getting the best out of bronchodilator therapy. Patient Management July: 155–185

Butler DS 1991 Mobilisation of the nervous system. Churchill Livingstone, Melbourne

Campbell AH, O'Connell JM, Wilson F 1975 The effect of chest physiotherapy upon the FEV_1 in chronic bronchitis. Medical Journal of Australia 1: 33–35

Campbell EJ, Baker D, Crites-Silver P 1988 Subjective effects of humidification of oxygen for delivery by nasal cannula. Chest 93: 289–293

Carr L, Pryor JA, Hodson ME 1995 Self chest clapping: patients' views and the effects on oxygen saturation. Physiotherapy 81: 753–757

Carr L, Smith RE, Pryor JA, Partridge C 1996 Cystic fibrosis patients' views and beliefs about chest clearance and exercise – a pilot study. Physiotherapy 82: 621–626

Cecins NM, Jenkins SC, Pengelley J, Ryan G 1999 The active cycle of breathing techniques – to tip or not to tip? Respiratory Medicine 93: 660–665

Cegla UH, Bautz M, Fröde G, Werner Th 1997 Physiotherapie bei patienten mit COAD und tracheobronchialer instabilität-verleich zweier oszillierender PEP-systeme (RC-CORNET®, VRP1 DESITIN). Pneumologie 51: 129–136

Chatburn RL 1987 Physiologic and methodologic issues regarding humidity therapy. Journal of Pediatrics 114: 416–420

Chatham K, Marshall C, Campbell IA, Prescott RJ 1993 The Flutter VRPI device in post-thoracotomy patients. Physiotherapy 79: 95–98

Chatham K, Baldwin J, Griffiths H, Summers L, Enright S 1999 Inspiratory muscle training improves shuttle run performance in healthy subjects. Physiotherapy 85(12): 676–683

Chatwin M, Hart N, Nickol AH, Heather S, Moxham J, Polkey MI 2000 Low frequency fatigue induced by a single inspiratory muscle training session. Thorax 55 (suppl 3): 107

Chen H, Dukes R, Martin BJ 1985 Inspiratory muscle training in patients with chronic obstructive pulmonary disease. American Review of Respiratory Disease 131: 251–255

Chevaillier J 1995 Autogenic drainage. In: Physiotherapy in the treatment of cystic fibrosis, 2nd edn. International Physiotherapy Group for Cystic Fibrosis (IPG/CF), pp 9–12

Chuter TAM, Weissman C, Starker PM, Gump FE 1989 Effect of incentive spirometry on diaphragmatic function after surgery. Surgery 105: 488–493

Chuter TAM, Weissman C, Mathews DM, Starker PM 1990 Diaphragmatic breathing maneuvers and movement of the diaphragm after cholecystectomy. Chest 97: 1110–1114

Clarke SW 1988 Inhaler therapy. Quarterly Journal of Medicine 67(253): 355–368

Clarke SW 1995 Physical defences. In: Brewis RAL, Corrin B, Geddes DM, Gibson GJ (eds) Respiratory medicine, vol 1, 2nd edn. WB Saunders, London

Cole P 1995 Bronchiectasis. In: Brewis RAL, Corrin B, Geddes DM, Gibson GJ (eds) Respiratory medicine, vol 2, 2nd edn. W B Saunders, London

Collis GG, Cole CH, Le Souëf PN 1990 Dilution of nebulised aerosols by air entrainment in children. Lancet 336: 341–343

Conway JH 1992 The effects of humidification for patients with chronic airways disease. Physiotherapy 78: 97–101

Conway JH, Fleming JS, Perring S, Holgate ST 1992 Humidification as an adjunct to chest physiotherapy in aiding tracheo-bronchial clearance in patients with bronchiectasis. Respiratory Medicine 86: 109–114

Coombs HC 1918 The relation of the dorsal roots of the spinal nerves and the mesencephalon to the control of respiratory movements. American Journal of Physiology 46: 459–471

Coombs HC, Pike FH 1930 The nervous control of respiration in kittens. American Journal of Physiology 95: 681–693

Cunningham S, Prasad SA, Collyer L, Carr S, Balfour-Lynn I, Wallis C 2001 Bronchoconstriction following nebulised Colistin in cystic fibrosis. Archives of Disease in Childhood 84 (5): 432–33

Currie DC, Munro C, Gaskell D, Cole PJ 1986 Practice, problems and compliance with postural drainage: a survey of chronic sputum producers. British Journal of Diseases of the Chest 80: 249–253

Dab I, Alexander F 1979 The mechanism of autogenic drainage studied with flow volume curves. Monographs of Paediatrics 10: 50–53

Dail CW 1951 'Glossopharyngeal breathing' by paralyzed patients. California Medicine 75: 217–218

Dail CW, Affeldt JE, Collier CR 1955 Clinical aspects of glossopharyngeal breathing. Journal of the American Medical Association 158: 445–449

David A 1991 Autogenic drainage – the German approach. In: Pryor JA (ed) Respiratory care. Churchill Livingstone, Edinburgh, pp 65–78

Davidson AGF, Wong LTK, Pirie GE, McIlwaine PM 1992 Long-term comparative trial of conventional percussion and drainage physiotherapy versus autogenic drainage in cystic fibrosis. Pediatric Pulmonology (suppl) 8: 298

De Troyer A 1997 Mechanics of the chest wall muscles. In: Miller AD, Bianchi AL, Bishop BP (eds) Neural control of the respiratory muscles. CRC Press, New York

De Troyer A, Peche R, Yernault J, Estenne M 1994 Neck muscle activity in patients with severe chronic obstructive disease. Journal of Respiratory Care Medicine 150: 41–47

Dean E 1985 Effect of body position on pulmonary function. Physical Therapy 65: 613–618

Dekhujzen PNR, Folgering HTM, van Herwaarden CLA 1991 Target flow inspiratory muscle training during pulmonary rehabilitation in patients with COPD. Chest 99: 128–133

DeVilbiss Oxygen Services 2000 Manufacturer's guidelines for oxygen concentrators. Sunrise Medical Ltd, West Midlands DY8 4PS, England

Dodd ME, Hanley SP, Johnson SC, Webb AK 1995 District nebuliser compressor service: reliability and costs. Thorax 50: 82–84

Dodd ME, Abbott J, Maddison J, Moorcroft AJ, Webb AK 1997 Effect of tonicity of nebulised colistin on chest tightness and pulmonary function in adults with cystic fibrosis. Thorax 52: 656–658

Dodd ME, Kellet F, Davis A et al 2000 Audit of oxygen prescribing before and after the introduction of a prescription chart. British Medical Journal 321: 864–865

Duron B, Bars P 1986 Effect of thoracic cutaneous nerve stimulations on the activity of the intercostal muscles and motoneurons of the cat. In: Euler C, Lagercrantz A (eds) Neurobiology of the control of breathing (Nobel conference series). Raven Press, New York

Duron B, Rose D 1997 The intercostal muscles. In: Miller AD, Bianchi AL, Bishop BP (eds) Neural control of the respiratory muscles. CRC Press, New York

Eng PA, Morton J, Douglass JA, Riedler J, Wilson J, Robertson CF 1996 Short-term efficacy of ultrasonically nebulized hypertonic saline in cystic fibrosis. Pediatric Pulmonology 21: 77–83

Enright S, Chatham K, Baldwin J, Griffiths H. 2000 The effect of inspiratory muscle training in the elite athlete: a pilot study. Physiotherapy in Sport 1: 1–5

Epstein SK. 1994 An overview of respiratory muscle function. Clinical Chest Medicine 15 (4): 619–639

Euler C 1986 Breathing behavior. In: Euler C, Lagercrantz A (eds) Neurobiology of the control of breathing (Nobel conference series). Raven Press, New York

European Respiratory Society 2000 European Respiratory Society nebulizer guidelines: clinical aspects. European Respiratory Review 10 (76)

Everard ML, Evans M, Milner AD 1994 Is tapping jet nebulisers worthwhile? Archives of Disease in Childhood 70: 538–539

Falk M, Andersen JB 1991 Positive expiratory pressure (PEP) mask. In: Pryor JA (ed) Respiratory care. Churchill Livingstone, Edinburgh, pp 51–63

Falk M, Kelstrup M, Andersen JB, Kinoshita T, Falk P, Støvring S, Gøthgen I 1984 Improving the ketchup bottle method with positive expiratory pressure, PEP, in cystic fibrosis. European Journal of Respiratory Diseases 65: 423–432

Fleck S 1994 Detraining: its effects on endurance and strength. National Strength and Conditioning Journal 2: 22–28

Flower KA, Eden RI, Lomax L, Mann NM, Burgess J 1979 New mechanical aid to physiotherapy in cystic fibrosis. British Medical Journal 2: 630–631

Frazier DT, Xu Fadi, Lee L-Y 1997 Respiratory-related reflexes and the cerebellum. In: Miller AD, Bianchi AL, Bishop BP (eds) Neural control of the respiratory muscles. CRC Press, New York

Freitag L, Bremme J, Schroer M 1989 High frequency oscillation for respiratory physiotherapy. British Journal of Anaesthesia 63: 44S–46S

Fung KP, Chow OK, So SY 1986 Attenuation of exercise induced asthma by acupuncture. Lancet 2: 1419–1422

Gallon A 1991 Evaluation of chest percussion in the treatment of patients with copious sputum production. Respiratory Medicine 85: 45–51

George RJD, Johnson MA, Pavia D, Agnew JE, Clarke SW, Geddes DM 1985 Increase in mucociliary clearance in normal man induced by oral high frequency oscillation. Thorax 40: 433–437

Gleeson JG, Price JF 1988 Nebuliser technique. British Journal of Diseases of the Chest 82: 172–174

Goldman M 1974 Mechanical coupling of the diaphragm and the rib cage. In: Pengelly LD, Rebuck AS, Campbell EJM (eds) Loaded breathing. Proceedings of an international symposium, 'The effects of mechanical loads on breathing'. Longman Canada, Don Mills, Ontario

Goldman JM, Teale C, Muers MF 1992 Simplifying the assessment of patients with chronic airflow limitation for home nebulizer therapy. Respiratory Medicine 86: 33–38

Goldstein RS 1993 Ventilatory muscle training. Pulmonary rehabilitation in chronic respiratory insufficiency. Thorax 48: 1025–1033

Gondor M, Nixon PA, Mutich R et al 1999 Comparison of flutter device and chest physical therapy in the treatment of cystic fibrosis pulmonary exacerbation. Pediatric Pulmonology 28(4): 255–260

Goodwin MJ 1994 Mechanical chest stimulation as a physiotherapy aid. Medical Engineering and Physics 16: 267–272

Gordon J 1991 Spinal mechanisms of motor coordination. In: Kandel ER, Schwartz JH, Jessel JM (eds) Principles of neural science. Appleton & Lange, Connecticut

Gormezano J, Branthwaite MA 1972 Pulmonary physiotherapy with assisted ventilation. Anaesthesia 27: 249–257

Gosselink R, De Leyn P, Troosters T, Deneffe G, Lerut A, Decramer M 1997 Incentive spirometry does not affect recovery after thoracic surgery. European Respiratory Journal 10 (suppl 25): 725

Grassino A 1974 Influence of chest wall configuration on the static and dynamic characteristics of the contracting diaphragm. In: Pengelly LD, Rebuck AS, Campbell EJM (eds) Loaded breathing. Proceedings of an international symposium, 'The effects of mechanical loads on breathing'. Longman Canada, Don Mills, Ontario

Grassino A 1989 Inspiratory muscle training in COPD patients. European Respiratory Journal (suppl) 7: 581s–586s

Gray's Anatomy 1973 Longman, Edinburgh

Green M, Moxham J 1985 The respiratory muscles. Clinical Science 68: 1–10

Gregersen GG, Lucas DL 1967 An in vivo study of the axial rotation of the human thoraco-lumbar spine. Journal of Bone and Joint Surgery 49A: 247–262

Gunawardena KA, Patel B, Campbell IA, Macdonald JB, Smith AP 1984 Oxygen as a driving gas for nebulisers: safe or dangerous? British Medical Journal 288: 272–274

Hall JC, Tarala R, Harris J, Tapper J, Christiansen K 1991 Incentive spirometry versus routine chest physiotherapy for prevention of pulmonary complications after abdominal surgery. Lancet 337: 953–956

Hansen LG, Warwick WJ, Hansen KL 1994 Mucus transport mechanisms in relation to the effect of high frequency chest compression (HFCC) on mucus clearance. Pediatric Pulmonology 17: 113–118

Harrison DA, Breen DP, Harris ND, Gerrish SP 1993 The performance of two intensive care humidifiers at high gas flows. Anaesthesia 48: 902–905

Hasani A, Pavia D, Agnew JE, Clarke SW 1994 Regional lung clearance during cough and forced expiration technique (FET): effects of flow and viscoelasticity. Thorax 49: 557–561

Henderson RC, Madsen CD 1996 Bone density in children and adolescents with cystic fibrosis. Journal of Pediatrics 128: 28–34

Henderson RC, Specter BB 1994 Kyphosis and fractures in children and young adults with cystic fibrosis. Journal of Paediatrics 125: 208–212

Hilaire G, Monteau R 1997 Brainstem and spinal control of respiratory muscles during breathing. In: Miller AD, Bianchi AL, Bishop BP (eds) Neural control of the respiratory muscles. CRC Press, New York

Hill SL, Barnes PK, Hollway T, Tennant R 1984 Fixed performance oxygen masks: an evaluation. British Medical Journal 288: 1261–1263

Hinds CJ, Watson D 1996 Intensive care, 2nd edn. WB Saunders, London, pp 33, 175

Hofmeyr JL, Webber BA, Hodson ME 1986 Evaluation of positive expiratory pressure as an adjunct to chest physiotherapy in the treatment of cystic fibrosis. Thorax 41: 951–954

Homnick DN, White F, De Castro C 1995 Comparison of effects of an intrapulmonary percussive ventilator to standard aerosol and chest physiotherapy in treatment of cystic fibrosis. Pediatric Pulmonology 20: 50–55

Homnick DN, Anderson K, Marks JH 1998 Comparison of the flutter device to standard chest physiotherapy in hospitalized patients with cystic fibrosis: a pilot study. Chest 114 (4): 993–997

Hutchinson GR, Parker S, Pryor JA et al 1996 Home-use nebulizers: a potential source of *Burkholderia cepacia* and other colistin-resistant, gram-negative bacteria in patients with cystic fibrosis. Journal of Clinical Microbiology 34: 584–587

Jacob W 1990 Physiotherapy in the ICU. In: Oh TE (ed) Intensive care manual, 3rd edn. Butterworths, Sydney, ch. 4, p. 24

Janda V 1994 Muscles and motor control in cervicogenic disorders: assessment and management physical therapy for the cervical and thoracic spine. In: Grant R (ed) Clinics in physical therapy, 2nd edn. Churchill Livingstone, New York

Jean A, Car A, Kessler JP 1997 Brainstem organization of swallowing and its interaction with respiration. In: Miller AD, Bianchi AL, Bishop BP (eds) Neural control of the respiratory muscles. CRC Press, New York

Jeffrey AA, Warren PM 1992 Should we judge a mask by its cover? Thorax 47: 543–546

Jenkins SC, Soutar SA, Moxham J 1988 The effects of posture on lung volumes in normal subjects and in patients pre- and post-coronary artery surgery. Physiotherapy 74: 492–496

Jessurun, GAJ, Tio, RA, De Jongste, MJL, Hautvast, RWM, Den Heijer P, Crijns HJGM 1998 Coronary blood flow dynamics during transcutaneous electrical nerve stimulation for stable angina pectoris associated with severe narrowing of one major coronary artery. American Journal of Cardiology 82(8): 921–926

Jobst K 1986 Controlled trial of acupuncture for disabling breathlessness. Lancet 2: 1416–1419

Kelleher WH, Parida RK 1957 Glossopharyngeal breathing. British Medical Journal 2: 740–743

Kendrick AH, Smith EC, Denyer J 1995 Nebulizers – fill volume, residual volume and matching of nebulizer to compressor. Respiratory Medicine 89: 157–159

Kenyon JN 1983 Modern techniques of acupuncture; vol. 1:a practical scientific guide to electro-acupuncture. Thorsons, Wellingborough

Kenyon JN 1988 Acupressure techniques. Healing Arts Press, Canada

Kieselmann R 1995 Modified AD. In: Physiotherapy in the treatment of cystic fibrosis, 2nd edn. International Physiotherapy Group for Cystic Fibrosis (IPG/CF), pp 13–14

Kim MJ, Larson M, Sachs P, Sharp JT 1984 Respiratory muscle training in patients with chronic obstructive pulmonary disease. American Review of Respiratory Disease 129: 129–131

Koepchen HP, Abel H-H, Klussendorf D, Lazar H 1986 Respiratory and cardiovascular rhythmicity. In: Euler C, Lagercrantz A (eds) Neurobiology of the control of breathing (Nobel conference series). Raven Press, New York

Komi PV, Hakkinen K 1991 Strength and power. In: Dirix A, Knuttgen HG, Tittel K (eds) The Olympic book of sports medicine. Blackwell, Oxford, pp 181–193

Konstan MW, Stern RC, Doershuk CF 1994 Efficacy of the Flutter device for airway mucus clearance in patients with cystic fibrosis. Journal of Pediatrics 124: 689–693

Kosterlitz NW, Hughes J, Smith TW, Fothergill LA, Morgan DA, Morris HR 1975 Identification of two related pentapeptides from the brain, with potent opiate agonist activity. Nature 258: 557–579

Langenderfer B 1998 Alternatives to percussion and postural drainage. A review of mucus clearance therapies: percussion and postural drainage, autogenic drainage, positive expiratory pressure, flutter valve, intrapulmonary percussive ventilation and high-frequency chest compression with the ThAIRapy vest. Journal of Cardiac and Pulmonary Rehabilitation 18: 283–289

Langlands J 1967 The dynamics of cough in health and in chronic bronchitis. Thorax 22: 88–96

Larson JL, Kim MJ, Sharp JT, Larson D 1988 Inspiratory muscle training with a pressure threshold device in patients with chronic obstructive pulmonary disease. American Review of Respiratory Disease 138: 689–696

Larson JL, Covey MK, Vitalo CA, Alex CG, Patel M, Kim MJ 1993 Maximal inspiratory pressure. Learning effect and test-retest reliability in patients with chronic obstructive pulmonary disease. Chest 104: 448–453

Lawler J, Powers S, Criswell D 1993 Inducibility of NADP-specific isocitrate dehydrogenase with endurance training in skeletal muscle. Acta Physiologica Scandinavica 149: 177–181

Lawrence R, Rosch PJ, Plowden J 1998 Magnet therapy, the pain cure alternative. Prima Publishing, USA, pp. 69–72

Leach RM, Bateman N T 1994 Domiciliary oxygen therapy. British Journal of Hospital Medicine 51: 47–54

Leak AM, Cooper J, Dyer S, Williams K, Turner-Stokes L, Frank OA 1994 The Northwick Park neck pain questionnaire, devised to measure neck pain and disability. British Journal of Rheumatology 33: 474–496

Leith DE, Bradley M 1976 Ventilatory muscle strength and endurance training. Journal of Applied Physiology 41: 508–516

Lewis RA, Fleming JS 1985 Fractional deposition from a jet nebuliser: how it differs from a metered dose inhaler. British Journal of Diseases of the Chest 79: 361–367

Lindemann H 1992 The value of physical therapy with VRP1 Desitin ('Flutter'). Pneumologie 46(12): 626–630

Lock SH, Blower G, Prynne M, Wedzicha JA 1992 Comparison of liquid and gaseous oxygen for domiciliary portable use. Thorax 47: 98–100

Lockwood S 1996 The variable parameters of transcutaneous electrical nerve stimulation (TENS) and their clinical use. New Zealand Journal of Physiotherapy April: 7–10

Loddenkemper R 1975 Dose- and time-response of Sch 1000 MDI on total (R_t) and expiratory (R_e) airways resistance in patients with chronic bronchitis and emphysema. Postgraduate Medical Journal 51(suppl 7): 97

Lopez-Vidriero MT, Reid L 1978 Bronchial mucus in health and disease. British Medical Bulletin 34(1): 63–74

Lunteren E, Dick TE 1997 Muscles of the upper airway and accessory respiratory muscles. In: Miller AD, Bianchi AL, Bishop BP (eds) Neural control of the respiratory muscles. CRC Press, New York

Macklem PT 1974 Physiology of cough. Transactions of the American Broncho-Esophalogical Association 150–157

Maddison J, Dodd M, Webb AK 1994 Nebulised colistin causes chest tightness in adults with cystic fibrosis. Respiratory Medicine 88: 145–147

Make BJ, Hill N S, Goldberg AL et al 1998 Mechanical ventilation beyond the intensive care unit. Report of a consensus conference of the American College of Chest Physicians. Chest 113 (Suppl 5): 289S–344S

Mannheimer JS, Lampe N 1984 Clinical transcutaneous electrical nerve stimulation. FA Davis, Philadelphia

Matthews HR, Hopkinson RB 1984 Treatment of sputum retention by minitracheotomy. British Journal of Surgery 71: 147–150

McCool FD 1992 Inspiratory muscle weakness and fatigue. RT/The Journal for Respiratory Care Practitioners 5(6): 32–41

McDonnell T, McNicholas WT, FitzGerald MX 1986 Hypoxaemia during chest physiotherapy in patients with cystic fibrosis. Irish Journal of Medical Science 155: 345–348

McGavin CR, Naoe H, McHardy GJR 1976 Does inhalation of salbutamol enable patients with airway obstruction to walk further? Clinical Science and Molecular Medicine 51: 12–13

McIlwaine PM, Wong LT, Peacock D, Davidson AG 1997 Long-term comparative trial of conventional postural drainage and percussion versus positive expiratory pressure physiotherapy in the treatment of cystic fibrosis. Journal of Pediatrics 131(4): 570–574

McIlwaine PM, Wong LT, Peacock D, Davidson AG 2001 Long-term comparative trial of positive expiratory pressure versus oscillating positive expiratory pressure (flutter) physiotherapy in the treatment of cystic fibrosis. Journal of Pediatrics 138(6): 845–850

Mead J, Turner JM, Macklem P T, Little JB 1967 Significance of the relationship between lung recoil and maximum expiratory flow. Journal of Applied Physiology 22: 95–108

Mead J, Takishima T, Leith D 1970 Stress distribution in lungs: a model of pulmonary elasticity. Journal of Applied Physiology 28: 596–608

Medic-Aid Ltd 1996 Nebulizer therapy training pack. Medic-Aid Ltd, Heath Place, Bognor Regis, W Sussex, UK

Medical Research Council Working Party 1981 Long term domiciliary oxygen therapy in chronic hypoxic cor pulmonale complicating chronic bronchitis and emphysema. Lancet 1: 681–686

Melzack R, Wall P 1988 The challenge of pain, 2nd edn. Penguin Books, London

Menkes HA, Traystman RJ 1977 Collateral ventilation. American Review of Respiratory Disease 116: 287–309

Mestitz H, Copland JM, McDonald CF 1989 Comparison of outpatient nebulized vs metered dose inhaler terbutaline in chronic airflow obstruction. Chest 96: 1237–1240

Miller AD, Bianchi AL, Bishop BP 1997 Overview of the neural control of the respiratory muscles. In: Miller AD, Bianchi AL, Bishop BP (eds) Neural control of the respiratory muscles. CRC Press, New York

Miller MR 2000 Peak expiratory flow meters. In: European Respiratory Society: the buyer's guide, volume 3, pp 12–14. ERS, Lausanne, Switzerland 3:12–14

Morgan MDL, Silver JR, Williams SJ 1986 The respiratory system of the spinal cord patient. In: Bloch RF, Basbaum M(eds) Management of spinal cord injuries. Williams and Wilkins, Baltimore, pp 78–115

Nakamura S, Mikami M, Kawakami M, Sudo E, App EM, King M 1998 Comparative evaluation of the flutter and the cornet in improving the cohesiveness of sputum from patients with bronchiectasis. European Respiratory Society Meeting (abstract)

Nathan H 1962 Osteophytes of the vertebral column. An anatomical study of their development according to age, race and sex with considerations as to their aetiology and significance. Journal of Bone and Joint Surgery 44A: 243

Nebuliser Project Group of the British Thoracic Society Standards of Care Committee 1997 Current best practice for nebuliser treatment. Thorax 52 (suppl 2): S1–S106

Nelson HP 1934 Postural drainage of the lungs. British Medical Journal 2: 251–255

Newman SP, Pellow PGD, Clarke SW 1986 Droplet size distributions of nebulised aerosols for inhalation therapy. Clinical Physics and Physiological Measurement 7: 139–146

Newman SP, Weisz AWB, Talaee N, Clarke SW 1991 Improvement of drug delivery with a breath actuated pressurised aerosol for patients with poor inhaler technique. Thorax 46: 712–716

Nikander K, Denyer J 2000 Breathing patterns. European Respiratory Review 10 (76): 576–579

Nocturnal Oxygen Therapy Trial Group 1980 Continuous or nocturnal oxygen therapy in hypoxemic chronic obstructive lung disease: a clinical trial. Annals of Internal Medicine 93: 391–398

Nogier PMF 1981 Handbook to auriculotherapy. Maisonneuve SA, France

Nomori H, Kobayashi R, Fuyuno G, Marinagaa S, Yashima H 1994 Pre-operative respiratory muscle training: assessment in thoracic surgery patients with special reference to post-operative pulmonary complications. Chest 105 (6): 1782–1788

Oberwaldner B, Evans JC, Zach MS 1986 Forced expirations against a variable resistance: a new chest physiotherapy method in cystic fibrosis. Pediatric Pulmonology 2: 358–367

Oberwaldner B, Theissl B, Rucker A, Zach MS 1991 Chest physiotherapy in hospitalized patients with cystic fibrosis: a study of lung function effects and sputum production. European Respiratory Journal 4: 152–158

O'Driscoll BR, Kay EA, Taylor RJ, Bernstein A 1990 Home nebulizers: can optimal therapy be predicted by laboratory studies? Respiratory Medicine 84: 471–477

Oh TE 1990 Humidification. In: Oh TE(ed) Intensive care manual, 3rd edn. Butterworths, Sydney, pp 169–173

Oikkonen M, Karjalainen K, Kähärä V, Kuosa R, Schavikin L 1991 Comparison of incentive spirometry and intermittent positive pressure breathing after coronary artery bypass graft. Chest 99: 60–65

O'Neill SO, McCarthy DS 1983 Postural relief of dyspnoea in severe chronic airflow limitation: relationship to respiratory muscle strength. Thorax 38: 595–600

Pardy RL, Rochester DF 1992 Respiratory muscle training. Seminars in Respiratory Medicine 13: 53–62

Partridge C, Pryor J, Webber B 1989 Characteristics of the forced expiration technique. Physiotherapy 75: 193–194

Pavia D, Webber B, Agnew JE, Vora H, Lopez-Vidriero MT, Clarke SW, Branthwaite MA 1988 The role of intermittent positive pressure breathing (IPPB) in bronchial toilet. European Respiratory Journal 1(suppl 2): 250S

Pedersen S 1996 Inhalers and nebulizers: which to choose and why. Respiratory Medicine 90: 69–77

Peiper A 1963 Cerebral function in infancy and childhood. Consultants Bureau, New York

Pendleton N, Cheesbrough JS, Walshaw MJ, Hind CRK 1991 Bacterial colonisation of humidifier attachments on oxygen concentrators prescribed for long term oxygen therapy: a district review. Thorax 46: 257–258

Pfleger A, Theissl B, Oberwaldner B, Zach MS 1992 Self-administered chest physiotherapy in cystic fibrosis: a comparative study of high-pressure PEP and autogenic drainage. Lung 170: 323–330

Pike SE, Machin AC, Dix KJ, Pryor JA, Hodson ME 1999 Comparison of flutter VRP1 and forced expirations (FE) with active cycle of breathing techniques (ACBT) in subjects with cystic fibrosis. Netherlands Journal of Medicine 54: S55–56

Pin I, Gibson PG, Kolendowich R et al 1992 Use of induced sputum cell counts to investigate airway inflammation in asthma. Thorax 47: 25–29

Powers S, Criswell D, Lieu F, Dodd S, Silverman H 1992 Diaphragm fibre type specific adaptation to endurance exercise. Respiratory Physiology 89: 195–207

Practical ear needling therapy 1980 Medicine & Health Publishing Co, Hong Kong

Prasad SA, Main E 1998 Finding evidence to support airway clearance techniques in cystic fibrosis. Disability and Rehabilitation 20 (6/7): 235–246

Preston IM, Matthews HR, Ready AR 1986 Minitracheotomy. Physiotherapy 72: 494–497

Pryor JA, Webber BA 1979 An evaluation of the forced expiration technique as an adjunct to postural drainage. Physiotherapy 65: 304–307

Pryor JA, Webber BA, Hodson ME, Batten JC 1979 Evaluation of the forced expiration technique as an adjunct to postural drainage in treatment of cystic fibrosis. British Medical Journal 2: 417–418

Pryor JA, Parker RA, Webber BA 1981 A comparison of mechanical and manual percussion as adjuncts to postural drainage in the treatment of cystic fibrosis in adolescents and adults. Physiotherapy 67: 140–141

Pryor JA, Wiggins J, Webber BA, Geddes DM 1989 Oral high frequency oscillation (OHFO) as an aid to physiotherapy in chronic bronchitis with airflow limitation. Thorax 44: 350P

Pryor JA, Webber BA, Hodson ME 1990 Effect of chest physiotherapy on oxygen saturation in patients with cystic fibrosis. Thorax 45: 77

Pryor JA, Webber BA, Hodson ME, Warner JO 1994 The Flutter VRP1 as an adjunct to chest physiotherapy in cystic fibrosis. Respiratory Medicine 88: 677–681

Putt MT, Paratz JD 1996 The effect of stretching pectoralis major and anterior deltoid muscles on the restrictive component of chronic airflow limitation. In: Proceedings of the National Physiotherapy Conference, Brisbane, Queensland. Australian Physiotherapy Association, Brisbane, Queensland

Reid WD, Samrai B 1995 Respiratory muscle training for patients with chronic obstructive pulmonary disease. Physical Therapy 75 (11): 996–1005

Reid WD, Huang J, Bryson S 1994 Diaphragm injury and myofibrillar structure induced by resistive loading. Journal of Applied Physiology 76: 176–184

Reisman JJ, Rivington-Law B, Corey M, Marcotte J, Wannamaker E, Harcourt D, Levison H 1988 Role of conventional physiotherapy in cystic fibrosis. Journal of Pediatrics 113: 632–636

Reynolds JEF(ed) 1996 Martindale. The extra pharmacopoeia, 31st edn. Royal Pharmaceutical Society, London, pp 1060–1063

Richler DW, Ballanyi K, Ramirez J-M 1997 Respiratory rhythm generation. In: Miller AD, Bianchi AL, Bishop BP (eds) Neural control of the respiratory muscles. CRC Press, New York

Ricksten SE, Bengtsson A, Soderberg C, Thorden M, Kvist H 1986 Effects of periodic positive airway pressure by mask on postoperative pulmonary function. Chest 89: 774–781

Rood M 1973 Unpublished lectures given at the University of Western Ontario, London, Ontario

Royal College of Physicians 1999 Domiciliary oxygen therapy services. Clinical guidelines and advice for prescribers. Royal College of Physicians, London

Ruffin RE, Fitzgerald JD, Rebuck AS 1977 A comparison of the bronchodilator activity of Sch 1000 and salbutamol. Journal of Allergy and Clinical Immunology 59: 136–141

Ryan DW 1990 Minitracheotomy. British Medical Journal 300: 958–959

Sanderson PJ 1984 Common bacterial pathogens and resistance to antibiotics. British Medical Journal 289: 638–639

Schoeffel RE, Anderson SD, Altounyan REC 1981 Bronchial hyperreactivity in response to inhalation of ultrasonically nebulised solutions of distilled water and saline. British Medical Journal 283: 1285–1287

Schöni MH 1989 Autogenic drainage: a modern approach to physiotherapy in cystic fibrosis. Journal of the Royal Society of Medicine 82(suppl 16): 32–37

Shah P, Dhurjon L, Metcalfe T, Gibson JM 1992 Acute angle closure glaucoma associated with nebulised ipratropium bromide and salbutamol. British Medical Journal 304: 40–41

Sharp JT, Drutz WS, Moisan T, Forster J, Machnach W 1980 Postural relief of dyspnea in severe chronic obstructive pulmonary disease. American Review of Respiratory Disease 122: 201–211

Shelly MP, Lloyd GM, Park GR 1988 A review of the mechanisms and methods of humidification of inspired gases. Intensive Care 14: 1–9

Shneerson J 1992 Transtracheal oxygen delivery. Thorax 47: 57–59

Sieck GC, Prakash YS 1997 The diaphragm muscle. In: Miller AD, Bianchi AL, Bishop BP (eds) Neural control of the respiratory muscles. CRC Press, New York

Sjolund, BH, Eriksson, MBE 1979 The influence of naloxone on analgesia produced by peripheral conditioning stimulation. Brain Research 173: 295

Sjolund, BH, Eriksson, M, Loeser, JD 1990 Transcutaneous nerve stimulation of peripheral nerves. In: Bonica J (ed) Management of pain, 2nd edn. Lea & Febiger Philadelphia, pp 1852–1861

Smaldone GC, Vinciguerra C, Marchese J 1991 Detection of inhaled pentamidine in health care workers. New England Journal of Medicine 325: 891–892

Smith K, Cook D, Guyatt GH, Madhavan J, Oxman AD 1992 Respiratory muscle training in chronic airflow limitation: a meta-analysis. American Review of Respiratory Disease 145: 533–539

Stainton MC, Neff EJ 1994 The efficacy of Seabands for the control of nausea and vomiting in pregnancy. Health Care for Women International 15 (6): 563–575

Starke ID, Webber BA, Branthwaite MA 1979 IPP Band hypercapnia in respiratory failure: the effect of different concentrations of inspired oxygen on arterial blood gas tensions. Anaesthesia 34: 283–287

Stock MC, Downs JB, Gauer PK, Alster JM, Imrey PB 1985 Prevention of postoperative pulmonary complications with CPAP, incentive spirometry, and conservative therapy. Chest 87: 151–157

Sukumalchantra Y, Park SS, Williams MH 1965 The effect of intermittent positive pressure breathing (IPPB) in acute ventilatory failure. American Review of Respiratory Disease 92: 885–893

Sumi T 1963 The segmental reflex relations of cutaneous afferent inflow to thoracic respiratory motoneurones. Journal of Neurophysiology 26: 478–493

Sutton PP, Parker RA, Webber BA et al 1983 Assessment of the forced expiration technique, postural drainage and directed coughing in chest physiotherapy. European Journal of Respiratory Diseases 64: 62–68

Sweet WH 1981 Some current problems in pain research and therapy (including needlepuncture, 'Acupuncture'). Part 2 of the second John J Bonica Lecture. Pain 10 (3): 297–309

Sykes MK, McNicol MW, Campbell EJM 1976 Respiratory failure, 2nd edn. Blackwell Science, Oxford, p 153

Thiagamoorthy S, Carter M, Merchant S et al 2000 Administering, monitoring and withdrawing oxygen therapy (letter). Respiratory Medicine 94: 1253

Thomas J, De Hueck A, Kleiner M et al 1995 To vibrate or not to vibrate: usefulness of the mechanical vibrator for clearing bronchial secretions. Physiotherapy Canada 47 (2): 120–125

Thompson B 1978 Asthma and your child, 5th edn. Pegasus Press, Christchurch, New Zealand

Thompson B, Thompson HT 1968 Forced expiration exercises in asthma and their effect on FEV1. New Zealand Journal of Physiotherapy 3: 19–21

Thoracic Society 1950 The nomenclature of bronchopulmonary anatomy. Thorax 5: 222–228

Tilling SE, Hayes B 1987 Heat and moisture exchangers in artificial ventilation. British Journal of Anaesthesia 59: 1181–1188

Tomashefski JF, Bruce M, Goldberg HI, Dearborn DG 1986 Regional distribution of macroscopic lung disease in cystic fibrosis. American Review of Respiratory Disease 133: 535–540

Tomkiewicz RP, Biviji A, King M 1994 Effects of oscillating air flow on the rheological properties and clearability of mucous gel simulants. Biorheology 31: 511–520

Tucker B, Jenkins S, Cheong D, Robinson P 1999 Effect of unilateral breathing exercises on regional lung ventilation. Nuclear Medicine Communications 20: 815–821

van der Schans CP 1997 Forced expiratory manoeuvres to increase transport of bronchial mucus: a mechanistic approach. Monaldi Archives of Chest Disease 52: 367–370

van der Schans CP, van der Mark Th W, de Vries G et al 1991 Effect of positive expiratory pressure breathing in patients with cystic fibrosis. Thorax 46: 252–256

van Hengstum M, Festen J, Beurskens C, Hankel M, van den Broek W, Corstens F 1990 No effect of oral high frequency oscillation combined with forced expiration manoeuvres on tracheobronchial clearance in chronic bronchitis. European Respiratory Journal 3: 14–18

Vater M, Hurt P G, Aitkenhead AR 1983 Quantitative effects of respired helium and oxygen mixtures on gas flow using conventional oxygen masks. Anaesthesia 38: 879–882

Veith I 1949 Huang Ti Nei Ching Su Wen: the Yellow Emperor's classic of internal medicine. University of California Press, Berkeley

Vibekk P 1991 Chest mobilization and respiratory function. In: Pryor JA (ed) Respiratory care. Churchill Livingstone, Edinburgh, pp 103–119

Vora V A, Vara DD, Walton R, Morgan MDL 1995 The assessment of nebulised bronchodilator treatment in COPD by shuttle walk test and breathing problems questionnaire. Thorax 50(suppl 2): A29

Walsh DM 1997 TENS: clinical applications and related theory. Churchill Livingstone, London

Wanner A 1977 Clinical aspects of mucociliary transport. American Review of Respiratory Disease 116: 73–125

Ward RJ, Danziger F, Bonica JJ, Allen GD, Bowes J 1966 An evaluation of postoperative respiratory maneuvers. Surgery, Gynecology and Obstetrics 123: 51–54

Watson D, Trott P 1993 Cervical headache – an investigation of natural head posture and upper cervical flexor muscle performance. Cephalgia 13: 272–284

Webb AK, Egan JJ, Dodd ME 1996 Clinical management of cystic fibrosis patients awaiting and immediately following lung transplantation. In: Dodge JA, Brock DJH, Widdicombe JH (eds) Cystic fibrosis – current topics, vol 3. John Wiley, Chichester, p 332

Webber BA 1988 The Brompton Hospital guide to chest physiotherapy, 5th edn. Blackwell Science, Oxford, p 43

Webber BA 1990 The active cycle of breathing techniques. Cystic Fibrosis News Aug/Sep: 10–11

Webber BA 1991 The role of the physiotherapist in medical chest problems. Respiratory Disease in Practice Feb/Mar: 12–15

Webber BA, Higgens JM 1999 Glossopharyngeal ('frog') breathing – what, when and how? Video available: telephone +44 (0)1494 725724

Webber BA, Shenfield GM, Paterson JW 1974 A comparison of three different techniques for giving nebulized albuterol to asthmatic patients. American Review of Respiratory Disease 109: 293–295

Webber BA, Parker R, Hofmeyr J, Hodson M 1985 Evaluation of self-percussion during postural drainage using the forced expiration technique. Physiotherapy Practice 1: 42–45

Webber BA, Hofmeyr JL, Morgan MDL, Hodson ME 1986 Effects of postural drainage, incorporating the forced expiration technique, on pulmonary function in cystic fibrosis. British Journal of Diseases of the Chest 80: 353–359

Wedzicha JA 2000 Long-term oxygen therapy vs long-term ventilatory assistance. Respiratory Care 45(2): 178–187

West JB 1997 Pulmonary pathophysiology, 5th edn. Williams and Wilkins, Baltimore, pp 7–9

Wheeler JB, Doleys DM, Harden RS, Clelland JA. 1984 Conventional TENS electrode placement and pain threshold. Physical Therapy 64 (5): 745

White AA, Panjabi MM 1990 Clinical biomechanics of the spine, 2nd edn. Lippincott, Philadelphia

White S, Sahrmann S 1994 Physical therapy for the cervical and thoracic spine. In: Grant R(ed) Clinics in physical therapy, 2nd edn. Churchill Livingstone, New York

Wilson AM, Nikander K, Brown PH 2000 Drug device matching. European Respiratory Review 10 (76): 558–566

Wilson GE, Baldwin AL, Walshaw MJ 1995 A comparison of traditional chest physiotherapy with the active cycle of breathing in patients with chronic suppurative lung disease. European Respiratory Journal 8 (suppl 19): 171S

Wilson R, Cole PJ 1988 The effect of bacterial products on ciliary function. American Review of Respiratory Disease 138: S49–S53

Wolf SL, Gersh MR, Rao VR 1981 Examining electrode placements and stimulating parameters in treating chronic pain with conventional transcutaneous electrical nerve stimulation (TENS). Pain 11: 37–47

Wolfsdorf J, Swift DL, Avery ME 1969 Mist therapy reconsidered: an evaluation of the respiratory deposition of labelled water aerosols produced by jet and ultrasonic nebulizers. Pediatrics 43: 799–808

Wollmer P, Ursing K, Midgren B, Eriksson L 1985 Inefficiency of chest percussion in the physical therapy of chronic bronchitis. European Journal of Respiratory Diseases 66: 233–239

Wurtemberger G, Hutter BO 2000 Health-related quality of life, psychological adjustment and compliance to treatment in patients on domiciliary liquid oxygen. Monaldi Archives for Chest Disease 55(3): 216–214

Zach MS, Oberwaldner B 1992 Effect of positive expiratory pressure breathing in patient's with cystic fibrosis. Thorax 47: 66–67

Zack MB, Pontoppidan H, Kazemi H 1974 The effect of lateral positions on gas exchange in pulmonary disease. American Review of Respiratory Disease 110: 49–55

Zocchi L, Fitting J, Majani C, Fracchia C, Rampula C, Grassino A 1993 Effect of pressure and timing of contraction on human rib cage muscle fatigue. American Review of Respiratory Disease 147: 857–864

Zusman M 1986 The absolute visual analog scale (AVAS): as a measure of pain intensity. Australian Journal of Physiotherapy 32: 244–246

FURTHER READING

Musculoskeletal dysfunction in respiratory disease

Biomechanics of the thoracic spine and ribs

Lee D 1994 Manual therapy for the thorax – a biomechanical approach. DOPC, Delta BC

White AA, Panjabi MM 1990 Clinical biomechanics of the spine, 2nd edn. Lippincott, Philadelphia

Disorders of the thoracic spine

Boyling JD, Palastanga N 1994 In: Grieve GP (ed) Modern manual therapy of the vertebral column, 2nd edn. Churchill Livingstone, Edinburgh

Grieve GP 1988 Common vertebral joint problems, 2nd edn. Churchill Livingstone, Edinburgh

Musculoskeletal assessment and treatment techniques

Grieve GP 1991 Mobilisation of the spine – a primary handbook of clinical method, 5th edn. Churchill Livingstone, Edinburgh

Janda V 1994 Muscles and motor control in cervicogenic disorders: assessment and management physical therapy for the cervical and thoracic spine. In: Grant R(ed) Clinics in physical therapy, 2nd edn. Churchill Livingstone, New York

Kendal FP, McCreary E 1983 Muscle testing and function, 3rd edn. Williams and Wilkins, Baltimore

Maitland GD 1986 Vertebral manipulation, 5th edn. Butterworths, London

White S, Sahrmann S 1994 Physical therapy for the cervical and thoracic spine. In: Grant R(ed) Clinics in physical therapy, 2nd edn. Churchill Livingstone, New York

7

Patients' problems, management and outcomes

Sue Jenkins   Beatrice Tucker

INTRODUCTION

This chapter discusses the problems commonly encountered by the physiotherapist when working with patients who have respiratory or cardiovascular dysfunction. These problems are identified by the analysis and interpretation of data obtained during patient assessment (see Ch. 1). The presence of pathology affecting the respiratory and cardiovascular systems affects normal physiological functioning and the signs and symptoms produced are the clinical manifestations of this pathophysiology. The physiotherapist therefore requires a thorough knowledge of normal physiology as well as the pathology and pathophysiology of the respiratory and cardiovascular systems.

PROBLEM SOLVING

The key to effective physiotherapy management of a patient is accurate identification of the patient's problems. The assessment will reveal clinical features that the physiotherapist considers important and these are used to determine the patient's main problem(s). The problems commonly encountered are:

- dyspnoea
- decreased exercise tolerance
- impaired airway clearance
- airflow limitation
- respiratory muscle dysfunction
- reduced lung volume
- impaired gas exchange
- abnormal breathing pattern

- pain
- musculoskeletal dysfunction – postural abnormalities, decreased compliance or deformity of the chest wall.

The problems identified in this chapter are specific to the physiotherapist and are not based on pathologies or derived in the same manner as the medical problem list. For example, a patient may be admitted to hospital with a diagnosis of chest infection associated with excess sputum. The physiotherapist is not able to treat infection per se but is able to manage the problem of impaired airway clearance. In order to determine the patient's problem(s) it is essential to identify the significant information gained from the subjective and objective examination. For example, wheezes on auscultation and a reduction in forced expiratory flow are important clinical features that indicate airflow limitation.

Some features may provide evidence of a number of patient problems; for example, reduced chest expansion may be a feature of reduced lung volume and impaired airway clearance (e.g. resulting from excess bronchial secretions). It is necessary to evaluate all the significant clinical features to differentiate and identify the problem(s).

Some of the clinical findings revealed during the assessment may not be features of any of the cardiopulmonary problems listed in this chapter (e.g. poor-self management skills, the presence of risk factors such as cigarette smoking, incorrect use of an inhaler or immobility in the early post-operative period). Patient assessment will also identify the presence of any important factors that must be considered when applying the principles of physiotherapy management for a particular problem to an individual patient. Examples of such factors include co-morbidities, for example diabetes mellitus, raised intracranial pressure or osteoporosis.

The problem-oriented approach to patient management not only assists with the identification of existing problems but also enables recognition of potential patient problems. For example, a high-risk surgical patient has the potential to develop problems of impaired airway clearance or reduced lung volume but if preventive treatment is started during the at-risk period, these problems may not develop.

Many patients will have more than one problem but physiotherapy management may be similar for the different problems. Further, some problems are not amenable to physiotherapy intervention or physiotherapy intervention may be detrimental. For the patient with more than one problem, it is essential to prioritize the problem list and to establish the short and long-term goals for each problem. Some problems may only be short term; for example, pain in the immediate postoperative period. Developing and prioritizing the problem list and developing the goals should, whenever possible, take place in consultation with the patient. For example, an individual who is considered to be at risk for the development of ischaemic heart disease (IHD) may seek physiotherapy assistance to develop an exercise programme designed to decrease the likelihood of IHD. Such a programme would be very different from one aimed at achieving and maintaining high levels of physical fitness.

Having identified the goals, the next stage is to identify the means of achieving these goals through physiotherapy intervention and the timeframe over which they are to be achieved. The appropriate intervention requires selecting the optimal physiotherapy management strategy and this should be evidence based where possible. When a patient has several physiotherapy problems, the physiotherapy techniques selected should ideally address more than one of the high-priority problems. When selecting a treatment approach, the potential risks to the patient (e.g. the possibility of causing adverse physiological responses) and methods to minimize such risks must be taken into consideration. Other factors to be considered include ensuring that the intervention is acceptable to the specific cultural group, is appropriate for the patient's age, ability and level of motivation and the presence of any psychosocial factors which may interfere with the treatment approach (e.g. anxiety or depression). It is important also to determine the patient's likes and dislikes; for example, patient preferences for types of activities are vital considerations when developing an exercise programme.

Common to the management of most problems is the education of the patient by the physiotherapist. This is essential to ensure that the patient takes responsibility for their own management and becomes actively involved in the management of their problem and the prevention of associated problems. Patient education is covered in Chapter 8. If the problem is amenable to physiotherapy, treatment should be commenced. With some problems, a stage will be reached when the natural rate of recovery will no longer be augmented by physiotherapy intervention and treatment should then be discontinued.

The selection and use of appropriate outcome measures are fundamental to the evaluation of physiotherapy intervention. Healthcare fundholders increasingly require data demonstrating the effects of physiotherapy intervention, using instruments that are reliable and valid. Other parties requiring outcome data include the patient, the patient's relatives and caregivers, employers of physiotherapists, clinicians, groups and associations of patients with particular conditions (e.g. cystic fibrosis), members of other healthcare professions and insurers. Thus, when selecting which outcome data to monitor it is important to consider the relevant stakeholders.

In this chapter the problems commonly encountered are discussed. The underlying pathophysiology for each problem is outlined and the clinical features that assist in the identification of the problem are described. The medical and physiotherapy management is listed alongside each problem. The discussion of each problem concludes with guidelines for the choice of clinical outcome measures to be used to evaluate physiotherapy intervention.

PROBLEM – DYSPNOEA

Dyspnoea is the clinical term used for describing shortness of breath or breathlessness. It is one of the most common and distressing symptoms experienced by patients with chronic respiratory or cardiac disease. The American Thoracic Society defines dyspnoea as 'a term used to char-

acterize a subjective experience of breathing discomfort that consists of qualitatively distinct sensations that vary in intensity' (Meek et al 1999, p 322). There are many factors that play a part in the generation of dyspnoea; these include physiological, psychological, social and environmental factors. Clinically, the terms breathlessness and dyspnoea are used interchangeably.

In addition to limiting physical and social functioning, the sensation of dyspnoea is often accompanied by fear and anxiety and, in some patients, may be perceived as life threatening. Dyspnoea is not tachypnoea (increased rate of breathing), hyperventilation (breathing in excess of metabolic needs) or hyperpnoea (increased breathing). These three terms all describe ventilation in response to different stimuli. Although a decrease in the partial pressure of oxygen in the arterial blood (PaO_2) and an increase in the partial pressure of carbon dioxide in arterial blood ($PaCO_2$) may give rise to increased ventilation, it is unclear whether the altered chemoreceptor stimulation can be directly perceived (Tobin 1990). The sensation of dyspnoea appears to originate with the activation of sensory systems involved with respiration (Meek et al 1999).

Dyspnoea is a frequent presenting complaint in patients seeking medical help. On occasions, it may be difficult to distinguish from the patient's account whether the symptoms are of respiratory or cardiovascular origin as in both situations the patient may complain of breathlessness on exertion, when lying down (orthopnoea, due to the increased work of breathing [WOB] in supine), breathlessness waking the patient at night (paroxysmal nocturnal dyspnoea) and of acute episodes of breathlessness at rest.

Although it can be readily appreciated how dyspnoea leads to decreased exercise tolerance and poor quality of life (QOL), the mechanisms responsible for the sensation of dyspnoea are poorly understood and the management of dyspnoea poses considerable difficulties (Stulbarg & Adams 2000).

Different terms used by patients to describe their breathlessness include 'my breathing requires effort', 'my chest feels tight', 'I feel out of breath', 'I cannot get enough air in' and it is likely that the term 'breathlessness' embraces several types of sensation (Mahler 1987).

There is only a weak correlation between dyspnoea and objective measures of pulmonary function (Eakin et al 1993, O'Donnell 1994). Similarly, the relationship between blood gas abnormalities and dyspnoea is weak in individual patients (Meek et al 1999). A moderately strong positive correlation exists between dyspnoea and level of physical function as measured by walking tests (Eakin et al 1993). The finding that the level of dyspnoea experienced for a given level of functional impairment varies considerably among patients may be due to the fact that dyspnoea is a subjective sensation and thus dependent on a variety of stimuli including behavioural influences and the ability of the patient to describe the unpleasant sensation of dyspnoea (Tobin 1990).

Clinically, dyspnoea results from several different pathophysiological mechanisms and in some patients more than one mechanism will be responsible (Table 7.1) (Burns & Howell 1969, Cheitlin et al 1993, Gardner 1996, Gift et al 1986, McCarren 1992, Meek et al 1999, Tobin 1990, Zadai & Irwin 1992).

Clinical features and assessment

The time course for the onset of dyspnoea gives important information as to the likely aetiology and is elicited from the subjective assessment.

Table 7.1 Pathophysiological basis for dyspnoea in respiratory and cardiovascular disease and clinical examples

Pathophysiological basis	Clinical examples
Added load on mechanics of breathing imposed by: 1. Increase in elastic WOB due to a. Decrease in C_L	Increases the inspiratory muscle work required to overcome the elastic recoil of the lungs. This work increases with increases in $\dot{V}_E$ which are achieved with a low V_T and high respiratory rate, e.g. ILD, breathing at low lung volumes, pulmonary congestion
b. Decrease in C_{CW} and /or compliance of the abdominal compartment	Increases the WOB, e.g. obesity, kyphoscoliosis, ankylosing spondylitis
2. Increase in airways resistance	Requires increased work on inspiration and expiration to effect airflow through narrowed airways.
Weakness or fatigue of the respiratory muscles	See Problem – respiratory muscle dysfunction
Increase in ventilatory requirements	Increase in metabolic rate due to fever or exercise Hypoxaemia
Low CO / ischaemia	Inadequate CO causes reflex medullary ventilatory stimulation when oxygen supply to exercising muscle is inadequate to meet metabolic needs, e.g. IHD, heart failure or in the presence of ventricular arrhythmias, valvular problems or cardiomyopathy
Blood gas abnormalities	Anaemia Carboxyhaemoglobin Carbon monoxide poisoning
Cardiovascular and respiratory deconditioning	May lead to dyspnoea with low-intensity exercise
Acute changes in permeability of pulmonary capillaries	Pulmonary oedema resulting from heroin overdose, exposure to toxic fumes
Perfusion limitation	The presence of a large $\dot{V}/\dot{Q}$ mismatch or shunt invariably causes dyspnoea, e.g. pulmonary embolus, pulmonary infarction, cyanotic heart disease, pulmonary congestion
Psychosocial factors	Anxiety and depression may heighten perception of breathlessness
Psychogenic factors	May contribute to the aetiology of hyperventilation disorders

Abbreviations: WOB, work of breathing; C_L, lung compliance; $\dot{V}_E$, minute ventilation; V_T, tidal volume; ILD, interstitial lung disease; C_{CW}, chest wall compliance; CO, cardiac output; IHD, ischaemic heart disease; $\dot{V}/\dot{Q}$, ventilation/perfusion ratio

The patient's account will often reveal that exercise tolerance is limited by breathlessness unless the patient has a chronic hyperventilation disorder in which case dyspnoea usually occurs at rest and is often accompanied by an excessive frequency of sighs (see Ch. 19 on hyperventilation disorders). Careful questioning should also ascertain whether the patient experiences any problems with bladder and bowel function (see Special case).

The patient will usually display an altered breathing pattern. This may include the use of the accessory muscles of respiration (including an increase in abdominal effort during expiration) and, in patients with chronic obstructive pulmonary disease (COPD), paradoxical breathing and pursed-lip breathing may be present. The rate and depth of breathing should be observed, as well as the symmetry of chest movements and the inspiratory to expiratory ratio. Characteristically, expiratory time will be prolonged in the presence of airflow limitation. The patient may complain of feeling hot and appear sweaty if the WOB is excessive. Assessment may reveal signs and symptoms of other problems, in particular airflow limitation, impaired airway clearance, impaired gas exchange or, in the case of cardiac disease, angina may accompany dyspnoea. If respiratory muscle weakness is known or suspected, maximum inspiratory and expiratory mouth pressures ($P_i$max and $P_e$max) should be measured. The chest radiograph may show signs of pleural involvement (e.g. effusion, pneumothorax), pulmonary oedema, lung hyperinflation, areas of collapse or consolidation and in some patients may be normal (e.g. chronic hyperventilation disorder, dyspnoea associated with angina). Hypoxaemia is not always present and $PaCO_2$ may be raised, normal or low. A laboratory-based incremental exercise test with measurement of ventilation and cardiovascular variables can be used to differentiate between dyspnoea from cardiovascular and respiratory origin.

Measurement of dyspnoea is useful to classify the severity of a patient's functional impairment due to dyspnoea, individualize rehabilitation programmes and monitor a patient's condition and response to therapy. Quantification of a sensation such as dyspnoea is difficult and a variety of methods are available (Box 7.1) (Eakin et al 1993, Garrod et al 2000, Guyatt et al 1987, 1989, Hyland et al 1994, Jones et al 1991, 1992, Lareau et al 1994, 1998, Stulbarg & Adams 2000, Walker

---

Box 7.1 Examples of scales for the assessment of dyspnoea

Dyspnoea intensity scales
Used to measure dyspnoea at a particular moment in time, e.g. before, during and after exercise

Visual analogue scale
Modified Borg (0–10) Category Scale

Dyspnoea threshold scales
These scales require the patient to rate the activity that is the threshold for provoking dyspnoea

Medical Research Council (MRC) Scale
American Thoracic Society (ATS) Scale
Oxygen Cost Diagram (OCD)
New York Heart Association Scale

Other tools for assessing dyspnoea
Included in this group are QOL scales that include assessment of dyspnoea and the impact of dyspnoea on functional status

Baseline and Transitional Dyspnoea Indexes (BDI, TDI)
Chronic Respiratory Disease Questionnaire (CRQ)
St George's Respiratory Questionnaire (SGRQ)
Chronic Heart Failure Questionnaire
Breathing Problems Questionnaire (BPQ)
University of California San Diego Shortness of Breath Questionnaire (UCSD SOBQ)
COPD Self-Efficacy Scale (SES)
Pulmonary Functional Status and Dyspnoea Questionnaire (PFSDM, PFSDQ)
London Chest Activity of Daily Living scale (LCADL)

Abbreviations: QOL, quality of life; COPD, chronic obstructive pulmonary disease

& Tan 1997, Weiser et al 1993, Wigal et al 1991). For example, assessment of dyspnoea in response to exercise is generally performed using either the modified Borg (0–10) Category Scale or a visual analogue scale (Borg 1982, Stulbarg & Adams 2000). When using either of these scales it is important to have standardized, simple written instructions that are used consistently and read aloud to the patient. New instruments are continually being developed and when selecting a scale it is important to ensure that the scale has adequate validity, reliability and sensitivity. Further, many scales can be time consuming to use and this poses a major limitation to their usefulness in the clinical setting.

Special case – problems with bladder and bowel function

Problems with continence may arise in the presence of dyspnoea, decreased exercise tolerance or impaired airway clearance (White et al 2000). Patients who are breathless often have a reduced appetite and fluid intake and difficulty with food preparation, leading to inadequate soluble fibre intake which may result in constipation. Added to this the breathless patient who is also constipated may have difficulty breath holding and assuming an adequate position which causes problems with in defaecation (Markwell & Sapsford 1995). Reduced fluid intake and frequent or 'just in case' toileting, to prevent stress or urge urinary incontinence, can result in the bladder becoming accustomed to accommodating smaller volumes of urine. This leads to an increased frequency to void and this requires more effort for the individual who is breathless. In the patient with respiratory disease, dyspnoea is exacerbated during functional tasks requiring the upper limbs, such as undressing, and this may make the symptom of urgency worse or even result in incontinence.

Medical management

Identification and management of the underlying cause of dyspnoea (e.g. airflow limitation, hypoxaemia, heart failure) and any associated problems are essential. Dyspnoea that persists despite such treatment should be managed by focusing on the symptom rather than the disease and, in particular, treatment should target the specific mechanisms (e.g. anxiety, respiratory muscle dysfunction) contributing to the individual's dyspnoea. Nutritional repletion has been shown to improve respiratory muscle function (Meek et al 1999) and may have a beneficial effect on dyspnoea.

Oxygen therapy may decrease exertional dyspnoea but it is difficult to predict an individual's response and there is only a weak correlation between hypoxaemia and dyspnoea (Meek et al 1999). Resting the respiratory muscles using non-invasive ventilation (NIV) may enhance respiratory muscle function and decrease dyspnoea (Turkington & Elliott 2000).

Psychotropic drugs including opiates and anxiolytics may be useful in anxious or depressed patients with chronic lung disease. Cognitive-behavioural approaches that attempt to modify the affective response (e.g. anxiety, distress or panic) to dyspnoea may be effective (Meek et al 1999, Stulbarg & Adams 2000).

Physiotherapy management

The following physiotherapy strategies are used in the patient with dyspnoea. Positioning and breathing control are used to decrease the WOB and eliminate unnecessary muscular activity (McCarren 1992, O'Neill & McCarthy 1983). Positions such as side lying (which reduces the load of the abdominal contents on the diaphragm) and supported crook lying or forward lean sitting may be useful for patients who are severely distressed. Relaxation techniques, which do not involve breath holding or the contraction of large muscle groups, are particularly useful for patients who are anxious (Hough 1996). Symptomatic relief may be achieved by increasing the movement of cold air onto the patient's face (e.g. sitting by an open window, use of a fan) via stimulation of mechanoreceptors on the face or a decrease in the temperature of the facial skin which, via the trigeminal nerve, may alter afferent feedback to the brain and the perception of dyspnoea (Meek et al 1999).

Pursed-lip breathing is often spontaneously adopted by patients with COPD and may be very effective in reducing the discomfort associated with dyspnoea. This technique has been shown to decrease respiratory rate and increase tidal volume (V_T) and in turn may improve gas exchange (Meek et al 1999). Recovery from dyspnoea following physical activity can be assisted by using positioning (e.g. forward lean) together with breathing techniques such as breathing control. Paced breathing during walking and exhalation during effort are other breathing strategies that may be helpful. Patients should be educated on the conservation of energy during activities of daily living.

Exercise training is an effective method of relieving dyspnoea in patients with stable chronic respiratory disease and in those with cardiac failure (Balady 1998, Lareau et al 1999). The underlying mechanisms responsible for the improvement are varied and for the individual may include any of the following:

- Physiologic training effect with decreased lactate production and thus decreased ventilation at a given submaximal workload.
- Decreased oxygen consumption and ventilation for a specific activity as a result of improved mechanical efficiency (e.g. increased stride length when walking).
- Reduced anxiety as a result of improved self-confidence and desensitization to the intensity of dyspnoea from repeated controlled exposure to a stimulus (e.g. as may occur with regular participation in supervised exercise classes) (Stulbarg & Adams 2000).

Supplementary oxygen may be used for patients who are dyspnoeic on exercise and demonstrate significant oxygen desaturation provided that oxygen therapy is shown to produce benefit. Walking aids that facilitate a forward lean position can result in an improved ability to exercise and may reduce dyspnoea and hypoxaemia (Honeyman et al 1996). The application of ventilatory support during exercise may improve exercise capacity and decrease dyspnoea following exercise (Bianchi et al 1998, Keilty et al 1994).

Extremes of temperature and humidity should be avoided as these tend to heighten dyspnoea perception in most individuals (Weiser et al 1993).

Vibration (100 Hertz) on the chest wall may decrease dyspnoea and alter breathing to a slower and deeper pattern in patients with severe chronic respiratory disease (Meek et al 1999, Sibuya et al 1994). The use of high-frequency oscillation and external chest wall compression to relieve dyspnoea is experimental (see Ch. 6 on physiotherapy techniques).

Clinical outcomes

Medical management of the underlying problem, for example, pulmonary oedema or pneumothorax, will often result in a rapid reduction in dyspnoea. This may be via self-report or measured using a scale.

Improvements in dyspnoea in response to exercise training can be measured using a dyspnoea intensity scale or self-efficacy scale (see Box 7.1). A reduction in dyspnoea occurring during everyday activities may be measured using QOL scales, measures of functional status or by assessing self-efficacy (i.e. the person's confidence in their ability to manage their breathlessness whilst undertaking the task).

PROBLEM – DECREASED EXERCISE TOLERANCE

Exercise capacity in patients with respiratory or cardiovascular disease is usually limited by dyspnoea, pain (chest or legs) or fatigue (general or local). This section outlines the pathophysiological basis for exercise limitation occurring in commonly encountered respiratory and cardiovascular conditions.

Many patients with respiratory or cardiovascular disease avoid exercise and become physically deconditioned (Hamilton et al 1995). In a deconditioned individual, the oxygen cost of exercise is higher at any given exercise intensity than in an individual who is physically fit. This is due to central and peripheral mechanisms which include an increased heart rate (HR) response to exercise, increase in cardiac afterload and a decrease in muscle capacity for aerobic exercise. In addition, failure to exercise may decrease the skill and efficiency of physical movements. Physical activities that were commonplace may, in the deconditioned individual, require a much higher level of cognitive function. These processes give rise to an increase in the oxygen cost of exercise.

A number of people with respiratory or cardiovascular disease are elderly. In addition to the age-related decline in physical work capacity, such individuals may have neurological or musculoskeletal conditions that limit the ability to exercise. Depression and anxiety often accompany chronic disease and further limit exercise capacity and decrease the motivation to exercise.

Respiratory disease

Patients with significant respiratory disease usually terminate exercise due to dyspnoea and fail to reach maximal heart rates. In a proportion of patients leg fatigue is also a limiting factor. A respiratory impairment to exercise may be due to dysfunction of any or all components of the respiratory system. Normally, the ventilation requirements for exercise are met by an increase in both V_T and respiratory rate. Physiological abnormalities present in respiratory disease limit the ability to increase V_T during exercise and thus minute ventilation ($\dot{V}_E$) is met by a disproportionate increase in respiratory rate. This occurs in COPD, interstitial lung disease (ILD), chest wall defects and respiratory muscle weakness. The excessive increase in respiratory rate is very costly in terms of the oxygen required by the respiratory muscles because of the much larger number of muscle contractions and the increase in wasted ventilation. In effect, the respiratory muscles use oxygen at the expense of the other skeletal muscles. Under resting conditions, healthy individuals use approximately 1–2% of total body oxygen consumption ($\dot{V}O_2$) for the task of respiration, increasing to 10–20% at maximal exercise. In contrast, patients with COPD, at rest, may require up to 15% of the total body $\dot{V}O_2$ for respiration, increasing to an estimated 35–40% during moderate exercise (Levison & Cherniack 1968, Pardy et al 1984). Airflow limitation reduces the ability to breathe as deeply and rapidly as required during exercise. The decrease in expiratory time, as a consequence of the increased respiratory rate, limits expiration and so functional residual capacity (FRC) rises. The associated lung hyperinflation serves to improve ventilation by decreasing airway resistance and increasing expiratory flow rates. However, the main disadvantage of this compensatory mechanism is the altered dynamics of the respiratory muscles and the increase in the elastic WOB. There is also a relative increase in dead-space ventilation and a reduction in alveolar ventilation.

With ILD, the reduction in peak $\dot{V}O_2$ has been shown to be due to abnormalities of the pulmonary circulation with accompanying gas exchange impairment (Hansen & Wasserman 1996).

The presence of fibrosis severely limits inspiratory capacity. Thus, the extent to which V_T can be increased with exercise is reduced and the patient has to breathe with a much higher rate in order to meet the ventilatory requirements.

In patients with respiratory muscle weakness, there is a decreased ability to generate the intrapleural pressures required to expand the lungs during exercise so V_T fails to increase normally with increasing workloads.

If asthma is not well controlled, exercise capacity may be limited by bronchoconstriction and exercise-induced asthma (EIA) may be the only symptom in young patients with mild disease. The response to exercise is variable and depends on the type and intensity of exercise, pre-existing lung function and the degree of hyper-responsiveness (Storms 1999). For most people with asthma, the bronchoconstriction mainly occurs within 5–10 minutes following cessation of exercise of a sufficient intensity. The mechanism responsible is thought to be due to the increase in ventilation during exercise, particularly in conditions of cold or dry air when increased airflow can cause an increase in the rate of water loss from the respiratory mucosa. The resultant hypertonicity of airway fluid and decreased temperature in the respiratory tract causes the release of mediators from the mast cells and consequent bronchoconstriction and bronchial oedema. Following exercise, there is a refractory period lasting 1–2 hours. When exercise is performed in repeated short bouts the exercise-induced bronchoconstriction is much less severe (Storms 1999).

One of the major problems experienced by many patients with moderate to severe respiratory disease is marked dyspnoea when performing activities of daily living which involve use of the upper limbs, especially when the upper limbs are unsupported (e.g. teeth cleaning, shaving, washing and hair combing). Patients with severe ventilatory limitation often fix their shoulder girdle so that the accessory muscles can exert an expanding force on the rib cage in an effort to shift more air in and out of the lungs. Activities involving the upper limbs may mean loss of these arm trunk muscles as muscles of elevation, thereby reducing their contribution to the generation of the intrapleural pressure needed for inspiration. The breathing pattern during unsupported upper limb exercise is often noticed to be rapid and irregular and dysynchronous thoracoabdominal movements may be observed (Celli 1994). A further stress is imposed when exercise involves raising the arms above the head. Lactate accumulates in the blood immediately with the onset of upper limb exercise. This leads to an increase in carbon dioxide (CO_2) production and thus ventilation.

Gas exchange may be abnormal during exercise and this may contribute to a decrease in exercise capacity. In COPD, different patterns of arterial blood gas changes occur with exercise and it is difficult to accurately identify patients likely to exhibit arterial desaturation. Patients with a less severe reduction in forced expiratory volume in one second (FEV_1) and diffusing capacity tend not to develop significant desaturation with exercise (Moss & Make 1993). In ILD, hypoxaemia may be very severe during physical activity and is thought to be due to an increase in ventilation perfusion ($\dot{V}/\dot{Q}$) mismatching and a loss of the alveolar-capillary surface area required for effective gas transfer (Wasserman et al 1987).

Cardiovascular impairment

Exercise intolerance is demonstrated in most patients with left ventricular dysfunction but the pathophysiological basis for the development of limiting symptoms such as dyspnoea and fatigue is somewhat controversial (Balady 1998). Abnormalities in the central circulation (left ventricular systolic and diastolic dysfunction), the peripheral vessels and in the skeletal muscles may be present. Leg blood flow is often lower than normal in patients with cardiac failure and intrinsic skeletal muscle abnormalities may be identified (Balady 1998). Many patients with cardiac failure report leg fatigue during exercise and this fatigue is associated with increased lactate release from the muscles.

Metabolic acidosis may develop at very low-intensity exercise and may even occur at rest. In order to rid the body of the excess CO_2 produced, breathing is stimulated and this may contribute to the sensation of dyspnoea.

In patients with peripheral arterial disease, the oxygen supply to the working muscles is decreased. This leads to a build-up of lactic acid and pain occurs during low-intensity exercise.

Other disorders

Obesity is present in many individuals with cardiovascular disease and decreases exercise capacity owing to the increase in resting metabolic requirements and the greater respiratory and cardiac work required by an obese individual when exercising. Similarly, diabetes mellitus is also associated with cardiovascular disease and, if poorly controlled, leads to chronic metabolic acidosis causing an increase in ventilation at any given workload. Cigarette smoking increases the level of carboxyhaemoglobin, thus reducing the oxygen-carrying capacity of the blood. When exercise is performed immediately after smoking a cigarette, cardiac work is increased due to the smoking-related rise in heart rate (HR) and blood pressure (BP).

Fatigue may be present in many acute and chronic conditions and is an important limiting factor to exercise. Fatigue may be cardiovascular (low cardiac output, anaemia), pulmonary (excessive WOB), metabolic (hyperglycaemia, hypothyroidism), neurologic, muscular (local muscle glycogen depletion, lactate accumulation in muscle and blood), psychogenic in origin (anxiety, depression) or simply due to poor patient motivation.

Clinical features and assessment

An incremental exercise test, including measurements of relevant physiologic and subjective measures before, during and following the test, is essential to identify the pathophysiological limitation to exercise (see Chs. 3, 14 and 15 on assessment, pulmonary rehabilitation and cardiac rehabilitation). These measures may include $\dot{V}O_2$, carbon dioxide production ($\dot{V}CO_2$), breathing pattern (V_T, respiratory rate), oxygenation (oxygen saturation [SpO_2], PaO_2), HR (electrocardiogram, polar monitor), pulse rate and strength, and BP and rate pressure product (RPP). The reason for termination of exercise (e.g. dyspnoea, leg fatigue/pain, abnormal physiological responses) should be recorded and symptom intensity measured using standard scales. Ratings of perceived exertion also may be useful. Alternative methods of assessing exercise capacity, when sophisticated equipment and relevant technical expertise are not available, include field walking tests (incremental shuttle walking test, 6–minute walk test), an incremental cycle ergometry test or endurance tests such as the endurance shuttle walking test (these tests are covered in detail in Chapter 3).

Peak expiratory flow rate or FEV_1 should be measured before and at intervals after exercise in patients with suspected EIA.

For the patient with acute cardiopulmonary dysfunction an exercise test is inappropriate. Information regarding the likely responses to measures aimed at improving oxygen transport will be obtained from knowledge of responses to nursing and medical interventions and observation of subjective and objective data over time. It is critical to consider the total patient picture and not rely on any one specific variable when assessing the patient with acute cardiopulmonary dysfunction (see Ch. 5 on the effects of positioning and mobilization on oxygen transport).

Medical management

Identification and management of the underlying cause of reduced exercise tolerance (e.g. COPD, IHD, valvular heart disease, heart failure, cardiomyopathy, metabolic abnormality) are essential. Optimizing management of associated conditions (e.g. diabetes mellitus, peripheral arterial disease) is necessary for patients to achieve their maximum exercise capacity.

Oxygen therapy is used to prevent a significant decrease in PaO_2 to maintain the metabolic needs, prevent the compensatory effects of chronic hypoxaemia, reduce dyspnoea and increase exercise tolerance.

Respiratory muscle strength is enhanced by ensuring that nutrition is optimal for patients who are malnourished (Lareau et al 1999, Weiser et al 1993). Weight reduction will reduce the increased load on the respiratory muscles which results from obesity. Resting the respiratory muscles using NIV may enhance respiratory muscle function, decrease dyspnoea and improve exercise tolerance (Turkington & Elliott 2000). Suppression of the associated psychoemotional problems such as anxiety and depression using psychotropic drugs (e.g. opiates, anxiolytics) may allow patients with chronic lung disease to increase their exercise capacity.

Physiotherapy management

An exercise programme should be designed to meet the specific requirements of the patient. The mode, intensity, duration and frequency of exercise should be individually selected for each patient based on assessment findings and established goals. The programme should consist of a warm-up, stretches, an aerobic component, resistive training (when appropriate) and a cool-down. Postural correction is also important (see Problem – musculoskeletal dysfunction – postural abnormalities, decreased compliance or deformity of the chest wall). The programme should include upper and lower limb activities including both supported and unsupported upper limb exercises (Celli 1994). Unsupported exercises are especially important for patients who have respiratory disease and complain of dyspnoea during arm movements (Lareau et al 1999). Although it is recognized that endurance training is beneficial for most patients, it may be more important for some patients to improve their speed of movement over a short distance (e.g. to cross a road or to improve their ability to reach the toilet because of urinary or faecal urgency) rather than focusing on improving the distance the patient can walk.

Intermittent exercise is useful to improve the exercise endurance of patients who are severely deconditioned, extremely breathless, excessively fatigued or have claudication pain and is necessary for critically ill patients and patients in whom severe arterial desaturation occurs on exercise. Oxygen, rest, energy conservation, positioning and breathing control and non-invasive ventilatory support may improve exercise tolerance (see Problem – dyspnoea).

Breathing strategies used to relieve dyspnoea (e.g. pursed-lip breathing, exhalation with effort, paced breathing) may be useful to improve exercise tolerance. Often patients have an increased exercise tolerance when the upper limbs are supported, for example by use of a gutter frame or on the handlebars of a bike. Specific respiratory muscle training results in an increased strength and capacity of these muscles to meet a respiratory load but improvement in symptoms and exercise capacity is still debated (Lareau et al 1999) (see Ch. 14 on pulmonary rehabilitation). Exercise testing and prescription for special cases, such as patients with diabetes mellitus, are covered elsewhere (American College of Sports Medicine 1998).

Patients should, when possible, exercise in an appropriate environment. Cold dry conditions, airborne irritants and pollutants and excessively windy conditions should be avoided. Patients should be encouraged to stay indoors during extreme conditions.

Coached training with appropriate emotional support and encouragement is beneficial for patients with fatigue, dyspnoea or anxiety.

Special case – exercise-induced asthma

Exercise training is beneficial to patients with EIA for several reasons. At a given workload, ventilation is reduced by training thereby reducing the prime trigger for EIA. Patients are thus able to train at a higher workload before symptoms occur. Individuals with symptoms may be reluctant to exercise and should be encouraged to participate in regular physical exercise to prevent deconditioning and gain psychological benefits. Symptoms of EIA may be reduced by:

- Administering an inhaled short-acting beta-2 agonist or non-steroidal antiinflammatory such as sodium cromoglycate prior to exercise.
- Adequately warming up prior to exercise and including intermittent exercise to provide and make use of the refractory period.
- Exercising in an appropriate environment. Cold dry environments should be avoided (e.g. by avoiding early morning or late night activity). Swimming is beneficial as a choice of exercise because of the humidity provided by the water (Storms 1999).

Clinical outcomes

Improved cardiorespiratory fitness should be expected in patients who are able to participate in an endurance training programme. A true training effect may occur in patients who are able to exercise above their anaerobic threshold. The physiologic benefits of endurance training include a reduction in cardiac and respiratory workload at a given intensity of submaximal exercise. This should be associated with a reduction in HR and RPP at rest and with submaximal exercise. Oxygen consumption, stroke volume, cardiac output, peripheral vascular resistance, muscle blood flow and oxygen extraction are all increased at maximal exercise. Following training, HR, BP and respiratory rate should return more rapidly to preexercise levels. Additional benefits may include an increase in muscle mass and loss of adipose tissue and an improved sense of well-being. In patients with more severe disease who are unable to exercise at a sufficient intensity to obtain a true training effect, exercise training is still beneficial and should be associated with an increase in walking distance and a decrease in dyspnoea. Such patients may report increased ease of performing activities of daily living. The patient may score lower on the rating of perceived exertion scale for a given physical activity.

Following an endurance training programme, patients with IHD may be able to exercise at a higher RPP before the onset of angina. Improved physical functioning should be reflected in improvements in QOL and self-efficacy.

The benefits from participation in cardiac or pulmonary rehabilitation programmes are discussed in detail in the relevant chapters in this book.

Benefits observed in the patient with acute cardiopulmonary dysfunction may include an improved tolerance to changes in body posture including tolerating prolonged periods sitting out of bed, the ability to ambulate with less support and to perform simple self-care activities.

PROBLEM – IMPAIRED AIRWAY CLEARANCE

Impaired airway clearance is an important physiotherapy problem because of the potential for the patient to develop an overwhelming infection, major atelectasis and other associated problems such as impaired gas exchange and airflow limitation. Further, untreated persistent infections may predispose to the development of chronic lung disease.

In the healthy lung up to 100 ml of mucus is produced each day, primarily from submucosal glands and goblet cells as well as clara cells and tissue fluid exudate (Clarke 1990).

The composition of mucus in health is at least 95% water. The remaining constituents are salts and other dialysable components, free protein, glycoproteins, carbohydrates, lipids, deoxyribonucleic acid, some cellular debris and foreign particles (Houtmeyers et al 1999).

Mucus is carried upwards on the mucociliary blanket, the major mechanism for clearing particles from the airways, and eventually swallowed. In situations where mucus secretion is greatly increased (e.g. very dusty environments), clearance of secretions is augmented by cough and expectoration. Absorptive mechanisms operating at the alveolar level are responsible for clearing some of the peripheral secretions. When the volume of mucus reaching the larynx and pharynx has increased to the extent that an individual becomes conscious of its presence on coughing or 'clearing the throat' then the mucus is defined as sputum; the presence of sputum is abnormal.

Whilst mucociliary transport is the major method of clearing mucus in healthy subjects, cough is an important mechanism, especially in people with lung disease (Irwin & Widdicombe 2000). The importance of cough as a means of airway clearance is evident from research in patients with chronic bronchitis where the clearance of sputum is increased by 20% with cough as compared to only a 2.5% increase with cough in healthy subjects (Puchelle et al 1980). The effectiveness of a cough is related to the volume and thickness of mucus and is most effective when a high linear velocity is achieved (i.e. small cross-sectional area of airway and high linear flow rate) (Irwin & Widdicombe 2000). An impairment of expiratory flow rates or ability to compress the airways dynamically may lead to an ineffective cough. Huffing, which involves relatively lower peak expiratory flow rates and intrapulmonary pressure gradients, has a similar effect on mucus clearance when compared to coughing (Bennett & Zeman 1994).

Vigorous coughing can cause a number of adverse effects including abnormal cardiovascular responses (e.g. arterial hypotension and cardiac rhythm disturbances), abnormalities of the genitourinary tract (e.g. urinary incontinence), gastrointestinal symptoms (e.g. gastro-oesophageal reflux, inguinal hernia), musculoskeletal problems (e.g. rupture of rectus abdominis, rib fractures), neurologic features (e.g. cough syncope, headache, stroke, seizures) and respiratory complications (e.g. airflow limitation, laryngeal trauma, pneumothorax, tracheobronchial trauma) (Irwin & Widdicombe 2000). These effects are largely due to the high intrathoracic pressures and expiratory velocities associated with vigorous coughing and the associated high energy consumption. Also affected will be the individual's QOL.

Table 7.2 lists the pathophysiological basis of impaired airway clearance and includes clinical examples (Clarke 1990, Foltz & Benumof 1987,

Table 7.2 Pathophysiological basis of impaired airway clearance

Pathophysiological basis	Comment and clinical examples
Increased or altered composition of mucus:	
1. Increase in production	Chronic bronchitis, asthma, cystic fibrosis, bronchiectasis, presence of an artificial airway Tracheal intubation may provoke reflex mucus secretion Pneumonia
2. Colonization of mucus, e.g. viral, bacterial and fungal organisms	Bypassing of upper respiratory tract – cuffed tube mechanically blocks mucociliary escalator and may lead to pooling and stagnation of secretions, promoting colonization and infection
3. Systemic dehydration	Leads to viscous secretions which are difficult to mobilize and expectorate May occur postoperatively especially if fluid restriction is imposed Excess fluid loss associated with prolonged very high respiratory rate
Abnormalities in cilia structure or function	Primary ciliary dyskinesia Endobronchial suctioning may lead to mucosal haemorrhage and erosions in the tracheobronchial tree slowing mucociliary transport by damaging ciliated epithelium
Impaired mucociliary clearance:	
1. Age	Rate of mucociliary clearance is decreased by as much as 60% in the elderly
2. Sleep	Reduces mucociliary clearance
3. Environmental pollutants	These may disturb clearance. The effects sometimes depend on dose
4. Drugs	Some general anaesthetics, morphine and other narcotics depress mucociliary transport
5. High inspired oxygen	May produce acute tracheobronchitis leading to loss of ciliated epithelium, mucus retention and slowed transport of mucus
6. Hypoxia and hypercapnia	Slow mucociliary clearance
7. Social factors	Failure to expectorate due to embarrassment
Abnormal cough reflex:	
1. Decreased	Decreased level of consciousness, general anaesthesia, narcotic analgesics Inhibition due to pain, e.g. following surgery, pleurisy, chest wall trauma Damage to the vagal or glossopharyngeal nerves Laryngectomy Paralysed vocal cords Denervated lungs (lung, heart-lung transplant)
2. Increased	Occurs especially in patients with poorly controlled asthma Cause uncertain but not thought merely to be due to bronchial hyper-reactivity. Viral infections also increase sensitivity
Ineffective cough due to the inability to generate sufficient expiratory airflow	Severe reduction in vital capacity Expiratory muscle weakness decreases the cough-induced dynamic compression of the airways Airflow limitation may cause the cough to be weak and/or ineffective Cough is ineffective in the presence of bronchiectatic segments due to lack of airflow through these segments
Abnormal cough:	
1. Post-nasal drip syndrome	Cough results from the stimulation of the cough reflex
2. Gastro-oesophageal reflux	May lead to chronic cough and aspiration of gastric contents May be associated with complaints of heartburn, sour taste, regurgitation

Houtmeyers et al 1999, Irwin & Widdicombe 2000, Johnson & Pierson 1986, Judson & Sahn 1994).

Infection may develop when there is stagnation and colonization of mucus. Once infection occurs, mucus retention is aggravated by oedema of the airway walls, bronchoconstriction due to irritation of the mucous membrane, extrinsic compression of the bronchial airways by secondary lymph node enlargement and an increase in mucus viscosity. The marked inflammatory response to infection is characterized by the persistent influx of neurophils which further contributes to the increase in mucus viscosity and

Table 7.3 Pathophysiological effects of mucus retention

Pathophysiological effect	Cause
Increase in airways resistance	Partial or complete airway obstruction from mucus in airway lumen. This may lead to atelectasis from absorption of gas (complete obstruction) or to air trapping and regional overdistension (partial obstruction)
Hypoxaemia	$\dot{V}/\dot{Q}$ mismatch due to premature airway closure in dependent lung regions and atelectasis Intrapulmonary shunting may occur with lobar collapse
Hypercapnia	May occur especially if sputum retention occurs in patients with chronic lung diseaseAbb

Abbreviation: $\dot{V}/\dot{Q}$ ventilation/perfusion ratio.

mucus retention. Destruction of bronchial airways may occur with chronic infection due to the production of toxic imflammatory mediators such as leukotreines, proteases and elastases (Hardy 1994). The problem of mucus retention is compounded by the increased mucus produced by the abnormal airways (Hardy 1994). The pathophysiological effects of mucus retention are given in Table 7.3.

Special case – postoperative patient with impaired airway clearance

Many factors either present preoperatively or arising in the peri- or postoperative period increase mucus secretion and/or impair mucociliary clearance and thus may be responsible for the development of postoperative pneumonia. It is therefore important for the physiotherapist to identify patients who have an increased risk of developing pneumonia.

Although mucociliary clearance may be impaired in the presence of atelectasis it is unclear whether atelectasis predisposes to more severe postoperative complications such as pneumonia (Platell & Hall 1997).

Studies show that pneumonia occurs in approximately 15–20% of patients after abdominal surgery (Celli et al 1984, Hall et al 1991) and in no more than 10% of patients following cardiac surgery or lung resection (Gosselink et al 2000, Jenkins et al 1989, Stiller et al 1994, Stock et al 1984). These values assume that preoperative lung function is within the normal range. Individuals who have a productive cough, especially when associated with purulent sputum, are at increased risk (Mitchell et al 1982) as are those

with respiratory disease when the airways are colonized with bacteria (Dilworth & White 1992, Smith & Ellis 2000).

The risk of developing postoperative pneumonia is significantly increased in patients who smoke or who have only recently ceased to smoke (Dilworth & White 1992, Jenkins et al 1990, Morran et al 1983, Warner et al 1989). The mechanisms responsible include mucus hypersecretion, impaired tracheobronchial clearance, bronchial hyper-reactivity and impairment of the immune system (Fairshter & Williams 1987, Pearce & Jones 1984).

Low serum albumin, protein depletion or malnutrition significantly increase the chance of developing postoperative pneumonia (Garibaldi et al 1981, Windsor & Hill 1988). The factors responsible in malnourished patients are ineffective cough secondary to expiratory muscle weakness and impaired function of the immune system (Arora & Gal 1981, Arora & Rochester 1982, Branson & Hurst 1988, Rochester & Esau 1984).

Preoperative hospitalization in excess of 7 days, prolonged mechanical ventilation (>2 days) and major surgery exceeding 4 hours have all been shown to increase the risk of postoperative pneumonia (Smith & Ellis 2000).

Microaspiration of gastric bacteria and the presence of a nasogastric tube for more than 24 hours postoperatively is associated with an increased frequency of postoperative pneumonia (Dilworth & White 1992, Mitchell et al 1982). Mucociliary clearance is slowed in intubated and ventilated patients, adding to the risk of infection.

The evidence of advanced age as a risk factor is controversial (Celli et al 1984, Dilworth & White 1992, Roukema et al 1988, Windsor & Hill 1988).

There appears to be no absolute threshold of pre-operative pulmonary function for predicting the occurrence of postoperative pulmonary complications. However, such information, when available, assists clinical decision making in the postoperative period (Gass & Olsen 1986, Tisi 1979).

Other factors which have not been studied extensively but which are considered to increase the risk include emergency surgery, systemic dehydration and patient motivation. High levels of neuroticism or trait anxiety are thought to slow the recovery from surgery (Mathews & Ridgeway 1981).

Ineffective cough in the postoperative period may occur as a result of a number of factors. These include: suppressed cough reflex; reduced expiratory flow rates; inability to coordinate chest wall motion and timing for an effective cough; diaphragm dysfunction; positioning in supine or a semi-recumbent position and pain. Also implicated are the presence of a nasogastric tube or artificial airway and preexisting cough impairment, for example airflow limitation as in COPD or reduced expiratory muscle strength (Smith & Ellis 2000).

Clinical features and assessment

The clinical features are usually those resulting from mucus retention. These include an abnormal breathing pattern due to increased WOB, hypoxaemia and on occasions hypercapnia. The presence of infection may produce fever and tachycardia. When the secretions cause marked airflow limitation, wheezing may be audible with the unaided ear (see Problem – airflow limitation). Auscultatory findings may include diminished or absent breath sounds, bronchial breath sounds, crackles and wheezes.

The following features of cough should be assessed: precipitating factors, the severity, the pattern of occurrence, sound of the cough and presence of accompanying sounds or complaints such as wheeze, stridor or hoarseness. Smoking history and occupational history are important in the assessment of a patient with impaired airway clearance. The quality of the cough should be assessed (e.g. dry, hacking, effectiveness).

Assessment should identify the presence of any adverse effects associated with cough. The examination of any sputum expectorated is important. In a patient with a chronic disease, assessment should include the pattern of daily sputum production, amount, type and consistency of the sputum and a review of the patient's physiotherapy regimen. Ease of sputum expectoration can be measured using a Likert scale or a VAS. Measurement of PeMax may be helpful with low values frequently being associated with difficulty in moving the secretions proximally.

Arterial blood gas analysis may show a lowered PaO_2 and arterial oxygen saturation (SaO_2). Arterial PCO_2 may be normal, increased or lowered (e.g. due to hyperventilation in the early stages of acute asthma). The chest radiograph may show signs of lung collapse, consolidation or hyperinflation. Other chest radiograph abnormalities may reflect the underlying disease process; for example, bronchiectatic changes. Pulmonary function tests may reveal signs of airflow limitation, gas trapping or reduced lung volumes.

Assessment may also reveal signs of associated problems, including dyspnoea, decreased exercise tolerance, airflow limitation, respiratory muscle dysfunction and impaired gas exchange.

It is often difficult to distinguish the clinical features of atelectasis from pneumonia in the postoperative patient. Features suggestive of pneumonia are present when the patient looks ill (is pale and clammy or flushed and sweaty), has abnormalities in conscious state (e.g. agitated, distressed or drowsy), tachycardia, increased respiratory rate, laboured breathing, oral temperature exceeding 38°C, auscultatory findings such as decreased breath sounds or bronchial breath sounds, added sounds (wheeze, crackles), hypoxaemia, abnormal chest X-ray, bacterial contamination of sputum or raised white cell count that is not otherwise explained (Stiller & Munday 1992, Stiller et al 1994).

Medical management

Recognition and management of the underlying cause of impaired airway clearance are essential.

The most common causes of chronic cough are postnasal drip syndrome, asthma, gastro-oesophageal reflux, chronic bronchitis, bronchiectasis and, less commonly, the administration of angiotensinogen-converting enzyme inhibitors (Irwin & Widdicombe 2000).

Antihistamines and decongestants administered orally or via a nasal spray are useful in postnasal drip syndrome. When inflammation is present a corticosteroid nasal spray may be used. Impaired cough due to pain is treated by analgesic drugs. Cough expectorants and mucolytics such as hypertonic saline and acetylcysteine may be used to decrease the viscosity of tenacious secretions. Inhaled beta-2 agonists and mucolytics such as recombinant human deoxyribonuclease (DNase), hypertonic saline and acetylcysteine have been shown to increase mucociliary clearance (Barnes 2000). Chronic, irritating, non-productive cough may be treated by non-specific antitussives such as ipratropium bromide (Irwin & Widdicombe 2000).

Infection (bronchial or nasal) is treated using appropriate antibiotic, antifungal or antiprotozoal therapy. Adequate fluid intake is essential. Patients who are at risk of developing recurrent infections should be immunized annually. All patients should be counselled to cease tobacco use. Avoidance of irritants or allergic precipitating factors is encouraged wherever possible.

Appropriate drug management combined with dietary control and head-up positioning during sleep is beneficial for the majority of patients with gastro-oesophageal reflux (Irwin & Widdicombe 2000).

Intubation, tracheostomy or minitracheostomy and humidification may be required to enable airway management, for example following depression of the central nervous system, damage to the glossopharyngeal or vagal nerves or surgical excision of the larynx.

Physiotherapy management

Physiotherapy has an important role in the management of impaired airway clearance but bronchial secretions only become a physiotherapy problem when they are excessive, retained or difficult to eliminate. Many patients expectorate a small amount of foul-smelling, tenacious sputum postoperatively but this is not a problem if the patient is conscious, able to cough effectively and self-ambulating.

Patients should be educated on the avoidance of environmental factors such as cigarette smoke and cold wet environments as these may trigger cough and predispose to infection. Education to enable early recognition of chest infection and treatment strategies to initiate early management are important.

A large range of airway clearance techniques is available (see Ch. 6 on physiotherapy techniques). Factors for consideration when selecting airway clearance techniques are listed in Box 7.2. Humidification is especially important when the upper airway is bypassed, when high concentrations of inspired oxygen are being delivered and in patients who have thick and tenacious secretions. Nebulizers containing saline (normal or hypertonic), water or mucolytics are used to liquefy secretions, enhance mucociliary clearance and increase sputum yield prior to airway clearance techniques (Conway et al 1992). Bronchodilators may be given to reduce airflow limitation and may improve mucociliary transport and hypoxaemia (Yeates & Mortensen 2000).

Mobilization of secretions may be achieved using ambulation, which enhances mucociliary

---

Box 7.2 Factors for consideration when selecting airway clearance techniques (adapted from Hardy 1994, p. 449)

- Evidence supporting the technique
- Potential adverse effects of the technique (i.e. contraindications, precautions or required modifications)
- Patient motivation
- Patient's goals
- Physiotherapist's/physician's goals
- Patient preferences
- Patient's age and ability to concentrate and learn technique
- Limitations of technique, e.g. time and equipment or assistance needed to use technique
- Ease of teaching technique
- Skill of physiotherapist with particular techniques

clearance, by spontaneous increases in V_T and flow rates (Wolff et al 1977). Despite increases in minute ventilation, patients may not increase V_T significantly during ambulation in the early postoperative period and deep breaths should be encouraged simultaneously (Orfanos et al 1999). Breathing techniques such as the active cycle of breathing techniques and autogenic drainage, body positioning including gravity-assisted drainage positions and continuous lateral rotation therapy, and manual techniques including percussion, shaking and vibrations are used to mobilize secretions. Devices such as the positive expiratory pressure mask, oscillating positive expiratory pressure (Flutter VRPI, Acapella) and intermittent positive pressure breathing (IPPB) are used for the mobilization of secretions as are devices using the principle of vibrations such as oral high-frequency oscillation and high-frequency chest wall compression. Manual hyperinflation may be required in some intubated patients. These techniques are discussed in Chapter 6.

Removal of secretions can be facilitated using the forced expiration technique, high lung volume huff or cough with support, where necessary and suctioning. Spontaneous cough may be elicited by physical activity. The cough reflex may be elicited using a tracheal rub or suctioning. Strengthening of the abdominal muscles and assisted cough techniques (e.g. abdominal support with an upward pressure) may be helpful for patients with impaired cough due to weakness of the abdominal muscles. Assisted cough techniques may also be necessary when treating the person with intellectual impairment who has retained secretions.

For patients with pain, adequate analgesia is essential prior to airway clearance techniques (see Problem – pain).

Patients who have stress incontinence or excess flatus should be encouraged to contract their pelvic floor muscles prior to, and during, forced expiratory manoeuvres.

In the postoperative patient it is essential to establish whether the patient has excess secretions and their ability to manage their own airway clearance. This determines the risk of the patient developing postoperative pneumonia. The techniques to assist sputum clearance in the postoperative patient include increasing alveolar ventilation and expiratory flow rates using, for example, upright positioning, ambulation with encouragement to take deep breaths, thoracic expansion exercises (sustained maximal inspirations), incentive spirometry and IPPB. Mobilization of secretions may also be assisted using an airway clearance technique, gravity-assisted drainage positions, vibrations, percussion and supported huff or cough. Manual hyperinflation and suctioning will be required for the ventilated patient.

Clinical outcomes

Short-term benefits should be observed by an increase in sputum expectorated, as measured by weight, volume or rate of expectoration. Another benefit may be increased ease of sputum expectoration. With acute conditions, resolution of chest radiograph abnormalities may be seen. Abnormal findings on auscultation may become less evident or resolve. Removal of excess bronchial secretions may improve or eliminate the associated problems such as impaired gas exchange, airflow limitation and dyspnoea. Radio-aerosol clearance may be used as an outcome measure in studies of airway clearance techniques. Long-term benefits in patients with chronic lung disease may include a reduction in the number of exacerbations per year, fewer courses of antibiotics, fewer and shorter periods of hospitalization and a reduction in the number of days lost from studies or work. Such benefits will also be demonstrated by cost savings. Measurable improvements in QOL should also be seen.

In the high-risk postoperative patient with excess bronchial secretions, benefits from physiotherapy intervention may be measured by the prevention of pneumonia.

Improved cough or huff technique may be associated with a reduction in associated problems such as fatigue, dyspnoea, syncope, airflow limitation, arterial oxygen desaturation or stress incontinence.

PROBLEM – AIRFLOW LIMITATION

Airflow limitation generally occurs in conjunction with other physiotherapy problems, such as dyspnoea, decreased exercise tolerance, impaired airway clearance and abnormal cough. The pathophysiological basis for airflow limitation is given in Table 7.4 (West 1998).

Special case – lung hyperinflation in chronic airflow limitation

Lung hyperinflation is a compensatory mechanism aimed at overcoming the increase in expiratory airflow resistance. In order to achieve adequate ventilation, most patients with COPD breathe with a smaller V_T and increased rate when compared to healthy individuals. The increased rate reduces expiratory time and may lead to the development of intrinsic positive end-expiratory pressure (PEEP). In order to initiate inspiratory airflow, the inspiratory muscles are required to generate a pleural pressure in excess of the intrinsic PEEP. The excessive lowering of the intrapleural pressure required to ventilate the lungs may cause indrawing of the intercostal spaces and supraclavicular fossae on inspiration.

The WOB on inspiration is also increased due to the decrease in lung compliance that occurs with lung hyperinflation. The diaphragm fibres are shortened and the altered length–tension relationship may decrease the ability to generate muscle tension and inspiratory pressure. In extreme cases, the diaphragm contracts isometrically (i.e. as a fixator) and at high lung volumes the function of the inspiratory intercostal muscles is markedly reduced. When acting as a fixator, the main effect of the diaphragm is to prevent transmission of the negative intrapleural pressure to the abdomen thereby preventing suction of the diaphragm into the thorax. Lung hyperinflation reduces the zone of apposition of the diaphragm. The net effect of this is a decreased ability of the diaphragm to elevate the lower rib cage. When hyperinflation is severe, the zone of apposition is lost and the diaphragm fibres are realigned in a horizontal direction. In this instance, contraction of the diaphragm pulls the lower rib cage inwards (Hoover's sign) and abdominal paradox may also been seen. At rest, the ribs are in a more horizontal position and, when the parasternal and intercostal muscles contract, there is little elevation of the ribs (Ferguson 1993).

Table 7.4 Pathophysiological basis of airflow limitation and clinical examples (West 1998)

Pathophysiological basis	Clinical examples
Changes in the airway wall:	
1. Smooth muscle contraction	Asthma
2. Smooth muscle hypertrophy and hyperplasia	Asthma
3. Inflammation of the mucosa	Asthma
4. Hypertrophy of mucous glands	Chronic bronchitis
5. Thickening of the bronchial wall	Chronic bronchitis, asthma
6. Dilatation and destruction of airway walls	Cystic fibrosis, bronchiectasis
7. Infiltration of the bronchial mucosa with eosinophils and mononuclear cells	Asthma
8. Changes in osmolarity of normal airway fluid produced by cooling	EIA. FEV_1 falls rapidly after cessation of exercise. EIA is exacerbated by exercise in cold, dry atmospheres
Factors outside the airway:	
1. Loss of radial traction due to a decrease in elastic recoil secondary to increases in lung compliance	Emphysema
2. Compression	Enlarged lymph node, neoplasm, peribronchial oedema as occurs with pulmonary oedema
Partial or total occlusion of airway lumen	Mucus, e.g. in chronic bronchitis, cystic fibrosis, bronchiectasis, asthma Inhaled foreign body

Abbreviations: EIA, exercise-induced asthma; FEV_1, forced expiratory volume in one second

Some patients with severe hyperinflation, especially during exercise, may use the abdominal release mechanism to decrease the work of the diaphragm while still maintaining its output. To effect this mechanism, the patient contracts the abdominal muscles at the end of expiration, thus pushing the contents of the abdomen up against the diaphragm and improving its length–tension relationship. The increase in lung volume during the subsequent inspiration occurs by a sudden release of the abdominal pressure that acts to passively pull the diaphragm downwards (McCarren 1992). Normally, expiration is passive, but with a decrease in expiratory airflow the patient may recruit the abdominal muscles and other expiratory and inspiratory (contracting with reversed origin) muscles in an attempt to augment expiration.

Clinical features and assessment

The patient with airflow limitation may complain of chest tightness, cough and breathlessness. Exercise tolerance is often limited. In asthma, cough and dyspnoea may be particularly evident at night and may lead to poor sleep patterns. Wheezing may be audible with the unaided ear. With long-standing disease, examination of the chest may reveal signs of hyperinflation. These signs include a barrel-shaped chest with an increase in the anteroposterior diameter, use of accessory muscles and a raised shoulder girdle. Indrawing of the intercostal spaces and supraclavicular fossae may be visible. Pursed-lip breathing is seen in some patients with severe airflow limitation. Auscultatory findings associated with hyperinflation include reduced breath sounds and the percussion note may be hyperresonant. Wheezes heard on auscultation in patients with airflow limitation are often multiple, polyphonic and widespread.

The chest radiograph may show signs of hyperinflation as well as signs consistent with the underlying condition; for example, the presence of emphysematous bullae or bronchiectatic changes.

Abnormalities in pulmonary function indicative of airflow limitation consist of a reduction in FEV_1, FEV_1/forced vital capacity (FVC) ratio, peak expiratory flow and forced expiratory flow over the middle half of the FVC manoeuvre ($FEF_{25-75\%}$). Characteristic patterns can be seen in the flow-volume loop and may help with identifying the cause and site of the airflow limitation. Functional residual capacity, residual volume (RV) and total lung capacity (TLC) are often increased. An absolute increase in TLC reflects hyperinflation whereas air trapping is the term used to describe increases in FRC and RV (Ruppel 1998). Gas exchange abnormalities may include hypoxaemia due to $\dot{V}/\dot{Q}$ mismatching. Arterial PCO_2 is often normal, especially in patients with a normal hypercapnic respiratory drive, and will be raised in those with type II respiratory failure. A lowered $PaCO_2$ may be present in the early stages of a severe asthma attack if the patient is acutely hyperventilating.

Medical management

Education of patients by health professionals includes explaining in simple terms the mechanism of airflow limitation, the importance of avoiding trigger factors including cigarette smoke, use and effects of medication and a self-management plan (e.g. the use of a peak flow meter for patients with variable airflow limitation and management of symptoms including a plan of action in the event of progressive symptoms).

Smoking cessation may be effective if patients are provided with adequate support in therapy groups and use nicotine replacement therapy (Raw et al 1998). Bronchodilators such as beta-2 agonists (long and short acting) and anticholinergic drugs are used to relieve the reversible elements of airflow limitation. For patients who do not demonstrate an improvement in spirometry, these drugs may provide relief from symptoms and are used for maintenance treatment. Methylxanthines are bronchodilators which may also be beneficial in some patients.

Patients who manifest with mild symptoms of reversible airflow limitation on rare occasions may only require symptomatic relief using short-acting inhaled bronchodilators. However, when patients with asthma begin to use inhaled bronchodilators on a regular basis, antiinflammatory agents such as inhaled corticosteroids are also usually required. In some patients with COPD, the number of exacerbations and rate of decline in QOL may be reduced when treated with inhaled corticosteroids (Calverley 1999). Non-steroidal anti-inflammatory drugs (NSAIDs) such as sodium cromoglicate are prophylactic drugs used in the management of some patients with asthma. Antileukotreines are a new anti-asthma agent used to achieve bronchodilatation and a reduction in symptoms (Barnes 1999). If airflow limitation is severe, oral or intravenous drugs are required. Beta-2 agonists and sodium cromoglicate are also used in the management of EIA (Storms 1999). Inhaled foreign bodies are generally removed by bronchoscopy. Surgical intervention, laser treatment, chemotherapy and/or radiotherapy may be indicated for the management of neoplasms compressing or occluding airways. The mechanical effects of severe hyperinflation may be improved with lung volume reduction surgery.

Physiotherapy management

Patient education is essential for optimal management and should include the factors outlined in the section on medical management.

Effective delivery of bronchodilators prior to airway clearance techniques or exercise is essential. A large range of devices is available for the delivery of inhaled respiratory medications (see Ch. 6 on physiotherapy techniques). The physiotherapist, in conjunction with the patient, doctor and pharmacist, should choose a suitable delivery device. Education of the patient in its use, including the appropriate breathing pattern, is necessary to ensure maximum penetration and deposition of the drug (Fink 2000).

Airway clearance techniques should be adapted to ensure that no increase in airflow limitation occurs (see Ch. 6).

For management of EIA, see 'special case' (p. 253).

Clinical outcomes

These may include a reduction in symptoms such as chest tightness, wheeze, cough and dyspnoea and an increase in exercise tolerance. With a reduction in airflow limitation, the abnormal findings observed in the breathing pattern may disappear (e.g. following recovery from an acute attack of asthma) or be reduced. Lung function and gas exchange abnormalities may be reversible depending on the underlying aetiology. Improved control of the symptoms of airflow limitation should lead to improved QOL.

PROBLEM – RESPIRATORY MUSCLE DYSFUNCTION

Weakness (the inability of rested muscles to generate the expected maximum force) and fatigue (the inability of muscle to sustain a given level of work or a loss in the capacity of a muscle to develop a force due to loaded muscle activity that is reversible by rest) of the respiratory muscles may occur in a wide range of conditions. Mild forms of dysfunction are often difficult to detect clinically and, in some patients, both weakness and fatigue may be present. Assessment of the respiratory muscles is important because:

- Dyspnoea in patients with no respiratory or cardiovascular disease may be due to respiratory muscle weakness.
- There may be few clinical signs of dysfunction even in patients with moderate to severe weakness.
- Respiratory muscle weakness is invariably present in patients with significant generalized neuromuscular disease and can be a compounding factor in many conditions, for example steroid myopathy and malnutrition (Polkey et al 1995).
- Respiratory muscle weakness may be the cause of ineffective cough.

The factors which predispose to respiratory muscle dysfunction can broadly be divided into three groups. The first group relates to factors that may depress respiratory drive (e.g. drug overdose, brainstem lesions, sleep-disordered breathing).

Impaired neuromuscular competence, for example neuromuscular disorders, myopathies and connective tissue disorders, electrolyte disorders, malnutrition and hypoxaemia, all of which may lead to a decrease in the force-generating ability of the respiratory muscles, constitute the second group. The third group of factors are those which increase respiratory muscle work by increasing the WOB (e.g. changes in lung and chest wall compliance or an increase in airway resistance) or where minute ventilation is increased as a result, for example, of fever, pulmonary embolus or excessive caloric intake (Schmidt et al 2000).

Clinical features and assessment

Respiratory muscle involvement is commonly associated with a widespread neurological or muscle disorder (Moxham 1999). The main features associated with respiratory muscle dysfunction are dyspnoea, a decrease in exercise tolerance and, in patients with more severe disease, type II respiratory failure.

The patient may report breathlessness, especially when lying down or when standing in water up to the chest, for example when entering the sea or a swimming pool. The weight of water causes pressure on the abdominal wall and thus the load on the diaphragm is increased. Daytime somnolence, early morning headaches and impaired mental function may be present if arterial desaturation and hypercapnia occur during sleep. In the dyspnoeic patient, the abnormalities in breathing pattern may include increased respiratory rate, decreased V_T, reduced chest expansion, use of accessory muscles, respiratory alternans (periods of breathing using only chest wall muscles alternating with periods of breathing using the diaphragm) and paradoxical movement of the rib cage or abdomen (Moxham 1999, Wilkins et al 1995). Profound diaphragm weakness or paralysis gives rise to paradoxical inward abdominal movement occurring during inspiration and is most easily seen with the patient in supine (Moxham 1999). This occurs due to the passive transmission of the negative intrapleural pressure generated by the other inspiratory muscles which causes the abdominal contents to be pulled upwards, unre-

sisted by the ineffectual diaphragm. When upright, recruitment of the abdominal muscles may occur during expiration in order to elevate the diaphragm so that gravity can assist diaphragm descent during inspiration. However, these clinical signs are often absent unless the diaphragm is paralysed or the strength of the diaphragm is significantly reduced. The patient may have a weak cough which may be due to inadequate inspired volume and/or weakness of the expiratory muscles, resulting in ineffective expiratory airflow. Weakness of the bulbar muscles may contribute to the impaired cough and may also contribute to aspiration of gastric contents. Physical examination may reveal signs of generalized muscle weakness and there may be marked weight loss.

The plain chest radiograph and fluoroscopic screening of the diaphragm during sniffing are useful diagnostic tools in hemidiaphragm weakness. The affected side is raised and moves paradoxically upwards on sniffing. Radiography and fluoroscopy are less useful when the problem is bilateral (Moxham 1999). Movement of the diaphragm can also be assessed using ultrasonography. The chest radiograph may show a reduction in lung volume and elevated hemidiaphragms.

Lung function

Lung function may be normal in the absence of marked weakness. The characteristic abnormalities of inspiratory muscle weakness are a reduced vital capacity (VC) and TLC. In the presence of severe bilateral diaphragm weakness, the VC is low when the patient is upright and typically falls by more than 50% when supine (Moxham 1999). This fall in VC is due to the weight of the abdominal contents in supine which push up against the diaphragm.

Measurement of VC is especially useful in the management of progressive disorders such as Guillain–Barré syndrome. Residual volume will be normal unless the expiratory muscles are also involved. The RV/TLC ratio is therefore normal or high but, in contrast to diseases characterized by airflow limitation, the FEV_1/FVC is not reduced. Carbon monoxide transfer coefficient is normal or raised in patients with reduced lung volume (Moxham 1999). FRC is decreased due to the loss of end-expiratory tone in the muscles that hold the chest wall out. Muscle weakness occurring acutely has no effect on lung compliance but with persistent weakness both lung and chest wall compliance are reduced (Moxham 1999). Global respiratory muscle strength can be assessed by measuring P_iMax and P_eMax but for quantification of diaphragmatic weakness the transdiaphragmatic pressure must be measured (see Ch. 3 on cardiopulmonary function testing). Phrenic nerve stimulation may also be used to measure diaphragm strength (Moxham 1999).

Since respiratory muscle weakness is often associated with generalized muscle weakness, it is useful to obtain an indication of limb muscle strength, for example by measuring hand grip or quadriceps strength. Respiratory muscle endurance can be assessed by measuring the maximal voluntary ventilation and the maximum sustained ventilation or by assessing the ventilatory response to added inspiratory loads (Clanton & Diaz 1995, Ferguson 1993). Exercise tolerance and QOL should also be assessed, when appropriate. The PaO_2 and the SaO_2 may be low due to microatelectasis and $\dot{V}/\dot{Q}$ mismatching. Hypercapnia, in the absence of co-existent lung disease, is uncommon until VC has fallen to 50% of normal or the P_iMax is reduced to 30% predicted (Moxham 1999).

Blood gas abnormalities

In the patient with severe weakness of the respiratory muscles, hypercapnia often develops insidiously at night. When healthy subjects sleep, a degree of hypoventilation occurs which results in an increase in $PaCO_2$ of 0.3–1 kPa (2–8 mmHg) and a fall in PaO_2 and SaO_2 of 0.4–1.3 kPa (3–10 mmHg) and 2–3% respectively (Hara & Shepard 1990). In the elderly, periods of apnoea, hypopnoea and desaturation frequently occur during sleep (Phillips et al 1992). Tidal volume is decreased by 15–25% and is shallower during rapid eye movement (REM) than non-REM sleep. In addition, hypercapnic and hypoxic ventilatory

responses are depressed (Hara & Shepard 1990). Further problems occur during REM sleep in patients with diaphragm dysfunction because a reduction in the tone of the intercostal and accessory muscles increases the work of the diaphragm. Nocturnal desaturation in patients with respiratory muscle weakness is mainly due to hypoventilation. An additional mechanism in some patients might be increased $\dot{V}/\dot{Q}$ mismatching arising from the small fall in FRC that occurs during sleep. With progressive hypoventilation, signs of type II respiratory failure develop.

Medical management

Patients with some types of neurological dysfunction may recover spontaneously (e.g. Guillain–Barré syndrome) or may require periods of assisted ventilation. For patients with a chronic disorder, assisted ventilation may be useful at night to rest the respiratory muscles, improve quality of sleep and symptoms of nocturnal hypoventilation, improve daytime blood gas tensions and increase long-term survival and QOL (Turkington & Elliott 2000). If the diaphragm is intact, pacing of the phrenic nerve may sustain ventilation. Adequate nutrition is essential for malnourished patients as is weight loss for obese patients. Correction of metabolic and electrolyte imbalance is necessary to reduce muscle weakness. Attempts have been made to improve respiratory muscle function with drugs. Methylxanthines may have a very small inotropic action and may be used in patients with impending respiratory failure (Fernandez et al 1993, Jenne 1993).

Physiotherapy management

Targeted respiratory muscle training may be an effective means of increasing the strength and endurance of the respiratory muscles (see Ch. 6 on physiotherapy techniques). Some benefits may be gained from unsupported upper limb exercise as this type of exercise may assist with improving the function of the accessory respiratory muscles. Patients may also benefit from general exercise training to enhance oxygen transport (Dean & Ross 1992).

The presence of fatigue, for example in a patient who is acutely unwell, will necessitate that treatments are short and interspersed with sufficient rest periods.

Clinical outcomes

These depend on the aetiology. Benefits may be seen fairly rapidly if the underlying cause is a metabolic abnormality that is easily corrected. In selected patients, the benefits from resting the respiratory muscles using assisted ventilation include physiological benefits of improved blood gas tensions, respiratory muscle function, restoration of normal sleep pattern and increased long-term survival. Functional benefits are reflected by an increased work capacity and increased ability to participate in exercise training. Exercise that incorporates intensive upper limb training and, in some patients inspiratory muscle training, may improve tolerance of dyspnoea, increase respiratory muscle strength and improve QOL (Turkington & Elliott 2000).

In some patients, the underlying cause of respiratory muscle dysfunction is progressive and benefit from physiotherapy may largely be seen by the successful management of associated and potential problems, such as impaired airway clearance and prevention of chest infection.

PROBLEM – REDUCED LUNG VOLUME

Reduced lung volumes occur in a variety of situations and may be short-lived (e.g. following major surgery) or chronic (e.g. ILD). On occasions the cause is a disease process affecting the lung parenchyma but in many situations the reduction in lung volume arises from processes affecting other structures, such as the respiratory muscles or the pleura. A decrease in FRC is an almost universal finding following upper abdominal surgery or cardiothoracic surgery. The physiotherapist does not always have a role in the management of the problem, for example when the cause is abdominal ascites or pregnancy unassociated with respiratory disease. The pathophysiological basis for a reduction in lung volume, clinical examples and examples of medical intervention are given in Table 7.5. (Johnson & Pierson 1986).

The main consequences of a decrease in lung volume are:

- Atelectasis in dependent lung regions.
- Impaired oxygenation due to $\dot{V}/\dot{Q}$ mismatching and, in some cases, intrapulmonary shunting. This occurs because the small airways in the dependent lung regions may close during quiet breathing. With acute lobar atelectasis, hypoxaemia may be absent or minimal if there is an accompanying decrease in perfusion to the affected area (i.e. if hypoxic pulmonary vasoconstriction occurs). Low tidal volume breathing may be associated with a failure to clear the anatomic dead space.
- Inefficient cough due to the reduction in VC which reduces the ability to generate an adequate expiratory airflow.
- Increased WOB as airway resistance is increased and lung compliance is reduced.
- Decreased exercise tolerance due to the inability to meet the ventilatory demands of exercise.

Special case – the surgical patient

Following upper abdominal or cardiothoracic surgery, a restrictive ventilatory defect and arterial hypoxaemia occur. The changes in lung function are most severe within the first 24–72 hours after surgery and are followed by a gradual return to preoperative levels. This may take up to 7 days after upper abdominal surgery and several weeks after cardiac surgery (Jenkins et al 1990, Locke et al 1990, Meyers et al 1975, Morran et al 1983). A rise in $PaCO_2$ is unusual unless marked respiratory depression occurs, for example following high doses of narcotic analgesics. However, in many patients these lung function abnormalities will resolve spontaneously with normal postoperative care.

Some degree of atelectasis is almost a universal consequence of major abdominal or cardiothoracic surgery but in many patients the atelectasis will resolve over time, provided that the patient

Table 7.5 Pathophysiological basis for reduced lung volume, clinical examples and examples of medical intervention

Pathophysiological basis	Clinical examples	Examples of medical interventions
Atelectasis:	Normal consequence of UAS and CT surgery due to the anaesthetic, operation and changes occurring in the postoperative period including a lack of periodic deep breaths	CPAP
1. Reduced function of surfactant	ARDS, smoke inhalation, high FiO_2	Mechanical ventilation (e.g. PPV)
2. Airway obstruction	Foreign body, mucus plugging	Removal of foreign body/mucus by bronchoscopy
	Hilar adenopathy, mediastinal masses	Surgical removal, laser treatment, radiotherapy, chemotherapy
3. Negative airway pressure	Endobronchial suctioning	
Compression of lung tissue:		
1. Pleural space encroachment	Effusion, empyema	Insertion of ICC; antibiotics or surgical decortication for empyema
2. Mediastinal structures	Tension pneumothorax causing mediastinal shift and compression of the contralateral lung	Insertion of ICC
3. Cardiomegaly	Decreases ventilation to left lower lobe when supine, e.g. left ventricular failure	Management of cause of cardiac failure
4. Abdominal distension	Obesity, ascites, following surgery, running-in phase of peritoneal dialysis, pregnancy	Dietary advice for the obese patient; drainage of ascites or peritoneal dialysis
Decrease in compliance:		
1. Lung	Restrictive diseases, e.g. ILD	Corticosteroids or immunosuppressants for some lung diseases. Mechanical ventilation or support using NIV
2. Thorax	Kyphoscoliosis, ankylosing spondylitis; disruption to the integrity of the chest wall due to trauma, e.g. rib fractures	Surgical correction; PPV for patients with fractured ribs
Decreased ability of respiratory muscles to generate sufficient negative pressure	Respiratory muscle dysfunction (see Problem – respiratory muscle dysfunction)	Mechanical ventilation or support using NIV
Posture	Supine position associated with a low resting lung volume due to increased thoracic blood volume	
Pain	May cause patient to take shallower breaths with the absence of sighs. Absence of sighs leads to atelectasis in dependent lung regions, reduces surfactant activity and decreases lung compliance	Pain control using analgesics administered orally, intramuscularly, intravenously, regional nerve blocks (epidural, intercostal nerve block), acupuncture/acupressure or hypnosis

Abbreviations: UAS, upper abdominal surgery; CT, cardiothoracic; CPAP, continuous positive airway pressure; ARDS, acute respiratory distress syndrome; FiO_2, fraction of inspired oxygen; ICC, intercostal catheter; ILD, interstitial lung disease; NIV, non-invasive ventilation; PPV, positive pressure ventilation

is assisted to adopt an upright position and to ambulate in the early postoperative period. In a minority of patients clinically significant atelectasis (i.e. atelectasis that in some way alters the normal postoperative course) may occur. The pathogenesis for the development of postoperative atelectasis is provided in Table 7.5. Factors predisposing to the development of postopera-tive pneumonia have been covered in the problem of impaired airway clearance.

Clinical features and assessment

Many patients with reduced lung volumes present with the problems of dyspnoea, decreased exercise tolerance or mucus retention due to an ineffective cough. Orthopnoea may also be present.

In general there will be an abnormal breathing pattern characterized by a small V_T and increased rate. In the presence of pain, or fear of pain (e.g. in the patient with a surgical incision or pleuritic pain), there will be absence of periodic deep breaths. Chest expansion will be reduced and this may be a localized finding, for example in the area overlying a collapsed lobe.

The cough will be weak, due mainly to the inability to generate adequate expiratory airflow because of the low V_T. Pain will inhibit effective coughing in some patients.

Symptoms resulting from acute lobar collapse depend on the extent of the collapse, the abruptness of onset and the underlying respiratory impairment. A slowly developing segmental or lobar collapse may produce few symptoms if the patient has otherwise normal lungs. If the same degree of collapse occurs suddenly in a patient with chronic lung disease, severe respiratory distress may develop.

On auscultation there will be absent, diminished or bronchial breath sounds. Over the area of a pneumothorax, the percussion note will be hyper-resonant.

Lung function testing will show a decrease in VC and all other lung volumes except when the expiratory muscles are weak, in which case the RV is raised. Peak inspiratory and expiratory mouth pressures may be reduced if there is weakness of the respiratory muscles. Hypoxaemia may be present, primarily as a result of $\dot{V}/\dot{Q}$ mismatching arising from changes in the FRC/closing volume relationship. Hypercapnia is often absent but will occur if there is associated hypoventilation.

Chest radiograph findings may be very helpful in identifying the cause of the reduction in lung volumes such as a pleural disorder, lobar or lung collapse.

Medical management

Medical management involves the management of the underlying cause of reduced lung volume. Examples of medical interventions are listed in Table 7.5.

Physiotherapy management

Optimization of lung volumes is achieved by upright positioning. As upright positions increase FRC, high sitting, sitting out of bed and ambulation are encouraged. The side-lying position is preferred to slumped or supine positions and may be modified by tilting the patient towards prone to further decrease compression on lung tissue. This is especially so in patients with abdominal distension (Jenkins et al 1988).

Tidal volume is increased using breathing exercises (e.g. thoracic expansion exercises, sustained maximal inspirations with or without the use of an incentive spirometer, IPPB) and manual hyperinflation. Ambulation increases $\dot{V}_E$ and is useful to assist with the reexpansion of lung tissue in patients with pleural disease or atelectasis. When ambulating, patients should be encouraged to take intermittent deep breaths to ensure that the increased $\dot{V}_E$ is not solely due to an increase in respiratory rate (Orfanos et al 1999). FRC may be increased with the use of CPAP. In patients with pain, treatment should be performed when pain management is optimal (see Problem – pain).

Patients at increased risk of developing clinically significant atelectasis following surgery should be identified and prophylactic physiotherapy commenced. Decreased lung volumes should be managed using the techniques listed earlier in this section.

Obese patients may benefit from exercise programmes designed to achieve weight reduction provided that exercise is accompanied by dietary control.

Clinical outcomes

Physiological improvements from physiotherapy intervention may include an increase in lung volumes and capacities, for example FRC and VC, and a rise in PaO_2 and SaO_2. Peak inspiratory and expiratory mouth pressures may increase if the cause is reversible weakness of the respiratory muscles. The physiological changes may be associated with an improvement in breathing pattern, a reduction in dyspnoea and an increase in exercise tolerance. Auscultation may reveal improved breath sounds to the affected area(s). Chest radiograph changes are not always a good indication of clinical progress; for example, following coronary artery surgery small pleural effusions may persist for a considerable time after the patient has recovered clinically.

In the high-risk surgical patient, the outcome will be prevention of clinically significant atelectasis.

In the obese individual, the abnormal physiological changes will be reversed with weight loss (Thomas et al 1989).

PROBLEM – IMPAIRED GAS EXCHANGE

Impaired gas exchange is common in patients with respiratory or cardiovascular disease. In some patients, abnormalities may only become evident when increased demands are imposed on the respiratory and cardiovascular systems such as during exercise, with an infective exacerbation or when changes in ventilation occur as a normal consequence of sleep. Gas exchange abnormalities rarely occur in the absence of one or more of the other problems discussed in this chapter. Although changes in ventilation arise in response to hypoxaemia and hypercapnia, dyspnoea is not necessarily present.

The physiotherapist does not always have a role in the management of impaired gas exchange; for example, in the patient with acute pulmonary embolus or in the postoperative patient who has minimal hypoxaemia but is self-ambulating and has no other problems which are amenable to physiotherapy intervention.

The following section outlines the pathophysiology, clinical features and assessment of hypoxaemia, hypercapnia and hypocapnia (Vas Fragoso 1993, West 2000).

Hypoxaemia

This is seen in a wide range of conditions. The pathophysiological basis and clinical examples of hypoxaemia are given in Table 7.6.

Hypercapnia

A raised $PaCO_2$ is the hallmark of type II respiratory failure and accompanies a decrease in PaO_2. The pathophysiological basis of hypercapnia and clinical examples are given in Table 7.7 (Vas Fragoso 1993).

Hypocapnia

In clinical practice, a low $PaCO_2$ is a far less common occurrence than a raised $PaCO_2$. An increase in rate or depth of breathing is not necessarily associated with hypocapnia. For example, a large V_T in conjunction with a slow rate may not reduce $PaCO_2$ below normal levels. Conversely, a low V_T and high rate, such as when panting, may not lower $PaCO_2$ or may even raise $PaCO_2$ if the V_T fails to clear the anatomic dead space. The pathophysiology of hyperventilation disorders is reviewed elsewhere (Gardner 1996).

Clinical features and assessment

Hypercapnia is a powerful respiratory stimulant and, under normal conditions, $PaCO_2$ is an important factor in the chemical control of ventilation. When the $PaCO_2$ is normal, there is little increase in ventilation until PaO_2 has fallen below 8 kPa (60 mmHg) (Weil et al 1975). When hypercapnia is present, the ventilatory response to hypoxia is enhanced (West 2000). The ventilatory response to hypoxia and hypercapnia varies considerably among subjects and is reduced with advanced age and during sleep (Hara & Shepard 1990, West 2000). In some patients with severe COPD, the ventilatory response to $PaCO_2$ is significantly decreased (West 1998). Patients may adapt to gradual changes in arterial blood gas tensions whereas acute hypoxia and hypercapnia are less well tolerated.

There are few clinical features associated with mild hypoxaemia. The features of moderate to severe hypoxaemia which develops acutely are restlessness, confusion, sweating, tachycardia, hypertension, skin pallor and cyanosis. As hypoxaemia worsens, pulmonary hypertension may develop and with severe hypoxaemia the cardio-

Table 7.6 Pathophysiological basis of hypoxaemia and clinical examples

Pathophysiological basis	Comment	Clinical examples
Hypoventilation	Site of abnormality:	
	1. Respiratory centre	Hypoxic and hypercapnic ventilatory drives depressed by drugs, anaesthesia and as a normal consequence of sleep
	2. Medulla	Trauma, neoplasm
	3. Spinal cord	Trauma, neoplasm
	4. Anterior horn cell	Poliomyelitis
	5. Innervation of the respiratory muscles	Phrenic nerve paralysis
	6 Disease of the myoneural junction	Myasthenia gravis
	7. Respiratory muscles	Weakness or fatigue from many causes (see Problem – respiratory muscle dysfunction)
	8. Upper airway obstruction	Foreign body, during sleep apnoea syndrome
	9. Excessive WOB	Variety of causes including added load on the mechanics of breathing such as in the patient with acute severe asthma who is exhausted
$\dot{V}/\dot{Q}$ mismatch	Low $\dot{V}/\dot{Q}$ ratio is the commonest cause of hypoxaemia in respiratory disease. $\dot{V}/\dot{Q}$ mismatch arises due to abnormalities in FRC/CV relationship, e.g.:	
	1. Decrease in FRC	Reduced lung volumes secondary to UAS or CT surgery, obesity, ascites, atelectasis, supine position, ILD
	2. Increase in CV	Small airway closure due to airflow limitation, cigarette smoking, pulmonary oedema, increased age
	Perfusion limitation	Pulmonary embolus pulmonary infarction
	Intrapulmonary shunt	Atelectasis, pneumonia, pulmonary oedema, ARDS
	Cardiac shunt	ASD, VSD
Diffusion limitation	Decrease in alveolar–capillary surface area	Emphysema
	Decrease in diffusion gradient	Low FiO_2 as occurs at high altitude
	Increased thickness of alveolar–capillary membrane	Scarring or fluid in the interstitial space, e.g. ILD, pulmonary oedema
	Decreased transit time of RBC in pulmonary capillary	May cause hypoxaemia on exercise in the presence of another cause of diffusion limitation
Decrease in F_iO_2	High altitude	
	Malfunctioning of respiratory equipment	Disconnection of gas supply
	Endobronchial suctioning	
Mixed causes	Combination of $\dot{V}/\dot{Q}$ mismatch, diffusion limitation, shunt and hypoventilation	Seen in severe chronic lung disease
Imbalance between $\dot{V}O_2$ and DO_2	This causes a reduction in PvO_2 which reflects greater oxygen extraction to compensate for inadequate DO_2 relative to $\dot{V}O_2$. Low PvO_2 magnifies the effects of $\dot{V}/\dot{Q}$ mismatch and shunt on a patient's level of oxygenation	Low cardiac output states, severe anaemia, severe hypoxaemia

Abbreviations: WOB, work of breathing; $\dot{V}/\dot{Q}$, ventilation perfusion; FRC, functional residual capacity; CV, closing volume; UAS, upper abdominal surgery; CT, cardiothoracic; ILD, interstitial lung disease; ARDS, acute respiratory distress syndrome; ASD, atrial septal defect; VSD, ventricular septal defect; FiO_2, fraction of inspired oxygen; RBC, red blood cell; PvO_2, mixed venous oxygen tension; DO_2, oxygen delivery; $\dot{V}O_2$, oxygen consumption

vascular system may respond with bradycardia and hypotension. Circulatory failure and shock occur when the PaO_2 falls to profoundly low levels (West 1998, Youtsey 1994). Hypoxaemia exacerbates cardiac arrhythmias and angina in patients with IHD and may predispose to heart failure. The long-term cardiovascular consequences of hypoxaemia are pulmonary hyperten-

Table 7.7   Pathophysiological basis of hypercapnia and clinical examples

Pathophysiological basis	Clinical examples
Hypoventilation: 1. Reduced central drive	Obesity-hypoventilation syndrome, depression of the respiratory centre due to reduced conscious state, anaesthesia, narcotics, barbiturates
2. Respiratory muscle dysfunction	Variety of causes, e.g. neuromuscular disorders (see Problem – respiratory muscle dysfunction)
3. Added load on the mechanics of breathing	Changes in compliance of the lung or chest wall, e.g. chest wall trauma, pulmonary oedema, large pleural effusion, ILD Increase in airways resistance e.g. severe COPD
Increased $\dot{V}CO_2$	Increased metabolism, e.g. fever, sepsis, trauma, burns, exercise Metabolic acidosis Nutritional supplements with excessive carbohydrate
Increased dead space as a fraction of V_T	COPD, pulmonary embolus, low lung volume breathing, e.g. with pain, respiratory muscle weakness

Abbreviations: ILD, interstitial lung disease; COPD, chronic obstructive pulmonary disease; $\dot{V}CO_2$, carbon dioxide production; V_T, tidal volume

sion and cor pulmonale. Raised levels of CO_2 in arterial blood cause vasodilatation. The patient has warm peripheries and the greatly increased cerebral blood flow is responsible for headache, raised cerebrospinal fluid pressure and sometimes papilloedema. A raised $PaCO_2$ may be associated with a flapping tremor of the outstretched hands (asterixis). The clinical features which result from a combination of hypoxia and hypercapnia on the central nervous system are restlessness, confusion, slurred speech and fluctuations of mood. High levels of $PaCO_2$ cause decreased levels of consciousness.

The signs and symptoms of hypocapnia are many and varied (Gardner 1996). They include tetany and paraesthesia in the hands, face and trunk. A reduction in central nervous system and cerebral blood flow may be responsible for dizziness, loss of consciousness, visual disturbances, headache, tinnitus, ataxia and tremor. With acute hypocapnia, arterial BP falls and HR increases. Peripheral vasoconstriction is thought to be responsible for the complaint of cold hands. Hyperventilation is a cause of atypical chest pain. Hyperventilation may be associated, but is not synonymous, with dyspnoea. The physiotherapy assessment of the patient with a hyperventilation disorder is detailed in Chapter 19 on hyperventilation disorders.

Assessment must include measures of oxygenation, commonly the PaO_2 or SaO_2, the $PaCO_2$ and the arterial hydrogen ion concentration. These can be measured by intermittent arterial blood sampling or monitored continuously using a pulse oximeter for SpO_2 and a transcutaneous electrode for $PaCO_2$. Nocturnal monitoring of SaO_2 and $PaCO_2$ may provide important information. For patients with a suspected hyperventilation disorder, measurement of expired CO_2 is useful.

The age of the patient is an important consideration in the interpretation of PaO_2 values. Average values for PaO_2 range from 11.2–13.9 kPa (84–104 mmHg) in individuals aged 25 years and from 9.5 to 12.1 kPa (71–91 mmHg) for those aged 65 years (Nunn 1987). For normal values for the paediatric population refer to Chapter 9. In addition, obesity decreases PaO_2 due to an increase in $\dot{V}/\dot{Q}$ mismatching (Jenkins & Moxham 1991). Interobserver reliability for the detection of central cyanosis is poor when SaO_2 is above 85%. Anaemia impairs the detection of central cyanosis whereas it is more easily diagnosed if polycythaemia is present (Flenley 1990).

Medical management

The recognition and management of the underlying cause of hypoxaemia are essential. Oxygen therapy is indicated whenever tissue oxygenation is impaired, in order to allow essential metabolic reactions to occur and to prevent complications attributed to hypoxaemia (Oh 1997). Nocturnal and ambulatory oxygen are useful in patients who desaturate during sleep or during physical activity and may prevent/reverse the consequences of chronic hypoxaemia (Wedzicha 2000). Assisted ventilation may be required and nitric oxide may be used as a selective pulmonary artery vasodilator to improve $\dot{V}/\dot{Q}$ matching (Schmidt et al 2000).

Impaired perfusion due to pulmonary emboli may only require thrombolytic therapy or surgical intervention.

Lung transplantation or lung volume reduction surgery may be the required treatment for selected patients with chronic respiratory failure.

Physiotherapy management

It is essential that the pathophysiological cause(s) is identified. Gas exchange may by optimized by positioning patients in an upright position to improve FRC. In spontaneously breathing adults with unilateral lung pathology, $\dot{V}/\dot{Q}$ matching may be improved by positioning in side lying with the unaffected lung dependent. The side-lying position may, however, increase $\dot{V}O_2$ and cause hypoxaemia in susceptible patients (Horiuchi et al 1997). Prone or semi-prone positioning may improve oxygenation in acutely ill patients who are mechanically ventilated and paralysed. Hypoxaemia due to hypoventilation may be worsened by positioning in lying.

Transient hypoxaemia is avoided by the correct application of techniques such as suctioning and can be avoided during periods of increased $\dot{V}O_2$ by using the correct oxygen therapy device and its correct application.

The use of breathing techniques (e.g. thoracic expansion exercises, sustained maximal inspirations, breathing control, pursedlip breathing) and assisted breathing devices (e.g. IPPB, NIV) may improve gas exchange. The elimination of excessive muscle activity may reduce $\dot{V}O_2$ in patients who are severely breathless.

Physical activity may improve gas exchange by improving oxygen transport or may result in desaturation in some patients with severe cardiopulmonary dysfunction.

Clinical outcomes

As restoration of blood gas tensions and arterial hydrogen ion concentration to normal levels occurs there should be a measurable improvement in cognitive function. Depending on the presence of associated problems, there may be a reduction in dyspnoea and an increase in exercise tolerance. Long-term domiciliary oxygen therapy has been shown to improve survival, cognitive function and QOL in patients with cor pulmonale by ameliorating the adverse cardiovascular effects of chronic hypoxaemia (Oh 1997).

PROBLEM – ABNORMAL BREATHING PATTERN

Abnormal breathing pattern is rarely identified in the physiotherapy problem list as it seldom occurs alone and is more usually associated with other problems, many of which are amenable to physiotherapy intervention. Such associated problems include dyspnoea, airflow limitation, reduced lung volumes, impaired airway clearance, impaired gas exchange and pain. Resolution of the associated problems is usually accompanied by improvement in breathing pattern. Many patients who have an abnormal breathing pattern will complain of breathlessness. The pathophysiological basis of an abnormal breathing pattern and clinical examples are given in Table 7.8 (MacIntyre 1990, Tobin 1990).

Clinical features and assessment

These include abnormalities in rate, depth, including excessive sighing or breath holding, and changes in the inspiratory to expiratory ratio. Observation and palpation may reveal limited or asymmetrical chest wall movement, asynchronous movements or respiratory alternans. The patient may use the accessory muscles of inspiration and fix the shoulder girdle in order to maximize accessory muscle function. Abdominal movements may be absent or significantly reduced and, on palpation, the anterior abdominal wall may be splinted. Increased abdominal effort during expiration may be present due to recruitment of the accessory

Table 7.8 Pathophysiological basis of abnormal breathing pattern and clinical examples

Pathophysiological basis	Clinical examples
Increase in elastic or resistive WOB due to abnormalities of the lung or thorax	Decrease in C_L or C_{CW}, e.g. ILD, kyphoscoliosis, ankylosing spondylitis, obesity Any factor causing airflow limitation (see Problem – airflow limitation)
Impaired ventilatory pump	Respiratory muscle dysfunction from a variety of causes (see Problem – respiratory muscle dysfunction)
Abnormal respiratory centre control	Depression of the respiratory centre due to loss of consciousness, anaesthesia, narcotics, barbiturates
CNS disorders	Ataxic (Biot's) breathing Irregular pattern. Variable V_T with periods of apnoea
Brainstem disorders	Apneustic breathing – sustained inspiratory effort with irregular and brief expirations
Cerebrovascular disorders	Cheyne–Stokes respiration – cyclical pattern of periods of deep breathing becoming progressively more shallow and then periods of apnoea. Seen in severe neurological disorders and occasionally in LVF, uraemia, drug-induced respiratory depression
Chemical control of breathing	Hypoxia, hypercapnia and acid-base disturbances (raised H^+) increase ventilation
Renal acidosis, diabetic ketoacidosis	Kussmaul breathing – large V_T, fast, normal or slow rate, high $\dot{V}_E$
Stimulation from intrapulmonary receptors	Irritant receptors (rapidly adapting) respond to chemical or physical stimuli Pulmonary stretch receptors (slowly adapting) respond to marked increases in lung volume C-fibre receptors deep within lung parenchyma (J receptors) and in bronchi respond to vascular engorgement and congestion, chemical stimuli and less so to mechanical stimuli
Voluntary factors	Inhibition of sighs due to pain from abdominal or thoracic incisions, pleural disorders, e.g. pleurisy, pneumothorax
Anxiety	May be associated with a variety of abnormal patterns including excessive sighing, rapid breathing, small V_T, breath holding

Abbreviations: WOB, work of breathing; C_L, lung compliance; C_{CW}, chest wall compliance; ILD, interstitial lung disease; CNS, central nervous system; V_T, tidal volume; LVF, left ventricular failure; H^+, hydrogen ions; $\dot{V}_E$, minute ventilation

expiratory muscles. Pursed-lip breathing may be seen if the cause of the abnormal breathing pattern is severe airflow limitation. Assessment may reveal signs of chronic lung hyperinflation (see Problem – airflow limitation). Arterial blood gas analysis, pulmonary function test results, auscultatory and chest radiograph findings may demonstrate abnormalities consistent with an underlying problem.

Medical management

Recognition of the underlying cause and amelioration where possible are essential. Management is mainly directed at reducing the WOB. Disorders of the brainstem or central nervous system may resolve spontaneously or as a result

of interventions aimed at decreasing intracranial pressure (e.g. diuretic therapy, sedation, paralysis, mechanical ventilation and surgery).

Physiotherapy management

It is rare that physiotherapy management is focused on changing breathing patterns as abnormal breathing patterns are often associated with strategies employed by the patient to reduce breathlessness. Thus, physiotherapy generally aims to try and eliminate the exaggerated muscle activity associated with increased WOB.

In some patients, abnormal breathing patterns such as pursedlip breathing and fixation of the shoulder girdle are necessary to optimize gas exchange (Breslin 1995). Breathing patterns should not be altered in these patients and breathing strategies such as pursed-lip breathing are often encouraged. The excessive use of muscle activity should be discouraged and positioning used to relieve dyspnoea and reduce $\dot{V}O_2$. Breathing strategies used to relieve dyspnoea (e.g. breathing control, exhalation with effort, paced breathing) may be useful to improve breathing patterns during activity and rest. When an abnormal breathing pattern results from anxiety, strategies such as relaxation and breathing control are encouraged (see Chapter 19 on hyperventilation).

Neurophysiological facilitation techniques may be used to alter rate and depth of breathing in some patients (see Chapter 6 on physiotherapy techniques).

Clinical outcomes

Benefits from physiotherapy intervention may be demonstrated by an improvement in the underlying problems of dyspnoea, airflow limitation, reduced lung volumes, impaired airway clearance, impaired gas exchange and pain. These improvements should result in an improved breathing pattern.

PROBLEM – PAIN

This section discusses pain of respiratory and cardiovascular origin as well as other causes of pain located in the chest.

Patients tend not to ignore chest pain unless it has a familiar and recurrent pattern. Thus, patients may be more likely to seek medical advice for chest pain than for chronic cough and sputum production, especially when cough and sputum occur in an individual who smokes cigarettes.

Chest pain of respiratory origin

Pain of respiratory origin arises from the parietal pleura and from stimulation of the mucosa of the trachea and main bronchus. The lung parenchyma and visceral pleura are insensitive to pain. However, inflammatory processes in peripheral regions of the lung that involve the overlying visceral pleura often lead to pain from involvement of the adjacent parietal pleura. The origin and characteristic features of pain of respiratory origin, together with clinical examples, are given in Table 7.9 (Murray & Gebhart 2000).

Table 7.9 Site and characteristic features of chest pain of respiratory origin

Origin	Characteristic features	Stimulus	Clinical examples
Pleura Tends to be limited to the affected region but may be referred to the ipsilateral neck or shoulder tip or to the upper abdomen or lower back	Sharp stabbing pain due to inflammation or stretching of the parietal pleura Described as sharp, dull, ache, burning or a catching pain	Exacerbated by deep inspiration, coughing and sneezing May be associated with dyspnoea	Pneumonia, carcinoma, pulmonary tuberculosis, pneumothorax, pleurisy, pulmonary infarction
Chest wall pain Commonly due to strain, inflammation, malposition of, or injury to, muscles, ligaments, cartilage or bone	Usually localized to affected area May be a dull ache or sharper pain	Usually increased on respiratory movements, including deep inspiration and cough Also exacerbated by trunk and shoulder movements	Often seen in patients with chronic cough or dyspnoea Post ICC insertion, CT surgery, fractured ribs, musculoskeletal disorders Tumours involving ribs or soft tissues
Tracheobronchial tree	Generally described as a raw, retrosternal discomfort or a dull ache	Deep inspiration, coughing	Usually acute inflammation from infection or from inhalation of irritant fumes May occur with oxygen therapy

Abbreviations: ICC, intercostal catheter; CT, cardiothoracic

Table 7.10 Causes and characteristic features of chest pain of cardiovascular origin

Cause	Characteristic features	Stimuli
Myocardial ischaemia: 1. Stable angina pectoris	Myocardial ischaemia does not always cause pain Described as severe pressure, squeezing, ache, tightness or retrosternal burning Maximal intensity is retrosternal or to the left of the sternum but may radiate to the neck, jaw, shoulder or down the inner aspects of the arms, more commonly the left Often associated with dyspnoea	Physical exertion – often occurs at the same RPP Emotional stimuli Heavy meal Inhalation of cigarette smoke With rest, the pain tends to subside within 2–10 minutes Relieved by nitroglycerin
2. Unstable angina pectoris 3. Myocardial infarction	As for stable angina Pain is similar to that of angina but is generally more severe and of longer duration	Unpredictable pattern and may occur at rest Usually requires large doses of opiates to control the pain
Pain mimicking angina is common in patients with aortic stenosis and occurs in some patients with mitral valve prolapse, myocarditis and hypertrophic cardiomyopathy		
Pericarditis due to inflammation of parietal pericardium from a variety of causes – bacterial, viral, neoplasm, post-MI	Sharp stabbing pain, central or left side of chest and left arm and may radiate to neck, back and upper abdomen May be associated with friction rub in the absence of effusion	Deep inspiration, supine and left side-lying positions Sitting and leaning forwards may decrease pain
Diseases of the aorta: 1. Aortic stenosis 2. Dissection of the aorta	Produces angina-like pain on exertion Searing severe pain of sudden onset May present in upper back and may radiate to neck and face	
Peripheral arterial disease	Cramp-like pain in the calves, thighs and buttocks May be accompanied by profound weakness in the legs	In the early stages pain occurs on exercise (claudication pain) and is relieved by rest With severe ischaemia, rest pain and paraesthesia occur, especially when in bed

Abbreviations: RPP, rate pressure product (systolic blood pressure x heart rate); MI, myocardial infarction

Cardiovascular origin

Table 7.10 outlines the main causes and characteristic features of pain due to cardiovascular origin

Clinical features and assessment

Clinical features are outlined in Tables 7.9. and 7.10. Associated with the pain may be signs of an abnormal breathing pattern and systemic signs such as sweating, pallor and tachycardia. In addition to the subjective history, pain scales, for example VAS, or pain questionnaires should

be used to quantify pain and its effects on function. In the patient with acute cardiopulmonary dysfunction asking for a verbal rating of pain severity on a 0–10 or 0–5 scale is more appropriate than presenting the patient with a scale. Measurement of the RPP at which pain develops may be useful in patients with angina undergoing exercise testing.

Chest pain which is unrelated to respiratory or cardiovascular disease

Neural, muscular or skeletal pain. Examples of causative factors are disc degeneration, bony metastases, muscle injuries, inflammation of soft tissues and disorders of the costal cartilages.

Oesophageal pain. The causes of pain arising from the oesophagus are:

1. spasm – when this occurs the pain may last up to one hour and there may not be an obvious provoking factor. The pain closely resembles that of unstable angina and is often relieved by nitroglycerin
2. oesophageal tear – this may occur in association with prolonged vomiting. The pain is felt centrally
3. gastro-oesophageal reflux gives rise to pain felt in the centre of the chest and the epigastrium. The pain is increased when lying down and relieved by sitting upright and by taking antacids. The commonest cause is hiatus hernia.

Peptic ulceration and gallbladder disease. Diseases of the stomach, duodenum or biliary system may give rise to pain felt in the chest although it is more commonly confined to the abdomen. With peptic ulceration the pain is burning in nature, occurs following meals and is relieved by antacids.

The postprandial pain occurring in gastric ulceration may resemble angina occurring after a heavy meal.

Pain of biliary origin is usually colicky in nature and felt on the right side of the abdomen, the front and back of the chest. The pain may be related to the ingestion of certain foods.

'Pseudoangina' due to hyperventilation syndrome. Hyperventilation may cause atypical chest pain which may mimic angina in some patients (Gardner 1996).

Medical management

Diagnosis and management of the underlying cause are essential.

Antiinflammatory agents or analgesics are used for musculoskeletal, pleuritic or pericardial pain. Pain relief may also be achieved using acupuncture/acupressure or hypnosis. Medical management of chest pain for coronary insufficiency is based on reducing myocardial oxygen demand.

Management of angina may include pharmacological therapy, angioplasty or coronary artery surgery. Antiarrhythmic drugs and anticoagulants may be indicated in some patients. Management of cardiac dysfunction may include insertion of a pacemaker or heart transplantation.

Methods to reduce risk factors may include education on smoking cessation, the benefits of regular physical exercise, dietary management and the use of lipid-lowering drugs to reduce hyperlipidaemia and body weight, counselling on lifestyle changes and hormone replacement therapy for menopausal women.

Patients and families often require psycho-emotional support especially when pain is of cardiac origin, as such pain is often associated with a fear of impending death.

Management of claudication pain includes the use of analgesics. In some patients, hyperbaric oxygen may be indicated. Revascularization procedures for significant stenosis include bypass surgery (e.g. aortofemoral and axillofemoral bypass) or transluminal angioplasty. Amputation may be necessary if repeated attempts at grafting fail and further grafting becomes impossible.

Physiotherapy management

Direct methods of pain management include heat modalities, interferential, transcutaneous electrical nerve stimulation (p. 231), entonox (p. 383), acupuncture (p. 233) and manual therapy (p. 161). Knowledge of pain management (drugs and their onset/duration of action, route of administration) is required so that treatment can be provided when pain management is optimal.

Education of the patient regarding risk factors for cardiovascular disease (described in the section on medical management) and the implementation of strategies to adopt lifestyle changes, including smoking cessation, dietary control and increasing levels of physical activity, are necessary for many patients with or at risk of cardiovascular disease. For the management of patients with stable angina and patients following myocardial infarction including risk factor modification and exercise training, see Chapter 15 on cardiac rehabilitation.

Special case – intermittent claudication

Exercise training for patients with claudication pain as the limiting factor to exercise is important. Aerobic exercise, such as walking or cycling combined with stretching, is most beneficial (American College of Sports Medicine 1998, Robeer et al 1998). This should take the form of intermittent exercise with the patient exercising to the point of pain intolerance. Progression to continuous aerobic activity is necessary to develop a higher mechanical efficiency for performance of the specific activity and a higher anaerobic capacity (tolerance to ischaemic pain and blood lactate). Improvement of leg muscle oxygenation following exercise training may be due to: increased blood flow through collateral vessels and the development of collaterals, higher arterial-venous oxygen difference locally, more local muscle capillary beds and higher levels of oxidative enzymes.

Education on foot care and hygiene for the prevention of gangrene includes the avoidance of minor trauma, poorly fitted footwear and the importance of regular toenail clipping.

Clinical outcomes

These should include a reduction in pain and an increase in function as measured using pain scales and from subjective questioning. There may be a decreased need for analgesics. In the patient with stable angina pectoris, endurance exercise training should be associated with an improved exercise tolerance and the onset of angina at a higher RPP. An increased distance walked before the onset of leg pain and fatigue, and a reduction in symptoms at rest should occur in the patient with claudication pain.

PROBLEM – MUSCULOSKELETAL DYSFUNCTION: POSTURAL ABNORMALITIES, DECREASED COMPLIANCE OR DEFORMITY OF THE CHEST WALL

The risk of developing chest wall stiffness and abnormal posture is greatest in patients with chronic respiratory disease especially when this is associated with lung hyperinflation. Also at risk are patients following sternotomy or thoracotomy and patients who receive mechanical ventilation for long periods. Changes in muscle length, strength and endurance will occur as a result of chest wall and postural abnormalities. As a number of these patients will be in the older age group they will, in addition, have age-related changes affecting the musculoskeletal system. With increased age, there is a decrease in the range of movement of the costovertebral joints and a decrease in the elasticity of the cartilage in the thoracic spine. These changes increase thoracic kyphosis.

Clinical features and assessment

The patient may present with an abnormal posture, reduced range of movement of the cervical spine, thoracic spine and glenohumeral joint and may complain of pain or stiffness resulting in decreased function.

The assessment of pain, associated functional limitation, posture, muscle length, strength and endurance and joint range of movement are covered in detail in Chapter 6 on physiotherapy skills and techniques.

Medical management

Management of chronic chest wall deformities may include the use of NSAIDs when pain is an accompanying feature. External bracing or surgical correction may be used to correct deformity (Adams & Hamblen 1995).

Physiotherapy management

Physiotherapy management should include, where appropriate, postural correction, stretching techniques (e.g. hold-relax) of tight muscles, mobilizations to the cervical spine and thoracic spine, costotransverse, costochondral and sternochondral joints, to the ribs and to the glenohumeral joint (Bray et al 1995, Vibekk 1991) and muscle-strengthening exercises. Postural correction and stretches to improve chest wall mobility should be incorporated into other active exercises and activities of daily living. Where possible, especially when chronic lung disease is present, patients should be taught to perform their own treatment, including mobilizations.

The patient's position during treatment will need to be carefully selected as many patients will not be able to lie prone or supine due to dyspnoea and mobilizations will have to be performed in sitting or forward lean sitting.

The physiotherapy management of this problem is covered in detail in Chapter 6 on physiotherapy techniques.

Clinical outcomes

These should include improved posture, an increase in VC and in the range of movement of the cervical spine, thoracic spine and glenohumeral joints. Associated with the increased range of movement should be an improvement in function and a decrease in pain. These changes may be associated with a decrease in dyspnoea. The psychosocial benefits may consist of enhanced self-esteem, as a result of improved physical appearance, and improved QOL.

REFERENCES

Adams JC, Hamblen DL 1995 Outline of orthopaedics, 12th edn. Churchill Livingstone, Edinburgh, ch 10

American College of Sports Medicine 1998 ACSM's resource manual for guidelines for exercise testing and prescription, 3rd edn, Williams and Wilkins, Baltimore

Arora NS, Gal TJ 1981 Cough dynamics during progressive expiratory muscle weakness in healthy curarized subjects. Journal of Applied Physiology 5(3): 494–498

Arora NS, Rochester DF 1982 Respiratory muscle strength and maximal voluntary ventilation in undernourished patients. American Review of Respiratory Disease 126(2): 5–9

Balady GJ 1998 Exercise training in the treatment of heart failure: what is achieved and how? Annals of Medicine 30 (suppl 1): 61–65

Barnes PJ 1999 Drugs for airways diseases. Medicine 37–45

Barnes PJ 2000 Airway pharmacology. In: Murray JF, Nadel JA (eds) Respiratory medicine, vol 1, 3rd edn. WB Saunders, Philadelphia, ch 11

Bennett WD, Zeman KL 1994 Effect of supramaximal flows on cough clearance. Journal of Applied Physiology 7: 1577–1583

Bianchi L, Foglio K, Pagani M, Vitacca M, Rossi A, Ambrosino N 1998 Effects of proportional assist ventilation on exercise tolerance in COPD patients with chronic hypercapnia. European Respiratory Journal 11: 422–427

Borg GAV 1982 Psychophysical basis of perceived exertion. Medicine and Science in Sports and Exercise 14: 377–381

Branson RD, Hurst JM 1988 Nutrition and respiratory function: food for thought. Respiratory Care 33(2): 89–92

Bray CE, Partridge JE, Banks SK 1995 Thoracic mobilisation in the management of respiratory and cardiac patients. Proceedings of the Australian Physiotherapy Association Cardiothoracic Special Group, 4th National Conference, 22–24 April, Melbourne

Breslin EH 1995 Breathing retraining in chronic pulmonary disease. Journal of Cardiopulmonary Rehabilitation 15: 25–33

Burns BH, Howell JBL 1969 Disproportionately severe breathlessness in chronic bronchitis. Quarterly Journal of Medicine 38: 277–294

Calverley PMA 1999 Management of chronic obstructive pulmonary disease. Medicine 73–78

Celli BR 1994 Physical reconditioning of patients with respiratory diseases: legs, arms, and breathing retraining. Respiratory Care 39(5): 481–495

Celli BR, Rodriguez KS, Snider GL 1984 A controlled trial of intermittent positive pressure breathing, incentive spirometry, and deep breathing exercises in preventing pulmonary complications after abdominal surgery. American Review of Respiratory Disease 130: 12–15

Cheitlin MD, Sokolow M, McIlroy MB 1993 Clinical cardiology, 6th edn. Prentice Hall, London, pp 39–41

Clanton TL, Diaz PT 1995 Clinical assessment of the respiratory muscles. Physical Therapy 75(11): 983–995

Clarke S 1990 Physical defences. In: Brewis RAL, Gibson GJ, Geddes DM (eds) Respiratory medicine. Baillière Tindall, London, pp 176–189

Conway JH, Fleming JS, Perring S, Holgate ST 1992 Humidification as an adjunct to chest physiotherapy in aiding tracheo-bronchial clearance in patients with bronchiectasis. Respiratory Medicine 86(2): 109–114

Dean E, Ross J 1992 Mobilisation and exercise conditioning. In: Zadai C C (ed) Pulmonary management in physical therapy. Churchill Livingstone, New York, ch 8

Dilworth JP, White RJ 1992 Postoperative chest infection after upper abdominal surgery: an important problem for smokers. Respiratory Medicine 86: 205–210

Eakin E G, Kaplan R M, Ries A L 1993 Measurement of dyspnoea in chronic obstructive pulmonary disease. Quality of Life Research 2: 181–191

Fairshter R D, Williams J H 1987 Pulmonary physiology in the postoperative period. Critical Care Clinics 3(2): 287–306

Ferguson GT 1993 Respiratory muscle function in chronic obstructive pulmonary disease. Seminars in Respiratory Medicine 14(6): 430–445

Fernandez E, Tanchoco-Tan M, Make BJ 1993 Methods to improve respiratory muscle function. Seminars in Respiratory Medicine 14(6): 446–465

Fink JF 2000 Aerosol device selection: evidence to practice. Respiratory Care 45(7): 874–885

Flenley DC 1990 Respiratory medicine, 2nd edn. Bailliére Tindall, London, p 56

Foltz BD, Benumof JL 1987 Mechanisms of hypoxemia and hypercapnia in the perioperative period. Critical Care Clinics 3(2): 269–286

Gardner WN 1996 The pathophysiology of hyperventilation disorders. Chest 109(2): 516–534

Garibaldi RA, Britt MR, Coleman ML, Reading JC, Pace NL 1981 Risk factors for post-operative pneumonia. American Journal of Medicine 70: 677–680

Garrod R, Bestall JC, Paul EA, Wedzicha JA, Jones PW 2000 Development and validation of a standardized measure of activity of daily living in patients with severe COPD: the London Chest Activity of Daily Living scale (LCADL). Respiratory Medicine 94: 589–596

Gass GD, Olsen GN 1986 Preoperative pulmonary function testing to predict postoperative morbidity and mortality. Chest 89(1): 127–135

Gift AG, Plant SM, Jacox A 1986 Psychologic and physiologic factors related to dyspnea in subjects with chronic obstructive pulmonary disease. Heart Lung 15(6): 595–601

Gosselink R, Schrever K, Cops P, et al 2000 Incentive spirometry does not enhance recovery after thoracic surgery. Critical Care Medicine 28(3): 679–683

Guyatt GH, Berman LB, Townsend M, Pugsley SO, Chambers LW 1987 A measure of quality of life for clinical trials. Thorax 42: 773–778

Guyatt GH, Nogradi S, Halcrow S, Singer J, Sullivan MJ, Fallen EL 1989 Development and testing of a new measure of health status for clinical trials in heart failure. General Internal Medicine 4: 101–107

Hall JC, Tarala R, Harris J, Tapper J, Christiansen K 1991 Incentive spirometry versus routine chest physiotherapy for prevention of pulmonary complications after abdominal surgery. Lancet 337: 953–956

Hamilton AL, Killian KJ, Summers E, Jones NL 1995 Muscle strength, symptom intensity, and exercise capacity in patients with cardiorespiratory disorders. American Journal of Respiratory and Critical Care Medicine 152: 2021–2031

Hansen JE, Wasserman K 1996 Pathophysiology of activity limitation in patients with interstitial lung disease. Chest 109(6): 1566–1576

Hara KS, Shepard JW 1990 Sleep and critical care medicine In: Martin RJ (ed) Cardiorespiratory disorders during sleep. Futura, Mount Kisco, pp 324–325

Hardy K A 1994 A review of airway clearance: new techniques, indications and recommendations. Respiratory Care 39(5): 440–452

Honeyman P, Barr P, Stubbing DG 1996 Effect of a walking aid on disability, oxygenation, and breathlessness in patients with chronic airflow limitation. Journal of Cardiopulmonary Rehabilitation 16: 63–67

Horiuchi K, Jordan D, Cohen D, Kemper MC, Weissman C 1997 Insights into the increased oxygen demand during chest physiotherapy. Critical Care Medicine 25: 1347–1351

Hough A 1996 Physiotherapy in respiratory care. A problem-solving approach to respiratory and cardiac management, 2nd edn. Chapman and Hall, London, pp 164–166

Houtmeyers E, Gosselink R, Gayan-Ramirez G, Decramer M 1999 Regulation of mucociliary clearance in health and disease. European Respiratory Journal 13: 1177–1188

Hyland ME, Bott J, Singh S, Kenyon CAP 1994 Domains, constructs and the development of the breathing problems questionnaire. Quality of Life Research 3: 245–256

Irwin RS, Widdicombe J 2000 Cough. In: Murray J F, Nadel JA (eds) Textbook of respiratory medicine, vol 1, 3rd edn. WB Saunders, Philadelphia, ch 21

Jenkins SC, Moxham J 1991 The effects of mild obesity on lung function. Respiratory Medicine 85: 309–311

Jenkins SC, Soutar SA, Moxham J 1988 The effects of posture on lung volumes in normal subjects and in patients pre- and post-coronary artery surgery. Physiotherapy 74(10): 492–496

Jenkins SC, Soutar SA, Loukota JM, Johnson LC, Moxham J 1989 Physiotherapy after coronary artery surgery- are breathing exercises necessary? Thorax 44: 634–639

Jenkins SC, Soutar SA, Loukota JM, Johnson LC, Moxham J 1990 A comparison of breathing exercises, incentive spirometry and mobilisation after coronary artery surgery. Physiotherapy Theory and Practice 6: 117–126

Jenne JW 1993 Pharmacology in the respiratory patient. In: Hodgkin JE, Connors GL, Bell WC (eds) Pulmonary rehabilitation. Guidelines to success, 2nd edn. Lippincott, Philadelphia, ch 9

Johnson NT, Pierson DJ 1986 The spectrum of pulmonary atelectasis: pathophysiology, diagnosis, and therapy. Respiratory Care 31(11): 1107–1120

Jones PW, Quirk FH, Baveystock CM 1991 The St George's Respiratory Questionnaire. Respiratory Medicine 85(suppl B): 25–31

Jones PW, Quirk FH, Baveystock CM, Littlejohns P 1992 A self-complete measure of health status for chronic airflow limitation. The St. George's respiratory questionnaire. American Review of Respiratory Disease 145: 1321–1327

Judson MA, Sahn SA 1994 Mobilization of secretions in ICU patients. Respiratory Care 39(3): 213–226

Keilty SEJ, Ponte J, Fleming TA, Moxham J 1994 Effect of inspiratory pressure support on exercise tolerance and breathlessness in patients with severe stable chronic obstructive pulmonary disease. Thorax 49: 990–994

Lareau SC, Carrieri-Kohlman V, Janson-Bjerklie S, Roos P 1994 Development and testing of the pulmonary functional status and dyspnea questionnaire. Heart Lung 23: 242–250

Lareau SC, Meek PM, Roos PJ 1998 Development and testing of the modified version of the pulmonary functional status and dyspnea questionnaire (PFSDQ-M). Heart Lung 27: 159–168

Lareau SC, ZuWallack R, Carlin B et al, 1999 Pulmonary rehabilitation – 1999. American Journal of Respiratory and Critical Care Medicine 159: 1666–1682

Levison H, Cherniack RM 1968 Ventilatory cost of exercise in chronic obstructive pulmonary disease. Journal of Applied Physiology 25: 21–25

Locke TJ, Griffiths TL, Mould H, Gibson GJ 1990 Rib cage mechanics after median sternotomy. Thorax 45: 465–468

MacIntyre N R 1990 Respiratory monitoring without machinery. Respiratory Care 35(6): 546–553

Mahler D A 1987 Dyspnea: diagnosis and management. Clinics in Chest Medicine 8(2): 215–230

Markwell S, Sapsford R 1995 Physiotherapy management of obstructed defaecation. Australian Journal of Physiotherapy 41(4): 279–283

Mathews A, Ridgeway V 1981 Personality and surgical recovery: a review. British Journal of Clinical Psychology 20: 243–260

McCarren B 1992 Dynamic pulmonary hyperinflation. Australian Journal of Physiotherapy 38(3): 175–179

Meek P M, Schwartzstein R M, Adams L et al 1999 Dyspnea. Mechanisms, assessment and management: a consensus statement. American Journal of Respiratory and Critical Care Medicine 159: 321–340

Meyers JR, Lembeck L, O'Kane H, Baue AE 1975 Changes in functional residual capacity of the lung after operation. Archives of Surgery 110: 576–583

Mitchell C, Garrahy P, Peake P 1982 Postoperative respiratory morbidity: Identification and risk factors. Australian and New Zealand Journal of Surgery 52(2): 203–209

Morran CG, Finlay IG, Mathieson M, McKay AJ, Wilson N, McArdle CS 1983 Randomized controlled trial of physiotherapy for post-operative pulmonary complications. British Journal of Anaesthesia 55: 1113–1116

Moss M, Make BJ 1993 Pulmonary response to exercise in health and disease. Seminars in Respiratory Medicine 14(2): 106–120

Moxham J 1999 Respiratory muscles. Medicine 126–129

Murray JF, Gebhart GF 2000 Chest pain. In: Murray JF, Nadel JA (eds) Textbook of respiratory medicine, vol 1, 3rd edn. WB Saunders, Philadelphia, ch 22

Nunn JF 1987 Applied respiratory physiology, 3rd edn. Butterworths, London

O'Donnell DE 1994 Breathlessness in patients with chronic airflow limitation. Mechanisms and management. Chest 106: 904–912

Oh TE 1997 Oxygen therapy. In: Oh TE (ed) Intensive care manual, 4th edn. Butterworths, Oxford, pp. 209–216

O'Neill S, McCarthy DS 1983 Postural relief of dyspnoea in severe chronic airflow limitation: Relationship to respiratory muscle strength. Thorax 38: 595–600

Orfanos P, Ellis ER, Johnston C 1999 Effects of deep breathing exercises and ambulation on pattern of ventilation in post-operative patients. Australian Journal of Physiotherapy 45: 173–182

Pardy RL, Hussain SNA, Macklem PT 1984 The ventilatory pump in exercise. Clinics in Chest Medicine 5(1): 35–49

Pearce AC, Jones RM 1984 Smoking and anaesthesia: preoperative abstinence and perioperative morbidity. Anesthesiology 61: 576–584

Phillips BA, Berry DTR, Schmitt FA, Magan LK, Gerhardstein DC, Cook YR 1992 Sleep-disordered breathing in the healthy elderly. Clinically significant? Chest 101(2): 345–349

Platell C, Hall JC 1997 Atelectasis after abdominal surgery. Journal of the American College of Surgeons 185: 584–592

Polkey MI, Green M, Moxham J 1995 Measurement of respiratory muscle strength. Thorax 50: 1131–1135

Puchelle E, Zahm JM, Girard F, Bertrand A, Polu J M, Aug F, Sadoul P 1980 Mucociliary transport in vivo and in vitro: relations to sputum properties in chronic bronchitis. European Journal of Respiratory Diseases 61(suppl): 254–264

Raw M, McNeill A, West R 1998 Smoking cessation guidelines for health professionals. Thorax 53(suppl 5, part 1): S1–S19

Robeer GG, Brandsma JW, Van Den Heuvel SP, Smit B, Oostendorp RA, Wittens CH 1998 Exercise therapy for intermittent claudication: a review of the quality of randomised clinical trials and evaluation of predictive factors. European Journal of Vascular and Endovascular Surgery 15(1): 36–43

Rochester DF, Esau SA 1984 Malnutrition and the respiratory system. Chest 85(3): 411–415

Roukema JA, Carol EJ, Prins JG 1988 The prevention of pulmonary complications after upper abdominal surgery in patients with noncompromised pulmonary status. Archives of Surgery 123: 30–34

Ruppel G 1998 Manual of pulmonary function testing, 7th edn. Mosby, St Louis, p 77

Schmidt GA, Hall JB, Wood LDH 2000 Ventilatory failure. In: Murray JF, Nadel JA (eds) Textbook of respiratory medicine, vol 2, 3rd edn. WB Saunders, Philadelphia, ch 93

Sibuya M, Yamada M, Kanamaru A et al 1994 Effect of chest wall vibration on dyspnea in patients with chronic respiratory disease. American Journal of Critical Care Medicine 149: 1235–1240

Smith MCL, Ellis ER 2000 Is retained mucus a risk factor for the development of postoperative atelectasis and pneumonia? Implications for the physiotherapist. Physiotherapy Theory and Practice 16: 69–80

Stiller KR, Munday RM 1992 Chest physiotherapy for the surgical patient. British Journal of Surgery 79: 745–749

Stiller K, Montarello J, Wallace M et al H 1994 Are breathing and coughing exercises necessary after coronary artery surgery? Physiotherapy Theory and Practice 10: 143–152

Stock MC, Downs JB, Cooper RB et al 1984 Comparison of continuous positive airway pressure, incentive spirometry, and conservative therapy after cardiac operations. Critical Care Medicine 12(11): 969–972

Storms WW 1999 Exercise induced asthma: diagnosis and treatment for the recreational or elite athlete. Medicine and Science in Sports and Exercise 31(1) (suppl): S33–S38

Stulbarg MS, Adams L 2000 Dyspnea. In: Murray JF, Nadel JA (eds) Textbook of respiratory medicine, vol 1, 3rd edn. WB Saunders, Philadelphia, ch 20

Thomas PS, Cowen ERT, Hulands G, Milledge JS 1989 Respiratory function in the morbidly obese before and after weight loss. Thorax 44: 382–386

Tisi GM 1979 Preoperative evaluation of pulmonary function. Validity, indications and benefits. American Review of Respiratory Disease 119: 293–310

Tobin MJ 1990 Dyspnea. Pathophysiologic basis, clinical presentation, and management. Archives of Internal Medicine 150: 1604–1613

Turkington PM, Elliott MW 2000 Rationale for the use of non-invasive ventilation in chronic ventilatory failure. Thorax 55: 417–423

Vas Fragoso CA 1993 Monitoring in adult critical care. In: Kacmarek RM, Hess D, Stoller JK (eds) Monitoring in respiratory care. Mosby, St Louis, ch 21

Vibekk P 1991 Chest mobilization and respiratory function. In: Pryor JA (eds) Respiratory care. Churchill Livingstone, Edinburgh, pp 103–119

Walker JM, Tan L-B 1997 Cardiovascular disease. In: Souhami RL, Moxham J (eds) Textbook of medicine, 3rd edn. Churchill Livingstone, Edinburgh, pp 381–505

Warner MA, Offord KP, Warner ME, Lennon RL, Conover MA, Jansson-Schumacher U 1989 Role of preoperative cessation of smoking and other factors in postoperative pulmonary complications: a blinded prospective study of coronary artery bypass patients. Mayo Clinic Proceedings 64: 609–616

Wasserman K, Hansen JE, Sue DY, Whipp BJ 1987 Principles of exercise testing and interpretation. Lea and Febiger, Philadelphia, pp 47–57

Wedzicha JA 2000 Long-term oxygen therapy. In: Donner CF, Decramer M (eds) Pulmonary rehabilitation. European Respiratory Monograph (vol 5, monograph 13), ch 13

Weil JV, McCullough RE, Kline JS, Sodal IE 1975 Diminished ventilatory response to hypoxia and hypercpania after morphine in normal man. New England Journal of Medicine 292: 1103–1106

Weiser PC, Mahler DA, Ryan KP, Hill KL, Greenspon LW 1993 Dyspnea:Symptom assessment and management. In: Hodgkin JE, Connors GL, Bell CW (eds) Pulmonary rehabilitation. Guidelines to success, 2nd edn. Lippincott, Philadelphia, ch 26

West JB 1998 Pulmonary pathophysiology – the essentials, 5th edn. Williams and Wilkins, Baltimore

West JB 2000 Respiratory physiology – the essentials, 6th edn. Williams and Wilkins, Baltimore

White D, Stiller K, Roney F 2000 The prevalence and severity of symptoms of incontinence in adult cystic fibrosis patients. Physiotherapy Theory and Practice 16: 35–42

Wigal JK, Creer TL, Kotses H 1991 The COPD self-efficacy scale. Chest 99: 1193–1196

Wilkins RL, Sheldon RL, Krider SJ 1995 Clinical assessment in respiratory care, 3rd edn. Mosby, St Louis, p 58

Windsor JA, Hill GL 1988 Risk factors for post-operative pneumonia. The importance of protein depletion. Annals of Surgery 208(2): 209–214

Wolff RK, Dolovich MB, Obminski G, Newhouse MT 1977 Effects of exercise and eucapnic hyperventilation on bronchial clearance in man. Journal of Applied Physiology 43(1): 46–50

Yeates DB, Mortensen J 2000 Deposition and clearance. In Murray JF, Nadel JA (eds) Textbook of respiratory medicine, vol 1, 3rd edn, WB Saunders, Philadelphia, ch 15

Youtsey JW 1994 Oxygen and mixed gas therapy. In: Barnes TA (ed) Core textbook of respiratory care practice, 2nd edn. Mosby, St Louis, p 150

Zadai CC, Irwin S 1992 Exercise pathophysiology: pulmonary impairment. In: Zadai CC (ed) Pulmonary management in physical therapy. Churchill Livingstone, New York, ch 3

8

Interpersonal aspects of care: communication, counselling and health education

Julius Sim

INTRODUCTION

The intention of this chapter is to provide an insight into the part that various features of interpersonal communication can play in the management of patients with cardiac and respiratory problems. In addition to a general account of the role of communication in the therapeutic relationship, particular attention will be given to two specialist applications of communication, namely counselling and health education. Some of the associated ethical issues will also be touched upon. Underlying the discussion in this chapter is the notion that the disability and handicap associated with illness – and chronic illness especially – occur within a social and interpersonal context and are not merely the result of a biological process. The effective care and rehabilitation of patients with cardiorespiratory dysfunction must acknowledge this.

In order to examine these aspects of the physiotherapist's work, it is necessary to explore the psychological and social aspects of cardiorespiratory dysfunction. Accordingly, it is to these topics that the first part of this chapter is directed.

PSYCHOSOCIAL DIMENSIONS OF CARDIORESPIRATORY DYSFUNCTION

Like all illnesses, those of cardiorespiratory origin have psychosocial as well as physiological dimensions. Thus, at a general level, social factors play a part in the aetiology of many chronic respiratory diseases and such patients come disproportionately from the lower social classes (French 1997, Williams 1989) and from areas characterized by industrialization. Psychological factors may be similarly implicated, either as aetiological factors in their own right or as significant co-factors. Once a cardiac or respiratory disease has become established in a particular individual, it impinges on the person's consciousness. The objective biological fact of dysfunction becomes a subjective experience (Nicholls 2000); a disease becomes an illness (Sim 1990a). This has ramifications beyond the biological to the psychosocial sphere. Figure 8.1 illustrates the way in which a physiological phenomenon such as bronchospasm may impinge on various levels of physical, psychological and social functioning. Subjective health perception will determine the individual's quality of life, often to a greater degree than objective disease severity (Staab et al 1998).

Consequently, a problem-oriented or problem-based assessment of the cardiorespiratory patient (see Ch. 1) should encompass psychosocial as well as physical factors. The problems identified in the course of the assessment will consist of those to do with the condition as it is subjectively experienced as well as its physical manifestations. Of course, the same clinical feature will very often represent problems of both types – for example, breathlessness – and there will be an interaction between the physical and the psychological factors. However, it should be noted that the degree to which patients experience subjec-tive problems may only be weakly related to the severity of such objective factors as airflow limitation (Guyatt et al 1987, Morgan et al 1983, Pinkerton et al 1985, Snadden & Brown 1992).

Some psychosocial features of cardiorespiratory illness

It will be useful to look briefly at just some of the specific social and psychological forces that operate in cardiorespiratory illness.

Anxiety

Many of the symptoms experienced by cardiac or respiratory patients are particularly distressing, e.g. breathlessness, palpitations, angina and bronchospasm. This is not only due to their inherent unpleasantness but also because their onset is frequently unexpected and unpredictable. The asthmatic patient may be prone to an attack with little warning. Suddenness of onset is perhaps the characteristic most associated with angina. The popular image of conditions such as these tends to exaggerate their more dramatic features; this is likely to have been internalized by the patient and may heighten feelings of anxiety. Stress and anxiety are also associated with the trajectory of the disease. In cystic fibrosis, for example, there may be a pervading sense of uncertainty regarding disease progression, prospects of cure, life expectancy and social reaction (Waddell 1982). Aspects of treatment and management can also

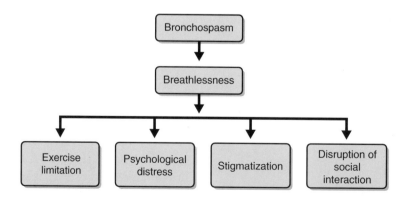

Figure 8.1 Relationship of bronchospasm to the functional, psychological and social aspects of respiratory dysfunction.

produce anxiety. Strange environments such as the intensive care unit can give rise to disorientation, loneliness, fear and helplessness (Hough 1996). According to a study by Williams, some patients find exercise tests not only distressing and anxiety provoking, but even 'unethical or punitive' (Williams 1993, p 37).

Fear

Closely linked to anxiety is fear. In conditions whose prognosis is unfavourable, such as cryptogenic fibrosing alveolitis or carcinoma of the lung, a sense of fear regarding the future may be a more or less constant emotion. In conditions such as asthma, angina or myocardial infarction, fear may manifest itself in the sense of panic that accompanies an attack (Bennett 1993, Snadden & Brown 1992). Fear of unpleasant symptoms may lead to a vicious cycle of inactivity (Gibson 1997).

Defence mechanisms

Patients may respond to crises, such as a diagnosis of heart disease or bronchial carcinoma, with a variety of responses. These may include maladaptive psychotic mechanisms such as denial, distortion and projection or less severe neurotic mechanisms such as displacement, intellectualization and repression (Porritt 1990). In cases of cystic fibrosis, where the family impact of the diagnosis is especially great (Dushenko 1981), these reactions may involve parents as well as patients themselves.

Depression

Reactive depression is relatively common in cases of chronic cardiac and respiratory impairment. Indeed, psychiatric morbidity has been reported in 42–50% of patients with chronic bronchitis (McSweeny et al 1982, Rutter 1977).

Stigmatization

Symptoms of cardiorespiratory dysfunction may become a source of stigma, owing to their disruptive effect on smooth social interaction (Sim

1990b). An awareness of others' discomfort at their breathlessness may cause patients with advanced emphysema to curtail social contact (Fagerhaugh 1973). Patients and families with cystic fibrosis may experience stigmatization (Waddell 1982) and this may arise from a number of the clinical features of this condition; for example, coughing, expectoration and flatus. Williams (1993, p 110) points out that such symptoms 'tend to violate tacit, yet culturally entrenched, social expectations, codes of etiquette and decorum, found deeply embedded within routine social interaction'. In addition, factors such as diminutive stature, underweight and delayed development of secondary sex characteristics may adversely affect body image (Johannesson et al 1998, Simmons et al 1985). Perceived lack of attractiveness may reduce social confidence and inhibit sexual and emotional relationships, leading to feelings of reduced self-worth. Many males with cystic fibrosis are infertile, which may undermine feelings of manhood.

Loss of self

Radley (1994) uses this term to describe the changes in self-concept imposed on a person with a chronic illness. The individual's world and his or her place within it, have to be reappraised and cognitively restructured, which may be painful and hard to accept. Similarly, Bury (1982) uses the term 'biographical disruption' to describe the life-changing impact of chronic illness.

Disruption of family relationships

Although in some cases illness can cause a strengthening of family ties, in other cases it can be a source of stress or conflict. The need to look after a disabled spouse, with the resulting toll on financial, personal and emotional resources, can place strain on the marital relationship (Williams 1993). Lask (2000) describes the effect of cystic fibrosis on the family as 'devastating'. There may be strong feelings of guilt in the parents, in view of the hereditary nature of the disease, and resentment in the child at the degree of dependency on his or her parents and the restrictions that treatment imposes on social activities and mixing with peers. Overprotectiveness on the part of the parents may keep the child from normal activities with those of the same age and lead to a degree of social isolation (Norman & Hodson 1983). Adolescence is a time when family relationships may be especially strained (Dushenko 1981). Beyond the confines of the family, social networks and peer groups can be important determinants of well-being (D'Auria et al 2000, Lask 2000, Snadden & Brown 1992). Clearly, an assessment of the patient that focuses solely on the individual and neglects his or her family and social context, will necessarily be incomplete.

Lay conceptions of health

As with all diseases and illnesses, patients (and, of course, non-patients) have their own cultural conceptions of cardiac and respiratory conditions (Helman 2000). These lay beliefs will determine how the aetiology, clinical features and treatment of these conditions are regarded and although they may depart considerably from orthodox biomedical explanations, such beliefs may be rational and internally consistent (Donovan et al 1989).

These, then, are some of the psychosocial features of cardiorespiratory dysfunction. An awareness of these aspects of the individual's illness is crucial to the success of subsequent management and treatment (Williams 1993). However, these are processes that have their own important psychosocial dimension and these too should be understood.

PSYCHOSOCIAL ASPECTS OF CARE AND TREATMENT

There are certain features of the physiotherapist–patient relationship that have an important bearing on issues to do with communication. Above all, it tends to be an unequal relationship, with a differential distribution of power. The physiotherapist has specialized technical knowledge that the patient usually lacks, thereby creating a competency gap, reinforced by the fact that, in the hospital setting at least, the physiotherapist is on 'home ground' whereas the patient is in an unfamiliar environment.

Coupled with this competency gap in many cases may be a status gap. One of the key features of the doctor–patient relationship is the difference in social status that may exist between the doctor and the patient; the same obtains, although to a less marked degree, in the case of the physiotherapist and the patient. When this status gap exists, the professional can use superior social status to enhance his or her standing as 'expert' to exert leverage on the client (Freidson 1962). Physiotherapists are not immune from such tendencies (Hugman 1991). In the process, patients or clients are likely to be inhibited in initiating or discussing their own agenda of topics or concerns (Tuckett et al 1985) and 'the transmission of information is likely to be halting and imperfect' (Thompson 1984, p 89). This is compounded by a tendency for patients (or parents) and practitioners to employ different terminology and frames of reference when communicating (Østergaard 1998).

There is also a tendency (perhaps more in hospital and acute care settings than in community healthcare) for the physiotherapist to act as an 'active initiator', leading the interaction and setting the agenda for treatment, while the patient assumes the role of 'passive responder'. As a result, the physiotherapist will tend to set the agenda for the encounter and direct the flow and pattern of communication. There may therefore be a neglect of issues which are of concern to the patient, but which the physiotherapist is unaware of or unconcerned with.

Finally, an element of professional distance or detachment characterizes the practitioner's role. This is reinforced by such factors as the wearing of uniform, the avoidance of certain kinds of informality and simple physical distance. There are, however, certain features of the physiotherapist's role that tend to reduce professional distance. Physiotherapists are generally in frequent and prolonged contact with their patients, which may allow a certain degree of informality to develop between them. In addition, they are usually in a position of close physical proximity, with varying degrees of direct physical contact. The determinants of professional distance can therefore be adjusted when appropriate in order to facilitate the communication process.

Categories of intervention

The physiotherapist's role with respect to the cardiorespiratory patient can be divided into three forms of involvement:

1. *Physical treatment* – this involves the direct use of various physical modalities, such as breathing exercises, airway clearance techniques, chest shaking.
2. *Psychological care* – given that most respiratory conditions have little prospect of ultimate cure, assisting the patient in coming to terms with the impact of respiratory impairment is an important part of the therapist's role. This may involve some form of counselling.
3. *Education* – by various forms of health education, the physiotherapist can help the patient adapt to the functional constraints imposed by cardiorespiratory impairment and can encourage preventive strategies that may limit further deterioration.

There is, of course, no real dividing line between these areas of involvement. Physical treatment can have direct psychological benefit; for example, anxiety and depression may respond favourably to pulmonary rehabilitation (Withers et al 1999). Equally, psychological care can enhance the effectiveness of physical treatment by lessening anxiety and increasing adherence (Bott 1997). Similarly, by fostering a sense of purpose, self-confidence and empowerment, health education can provide the patient with psychological support. Above all, these facets of the therapist's role have in common the need for effective communication and it is to this that we will now turn.

COMMUNICATION

A model of the communication process

Communication is a complex process, involving both verbal and non-verbal elements. Verbal communication can be either oral or written. Non-verbal communication incorporates such factors as facial expression, body language, spatial factors such as the relative position of the participants and ecological factors relating to the environment in which communication occurs, with its various visual, olfactory and other exteroceptive stimuli. Verbal and non-verbal elements of communication exist in a mutual relationship, such that they can either reinforce or counteract one another. Northouse & Northouse (1992, p 118) suggest four reasons why non-verbal elements of communication may be particularly important in the context of healthcare:

1. To lessen feelings of uncertainty and anxiety, patients become particularly sensitive to non-verbal cues from health professionals.
2. Patients may not wholly trust or believe the explicit information given to them by healthcare staff and may seek to discern the 'true' message from non-verbal communication on the part of the professional.
3. Patients may rely on non-verbal cues for information before any verbal interaction has occurred.
4. If a practitioner seems to be busy or unapproachable, patients may rely heavily on non-verbal messages.

For a single communication act, there will be an *initiator*, who encodes the intended meaning into a message of a certain form (e.g. a sentence with a certain grammatical structure) that is then transferred by means of a *medium* (e.g. the spoken word) to a *recipient*, who decodes the message. This process is subject to slippage at virtually any point: the process of encoding can distort the intended message; the medium can lend changes in emphasis or undertones of meaning (e.g. tone of voice or its absence in the case of written communication); there can be further distortion as the recipient decodes the message (e.g. words may be taken to have a different meaning or connotation from that intended or may even be unintelligible); or non-verbal behaviour can be taken as a gloss on the message which may or may not accord with the desired meaning.

Moreover, just as the recipient responds to the message, so the initiator monitors and reacts to the recipient's response in an ongoing feedback process (e.g. signs of non-comprehension are likely to prompt elaboration, whereas apparent understanding will probably encourage the initiator to encode a fresh message). Although it is helpful for the purposes of analysis to look at single communication acts, they are of course not discrete events, like shots in a game of tennis. There is, rather, a constant interplay within as well as between communication acts – the initiator relies on constant feedback from the recipient during the process of encoding, while the recipient similarly relies on various cues from the initiator while decoding. The roles of initiator and recipient are held simultaneously, not sequentially.

For purposes of clarity, the communication process so far has been seen as involving just two participants; needless to say, the intricacy and essential vulnerability of the process increase when more than two participants are involved. The complexity of the communication process suggests:

- that it is likely to take different forms in different contexts and to serve different purposes
- that it requires a considerable degree of skill in the participants if it is to be effective
- that there are a large number of diverse factors which are capable of enhancing or detracting from the process.

Purposes of communication

In a therapeutic setting, there are many possible purposes of communication, of which perhaps the foremost are to:

- pass on information
- gain or extract information
- establish interpersonal relationships
- influence another's attitudes, opinions or behaviour
- express feelings or emotions

- gain an understanding of others' feelings, emotions, attitudes, etc.
- create or maintain personal identity.

Any of these purposes can, of course, be held by either physiotherapist or patient and can exist in virtually any combination. Moreover, they can be held either consciously or subconsciously. They can also be characterized as predominantly either instrumental or expressive. Instrumental communication is that which aims to secure a particular outcome or accomplish a specific task, such as when a physiotherapist asks a patient to take a deep breath or requests a specific item of factual information. Expressive communication has to do with the communication of emotions or states of mind and does not require (though of course it often obtains) a response from the other participant. Expressive communication is often referred to as 'consummatory', in that 'the goal is achieved by the act of communicating' (Dickson et al 1989, p 10). Expressive and instrumental aspects of communication often come together in a single communication act. Thus, a physiotherapist may smile at a patient to convey a feeling of caring (expressive goal) or to reassure the patient (instrumental goal) or, of course, for both reasons.

Detractors from effective communication

There are a number of factors that can undermine effective physiotherapist–patient communication.

Inappropriate attitudes. If viewed as a set of skills or techniques alone, communication will be ineffective. MacWhannell (1992) contends that a prerequisite for effective communication is a willingness to form a relationship and an accompanying quality of 'openness'. Negative attitudes to the other person, an unwillingness to listen to unwelcome or unpleasant messages or an impatience to speak oneself will all impede good communication (Inman & Katz 1997).

Inadequate skills. A disproportionate focus on the acquisition of motor skills and manual techniques during their training may cause physiotherapists to overlook the fact that communication is a skill that can be learnt like any other. Listening skills are just as important as those concerned with the delivery of messages (Nelson-Jones 1990). In particular, the therapist should acquire the skills of 'active listening', in which the listener overtly displays the fact that he or she is paying attention to what is being said (Hargie et al 1994). Ramsden (1999) points out that special skills are required for effective communication in health-care and one cannot simply rely on the habits of everyday interaction.

Language-related factors. As part of the competency gap identified earlier, health professionals are in possession of a specialized vocabulary that is likely to be unfamiliar to most patients. The inappropriate use of jargon fosters 'unshared meanings' and hinders effective communication (Northouse & Northouse 1992); therapists should learn 'when and how to use professional jargon and translate it into lay terms' (Purtilo 1990, p 124). Syntax is equally important; complex, lengthy sentences may obscure meaning and confuse the recipient. The term 'register' is defined as 'a variety of the use of language as used by a particular speaker or writer in a particular context' (Darbyshire 1967, p 23); the choice of inappropriate register in a therapeutic context will clearly detract from communication.

Emotional factors. Various emotions on the part of one or both participants may obscure or distort intended meanings. Fear, anxiety, defencelessness, embarrassment, hostility and depression are common emotional responses in healthcare contexts which may prevent good communication, particularly if they are unacknowledged by one or both parties.

Cultural factors. Certain features of verbal and non-verbal communication carry different meanings from culture to culture. As an example, the degree of touch or eye contact acceptable in Latin cultures is greater than in Western Europe (Hyland & Donaldson 1989). Argyle (1988) notes that, during conversation, Arabs will exhibit a far higher degree of mutual gaze than British or American interlocutors and that black Americans exhibit less eye contact, during both talking and listening, than white Americans. If one does not make proper allowance for such cultural variations, communication is likely to be misinterpreted.

Noise. The term 'noise' is applied to any form of extraneous interference to the communication process. It may take the form of: visual, auditory or olfactory distractions; impairment of visual cues between participants; concurrent activity that diverts attention; physical discomfort; unconducive positioning of participants, etc. It is not hard to imagine how all of these could simultaneously detract from communication in a setting such as an intensive care unit.

Physiological factors. In advanced chronic obstructive airways disease, dyspnoea and hypoxia may cause communication difficulties (Gibson 1997), making it difficult both to talk and to listen.

Facilitators of communication

To a large extent, factors that facilitate communication are the obverse of those that detract from it. Thus, the appropriate choice of register, judicious selection of vocabulary, absence of 'noise' and appropriate attitudes will all make for good communication. However, there are also some more specific considerations that will allow positive steps to improve communication.

Positioning. It is important to consider the appropriate use of physical distance. Hall (1966) has defined four basic distances for social interaction, ranging from 'intimate distance' (from direct contact to 18 inches between participants) to 'public distance' (12–25 feet or more between participants). It is clear that many of the physiotherapist's activities will bring him or her into the intimate distance, with the risk of invading the patient's personal space. At times, such as when implicit permission has not been gained, such intimacy may be a barrier to communication. On other occasions, when more expressive purposes are concerned, such proximity can instil confidence and a sense of caring and thereby enhance communication; use of public distance in such a case would be clearly inappropriate. Exaggerated physical distance from a patient who is expectorating can easily convey a sense of discomfort or distaste. The relative height of participants is also important. MacWhannell (1992) points out that an action such as sitting on the patient's bed facilitates eye contact and promotes a feeling of equality. It also counteracts the feeling of hurriedness that can often seem to characterize therapeutic activities.

Posture and gestures. For the purposes of analysing communication, there are two fundamental types of bodily posture. A closed posture is one that indicates that social interaction is not desired, whereas an open posture signals a willingness to interact (Hyland & Donaldson 1989). Sitting back in a chair with legs closely crossed and arms folded defensively would be a typical closed posture. Gestures, used appropriately, can illustrate meaning and be used as a form of emphasis. Excessive gesturing can, however, constitute a source of 'noise'. Posture and gestures can convey strong messages regarding the attitudes, emotions and status of the individual (Niven 2000) and should therefore be considered carefully when communicating with patients.

Facial expression and eye contact. Appropriate use of facial expression and eye contact can reinforce communication. Signs of attentiveness on the part of the physiotherapist provide positive feedback and encourage the patient to communicate more openly. The phenomenon of 'turn-taking' in conversation is partially governed by the participants' control of eye contact (Hargie et al 1994). Although in some situations it can connote hostility, eye contact is often a sign of affinity between individuals and can therefore be used by the therapist to create empathy. It can also be used to counteract various emotional detractors from communication. Avoiding eye contact can help to eliminate inappropriate levels of arousal and thus defuse aggression and hostility (Hyland & Donaldson 1989). When engaged in intimate procedures that might cause embarrassment to the patient, minimizing eye contact can help to define the procedure as instrumental rather than expressive and thus reduce embarrassment. Argyle (1983) notes that excessive eye contact, in the form of 'mutual gaze', can be distracting.

Context. Certain situations are more conducive to communication than others. An environment that is perceived as private, comfortable and calm is liable to facilitate the exchange of information and its retention. Similarly, the nature of concurrent activity may determine the ease with which a patient may ask questions (Alder 1995).

Touch. Judicious use of touch can convey liking and a sense of caring (Swain 1997). Porritt (1990, p 8) notes that the 'laying on of hands has always been synonymous with healing and these days is an important counter-balance to the technology of health care'. However, bodily touching can carry powerful emotional, sexual and cultural undertones (Lawler 1991). There is, therefore, a risk that touch may be perceived as inappropriate. Purtilo (1990, p 145) notes that the health professional, who is accustomed to touching patients, 'probably has so firm a concept of his or her good intentions that the question of inappropriateness or improper familiarity never arises'. Accordingly, Hargie et al (1994) emphasize the necessity of ensuring that touch on the part of health professionals is not misinterpreted. Hyland & Donaldson (1989) point out that touching often connotes dependency on the part of the person touched and that this may not be welcomed. Men and women may react differently to touch (Whitcher & Fisher 1979). Hargie et al (1994) note that certain groups of individuals, such as elderly people with no close relatives or those who have been widowed (categories which are likely to include many patients with chronic respiratory illness), may rarely experience touch from others and to this extent are deprived of a certain degree of emotional fulfilment. They point out that health professionals, by the appropriate use of touch, can help to redress this deficiency.

Memory

An important feature of effective communication is the ability of participants to retain information that is imparted. Although it is crucial that communication in the physiotherapist–patient relationship should be a two-way process, specific problems of recall seem to occur most often on the part of the patient. Reflecting this concern, extensive research has been conducted within health-

Box 8.1 Strategies to facilitate memory	
Utilizing primacy and recency effects	Information given either at the beginning or the end of the encounter tends to be retained best
Limiting the number of items of information given	Too many items can lead to 'overcrowding' of the short-term memory
Emphasizing the key points	This can be done by using repetition or by explicitly highlighting items
Categorization	Information is placed into separate categories, which are explicitly identified to the patient
Simplification	Short words and sentences are generally better and jargon should be avoided; the content of information should also be simple; whilst patients may comprehend complex ideas, they are likely not to retain them
Being specific	Instructions in particular should be specific rather than general
Providing feedback	This can be either positive or negative
Using written reinforcement	This gives the patient a source of subsequent reference
Making use of 'dual encoding'	The use of both concrete and abstract concepts brings into play both hemispheres of the brain when the information is processed by the listener
Contextualization	Information or instructions should be conveyed in the context in which they need to be recalled; alternatively, a variety of contexts should be used if information needs to be generalized
Cueing	Especially when behaviour has to be remembered (e.g. exercises or postural drainage), specific regular cues for recall, such as a radio programme or a meal, can be suggested

care on factors that may either hinder or facilitate memory and thus determine the degree of subsequent adherence (Ley 1988). Box 8.1 summarizes some of the principal steps that can be taken to maximize the information that patients will retain and recall; Ley (1988) provides further discussion of these and other factors. Baddeley (1997) contains a comprehensive coverage of this topic. It is important to stress that such techniques, useful though they are, should not be seen as a substitute for the less tangible interpersonal skills and attitudes that help to create the sort of relationship with the patient that is a prerequisite for good communication.

The importance of communication

As Thompson (1984, p 88) points out, 'dissatisfaction with medical communications remains the most prominent of patient complaints and a major factor in the move to alternative medicine'. Moreover, it is not merely a question of patients'

perceptions; ever since Egbert and colleagues' seminal study (Egbert et al 1964), the direct therapeutic value of good communication has repeatedly been demonstrated. It is, moreover, important not to take too restricted a view of the role of communication in healthcare:

First and foremost, all health professionals need to enlarge their repertoire of communication skills. In some circumstances 'controlling' and 'managerial' communication may be required and appropriate, particularly in a crisis, but the other more sensitive communication skills, associated with 'counselling' and 'helping' patients to sort out their own problems and take their own decisions, require quite different training and the development of quite different skills. (Thompson et al 1988, p 161)

These authors go on to argue that traditional forms of education and training for health professionals do little to instil these additional skills.

Therefore, good communication on the part of physiotherapists is not only a means of securing patient satisfaction, but is also an essential component of effective care and treatment. The quality of communication is at a particularly high premium in two specialist areas of the cardiorespiratory physiotherapist's work (counselling and health education) to which we will shortly turn. Before doing so, however, it is important to emphasize that communication also has moral significance. Good communication is required not only for the *effectiveness* of the relationship between therapist and patient, but also for the *ethics* of this relationship. In the course of caring for a patient, therapists may come into possession of information which, they may feel, the patient has a right to know (Sim 1986a). For example, it may be found that a man with unexplained unilateral pneumonia is suffering from previously undiagnosed bronchial carcinoma. Should this be made known to him, if it has not hitherto? Alternatively, a young woman with cryptogenic fibrosing alveolitis may seem to have unrealistic beliefs as to the prospects of cure. Should she be given a more accurate picture of her future?

Ethical issues also surround consent. Informed consent can be defined as 'the voluntary and revocable agreement of a competent individual to participate in a therapeutic or research procedure, based on an adequate understanding of its nature, purpose and implications' (Sim 1986b, p 584). In some instances, gaining consent to treatment procedures can be accomplished straightforwardly. However, in the case of nasopharyngeal suction, the patient may not be in a state of consciousness that permits explicit consent. Alternatively, the patient may seem to be withholding consent and a decision must be made whether or not to proceed nonetheless, on the grounds that the patient is expressing a wish that is not fully autonomous, or perhaps on the basis that the therapeutic benefits likely to accrue justify disregarding a lack of consent. Presumably with this latter argument in mind, Hough (1996, p 140) argues that '[f]orcible suction is unethical, usually illegal and acceptable only in life-threatening situations'. In children, competence to give, or to refuse, consent may be absent. If treatments such as suction are considered necessary, they may have to be given even if the child is unwilling – though only after a thorough and sensitive explanation to the child and his or her carers. Further discussion of ethical principles can be found in Beauchamp & Childress (1994) and Sim (1997).

COUNSELLING

Henry is a middle-aged man with emphysema who is suffering increasing restriction on his activities due to breathlessness, to the extent that he is unable to participate fully in running the family business. He is experiencing feelings of inadequacy and guilt and finds that he is losing what he perceives to be his role within the family.

Karla, an 18-year-old woman with cystic fibrosis, recently discovered that another patient of the same age, whom she had got to know very well during the course of several inpatient admissions, has died of the disease. The sense of purpose and hopefulness with which Karla previously pursued her treatment now seems to be weakening and she is becoming increasingly fatalistic about her future.

Gary is a young man with asthma who is subject to acute attacks of moderate severity. He is increasingly unwilling to engage in social activities, anticipating the disruption and alarm that a sudden attack may cause and fearful of straying from the support of his family, who 'know what to do'.

Each of these vignettes demonstrates the way in which the psychosocial features of respiratory disease may affect the patient. They equally show how the physiotherapist will require skills other than those of direct physical treatment in order to help. The focus here is on the second category of intervention identified earlier (psychological care) and in order to accomplish this the physiotherapist may feel the need to assume the role of counsellor in situations such as these. However, it is important first to be clear about what counselling is and what it is not. In general terms, counselling is the establishment of a helping relationship between practitioner and client, in which communication and other skills are used to assist the client to clarify and find meaning in his or her thoughts, emotions and behaviour, recognize and define problems and formulate a plan of action for the future. Counselling usually occurs on a one-to-one basis, but may be carried out in groups (Nelson-Jones 1982).

Counselling is not just being a passive receptacle for people's anxieties, fears, emotions, problems, etc. Nor does it consist in providing specific pieces of advice, guidance or reassurance; indeed, in his classification of helping strategies, Griffiths (1981) explicitly separates counselling from strategies such as 'giving information', 'teaching' and 'giving advice'. Burnard (1994) suggests that giving advice is rarely helpful in a counselling context. Equally, counselling, even of a psychodynamic nature, is not synonymous with psychoanalysis (Jacobs 1988). Rather, it is a process whereby the patient (or 'client' in counselling parlance) is assisted towards insight and an understanding of his or her own emotional, attitudinal and social situation. Emotions are not suppressed by the counsellor, nor are they permitted to flow in a totally free and unrestrained manner – they are clarified. Instead of providing ready-made strategies, the counsellor helps the client in setting his or her own goals. The counsellor frequently acts as a catalyst (Nichols 1993).

This all requires specific communication skills, which are as much to do with listening as with talking. The ability to understand and engage with others' experience and provide empathic feedback is central to the counselling role (Bennett 1993). Physiotherapists must assess carefully the extent to which they possess such skills. While some sort of counselling role is well within the capabilities of most, if not all, physiotherapists, it is important to recognize the limit of one's expertise and to refer patients to a more fully trained counsellor or even to a clinical psychologist, when the case demands (Nichols 1993).

Essential elements in counselling

Naturally, it is not possible to provide here a practical account of the skills required in counselling. The precise skills required will, in any case, differ somewhat between the various psychological approaches to counselling (Nelson-Jones 1982). However, it is perhaps worth looking briefly at some of what are generally agreed to be the essential ingredients of effective counselling.

Genuineness. Genuineness, or authenticity, has been defined as '[t]he degree to which we are freely and deeply ourselves and are able to relate to people in a sincere and undefensive manner' (Stewart 1992, p. 100). This quality is important in encouraging trust and disclosure on the part of the client.

Positive regard. The counsellor should show some degree of detachment. On the one hand, there should be no sign of disapproval, censure or blame. The counsellor should display 'unconditional positive regard' for the client (Burnard 1994), i.e. positive feelings towards the client which do not need to be 'earned', will not be affected by what the client may say or may have done and which the client should not necessarily feel obliged to reciprocate. Without such openness, acceptance and apparent liking, the client is unlikely to be forthcoming and confide in the counsellor. In the case of Gary, for example, any suggestion by the therapist that his anxieties are inappropriate or exaggerated would be likely to inhibit a counselling relationship. On the other hand, undue sympathy or emotional closeness should be avoided. Explicit emotional identification ('I know just how you feel') may threaten the essential privacy and uniqueness of the client's state of being and may accordingly be resented.

Non-possessiveness. A young female physiotherapist may be able to identify strongly with a patient such as Karla and feel that she understands the emotions that Karla is experiencing. Because of this powerful sense of empathy, she may experience an intense desire to help. However, the counsellor should not become possessive with regard to the client. Undue sympathy for the client may cause the counsellor to seek to impose what he or she sees as the optimum solution to the individual's problems, without due regard for what the client would regard as optimum. Dickson et al (1989) see altruism as an essential attribute for the counsellor and one result of this is that it is all too easy for the counsellor to become paternalistic. Just because the client has permitted access to what are often private and sensitive aspects of his or her life, this does not mean that the client has in any way surrendered personal control. The professional has to balance feelings of benevolence and a desire to help against respect for the client's autonomy. Above all, the therapist should be wary of what Swain (1995) calls exploitation – a process whereby the counselling relationship is used more to serve the counsellor's psychological needs and emotional interests than those of the client.

Willingness to yield control. The counsellor should not control the encounter excessively. Indeed, counsellors generally adopt a 'non-directive' approach and try to ensure that the course taken by the consultation is, as far as possible, in the control of the client. At the same time, skilful use of probing questions can facilitate this process and confrontation techniques may be required if the consultation seems to have reached an impasse, with the client 'going over the same ground without any new insights' (Brearley & Birchley 1994, p. 8). What are termed 'prescriptive interventions' do have a part to play in counselling but Burnard (1994) warns that they can very easily be overused. Specific practical advice might seem to be useful in the case of someone like Henry. However, it is often only of short-term usefulness and may encourage dependency. Moreover, if a suggested strategy does not work, the counsellor may be blamed and the relationship may be broken, depriving the counsellor of the opportunity to help further.

Orientation to action. Greater self-understanding on the part of the client is an important aim of counselling, but this is only of value if it in turn leads to a solution (whether partial or total) of the individual's problems (Munro et al 1989). According to Burnard (1994), immediacy is an essential quality in the counselling relationship; that is, the counsellor should have a concern with the here-and-now and should discourage the client from undue reminiscing about the past, which may remove the focus from issues of immediate practical concern. Accordingly, many counsellors feel that the client should always leave a consultation with some definite course of action to pursue, however minimal it may appear to be.

Establishing a contract. It is important to clarify mutual expectations. The counsellor should make it understood what sort of help is likely to be forthcoming, so that the client does not bring

unrealistic hopes to the relationship (Brearley & Birchley 1994). Similarly, boundaries should be set. The client should understand that, whilst help is freely given, this can only be for a certain period of time and that the counsellor may not necessarily be available at unarranged times between sessions. Setting a time limit to the session assists both counsellor and client (Brearley & Birchley 1994). It is important, however, not to undertake counselling if the necessary time is not likely to be available (Burnard 1994). As part of an effective working relationship, the client will be expected to confide information relating to often private and intimate aspects of his or her life. The client can only be expected to do so with an assurance of confidentiality on the part of the counsellor – indeed, it is unlikely that information will be freely disclosed otherwise (Sim 1996). A degree of privacy is surrendered on the understanding of an implicit assurance of discretion and confidentiality on the part of the counsellor (and of other clients in the case of group counselling). If it is felt that other professionals need to be consulted in order adequately to help the client, the counsellor will need to explain this to the client and obtain consent for information to be revealed to another party. In such a case, the benevolent aim of helping the client does not override the ethical requirement to respect privacy. It should also be remembered that patients may have legal redress in certain cases of breach of confidentiality (Mason & McCall Smith 1999).

Assuming the counselling role

It is fair to say that not all physiotherapists take readily to the role of counsellor. In common with many other practitioners, they may often be 'reluctant to deal with emotional and psychological dimensions of patients' problems' (Dickson et al 1989, p.126). There may be an unwillingness to explore aspects of patients' lives to do with such areas as intensely felt emotions, their personal fears, and feelings related to their sexuality.

More specifically, the predominant accent within physiotherapy training and education on physical treatment strategies may cause physiotherapists to feel, albeit unconsciously, that they are not performing their proper role if they are apparently 'just talking' to patients. It should be accepted that the process of 'problem solving' is likely to take a very different form in psychological care from that undertaken in physical treatment. The strategies adopted will often be far less tangible and may involve, in comparison, little active participation by the physiotherapist. Frequently, the therapist engaged in psychological care will not be providing specific, concrete interventions but will be involved in a more passive, facilitatory role, involving considerably more response than initiation. Any action to be taken is generally for the client rather than the therapist. Thus, Griffiths describes counselling as 'helping someone to explore a problem, clarify conflicting issues and discover alternative ways of dealing with it, so that they can decide what to do about it; that is, helping people to help themselves' (Griffiths 1981, p. 267).

In a similar way, the sort of dialogue which is likely to be engaged in may often appear to be less purposeful than that to which physiotherapists have become accustomed in the course of physical treatment. Pauses and even considerable periods of silence are often not only acceptable but positively beneficial in counselling and other forms of psychological care (Swain 1995); however, they may initially be a source of unease to therapists who are used to more 'business-like' exchanges with their patients.

Counselling, if it is to be effective, involves a new set of skills for many physiotherapists and, just as important, a new perspective on their professional role. However, appropriate training in counselling skills and a fuller understanding of the psychosocial dynamics of cardiorespiratory illness, will reveal a wider and more holistic approach to the management of these patients.

HEALTH EDUCATION

Health education and health promotion

The terms 'health education' and 'health promotion' are sometimes used almost interchangeably.

However, a valuable distinction can be drawn between them. 'Health promotion' is used to cover a broad spectrum of activities that seek to improve or restore health. The term has been defined by Downie et al (1996, p. 60) as follows: 'Health promotion comprises efforts to enhance positive health and reduce the risk of ill-health, through the overlapping spheres of health education, prevention and health protection'. Health promotion is about more than healthcare; hence, Hollis (2000, p. 356) argues that health promotion is about 'providing a strategy for better health as opposed to a strategy for better health services'.

This model of health promotion incorporates three key elements, identified by Tannahill (1985). One of these is *health education*, which we will return to in due course. The second element, *prevention*, concerns activities that are designed to reduce the incidence or risk of occurrence of any undesirable health-related state of being, whether this is physical illness, mental illness, physical injury, physical disability or handicap. Traditionally, prevention has been classified into three types (Farmer et al 1996). Primary prevention seeks to prevent the disease process from starting, while secondary prevention aims to detect disease at an early stage and forestall further progression. Tertiary prevention, meanwhile, 'aims at "damage limitation" in persons with manifest disease by modifying continuing risk factors such as smoking and the implementation of effective rehabilitation' (Farmer et al 1996, p. 137).

Downie et al (1996) criticize this typology for being unduly centred in the narrow concept of disease and for identifying prevention with the idea of treatment. They also note the lack of unanimity with which these three phases are used by various commentators. Downie et al (1996, p. 51) propose, instead, what they call 'four foci of prevention', which give a rather fuller idea of the potentialities of prevention:

- Prevention of the onset or first manifestation of a disease process or some other first occurrence, through risk reduction.
- Prevention of the progression of a disease process or other unwanted state, through early detection when this favourably affects outcome.

- Prevention of avoidable complications of an irreversible, manifest disease or some other unwanted state.
- Prevention of the recurrence of an illness or other unwanted phenomenon.

The third key element in health promotion is that of *health protection*. This comprises various legal controls, policy initiatives, codes of practice and other regulatory mechanisms that are designed to improve or restore health.

Health education is therefore just one of the ways in which the goals of health promotion can be pursued. There is, of course, a large degree of interrelation between the three elements; for example, a considerable proportion of health education may concern itself with prevention.

The scope of health education

Downie et al (1996, p. 28) define health education as: 'communication activity aimed at enhancing positive health and preventing or diminishing ill-health in individuals and groups, through influencing the beliefs, attitudes and behaviour of those with power and of the community at large'.

Thus, health education, like education in other contexts, has three main targets: beliefs (or knowledge), attitudes and behaviour. By seeking to influence one or more of these factors, the health educator hopes to enhance or restore health. In achieving this objective, the health educator is not restricted to activities centred on individuals. Ewles & Simnett (1999, p. 42) describe a 'societal change approach' which aims to 'effect changes on the physical, social and economic environment, to make it more conducive to good health' and Kiger (1995) draws attention to the role of political action within health promotion and education (which may involve the physiotherapist taking such action or encouraging and empowering patients to do so for themselves). Thus, although physiotherapists may spend most of their time dealing with individual patients, they should not neglect opportunities to take a broader approach to health. For example, in the case of children with cystic fibrosis, health education may extend to advising schools of the

need for treatment facilities or special diets. In the case of persons with acquired immune deficiency syndrome (AIDS), it may involve attempts to dispel misconceptions and to foster more tolerant attitudes in the wider community (Sim & Purtilo 1991). Furthermore, it is not only important that the wider community should be educated about health-related matters; patients themselves need to know about the broader context into which their health (or lack of it) fits.

Draper et al (1980, p. 493) emphasize this wider remit for health education in their description of three types of health education:

The first and most common is education about the body and how to look after it … The second is about health services – information about available services and the 'sensible' use of health care resources. But the third, about the wider environment within which health choices are made, is relatively neglected. It is concerned with education about national, regional and local policies, which are too often devised and implemented without taking account of their consequences for health.

They argue that health education that is restricted to the first two types is 'partial to the point of being socially irresponsible'.

At the heart of health education is the notion of empowerment. 'True health education should work to enable people to understand better what they are, what they believe and what they know' (Seedhouse 1986, p.91). Of equal, and related, importance is the idea of partnership between patient and health professional; effective health education cannot be a unilateral activity. 'The key to full partnership is continual patient/health professional communication' (Lorig 1996, p. xiv).

Health education and the physiotherapist

The question now arises as to how, and to what extent, the physiotherapist should incorporate the role of health educator in the management of patients with cardiac and respiratory conditions. A number of factors suggest that this is a highly appropriate role. First, it must be recognized that, with some exceptions (e.g. acute lobar pneumonia, hyperventilation syndrome), most of these conditions are not amenable to cure. There is, therefore, a need for a programme of long-term management, in addition to any short-term treatment. Second, any physical treatment that is administered is generally only beneficial for these conditions if it is continued between periods of direct contact with the therapist and, in addition, is augmented by self-care strategies on the part of the patient. Effective management of these patients consists therefore as much in what takes place in the patient's personal, domestic and social life as in what occurs in the healthcare setting. Third, cardiorespiratory disease offers full scope for prevention, under each of the four foci identified by Downie et al (1996) and health education is an important means of implementing preventive health measures. Finally, there are many areas of the individual's life in which changes in behaviour can have a beneficial effect on cardiorespiratory dysfunction, e.g. dietary adjustments, avoidance of possible sources of infection or allergic reaction, the taking of exercise, etc. Here, too, health education has a clear contribution to make.

Accordingly, the physiotherapist involved in the care of patients with cardiorespiratory problems can fulfil the role of health educator in a wide variety of ways, by:

- explaining the underlying pathological processes and the significance of these in terms of prevention and treatment
- advising on means by which general health may be maintained (e.g. adequate nutrition, appropriate balance of rest and activity)
- teaching treatment modalities which can be carried out independently, such as airway clearance techniques and strategies for coping with the physiological demands of the disease, such as breathing control and activity pacing
- instructing patients in the use of items of equipment, such as air compressors, nebulizers and oxygen concentrators
- providing information on appropriate health and social services available, including information on patients' statutory rights
- putting patients in contact with self-help groups and patients' organizations such as those that exist in many countries for patients with cystic fibrosis
- helping to create attitudes of confidence, self-worth and confidence, thereby empowering patients in their efforts to cope with disability.

In order to achieve such goals, the physiotherapist will need highly developed communication skills and an awareness of the factors identified previously that may either enhance or detract from the communication process. The therapist should also consider the psychological dynamics of the patient's illness and the stage of potential behaviour change that has been reached (a factor developed in the transtheoretical model of behaviour; Prochaska & Di Clemente 1984). There are, however, some specific points that should be considered. The first is that health education should not consist of unilateral giving of instruction and advice. It is essential that goals be mutually negotiated, otherwise patients will not see themselves as a partner in the overall process and will be poorly motivated to carry through recommended courses of action. Second, the therapist must gain a sound insight into the patient's psychological profile and social environment. For it to be effective, the content and manner of delivery of a message should be geared to the psychological, emotional and educational characteristics of the recipient. Hence, patients with a primarily internal locus of control (i.e. those who broadly regard themselves as capable of determining their own destiny) will respond to different forms of goal setting compared with patients who have an external locus of control (i.e. those who see themselves as subject to more fatalistic, external influences; see Wallston & Wallston 1982). Bennett & Murphy (1997) discuss some of the empirical research relevant to this issue.

Similarly, ignorance of the patient's social situation may lead the therapist to advocate inappropriate strategies that are incompatible with the individual's lifestyle. Cott (1999) notes that, in some cases, treatment interventions may be more burdensome to the patient than the symptoms they are intended to relieve. Furthermore, patients may face barriers to implementing self-management prescribed by practitioners that go beyond notions of willingness or motivation (Buston & Wood 2000). In the light of this, talk of 'non-compliant' patients is unhelpful. Locating failures of compliance in the patient is to overlook the fact that adherence is a property of a relationship, not of an individual. If adherence is not achieved, the relevant shortcomings reside in the rapport and understanding that exist (or perhaps do not exist) between therapist and patient. Such rapport and understanding are a shared responsibility. Patients and professionals may have very different notions of what compliance is or should be (Coy 1989, Roberson 1992); these should be explored carefully and sensitively. Increasingly, the terms 'compliance' and 'adherence' are being replaced by 'concordance', to reflect the shared nature of the decision making involved (Mullen 1997).

The third important consideration is that effective health education, like all areas of health work, relies on sound liaison and teamwork. It is important that messages are echoed and reinforced by all those with whom the patient comes into contact. Above all, it should be remembered that team members each have their own agenda and some sort of compromise must be effected in order that a shared set of priorities can be drawn up. Needless to say, the patient has his or her own agenda and this should be given full consideration in the process.

This leads us to the final consideration, which concerns a respect for the individual's autonomy. The concept of autonomy is a crucial one in healthcare ethics and relates to the individual's ability to make decisions and act upon them without unwarranted interference from others (Sim 1997). Here, it is important for the physiotherapist to consider carefully the nature and extent of professional expertise. In many instances, the therapist's expertise may allow him or her to identify authoritatively the best means of achieving a certain health-related goal. However, this does not mean that the therapist is in a privileged position to identify this as a valuable goal in the first instance. Such goals only have value in the context of the person's total

---

Box 8.2

Therapist's perspective
A way of life characterized by dietary control, use of antibiotics, abstention from smoking, and conscientious and regular physiotherapy.

Patient's perspective
A way of life characterized by participation with peers in social activities, including 'unhealthy' behaviours and independence from imposed routines and restrictions.

---

state of being and the ultimate authority on what matters to a given individual is, necessarily, that individual. The patient and the practitioner are likely to have fundamentally different perspectives on illness and disability, which go far beyond the concept of a 'knowledge gap' (Toombs 1993). Accordingly, the patient's values and priorities are liable to differ from the therapist's. In cystic fibrosis, for example, there may be a mismatch in conceptions of appropriate lifestyle and behaviour between the therapist and the patient (see Box 8.2).

Although the physiotherapist should advise the patient on actions and behaviour that are appropriate from a professional perspective, the patient must ultimately be allowed to make his or her own choices, however imprudent they may seem. The therapist's role is that of providing the information upon which such choices can be based, not of usurping the patient's right to choose. The physiotherapist must recognize the dividing line between education and indoctrination (Campbell 1990).

CONCLUSION

This chapter has attempted to highlight the role that communication and other interpersonal processes can play in the management of patients with cardiorespiratory problems. Communication skills are fundamental to the three main categories of intervention – physical treatment, psychological care and health education – and, like other professional skills, can be learnt and further developed in order to improve the quality of patient care.

REFERENCES

Alder B 1995 Psychology of health: applications of psychology for health professionals. Harwood Academic Publishers, Reading

Argyle M 1983 The psychology of interpersonal behaviour, 4th edn. Penguin, Harmondsworth

Argyle M 1988 Bodily communication, 2nd edn. Methuen, London

Baddeley AD 1997 Human memory: theory and practice, 2nd edn. Psychology Press, Hove

Beauchamp TL, Childress JF 1994 Principles of biomedical ethics, 4th edn. Oxford University Press, New York

Bennett P 1993 Counselling for heart disease. British Psychological Society, Leicester

Bennett P, Murphy S 1997 Psychology and health promotion. Open University Press, Buckingham

Bott J 1997 Physiotherapy. In: Morgan M, Singh S (eds) Practical pulmonary rehabilitation. Chapman and Hall, London

Brearley G, Birchley P 1994 Counselling in disability and illness, 2nd edn. Mosby, London

Burnard P 1994 Counselling skills for health professionals, 2nd edn. Stanley Thornes, Cheltenham

Bury M 1982 Chronic illness as biographical disruption. Sociology of Health and Illness 4: 167–182.

Buston KM, Wood S F 2000 Non-compliance among adolescents with asthma: listening to what they tell us about self-management. Family Practice 17: 134–138

Campbell A V 1990 Education or indoctrination? The issue of autonomy in health education. In: Doxiadis S (ed) Ethics in health education. Wiley, Chichester

Cott C 1999 Long-term care: living with chronic illness. In: Ramsden EL (ed) The person as patient: psychosocial perspectives for the health care professional. WB Saunders, London

Coy JA 1989 Philosophic aspects of patient noncompliance: a critical analysis. Topics in Geriatric Rehabilitation 4: 52–60

Darbyshire AE 1967 A description of English. Edward Arnold, London

D'Auria JP, Christian BJ, Henderson ZG, Haynes B 2000 The company they keep: the influence of peer relationships on adjustment to cystic fibrosis during adolescence. Journal of Pediatric Nursing 15: 175–182

Dickson DA, Hargie O, Morrow NC 1989 Communication skills training for health professionals: an instructor's handbook. Chapman and Hall, London

Donovan JL, Blake DR, Fleming W G 1989 The patient is not a blank sheet: lay beliefs and their relevance to patient education. British Journal of Rheumatology 28: 58–61

Downie RS, Tannahill C, Tannahill A 1996 Health promotion: models and values, 2nd edn. Oxford University Press, Oxford

Draper P, Griffiths J, Dennis J, Popay J 1980 Three types of health education. British Medical Journal 281: 493–495

Dushenko TW 1981 Cystic fibrosis: a medical overview and critique of the psychological literature. Social Science and Medicine 15E: 43–56

Egbert LD, Battit GE, Welsh CE, Bartlett MK 1964 Reduction of postoperative pain by encouragement and instruction of patients. New England Journal of Medicine 270: 825–827

Ewles L, Simnett I 1999 Promoting health: a practical guide, 4th edn. Baillière Tindall, Edinburgh

Fagerhaugh SY 1973 Getting around with emphysema. American Journal of Nursing 73: 94–99

Farmer R, Miller D, Lawrenson R 1996 Lecture notes on epidemiology and public health medicine, 4th edn. Blackwell Science, Oxford

Freidson E 1962 Dilemmas in the doctor–patient relationship. In: Rose AM (ed) Human behaviour and social processes: an interactionist approach. Routledge and Kegan Paul, London

French S 1997 Inequalities in health. In: French S (ed) Physiotherapy: a psychosocial approach, 2nd edn. Butterworth-Heinemann, Oxford

Gibson S 1997 Lifestyle management: relaxation, coping, sex, benefits and travel. In: Morgan M, Singh S (eds) Practical pulmonary rehabilitation. Chapman and Hall, London

Griffiths D 1981 Psychology and medicine. British Psychological Society/Macmillan, London

Guyatt GH, Townsend M, Berman LB, Pugsley SO 1987 Quality of life in patients with chronic airflow limitation. British Journal of Diseases of the Chest 81: 45–54

Hall ET 1966 The hidden dimension: man's use of space in public and private. Bodley Head, London

Hargie O, Saunders C, Dickson D 1994 Social skills in interpersonal communication, 3rd edn. Routledge, London

Helman CG 2000 Culture, health and illness, 4th edn. Butterworth-Heinemann, Oxford

Hollis V 2000 Health promotion. In: Kumar S (ed) Multidisciplinary approach to rehabilitation. Butterworth-Heinemann, Boston

Hough A 1996 Physiotherapy in respiratory care: a problem-solving approach to respiratory and cardiac management, 2nd edn. Chapman and Hall, London

Hugman R 1991 Power in caring professions. Macmillan, London

Hyland ME, Donaldson ML 1989 Psychological care in nursing practice. Scutari Press, Harrow

Inman C, Katz J 1997 Developing effective communication. In: Katz J, Peberdy A (eds) Promoting health: knowledge and practice. Macmillan, Basingtoke

Jacobs M 1988 Psychodynamic counselling in action. Sage, London

Johannesson M, Carlson M, Brucefors AB, Hjelte L 1998 Cystic fibrosis through a female perspective: psychosocial issues and information concerning puberty and motherhood. Patient Education and Counselling 34: 115–123

Kiger AM 1995 Teaching for health, 2nd edn. Churchill Livingstone, Edinburgh

Lask B 2000 Psychological aspects of cystic fibrosis. In: Hodson M, Geddes D M (eds) Cystic fibrosis, 2nd edn. Arnold, London

Lawler J 1991 Behind the screens: nursing, somology and the problem of the body. Churchill Livingstone, Melbourne

Ley P 1988 Communicating with patients: improving communication, satisfaction and compliance. Chapman and Hall, London

Lorig K 1996 Patient education: a practical approach. Sage, Thousand Oaks

McSweeny AJ, Grant I, Heaton RK, Adams KM, Timms RM 1982 Life quality of patients with chronic obstructive pulmonary disease. Archives of Internal Medicine 142: 473–478

MacWhannell DE 1992 Communication in physiotherapy practice (1). In: French S (ed) Physiotherapy: a psychosocial approach. Butterworth-Heinemann, Oxford

Mason JK, McCall Smith R A 1999 Law and medical ethics, 5th edn. Butterworths, London

Morgan AD, Peck DF, Buchanan DR, McHardy GJ 1983 Effect of attitudes and beliefs on exercise tolerance in chronic bronchitis. British Medical Journal 286: 171–173

Mullen PD 1997 Compliance becomes concordance. British Medical Journal 314: 691

Munro A, Manthel B, Small J 1989 Counselling: the skills of problem-solving. Routledge, London

Nelson-Jones R 1982 The theory and practice of counselling psychology. Cassell, London

Nelson-Jones R 1990 Human relationship skills: training and self-help, 2nd edn. Cassell, London

Nichols KA 1993 Psychological care in physical illness, 2nd edn. Chapman and Hall, London

Nicholls D 2000 Breathlessness: a qualitative model of meaning. Physiotherapy 86: 23–27

Niven N 2000 Health psychology for health care professionals. Churchill Livingstone, Edinburgh

Norman AP, Hodson ME 1983 Emotional and social aspects of treatment. In: Hodson ME, Norman AP, Batten JC (eds) Cystic fibrosis. Baillière Tindall, London

Northouse PG, Northouse LL 1992 Health communication: strategies for health professionals, 2nd edn. Appleton and Lange, Norwalk

Østergaard MS 1998 Childhood asthma: parents' perspective – a qualitative interview study. Family Practice 15: 153–157

Pinkerton P, Trauer T, Duncan F, Hodson ME, Batten JC 1985 Cystic fibrosis in adult life: a study of coping patterns. Lancet 2: 761–763

Porritt L 1990 Interaction strategies: an introduction for health professionals. Churchill Livingstone, Melbourne

Prochaska JO, Di Clemente CC 1984 The transtheoretical approach: crossing traditional boundaries of change. Irwin, Homewood

Purtilo RB 1990 Health professional and patient interaction, 4th edn. WB Saunders, Philadelphia

Radley A 1994 Making sense of illness: the social psychology of health and disease. Sage, London

Ramsden E 1999 Communication in the therapeutic context. In: Ramsden EL (ed) The person as patient: psychosocial perspectives for the health care professional. WB Saunders, London

Roberson MHB 1992 The meaning of compliance: patient perspectives. Qualitative Health Research 2: 7–26

Rutter BM 1977 Some psychological concomitants of chronic bronchitis. Psychological Medicine 7: 459–464

Seedhouse D 1986 Health: the foundations for achievement. John Wiley, Chichester

Sim J 1986a Truthfulness in the therapeutic relationship. Physiotherapy Practice 2: 121–127

Sim J 1986b Informed consent: ethical implications for physiotherapy. Physiotherapy 72: 584–587

Sim J 1990a The concept of health. Physiotherapy 76: 423–428

Sim J 1990b Stigma, physical disability and rehabilitation. Physiotherapy Canada 42: 232–238

Sim J 1996 Client confidentiality: ethical issues in occupational therapy. British Journal of Occupational Therapy 59: 56–61

Sim J 1997 Ethical decision making in therapy practice. Butterworth-Heinemann, Oxford

Sim J, Purtilo RB 1991 An ethical analysis of physical therapists' duty to treat persons with AIDS: homosexual patients as a test case. Physical Therapy 71: 650–655

Simmons RJ, Corey M, Cowen L, Keenan N, Robertson J, Levison H 1985 Emotional adjustment of early adolescents with cystic fibrosis. Psychosomatic Medicine 47: 111–122

Snadden D, Brown J B 1992 The experience of asthma. Social Science and Medicine 34: 1351–1361

Staab D, Wenninger K, Gebert N, et al 1998 Quality of life in patients with cystic fibrosis and their parents: what is important besides disease severity? Thorax 53: 727–731

Stewart W 1992 An A–Z of counselling theory and practice. Chapman and Hall, London

Swain J 1995 The use of counselling skills: a guide for therapists. Butterworth-Heinemann, Oxford

Swain J 1997 Interpersonal communication. In: French S (ed) Physiotherapy: a psychosocial approach, 2nd edn. Butterworth-Heinemann, Oxford

Tannahill A 1985 What is health promotion? Health Education Journal 44: 167–168

Thompson IE, Melia KM, Boyd KM 1988 Nursing ethics, 2nd edn. Churchill Livingstone, Edinburgh

Thompson J 1984 Communicating with patients. In: Fitzpatrick R, Hinton J, Newman S, Scambler G, Thompson J (eds) The experience of illness. Tavistock, London

Toombs SK 1993 The meaning of illness: a phenomenological account of the different perspectives of physician and patient. Kluwer, Dordrecht

Tuckett D, Boulton M, Olson C, Williams A 1985 Meetings between experts: an approach to sharing ideas in medical consultations. Tavistock, London

Waddell C 1982 The process of neutralisation and the uncertainties of cystic fibrosis. Sociology of Health and Illness 4: 210–220

Wallston KA, Wallston BS 1982 Who is responsible for your health? The construct of health locus of control. In: Sanders GS, Suls J (eds) Social psychology of health and illness. Lawrence Erlbaum, Hillsdale

Whitcher SJ, Fisher JD 1979 Multidimensional reaction to therapeutic touch in a hospital setting. Journal of Personality and Social Psychology 37: 87–96

Williams SJ 1989 Chronic respiratory illness and disability: a critical review of the psychosocial literature. Social Science and Medicine 28: 791–803

Williams SJ 1993 Chronic respiratory illness. Routledge, London

Withers NJ, Rudkin ST, White RJ 1999 Anxiety and depression in severe chronic obstructive pulmonary disease: the effects of pulmonary rehabilitation. Journal of Cardiopulmonary Rehabilitation 19: 362–365

Physiotherapy and medical management

9

Mechanical support

Adults

John S Turner

Paediatrics

Robert C Tasker

ADULTS

INTRODUCTION

Medical technology has advanced to the point where efficient mechanical support of lungs, heart and kidneys is now available. The gastro-intestinal tract may be supported by means of total parenteral nutrition and the haemo-poietic system by cell transfusion and colony-stimulating factors (such as granulocyte–macrophage colony-stimulating factor). There is as yet no effective form of hepatic support, although liver transplantation is being performed in the acute setting, as is heart and lung transplantation. The indications for these dramatic and heroic measures are, however, limited.

This section covers respiratory, cardiac and renal support, with most of the emphasis being placed on respiratory support, including newer forms of ventilation and weaning.

RESPIRATORY SUPPORT

Respiratory failure is usually defined as the inability to maintain a PaO_2 of more than 8 kPa (60 mmHg) or a $PaCO_2$ of less than 6 kPa (45 mmHg). The causes are numerous and some of the more common ones are listed below in the section on indications for mechanical ventilation. Respiratory support aims to correct these biochemical abnormalities. This can be performed in a number of ways.

Oxygen therapy

Oxygen is delivered by means of facemask or nasal cannulae. Oxygen therapy will correct the majority of less severe cases of hypoxia, but obviously cannot correct hypercarbia.

Continuous positive airway pressure

In the technique of continuous positive airway pressure (CPAP), oxygen is delivered by a system that maintains a positive pressure in the circuitry and airways throughout inspiration and expiration. CPAP is useful in cases where lung volumes are reduced, in particular the functional residual capacity (Fig. 9.1). Examples of this include subsegmental lung collapse, pneumonia and acute respiratory distress syndrome. Again, hypercarbia cannot be corrected and may be worsened as dead-space ventilation may be increased. CPAP usually improves ventilation/perfusion $(\dot{V}/\dot{Q})$ mismatch and, by improving lung compliance, it may reduce the work of breathing.

There are two basic methods of providing CPAP: continuous-flow or demand-flow. Continuous-flow systems have gas flowing through the circuit throughout the respiratory cycle. A high gas flow (50–100 l/min) is necessary to maintain this flow during the initial phase of inspiration. There is no demand valve to open, but the system is noisy and uses large volumes of

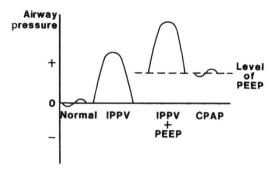

Figure 9.2 Pressure–time curves of various modes of ventilation.

oxygen and air. On the other hand, demand-flow systems (including the CPAP mode on ventilators) allow gas to flow only when inspiration is initiated and a demand valve is thereby opened. This is a quieter system and uses less gas, but a certain amount of work is required of the patient in order to open the demand valve. Some systems are worse than others in this regard, although a modification of the demand-flow system known as 'flow-by' seems to present the patient with little additional work. This system is becoming more widely available. When CPAP is combined with positive pressure ventilation, it is generally known as 'positive end-expiratory pressure' (PEEP) (Fig. 9.2).

Conventional mechanical ventilation

Mechanical ventilation has evolved from negative pressure ventilators used in the polio epidemic of the 1950s. Positive pressure ventilators that followed are now controlled by sophisticated microprocessor technology. The physiology, principles and practice of mechanical ventilation have been reviewed in detail (Hubmayr et al 1990, Schuster 1990).

The basic principles of how a ventilator works remain unchanged. Very simply, *inspiration* may be generated by application of either a constant pressure or a constant flow of gas to the lungs and *expiration* may be allowed when either a set pressure has been reached, a set volume has been delivered or a set time has passed. A recent paper explains the terminology well (Kapadia 1998). Modern ventilators have a variety of ventilation

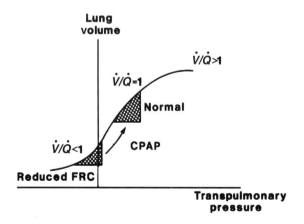

Figure 9.1 Continuous positive airway pressure (CPAP) increases a reduced functional residual capacity (FRC).

modes which allow for comfortable patient–ventilator interaction. Ventilation modes commonly employed and available on most modern ventilators include:

1. *Controlled mandatory ventilation* (CMV) – here the patient has no control over ventilation. Breaths are delivered at a rate and volume that are determined by adjusting the ventilator controls, regardless of the patient's attempts to breathe. If the patient is not unconscious or paralysed, CMV may be uncomfortable.
2. *Intermittent mandatory ventilation* (IMV) – here respiratory rate and tidal volume are set as above, but the patient may breathe spontaneously between the mandatory breaths, which still are delivered at the preset regular intervals.
3. *Synchronized intermittent mandatory ventilation* (SIMV) – the mandatory breaths are delivered in synchrony with the patient's breathing. Again the patient may breathe on his own, but the mandatory breaths will be delivered at a time in the ventilatory cycle that is convenient for the patient (a breath will therefore not be delivered while the patient is breathing out). Patient comfort is improved.
4. *Inspiratory pressure support* (IPS) – this is a pressure-limited form of ventilation, with each breath being triggered by the patient. Once a breath is triggered, a flow of gas enters the circuit, with the pressure rapidly reaching the preset level. This pressure is maintained until the flow decreases to a ventilator-specific level, at which time expiration is allowed. The patient has full control over the respiratory rate. IPS can deliver the same level of ventilation (as assessed by gas exchange) as SIMV, often with lower peak airway pressures, as long as the patient has an adequate respiratory drive. Alone or in combination with SIMV, it can make ventilation more comfortable for the patient. Theoretically, by allowing some degree of muscle training without permitting fatigue, IPS would be helpful in weaning patients from mechanical ventilation. To date, clinical trials addressing this issue have shown conflicting results.
5. *Inverse ratio ventilation* – this is ventilation where the inspiratory phase is longer than the expiratory phase. It may be volume or pressure regulated, the latter (pressure-controlled inverse ratio ventilation or PCIRV) being the most widely used. The technique has been well described (Tharratt et al 1988) but there are no clinical trials comparing it with other simpler forms of ventilation. It is now widely used but requires expertise and careful monitoring of haemodynamic and respiratory parameters.

Non-invasive ventilation

Non-invasive ventilation (ventilation without an endotracheal tube or tracheostomy) can be delivered by negative or positive pressure techniques. Negative pressure ventilation is epitomized in the large and frightening 'iron lung', used in the 1950s for the ventilation of patients with poliomyelitis. Newer and much more compact and comfortable negative pressure ventilators are now available (Shneerson 1991) and domiciliary ventilation with them is feasible. A review by Branthwaite (1991) covers the practical aspects of this form of ventilation. Non-invasive ventilation is considered further in Chapter 10.

Indications for mechanical ventilation

The indications for ventilation vary for different disorders and are rarely absolute. In practical (and somewhat simplistic) terms they include the following.

Acute respiratory distress syndrome. A patient who has a PaO_2 of less than 8 kPa (60 mmHg) on oxygen and CPAP.

Pneumonia. A patient who is unable to clear secretions or who has a PaO_2 of less than 8 kPa (60 mmHg) on oxygen and CPAP.

Asthma. A patient who is becoming exhausted or confused, usually with a rising $PaCO_2$.

Chronic obstructive airways disease. Similar to asthma, but a higher $PaCO_2$ may be normal for the patient. Non-invasive ventilation may be an option in these patients (Elliott et al 1990) in selected circumstances and with the necessary expertise.

Respiratory muscle weakness. A patient who is unable to clear secretions, who has lost bulbar function or who cannot produce a vital capacity of more than 15 ml/kg.

Blunt chest trauma. A patient who, despite adequate analgesia, cannot produce a vital capacity of more than 15 ml/kg or is unable to clear secretions or who has a PaO_2 of less than 8 kPa (60 mmHg) on oxygen and CPAP.

Pulmonary oedema. This is largely a clinical decision, as pulmonary oedema tends to improve very quickly with appropriate medical treatment. Patients who are moribund or not responding to treatment will need ventilation, as will patients who have had a large myocardial infarct.

Other system involvement. This is largely a clinical decision, as pulmonary oedema tends to improve very quickly with appropriate medical treatment.

Elective postoperative ventilation. Some patients may be electively ventilated postoperatively, either because of the magnitude of the surgery or because they have impaired pulmonary function.

Aims and complications of respiratory support

The first and most important aim of respiratory support is to oxygenate the patient. This is initially done by increasing the inspired oxygen concentration. Oxygen concentrations of above 50% are toxic to the lungs if used for any length of time, with toxicity increasing exponentially as the concentration rises further. PEEP may be added to improve oxygenation. PEEP may depress cardiac output more than it improves oxygenation and oxygen delivery may therefore be compromised. Increasing the inspiratory time to allow for higher mean airway pressures but lower peak inspiratory pressure (PIP) may improve oxygenation. Sedation and occasionally muscle relaxants may be necessary to ventilate a critically ill patient. Lower tidal volumes and higher PEEP levels have recently been shown to be beneficial in acute respiratory distress syndrome (ARDSnet).

Barotrauma, which is related to PIP, needs to be avoided. There is no pressure which is absolutely safe, but barotrauma occurs with significant

frequency once the PIP exceeds 50 cmH_2O and increases exponentially as pressures rise above this level. Manoeuvres to lower PIP include reducing the tidal volume, reducing PEEP and allowing a longer inspiratory time (even to inverse ratio ventilation).

The importance of carbon dioxide removal has decreased recently. Patients with severe respiratory failure have been ventilated in a way that allows the $PaCO_2$ to rise to up to 8 kPa (60 mmHg) or more (Hickling et al 1990). This concept of 'permissive hypercapnia' has been used in a variety of situations and generally allows a smaller tidal volume and minute volume to be used, reducing the incidence of barotrauma and oxygen toxicity.

Patient comfort and acceptability can be achieved by carefully matching patient and ventilator. Tidal volume, rate and inspiratory time can be manipulated to make the patient comfortable. This is an art and demands patience and understanding. Occasionally, sedation is needed, but this should be a last resort.

Respiratory support is not without complications, some of which are minor and some of which may be lethal. The more commonly occurring complications include barotrauma, haemodynamic disturbances, nosocomial infections, alteration in gastrointestinal motility and a positive fluid balance (Pingleton 1988).

Weaning from respiratory support

Criteria for weaning from mechanical ventilation were first described in the 1970s. They are adequate in most cases, but their relatively high failure rate has led investigators to look at other predictors of a successful wean. These include work of breathing (Fiastro et al 1988) and more recently the 'CROP index' and rapid shallow breathing index (Yang & Tobin 1991). The latter is simple to perform and is by far the most practically useful of the above. It is calculated by allowing the patient to breathe room air through a spirometer for one minute while the respiratory rate is counted. The minute volume (measured on the spirometer) is divided by the respiratory rate to give an average tidal volume. The index is calculated by dividing the respiratory rate by the tidal volume (in litres). Weaning is unlikely with an index above 100 and likely with an index below 100.

Conventional weaning criteria involve clinical, mechanical and biochemical parameters.

Clinical

- The clinical condition of the patient is improving.
- The patient is cooperative and alert and able to clear secretions.
- There is no abdominal distension, cardiovascular instability or likelihood of prolonged immobility.
- The respiratory rate is less than 30 breaths/min.

Mechanical

- Vital capacity is more than 15 ml/kg.
- Maximal inspiratory mouth pressure is more than 20 cmH_2O.
- Minute volume is less than 10 l/min.

Biochemical

- Normal pH and $PaCO_2$.
- PaO_2 more than 8 kPa (60 mmHg) on no more than 40% oxygen and 5 cm PEEP.

Once the above criteria are satisfied, weaning may be started. Before and during the weaning period, meticulous attention needs to be paid to nutrition, electrolyte status, control of infection and bronchospasm and mobilization of the patient. The last factor is probably the most important and the physiotherapist will be very involved in sitting and then standing and walking the patient. Even patients with many lines, tubes and catheters can be mobilized with a little ingenuity.

Weaning can be performed in two different ways. Either the proportion of breathing performed by the ventilator can be gradually reduced, letting the patient perform a greater and greater amount of breathing until he is independent of the ventilator (IMV was the first ventilatory mode to allow this) or the patient can be allowed to breathe spontaneously for progres-

sively longer periods with full ventilation between them (the so-called 'T-piece method'). Both methods have their proponents, although there is probably little to choose between them. The latter method is commonly used in difficult weans.

Common problems which may cause difficulties with weaning (Branthwaite 1988) include:

- impaired ventilatory drive
- upper and lower airway incompetence, obstruction or secretions
- lung parenchymal fluid or infection
- pleural effusion or pneumothorax
- chest wall abnormality, instability or respiratory muscle weakness
- electrolyte or nutritional problems
- cardiovascular insufficiency.

Other modes of respiratory support

Less conventional modes of respiratory support include extracorporeal membrane oxygenation (ECMO), extracorporeal carbon dioxide removal (ECCO$_2$R), intravenacaval oxygenation (IVOX) and high-frequency jet ventilation (HFJV). These modes are only available in major centres, are costly and extremely labour intensive and have not yet been shown in controlled studies to hold any advantage over conventional ventilation (Evans & Keogh 1991). They have their enthusiasts, however, and in their hands the results are impressive.

Extracorporeal membrane oxygenation

This is a well-established and useful technique in neonatal respiratory distress syndrome, but has not shown advantages over conventional ventilation in controlled trials in adults. However, it may still be a useful technique for short periods, especially as a bridge to transplantation, an indication for which it has been used successfully. The technique involves a high-flow extracorporeal circuit from the inferior vena cava to the aorta using cannulae in the femoral vein and artery. A membrane oxygenator is used in the circuit to provide oxygenation and carbon dioxide removal. The extracorporeal blood flow is up to 80% of the cardiac output and vital organs may be poorly perfused with non-pulsatile blood flow.

Extracorporeal carbon dioxide removal

An uncontrolled trial showed startling results with the ECCO$_2$R technique (Gattinoni et al 1986), with a survival rate of 47% in 55 patients with ARDS in whom the mortality was predicted to be more than 90%. A low flow venovenous circuit is used with a membrane oxygenator and the patient is ventilated at a slow rate with very small tidal volumes. Complications are less common than with ECMO. A controlled trial comparing ECCO$_2$R with conventional ventilation has shown the newer mode to be no better (Morris et al 1994). Enthusiasts may still get excellent results, however.

Complications of extracorporeal gas exchange (ECMO and ECCO$_2$R) include haemorrhage, thrombosis and thromboembolism, sepsis and multiple organ failure, although the latter complication may merely reflect the organ failure associated with the respiratory failure for which the technique is used.

Intravenacaval oxygenation

Intravenacaval oxygenation (IVOX) has been recently developed (Conrad et al 1993) and clinical trials have shown it to be a useful adjunctive therapy. A catheter with multiple fine tubes within it is placed in the inferior vena cava. Oxygen is passed through these at subatmospheric pressure and gas exchange takes place by passive diffusion. This technique is falling out of favour.

High-frequency jet ventilation

In high-frequency jet ventilation (HFJV), small pulses of gas at a rate of 60–600 per minute are delivered from a jet nozzle at the proximal end of the endotracheal tube, with humidified warmed air being entrained from a bias gas source. Lung volume is maintained with a higher mean airway pressure, thereby improving oxygenation. There are several theories as to how gas exchange can occur with such an unphysiological method of ventilation. Diffusion of gas and regional convective currents seem to play a major role. Although a controlled clinical trial has shown no advantage over conventional ventilation (Carlon et al 1983), the technique has been shown to be safe and newer computer-controlled prototypes are showing promise.

Nitric oxide administration

Administration of this gas via the ventilator was shown to reduce pulmonary artery pressures and improve arterial oxygenation in patients with severe respiratory failure (Rossaint et al 1993). It appears that ventilation/perfusion matching is improved without systemic vasodilatation. A mortality benefit has not been shown.

Prone position

A surprisingly simple and low-tech manouevre, turning the patient prone has been shown to dramatically improve oxygenation in a number of patients. There are logistic difficulties inherent in the technique and it does not always work, but when used early in severe respiratory failure, results are often impressive. The mechanism by which it works is complex (see also Chapter 5). A recent controlled study (Gattinoni et al 2001) has shown no mortality benefit.

CARDIAC SUPPORT

Even before heart transplantation was pioneered in 1967, the need for an artificial heart had been identified. This could be used for short-term support of the heart while waiting for it to recover from an acute insult (such as myocardial infarction or cardiac surgery) or for a donor heart to become available for transplantation or for long-term cardiac support. There are modalities available which provide partial to complete support, but they are expensive and may have significant side effects.

Intra-aortic balloon pump

The intra-aortic balloon pump (IABP) comprises a sausage-shaped balloon (15 mm × 280 mm and inflated by 40 ml of gas) mounted on a dual-lumen catheter. The balloon is introduced via the femoral artery, either percutaneously or by surgical dissection and direct vision, to the thoracic aorta (Fig. 9.3). Correct positioning of the catheter is confirmed by fluoroscopy or chest radiography. The catheter is attached to a console with a helium gas source for balloon inflation. The IABP is triggered by the electrocardiogram (ECG) to deflate during ventricular systole and to inflate during diastole. By so doing it improves cardiac performance (the left ventricle ejects into an 'empty' aorta) and improves myocardial perfusion (which occurs during diastole and is enhanced by the blood not running off into the aorta).

Indications for the use of the IABP include cardiogenic shock (after myocardial infarction), unstable angina, weaning from cardiopulmonary bypass and stabilization of patients with acute mitral regurgitation or ventricular septal defect following myocardial infarction. In these cases it is used as a bridge to definitive surgery, although the mortality for these defects remains in the region of 50%. The IABP cannot generate a cardiac output independent of the heart and a minimum cardiac output of about 1.5 l/min is needed for it to be effective.

The IABP is clearly a major invasive device and complications may be serious. They include aortic dissection, arterial perforation, limb ischaemia, thrombocytopenia and dislodgement of atherosclerotic emboli. Air embolism may occur if the balloon bursts. Major bleeding may occur following removal of the IABP.

Ventricular assist device

A ventricular assist device (VAD) is simply a pump that functions in parallel with the heart. Blood is withdrawn from the venous side of the circulation and returned to the arterial side, usually with a catheter in the left atrium and the left ventricle (left ventricular assist device or LVAD). Occasionally, both sides of the heart need support and this is achieved with a biventricular assist device (BIVAD). The VAD can provide most of the cardiac output, but the flow it delivers is not pulsatile, which may adversely affect vital organs such as the kidneys. Newer units may provide pulsatile flow and may be used for months. A total implantable unit may be placed in the upper abdomen. Indications for its use include failure to wean from cardiopulmonary bypass and bridging to heart transplantation or recovery from myocarditis. It is not without significant complications, with haemorrhage, thromboembolism and septicaemia being the most common.

RENAL SUPPORT

Before the advent of dialysis and transplantation, chronic renal failure (CRF) was invariably fatal and acute renal failure (ARF) usually fatal. Today, although ARF still carries a high mortality rate, especially when part of the complex of multiple organ failure, CRF can be effectively managed in dialysis and renal transplantation programmes.

The aims of renal support are very simple. They include control of fluid, electrolytes and acid–base status and elimination of uraemic toxins and drugs. These aims can be carried out in a number of ways which are detailed below.

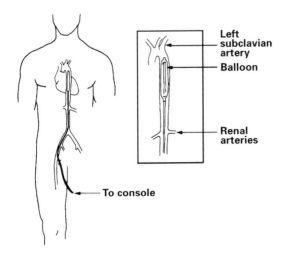

Figure 9.3   Placement of the intra-aortic balloon pump.

General principles of dialysis

All forms of dialysis involve diffusion of solute across a semipermeable membrane and down a concentration gradient. In peritoneal dialysis the membrane is the peritoneum and the blood flow is provided by the capillaries supplying it. In all forms of haemodialysis, the membrane is composed of cellophane or cuprophane and blood flow is provided by an extracorporeal circuit.

Conventional haemodialysis

Haemodialysis (HD) was first described in 1960 and is now the most commonly used dialysis therapy for both ARF and CRF. Blood is pumped through an extracorporeal system which includes a filter with a semipermeable membrane and dialysate (usually water mixed with predetermined concentrations of electrolytes and buffer) flows in a countercurrent direction through the filter, on the other side of the membrane. A gradient is thus created for electrolytes and metabolic waste products to diffuse across the membrane and fluid is driven across by hydrostatic pressure.

Vascular access is obtained by intravenous catheters or by the surgical creation of arteriovenous fistulae or shunts. HD is generally performed for 4–6 hours at a time, either daily or on alternate days. Although HD allows rapid correction of fluid and electrolyte abnormalities, it may not be well tolerated in critically ill, haemodynamically unstable patients. Hypotension may develop and cause further ischaemic insult to the kidney. Hypoxaemia almost invariably occurs; it is caused by neutrophil aggregation in the lungs and complement activation in the filter membrane.

Continuous forms of renal support

Conventional haemodialysis is not well tolerated in critically ill patients as it may produce rapid changes in intravascular volume, blood pressure, PaO_2 and pH. Slower but continuous forms of haemodialysis were developed to address this problem. Outcome data are impressive when compared with historical controls (Bellomo & Boyce 1993). The terminology is confusing; terms such as CAVH, CAVHD, CVVH and CVVHD (see below) perplex the uninitiated. The treatment choices differ in several ways (Schetz et al 1989). Access to the circulation may be by both arterial and venous cannulae (arteriovenous) or by venous cannulae (venovenous). The blood flow through the circuit may be pumped by an external pump or by the patient's own arterial pressure, as in arteriovenous systems. Pure haemofiltration may be performed or may be combined with dialysis (Fig. 9.4). Whatever the method, the extracorporeal circuit needs to be anticoagulated to prevent the blood from clotting.

Continuous haemofiltration

In continuous haemofiltration, blood flow in the extracorporeal circuit may be driven by a pump with vascular access provided by venous catheters (continuous venovenous haemofiltra-

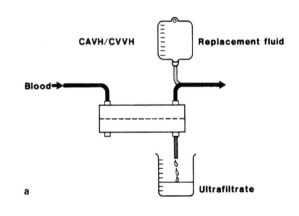

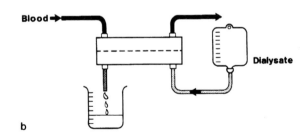

Figure 9.4 Continuous renal support: the concepts of filtration and dialysis. **a** Haemofiltration alone. **b** Haemofiltration with dialysis.

tion or CVVH) or may be driven by the patient's own arterial pressure with an arterial and a venous catheter (continuous arteriovenous haemofiltration or CAVH). The hydrostatic pressure created in either system drives filtrate through the semipermeable membrane. This filtrate is essentially plasma water, but as it moves across the membrane it drags solutes with it by the process of convection. Large amounts of filtrate may be removed (up to 1 l/hour) and this fluid (the ultrafiltrate) is replaced with a fluid that has an electrolyte composition similar to plasma.

Continuous haemofiltration with dialysis

The terminology for continuous haemofiltration with dialysis is similar to the above, with the variants being continuous venovenous haemofiltration with dialysis (CVVHD) and continuous arteriovenous haemofiltration with dialysis (CAVHD). Here dialysis fluid is pumped through the filter in a countercurrent direction to the blood flow (similar to HD outlined above). Greater solute clearance can be achieved and as the hydrostatic pressure does not need to be as high as in CVVH, less ultrafiltrate is formed and less replacement fluid is needed. As CAVHD does not involve actively pumping blood into the extracorporeal circuit, it can be used in haemodynamically very unstable patients and may be the technique of choice in that situation.

Peritoneal dialysis

The peritoneum is an excellent semipermeable membrane and is used as such in peritoneal dialysis (PD). A catheter is inserted percutaneously into the peritoneal cavity and dialysate (usually 1–2 l) is allowed to run in, remain in the peritoneal cavity for a period of time and then run out. Dialysate comes in premixed bags and its composition allows for the removal of electrolytes and uraemic waste products. Solute clearance is determined by dialysate flow rate, peritoneal permeability, peritoneal vascularity and blood flow. Dialysate with a high glucose concentration allows large amounts of fluid to be removed by osmosis.

The most common complication of PD is abdominal discomfort caused by raised intra-abdominal pressure and splinting of the diaphragm; this may result in basal subsegmental lung collapse and hypoxaemia. Peritonitis is a more serious problem and usually relates to contamination of the dialysate at the time of bag changes. Prompt recognition and the instillation of intraperitoneal antibiotics are the mainstays of treatment. Other complications include bowel perforation (usually at the time of catheter insertion) and hyperglycaemia.

The main advantage of PD is that correction of fluid and metabolic abnormalities is gradual and there is minimal haemodynamic disturbance (although ventilation may be compromised by the intra-abdominal fluid). However, clearance of uraemic toxins is generally less efficient than with HD and this may be a problem in critically ill hypermetabolic patients. In addition, PD cannot be used in patients with acute intraabdominal pathology or recent abdominal surgery.

Indications for renal support

Acute renal failure

The indications for renal support in acute renal failure are generally based on clinical parameters rather than on biochemistry alone. They include the speed of deterioration of renal function, the general clinical scenario and the likely rapidity of recovery. Absolute indications for urgent renal support are fluid overload, hyperkalaemia or acidosis unresponsive to conventional treatment. The urea and creatinine values are useful as a guide to starting renal support, but absolute values are controversial. As a rough rule, dialysis is often started when urea is greater than 40 mmol/l, creatinine is greater than 500 µmol/l or when potassium is greater than 6 mmol/l.

Chronic renal failure

The decision to initiate renal support in a patient with chronic renal failure is usually made by the renal unit in a major hospital. It is almost always coupled with entering the patient onto a waiting list for renal transplantation, using renal support as a bridge until a live related or cadaver transplant can be performed. Patients are fully assessed for their suitability to enter such a programme by a team that generally includes physicians, nurses, a social worker and a psychiatrist.

Potential hazards for physiotherapists

Mechanical problems

These include kinking of support lines, disconnection of different parts of the circuit and, worst of all, displacement of catheters from artery or vein. The former will cause the system to stop functioning or to function less well, but the latter can cause spectacular haemorrhage which may be fatal if not noticed immediately. Disconnection may also cause air embolism. Great care should therefore be taken when moving patients on dialysis.

Haemodynamic

Patients on renal support may be relatively depleted of intravascular fluid and changes in posture may produce hypotension and, occasionally, cardiac arrhythmias.

Infection

Renal failure produces a state of relative immunosuppression with patients being more susceptible to infection. Meticulous care therefore needs to be taken with sterile techniques such as suctioning and even manual hyperinflation.

Respiratory

Patients on dialysis are prone to hypoxaemia (for the reasons mentioned above) and may desaturate rapidly during suctioning or turning.

PAEDIATRICS

INTRODUCTION

The practice of mechanical ventilation in children needs to be informed by an understanding of age-related pathophysiology if treatment is to be effective. In contrast to adults, the most common causes of respiratory failure in children differ with age. In the newborn infant, prematurity, hyaline membrane disease, asphyxia and aspiration pneumonia are the most common aetiologies. Under 2 years of age, bronchopneumonia, bronchiolitis, croup, status asthmaticus, foreign body inhalation and congenital heart and airway anomalies are important, compared with asthma, accidental poisoning and central nervous system infection, trauma and cerebral hypoxia/ischaemia in the over 2 year olds. Although the principles of when and how mechanical support should be undertaken in such patients are, broadly speaking, similar to those applied in adults, there are differences in epidemiolology and pathophysiology which warrant consideration. The emphasis, therefore, of this section will be a paediatric perspective of respiratory supportive therapy which builds on the previous discussion about adults.

EPIDEMIOLOGY OF ACUTE RESPIRATORY FAILURE IN CHILDREN

Epidemiologically, there is little information in children about the incidence of acute respiratory failure. Adult definitions using blood gas parameters may be appropriate for certain age-groups but in others they may not be useful. For example, in infants with acute bronchiolitis, acute respiratory failure is usually defined as: $PaCO_2 = 8$ kPa (60 mmHg) with, in addition, $PaO_2 = 60$ mmHg (8 kPa) when using $F_iO_2 = 0.6$; or, in the case of patients with respiratory arrest, a preceding history of severe respiratory distress accompanied by cyanosis.

However, when trying to look at large populations, in the absence of blood gases, a more pragmatic definition for acute respiratory failure is needed. For example, when using the definition of 'acute airway management necessitating endotracheal tube intubation' it is possible to explore issues such as the pattern and timecourse of paediatric disease (Tasker 2000) which, clearly, have some bearing on how mechanical support should be undertaken.

Pattern of and timecourse of disease

Table 9.1 summarizes a retrospective analysis of 1000 infants and children (aged older than 28 days and younger than 17 years) who required endotracheal intubation for acute respiratory failure complicating acutely acquired medical, rather than surgical, disease (Tasker 2000). These children were cared for on a general medical intensive care unit in London (Great Ormond Street Hospital for Children) prior to 1996. The three major categories relate to the system or problem underlying respiratory failure (respiratory tract disorder, central nervous system disorder or systemic disorder) and the subcategories relate to the clinical diagnostic entities commonly encountered in intensive care. Respiratory tract problems due to infection are, not surprisingly, the most common problems seen. The timecourse of recovery in survivors is influenced by the site within the airways that infection has reached. This is reflected by an increase in the length of stay in the ICU with more distally affected tissues (i.e upper airway compared with lower airway). In relating such information to clinical practice one can use the expected timecourse to decide on an agenda for treatment or 'care pathway'. For example, given that the expected timecourse for intensive care recovery in pneumonia necessitating intubation is around 8 days (interquartile range 5–12 days) one can then predict when certain targets should be met. The same applies to the other 11 distinct diagnosis-related entities. This idea will be revisited later in this chapter where three clinical examples are discussed.

Acute hypoxaemic respiratory failure

Acute hypoxaemic respiratory failure (AHRF) signifies respiratory failure at the more severe end of the pathophysiological spectrum, irrespective of underlying aetiology. For paediatric practice we identify this state by using diagnostic criteria which have been modified from the American-European Consensus Conference diagnostic criteria for acute respiratory distress syndrome (ARDS) (Bernard et al 1994). These criteria include:

- acute onset of respiratory failure over less than 48 hours

Table 9.1 Diagnostic distribution of 1000 children requiring endotracheal tube intubation during acute medical illness ordered by number (n), age and length of stay on the intensive care unit in survivors. (IQR, interquartile range: LRTD, lower respiratory tract disease)

System disorder	n	Age in months median (IQR)	Length of stay in survivors median (IQR) days, m : f
Respiratory tract	**521**	**13 (4–40)**	
Upper airway infection	80	21 (12–35)	4 (3–5) : 3 (3–5)
Bronchiolitis	89	3 (2–6)	5 (4–9) : 6 (3–9)
Asthma	25	37 (21–86)	4 (3–5) : 4 (3–5)
Pneumonia	90	10 (4–40)	8 (5–12) : 9 (4–14)
Pneumonia and immunodeficiency	120	16 (5–51)	9 (5–16) : 9 (7–14)
Neuromuscular disease	66	22 (7–88)	10 (5–19) : 8 (5–20)
Non-infective LRTD	51	16 (7–69)	5 (3–8) : 6 (4–10)
Central nervous	**342**	**18 (6–62)**	
Infection	117	22 (8–65)	4 (2–6) : 4 (3–7)
Hypoxia-ischaemia	78	14 (4–34)	5 (2–10) : 3 (1–8)
Other encephalopathy	147	17 (6–70)	5 (3–8) : 5 (2–8)
Systemic	**137**	**19 (6–52)**	
Septicaemia	90	19 (4–69)	6 (4–10) : 6 (4–12)
Inflammatory syndromes	47	19 (6–32)	4 (3–9) : 5 (3–8)

- evidence of a severe defect in oxygenation (PaO_2/F_iO_2 of less than 26.7 kPa, 200 mmHg) for at least 6 consecutive hours on the day of admission
- no evidence of left atrial hypertension
- four-quadrant interstitial shadowing on chest radiograph.

Children meeting all the above criteria except the characteristic chest X-ray appearances of ARDS (last criterion) are described as cases of AHRF.

The significance of AHRF is that it implies a certain severity of illness and risk of mortality, factors which are important when it comes to deciding which ventilatory strategy should be adopted and the use of adjunctive therapies (see section on 'ventilation strategies for specific disease'). For example, in a recent prospective, epidemiological study, conducted on a general medical paediatric intensive care unit in London, Peters and colleagues (1998) found that out of 850 mechanically ventilated infants and children, AHRF occurred in 118 patients (14%, 95% confidence interval (CI) 12–16%). Of these 118 patients, 52 met the criteria for ARDS (44%, 35–53%). In all 850 patients, mortality was 26/118 (22%, 18–26%) for those with AHRF, which was four times higher than the mortality seen in those patients without AHRF (39/732; 5%, 4–7%). In the 118 AHRF patients, mortality was 19/52 (37%, 24–51%) for those with ARDS, which was three times higher than the mortality seen in those patients without ARDS (7/66; 11%, 4–21%). Therefore, identifying these entities (i.e. AHRF and ARDS) at an early stage is important, not least because patterns of response – or failed response – to respiratory support seem to follow a predictable pattern and timecourse (Peters et al 1998).

INDICATIONS FOR SUPPORTIVE RESPIRATORY THERAPY

For practical purposes we can consider the treatment of respiratory dysfunction in terms of treating hypoxia and hypercarbia. Appropriate management is aimed first at prevention, second at early diagnosis and third at a clear under-

standing of the pathophysiology and way in which the proposed treatment works to maintain or restore good lung function.

Hypoxia

Hypoxia must be treated by the administration of supplemental oxygen. At the same time attempts should be made to correct the underlying problem. Local processes such as atelectasis and bronchopneumonia can result in a portion of the pulmonary blood flow perfusing unventilated alveoli, so-called intrapulmonary shunt, which in some cases may be effectively treated by pulmonary toilet and postural change. With a large shunt fraction (i.e. greater than 25% of pulmonary blood flow), PaO_2 is not significantly improved by solely increasing the FiO_2. In these cases a diffuse pulmonary process is usually present and a form of assisted positive airway pressure is required. Such assistance may also be required for severe impairment of chest wall mechanics from rib fractures, pain, weakness, etc., even in the absence of pulmonary parenchymal disease.

In infants and children, there are several methods of administering oxygen (Table 9.2). Nasal catheters and cannulae are not usually tolerated by younger patients. Oxygen delivered via the oxygen inlet of an incubator rarely exceeds an FiO_2 of 0.4. When oxygen is delivered into a tent the concentration varies depending on leaks. Regardless of the technique, it is essential

Table 9.2 Methods of oxygen administration

	Maximum achievable FiO_2 at 6–10 l/min of oxygen (%)
Nasopharyngeal catheter	50
Nasal prongs	50
Masks:	
without reservoir bag	50
with reservoir bag (partial rebreathing)	70
with reservoir (non-rebreathing)	95
Venturi	24, 28, 35, 40
Incubator	40
Canopy tent	50
Head box	95

that the administered oxygen is heated and humidified. To avoid damage to the lungs, oxygen administration should be discontinued as soon as possible (as indicated by blood gas measurements). An FiO_2 below 0.6 is preferred so as to minimize the risk of oxygen toxicity. Reduction in the FiO_2 should be carried out cautiously in a stepwise manner. To facilitate this process both the concentration and duration of oxygen therapy must be recorded accurately. A well-calibrated oxygen analyser must be used to check the inspired concentration at least every 2 hours. The necessity for monitoring PaO_2 in preterm newborn infants is related to both the potential for pulmonary oxygen toxicity and the danger of retrolental fibroplasia. In any patient, oxygen should be administered at the lowest concentration sufficient to maintain the PaO_2 between 6.7 and 13.3 kPa (50–100 mmHg). In this regard, continuous measurement or monitoring of transcutaneous partial pressure of oxygen or pulse oximetry arterial oxygen saturation (SpO_2) are essential additions to the direct, and intermittent, measurement of arterial blood gases.

Lastly, it should also be remembered that supplemental oxygen may cause further respiratory depression if there has been chronic respiratory failure and a loss of sensitivity to CO_2. This phenomenon is generally uncommon in paediatric practice, but has been encountered in children with cystic fibrosis and bronchopulmonary dysplasia.

In addition to oxygen, PEEP may be useful in the management of hypoxia. PEEP or CPAP has been shown to increase lung compliance by recruiting additional areas of the lung for ventilation. Also, PEEP or CPAP improves oxygenation by decreasing intrapulmonary shunt. The addition of some PEEP to all mechanical ventilation modes is a common practice in maintaining an adequate functional residual capacity. However, PEEP may adversely affect lung mechanics if hyperinflation occurs, which results in impaired pulmonary perfusion, further accentuating any ventilation-perfusion mismatch. Therefore PEEP above 4 cmH_2O is generally not indicated when there is already regional hyperinflation, such as occurs in bronchopulmonary dysplasia (Box 9.1).

Box 9.1 Positive end-expiratory pressure

Advantages
Increased functional residual capacity
Recruits additional lung units, improving compliance
Reduces pulmonary shunt fraction
Allows for a decrease in FiO_2

Disadvantages
Increases mean airway pressure, leading to reduced venous return
Can increase 'dead space' by impairing perfusion to hyperinflated regions
Can increase pulmonary vascular resistance and right heart dysfunction
Altered renal blood flow with increase in antidiuretic hormone release
Barotrauma caused by increased airway pressure

Box 9.2 Initial treatment of hypoxia

1. Increase FiO_2 to maintain SaO_2 > 90% (see Table 9.2)
2. Consider positve pressure and PEEP, if large shunt. Indications:
   hypoxaemia with FiO_2 > 0.5
   diffuse lung disease
   maintain lung volume
3. Initiate aggressive pulmonary toilet
4. Eliminate the underlying cause:
   pain
   fluid overload
   atelectasis
   bronchopneumonia
5. Correct systemic abnormalities:
   hypovolaemia
   sepsis
   carbon monoxide poisoning

In this context a strategy for treating hypoxia is outlined in Box 9.2.

Hypercarbia

When shallow (or ineffectual) breathing is present, the dead space (i.e. ventilated but non-perfused regions) becomes a larger fraction of each breath. This change results in a decrease in alveolar ventilation, even if the lung parenchyma is normal. When hypercarbia has been found and its cause considered, the most appropriate treatment can be effectively initiated. Increasing alveolar ventilation is relatively easy with mechanical ventilation, but an increase in mean airway pressure occurs, with its potential detrimental effects.

If the patient is already being treated with full mechanical ventilation the first step is to make sure that the patient is actually receiving an appropriate tidal volume and minute ventilation. Ventilatory system leaks and loss of a portion of the tidal volume through compression loss in the tubing, as well as abnormalities in endotracheal tube function, are common causes. Having excluded mechanical factors, the other causes of hypercarbia may be related to an increase in CO_2 production or an increase in dead-space ventilation. In the latter case, an increase in dead space due to excessive PEEP (particularly when there is already hyperinflation or hypovolaemia) can be corrected by intravenous volume loading.

Endotracheal intubation

There are four absolute indications for controlling the airway by endotracheal intubation. First, maintaining the patency of the airway where problems are present or anticipated (e.g. direct airway trauma, oedema or infection). Second, to protect the airway from aspiration in states of altered consciousness, where airway-protective mechanisms may be lost or impaired. Third, to facilitate pulmonary toilet and avoid airway obstruction when there is marked atelectasis and pulmonary infection – an inadequate cough might necessitate more direct access to the airways for suctioning. Fourth, when positive pressure breathing is indicated because of inadequate spontaneous ventilation.

In practice, establishing airway and respiratory support for the acutely ill child should be carried out by experienced staff, because such patients can deteriorate rapidly, particularly at the time of inducing anaesthesia. Following pre-oxygenation with 100% inspired oxygen, a variety of agents are used to facilitate endotracheal intubation including: intravenous induction with drugs such as fentanyl, midazolam and suxamethonium or inhalational induction with gases such as halothane or isoflurane. Table 9.3 provides a guide to the appropriate endotracheal tube size, length and suction catheter used in the

Table 9.3 Endotracheal tube size and suction catheters

Age	Weight (kg)	Endotracheal tube (mm)	Length at lip (cm)	Length at nose	Suction catheter (Fr gauge)
Newborn	<0.7	2.0	5.0	6.0	5.0
	<1	2.5	5.5	7.0	5.0
	1	3.0	6.0	7.5	6.0
	2	3.0	7.0	9.0	6.0
	3	3.0	8.5	10.5	6.0
	3.5	3.5	9.0	11	7.0
3 months	6.0	3.5	10	12	7.0
1 year	10	4.0	11	14	8.0
2 years	12	4.5	12	15	8.0
3 years	14	4.5	13	16	8.0
4 years	16	5.0	14	17	10
6 years	20	5.5	15	19	10
8 years	24	6.0	16	20	12
10 years	30	6.5	17	21	12
12 years	38	7.0	18	22	12–14
14 years	50	7.5	19	23	14

paediatric age range and Figure 9.5 illustrates two commonly used methods of endotracheal tube fixation.

MECHANICAL VENTILATION

In children, mechanical ventilatory support using positive pressure ventilation is more frequently used than negative pressure support.

General ventilatory care

A variety of ventilators are used in paediatric mechanical ventilation (Fig. 9.6). The effectiveness of a particular ventilator depends not least on the skill and experience of those administering this form of therapy though, of course, the functional characteristics of the machine itself are also an important factor. One type may best suit a particular age group under certain conditions (Table 9.4). The volume-cycled (pressure-limited) machine is effective when airway resistance is markedly increased and lung compliance is decreased, because even under these circumstances the appropriate tidal volume will continue to be delivered to the patient. However, a sudden increase in lung compliance may lead to intrathoracic air leak or pneumothorax, which is difficult to detect unless inspiratory pressure is

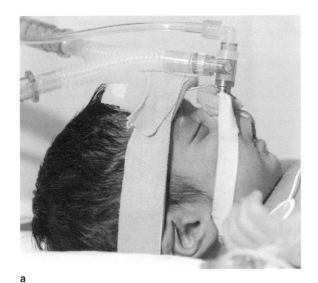

a

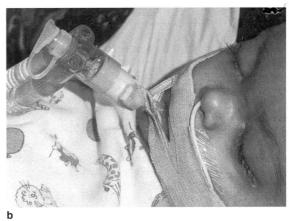

b

Figure 9.5 Endotracheal tube fixation for (**a**) nasal and (**b**) oral tubes.

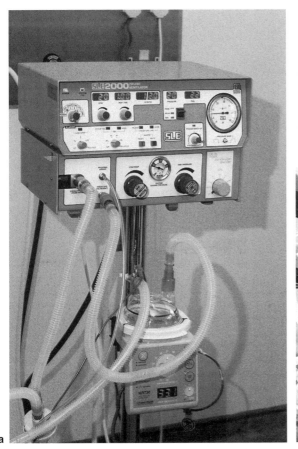

a

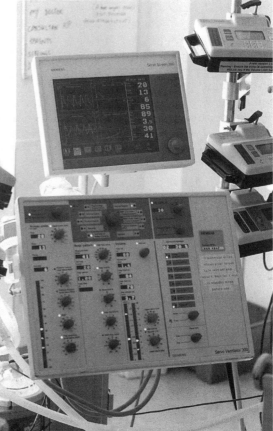

b

Fig. 9.6 (**a**) The SLE 2000 infant ventilator and (**b**) the Servo 300 ventilator.

Table 9.4 Advantages and disadvantages of pressure-limited and volume-limited ventilation

	Pressure-limited	Volume-limited
Advantages	Avoids excessive inflating pressures Decreased risk of barotrauma	Constant volume delivered High inflating pressures reflect changes in mechanics
Disadvantages	Variable volume delivered No signs of altered mechanics	Capable of generating very high inflating pressures Increased risk of barotrauma

monitored. In contrast, use of the pressure-cycled (flow rate-limited) ventilator in the presence of leaks disturbs the attainment of the preset pressure and thereby alters the cycling pattern. However, a decrease in lung compliance, such as that caused by accumulation of secretions, may be associated with a decrease in tidal volume. This situation may go unrecognized because the ventilator will continue to cycle at the preset pressure.

In conditions associated with low lung volumes, such as hyaline membrane disease, atelectasis and severe pneumonia (e.g. viral, *Pneumocystis carinii*), alveolar collapse may be alleviated or prevented by the use of PEEP. Alveolar pressure is not allowed to return to zero or atmospheric pressure but is held at 3–5 cmH$_2$O above atmospheric pressure during expiration.

Complications of ventilator therapy occur frequently and all intensive care staff should be continually aware of the potential hazards (Box 9.3). Aseptic technique is important for tracheal airway care because nosocomial infection constitutes a large and preventable problem. The application of PEEP, increased tidal volumes and increased airway pressure can also produce complications. Potential disruption of the normal ventilation perfusion matching seen with spontaneous breathing can occur with lung over-expansion and leads to regional hypoperfusion. Cardiac output and oxygen delivery can be impaired by a decrease in venous return, an increase in pulmonary vascular resistance and a decrease in left ventricular output. The more compliant the lung or the less compliant the chest wall, the greater the transmission of positive airway pressure to the mediastinum and the greater the negative effect on cardiac function. The concomitant decrease in cardiac output, in

---

Box 9.3 Complications associated with mechanical ventilation

Respiratory
Tracheal lesions, e.g. erosions, oedema, stenosis, granuloma, obstruction
Accidental endotracheal tube displacement into bronchus, oesophagus or hypopharynx
Infection
Air leaks, e.g. pneumothorax, pneumomediastinum, interstitial emphysema
Air trapping causing hyperinflation
Excessive secretions resulting in atelectasis
Oxygen hazards, e.g. depression of ventilation, bronchopulmonary dysplasia
Pulmonary haemorrhage

Circulatory
Impaired venous return resulting in decreased cardiac output and systemic hypotension
Oxygen hazards, e.g. retrolental fibroplasia, cerebral vasoconstriction
Septicaemia
Intracranial haemorrhage, e.g. intraventricular, subarachnoid
Hyperventilation leading to decreased cerebral blood flow

Metabolic
Increased work of breathing because of 'fighting' the ventilator
Alkalosis due to potassium depletion or excessive bicarbonate therapy

Renal and fluid balance
Antidiuresis
Excess water in the inspired gas

Equipment malfunction (mechanical)
Ventilator leaks or valve dysfunction
Overheating of inspired gases
Kinked or disconnected tubes

---

large part, can be overcome by volume loading or inotropic support.

Barotrauma is the result of high airway inspiratory pressure causing alveolar disruption. Airway pressure may be reduced by decreasing the tidal volume, PEEP or peak inspiratory pressure (PIP) or by paralysing the already sedated patient. Pulmonary interstitial emphysema, pneumomediastinum, pneumoperitoneum and subcutaneous emphysema do not require specific treatment unless there is significant haemodynamic impairment. Poor renal function, as exhibited by decreased glomerular filtration rate, urine production and sodium excretion, can be a consequence of hypoxia and hypercarbia. This may be further compounded by the effects of mechanical ventilation with PEEP on producing an antidiuretic hormone-mediated salt and water retaining effect (probably secondary to decreased cardiac output), an increased renal vein pressure and a neural reflex from the pressure-distorted atrial wall.

Acute deterioration and 'troubleshooting'

The adequacy of gas exchange and ventilation should be assessed frequently in mechanically ventilated patients, with therapy titrated against expected parameters or targets (Table 9.5). When acute deterioration during mechanical ventilation occurs 'troubleshooting' should begin with disconnecting the patient from the ventilator and bagging with an F_iO_2 of 1.0. Easy ventilation with the bag and patient stabilization suggests a ventilator problem, which should be systematically addressed (e.g. checking the circuit for leaks, checking ventilator function, checking gas flow). However, it should be remembered that 'handbagging' can result in an increased tidal volume,

which can also be responsible for the patient's improvement. Patients with stiff lungs are frequently dyspnoeic, despite adequate gas exchange. Increasing the tidal volume will correct this subjective feeling and may also account for patient improvement. Difficult bagging at the time of disconnecting the ventilator strongly suggests a problem with the endotracheal tube or the lung to chest-wall complex. A suction catheter (Table 9.3) should be passed down the endotracheal tube to check for narrowing or blockage. Chest examination, blood gases and chest radiography should be ordered. A blocked endotracheal tube should be replaced. A pneumothorax requires chest tube placement. If neither of these is the cause for deterioration, then the possibilities may include new problems such as an increased oxygen demand due to sepsis, impaired oxygen delivery due to heart failure or acute pulmonary injury due to gastric aspiration. These and other causes need to be sought and treated appropriately.

Newer ventilatory support techniques

High-frequency ventilation techniques, including high-frequency positive pressure ventilation, high-frequency jet ventilation and high-frequency oscillatory ventilation (HFOV), achieve adequate ventilation by employing tidal volumes that are often less than actual dead space and respiratory rates of 60–3000 cycles/minute (Fig. 9.7). The high-velocity ventilations result in increased mixing by Brownian motion, which enhances gas

Table 9.5 Normal values

	Newborn	Up to 3 years	3–6 years	> 6 years
Respiratory rate (breaths/minute)	40–60	20–30	20–30	15–20
Arterial blood pH	7.30–7.40	7.30–7.40	7.35–7.45	7.35–7.45
$PaCO_2$ (mmHg) (kPa)	30–35 4.0–4.7	30–35 4.0–4.7	35–45 4.7–6.0	35–45, 4.7–6.0
PaO_2 (mmHg) (kPa)	60–90 8.0–12.0	80–100 10.7–13.3	80–100 10.7–13.3	80–100 10.7–13.3
Heart rate (beats/minute)	100–200	100–180	70–150	70–150
Systolic blood pressure (mmHg)	60–90	75–130	90–140	90–140
Diastolic blood pressure (mmHg)	30–60	45–90	50–80	50–80

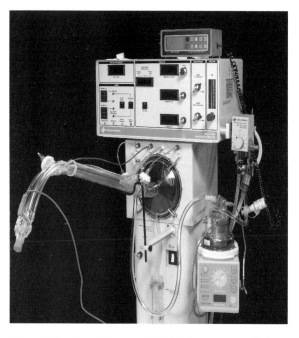

Figure 9.7 A ventilator used for high-frequency oscillation.

diffusion and exchange. In theory, ventilation is more evenly distributed with the use of decreased airway pressures (Gertsmann et al 1991). Indications for this form of ventilation may include bronchopleural fistula and refractory hypoxaemia. The decision on when to initiate such therapy has to be based on the full clinical picture. The experience reported by Watkins and colleagues (2000) in 100 courses of such ventilation would suggest that, in the presence of AHRF or ARDS, a threshold mean airway pressure of 16 cmH$_2$O would be an appropriate indication.

Extracorporeal membrane oxygenation (ECMO) is designed to provide a variable degree of cardiopulmonary support for a predetermined period of time over which the underlying pulmonary disorder is expected to recover. Potentially, ECMO allows recovery without subjecting the lungs to the risks of barotrauma or oxygen toxicity. Venoarterial systems may be used to completely take over the child's own heart and lung function (Fig. 9.8), although in practice extracorporeal flows

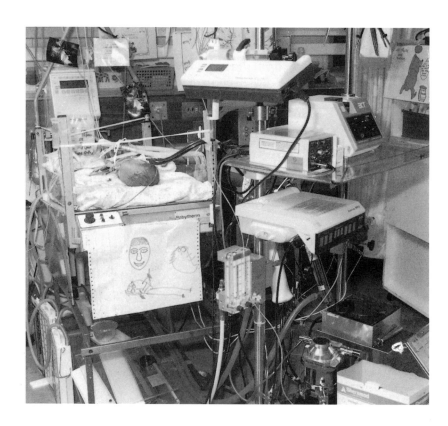

Figure 9.8 Extracorporeal membrane oxygenation.

may be limited by venous drainage (usually from the right internal jugular vein). Venovenous systems have been used for CO_2 removal and, in the complete absence of pulmonary function, will provide SpO_2 of 80%. Using extracorporeal support, success has been achieved in neonates with persistent pulmonary hypertension who have failed to respond to conventional mechanical ventilation (Bartlett et al 1982), and some children with acute lung injury (Pearson et al 1993). However, appropriate patient selection is a critical and contentious issue. One method, proposed by Bartlett (1990), is to identify neonates at high risk for failing to respond to conventional therapy by applying an index of oxygenation, which is related to the mean airway pressure and the FiO_2 used during mechanical ventilation, and the achieved PaO_2:

$$\text{Oxygenation index (OI)} = \text{mean airway pressure} \times FiO_2 \times 100 / PaO_2 \text{ (mmHg)}$$

In Bartlett's proposal (1990), an OI greater than 25 predicted a 50% mortality rate and an OI greater than 40 predicted an 80% mortality rate. Given this background, prospective trials have documented an 83% survival rate with ECMO in neonates, but convincing data in older children and adults are lacking. Anecdotally, Goldman and colleagues (1997) have found that, in the setting of meningococcal sepsis, ARDS which fails to respond to high-frequency oscillation may be reasonably treated with ECMO.

VENTILATION STRATEGIES FOR SPECIFIC DISEASE

In paediatric practice there are some specific diseases or problems which do require a specific ventilatory strategy. These issues are illustrated by the examples which follow.

Acute bronchiolitis

The typical features of bronchiolitis are:

- acute generalized peripheral airway obstruction ('air trapping'), as recognized by tachypnoea, decreased breath sounds and low diaphragms on chest radiograph

- occurrence in the infant less than 2 years of age, because their airways are smaller and contribute a larger fraction of airway resistance
- usually the first episode, with little or no evidence of past similar episodes.

This syndrome is usually caused by viral infection. Respiratory syncytial virus (RSV) is the most frequent viral aetiology and occurs primarily in infants under 6 months of age, usually with less fever or leucocytosis than is observed with RSV-negative disease. Other viral causes include adenovirus, influenza and parainfluenza viruses and rhinovirus. Cytomegalovirus can produce a bronchiolitis or pneumonitis-like illness in immunocompromised children. Rare non-viral causes of the bronchiolitis syndrome include *Mycoplasma pneumoniae* and *Bordetella pertussis* infection.

Pathologically, RSV infection in the nasopharynx progresses to involve the lower respiratory tract. There is bronchiolar epithelial cell necrosis and peribronchiolar infiltration with lymphocytes, plasma cells and macrophages. Although there is submucosal oedema, there are no obvious changes in elastic tissue or smooth muscle. Within the airway, there are mucus plugs laden with cellular debris. The combined effect of these changes in the lung is the production of areas of partial or complete airway obstruction, which results in hyperinflation (ball-valve inflow obstruction) and atelectasis (stop-valve or ball-valve outflow obstruction).

Sixteen percent of infants hospitalized for RSV have apnoea and its course is usually shortlived. Clinically the episodes are diaphragmatic or non-obstructive with complete absence of respiratory effort. The mechanism is unclear but may be related to stimulation of laryngeal chemoreceptors, sensitization of airway receptors or respiratory muscle fatigue. Whatever the cause, there is an association with immature mechanisms responsible for respiratory control. In these cases, endotracheal intubation with minimal support is required until the problem of apnoea resolves.

In patients with worsening respiratory distress due to pulmonary parenchymal changes, mechanical support does not necessarily require endotracheal intubation. In some instances, nasopharyngeal prong CPAP, which maintains positive transpulmonary pressure during spontaneous breathing, can be used in bronchiolitis to avoid, perhaps, the need for mechanical ventilation or as an adjunct to weaning from ventilatory support in the very young infant. However, when infants with RSV infection require mechanical ventilation, there are many similarities with mechanical ventilation of adults with status asthmaticus (Box 9.4). Clinical observation of inspiratory and expiratory chest excursion as well as regular auscultation are important if overventilation, with associated hyperinflation and barotrauma, is to be avoided. The aim is to maintain or achieve adequate arterial oxygenation and control of respiratory acidosis with masterly con-

trolled mechanical hypoventilation. This may even necessitate ventilating at slow rates with prolonged expiratory times to permit adequate CO_2 clearance. Low levels of PEEP are also sometimes used to decrease airway resistance and improve gas exchange, although in studies of lung mechanics this has not been verified. With pressure-limited ventilation, the presence of inadvertent or auto-PEEP requires that inspiratory pressures be raised above the trapped alveolar pressure before inspiratory flow can begin. With volume-controlled ventilation, observed peak inflation pressures will rise.

In patients with hyperinflation the ventilatory strategy adopted should aim to limit ventilator-associated dynamic hyperinflation and impaired minute ventilation by ventilation at slow rates (10–15 breaths/minute) and prolonged expiratory times. A time-cycled, pressure-limited mechanical ventilator is used in this instance while aiming for an arterial pH > 7.25 and a SpO_2 88–92%. When indicated, neuromuscular blockade and antibiotics will need to be prescribed. All patients should receive adequate analgesia and sedation during mechanical ventilation. Bronchodilators can be administered if patients demonstrate a therapeutic response to an initial trial dose. In the acute phase of illness, fluids, electrolytes and hydration must be closely monitored while generally restricting fluid to 67–75% of maintenance requirements. In the weaning phase, patients can be removed from ventilatory support when safe to do so. In regard to blood gas parameters this means, in general, adequate oxygenation in a FiO_2 < 0.4 and normal pH, with good respiratory drive, in the absence of hypercarbia. Discharge from the intensive care unit can then be considered once the patient has managed at least 12–24 hours without any respiratory assistance. Overall these patients will, on average, spend about 7 days (interquartile range 4–8 days) on the intensive care unit (Tasker et al 2000).

In about one-fifth of mechanically ventilated patients with RSV more severe disease is seen (Tasker et al 2000). In this instance, more extensive pulmonary pathology results in a picture of pneumonitis with diffuse alveolar consolidation rather than bronchiolitis with lung hyperinflation. These

---

Box 9.4   Ventilation of acute bronchiolitis

Oxygenation
Aim: PaO_2 9–10 kPa

		Using PEEP and supplemental oxygen
If	FiO_2 ≥ 0.6	Increase PEEP
If	PaO_2 ≥ 11.3 kPa	Decrease FiO_2 to 0.6: – then decrease PEEP to 4 cmH_2O – then decrease FiO_2

Carbon dioxide
Aim: $PaCO_2$ 5.3–6.5 kPa

		Using rate 10–15/min, tidal volume 15 ml/kg or whatever PIP to achieve adequate chest movement If PIP ≥ 30 cmH_2O or if agitated then paralyse
If	$PaCO_2$ ≥ 7 kPa	Pressure-limited ventilation: – increase PIP before rate if chest excursion inadequate Volume ventilation: – increase minute ventilation with rate up to 20/min
If	$PaCO_2$ ≤ 4.7 kPa	Lower tidal volume to 10 ml/kg: – then PIP to 25 cmH_2O – then rate

Extubation criteria

PaO_2 ≥ 9.3 kPa		PEEP/CPAP ≤ 4 cmH_2O FiO_2 ≤ 0.4
$PaCO_2$ ≤ 6 kPa		Rate ≤ 6/min

Continue with supplemental oxygen until SpO_2 ≥ 0.95 in room air infants have the clinical features of ARDS as they exhibit four-quadrant consolidation on chest radiograph. Oxygenation is compromised with best achievable alveolar arterial oxygen gradients ($AaDO_2$, torr) and mean airway pressure (MAP, cmH_2O) values as follows: first 24 hours of mechanical ventilation, $AaDO_2 > 400$ and MAP > 10; second 24 hours, $AaDO_2 \geq 300$ and MAP > 10. In regard to mechanical support, the aim should be to recruit lung volume with the addition of PEEP. Sometimes high-frequency oscillatory ventilation or ECMO is required if lung injury becomes more extensive with likely development of interstitial emphysema and pneumothoraces. The timecourse of this problem is very different to the usual course of bronchiolitis and, on average, patients spend at least 2 weeks on the intensive care unit (Tasker et al 2000).

Acute hypoxaemic respiratory failure

In patients with AHRF or ARDS there is a widely accepted ventilatory strategy which should be employed. In children the strategy of permissive hypercarbia using low tidal volumes translates into accepting $PaO_2 \sim 8$ kPa (60 mmHg) provided the arterial pH is ≥ 7.25. Practically, the ventilator is set so that peak inspiratory pressures are limited to below 35 cm H_2O while employing high mean airway pressures to ensure maximum lung volume recruitment via the use of PEEP and inverse inspiratory-to-expiratory ratios. If oxygenation is inadequate with a mean airway pressure of 16 cm H_2O or greater, then high-frequency oscillatory ventilation should be considered, particularly if the problem is one of diffuse parenchymal changes or consolidation.

Recently, adjunctive therapy with inhaled nitric oxide has been considered in this population. Unfortunately, in children with significant intrapulmonary shunting (i.e. AHRF or ARDS), a randomized controlled trial of its use has not demonstrated any beneficial effect on outcome (Dobyns et al 1999).

Non-invasive support

In children with neuromuscular disease there is a risk of chronic alveolar hypoventilation. Once further compromised by an episode of pneumonia, aspiration or general anaesthesia, many such patients require a period of mechanical ventilation. Their problems are then further exacerbated by the need for sedative and analgesic drugs (administered in order to tolerate the endotracheal tube) and the presence of an abnormal central respiratory response to hypercapnia. All of these, taken together, can make it extremely difficult to wean mechanical ventilation once it has been initiated.

However, one technique, which has historically been used effectively in children with poliomyelitis, is extrathoracic negative pressure ventilation with a cuirass (Lassen 1953). In the past decade there has been renewed interest in this form of ventilation (Meessen et al 1994). There are many physiological reasons why negative pressure support should be beneficial, such as its ability to increase tonic activity in the diaphragm and intercostal muscles. In children with neuromuscular disease who are on positive pressure mechanical support we have found that, when it comes to weaning, extubation and the introduction of negative pressure support means that analgesia and sedation can be discontinued quite quickly (Chisakuta & Tasker 1998). This approach should limit the unavoidable iatrogenic worsening of respiratory drive which results from the co-administration of analgesia and sedation (which is invariably necessary for children in order that they may tolerate the endotracheal tube). In myasthenic patients we have found that the timecourse of mechanical ventilatory support can be more than halved by using this technique.

REFERENCES

ARDSnet Online. http://hedwig.mgh.harvard.edu/ardsnet/index.html

Bartlett, RH 1990 Extracorporeal life support for cardiopulmonary failure. Current Problems in Surgery 27: 623

Bartlett RH, Andrews AF, Toomasian JM 1982 Extracorporeal membrane oxygenation (ECMO) for newborn respiratory failure: 45 cases. Surgery 92: 425

Bellomo R, Boyce N 1993 Acute continuous hemodiafiltration: a prospective study of 110 patients and a review of the literature. American Journal of Kidney Disease 21: 508–518

Bernard GR, Artigas A, Brigham KL, et al 1994 The American-European consensus conference on ARDS: Definitions, mechanisms, relevant outcomes and clinical trial coordination. American Journal of Respiratory and Critical Care Medicine 149: 818

Branthwaite MA 1988 Problems in practice. Getting a patient off the ventilator. British Journal of Diseases of the Chest 82: 16–22

Branthwaite MA 1991 Non-invasive and domiciliary ventilation: positive pressure techniques. Thorax 46: 208–212

Carlon GC, Howland WS, Ray C et al 1983 High frequency jet ventilation. A prospective randomised evaluation. Chest 84: 551–559

Chisakuta A, Tasker RC 1998 Respiratory failure in myasthenia gravis and negative pressure support. Pediatric Neurology 19: 225

Conrad SA, Eggerstede JM, Morris VF, Romero MD 1993 Prolonged intracorporeal support of gas exchange with an intravenacaval oxygenator. Chest 103: 158–161

Dobyns EL, Cornfiel DN, Anas NG, et al 1999 Multicenter randomized controlled trial of the effects of inhaled nitric oxide therapy on gas exchange in children with acute hypoxemic respiratory failure. Journal of Pediatrics 134: 406

Elliott MW, Steven MH, Phillips GD, Branthwaite MA 1990 Non-invasive mechanical ventilation for acute respiratory failure. British Medical Journal 300: 358–360

Evans TW, Keogh BF 1991 Extracorporeal membrane oxygenation: a breath of fresh air or yesterday's treatment? Thorax 46: 692–694

Fiastro JF, Habib MP, Shon BY, Campbell SC 1988 Comparison of standard weaning parameters and the mechanical work of breathing in mechanically ventilated patients. Chest 94: 232–238

Gattinoni L, Tognoni G, Pesenti A et al 2001. Effect of prone positioning on the survival of patients with acute respiratory failure. New England Journal of Medicine 345: 568–573

Gattinoni L, Pesenti A, Mascheroni D et al 1986 Low frequency positive pressure ventilation with extracorporeal CO_2 removal in severe acute respiratory failure. Journal of the American Medical Association 256: 881–886

Gertsmann DR, De Lemos, RA, Clark RH 1991 High frequency ventilation: issues of strategy. Clinics in Perinatology 18(3): 563

Goldman AP, Kerr SJ, Butt W, et al 1997 Extracorporeal support for intractable cardiorespiratory failure due to meningococcal disease – United Kingdom and Australian experience. Lancet 349: 466

Hickling KG, Henderson SJ, Jackson R 1990 Low mortality associated with low volume pressure limited ventilation with permissive hypercapnia in severe adult respiratory distress syndrome. Intensive Care Medicine 16: 372–377

Hubmayr RD, Abel MD, Rehder K 1990 Physiologic approach to mechanical ventilation. Critical Care Medicine 18: 103–113

Kapadia F 1998 Classic therapies revisited. Mechanical ventilation: simplifying the terminology. Postgraduate Medical Journal 74: 330–335

Lassen, H.C.A. 1953 A preliminary report on the 1952 epidemic of poliomyelitis in Copenhagen with special reference to the treatment of acute respiratory insufficiency. Lancet 1: 37

Meessen NE, Van der Grinten CP, Luijendijk SC, et al. 1994 Continuous negative airway pressure increases tonic activity in diaphragm and intercostal muscles in humans. Journal of Applied Physiology 77: 1256

Morris AH, Wallace CJ, Menlove RL et al 1994 Randomized clinical trial of pressure-controlled inverse ratio ventilation and extra-corporeal CO_2 removal for adult respiratory distress syndrome. American Journal of Respiratory and Critical Care Medicine 149: 295–305

Pearson GA, Grant, J., Fields, D. et al. 1993 Extracorporeal life support in paediatrics. Archives of Diseases in Childhood 68: 94

Peters MJ, Tasker RC, Kiff KM, Yates R, Hatch DJ 1998 Acute hypoxemic respiratory failure in children: case mix and the utility of respiratory severity indices. Intensive Care Medicine 24: 699

Pingleton SK 1988 State of the art. Complications of acute respiratory failure. American Review of Respiratory Disease 137: 1463–1493

Rossaint R, Falke KJ, Lopez F et al 1993 Inhaled nitric oxide for the adult respiratory distress syndrome. New England Journal of Medicine 328: 399–405

Schetz M, Lauwers PM, Ferdinande P 1989 Extracorporeal treatment of acute renal failure in the intensive care unit: a critical view. Intensive Care Medicine 15: 349–357

Schuster DP 1990 A physiologic approach to initiating, maintaining, and withdrawing ventilatory support during acute respiratory failure. American Journal of Medicine 88: 268–278

Shneerson JM 1991 Non-invasive and domiciliary ventilation: negative pressure techniques. Thorax 46: 131–135

Tasker RC 2000 Gender differences and critical medical illness. Acta Paediatrica 89: 621

Tasker RC, Gordon I, Kiff K 2000 Time course of severe respiratory syncytial virus infection in mechanically ventilated infants. Acta Paediatrica 89: 938

Tharratt RS, Allen RP, Albertson T E 1988 Pressure controlled inverse ratio ventilation in severe adult respiratory failure. Chest 94: 755–762

Watkins SJ, Peters MJ, Tasker RC 2000 One hundred courses of high frequency oscillatory ventilation: what have we learned? European Journal of Pediatrics 159: 134

Yang KL, Tobin MJ 1991 A prospective study of indexes predicting the outcome of trials of weaning from mechanical ventilation. New England Journal of Medicine 324: 1445–1450

10

Non-invasive ventilation

Amanda J. Piper   Elizabeth R Ellis

INTRODUCTION

The application of non-invasive ventilatory support to improve ventilation is not a new idea. The tank ventilator or 'iron lung', which provides negative pressure to the chest wall, was first developed in the 19th century (Woollam 1976). Further developments and modifications occurred, but it was not until the poliomyelitis outbreaks of the 1940s and 1950s that such devices became widely used. Continuous positive airway pressure through a facemask for patients with pulmonary oedema and other forms of acute respiratory failure was extensively described in the 1930s (Barach et al 1938, Poulton & Oxon 1936). However, with the development of positive pressure ventilators and the introduction of the endotracheal tube in the 1960s, use of non-invasive forms of ventilatory support for acute respiratory failure declined. Negative pressure devices continued to be used in patients with severe respiratory muscle impairment following poliomyelitis and in other patient groups presenting with chronic respiratory failure where long-term ventilatory support in the home was required (Garay et al 1981, Weirs et al 1977).

Since the mid-1980s, interest in non-invasive ventilatory support has again flourished, specifically the use of positive airway pressure devices and facemask interfaces. Although this interest had its genesis in the area of sleep-disordered breathing and chronic respiratory failure, clinicians have rapidly recognized the value of this therapy in acute medical and surgical conditions where respiratory failure develops, in weaning from conventional ventilatory support and as an adjunct to established respiratory care programmes. In this chapter we will outline the mechanisms by which abnormal sleep-breathing contributes to the development of awake respiratory failure and the role nocturnal ventilatory support plays in reversing this. We will also look at the potential application of this technique in a broadening range of clinical conditions.

BREATHING, SLEEP AND RESPIRATORY FAILURE

It has been recognized for many years that significant changes in breathing and ventilation can occur during sleep (Gastaut et al 1966). However, it has only been in the past 15 years or so that the contribution abnormal breathing during sleep can play in the development of awake hypercapnia has been more fully appreciated. Our understanding of what happens to breathing during sleep has been greatly enhanced by three major developments in technology. The first is the routine use of accurate oximeters (Saunders et al 1976, Trask & Cree 1962), which have allowed the continuous monitoring of arterial oxygenation over prolonged periods of time. Secondly, the development of a comfortable and acceptable nasal mask interface (Sullivan et al 1981) has provided a simple but effective means by which abnormalities of breathing can be reversed. The last is the relatively recent development of portable ventilatory support systems for home use. These developments made it possible to continuously monitor changes in breathing associated with sleep state and to provide patients with a treatment intervention which was both effective and acceptable on a long-term basis.

Changes in breathing during sleep

Sleep is associated with a number of normal physiological events that have little effect on individuals with normal respiratory drive and mechanics. However, in patients with a range of respiratory abnormalities, sleep can lead to worsening respiratory function and gas exchange.

The awake state itself is associated with an additional stimulus to breathe, over and above that determined by the metabolic control system. This is known as the wakefulness drive to breathe and is lost with the onset of sleep. General postural muscle tone is also reduced at sleep onset, resulting in increases in upper airway resistance and reductions in ventilatory drive. At the same time, ventilatory responses to both hypoxia and hypercapnia are reduced so that there is an attenuated response to changes in gas exchange compared to wakefulness. As a result, a small fall in ventilation occurs with sleep in the range of 10–15% (Douglas et al 1982).

Although reduced, ventilation during non-rapid eye movement (NREM) sleep is steady, particularly during periods of slow-wave sleep. However, even in normal subjects there is substantial variation in breathing during rapid eye movement (REM) sleep, most pronounced during periods of phasic eye movements. During these episodes, alveolar ventilation may fall by as much as 40% (Douglas et al 1982, Gould et al 1988). REM sleep is also associated with alterations in respiratory control, caused by descending inhibition of alpha and gamma motor neurons. This produces hypotonia of postural muscles, including the intercostal and accessory respiratory muscles and a reduction in the rib cage contribution to ventilation. As a result, ventilation during REM sleep becomes heavily reliant on diaphragmatic activity.

In patients with severely compromised lung function or significant inspiratory muscle weakness, recruitment of other inspiratory and accessory muscles, including the abdominals, may occur to augment breathing. By this compensatory mechanism, individuals are usually able to maintain adequate ventilation during wakefulness and NREM sleep for prolonged periods. In those with significant lung disease, recruitment of the intercostal muscles occurs not only to augment ventilation but to maintain end-expiratory lung volume, thereby preventing small airway closure. With the transition into REM sleep, this postural muscle activity will be lost, resulting in a reduction in minute ventilation, worsening ventilation perfusion relationships and a deterioration in gas exchange. Falls in saturation will be more severe in those patients with awake saturation values already near the steep portion of the oxyhaemoglobin dissociation curve. The degree of abnormal breathing which then occurs will depend upon the patient's arousal response. Arousal causes a change in state from sleep to transient wakefulness, permitting the re-emergence of accessory muscle activity and restoration of ventilation, albeit briefly. In this way, arousal acts as a defensive mechanism, limiting the degree of gas exchange abnormality that is permitted to occur. However, this response also leads to sleep fragmentation, which in itself can alter respiratory drive and arousal thresholds, so that eventually more extreme blood gas derangement must occur before the arousal response is activated.

The role of sleep in the development of awake hypercapnic respiratory failure

It is now well recognized that decompensated breathing first becomes apparent in REM sleep (Bye et al 1990). However, as REM sleep takes up only a relatively small proportion of total sleep time, patients with REM hypoventilation, even if severe, may remain clinically stable for months or even years before significant daytime hypercapnia becomes apparent. Initially, ventilation and sleep between periods of REM hypoventilation are usually normal, often through the recruitment of accessory respiratory muscles. In addition, the arousal mechanism operates to defend ventilation by limiting the amount of time spent in REM sleep and therefore the degree of abnormal gas exchange that occurs. Characteristically, awake blood gases remain normal during this initial stage.

Progression of abnormal breathing into NREM sleep heralds the second stage in the evolution of sleep-induced respiratory failure (Piper & Sullivan 1994a). Mechanisms responsible for this progression include not only a deterioration of the underlying disease itself but the appearance of other factors which may load breathing such as ageing, weight gain, upper airway dysfunction or the development of an intercurrent illness such as a chest infection. Sleep fragmentation from abnormal breathing events has the capacity to further alter respiratory control and depress arousal. These factors allow more severe sleep-disordered breathing to occur, with less arousal between events. This begins a vicious cycle whereby resetting the sensitivity of the ventilatory control system occurs so that higher levels of carbon dioxide and lower levels of oxygen are tolerated without stimulating a change in respiration, not only asleep but during wakefulness as well. During this stage, daytime CO_2 retention becomes apparent (Fig. 10.1).

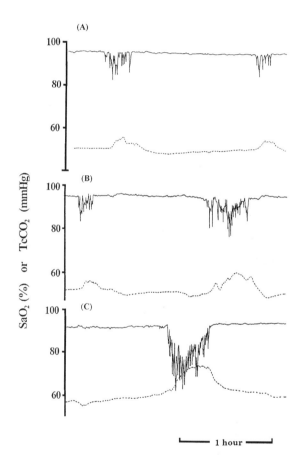

Figure 10.1 Serial recordings of oxygen saturation (SaO_2) and transcutaneous carbon dioxide ($TcCO_2$) from a patient with Duchenne muscular dystrophy showing progressive nocturnal respiratory failure. Panel (A) illustrates mild sleep-disordered breathing, with modest falls in SaO_2. Eight months later (B), more substantial oxygen desaturation was apparent during REM sleep, with rises in carbon dioxide. By panel (C), severe REM desaturation was occurring, with failure of SaO_2 to return to baseline values between periods of abnormal breathing. This was accompanied by large rises in CO_2. Over the same period, awake CO_2 had risen from 40 to 45 mmHg (5.3 to 6.0 kPa), with no change in inspiratory muscle pressures.

The final stage in the development of sleep-induced hypercapnia is characterized by unstable respiratory failure both awake and asleep. During this stage, changes in blood gases during sleep are extreme and sleep architecture may be profoundly disturbed. By this stage, the clinical condition of the patient may deteriorate considerably, which can be mistaken for a progression of the underlying disease process. However, by supporting breathing during sleep, significant improvements in awake blood gases, reduction in hospital admissions, improved exercise tolerance and improved quality of life can be achieved.

INDICATIONS FOR NON-INVASIVE VENTILATION

Chronic respiratory failure

From the above analysis it is clear that sleep-disordered breathing causing unstable respiratory failure and severe daytime symptoms is an obvious indication for non-invasive ventilatory support. There are a number of disorders where nocturnal respiratory failure occurs, producing awake hypercapnia (Box 10.1). The following features are indicators that sleep hypoventilation may be occurring and where nocturnal ventilatory support should be considered:

- daytime hypercapnia $PaCO_2 > 6$ kPa (45 mmHg)
- severe nocturnal hypoxaemia
- excessive daytime sleepiness
- severe early morning headaches.

However, for many patients the onset of nocturnal respiratory failure occurs over an extended period of time, in some cases even years. With such an insidious onset, the signs and symptoms of chronic hypoventilation may be overlooked or incorrectly attributed to the ongoing progression of the primary disease process.

More difficult questions arise in patients with milder conditions and there are specific issues that affect individuals with particular diseases or syndromes. In all cases the feasibility of non-invasive ventilation (NIV) depends on whether

Box 10.1 Conditions where nocturnal hypercapnic respiratory failure is likely to occur

Neuromuscular	Myopathies
	    Duchenne muscular dystrophy
	    Acid maltase deficiency
	Neuropathies
	    Poliomyelitis
	    Motor neurone disease
	    Bilateral phrenic nerve palsy

Chest wall	Kyphoscoliosis Thoracoplasty
Impaired ventilatory control	Obesity hypoventilation syndrome Brainstem injury Primary alveolar hypoventilation
Airway obstruction	Severe obstructive sleep apnoea
Lung disease	Chronic obstructive pulmonary disease Cystic fibrosis Bronchiectasis

the presentation is acute or chronic. The capacity of an individual to maintain adequate ventilation during sleep depends on a balance between the respiratory load placed on the respiratory muscles and the ability of the respiratory muscles to sustain that load. Chronic adaptations (as described earlier) which occur in response to the failure to maintain adequate ventilation can complicate this balance. The kinds of loads that are placed on the respiratory muscles include those that occur during sleep, such as upper airway resistance, which may be considerable and the relative inefficiency of the rib cage when the intercostal muscles are inhibited during REM. These changes may occur on a background of high work of breathing from increased airways resistance, from decreased respiratory compliance from chest wall deformities or lung disease or from the relative inefficiency of muscle contraction from hyperinflation.

On the other hand, the respiratory muscles may be unable to sustain the work of breathing because of inherent problems of their own. Respiratory muscle performance can be adversely affected by hypoxaemia, hypercapnia, malnutrition, biomechanical alterations, trauma or disease.

Factors affecting muscle performance and respiratory load can present differently in each patient. Therefore, it is important to analyse each case as it helps to predict how effective different types of intervention are likely to be. For example, a patient may have a normal work of breathing but very weak muscles, as occurs in neuromuscular disease. The condition of these patients is often complicated by lung and chest wall stiffness as a chronic adaptation to low lung volumes. Alternatively, a patient may have normal muscles but a very high work of breathing. This high work of breathing may be generalized throughout the respiratory system, as in restrictive lung disease, or it may be localized, as in upper airway obstruction. In other instances, the patient may have 'weak' muscles with an increase in the work of breathing, such as in obstructive lung disease with significant hyper-inflation, hypoxaemia and malnutrition.

Assessment of chronic hypoventilation

Although a number of investigators have tried to use daytime pulmonary function tests as a predictor of the degree of abnormal breathing occurring during sleep, no strong correlation has been found (Bye et al 1990). However, we do know that a low vital capacity, a significant fall in vital capacity from erect to supine or a maximum inspiratory pressure of less than 30 cmH$_2$O are all indicators that sleep-disordered breathing and hypoventilation may be present (Bye et al 1990). Each of these tests can be easily carried out at the bedside as part of the overall assessment of a patient presenting in respiratory failure. Strong use of the accessory respiratory muscles at rest, including the sternomastoid and the abdominal muscles, should raise the possibility that respiratory function may worsen during sleep.

In general, if there is awake hypercapnia then there will be substantial sleep-linked worsening of respiratory failure (Piper & Sullivan 1994a), although the converse does not necessarily hold true. Many subjects with awake CO$_2$ within the normal range will have significant sleep-linked respiratory failure.

The limitations of daytime indices as predictors of nocturnal hypoventilation mean that detailed sleep studies are required in order to accurately assess the severity and nature of the disorder. Sleep studies should include measurement of the standard sleep parameters such as electroencephalogram (EEG), electrooculogram (EOG) and submental electromyogram (EMG). The extent and quality of sleep is essential information for gauging the likely impact that the disordered breathing may have on cognitive and other functions. In addition, comprehensive cardiac and respiratory monitoring should be carried out, including electrocardiogram (ECG), oximetry, airflow, diaphragm EMG, rib cage and abdominal movement and transcutaneous CO$_2$.

Kyphoscoliosis

The final stages of severe kyphoscoliosis have been characterized by progressive respiratory failure associated with severe nocturnal hypoventilation (Ellis et al 1988). The REM hypoventilation is probably caused by a combination of a very high work of breathing for a diaphragm that is at a significant mechanical disadvantage. In some patients sleep-disordered breathing is also complicated by upper airway obstruction. Nose mask ventilation is particularly suitable for these patients as other methods of assisted ventilation are very difficult. Tracheostomy can be difficult because of the loss of the extrathoracic trachea and the fitting of a cuirass is made exceptionally difficult by the chest wall deformity. Non-invasive ventilation can be readily achieved with a nose mask in this group despite the stiffness of the chest wall and the additional requirement of positive expiratory pressures (Ellis et al 1988).

Cystic fibrosis

Although low-flow oxygen therapy has been the mainstay of treatment for patients with cystic fibrosis (CF) developing respiratory failure, several reports have shown that, at least acutely during sleep, oxygen therapy can promote CO$_2$ retention (Gozal 1997, Milross et al 2001). The beneficial effects of nocturnal non-invasive ventilation for patients with end-stage CF are beginning to be recognized. Non-invasive ventilation has been shown to be of value during periods of acute deterioration, where marked pulmonary deterioration occurs despite maximum conventional therapy (Hill et al 1998, Piper et al 1992). Use of nasal ventilatory support in this setting can correct hypoxaemia without inducing additional CO_2 retention. In addition, this technique may also be utilized to stabilize the patient in the short term while donor organs become available (Hodson et al 1991) or on a longer term basis, allowing the patient to return home (Hill et al 1998, Piper et al 1992). Although in initial reports volume preset machines were used, bilevel pressure devices are now being increasingly used with similar outcomes (Gozal, 1997; Milross et al 2001).

Some patients report improved sputum clearance after initiation of nasal ventilatory support, possibly related to better tolerance of longer chest physiotherapy sessions (Piper et al 1992). Improved lung expansion and chest wall excursion while on the machine may also play a role. One study has shown that use of nasal ventilatory support during chest physiotherapy was able to ameliorate adverse effects such as reduced respiratory muscle performance and oxygen desaturation (Fauroux et al 1999).

Duchenne muscular dystrophy

Ventilatory support is often reluctantly prescribed for patients with progressive neuromuscular disease, owing to a perceived lack of quality of life for these patients. However, quality of life is often underestimated in such patients. The use of long-term non-invasive ventilation has been shown to stabilize pulmonary function and prolong life expectancy in patients with Duchenne muscular dystrophy (DMD) and awake hypercapnia (Simonds et al 1998). In contrast, Raphael and co-workers (1994) trialled non-invasive ventilation as a preventive measure in DMD patients free of daytime respiratory failure. They found no benefit from early intervention with this technique, with the treated group showing a similar rate of deterioration in blood gases and pulmonary function as a control group. Further, there was a higher death rate in the treated group, although the reasons for this were not entirely clear.

Chronic obstructive pulmonary disease

Nocturnal nasal ventilation has been used effectively in selected patients with stable chronic obstructive pulmonary disease (COPD). However, this form of therapy is not tolerated as well as in other diagnostic groups (Strumpf et al 1991) and longer term outcomes are not as favourable as in patients with neuromuscular and chest wall disorders (Simonds & Elliott 1995). Those patients most likely to benefit from nocturnal ventilatory support appear to be those with significant daytime hypercapnia, who have symptomatic sleep problems and in whom nocturnal hypercapnia can be successfully reduced by overnight ventilation. Meecham Jones et al (1995) reported a randomized crossover study of nasal pressure support ventilation plus oxygen therapy compared with domiciliary oxygen therapy alone in 18 hypercapnic patients with COPD. Improvements in daytime arterial blood gas tensions, overnight transcutaneous carbon dioxide ($TcCO_2$), total sleep time and sleep efficiency were seen during non-invasive ventilation and oxygen therapy compared with oxygen therapy alone, suggesting that control of hypoventilation with non-invasive ventilation can be achieved. Importantly, these authors found that those who showed the greatest reduction in nocturnal hypercapnia with ventilation were likely to gain the greatest benefit from the treatment.

Motor neurone disease

Respiratory insufficiency usually occurs as a late manifestation of this disorder, when global peripheral and respiratory muscle weakness has occurred. However, in a small number of patients, presentation with hypercapnia, severe orthopnoea and sleep fragmentation may be seen. Although nasal ventilatory support has been shown to be effective in relieving these symptoms in this group (Escarrabill et al 1998), its use also raises some ethical and clinical concerns that need to be discussed with the patient and their caregiver (Polkey et al 1999). There has been reluctance to initiate such therapy for a condition that is known to be relatively rapidly progressive and where many will experience involvement of the bulbar muscles and swallowing difficulties (Meyer & Hill 1994). However, in an observational cohort study following 39 patients with motor neurone disease (MND), Aboussouan and colleagues (1997) found that those who tolerated non-invasive positive pressure ventilation (NPPV) had a significant survival advantage compared to those who did not. Furthermore, 30% of patients with moderate to severe bulbar symptoms tolerated mask ventilation and benefited from it.

Non-invasive ventilation appears to have a place as a management alternative in motivated patients with appropriate home supports, where established respiratory failure is present or where quality of life is impaired by sleep disruption or severe orthopnoea (Polkey et al 1999). However, before undertaking such therapy in this group, frank discussion with the patient and carer needs to occur. Potential benefits of NIV in palliating symptoms should be discussed as well as its limitations in the face of progressively worsening respiratory and general muscle strength and disability.

Acute respiratory failure

In order to reduce the problems associated with endotracheal intubation and ventilation, an increasing number of centres are now using non-invasive ventilation as a treatment alternative for patients with acute respiratory failure. It avoids the complications of endotracheal intubation, is more comfortable for the patient, allowing speech and swallowing and avoids the need for sedation and immobilization. Treatment does not have to be instituted in the intensive care or emergency department environment and is increasingly commenced on general medical or surgical wards (Bott et al 1993, Piper & Willson 1996, Plant et al 2000, Servera et al 1995).

Appropriate patient selection is essential for a successful treatment outcome. Non-invasive ventilation should be seen as a therapy to prevent the need for intubation rather than an alternative to it. Therefore, when undertaking this therapy it is important to be able to identify those patients who are unlikely to respond well, in order that a

---

> **Box 10.2** Characteristics of patients with acute respiratory failure unlikely to do well on non-invasive ventilation (Vitacca et al 1993, Soo Hoo et al 1994, Brochard et al 1995, Kramer et al 1995)
>
> - Agitation, encephalopathic, uncooperative
> - Severe illness, including extreme acidosis (pH <7.2)
> - Presence of excessive secretions or pneumonia
> - Multiple organ failure
> - Haemodynamic instability
> - Inability to maintain a lip seal
> - Inability to protect the airway
> - Overt respiratory failure requiring immediate intubation

---

delay in mandatory intubation does not occur (Box 10.2). The ideal patient should be cooperative enough to tolerate a mask and to follow simple instructions. A successful outcome depends to a large degree on the ability to rapidly correct acidosis, decrease CO_2 and reduce respiratory rate (Soo Hoo et al 1994). This in turn will be influenced by the ability of the patient and the therapist to minimize mouth leaks and to coordinate breathing with the ventilator. If hypercapnia and acidosis fail to improve within the first few hours of treatment, longer term success is unlikely (Ambrosino et al 1995, Anton et al. 2000, Soo Hoo et al 1994).

In patients who are hypoxaemic but retain carbon dioxide, the use of non-invasive ventilation permits higher levels of inspired oxygen to be introduced without unduly worsening hypercapnia. Under these circumstances, the use of non-invasive ventilation supports patients until their acute deterioration can be reversed (Conway et al 1993).

The majority of studies reported to date have involved patients with COPD during an acute exacerbation. It appears that the type of ventilator (volume preset or bilevel pressure support) or the type of interface chosen (nose or full face mask) is not pivotal in determining the success of treatment. However, results will be influenced by the patient's tolerance and adaptation to the machine and some patients may find the bilevel pressure support devices easier to adapt to (Vitacca et al 1993). Very dyspnoeic patients tend to be mouth breathers and where it is not possible for the patient to maintain lip closure, a full facemask needs to be used to ensure machine–patient synchronization and that an effective tidal volume is delivered.

Use of non-invasive ventilatory support in COPD patients during acute respiratory failure has shown very encouraging outcomes. In a large study by Brochard and colleagues (1995), only 26% of the non-invasive ventilation group required intubation compared to 74% of the standard treatment group. Further, hospital stay was significantly longer and the mortality and complication rate higher in the group receiving standard treatment. However, an important caveat exists when interpreting these data. Only 31% of all patients with COPD admitted during the study period were considered suitable for enrolment, emphasizing that success with this form of therapy relies heavily on appropriate patient selection. Several recent studies have also provided data that suggest that the early administration of non-invasive ventilatory support during episodes of acute respiratory failure may improve the long-term outcome in patients with COPD. Improved 12-month survival and a reduction in the number of further intensive care unit (ICU) or hospital admissions have been reported in patients treated with mask ventilation compared to those undergoing either conventional therapy (Bardi et al 2000) or intubation and ventilation (Vitacca et al 1996).

Patients with acute exacerbations of COPD have been the group most widely studied and successfully treated with NIV. However, recent randomized controlled trials have provided evidence that NIV can provide similar benefits in patients presenting with hypoxaemic respiratory failure and community-acquired pneumonia (Antonelli et al 1998, 2000, Confalonieri et al 1999).

Cardiogenic pulmonary oedema also responds well to mask positive pressure therapy, either in the form of continuous positive airway pressure (CPAP) (Bersten et al 1991) or bilevel ventilatory support (Masip et al 2000, Mehta et al 1997). However, in a study comparing bilevel with CPAP therapy, there was a higher incidence of myocardial infarction in those treated with

bilevel therapy (Mehta et al 1997). Therefore, the current evidence suggests that mask CPAP should be the first mode of therapy in these patients, changing to mask bilevel ventilatory support if significant hypercapnia remains (Rusterholtz et al 1999). We are increasingly seeing patients who develop postoperative respiratory failure following major surgery. Many of these patients are overweight and probably have pre-existing sleep-disordered breathing. The affects of anaesthesia and analgesia may worsen an already compromized upper airway, producing apnoea and its sequelae such as hypoxaemia and blood pressure fluctuations. In addition, diaphragm inhibition after upper abdominal surgery can exacerbate REM hypoventilation. These patients generally respond well and rapidly to bilevel pressure support, improving gas exchange and pulmonary function.

Another group which responds very rapidly and positively to non-invasive ventilation are those patients with obesity hypoventilation. This syndrome is characterized by obesity, a long history of snoring, excessive daytime sleepiness and severe derangement of awake blood gases. These patients frequently present as grossly decompensated with right heart failure, lower limb oedema and hypercapnia. Use of non-invasive ventilatory support in these patients results in improved awake blood gases and clinical condition within days of commencing therapy, without the need for intubation and its associated complications. In most patients, transfer to more simple devices such as CPAP can be achieved for long-term domiciliary use (Piper & Sullivan 1994b).

Although some investigators have described nasal ventilation in the acute phase as a time-consuming procedure (Chevrolet et al 1991), more recent experience suggests that this is not necessarily the case (Bott et al 1993, Kramer et al 1995). It has also been shown that the use of this technique can be transferred to the general ward environment without a reduction in efficacy (Brown et al 1998, Plant et al 2000). However, training of staff regarding the management of patients undergoing this therapy is essential. This includes the need for continuous monitoring, not only to check the efficacy of the technique but also to ensure the safety of the patient. Sudden death may occur if an accidental disconnection from the ventilator takes place (Kramer et al 1995).

Non-invasive ventilation is usually continued until blood gases have stabilized for several hours, then trial periods off the mask are commenced. The patient's response to spontaneous ventilation is monitored and mask ventilatory support reinstituted if breathing deteriorates. In some cases, almost continuous use of the mask during the first day or two may be necessary. There is then a gradual withdrawal of awake ventilatory support to nocturnal use only. Prior to hospital discharge, investigation into the need for domiciliary therapy and the type of therapy required will be needed.

Weaning and early extubation

Although most patients can be weaned from mechanical ventilation without incident, a small number will require a prolonged weaning period. In many cases, a history of underlying lung, chest wall or neuromuscular disease will be found. Although a number of weaning strategies have been developed to facilitate the resumption of spontaneous breathing, some patients will not tolerate removal of ventilatory support without developing unacceptably high levels of carbon dioxide retention. Non-invasive ventilatory support can be a useful tool in the weaning of such patients from conventional mechanical ventilation, permitting the earlier removal of the endotracheal tube than with conventional invasive pressure support techniques (Girault et al 1999). In a randomized trial, Nava and colleagues (1998) showed that early extubation and use of NIV in patients presenting with hypercapnic respiratory failure not only reduced the duration of mechanical ventilation and the duration of ICU stay, but was also associated with a lower incidence of nosocomial pneumonia. Further, the 60-day survival rate was better in those treated with early extubation and mask ventilation than those continuing on conventional mechanical ventilation and weaning.

In patients already tracheostomized and on partial ventilatory support, nasal mask ventilation can be substituted for tracheal support (Restrick et al 1993). This is usually commenced on a continuous basis, with the patient removing the mask for short periods for eating, speaking and coughing. Periods of spontaneous breathing are then interspersed with periods on the nasal mask, the balance being determined by patient tolerance and clinical response. Once nasal ventilatory support has been shown to be acceptable and to effectively support ventilation, the tracheostomy tube is removed. Non-invasive ventilation is then used nocturnally and for any rest/sleep period during the day as required. Although many patients may be weaned entirely from the mask, some will have an underlying process which features sleep-disordered breathing. Therefore, investigation into the presence of nocturnal breathing abnormalities and discharge home on nocturnal ventilatory support should be considered.

PRACTICAL ISSUES IN THE APPLICATION OF NON-INVASIVE VENTILATION
Criteria for choosing a ventilator

A number of factors need to be considered when choosing a machine and mode of ventilatory support. These include the clinical condition of the patient on presentation, the diagnosis, the patient's respiratory drive, the compliance of the lungs and chest wall, the degree of synchronization that can be achieved between the patient and the device and the familiarity of the staff with the equipment. Sleep study data are useful in patients requiring long-term ventilation in identifying any degree of upper airway dysfunction which may be present as well as determining the patient's respiratory drive during sleep. Understanding the features and limitations of the various machines available and the modes of ventilatory support in which they can operate will assist in selecting the appropriate system to meet the patient's needs. In some centres, the choice of device will also be influenced by cost. However, the final decision should come down to how effective the device is in supporting ventilation and maintaining gas exchange in the individual.

Type of ventilator

There are currently two types of ventilator systems available for mask ventilation: volume-preset and pressure-preset devices. Each type of device has its own advantages and limitations. A successful outcome using mask ventilation will depend upon the clinician's understanding of the underlying pathological processes which have contributed to the patient's respiratory deterioration and choosing a machine and mode of ventilatory support which best meet the respiratory needs of the patient.

Volume-preset machines such as the PLV 100 (Lifecare, Lafayette, Colorado, USA), the PV 501 (Breas, Sweden) or the Bromptonpac (PneuPAC Ltd, Luton, Beds, UK) operate as time cycled flow generators and deliver a fixed tidal volume irrespective of the airway pressure generated, as long as leaks from the system are minimized. Pressure-preset systems include bilevel positive pressure devices, the most widely recognized being the BiPAP machine (Respironics, Murrysville, Pennsylvania, USA). Other pressure-preset devices include the DP90 (Taema, France) and the VPAP II (ResMed, Australia). With these devices, tidal volume will vary according to the inspiratory pressure set, the inspiratory–expiratory pressure difference and the chest wall/lung compliance of the patient.

In studies comparing the efficacy of these two systems, little difference has been found either in acute (Vitacca et al 1993) or chronic respiratory failure (Meecham Jones & Wedzicha 1993). However, there may be differences in patient acceptance, particularly during acute respiratory failure (Vitacca et al 1993), with many patients finding the bilevel pressure support devices easier to tolerate. Poor tolerance to volume-preset devices may be related to an increase in airway resistance causing an elevation of inspiratory pressure in the mask which may be uncomfortable or may cause leaks, thus limiting the effectiveness of ventilation (Soo Hoo et al 1994). On the other

hand, in patients with low chest wall compliance higher airway pressures may be needed to maintain optimal ventilation, particularly during REM sleep. In these patients, volume-preset ventilators can prove more reliable and effective in delivering a stable tidal volume despite changing chest wall mechanics. A change to a volume-preset device should always be considered if hypoventilation persists on bilevel ventilatory support (Schonhofer et al 1997).

Bilevel devices are said to compensate better for mild to moderate leaks from the mask and mouth than volume-preset devices. Clinical experience has shown that mouth leaks are common during mask ventilation, particularly during sleep and that these leaks may adversely affect the quality of ventilation and sleep architecture even with bilevel positive pressure devices (Meyer et al 1997, Piper & Willson 1996; Teschler et al 1999)

Settings

The mode of support needs to be set so that the breaths delivered will be either machine triggered or patient triggered. With the bilevel devices, a spontaneous mode of support is available, where the machine cycles into inspiration in response to the patient's spontaneous inspiratory effort. The volume-preset and a number of the bilevel devices can also be set to deliver a preset respiratory rate should the patient fail to trigger the device. Titration of inspiratory positive airway pressure (IPAP) for a patient on a bilevel device or tidal volume for a patient using a volume-preset one is made on the basis of patient tolerance and the effect such a pressure has on ventilation and gas exchange. However, when setting pressures or volumes it should be borne in mind that excessively high inspiratory pressures will promote leakage of air from the mouth, reducing the effectiveness of ventilatory support. Excessive hyperventilation can also occur, which may induce upper airway obstruction and the appearance of central apnoea. More recent evidence suggests that the timed mode of ventilation using bilevel devices is less predictable and less stable than nasal ventilation with volume-preset devices and may produce periodic breathing during both wakefulness and sleep, related to glottic closure (Parreira et al 1996).

The use of expiratory positive airway pressure (EPAP) may be advantageous in a number of clinical conditions, including controlling upper airway closure, recruiting collapsed alveoli or to overcome intrinsic end-expiratory pressure. Bilevel positive pressure devices are more reliable in maintaining end-expiratory pressure than volume-preset machines. However, setting of the EPAP reduces the differential pressure between inspiration and expiration, which may affect the degree to which minute ventilation is augmented. Elliott & Simonds (1995) found that the addition of 5 cmH_2O of EPAP in patients with neuromuscular disease reduced the severity of gas exchange abnormalities during sleep, but had no effect in patients with COPD. Further, they found the use of EPAP had deleterious effects on sleep quality in some patients. Similarly, the use of expiratory pressure in patients with COPD during acute exacerbations did not confer any additional benefit and was found to be poorly tolerated (Meecham Jones et al 1994).

In some cases the bilevel device may fail to adequately reduce CO_2 despite increasing minute ventilation and decreasing respiratory effort. This has been explained by CO_2 rebreathing in patients with exhaled flow rates that exceed the leak rate of the exhalation port at the set expiratory pressure (Ferguson & Gilmartin 1995). This is most likely to occur in patients with high respiratory rates where the duration of expiration is short. Although this can be eliminated by using EPAP pressures of 8 cmH_2O or more (Ferguson & Gilmartin 1995), the majority of patients are unlikely to need or tolerate these pressures. Further, IPAP pressure would need to be increased to maintain the IPAP–EPAP pressure difference, which may not produce greater ventilatory support because of increased mouth leaks (Fernandez et al 1993). There are now a number of different types of expiratory valves available such as the Plateau exhalation device or the non-rebreathing valve (Respironics, USA) which are effective in minimizing CO_2 rebreathing (Ferguson & Gilmartin 1995).

These considerations regarding ventilator settings highlight the need for monitoring of the patient during initial trials of non-invasive ventilation in order to determine response to therapy. In this way a change in the mode or type of ventilator can be made if ventilation is not being adequately supported. Although some centres have based machine settings on ventilation achieved during wakefulness (Strumpf et al 1991), such settings may not be adequate during sleep. This may relate to changes in the behaviour of the glottis, mouth leaks, alteration in respiratory drive or compliance of the respiratory system associated with changes in sleep state. It is recommended that ventilator parameters are based on patient tolerance and gas exchange while awake and then nocturnal monitoring is used to ensure that such settings are also appropriate to maintain adequate sleep ventilation (see 'Initiating therapy' below).

Humidification and oxygen therapy

In some patients, the high flows of cold dry air across the nasal passages can cause distressing nasal symptoms which may affect compliance with therapy or increase nasal resistance (Richards et al 1996) which will affect the amount of ventilation delivered. Patients may report sneezing, nasal stuffiness or rhinorrhoea and erroneously believe they are developing a head cold. The use of an in-line humidifier such as an HC-150 (Fisher & Paykel, New Zealand), that can both warm and moisten the air, will largely improve these symptoms. However, as nasal symptoms frequently point to the presence of significant mouth leaks, this should be attended to, as leaks may reduce the effectiveness of ventilation. In patients with bronchial hypersecretion, such as CF or bronchiectasis, the addition of in-line humidification whilst using nasal ventilatory support may be useful in ensuring secretions are well hydrated. Patients with acute respiratory failure may become dehydrated and can also benefit from additional humidification of the airways (Wood et al 2000).

In patients who require ventilatory support on a continuous basis, nebulized bronchodilators and normal saline can be given during mask ventilatory support, either via a mouthpiece whilst the nasal mask is in place or added in-line to the system close to the nasal mask. Bilevel ventilatory support devices have been used to deliver beta 2-agonists in the emergency department for patients with bronchospasm and have been shown to be associated with a greater increase in the peak expiratory flow rates compared to aerosols delivered by small-volume nebulizers alone (Pollack et al 1995).

Generally, supplemental oxygen is not required in those patients with chronic respiratory failure from neuromuscular or chest wall disorders. However, in patients with parenchymal disease or those with acute respiratory failure, additional oxygen is likely to be needed and can be added either into the ventilator tubing or into a port on the mask itself. The flow rate needed will be determined by the oxygen saturation achieved.

Interfaces

Either nasal or full facemasks may be used to deliver ventilatory support (Figs 10.2, 10.3) and advances in design of both types have meant a greater degree of comfort due to a more effective pressure distribution across a larger surface area.

It is recommended that a nasal mask be tried initially, transferring to a full facemask if mouth leaks cannot be controlled adequately with a chin strap (Figs 10.4, 10.5). A review of the available literature suggests that successful outcomes in acute respiratory failure can be achieved with both types of interface (Bott et al 1993, Soo Hoo et al 1994), although the full facemask has been preferred by some groups in the acute setting to better control mouth leaks (Fernandez et al 1993). Nasal masks tend to be more comfortable, have a lower dead space and allow easier access for secretion removal and speech. Individually moulded masks can be constructed for those patients difficult to fit with standard commercial masks or those using mask ventilation on a long-term basis. However, a high degree of skill and experience is needed to ensure comfort and fit and frequent refitting may be necessary.

Initiating therapy

At present there is no consensus as to when non-invasive ventilatory support should be com-

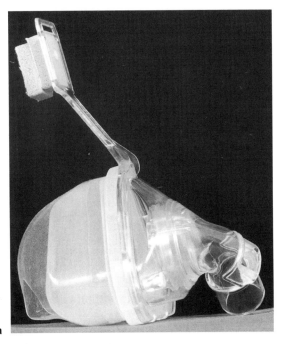 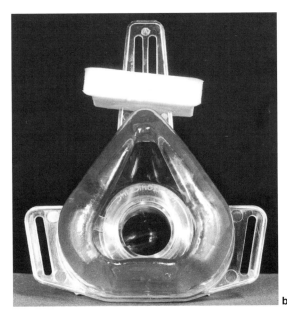

a   b

Figure 10.2 Examples of commercially available nasal mask systems. **a** The Series 2 Bubble Mask (ResMed, Australia); **b** the Gel Mask (Respironics, USA).

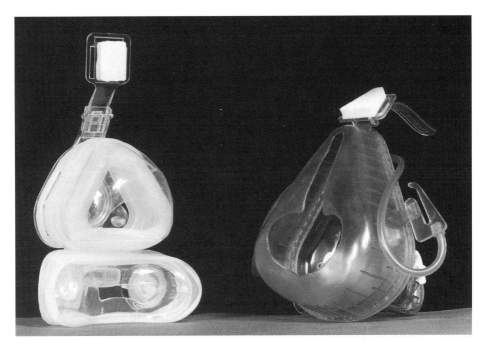

Figure 10.3 Two types of full facemask suitable for non-invasive ventilatory support. The nose-mouth mask (ResMed, Australia) on the left, and the Spectrum Face Mask (Respironics, USA) on the right.

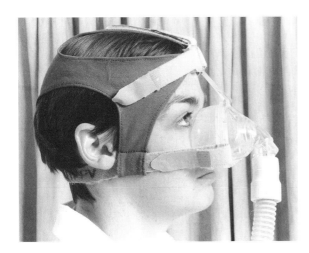

Figure 10.4 Nasal mask and headgear system (ResMed, Australia).

menced in patients with documented nocturnal hypoventilation. The decision is not a difficult one if a patient presents with awake hypercapnia or has overt symptoms of sleep-disordered breathing. However, the identification of isolated REM desaturation may be more difficult. Intervening too early may result in the patient rejecting therapy. Patients may need time to adapt to the idea of assisted ventilation as it may signal to them the 'beginning of the end'. The difficulty is that in some patients who are deteriorating rapidly, this may indeed be the case. With most, however, it should signal a new beginning. There are many reasons for rejecting the idea of the ventilator. Some patients do not believe in altering the natural course of events. Some may find it beyond their resources and capabilities to acquire and manage the technology. Some find the thought of sleeping with a machine totally foreign or too disruptive to their circumstances. Some believe that they will become ventilator dependent or that it will weaken their muscles.

Each of these beliefs needs to be explored and discussed without judgement. They can be resolved in a number of ways. Patients need to be allowed to make their own choice and when the symptoms of respiratory failure or sleep deprivation become severe enough they may then seek relief. Alternatively patients can be counselled, often with the help of other patients, that the benefits outweigh any real or perceived detriments. Patients have to be willing for trials to be successful and it is helpful if a member of the family or someone in the household can manage the equipment. For most patients, compliance is usually dependent on relief of symptoms. Paulus & Willig (1993) surveyed 34 patients with neuromuscular disorders ventilated nasally. Over half the patients considered nocturnal ventilation to be constraining, but felt that these constraints were more than acceptable if the benefits outweighed any inconveniences.

Kramer et al (1995) reported that approximately 18% of patients are intolerant of non-invasive therapy during acute respiratory failure, although compliance appears to be slightly better with bilevel pressure support devices than volume-preset (Vitacca et al 1993). Failure rates in patients with chronic respiratory failure have been reported at between 19% and 36% (Gay et al 1991, Strumpf et al 1991). However, acceptance of therapy may differ depending on the underlying pathology, the patient's response to therapy and relief of symptoms. Initial experience with mask ventilation may also influence outcome. A number of groups commence ventilation on an inpatient basis to provide the patient with maximum support whilst minimizing problems (Meecham Jones et al 1995, Piper & Willson 1996). This permits intensive coaching of patients to enable them to synchronize with the ventilator and to adjust the ventilator settings so there is better matching with the patient's own breathing pattern (Box 10.3). It also provides the opportunity to determine any problems arising, which could affect patient response to therapy and adversely affect their acceptance of treatment. After acclimatizing the patient to the mask and flow from the ventilator, the ventilator is then adjusted to match the patient's own respiratory pattern and timing. Further adjustments are then made to ensure blood gases are maintained or improved. Where inspiratory time or flow can be set, this will be based on the patient's own respiratory pattern, taking into account the effect short inspiratory times can have on gas exchange. In

---

Box 10.3   Steps in initiating therapy

- Introduce the patient slowly to the equipment and all its parts
- Ensure the mask fits comfortably and that the patient can experience the mask on their face without the ventilator connected
- Allow the patient the opportunity to feel the operation of the machine through the mask on their hand or cheek before applying it over their nose or mouth
- Allow the patient the opportunity to practise breathing with the ventilator, either holding the mask in place or allowing them to hold it in place before applying the straps
- Adjust settings initially for comfort and establish whether the patient can relax comfortably in a sleeping posture
- Provide opportunities for the patient to feed back any discomfort or uncertainty with regard to the use of the equipment
- Assess and adjust the performance of the ventilator during an afternoon nap to optimize gas exchange and patient comfort
- Progress to an overnight study, continuing to monitor and optimize gas exchange and sleep quality

---

patients where the compliance of the alveoli is heterogeneous, much of the delivered tidal volume will be directed towards those alveoli with short filling times, producing an overdistension of already inflated units and not contributing to improved gas exchange. Prolonging the inspiratory time allows the recruitment of alveoli with slower filling times, so that increased ventilation can contribute to improved gas exchange.

Adverse effects

There are many complications or adverse effects that can arise during attempts to establish patients on non-invasive ventilation. Mouth leaks during the inspiratory phase of the ventilator cycle are probably the most common problem and probably occur in all patients at some time but remain a significant problem in approximately 60% of patients. This leak can reduce effective ventilation and may only be obvious during certain sleep stages. Leaks may be seen in the presence of upper airway obstruction, if asynchrony between the patient and the ventilator develops or if the lips and palate fail to provide a seal. If the leak is significant it can usually be remedied by the use of a chin strap which should cradle the chin and hold the lower jaw up. The chin strap is designed to have elastic sections on the sides so that patients can still move their jaw comfortably and call out and breathe should their nose become blocked or the ventilator fail. Other solutions for this problem include repositioning of the neck, taping the lips, mouth guards and full facemasks. Full facemasks are usually preferred once the patient's confidence has been established. The presence of leaks will not only reduce the degree of effective ventilation reaching the lungs but may also cause sleep fragmentation. Upper airway obstruction can occur particularly if the cycling pressure is allowed to drop below the closing pressure of the upper airway. It is very difficult to establish effective ventilation when this occurs, although it can, in some very mild cases, be reduced by positioning the patient's head so that the neck is slightly more extended. Sometimes a chin strap alone is effective in lifting the jaw and thereby opening the upper airway. An increase in end-expiratory pressure usually ensures adequate ventilation. For some patients, the added expiratory pressures are only required in the first few days of assisted ventilation until there is some restoration of upper airway tone.

Mask leaks commonly occur on either side of the bridge of the nose and can cause significant irritation to the eyes. If the leak is small it can be compensated for by the machine and this is preferable to pulling the mask too tightly onto the face. Patients usually learn to eliminate the leaks by repositioning the mask or by adjusting the strap alignment. Elastic straps of the head harnesses usually need regular replacement to ensure effective mask pressures. Other solutions include custom-built masks and a change in sleeping posture.

Mask pressure can cause pressure sores or pressure marks on the bridge of the nose or across the top lip in particular. These are best prevented by careful selection of mask for size and skin sensitivity. The areas respond well to standard pressure care including gentle massage, being left clean, dry and open and getting a regular amount of sunshine. The bridge of the nose often becomes thick and tough with time, although some people have recurring problems. For these patients the bridge of the nose can be protected with special pressure-absorbing materials that are commonly used with prostheses. The mask can be adapted to reduce pressure by inserting a spacer on the top bar of the mask. Alternatively the patient may need to use a mouthpiece or nasal plugs (e.g. Puritan Bennett, Lenexa, KS, USA) which fit securely into the nares without pressure on the nasal bridge, permitting pressure areas to heal. Head harness or strap pressure can cause abrasions over the back of the neck or over the ears. This can be simply relieved by redesigning the head harness to realign the straps or to include cotton wadding or a pad over the tender parts.

Abdominal distension can be caused by air in the stomach particularly when high cycling pressures are required for effective ventilation. This problem is less frequent now but would be more likely with volume-cycled ventilators. It appears that air can track through the stomach to the bowel and cause considerable discomfort. Every effort should be made to lower the cycling pressure without compromising effective ventilation. Some patients find relief from lying on their left side at night, some from having an empty stomach and some resort to medications including charcoal tablets and acidophilus tablets.

Monitoring

When commencing mask ventilation in the acute situation, careful monitoring is mandatory in order to gauge the effectiveness of ventilatory support. Oximetry and transcutaneous carbon dioxide should be used to monitor trends in gas exchange continuously (Fig. 10.5). Direct measurements of arterial blood gases should be taken prior to commencing ventilation, then again at 1 hour, 6 hours, 24 hours and as needed depending on the patient's clinical condition. In addition, heart rate, respiratory rate and FiO_2 should be recorded hourly for the first few hours until the patient is stable. Blood pressure measurements may also be necessary, particularly if there is any question of the patient's haemodynamic stability.

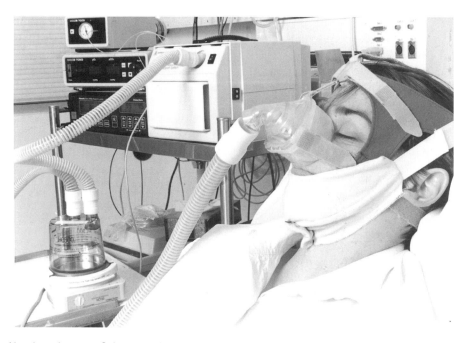

Figure 10.5 Nasal mask set-up. Oximeter and transcutaneous carbon dioxide monitors in the background are used to measure the physiological response to nasal ventilatory support. An active humidifier has been placed in the circuit between the bilevel ventilator and the patient (bottom left-hand corner).

These monitored trials are the only way of differentially diagnosing problems and resolving them promptly. In patients with chronic respiratory failure, acclimatization to the mask and machine can be carried out during the day, with monitoring of oxygen saturation and preferably CO_2, either end-tidal or transcutaneous. Frequently the patient will fall asleep during these initial trials and problems such as mouth leaks or the development of upper airway obstruction may be identified at this time. Once the patient is able to sleep for a number of hours on the machine, a sleep study, if possible, is performed to gauge the degree to which the patient and machine are synchronized, the stability in gas exchange, any technical problems which may occur and the effect of therapy on sleep. During these studies, a number of respiratory variables will be monitored in addition to the signals needed for sleep staging. Various centres will measure mask pressure, chest wall motion, diaphragmatic and other respiratory muscle electromyograms or inspiratory/expiratory tidal volumes to provide information about the efficacy of ventilatory support.

Ideally, the initial trials should have full polysomnography, respiratory monitoring and an expert therapist in attendance. After this the degree of monitoring can be reduced and the patients encouraged to manage the equipment themselves and solve any problems that may arise. Patients should be independent and confident in managing the equipment and their own care throughout the night prior to discharge from hospital. Alternatively, if individuals remain dependent on some assistance the home carers should be brought in for at least part of the night to develop skills in setting up and troubleshooting.

Home management

Most ventilator users adapt well to ongoing ventilatory support in the home and would choose ventilation again if required to do so (Goldstein et al 1995). However, it is important to provide full information to patients and families at the time of considering ongoing ventilation to ensure that an informed choice is made, especially in patients with progressive disorders. Family and community support is extremely valuable for a patient on nocturnal ventilatory support. Family acceptance of the therapy is important for ongoing compliance and for adequate maintenance of the equipment. Many patients report that they feel very isolated because there are so few people within the community with the same problem. This can manifest itself in at least two ways. First, they feel that no one in their peer group really understands what they are experiencing and second, they feel that healthcare providers in their local community do not understand their condition or their needs.

While patients are able to travel and stay with family and friends, they are often reluctant to do so because of the extra demands in terms of noise and setting up the ventilator. This can be particularly difficult for young people who wish to stay with friends and yet dread the consequences of being different. The noise of the equipment can be dampened with a soundproof casing that should be designed to allow adequate air into the inlet port and prevent overheating.

Care and maintenance of equipment

While patients are not ventilator dependent, many express considerable anxiety about the risk of being without the ventilator even for one night. They are anxious about the symptoms of sleep deprivation and hypercapnia. Those who are geographically isolated or live alone are particularly vulnerable to equipment failure. Back-up systems and emergency plans are valuable and need to be worked out with each individual. Patients should be encouraged to enter into a regular maintenance agreement with the companies or hospitals supplying the equipment. All relevant instructions for cleaning and maintenance should be provided in writing and in their preferred language.

NON-INVASIVE VENTILATION IN CHILDREN

Although non-invasive ventilatory support is now seen as a first-line therapy for adults with hypercapnic respiratory failure, this technique has, to date, been less commonly used by paediatric centres. To some extent this is due to a lack of randomized controlled trials of NIV in children, with some still considering mask ventilation to be an investigational technique in this population (Make et al 1998). In addition, some reports have suggested that infants and young children may not be tolerant of mask therapy (Heckmatt et al 1990), limiting the application of this technique. However, one of the earliest reports of mask ventilation use involved a 6-year-old child with congenital central hypoventilation syndrome (Ellis et al 1987b). Since that time, a number of studies have appeared in the literature describing the successful use of nasal masks for both CPAP and NIV in more than 200 children. Many of those described were under 6 years of age, yet tolerated therapy well both in the short and long-term (Fortenberry et al 1995, Simonds et al 2000, Villa et al 1997, Waters et al 1995).

Reports of nasal ventilation use in paediatric patients have included children with upper airway obstruction, cystic fibrosis, congenital central hypoventilation syndrome and neuromuscular disorders (Ellis et al 1987b, Padman et al 1994, Simonds et al 2000). Prior to the introduction of mask ventilation, children with chronic respiratory failure from these disorders were managed with tracheostomy in order to deliver positive pressure to the lungs. Although effective, the tracheostomy tube can also interfere with speech development and may predispose the child to chest infections. While mask ventilation can also be associated with side effects, most commonly skin breakdown and leak, these problems are generally minor or manageable. In the largest study of its kind to date, Simonds and colleagues (2000) reported the use of domiciliary mask ventilation in 40 children with respiratory failure secondary to congenital neuromuscular and skeletal disorders. The youngest child commenced on therapy at 9 months of age. Thirty-eight tolerated mask ventilatory support in the long term, resulting in reversal of nocturnal hypoventilation and significant improvements with daytime spontaneous CO_2 and O_2 levels.

Mask ventilation has also been used in children presenting with acute hypoxaemic or hypercapnic respiratory failure (Fortenberry et al 1995, Padman et al 1998). As with adults, therapy has been instituted to improve gas exchange, reduce the work of breathing and avoid intubation. It has also been used successfully to wean patients who failed attempted extubation or to facilitate extubation in those likely to have difficulty resuming spontaneous ventilation (Brinkrant et al 1997). In circumstances where there are ethical or medical concerns about the use of invasive ventilation techniques in children with severe neurological dysfunction or terminal diseases, mask ventilation offers a realistic active treatment alternative (Marino et al 1997). Although randomized trials are lacking, mounting clinical evidence suggests mask ventilation in children with acute respiratory failure is both feasible and safe.

Increasingly, bilevel devices rather than volume preset are used in this population due to simplicity, portability and cost. In addition, bilevel devices are flow initiated and therefore can be easier to trigger and more comfortable than volume-preset devices. In addition, the availability of setting EPAP with bilevel devices can be valuable in patients requiring stabilization of the upper airway as well as ventilatory support. The principles of adjusting settings for NIV in children are no different from those used with adults. Initial IPAP and EPAP pressures are set to achieve both patient comfort and the goals of ventilatory support, and are altered later depending on clinical response and patient acceptance. As the majority of bilevel devices do not have internal alarms, external alarm systems may be needed to alert carers to the loss of airway pressure associated with mask removal or machine malfunction.

Generally, children tolerate masks well although initially, extra time and effort may be needed to encourage the child to keep the mask in place. Imagination and patience, from both the clinician and the child, help. Compared to adult masks, there is a limited range for children and even fewer for neonatal use. Most 'children's' masks are simply scaled-down versions of the adult model. Although this is not much of a problem for the older, larger child, it can make fitting a mask for the younger patient (<2 years) a little more challenging. Medium-sized adult nasal masks can be used as full facemasks for the smaller child

(Simonds et al 2000). Care needs to be taken when choosing a mask to ensure dead space is minimized and sufficient carbon dioxide washout is occurring. However, as the technique becomes more widely accepted for this population, a larger choice of mask should become available.

A specific problem that could arise in children using long-term mask therapy is that of altered facial skeletal development resulting from the application of tightly fitting headgear and nasal mask. Although this has only been occasionally reported (Li et al 2000, Simonds et al 2000), the impact of mask therapy on craniofacial development should be taken into consideration when choosing and fitting mask equipment. Simonds and colleagues (2000) reported four cases of mild mid-facial hypoplasia in their series of 40 children treated long-term with mask ventilation. This problem was managed by using different masks rotated on a weekly basis to reduce and vary the pressure over the maxillary region.

In those patients requiring long-term therapy, frequent review is necessary to ensure the ventilator settings and the mask size remain adequate as the child grows and develops. Effective long-term therapy requires acclimatization and education of the child. In addition, the child's parents/carers need to be trained to supervise therapy and solve problems as they arise.

There is no doubt that as clinicians become more experienced and confident with the technique, more paediatric centres will come to accept mask ventilation as a suitable modality for children. As a consequence, increasingly more children will be offered mask ventilation as first-line therapy for the management of respiratory failure, in hospital as well as in the home. The success of this therapy relies heavily on initiation of treatment by skilled therapists and training both the child and family in its use.

PHYSIOTHERAPY INTERVENTION DURING NON-INVASIVE VENTILATION

Physiotherapists have been involved in the application of non-invasive ventilation since the polio epidemics of the 1950s. Through until the mid-1970s physiotherapists routinely administered respiratory medications by intermittent positive pressure breathing (IPPB) through a mask or mouthpiece. This mode of treatment was also used by physiotherapists to improve ventilation or reduce dyspnoea associated with a high work of breathing. A considerable amount of research has been done and reviewed by physiotherapists which contributed to rationalizing the use of this technique (Bennett et al 1976, Berend et al 1978). By the late 1970s and through the 1980s IPPB was being used predominantly to increase ventilation in patients with severe pain or with poor ventilatory control. It was also an excellent tool to provide hyperoxygenation and hyperinflation before and after nasopharyngeal or oropharyngeal suctioning. It has also been effective for sputum removal and for improving ventilation in specific groups (Starke et al 1979), particularly those who do not have sufficient conscious control of ventilation to increase their tidal volume independently. CPAP and bilevel positive pressure devices have replaced IPPB in many centres, being used on both medical and surgical wards as part of an overall strategy to increase ventilation, clear secretions and improve gas exchange.

By the mid to late 1980s the potential advantages of non-invasive ventilation in the management of chronic respiratory failure began to be realized (Grunstein et al 1991). Since that time physiotherapists have been closely involved in the application of this technique and investigation into its role in a wide range of clinical situations (Bott et al 1993, Conway et al 1993, Ellis et al 1987a, 1988, Keilty et al 1994, Milross et al 2001, Piper & Willson 1996, Piper et al 1992).

Physiotherapists may become involved with the application of this technique at a number of different levels (Box 10.4). Their skills and knowledge base regarding respiratory disease and its management place them in a good position to be key members in any non-invasive ventilation service. Physiotherapists are experienced in assessing breathing patterns and coaching patients to alter breathing in order to improve ventilation. When implementing non-invasive ventilatory support, training of the patient to

---

Box 10.4   Role of the physiotherapist

Assessment of the patient
- Identification of symptoms of sleep-disordered breathing
- Bedside pulmonary function testing including respiratory muscle strength
- Exercise tolerance (e.g. 6-minute walking test, shuttle test)
- Level of dyspnoea during daily activities

Initiating therapy
- Choice of device and setting
- Acclimatizing patient to mask and machine
- Education of patient and family regarding therapy
- Monitoring response to therapy

Planning a concurrent rehabilitation programme
- Need for oxygen and the level required during activities
- Upper limb and whole body training
- Lifestyle modification
- Use of ventilatory support as part of secretion clearance

Discharge planning
- Training patient and/or caregivers in the care and operation of the equipment
- Home exercise programme
- Ongoing appointments and emergency plans

Follow-up
- Pulmonary function testing
- Exercise tolerance
- Troubleshooting problems: technical problems versus changes in clinical condition

---

accept the mask and flow from the device is essential for eventual acceptance. There is also the need for close bedside monitoring of the patient, with ongoing ventilator adjustments to optimize ventilatory support and maximize patient comfort. Such adjustments require a solid understanding of respiratory physiology as well as good clinical skills in assessing the response of the patient to therapy. The use of non-invasive ventilation should be seen as an adjunct to other physiotherapeutic techniques as part of an overall rehabilitation programme.

Use of this modality has been reported to improve secretion clearance and increase tolerance to other physiotherapy procedures (Fauroux et al 1999, Piper et al 1992). It permits patients to adopt positions for postural drainage that they would otherwise not be able to adopt due to breathlessness. In patients with severe muscle weakness and poor cough, mask ventilation may be used to assist deep breathing and mobilization of secretions. Anecdotally, patients report being able to tolerate longer physiotherapy sessions when using ventilatory support, which is important in patients who tire easily but who have retained or copious secretions. The tidal volume or inspiratory pressure of the device may be increased during physiotherapy sessions to aid chest wall expansion and assist the mobilization of secretions (Fauroux et al 1999). The use of mask ventilation in this situation should be seen as an integral part of the patient's respiratory care regimen and used in conjunction with other physiotherapeutic techniques.

By the time patients with chronic respiratory failure present for nocturnal ventilatory support they are usually severely debilitated. Their presentation is usually characterized by severe shortness of breath on exertion, excessive daytime sleepiness, fatigue, prolonged illness and regular hospitalization. Because of all these factors it is very likely that significant peripheral deconditioning has occurred which limits their tolerance to daily activities and exercise perform-ance. After a period of nocturnal ventilatory support, patients are able to perform a great deal more work without fatigue and are capable of a reconditioning programme that should improve their quality of life further.

The beneficial effects of positive pressure during exercise in patients with severe lung disease have been reported (Keilty et al 1994, Kyroussis et al 2000). Benefits include reduced breathlessness, increased exercise time and improved oxygen saturation. However, the benefits of routine application of this technique during exercise training remain unclear and await further investigation.

SUMMARY

Non-invasive ventilation is a technique which can improve gas exchange and reduce the work of breathing and is becoming increasingly used to manage both chronic and acute respiratory failure. Physiotherapists will continue to have a significant role in the effective management of these patients.

REFERENCES

Aboussouan LS, Khan SU, Meeker DP, Stelmach K, Mitsumato H 1997 Effect of noninvasive positive pressure ventilation on survival in amyotrophic lateral sclerosis. Annals of Internal Medicine 127: 450–453

Ambrosino N, Foglio K, Rubini F, Clini E, Nava S, Vitacca M 1995 Noninvasive mechanical ventilation in acute respiratory failure due to chronic obstructive pulmonary disease: correlates for success. Thorax 50: 755–757

Anton A, Guell R, Gomez J, Serrano J, Castellano A, Carrasco JL, Sanchis J 2000 Predicting the result of noninvasive ventilation in severe acute exacerbations of patients with chronic airflow limitation. Chest 117: 828–833

Antonelli M, Conti G, Rocco M et al 1998 A comparison of noninvasive positive pressure ventilation and conventional mechanical ventilation in patients with acute respiratory failure. New England Journal of Medicine 339: 429–435

Antonelli M, Conti G, Bufi M et al 2000 Noninvasive ventilation for treatment of acute respiratory failure in patients undergoing solid organ transplantation. Journal of the American Medical Association 283: 235–241

Barach AL, Martin J, Eckman M 1938 Positive-pressure respiration and its application to the treatment of acute pulmonary edema. Annals of Internal Medicine 12: 754–795

Bardi G, Pierotello R, Desideri M, Valdisserri L, Bottai M, Palla A 2000 Nasal ventilation in COPD exacerbations: early and late results of a prospective, controlled study. European Respiratory Journal 15: 98–104

Bennett L, Heath J, Mitchell R 1976 An inpatient observation and comparison of the Bennett's IPPB and aerosol methods of administering salbutamol. Australian Journal of Physiotherapy 23: 111–113

Berend N, Webster J, Marlin EE 1978 Salbutamol by pressure-packed aerosol and by intermittent positive pressure ventilation in chronic obstructive bronchitis. British Journal of Diseases of the Chest 72: 122–124

Bersten AD, Holt AW, Verdig AE, Skowronski GA, Baggoley CJ 1991 Treatment of severe cardiogenic pulmonary oedema with continuous positive pressure delivered by face mask. New England Journal of Medicine 325: 1826–1830

Bott J, Carroll MP, Conway JH et al 1993 Randomized controlled trial of nasal ventilation in acute ventilatory failure due to chronic obstructive airways disease. Lancet 341: 1555–1557

Brinkrant DJ, Pope JF, Eiban RM 1997. Pediatric noninvasive nasal ventilation. Journal of Child Neurology 12: 231–236

Brochard L, Mancebo J, Wysocki M et al 1995 Noninvasive ventilation for acute exacerbations of chronic obstructive pulmonary disease. New England Journal of Medicine 333: 817–822

Brown JS, Meecham Jones DJ, Mikelsons C, Paul EA, Wedzicha JA 1998. Using nasal intermittent positive pressure ventilation on a general respiratory ward. Journal of the Royal College of Physicians London 32: 219–224

Bye PTP, Ellis ER, Issa FG, Donnelly PD, Sullivan CE 1990 The role of sleep in the development of respiratory failure in patients with neuromuscular disease. Thorax 45: 241–247

Chevrolet JC, Jolliet P, Abajo B, Toussi A, Louis M 1991 Nasal positive pressure ventilation in patients with acute respiratory failure. Difficult and time-consuming procedure for nurses. Chest 100: 775–782

Confalonieri M, Potena A, Carbone G, Della Porta R, Tolley EA, Meduri GU 1999 Acute respiratory failure in patients with severe community acquired pneumonia: a prospective randomized evaluation of non-invasive ventilation. American Journal of Respiratory and Critical Care Medicine 160: 1585–1591

Conway JH, Hitchcock RA, Godfrey RC, Carroll MP 1993 Nasal intermittent positive pressure ventilation in acute exacerbations of chronic obstructive pulmonary disease – a preliminary study. Respiratory Medicine 87: 387–394

Douglas NJ, White DP, Pickett CK, Weil JV, Zwillich CW 1982 Respiration during sleep in normal man. Thorax 37: 840–844

Elliott MW, Simonds AK 1995 Nocturnal assisted ventilation using positive airway pressure: the effect of expiratory positive airway pressure. European Respiratory Journal 8: 436–440

Elliott MW, Mulvey DA, Moxham J, Green M, Branthwaite MA 1991 Domiciliary nocturnal nasal intermittent positive pressure ventilation in COPD: mechanisms underlying changes in blood gas tensions. European Respiratory Journal 4: 1044–1052

Ellis ER, Bye PTP, Bruderer JW, Sullivan CE 1987a Treatment of respiratory failure in patients with neuromuscular disease. American Review of Respiratory Disease 135: 148–152

Ellis ER, McCauley VB, Mellis C, Sullivan CE 1987b Treatment of alveolar hypoventilation in a six-year-old girl with intermittent positive pressure ventilation through a nose mask. American Review of Respiratory Disease 136: 188–91

Ellis ER, Grunstein RR, Chan CS, Bye PTP, Sullivan CE 1988 Treatment of nocturnal respiratory failure in kyphoscoliosis. Chest 94: 811–815

Escarrabill J, Estopa R, Farrero E, Monasterio C, Manresa F 1998 Long-term mechanical ventilation in amyotrophic lateral sclerosis. Respiratory Medicine 92: 438–441

Fauroux B, Boule M, Lofaso F, Zerah F, Clement A, Harf A, Isabey D 1999 Chest physiotherapy in cystic fibrosis: improved tolerance with nasal pressure support ventilation. Pediatrics 103: E32

Ferguson GT, Gilmartin M 1995 CO2 rebreathing during BIPAP ventilatory assistance. American Journal of Respiratory and Critical Care Medicine 151: 1126–1135

Fernandez R, Blanch L, Valles J, Baigorri F, Artigas A 1993 Pressure support ventilation via face mask in acute respiratory failure in hypercapnic COPD patients. Intensive Care Medicine 19: 456–461

Fortenberry JD, Del Toro J, Jefferson LS, Evey L, Haase D 1995 Management of pediatric acute hypoxemic

respiratory failure with bilevel positive pressure (BiPAP) nasal mask ventilation. Chest 108: 1059–1064

Garay SM, Turino GM, Goldring RM 1981 Sustained reversal of chronic hypercapnia in patients with alveolar hypoventilation syndromes: long-term maintenance with noninvasive mechanical ventilation. American Journal of Medicine 70: 269–274

Gastaut H, Tassinari CA, Duron B 1966 Polygraphic study of the episodic diurnal and nocturnal manifestations of the Pickwick syndrome. Brain Research 1: 167–186

Gay PC, Patel AM, Viggiano RW, Hubmayr RD 1991 Nocturnal nasal ventilation for treatment of patients with hypercapnic respiratory failure. Mayo Clinic Proceedings 66: 695–703

Girault C, Daudenthun I, Chevron V, Tamion F, Lekay J, Bonmarchand G 1999 Noninvasive ventilation as a systematic extubation and weaning technique in acute-on-chronic respiratory failure. American Journal of Respiratory and Critical Care Medicine 160: 88–92

Goldstein RS, Psek JA, Gort EH 1995 Home mechanical ventilation. Demographics and user perspectives. Chest 108: 1581–1586

Gould GA, Gugger M, Molloy J, Tsara V, Shapiro CM, Douglas NJ 1988 Breathing pattern and eye movement density during REM sleep in humans. American Review of Respiratory Disease 138: 874–877

Gozal D 1997 Nocturnal ventilatory support in patients with cystic fibrosis: comparison with supplemental oxygen. European Respiratory Journal 10: 1999–2003

Grunstein RR, Ellis ER, Hillman D, McEvoy RD, Robertson CF, Saunders NA 1991 Treatment of sleep disordered breathing. Medical Journal of Australia 154: 355–359

Heckmatt JZ, Loh L, Dubowitz V 1990 Night-time nasal ventilation in neuromuscular disease. Lancet 335: 579–582

Hill AT, Edenborough FP, Cayton KM, Stableforth DE 1998 Long-term nasal intermittent positive pressure ventilation in patients with cystic fibrosis and hypercapnic respiratory failure (1991–1996). Respiratory Medicine 92: 523–526

Hodson ME, Madden BP, Steven MH, Tsang VT, Yacoub MH 1991 Non-invasive mechanical ventilation for cystic fibrosis patients – a potential bridge to transplantation. European Respiratory Journal 4: 524–527

Keilty SEJ, Ponte J, Fleming TA, Moxham J 1994 Effect of inspiratory pressure support on exercise tolerance and breathlessness in patients with severe stable chronic obstructive pulmonary disease. Thorax 49: 990–994

Kramer N, Meyer TJ, Mehang J, Cece RD, Hill NS 1995 Randomized, prospective trial of noninvasive positive pressure ventilation in acute respiratory failure. American Journal of Respiratory and Critical Care Medicine 151: 1799–1806

Kyroussis D, Polkey MI, Hamnegard CH, Mills GH, Green M, Moxham J 2000 Respiratory muscle activity in patients with COPD walking to exhaustion with and without pressure support. European Respiratory Journal 15: 649–655

Li KK, Riley RW, Guilleminault C 2000 An unreported risk in the use of home nasal continuous positive airway pressure and home nasal ventilation in children: mid-face hypoplasia. Chest 117: 916–918

Make BJ, Hill NS, Goldberg AI et al 1998 Mechanical ventilation beyond the intensive care unit. Report of a consensus conference of the American College of Chest Physicians. Chest 113 (suppl): 289S–344S

Marino P, Rosa G, Conti G, Coglioti AA 1997 Treatment of acute respiratory failure by prolonged non-invasive ventilation in a child. Canadian Journal of Anaesthesia 44: 727–731

Masip J, Betbese AJ, Paez J et al 2000. Non-invasive pressure support ventilation versus conventional oxygen therapy in acute cardiogenic pulmonary oedema: a randomized trial. Lancet 356: 2126–2132

Meecham Jones DJ, Wedzicha JA 1993 Comparison of pressure and volume preset nasal ventilator systems in stable chronic respiratory failure. European Respiratory Journal 6: 1060–1064

Meecham Jones DJ, Paul EA, Grahame-Clarke C, Wedzicha JA 1994 Nasal ventilation in acute exacerbations of chronic obstructive pulmonary disease: effect of ventilation mode on arterial blood gas tensions. Thorax 49: 1222–1224

Meecham Jones DJ, Paul EA, Jones PW, Wedzicha JA 1995 Nasal pressure support ventilation plus oxygen compared with oxygen therapy alone in hypercapnic COPD. American Journal of Respiratory and Critical Care Medicine 152: 538–544

Mehta S, Jay GD, Woolard RH et al 1997 Randomized, prospective trial of bilevel versus continuous positive airway pressure in acute pulmonary edema. Critical Care Medicine 25: 620–628

Meyer TJ, Hill NS 1994 Noninvasive positive pressure ventilation to treat respiratory failure. Annals of Internal Medicine 120: 760–770

Meyer TJ, Pressman MR, Benditt J, McCool FD, Millman RP, Natarajan R, Hill NS 1997 Air leaking through the mouth during nocturnal nasal ventilation: effect on sleep quality. Sleep 20: 561–569

Milross MA, Piper AJ, Norman M et al 2001 Low-flow oxygen and bilevel ventilatory support. Effects on ventilation during sleep in cystic fibrosis. American Journal of Respiratory and Critical Care Medicine 163: 129–134

Nava S, Ambrosino N, Clini E et al 1998 Noninvasive mechanical ventilation in the weaning of patients with respiratory failure due to chronic obstructive pulmonary disease. Annals of Internal Medicine 128: 721–728

Padman R, Nadkarni VN, Von Nessen S et al 1994 Noninvasive positive pressure ventilation in end-stage cystic fibrosis: a report of 7 cases: Respiratory Care 39: 436–439

Padman R, Lawless ST, Kettrick RG 1998 Noninvasive ventilation via bilevel positive airway pressure support in pediatric practice. Critical Care in Medicine 26: 169–173

Parreira VF, Jounieaux V, Aubert G, Dury M, Delguste PE, Rodenstein DO 1996 Nasal two-level positive-pressure ventilation in normal subjects. Effects on the glottis and ventilation. American Journal of Respiratory and Critical Care Medicine 153: 1616–1623

Paulus J, Willig TN 1993 Nasal ventilation in neuromuscular disorders: respiratory management and patient's experience. European Respiratory Review 3: 245–249

Piper AJ, Sullivan CE 1994a Sleep breathing in neuromuscular disease. In: Saunders N, Sullivan CE (eds) Sleep and breathing, 2nd edn. Marcel Dekker, New York, pp 761–821

Piper AJ, Sullivan CE 1994b Effects of short-term NIPPV in the treatment of patients with severe obstructive sleep apnea and hypercapnia. Chest 105: 434–440

Piper AJ, Willson G 1996 Nocturnal nasal ventilatory support in the management of daytime hypercapnic respiratory failure. Australian Journal of Physiotherapy 42(1): 17–29

Piper AJ, Parker S, Torzillo PJ, Sullivan CE, Bye PTP 1992 Nocturnal nasal IPPV stabilizes patients with cystic fibrosis and hypercapnic respiratory failure. Chest 102: 846–850

Plant PK, Owen JL, Elliott MW 2000 Early use of non-invasive ventilation for acute exacerbations of chronic obstructive pulmonary disease on general respiratory wards: a multicentre randomized controlled trial. Lancet 355: 1931–1935

Polkey MI, Lyall RA, Davidson AC, Leigh PN, Moxham J 1999 Ethical and clinical issues in the use of home non-invasive mechanical ventilation for the palliation of breathlessness in motor neurone disease. Thorax 54: 367–371

Pollack CV, Fleisch KB, Dowsey K 1995 Treatment of acute bronchospasm with beta-adrenergic agonist aerosols delivered by a nasal bilevel positive airway pressure circuit. Annals of Emergency Medicine 26: 552–557

Poulton EP, Oxon DM 1936 Left-sided heart failure with pulmonary edema – its treatment with the 'pulmonary plus pressure machine'. Lancet 231: 981–983

Raphael JC, Chevret S, Chastang C, Bouvet F 1994 Randomized trial of preventive nasal ventilation in Duchenne muscular dystrophy. Lancet 343: 1600–1603

Restrick LJ, Scott AD, Ward EM, Feneck RO, Cornwell WE, Wedzicha JA 1993 Nasal intermittent positive-pressure ventilation in weaning intubated patients with chronic respiratory failure from assisted intermittent, positive-pressure ventilation. Respiratory Medicine 87: 199–204

Richards GN, Cistulli PA, Ungar G, Berthon-Jones M, Sullivan CE 1996 Mouth leak with nasal continuous positive airway pressure increases nasal airway resistance. American Journal of Respiratory and Critical Care Medicine 154: 182–186

Rusterholtz T, Kempf J, Berton C et al 1999 Noninvasive pressure support ventilation (NIPSV) with face mask in patients with acute cardiogenic pulmonary edema (ACPE). Intensive Care Medicine 25: 21–28

Saunders NA, Powles ACP, Rebuck AS 1976 Ear oximetry: accuracy and practicability in assessment of arterial oxygenation. American Review of Respiratory Disease 113: 745–749

Schonhofer B, Sonneborn M, Haidl P, Bohrer H, Kohler D 1997 Comparison of two different modes for noninvasive mechanical ventilation: volume vs pressure controlled device. European Respiratory Journal 10: 184–191

Servera E, Perez M, Marin J, Vergara P, Castano R 1995 Noninvasive nasal mask ventilation beyond the ICU for an exacerbation of chronic respiratory insufficiency. Chest 108: 1572–1576

Simonds AK, Elliott MW 1995 Outcome of domiciliary nasal intermittent positive pressure ventilation in restrictive and obstructive disorders. Thorax 50: 604–609

Simonds AK, Muntoni F, Heather S, Fielding S 1998 Impact of nasal ventilation on survival in hypercapnic Duchenne muscular dystrophy. Thorax 53: 949–952

Simonds AK, Ward S, Heather S, Bush A, Muntoni F 2000 Outcome of paediatric domiciliary mask ventilation in neuromuscular and skeletal disease. European Respiratory Journal 16: 476–481

Soo Hoo GW, Santiago S, Williams AJ 1994 Nasal mechanical ventilation for hypercapnic respiratory failure in chronic obstructive pulmonary disease: determinants of success and failure. Critical Care Medicine 22: 1253–1261

Starke ID, Webber BA, Branthwaite MA 1979 IPPB and hypercapnia in respiratory failure. Anaesthesia 34: 283–287

Strumpf DA, Millman RP, Carlisle CC, Grattan LM, Ryan SM, Erickson AD, Hill NS 1991 Nocturnal positive-pressure ventilation via nasal mask in patients with severe chronic obstructive pulmonary disease. American Review of Respiratory Disease 144: 1234–1239

Sullivan CE, Berthon-Jones M, Issa FG, Eves L 1981 Reversal of obstructive sleep apnea by continuous positive airway pressure applied through the nose. Lancet 1: 862–865

Teschler H, Stampa J, Ragette R, Konietzko N, Berthon-Jones M 1999 Effect of mouth leak on effectiveness of nasal bilevel ventilatory assistance and sleep architecture. European Respiratory Journal 14: 1251–1257

Trask CH, Cree EM 1962 Oximeter studies on patients with chronic obstructive emphysema, awake and during sleep. New England Journal of Medicine 266: 639–642

Villa MP, Datta A, Castello D, Silvana P, Pagani J, Palamides S, Ronchetti K 1997 Bilevel positive airway pressure (BiPAP)

ventilation in an infant with central hypoventilation syndrome. Pediatric Pulmonology 24: 66–69

Vitacca M, Rubini F, Foglio K, Scalvini S, Nava S, Ambrosino N 1993 Noninvasive modalities of positive pressure ventilation improve the outcome of acute exacerbations in COLD patients. Intensive Care Medicine 19: 450–455

Vitacca M, Clini E, Rubini F, Nava S, Foglio K, Ambrosino N 1996 Non-invasive mechanical ventilation in severe chronic obstructive lung disease and acute respiratory failure: short- and long-term prognosis. Intensive Care Medicine 22: 94–100

Waters KA, Everett FM, Bruderer JW et al 1995 Obstructive sleep apnea: the use of nasal CPAP in 80 children. American Journal of Respiratory and Critical Care Medicine 152: 780–785

Weirs PWJ, LeCoultre R, Dallinga OT, Van Dijl W, Meinesz AF, Sluiter HJ 1977 Cuirass respirator treatment of chronic respiratory failure in scoliotic patients. Thorax 32: 221–228

Wood KE, Flaten AL, Backes WJ 2000 Inspissated secretions: a life-threatening complication of prolonged non-invasive ventilation. Respiratory Care 45: 491–493

Woollam CHM 1976 The development of apparatus for intermittent negative pressure respiration (1) 1832–1918. Anaesthesia 31: 537–547

FURTHER READING

Brochard L 2000 Non-invasive ventilation for acute exacerbations of COPD: a new standard of care. Thorax 55: 817–818

Meduri GU 1996 Noninvasive positive pressure ventilation in patients with acute respiratory failure. Clinics in Chest Medicine 17: 513–553

Simonds AK 1996 Non-invasive respiratory support. Chapman and Hall, London

Turkington PM, Elliott MW 2000 Rationale for the use of non-invasive ventilation in chronic ventilatory failure. Thorax 55: 417–423

11

Intensive care for the critically ill adult

Fran H Woodard   Mandy Jones

INTRODUCTION

The intensive care unit (ICU) is perceived as a
daunting environment to the undergraduate or
newly qualified physiotherapist (Fig. 11.1). The
patients present with a complexity of problems
which may be multisystem in origin and the
technology used in their treatment is continually
being updated and advanced. Illness severity
scoring systems such as the Acute Physiology
and Chronic Health Evaluation II (APACHE II)
are used to quantify the severity of illness, to
determine the success of different forms of treatment and to predict mortality (Knaus et al 1985).

The physiotherapist has a vital role to play in
the ICU. Once the initial fear has been conquered, this area provides a forum in which skills
and knowledge acquired from all the different
specialist areas can be utilized. The physiotherapist must consider the general condition of the
patient and must remember the possible feelings
and fears that he may have in his unnatural surroundings. Areas of concern are an inability to
speak and a loss of perception of time. The
patient will also probably suffer from chronic
sleep deprivation.

There is no place for routine physiotherapy
in the ICU. A thorough analytical assessment
will highlight physiotherapy problems which
may respond to treatment and associated contraindications.

This chapter attempts to guide the physiotherapist through this assessment and the implications of its findings, the problems associated with
mechanical ventilation and patient groups with

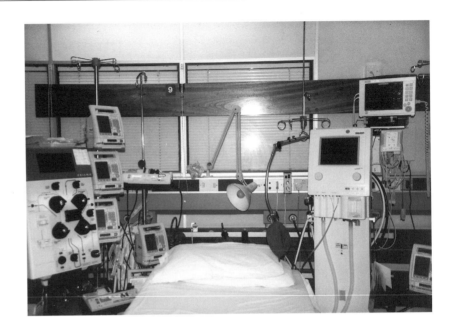

Figure 11.1 A typical ICU bed space.

specific needs. Once all appropriate information has been gathered, the relevant physiotherapy treatment can be selected.

ASSESSMENT OF THE CRITICALLY ILL PATIENT IN THE INTENSIVE CARE UNIT

Although the respiratory physiotherapist may be primarily concerned with the patient's respiratory system, an analytical assessment must be conducted on other related systems to allow a full overview of the patient's medical stability and suitability for treatment. This holistic approach must incorporate an understanding of both the implications and use of drug therapy (Pearson & Parr 1993).

Neurological system

The early stages of the management of the acute head injury and the neurosurgical patient involve sedation and frequently paralysis. Adequate sedation and/or paralysis are essential in the maintenance of stable intracranial pressure. Fluctuating intracranial pressures will occur as a result of environmental stimuli,

including physiotherapeutic intervention in the poorly sedated patient.

Important factors in assessment

Level of consciousness. The most widely used and accepted scoring system of the neurological patient is the Glasgow Coma Scale (GCS). Neurological centres may use their own scoring system in addition to the GCS (Frisby 1990) (see p. 10).

Pupils

- *Size.* The pupils are graded either numerically or by description ranging from pinprick to dilated. The most significant cause of sudden pupil dilatation is neurological deterioration (e.g. cerebral oedema). Pharmacological treatment can alter pupil size (e.g. reduced or pinprick as a result of opioid use or dilated after administration of atropine or adrenaline).
- *Reactivity.* The pupils' reaction to light indicates optic and oculomotor nerve function. Fixed dilated pupils may indicate severe neurological impairment or be caused by drug treatment, hypoxia or biochemical abnormalities.
- *Equality.* Each pupil is tested individually, as inequality may be an important localizing sign.

Cerebral perfusion pressure (CPP). This is the critical pressure required to ensure adequate blood supply to the brain and prevent acidosis, hypoxia and damage. The brain attempts to maintain a constant cerebral blood flow, despite variations in blood pressure, by a process of autoregulation. The range of blood pressure over which it is effective varies with the individual. Autoregulation may be impaired by a severe head injury or other neurological insults.

CPP = mean arterial pressure (MAP) *minus* intracranial pressure (ICP)

Normal value	>70 mmHg
Critical value	<50 mmHg

Intracranial pressure (ICP). The components influencing ICP are the blood, brain and CSF within the rigid skull. The blood component can be influenced by changes in $PaCO_2$ and venous drainage. Rises in ICP from normal levels correlate with a worse outcome (Miller et al 1977). ICP measurement is used as a diagnostic tool and to guide and assess the effectiveness of medical treatment. It can be measured by an extradural, subdural or subarachnoid bolt, intraparenchymal sensor or ventricular drain (Fig. 4.5, p. 134) (German 1994).

Normal value	<10 mmHg
Critical value	>25 mmHg

Drugs. See Table 11.1.

Considerations for physiotherapy

- Consistent levels of ICP (below the critical level) suggest a patient may be stable enough to tolerate intervention, whereas a fluctuating ICP indicates neurological instability which may be magnified by any physiotherapeutic intervention. It is worth noting that a sudden rise in ICP (which will reduce CPP) can be caused by hypercapnia secondary to respiratory complications such as atelectasis or sputum retention.

- In situations of increased or unstable ICP it may be necessary to use inotropic support to maintain MAP at a level to preserve CPP.
- The patient's level of sedation needs to be considered. It is well documented that sedation leads to a lowering of blood pressure. Therefore, it is essential that the patient's cardiovascular system is assessed thoroughly and any necessary drugs given before physiotherapy. It is important to note that when sedation is being weaned, the patient may become agitated and self-extubation is a risk.

Cardiovascular system

The cardiovascular stability of the critically ill patient is influenced by many interrelated factors. In some situations physiotherapeutic intervention may be contraindicated. A thorough assessment is therefore essential before any treatment is instigated.

Important factors in assessment

Heart rate (HR) and rhythm. The critically ill patient may develop a multitude of arrhythmias. There are many possible causes (e.g. electrolyte imbalance, action of drugs), but physiotherapy intervention in the unstable patient may precipitate or worsen them. The arrhythmias that may be encountered vary from severe rhythm disturbances causing cardiovascular compromise (e.g. decreased blood pressure potentially leading to reduced urine output) to more benign disturbances, but even ventricular ectopics may be a precursor of more serious arrhythmias (p. 96).

Normal value	50–100 bpm
Bradycardia	<50 bpm
Tachycardia	>100 bpm

Arterial blood pressure (BP). Blood pressure is dependent on various parameters. Blood pressure is equal to the rate of blood flow multiplied by the resistance produced by the vessels. Therefore in the cardiovascular system:

Table 11.1 Drugs in the ICU: the neurological system

Drug		Action	Considerations for physiotherapy
Hypnovel / Versed	midazolam	Sedatives	May need to be increased prior to physiotherapy intervention to prevent acute rises in ICP or BP. Care with manual hyperinflation as sedation can cause a drop in BP. Causes impairment of cough reflex, therefore difficulty in clearing secretions
Chloractil / Ormazine	chlorpromazine		
Diprivan	propofol		
Ketalar	ketamine		
Durogesic	fentanyl	Sedatives and analgesics	
Rapifen / Alfenta	alfentanil		
MST / Astramorph	morphine		
Pavulon	pancuronium	Muscle relaxants	Used by continuous infusion. Usually reflects either severe respiratory failure with difficulty in ventilation or neurological instability. Care with manual hyperinflation as it may not be tolerated. Absence of cough reflex. Care with positioning as reduced muscle tone leads to joint vulnerability
Tracrium	atracurium		
Norcuron	vecuronium		
Intraval / Pentothal	thiopentone	Sedative	Main indication for use is intractable fitting or very unstable ICP. Closely monitor CPP, ICP and MAP during treatment
Nimotop	nimodipine	Specific cerebral artery vasodilator	Usually used in patients whose ICP is raised and/or unstable. If physiotherapy is absolutely essential, monitor parameters carefully throughout treatment
Osmitrol	mannitol	Osmotic diuretic	
Decadron / Aerosels–Dex	dexamethasone	Corticosteroid–reduces cerebral oedema	
Epanutin / Dilantin	phenytoin	Anticonvulsant	If fitting is well controlled there is no contraindication for treatment

Mean BP = systemic vascular resistance (SVR) × cardiac output (CO)

CO = stroke volume (SV) × HR

Therefore:

BP = SVR × SV × HR

Normal value: 95/60–140/90 mmHg

Mean arterial

pressure (MAP) = Diastolic + $\dfrac{\text{(Pulse pressure)}}{3}$

Pulse pressure = the difference between systolic and diastolic pressures

The critically ill patient may develop hypotension because of hypovolaemia, sepsis, excessive use of sedative or vasodilatory drugs or a primary cardiac dysfunction. Hypertension may reflect, for example, inadequate sedation and analgesia or a Cushing's response to a raised ICP (Ganong 1995). If uncontrolled, both of these may be a contraindication to physiotherapy. The management of hypotension may require a fluid challenge or inotropic support. Increasing doses of inotropes indicate escalating cardiovascular instability.

Central venous pressure (CVP). In the absence of cardiovascular or pulmonary disease, CVP is a reflection of circulatory volume and therefore has a direct correlation with fluid balance. It is measured via a central venous catheter situated in a central vein (see p. 130).

Normal value   3–15 cmH$_2$O

Pulmonary artery pressure (PAP) and pulmonary capillary wedge pressure (PCWP). A normal PAP is approximately one-sixth of systemic pressure (West 1995). High PAPs may be seen in severe respiratory disease.

PCWP pressure gives an indirect measurement of left arterial pressure and left ventricular filling pressure. A high PCWP may be caused by poor left ventricular function, fluid overload, mitral valve disease and positive pressure ventilation. A low PCWP may be caused by hypovolaemia.

The pulmonary artery catheter (Swan–Ganz) may be used to derive numerical values for cardiac output, stroke volume and ventricular workload and may guide the use of inotropic support and fluid balance.

Normal values:

Mean pulmonary artery pressure (PAP)
10–20 mmHg (1.3–2.7 kPa)

Pulmonary capillary wedge pressure (PCWP)
6–15 mmHg (0.8–2 kPa)

Cardiac output (CO) 5 l/min

Drugs. See Table 11.2.

Considerations for physiotherapy

- The presence of arrhythmias must be assessed. Some arrhythmias can be essentially stable (e.g. slow atrial fibrillation). In this situation if the rhythm is normal for the patient or no cardiovascular compromise is present, physiotherapy may be carried out if indicated. Fast atrial fibrillation and many other supraventricular and ventricular tachycardias are unstable rhythms and therefore physiotherapy is contraindicated.
- A high PAP may indicate high pulmonary vascular resistance which would be exacerbated during manual hyperinflations. Manual hyperinflations must also be used with caution in patients with a low cardiac output (p. 368).

Respiratory system

The patient is assessed for the level of ventilatory support required, i.e. full, assisted or spontaneous ventilation. The presence of an endotracheal or tracheostomy tube, nasal mask or full facemask should be noted.

Important factors in assessment

Mode of ventilation/PEEP/CPAP. See also Chapter 9.

Humidification. The ability to clear secretions effectively must be assessed. If compressed dry air has been given, the need for humidification must be assessed. The alternatives are heat moisture exchangers (HME) or heated humidification (p. 228) (Branson et al 1993).

Oxygen therapy. An increase in oxygen requirement may reflect a deteriorating primary respiratory problem or impaired gas exchange as a result of a multisystem disorder. The level of therapeutic oxygen available ranges from room air at 21% (FiO_2 0.21) to 100% oxygen (FiO_2 1.0).

Respiratory rate (RR). The respiratory rate will vary depending on the type and amount of ventilatory support. In a fully ventilated patient, the rate is set and only originates from the ventilator. The rate may be set to achieve a specific goal in the individual patient. For example, a high respiratory rate may be desirable in a neurological patient to lower $PaCO_2$ (and thus ICP) or a lower respiratory rate may be preferred to produce a high normal $PaCO_2$ (permissive hypercapnia) in a patient with chronic airflow limitation (CAL).

In assisted modes, a proportion of the rate is delivered by the ventilator with patients able to initiate their own additional respiratory rate. The ventilator rate may be gradually reduced to encourage weaning (p. 304).

Patients who are breathing spontaneously may have abnormally high respiratory rates because of exhaustion, neurological impairment, anxiety, pain or biochemical abnormalities. The pattern of respiration in the spontaneously breathing patient is also important because it may reflect mechanical obstruction, poor coordination (e.g. residual muscle relaxation) and neurological impairment (e.g. periods of apnoea, p. 15).

Airway pressures. In the ventilated patient, although no pressure is totally safe, barotrauma is unlikely to occur in patients whose peak inspiratory pressure (PIP) is less than 40cmH$_2$O. Raised PIPs may be indicative of many differing clinical situations, e.g. reduced compliance, fibrosis, acute respiratory distress syndrome (ARDS), pulmonary oedema, sputum plugging or bronchospasm. Both mean and peak airway pressures can be displayed throughout the respiratory cycle on monitors.

Table 11.2 Drugs in the ICU: the cardiovascular system

Drug		Action	Considerations for physiotherapy
Inotropes			
Epifrin	adrenaline	↑ Heart rate ↑ Cardiac output	
Levophed	noradrenaline	Peripheral vasoconstriction ↑ Systemic vascular resistance	
Medihaler-Iso	isoprenaline	↑ Heart rate ↑ Cardiac output	
Dobutrex	dobutamine	↑ Myocardial contractility ↑ Heart rate	Inotropes are used to support blood pressure. Evaluation of cardiovascular stability and effect of inotropic support must be noted. Care with hyperinflations as blood pressure may be labile

Intropin	dopamine	Low doses < 5 µ/kg/min
		    ↑ Myocardial contractility
		    ↑ Renal perfusion
		Higher doses > 5 µ/kg/min
		    ↑ Systemic vascular resistance	

Dopacard	dopexamine	↑ Heart rate ↑ Renal perfusion ↑ Splanchnic perfusion	
Perfan	enoximone	↑ Myocardial contractility ↑ Peripheral dilatation	
Primator	milrinone	↓ Systemic vascular resistance	
Hypertensin	angiotensin	Potent vasoconstriction	Used in some centres in the severely unstable patient
Other relevant cardiac drugs			
Adalat	nifedipine	Vascular smooth muscle relaxant Coronary and peripheral artery dilator Antihypertensive	Used primarily in control of hypertension especially those at risk of myocardial ischaemia. Monitor BP and ECG during treatment
Coro-Nitro Tridil Angeze Imdur	GTN–glyceryl trinitrate ISMN–isosorbide mononitrate	Vasodilator	
Lanoxin	digoxin	Control of supraventricular tachycardia, atrial fibrillation or flutter	
Cordarone	amiodorone		Stable arrhythmias are not a direct contraindication to treatment. Monitor rhythm throughout intervention
Adenocor Adenocord	adenosine		
Berkaten Cordilox	verapamil	Anti-arrhythmic	
Laryng-o-Jet Anestacon	lignocaine		
Calciparine Hep-Lock	heparin		If over-anticoagulated, bleeding is a risk. Care during suction
Marevan Coumadin	warfarin	Anticoagulant	

Auscultation. In the ventilated patient normal breath sounds tend to be more harsh. This can be attributed to transmitted noises originating from the ventilator itself or to accumulated water in the tubes. During assessment it is important to compare zones on each side of the chest. The bases of a ventilated patient are difficult to access in the supine position but essential to auscultate (p. 17).

Percussion note. This is an extremely useful technique in the assessment of the ICU patient. The information gained from percussion may help to differentiate between pathologies, e.g. pleural effusion (stony dull), atelectasis or consolidation (dull). In an emergency, percussion can be used to distinguish quickly between a patient who has collapsed a lung (dull) and one who has sustained a pneumothorax (hyper-resonant).

Expansion. Equality of expansion may be felt by palpating a patient's chest. Palpation is also useful as an indicator of any underlying secretions, bronchospasm or surgical emphysema.

Chest radiograph (CXR). Chest radiographs are used as an adjunct in the respiratory assessment. In the intensive care setting portable anteroposterior (AP) radiographs are taken. AP films can produce magnification of certain structures such as the heart. Correct interpretation of the chest radiograph can be difficult because optimal positioning of the patient is limited and the film is rarely taken at full inspiration. Accurate day-to-day comparison between films can only be used as a rough guide as portable radiographs are taken at differing distances and exposures. It is important to note that in some conditions such as pneumonia, radiological appearances may lag behind the clinical situation (see Ch. 2).

Arterial blood gases (ABGs). ABG analysis and interpretation are used to ascertain the state of a patient's respiratory and metabolic function and acid–base balance (Table 11.3). It is measured by a blood sample from a line sited in any available artery or from an arterial stab (pp. 75, 137). To gain a full picture of a patient's condition, it is beneficial to observe trends or a series of arterial blood gas samples rather than one set of results in isolation.

Normal values:	
pH	7.35–7.45
$PaCO_2$	4.7–6.0 kPa (35–45 mmHg)
PaO_2	10.7–13.3 kPa (80–100 mmHg)
HCO_3^-	22–26 mmol/l
Base excess	−2 to +2

Sputum/haemoptysis. The presence of tenacious secretions which may potentially lead to plugging is an indication for urgent assessment and treatment. The analysis of a sputum specimen can be used as a guide for antibiotic therapy.

Evidence of fresh blood in the respiratory tract (e.g. pulmonary haemorrhage) may be a direct contraindication to some types of physiotherapy. However, bleeding may occur with some pneumonias and in this situation physiotherapy may be appropriate.

Drugs. See Table 11.4.

Considerations for physiotherapy

- A full assessment of the respiratory system will indicate a patient's ability to tolerate physiotherapeutic intervention. It is important to know the cause of raised airway pressures in a patient as some causes are an indication for treatment, whereas in others treatment would

Table 11.3 Arterial blood gases

Imbalance	Indicator	Clinical situation	Compensatory mechanisms
Respiratory acidosis	↓ pH ↑ $PaCO_2$	Sputum retention Atelectasis Hypoventilation V̇Q inequalities	↑ HCO_3^- ↑ H^+ ions excreted
Respiratory alkalosis	↑ pH ↓ $PaCO_2$	Hyperventilation, e.g. pain, anxiety Mechanical ventilation Neurogenic	↓ HCO_3^- via excretion
Metabolic acidosis	↓ pH ↓ HCO_3^-	Myocardial infarction Sepsis Gastrointestinal bleed Overaggressive diuretic therapy	↑RR→↓ $PaCO_2$
Metabolic alkalosis	↑ pH ↑ HCO_3^-	Profuse vomiting Profuse diarrhoea	↓ RR→↑ $PaCO_2$

Table 11.4 Drugs in the ICU: the respiratory system

Drug			Action	Considerations for physiotherapy
β₂-adrenoceptor agonists				
Aerolin/Ventolin	}	salbutamol	} Bronchodilatation	} Assess the degree of bronchospasm by auscultation and airway pressures. May be beneficial to use bronchodilatation therapy pre- and post-physiotherapy intervention
Airet				
Bricanyl	}	terbutaline		
Brethine				
Anticholinergics				
Atrovent		ipratropium bromide		
Smooth muscle relaxants				
Biophylline+	}	theophylline	} Bronchodilatation	High doses can lead to arrhythmias
Accurbron				
Amnivent	}	aminophylline		
Phyllocontin				
Corticosteroids				
Anflam+	}	hydrocortisone	Anti-inflammatory	Increased risk of infection. Used in patients with irritable airways
Acticort				
Respiratory stimulants				
Dopram		doxapram	Central respiratory stimulant	Can be used in patients with rising $PaCO_2$. Can produce fatigue such that physiotherapy is not tolerated. Patients may become agitated and uncooperative during treatment

be strongly contraindicated. For example, raised airway pressures due to gross sputum retention or plugging can be relieved with appropriate physiotherapeutic intervention. However, acute bronchospasm could be exacerbated by physiotherapy. A sudden increase in airway pressure may be indicative of a sputum plug, gross atelectasis, pneumothorax, airway occlusion or a kink in the ventilator tubing.

Renal system

The kidneys have a vital role in homeostasis. They are responsible for excretion of the waste products of metabolism, including drugs, production of hormones, control of the extracellular fluid composition which influences intracellular volume, osmolarity and acid–base status.

Important factors in assessment of fluid balance

- Measures of intravascular volume – HR/MAP/CVP/PCWP

- Urine output
- Assessment of peripheral perfusion and tissue turgor
- Daily weight
- Serum and urinary electrolytes
- Arterial blood gases
- Daily chest radiograph
- Net fluid balance

Acute renal failure (ARF) is associated with a rapidly rising urea and creatinine concentration, usually with a falling urine output. Hyperkalaemia, acidosis and fluid overload are common problems. ARF is often precipitated by hypotension, hypoxia and sepsis in the critically ill patient. Patients whose underlying renal function has already been compromised by diabetes, hypertension and vascular problems are particularly at risk. Renal replacement therapy is usually instigated when measures such as fluid resuscitation, cardiovascular support and the use of diuretics (Table 11.5) fail to improve function (Kirby & Davenport 1996). See Table 11.6.

Table 11.5   Drugs in the ICU: the renal system

Drug		Action	Considerations for physiotherapy
Inopin	dopamine	See Table 11.2	
Frusid	frusemide	Loop of Henlé diuretic	Over-diuresis can cause hypotension and dried secretions. Monitor BP. Hypokalaemia can be a problem. Care with arrhythmias
Lasix			
Osmitrol	mannitol	Osmotic diuretic	

Table 11.6   Types of renal support

Replacement therapy	Applications	Considerations for physiotherapy
Continuous haemofiltration/haemodiafiltration Requires vascular access to divert blood through an extracorporeal circuit, passing the blood continually via a filter (haemofiltration) which can be itself bathed in dialysis fluid (haemodiafiltration)	More effective correction of biochemical abnormalities May require anticoagulation Cardiovascular upset usually avoidable	Use of anticoagulation may cause bleeding, therefore care with suction Good for patients who are relatively unstable Care needs to be taken with large IV lines during changes of position
Intermittent haemodialysis Also requires access to the circulation but the treatment is carried out for only 3–5 hours every 24–48 hours	Large fluid shifts may cause severe cardiovascular disturbance Rapid correction of biochemistry	As above although physiotherapy can continue when patients are not on haemodialysis
Peritoneal dialysis Uses the peritoneum as a dialysis membrane Involves instillation of large volumes of fluid into the abdomen (1–2 litres)	Simple Little cardiovascular disturbance More suitable for chronic use Slow to alter biochemical abnormalities	Good positioning is essential to facilitate breathing as fluid leads to splinting of the abdomen. Ventilator weaning is more difficult because of diaphragmatic splinting

Haematological/immunological system

The haematological and immunological stability of a patient is often overlooked during the physiotherapy assessment. However, these systems may produce strong contraindications for physiotherapy. Patients with sepsis are often complicated by abnormal coagulation. Prolonged clotting times coupled with low platelet counts may lead to spontaneous bleeding from both mucous membranes and the respiratory tract. Physiotherapy may aggravate bleeding.

Patients who are immunocompromised through primary disease processes (e.g. malignancy), drug therapy (e.g. use of steroids) or as a complication of sepsis are particularly at risk from nosocomial infections (hospital acquired) and cross-infection.

Considerations for physiotherapy

- Appropriate care must be taken to minimize cross-infection with respect to local health and safety recommendations. Most ICUs advocate the use of a clean apron and gloves for each patient. Masks may be worn if indicated (e.g. open tuberculosis). While suctioning (p. 369), a sterile or second glove should be worn and goggles may be recommended.

Gastrointestinal system

A patient who has sustained a large gastrointestinal bleed may become hypovolaemic due to blood loss. A metabolic acidosis may be evident from arterial blood gas analysis. The patient may adopt an abnormal breathing pattern in an attempt to 'blow off' carbon dioxide and therefore reduce overall acidity.

Nutritional support is an important aspect of the care of the critically ill patient. Adequate nutrition is essential to prevent the loss of lean body tissue, provide material for repair and to facilitate recovery. Poor nutritional status, particularly deficits of magnesium and phosphates, may contribute to respiratory muscle weakness and delayed weaning from the ventilator (Rapper & Maynard 1992).

Routes of administration.

- Enteral – tube feeds directly into the gastrointestinal tract, e.g. nasogastric feeds or gastrostomy/jejunostomy
- Parenteral – intravenous feeding via central or peripheral line
- Oral – usually with supplementation.

Considerations for physiotherapy

- Ventilated patients with a reduced level of consciousness and a poor gag reflex may be prone to pulmonary aspiration if the endotracheal tube is uncuffed or the cuff deflated. Overfeeding may result in increased CO_2 production especially in patients with respiratory failure (Browne 1988a). In some circumstances it may be appropriate to stop feeding a patient during physiotherapy treatment. Feeding regimens can be altered to allow for interventions in liaison with the dietitian.

Musculoskeletal system

It is beneficial to know the patient's state of preadmission mobility. It is unlikely that a patient who does not have musculoskeletal complications will require regular passive movements but it is important to assess this regularly as the critically ill patient may develop musculoskeletal problems. Patients who have sustained musculoskeletal trauma, have pre-existing pathology or who have been ventilated for a prolonged time will require an in-depth assessment and appropriate treatment.

Positioning. The frequent turning of a patient will not only benefit the musculoskeletal system

and aid pressure relief, but will also enhance the respiratory system. A change of position may have several effects including assisting the drainage of secretions, improving ventilation/perfusion relationships and increasing functional residual capacity.

Beds. A wide variety of specialist beds are available to assist in the turning and positioning of the critically ill patient (Birtwistle 1994). It is essential for any patient, but imperative for the multi-trauma patient, to be assessed adequately for the appropriate specialist bed.

Considerations for physiotherapy

- The unstable patient may not tolerate a change in position.

MECHANICAL VENTILATION: IMPLICATIONS FOR PHYSIOTHERAPY

Mechanical ventilation is used in patients undergoing a general anaesthetic and in most patients requiring intensive care. Modern ventilators provide a wealth of different modalities to cater for patients from the most critically ill through the weaning process to extubation. At every different stage, a full assessment must be undertaken to identify the presence of any physiotherapy problems. Physiotherapy may need to be modified depending on a patient's ventilatory requirements and during the weaning process.

Intubation

The decision to intubate and ventilate a patient is never taken lightly, as this procedure in itself has an associated level of morbidity and mortality. Endotracheal tubes come in a variety of types and sizes. Most of those routinely used for adults have a high-volume, low-pressure cuff to limit tracheal damage. Paediatric tubes are often uncuffed and tracheostomy tubes vary (Table 11.7).

Considerations for physiotherapy

- When assessing the mechanically ventilated patient, it is important to note the ventilation

Table 11.7 Intubation

Site of tube	Indications and advantages	Type of tube
Oral	Most commonly used in adults Used in emergency situations	Endotracheal tube – cuffed (adults) – uncuffed (paediatrics)
Nasal	Used when oral intubation impossible or impractical, e.g. trauma Commonly used in paediatrics	
Tracheostomy – temporary – permanent	Used for long-term ventilation Improves comfort, reduces need for sedation, facilitates normal eating and drinking Maintains and protects airway where a neurological or anatomical abnormality is present	Portex® – cuffed or uncuffed – single lumen – speaking valve Shiley® – cuffed or uncuffed – fenestration for speech – long-term use – inner cannulae Silver – uncuffed – permanent use – single lumen – phonation tube

requirements and to understand their implication. The level of stability of both the cardiovascular and respiratory systems must be established. A patient with an unstable respiratory system requiring high levels of oxygen (FiO_2 >0.6) and/or high levels of PEEP (>10 cmH_2O) should have an absolute indication for treatment before physiotherapy is undertaken.

● If manual hyperinflations are indicated in a patient requiring a high level of PEEP, a PEEP valve should be used (p. 368).

● The inspiratory: expiratory (I:E) ratio can be altered in mechanical ventilation to meet an individual patient's needs. A prolonged expiratory time or an expiratory pause can be used in patients with chronic airflow limitation. A prolonged inspiratory time (inverse ratio ventilation) improves oxygenation in ARDS. An altered I:E ratio may be vital to maintain good oxygenation. In this situation, manual hyperinflation may not be tolerated.

● When positioning the mechanically ventilated patient it must be remembered that the physiological factors affecting ventilation/perfusion matching are altered. The application of positive pressure leads to non-dependent areas of lung being preferentially ventilated. Therefore, as perfusion is influenced by gravity some degree of inequality is always present.

For example, in right side lying, the right lung is dependent and therefore preferentially perfused, whereas the left lung is non-dependent and thus preferentially ventilated. As this mismatching occurs in all positions, frequent changes of position are essential. Use of the prone position has been shown to be of benefit in some patients with severe lung disease (Pappert et al 1994).

● When assessing a patient who requires an unconventional form of ventilation, e.g. high-frequency ventilation and/or nitric oxide (p. 305) and in whom physiotherapy is indicated, it is advantageous to discuss the plan of treatment with the medical staff.

Weaning

Weaning is the process of reducing or removing ventilatory support. As soon as the patient's condition stabilizes, weaning can start.

Influences on the weaning process

Neurological system. A reduced level of consciousness is not a direct contraindication to weaning as airway patency and protection can be maintained with an endotracheal or tracheostomy tube. The patient must be able to sustain adequate spontaneous ventilation. Sedative drugs need to be reduced during the weaning process.

Pathology such as Guillain–Barré syndrome and myasthenia gravis may require weaning to take place during the daytime as fatigue and poor diaphragmatic function may lead to nocturnal hypoventilation.

Cardiovascular system. A stable cardiovascular system is necessary for successful weaning. Reduced cardiac output due to hypovolaemia or arrhythmias may potentially result in respiratory muscle oxygen deprivation.

Respiratory system. The patient must be able to initiate an adequate respiratory drive during each stage of the weaning process. Any primary lung pathology should have resolved significantly to allow for improved respiratory function.

It is necessary that adequate oxygenation can be sustained with reducing levels of oxygen and PEEP. In the final stages of weaning, patients must be able to generate adequate minute volumes to maintain their $PaCO_2$ within the normal range.

Acid–base balance. It should be noted that the weaning process can be complicated in patients with an abnormal acid–base balance, e.g. severe metabolic acidosis will induce a raised respiratory rate, whereas metabolic alkalosis may lead to hypoventilation.

Renal system. Electrolyte balance is imperative to prevent excessive respiratory muscle fatigue. Acute renal failure with fluid overload will make weaning more difficult.

Nutrition. Adequate nutritional support is essential during weaning to help prevent muscle weakness and fatigue.

Infection. Overwhelming sepsis can cause impaired gas exchange with an increased O_2 consumption and CO_2 production which may delay weaning (Browne 1988a).

Methods of weaning

In the uncomplicated postoperative situation the whole process of weaning may only take a short period. As the patient regains consciousness and breathes spontaneously, rapid extubation can take place. In the long-term ventilated patient, the weaning process is started by reducing seda-

tion and positioning for optimal diaphragmatic excursion. Modern ventilators have an extensive range of weaning modalities. The patient is encouraged to self-ventilate on an assisted mode, e.g. synchronized intermittent mandatory ventilation (SIMV), while still receiving additional support for each spontaneous breath, e.g. inspiratory pressure support (IPS) (p. 303).

Gradually the IPS can be reduced together with the number of mandatory breaths. Once the patient can maintain adequate oxygenation and normal $PaCO_2$ levels, progression to either CPAP or a T-piece is achieved. At each stage ABG analysis will indicate whether adequate ventilation is being maintained. Weaning may be very protracted in some patients and the use of individualized programmes will smooth progress and maintain patients' morale (Browne 1988b).

In chronic respiratory patients a tracheostomy tube may aid the weaning process by reducing the anatomical dead space.

The patient who is difficult to wean because of pre-existing chronic lung pathology may benefit from the use of non-invasive positive pressure ventilation (Chapter 10).

Considerations for physiotherapy

- In the weaning phase a patient on assisted ventilation may have a high spontaneous respiratory rate. Manual hyperinflation may cause the patient distress and may be ineffective if only small tidal volumes are achieved. If a primary respiratory problem is causing the high respiratory rate, physiotherapy is indicated. It is important to start manual hyperinflation, matching the patient's own respiratory rate and depth. By slowly increasing the tidal volume, the $PaCO_2$ levels can be lowered, temporarily inhibiting the patient's respiratory drive and allowing effective manual hyperinflations.

- When a patient has been weaned on to CPAP, it is important that adequate physiotherapy input continues. Good positioning is essential to maximize further weaning potential. If sputum is present airway clearance techniques should be utilized.

Extubation

Although successful weaning culminates in extubation, the two processes must be assessed independently. Extubation should not be considered until the patient can protect his own airway and can cough and swallow (Browne 1988b).

Minitracheostomy tube

The sole purpose of the minitracheostomy is access for the removal of excess bronchial secretions. It can also be used in the decannulation process of a tracheostomy tube. It is important to remember that a minitracheostomy offers no airway protection (p. 214).

MUSCULOSKELETAL PROBLEMS

The critically ill patient in the ICU will require a musculoskeletal assessment. A short-term ventilated patient with no pre-existing musculoskeletal pathology should require minimal intervention. This should be reviewed regularly. However, any patient will benefit from sitting out of bed during the weaning process (Ciesla 1996) (see p. 147).

A patient requiring long-term ventilation or who presents with preexisting musculoskeletal or neurological pathologies will require an indepth assessment and identification of specific problems. Special attention should be given to the following areas: head and neck, shoulder girdle (Fig. 11.2a), hip extension and adduction, knee extension and Achilles tendon length (Fig. 11.2b). Muscle length and joint range of movement can be maintained by good positioning incorporating joint alignment, passive range of movements and muscle stretches. Liaison with the nursing staff will allow coordination of physiotherapy and nursing intervention, especially turning, to maximize patient care. A regular change of position will not only relieve pressure, but provide proprioceptive input. Once medical stability has been achieved and it is appropriate, the patient should be sat out of bed (Fig. 11.3a). It may be necessary to use a hoist or an assisted transfer. The progression of sitting in a chair, standing and ultimately walking (Fig. 11.3b) is

not only of great physiological benefit but also a psychological boost (Sciaky 1994).

Considerations for physiotherapy

- *Multiple trauma.* The injuries sustained during multiple trauma require a detailed assessment as each problem can be unique in presentation. It is important to discuss the management with the relevant medical team. Fixation of unstable joints or fractures may be difficult in the early stages until cardiovascular stability has been established. Any spinal injury, particularly of the cervical spine, must be considered unstable until it has been reviewed by a specialist. If external fixators have been applied, it is necessary to maintain range of movement and muscle length to the adjacent areas. The opinion of the relevant physiotherapy specialist should be sought (e.g. orthopaedic or plastics specialist).

- *Acute neurology.* While the patient is neurologically unstable, musculoskeletal intervention is not indicated. However, once neurological stability is achieved, early rehabilitation is essential for successful outcomes. It is important to assess the range of joint movement, two-joint muscle lengths, volitional and non-volitional motor activity and the presence of any prevalent patterns. Treatment is aimed at maintenance of passive range of joint movement, two-joint muscle stretches, maintaining anatomical alignment and inhibiting reflex activity by positioning. Plaster casting may be indicated to prevent significant shortening of tendons and muscle length and to assist in reduction of tone (Connine et al 1990). A change of position will aid proprioceptive input.

  Rehabilitation is progressed to sitting and standing. This will assist in gaining trunk control and pelvic alignment. This can be started while the patient is still requiring ventilatory support. It is advisable to turn a ventricular drain off before moving the patient. Close liaison with the nursing staff and the multidisciplinary team is essential to ensure effective ongoing rehabilitation. Early referral to the specialist physiotherapist and rehabilitation team will maximize potential recovery.

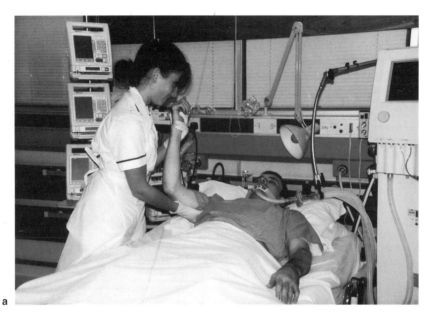

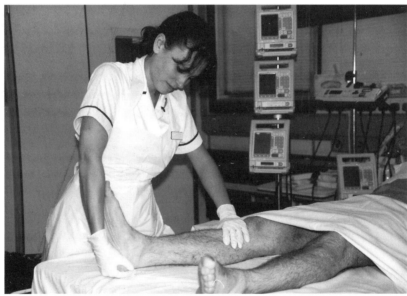

Figure 11.2 **a** Passive movements to upper limb. **b** Passive stretch to Achilles tendon.

PATIENT GROUPS WITH SPECIFIC NEEDS

The critically ill patient requiring intensive care may develop complications secondary to the primary diagnosis. The nature of these secondary complications may alter or even contraindicate physiotherapeutic intervention. An understanding of the commonly encountered complications is essential for complete assessment of these potentially unstable patients.

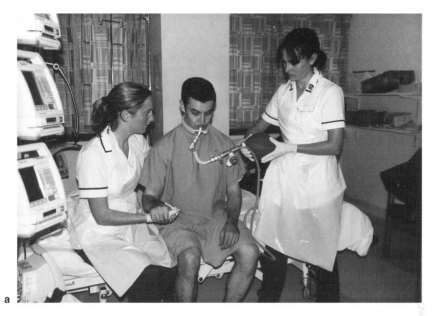

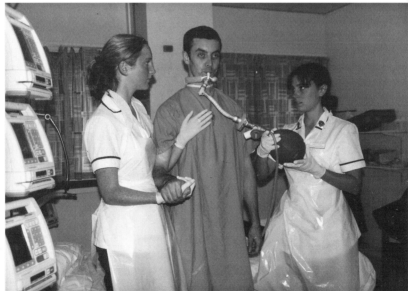

Figure 11.3 **a** Assisted ventilation while sitting. **b** Assisted ventilation while walking.

Systemic inflammatory response syndrome (SIRS) and sepsis

SIRS

Various insults to the body may lead to an exaggerated, generalized inflammatory response called systemic inflammatory response syndrome (SIRS). This inflammatory response involves highly complex interactions between several cell groups (macrophages, neutrophils, etc.), inflammatory mediators (TNF, IL-1) and internal regulatory pathways (fibrinolytic, clotting, complement) (Emery & Salmon 1991).

In its worst form there is severe disruption of vascular homeostasis with impairment of the endothelial barriers in many organs. This causes increased capillary permeability, often resulting in organ failure. There may be an associated loss of normal vascular tone causing hypotension in the systemic circulation and intrapulmonary shunting in the pulmonary circulation. Breakdown of the normal clotting/fibrinolytic pathways may result in prolonged clotting, intravascular thrombosis and thrombocytopenia.

If this inflammatory response is secondary to an infective cause, it is termed 'sepsis'. Causative organisms implicated in sepsis include bacteria, fungi, rickettsiae and other parasites. Sepsis is the major cause of mortality in the ICU.

SIRS can be defined clinically as the presence of two or more of the following criteria:

Temperature	>38° or < 36°C
Tachycardia	>90 bpm
Tachypnoea	>20/min or $PaCO_2$ <4.3 kPa (32.3 mmHg)
WBC	>12 × 10^9/litre
	or <4 × 10^9/litre
	or <10% immature neutrophils

Sepsis

Sepsis can be classified into three groups.

- *Sepsis.* The presence of SIRS, with a documented cultured infection.
- *Severe sepsis.* Sepsis with organ dysfunction, hypotension and hypoperfusion (e.g. hypoxaemia, lactic acidosis, oliguria).
- *Septic shock.* Severe sepsis with hypotension despite fluid resuscitation. The development of secondary abnormalities due to hypotension (e.g. cardiovascular instability, acute renal failure) (Kulkarni & Webster 1996).

Generalized management of SIRS and sepsis

If sepsis is suspected, every attempt should be made to identify the causative organisms. Cultures are taken from blood, urine, line sites and open wounds, etc. Imaging may include a chest radiograph and an ultrasound of the abdomen and pelvis. Possible sources of infection such as lines and abscesses must be eliminated. If a causative organism can be identified, appropriate antimicrobials are started. The mainstay of treatment in severe SIRS or sepsis is supportive.

Cardiovascular system. Fluid resuscitation, inotropes and vasopressors are used to maintain mean arterial blood pressure and adequate tissue perfusion.

Respiratory system. Ventilatory support is used to ensure adequate gaseous exchange.

Renal system. Adequate fluid resuscitation is paramount. The place of diuretics and dopamine is controversial. Haemofiltration or haemodialysis may become necessary as the septic process advances.

Haematological system. Blood, blood products and clotting factors can be given to assist the correction of abnormalities.

Gastrointestinal system. Adequate nutrition is essential in the septic patient. Enteral feeding is the preferred route, as there is evidence that it maintains gut mucosal integrity and decreases bacterial translocation which might otherwise perpetuate the ongoing inflammatory insult. In addition, parenteral nutrition is associated with an increase in line complications/infections. The risk of stress ulceration can be minimized by the use of histamine receptor antagonists (Rapper & Maynard 1992).

Musculoskeletal system. Pressure area care is essential to prevent further foci of infection. The use of a specialist mattress and/or bed may be advantageous.

Considerations for physiotherapy

- The septic patient will require extensive monitoring of simple parameters such as temperature, blood pressure, urine output and arterial blood gases, as well as haemodynamic factors such as pulmonary artery pressure, pulmonary artery wedge pressure and central venous pressure. Measurements of cardiac output and the calculation of pulmonary vascular resistance can be used to guide medical management. Physiotherapeutic intervention should only be undertaken in a situation where there is a strong indication and the patient is cardiovascularly stable (see p. 349). If manual hyperinflation is indicated, additional inotropic support and increased fluids may be required. Close monitoring of all parameters throughout treatment is essential.

Acute respiratory distress syndrome (ARDS)

ARDS represents the severe end of the spectrum of acute lung injury. This syndrome results from the disruption of the alveolar–capillary membrane, secondary to either local or distant injury. It is characterized by three features:

- hypoxaemia – this may vary in level of severity
- diffuse radiographical infiltrates
- reduced respiratory system compliance.

The acute phase is characterized by increased capillary permeability. This leads to the development of non-cardiogenic oedema. In those patients that survive there is subsequent repair, involving regeneration of the alveolar epithelium, producing varying degrees of lung fibrosis. The aetiology of ARDS is diverse ranging from direct lung trauma (e.g. aspiration, inhalation and near drowning) to systemic disorders (e.g. poisoning, obstetric complications, sepsis, major haemorrhage, etc.) (Murray 1996).

The management of patients with ARDS is essentially supportive. Where possible the identification and treatment of the underlying cause are paramount. Haemodynamic monitoring and support are necessary to maintain an adequate blood pressure and cardiac output, while monitoring and preventing fluid overload in the lungs.

Ventilatory strategies are aimed at improving alveolar recruitment, while avoiding further injury to the lungs. Present 'protective' ventilatory strategies aim to limit inspiratory pressure, accepting a lower tidal volume and often a concomitant rise in PCO_2 – *permissive hypercapnia* (Dakin & Evans 2001). The level of PEEP is often higher than conventionally used in an attempt to limit end-expiratory derecruitment of alveoli. In addition the normal ratio of inspiration to expiration may be prolonged – *inverse ratio ventilation.* Such ventilatory strategies are non-physiological and require the use of adequate levels of sedation and often muscle relaxants. It should be noted that a high level of PEEP may compromise cardiac output.

Alternative techniques include inhaled nitric oxide, high-frequency jet ventilation, extracorporeal gas exchange systems and exogenous surfactant.

Changes of position from supine to prone and/or prone to supine may improve ventilation/perfusion matching as dependent oedema is redistributed (Pappert et al 1994). Care must be taken with the position of the arms, head and neck. The use of continuous rotation on a specialist bed (kinetic therapy) may also be beneficial. As yet none of the above have been proven to have a positive effect on outcome (Mulnier & Evans 1995).

Considerations for physiotherapy

- In the early stages of ARDS when the main manifestation is interstitial oedema, physiotherapy has very little to offer. As the syndrome progresses and fibrosis is the most prominent feature, physiotherapy may assist in preventing areas of atelectasis and sputum plugging. Patients with ARDS frequently develop pneumothoraces due to decreased compliance. It should be noted that if several chest drains are in position, manual hyperinflation is of no benefit, as air escapes through the chest drains. In the later stages, if physiotherapy is indicated in a PEEP-dependent patient, a PEEP valve is recommended (p. 369). When suction is required, a closed-circuit suction system should be used (p. 371).

Disseminated intravascular coagulation (DIC)

DIC is a condition in which there is increased activation of both the normal procoagulant and anticoagulant pathways. It may be triggered by a variety of disorders including infection, trauma, malignancy and vasculitis. The increased activity leads to abnormal consumption of platelets, clotting factors and associated regulating factors. Initially the release of stored platelets and factors may maintain the balance of these two pathways. However, in severe conditions this compensation is lost and the situation is worsened as fibrinolysis produces fibrin degradation products which act as anticoagulants (Kesteven & Saunders 1993).

Also abnormal fibrin formation in the vasculature causes occlusion and is closely related to development of multiorgan failure. Treatment is aimed at eliminating the trigger, arresting intravascular clotting and replacement of clotting factors (Hambley 1995).

Considerations for physiotherapy

- DIC can be mild, moderate or severe. As it is a marker of severe illness, the overall stability of the patient must be assessed. In the mild situation where bleeding is minimal, physiotherapy can continue. In the severe state, blood loss may be considerable and the patient may become unstable. Any intervention which may exacerbate bleeding, e.g. suction, should be avoided unless it is essential.

Inhalation burns

15–25% of patients who suffer significant burns will present with respiratory complications. Respiratory failure and infection account for the majority of mortalities associated with burns (Bordow & Landers 1985). Smoke inhalation is suggested by soot around the nostrils and mouth. Initially hypoxia is caused by the high affinity of carbon monoxide for haemoglobin (210–250 times greater than oxygen). The oxygen dissociation curve shifts to the left (Murray 1976), greatly reducing the oxygen-carrying capacity of haemoglobin and thus reducing oxygen delivery to the tissues. Toxic elements in smoke can cause oedema of the mucosa, bronchospasm, destruction of cilia and loss of surfactant.

Thermal injury can be isolated to the pharynx and upper airway or if steam is inhaled there may be significant alveolar damage. Toxic elements (e.g. noxious gas) and thermal injury contribute to 'ongoing' hypoxia.

Considerations for physiotherapy

- Patients with either significant facial burns or inhalation injury will require intubation and ventilation. Following inhalation burns, patients can present with thick, tenacious, soot-stained secretions. These will require adequate humidification. Nebulized bronchodilators are essential in the presence of bronchospasm.
- Suction should be carried out with care to prevent further trauma to damaged airways. Careful consideration must be given to soft tissue damage and positioning of the patient (Keilty 1993).

Trauma

Injury in the trauma patient can result from many different mechanisms, ranging from a high-impact insult following a road traffic accident to assault or merely a fall. The patient may sustain multiple injuries which are often complex and interrelated. The scale of these injuries may predispose this group of patients to developing secondary associated problems such as ARDS or DIC (Antonelli et al 1994).

Head injury

Trauma to the head may involve a haemorrhage or contusion which may be focal or diffuse. Diagnosis is assisted by CT scanning. Primary damage sustained at the time of insult cannot be reversed. However, subsequent secondary damage (e.g. hypoxia and hypotension) can be minimized. Surgical intervention may be indicated as first-line management (e.g. evacuation of a clot or insertion of a ventricular drain or shunt). Patients who have undergone extensive surgery and remain critical or unstable will require continued care in the ICU. Patients not suitable for surgical intervention are conservatively managed in the ICU (e.g. gross cerebral oedema). Close monitoring is essential as neurological vital signs can change very suddenly. ICP and CPP valves are used to guide medical management (p. 349).

These patients are sedated and often paralysed in order to prevent fluctuating ICPs rising to critical levels (see Table 11.1). Intubation and ventilation are essential not only for airway protection but to enable manipulation of $PaCO_2$ levels. Carbon dioxide can have vasodilatory effects on blood vessels. By maintaining low carbon dioxide levels with hyperventilation, cerebral vasodilatation may be reduced, thus lowering cerebral blood flow and so reducing ICP. This approach is only used for the first 48 hours as after this time it is less effective (Eisenhart 1994).

These patients are nursed in 15–30° head elevation with their head in midline (i.e. nose in line with sternum). This will ensure maximal venous drainage from the cerebral circulation.

Inotropic support may be necessary to maintain adequate MAP and therefore CPP. Diuretic therapy such as mannitol is used to assist in the reduction of cerebral oedema. The use of steroids in head-injured patients remains controversial.

In extreme circumstances, when the brainstem is irreversibly damaged, the patient cannot sustain spontaneous ventilation. This is defined as brainstem death. This is assessed by specific tests. Some patients may be suitable for organ donation (Thomas 1991).

Considerations for physiotherapy

- Critically ill patients should always be closely assessed and monitored during any intervention, but this is paramount in the neurologically impaired patient as vital signs can fluctuate rapidly (e.g. ICP, CPP, MAP).
- A thorough assessment will demonstrate an indication for physiotherapy treatment of the acute neurological patient. It is important to distinguish between a neurological cause of deterioration and an underlying respiratory problem.
- Before physiotherapy the patient's level of consciousness and sedation should be reviewed and a bolus of sedation may be given as appropriate to prevent excessive rises in ICP. If indicated, the patient's position can be altered for treatment purposes. During movement the head must be maintained in the midline position at all times. Direct pressure should not be applied to the bolt, drain or shunt site.

- Ventricular drains should either be closed during excessive movement and physiotherapy and opened immediately after treatment, or raised. In patients where the drain must remain open (e.g. unclipped aneurysms or hydrocephalus), the drain may be raised 10–20 cm above the head when making a patient cough. This ensures that the drain still acts as a pressure-relieving device without allowing overdrainage. After a craniotomy, if the bone flap is not replaced, the patient can be repositioned provided that pillows are arranged to prevent direct pressure on the unprotected brain.
- The use of sedation and paralysing agents may result in a poor cough reflex and lead to the retention of secretions or atelectasis. Both these can lead to hypoxia and hypercapnia which in turn will cause cerebral vasodilatation and raised ICP (Garradd & Bullock 1986). Physiotherapy intervention may be essential. If manual hyperinflation is indicated, small rapid breaths should be interspersed between hyperinflations to maintain the low $PaCO_2$. It is important to note that manual hyperinflation may reduce cardiac output and therefore compromise CPP. As the cerebral and thoracic venous systems are in open communication, the increased intrathoracic pressure during manual hyperinflation may increase ICP. The increased intrathoracic pressure may also compromise cerebral venous drainage (Paratz & Burns 1993).
- Suction should only be used when absolutely indicated as it has been well documented to dramatically increase ICP. This is thought to be due to direct tracheal stimulation and increased intrathoracic pressure causing reduced venous return during a cough (Rudy et al 1991). It may be necessary to preoxygenate the unstable patient before suction. Excessive stimulation from manual techniques may increase ICP.
- In the early stages patients should be reassessed regularly but treatment should be restricted and of limited duration. It is important to remember that during the initial stages of reducing sedation, the patient may become agitated and self-extubation is a potential hazard. Similarly, in the first 48–72 hours, good positioning is adequate in the absence of tonal change. As soon as the patient is medically stable, intensive

rehabilitation should start. Despite ventilatory support the patient can sit or stand as indicated.

- Patients suitable for organ donation will require ongoing physiotherapy assessment and treatment to maintain optimum respiratory function.

Flail chest injury and pulmonary contusion

See Chapter 12, p. 405.

Pulmonary emboli. Pulmonary embolism is one of the potential complications of the trauma patient. It is a complication of deep vein thrombosis in which fragments of thrombus enter the pulmonary circulation and cause obstruction.

Considerations for physiotherapy

- Once anticoagulation therapy has been started and the risk of thrombus formation minimized, physiotherapy can continue as indicated. Anticoagulation therapy must be strictly monitored as excess use may lead to bleeding problems, therefore care must be taken with suction.

Fat emboli. Fat embolism is a complication of the multitrauma patient. The release of fat may be associated with fractures particularly of the pelvis or long bones or entry of fat globules into the venous circulation with massive trauma or extensive burns. These emboli may obstruct the pulmonary and/or cerebral circulation.

Considerations for physiotherapy

- Treatment is supportive and aimed at maximizing oxygen delivery to peripheral tissues. In the acute phase musculoskeletal intervention is contraindicated until any long bone fractures are stabilized. Chest physiotherapy can be complicated by the development of DIC.

Neurological conditions requiring intensive care

Myasthenia gravis

Myasthenia gravis is a disease which is due to a transmission defect at the neuromuscular junction (Scadding 1990). It is characterized by fatiguable weakness occurring in striated muscle. This may be local or generalized.

Considerations for physiotherapy

- Severe progression of the disease will necessitate ventilation. Treatment involves the administration of anticholinesterase drugs which help to maximize muscle function. These drugs frequently lead to excess secretions. Where possible, physiotherapy should be timed to occur after administration of the drug. Nocturnal ventilation may be required even after daytime weaning has been successful. A progressive rehabilitation programme should be instigated as soon as possible.

Guillain–Barré syndrome

Guillain–Barré syndrome is an acute demyelinating polyradiculoneuropathy affecting predominantly motor neurons (Hughes & Rees 1994, Tharakan et al 1989). Although prognosis is excellent for the majority of patients, 10–20% have significant residual disabilities as a result of muscle weakness, contracture, sensory dysfunction and psychological factors (Ferner et al 1987, Lennon et al 1993, van der Meche & Schmitz 1992). The course of the disease is divided into three stages (Karni et al 1984, Watson & Wilson 1989): initial acute stage, plateau stage and recovery stage. In the acute stage respiration may be compromised as a result of respiratory muscle weakness and bulbar palsy and mechanical ventilation may be indicated (Ferner et al 1987, Scadding 1990, Watson & Wilson 1989). Plasma exchange and intravenous immunoglobulin therapy are the main treatments available, both resulting in decreased morbidity and improved final outcome (Guillain–Barré Syndrome Study Group 1985, Hughes & Rees 1994, Rees 1993).

Considerations for physiotherapy

- From the onset of paralysis, physiotherapy intervention must be aimed at prevention of atelectasis and chest infection and maintenance of ventilation; in addition to maintenance of joint range and soft tissue length (Rees 1993). Treatments for the musculoskeletal system include passive/active-assisted/ strengthening exercises, stretches, positioning, splinting, standing using a tilt table or standing frame and provision of suitable seating (Edwards 1996, Ferner et al 1987, Fowler & Falkner 1992). Pain can be quite severe in all stages of the disease. Analgesia such as opiates, non-steroidal anti-inflammatories or Entonox may be administered prior to physiotherapy intervention to provide adequate pain control (Clark 1985, Ferner et al 1987, Fowler & Falkner 1992).

- As muscle function improves, an active weaning programme should be devised. The patient is encouraged to breathe spontaneously for increasing periods during the day, but is often given ventilatory support at night to ensure adequate rest (Ferner et al 1987). Once the patient is off ventilatory support, treatment is usually continued in a multidisciplinary rehabilitation unit.

Tetanus

Tetanus is a disease caused by a neuromuscular toxin produced by spores causing general muscle rigidity and convulsions. The respiratory muscles can be affected and paralysis and mechanical ventilation are necessary (Oh 1990).

Considerations for physiotherapy

- Adequate sedation and muscle relaxants must be given to ensure effective physiotherapy. Rehabilitation should start once the condition is stabilized.

Poliomyelitis

This virus attacks the grey matter of the spinal cord, brainstem and cortex. In particular, damage is sustained by anterior horn cells, especially those of the lumbar segments (Macleod et al 1987). The disease varies from influenza-like symptoms to severe paralysis, including the respiratory muscles. Intubation and ventilation may be necessary using intermittent positive pressure ventilation, although the use of negative pressure ventilation (iron lung) may still be seen (Higgens 1966) or non-invasive ventilation can be used.

Considerations for physiotherapy

- Irrespective of the method of ventilation, chest physiotherapy will be indicated in the presence of excess bronchial secretions and/or lung collapse. Early instigation of a rehabilitation programme is essential.

PHYSIOTHERAPY TECHNIQUES

Once a thorough assessment has been completed, the findings must be analysed to identify relevant physiotherapeutic problems. For each problem a suitable treatment plan must be formulated taking into consideration any potential influencing factors. Again, it should be emphasized that because of the complex nature of the ICU patient, there is no place for routine chest physiotherapy. It must be remembered that there will be situations when an indication for treatment exists but the patient's overall instability would result in the treatment having a negative effect. ICU patients may become 'end stage' and not for resuscitation, but this does not preclude them from a daily assessment and treatment as indicated (Pearson & Parr 1993).

Despite the fact that the ICU patient is often sedated and paralysed, communication is of paramount importance. As with a conscious patient, an introduction must be made together with an explanation of the planned treatment. This not only will ensure that the patient is informed of procedures but will provide an explanation and involve the relatives with the physiotherapy.

Gravity-assisted positioning

These positions use gravity to assist in the drainage of a specific bronchopulmonary segment and/or improve ventilation and perfusion (p. 200). When positioning the patient, care must be taken with tubes, drains and lines. The patient's cardiovascular stability must be assessed before any change of position. Modified positioning may be indicated.

Ventilation perfusion ratios $(\dot{V}/\dot{Q})$ during mechanical ventilation are not the same as those during spontaneous breathing (p. 147). After physiotherapy the patient can be positioned to optimize $\dot{V}/\dot{Q}$ matching. Mechanically ventilated patient, where there will always be a $\dot{V}/\dot{Q}$ mismatch, should be assessed individually to ascertain the most beneficial position (Pearson & Parr 1993).

Manual hyperinflation

'Bagging' can be used as a technique to hand ventilate a patient or during physiotherapy. When hand ventilating, normal tidal volumes are generally delivered whereas to facilitate physiotherapy, larger breaths or hyperinflations are necessary. Manual hyperinflation can be given using either a Water's bag circuit or an Ambu-bag. A greater range of volume is available with a Water's bag. For an adult a 2 or 3 litre Water's bag, connected to a flow of 10–15 litres of oxygen, is commonly used (Fig. 11.4). By altering the expiratory valve, volume and therefore inspiratory pressure can be manipulated. The use of a manometer acts as a guide to inflation pressures which are recommended to be less than 40 cmH$_2$O (Pearson 1996). If manual hyperinflation is indicated in a PEEP-dependent patient, a PEEP valve must be used to maintain positive end-expiratory pressure during treatment (Jones et al 1992).

Indications (Jones et al 1992, Hodgson et al 1996)

- To aid removal of secretions
- To aid reinflation of atelectatic segments
- To assess lung compliance
- To improve lung compliance

Therapeutic effects of manual hyperinflation

The most common technique used is a slow inspiration and inspiratory hold followed by quick expiratory release (Clement & Hübsch 1968). A prolonged inspiratory hold is contraindicated in a patient who is already hyperinflated (e.g. emphysema).

Slow deep inspiration

- Recruits collateral ventilation thus promoting mobilization of secretions
- Enhances interdependence to aid re-expansion of atelectatic segments
- Improves gaseous exchange
- Assesses and potentially improves compliance

Inspiratory hold (at full inspiration)

- Further utilizes collateral ventilation and interdependence as at higher volume; therefore maximizes pressure distribution.

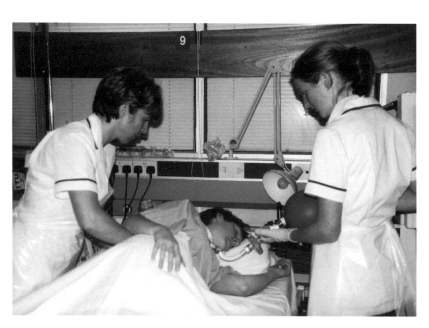

Figure 11.4 Manual hyperinflation with chest shaking.

Fast expiratory release

- Mimics a forced expiration (huff or cough)
- Stimulates a cough

Hand-held PEEP

- By grasping and holding the end of a semi-filled bag throughout inspiration and expiration it is possible to maintain a low level of PEEP.

Hazards of manual hyperinflation

Reduction in blood pressure. During manual hyperinflation the normal mechanism which 'sucks' the remaining blood from the inferior vena cava to the right atrium during negative pressure inspiration is lost. In addition, the positive pressure generated during manual hyperinflation increases intrathoracic pressure. Both mechanisms compromise venous return. The resultant effect could be a reduction in stroke volume and therefore a drop in blood pressure. This risk is potentially increased when using a PEEP valve or during prolonged inspiratory holds. It should be noted that if a bolus of sedation is given before treatment, this may lower the blood pressure through vasodilatation (Singer et al 1994).

Considerations for physiotherapy

- If the blood pressure drops during treatment, smaller tidal breaths should be given. If blood pressure remains compromised, the patient should be put back on to the ventilator, positioned appropriately and a medical review requested.
- The effects physiotherapy may have on respiratory parameters (Patman et all 2000).

Reduced saturations. Oxygen saturations can be compromised by sputum plugging, collapse, pneumothorax, bronchospasm and $\dot{V}/\dot{Q}$ mismatching.

Considerations for physiotherapy

- Reassessment will highlight the cause. Intermediate measures such as increasing the FiO_2 can be used.

Raised intracranial pressure. The presence of increased levels of $PaCO_2$ in cerebral blood vessels may lead to vasodilatation. The resultant increased cerebral blood flow may increase ICP (Eisenhart 1994).

Considerations for physiotherapy

- To prevent fluctuations in ICP during manual hyperinflation, small fast breaths should be interspersed between hyperinflations.

Reduced respiratory drive. $PaCO_2$ levels may be reduced during effective treatment. This may reduce the patient's respiratory drive.

Considerations for physiotherapy

- After finishing manual hyperinflation, the patient's spontaneous respiratory effort should be monitored.

Contraindications to manual hyperinflation

- Undrained pneumothorax (presence of patent intercostal drain – treat as normal)
- Potential bronchospasm
- Severe bronchospasm
- Gross cardiovascular instability inducing arrhythmias and hypovolaemia
- Unexplained haemoptysis
- An absolute indication for treatment should be present before manual hyperinflation is used on patients requiring PEEP levels greater than 15 cmH$_2$O plus maximal ventilatory support or patients with high peak and mean inspiratory pressures.

Suctioning the intubated patient

Each day, the normal person generates an average of 100 ml of bronchial secretions. If the normal mechanisms such as ciliary action are compromised, alveolar ventilation may be impaired. Suction may be indicated to remove these secretions. The suction catheter used must be less than half the diameter of the endotracheal tube. Trauma can be further minimized by the use of a catheter with an atraumatic end and a Y-connector. The vacuum pressure should be as low as possible (e.g. 8–20 kPa, 60–150 mmHg). Suction should never be routine, only when there is an indication. A full explanation of the procedure reduces patient anxiety (Copnell & Fergusson 1995).

Indications

- Inability to cough effectively
- Sputum plugging
- To assess tube patency

Technique

The technique (Fig. 11.5) should either be sterile or clean, depending on the hospital's infection control policy. Before suctioning, an explanation of the procedure is given to the patient and equipment is made ready. Pre- and post-oxygenation can be used as required. In the majority of patients, the depth of insertion is that sufficient to elicit a cough reflex. In the paralysed patient, insertion must be done with great care. Once the endpoint is reached (e.g. mucosa) the catheter must be withdrawn 1 cm before suction is applied to prevent mucosal invagination and trauma. The duration in adults should be limited to 10–15 seconds. Suction should be applied constantly while removing the catheter. Intermittent

suction should only be used when removing a sticky plug. Saline can be used as an aid in suctioning. The use of a sputum trap to obtain a specimen for microbiological assessment will assist with the correct antibiotic therapy (Ciesla 1996).

Hazards of suctioning

Mucosal trauma. Mucosal trauma is reduced by using an atraumatic catheter, good suctioning technique and the correct pressures.

Cardiac arrhythmias. Direct tracheal stimulation causing a vasovagal reflex can cause arrhythmias (Young 1984). Pre- and post-oxygenation can minimize this effect. If suction is necessary in patients who demonstrate arrhythmias on suctioning, it is advisable to discuss with medical staff regarding the use of pharmacological agents to prevent arrhythmias (e.g. atropine).

Hypoxia. Hypoxia can be caused by the interruption of ventilation, reflex bronchospasm and the removal of the oxygen supply. Pre- and post-oxygenation can minimize this effect.

Raised intracranial pressure. Suction has been proven to increase ICP dramatically, therefore

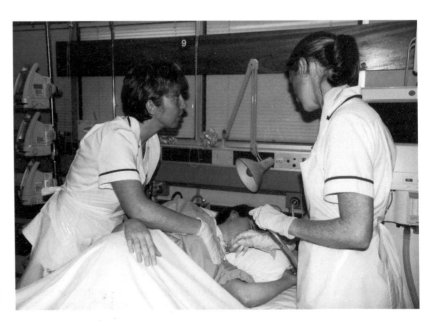

Figure 11.5 Endotracheal suction (with chest support).

suction should be used only when indicated (Young 1984).

Contraindications to suctioning the intubated patient

- Frank haemoptysis
- Severe bronchospasm
- Undrained pneumothorax
- Compromised cardiovascular system

Closed-circuit suction

Closed-circuit suction systems are available and consist of a catheter in a protective closed sheath which remains attached to the endotracheal or tracheostomy tube for 24 hours (Crimlisk et al 1994) or longer. The indications for use are: immunosuppressed patients, actively infectious patients (e.g. open tuberculosis) and patients with severe refractory hypoxaemia on high levels of PEEP.

Nasal and oral suction

Sedated and/or paralysed patients with a loss of gag and swallowing reflexes may need nasal and oral suction. A soft catheter (size 12 or 10 in adults) can be used for the nose, but a rigid sucker (Yankauer) may be necessary for the mouth or a catheter passed through an oral airway. To minimize trauma to the nasal passages a nasal airway (nasal trumpet) may be used. For suction of the non-intubated patient, see p. 213.

Saline administration

The administration of normal saline as a physiotherapy adjunct is widespread, although the evidence for its efficacy is not established (Raymond 1995). It is usual to use up to 5 ml of normal saline (0.9%), but on occasions it may be necessary to use greater volumes (e.g. removal of a large plug occluding the endotracheal tube). As with any adjunct to physiotherapy the use of normal saline should not be routine. If it is difficult to loosen and clear tenacious secretions on suction, the use of normal saline is indicated.

It is important to assess a patient's overall level of hydration as systemically dehydrated patients are at greater risk of plugging. Additional continuous heated humidification may be necessary and reduce the need for normal saline. Normal saline nebulizers can be incorporated into the ventilator circuit when indicated.

Considerations for physiotherapy

- Normal saline can be used to assist the removal of tenacious secretions during physiotherapy and/or to assess and maintain patency of an endotracheal tube. Normal saline can be administered just prior to treatment to stimulate a cough and to maximize the clearance of secretions. If normal saline is to be introduced at the beginning of a treatment, the use of short sharp hyperinflations can potentially aid dispersal of the fluid and heighten the stimulation of a cough.
- In the event of acute lobar collapse, it can be beneficial to administer normal saline at the beginning of treatment with the patient positioned with the 'collapsed' area in the dependent position. Gravity will then assist the passage of the saline. Once the saline has been administered and a few breaths by manual hyperinflation have been given, the patient should be repositioned in the correct gravity-assisted position. Manual hyperinflation in conjunction with manual techniques will aid in reinflation of the collapsed area.

Manual techniques

There are a variety of manual skills. Shaking and vibrations during the expiratory phase increase expiratory flow and aid the removal of secretions. Chest clapping may be indicated to assist in the mobilization of tenacious secretions.

Considerations for physiotherapy

- After assessment, if a patient is considered too unstable to tolerate manual hyperinflation, shaking and/or vibrations can be performed during the expiratory phase of the respiratory cycle in synchrony with the ventilator. This may aid removal of secretions.

Intermittent positive pressure breathing (IPPB)

IPPB can be used in the treatment of an intubated patient. The appropriate catheter mount is used in place of a mouthpiece or mask to connect the circuit to an endotracheal or tracheostomy tube (see p. 209).

Considerations for physiotherapy

- IPPB is extremely useful for physiotherapy in the weaning process. The positive pressure augments tidal volume in an essentially self-ventilating patient with respiratory muscle weakness or fatigue. A patient who has a depressed cough reflex following long-term intubation can be assisted with the use of IPPB. The increased tidal volume utilizes collateral ventilation and assists the mobilization of secretions. These patients often fatigue easily and IPPB reduces the work of breathing.

Periodic continuous positive pressure ventilation (PCPAP)

PCPAP is a useful adjunct in patients presenting with reduced lung volumes and/or areas of atelectasis. The circuit can be attached directly to an endotracheal or tracheostomy tube or via a facemask or mouthpiece in an extubated patient.

Considerations for physiotherapy

- PCPAP can be used to maximize functional residual capacity and to aid reinflation of areas of atelectasis immediately following extubation. In the multiproblematic patient CPAP or PCPAP can be used in conjunction with IPPB.

EMERGENCY SITUATIONS

Box 11.1 lists a few commonly encountered problem situations, together with some physiotherapy action guidelines. It must be remembered that in an emergency or potential crisis, help must be sought immediately. In the intensive care setting help is never far away. The patient's nurse should be alerted immediately. If the situation continues to be problematic, the medical team should be asked to review the patient urgently.

Acknowledgements

We would like to acknowledge the assistance of Dr Mark Evans, Dr Andrew Jones, Moira O'Connell and the Physiotherapy Department of St Mary's NHS Trust.

Box 11.1 Commonly encountered problem situations

Cardiopulmonary arrest
- Alert help immediately
- Follow 'arrest' procedure

Sudden drop in blood pressure
- Stop manual hyperinflations – give tidal breaths
- Check arterial line
  - correct reading
  - correct trace
- Alert help
- Terminate treatment – put patient back on to ventilator
- Put patient supine
- Monitor vital signs

Cardiac arrhythmias
- Check chest leads
  - attached
  - reading accurately
- Alert help
- Terminate treatment immediately and put patient back on to ventilator

Sudden rise in intracranial pressure
- Check ICP tracing
- Alert help
- Give rapid shallow breaths with bag – hyperventilate
- Terminate treatment and put patient back on to ventilator
- Check head and neck alignment and position

Dislodged endotracheal tube
- Alert help immediately
- If effective, continue to hand ventilate with tidal volumes until help arrives
- If ineffective – urgent help imperative
- Monitor vital signs especially saturation

Self-extubation
- Alert help immediately
- Assist ventilation with a resuscitation bag (e.g. Ambu) with face mask
- Closely monitor vital signs especially saturations
NB: If patient appears to be making adequate spontaneous effort with good saturations, administer high level of oxygen via a face mask and monitor closely

Fully blocked endotracheal or tracheostomy tube
- Alert help immediately
- Check positioning of endotracheal tube
- Attempt suction with saline
- Deflate cuff
- Assist ventilation with a resuscitation bag (e.g. Ambu) with face mask until help arrives
- Monitor vital signs especially saturations

Partially blocked endotracheal or tracheostomy tube
- Notify nursing staff
- Continue manual hyperinflations, saline administration and suction
- If unable to clear – inform medical staff
- Monitor vital signs especially saturations

Accidental removal of chest drain
- Apply immediate constant pressure to drain site occluding the hole
- Alert help immediately
- Terminate treatment immediately and put patient back on to ventilator
- Monitor vital signs
NB: If patient awake and making spontaneous effort, ask patient to exhale prior to applying pressure to drain site

Sudden desaturation
- Check saturation probe – accurate reading
- Notify nursing staff
- Assess cause (e.g. pneumothorax, 'plugging off', collapse, bronchospasm, cardiovascular instability)
- If physiotherapy will relieve problem – continue treatment
- Monitor vital signs – especially saturation
- Medical problem – alert help immediately
- Terminate treatment and put patient back on to ventilator

Sudden onset no breath sounds one lung
- Assess cause (e.g. collapse, sputum plug, pneumothorax, misplaced tube)
- If physiotherapy will relieve problem – continue treatment
- Monitor vital signs especially saturations and blood pressure
- Medical problem – alert help immediately
- Terminate treatment and put patient back on to ventilator

Sudden reduction in level of consciousness
- Alert help immediately
- Terminate treatment and put patient back on to ventilator
- Monitor vital signs

Accidental removal of vascular catheter or arterial line
- Apply constant pressure to site immediately
- Alert help

Accidental removal or dislodging of CVP line or PA catheter
- Apply constant pressure to site if removed
- If dislodged, prevent further traction on line
- Notify nursing staff

REFERENCES

Antonelli M, Moro ML, Capelli O et al 1994 Risk factors for early onset pneumonia in trauma patients. Chest 105: 224–228

Birtwistle J 1994 Pressure sore formation and risk assessment in intensive care. Care of the Critically Ill 10: 154–159

Bordow RA, Landers CF 1985 Pulmonary injury. In: Bordow RA, Moser KM (eds) Manual of clinical problems in pulmonary medicine, 2nd edn. Little Brown, Boston

Branson RD, Davis K, Campbell RS, Johnson DJ, Porembka DT 1993 Humidification in the intensive care unit. Prospective study of a new protocol utilizing heated humidification and a hygroscopic condenser humidifier. Chest 104: 1800–1805

Browne DRG 1988a Weaning patients from ventilators 1. Hospital Update July: 1809–1817

Browne DRG 1988b Weaning patients from ventilators 2. Hospital Update August: 1898–1906

Ciesla ND 1996 Chest physical therapy for patients in the intensive care unit. Physical Therapy 76: 609–625

Clark KJ 1985 Coping with Guillain–Barré syndrome. Intensive Care Nursing 1: 13–18

Clement AJ, Hübsch SK 1968 Chest physiotherapy by the 'bag squeezing' method. Physiotherapy 54: 355–359

Connine T, Sullivan T, Mackie T, Goodman M 1990 Effect of serial casting for the prevention of equinus in patients with acute head injury. Archives of Medical Rehabilitation 71: 310–312

Copnell B, Fergusson D 1995 Endotracheal suctioning: time-worn ritual or timely intervention? American Journal of Critical Care 4: 100–105

Crimlisk JT, Paris R, McGonagle EG, Calcutt JA, Farber HW 1994 The closed tracheal suction system: implications for critical care nursing. Dimensions of Critical Care Nursing 13: 292–300

Dakin J, Evans TW 2001 Progress in ARDS research: a protection racket? Thorax 56: 2–3

Denehy L 1999 The use of manual hyperinflation in airway clearance European Respiratory Journal 14: 958–965

Edwards S 1996 Neurological physiotherapy, a problem-solving approach. Churchill Livingstone, Edinburgh

Eisenhart K 1994 New perspectives in the management of adults with severe head injury. Critical Care Nursing 17: 1–12

Emery P, Salmon M 1991 Systemic mediators of inflammation. British Journal of Hospital Medicine 45: 164–168

Ferner R, Barnett M, Hughes RAC 1987 Management of Guillain–Barré syndrome. British Journal of Hospital Medicine Dec: 526–530

Fowler R, Falkner T 1992 The use of hypnosis for pain relief for patients with polyradiculoneuritis. Australian Physiotherapy 38: 217–221

Frisby JR 1990 Predicting outcome of critical illness. In: Oh TE (ed) Intensive care manual, 3rd edn. Butterworths, Sydney, pp 7–12

Ganong WF 1995 Review of medical physiology, 17th edn. Appleton and Lange, Norwalk, pp 482–496

Garradd J, Bullock M 1986 The effect of respiratory therapy on intracranial pressure in ventilated neurosurgical patients. Australian Journal of Physiotherapy 32: 107–111

German K 1994 Intracranial pressure monitoring in the 1990s. Critical Care Nursing 17: 21–32

Guillain–Barré Syndrome Study Group 1985 Plasmapheresis and acute Guillain–Barré syndrome. Neurology 35: 1096–1104

Hambley H 1995 Coagulation (II) – clinical problems in coagulation disorders. Care of the Critically Ill 11: 203–205

Higgens JM 1966 The management in cabinet respirators of patients with acute or residual respiratory muscle paralysis. Physiotherapy 52: 425–430

Hodgson C, Denehy L, Ntoumenopoulos G, Santamaria J 1996 The acute cardiorespiratory effects of manual lung hyperinflation on ventilated patients. European Respiratory Journal 9 (suppl 23): 37s

Hughes RAC, Rees JH 1994 Guillain–Barré syndrome current opinion. Neurology 7: 386–392

Jones AJM, Hutchinson RC, Oh TE 1992 Effects of bagging and percussion on total static compliance of the respiratory system. Physiotherapy 78: 661–666

Karni Y, Archdeacon L, Mills KR, Wiles CM 1984 Clinical assessment and physiotherapy in Guillain–Barré syndrome. Physiotherapy 70: 288–292

Keilty SEJ 1993 Inhalation burn injured patients and physiotherapy management. Physiotherapy 79: 87–90

Kesteven P, Saunders P 1993 Disseminated intravascular coagulation. Care of the Critically Ill 9: 22–27

Kirby S, Davenport A 1996 Haemofiltration/dialysis treatment in patients with acute renal failure. Care of the Critically Ill 12: 54–58

Knaus WA, Draper EA, Wagner DP, Zimmerman JE 1985 APACHE II: a severity of disease classification system. Critical Care Medicine 13: 818–829

Kulkarni V, Webster N 1996 Management of sepsis. Care of the Critically Ill 12: 122–127

Lennon SM, Koblar S, Hughes RAC, Goellar J, Riser AC 1993 Reasons for persistent disability in Guillain–Barré syndrome. Clinical Rehabilitation 7: 1–8

Macleod J, Edwards C, Bouchier I (eds) 1987 Davidson's principles and practice of medicine, 15th edn. Churchill Livingstone, Edinburgh, ch 15, p 644

Miller JD, Becker DP, Ward JD et al 1977 Significance of intracranial hypertension in severe head injury. Journal of Neurosurgery 47: 503–516

Mulnier C, Evans T 1995 Acute respiratory distress in adults (ARDS). Care of the Critically Ill 11: 182–186

Murray JF 1996 ARDS introduction and definition. In: Evans TW, Haslett C ARDS acute respiratory distress in adults. Chapman & Hall, London, pp 3–12

Murray JS 1976 The normal lung: the basis of diagnosis and treatment of pulmonary disease. W B Saunders, Philadelphia

Oh TE 1990 Tetanus. In: Oh T E (ed) Intensive care manual, 3rd edn. Butterworths, Sydney, ch 45, pp 305–309

Pappert D, Rossaint R, Salma K, Gruning T, Falke KJ 1994 Influence of positioning on ventilation–perfusion relationships in severe adult respiratory distress syndrome. Chest 106: 1511–1516

Paratz J, Burns Y 1993 The effect of respiratory physiotherapy on intracranial pressure, mean arterial pressure, cerebral perfusion pressure and end tidal carbon dioxide in ventilated neurosurgical patients. Physiotherapy Theory and Practice 9: 3–11

Patman S, Jenkins S, Stiller K 2000 Manual hyperinflation – effects on respiratory parameters. Physiotherapy Research International 5 (3): 157–171

Pearson SJ 1996 Peak airway pressures exerted during manual hyperinflation by physiotherapists and nursing staff. British Journal of Therapy and Rehabilitation 3: 261–266

Pearson S, Parr S 1993 Physiotherapy in the critically ill patient. Care of the Critically Ill 9: 128–131

Rapper S, Maynard N 1992 Feeding the critically ill patient. British Journal of Nursing 1: 273–280

Raymond S 1995 Normal saline instillation before suctioning: Helpful or harmful? A review of the literature. American Journal of Critical Care 4: 267–271

Rees J 1993 Guillain–Barré syndrome: the latest on treatment. British Journal of Hospital Medicine 50: 226–229

Rudy EB, Turner BS, Baun M, Stone KS, Brucia J 1991 Endotracheal suctioning in adults with head injury. Heart and Lung 20: 667–674

Scadding JW 1990 Neurological disease. In: Souhami RL, Moxham J (eds) Textbook of medicine. Churchill Livingstone, Edinburgh, ch 23

Sciaky AJ 1994 Mobilising the intensive care unit patient. Physical Therapy Practice 3: 69–80

Singer M, Vermaat J, Hall G 1994 Haemodynamic effects of manual hyperinflation in critically ill mechanically ventilated patients. Chest 106: 1182–1187

Tharakan J, Ferner RE, Hughes RAC, Winer J, Barnett M, Brown ER, Smith G 1989 Plasma exchange for Guillain–Barré syndrome. Journal of the Royal Society of Medicine 82: 458–461

Thomas S 1991 The gift of life. Nursing Times 87: 28–31

van der Meche FG, Schmitz PI 1992. A randomised trial comparing intravenous immune globulin and plasma exchange in Guillain-Barré syndrome. New England Journal of Medicine 326: 1123–1129

Watson GR, Wilson FM (1989) Guillain–Barré syndrome: an update. New Zealand Journal of Physiotherapy Dec: 17–24

West JB 1995 Respiratory physiology, 5th edn. Williams and Wilkins, Baltimore, p 35

Young CS 1984 A review of the adverse effects of airway suction. Physiotherapy 70: 104–106

FURTHER READING

Adam S, Forrest S 1999 ABC of intensive care: other supportive care. British Medical Journal 199; 319: 175–178.

American Association for Respiratory Care (AARC) 1993 Clinical practice guidelines. Endotracheal suctioning of mechanically ventilated adults and children with artificial airways. Respiratory Care 38: 500–503

Bennett D, Bion J 1999 ABC of intensive care: organisation of intensive care British Medical Journal 318: 1468–1470

Burton A, Conway JH, Holdate ST 1999 Weaning adults from mechanical ventilation. Physiotherapy 85: 12, 652–661

Dulguerov P, Gysin C, Perneger TV, Chevrolet JC 1999 Percutaneous or surgical tracheotomy: a meta-analysis. Critical Care Medicine 27: 1617–1625

Edwards S 1996 Neurological physiotherapy, a problem-solving approach. Churchill Livingstone, Edinburgh

Ellis E, Alison J (eds) 1994 Key issues in cardiorespiratory physiotherapy. Butterworth-Heinemann, Oxford

Evans TW, Haslett C 1996 ARDS acute respiratory distress in adults. Chapman and Hall, London

Evans TW, Smithies M 1999 ABC of intensive care: organ dysfunction. British Medical Journal 318: 1606–1609.

Fiddler H, Williams N 2000 ECMO: a physiotherapy perspective, Physiotherapy 86 (4): 203–208

Ganong WF 1995 Review of medical physiology, 17th edn. Appleton and Lange, Norwalk

Gower P 1991 Handbook of nephrology, 2nd edn. Blackwell Science, Oxford

Griffiths RD, Jones C 1999 ABC of intensive care: recovery from intensive care. British Medical Journal 319: 501–504

Gunning K, Rowan K 1999 ABC of intensive care: outcome date and scoring systems. British Medical Journal 319: 241–244

Hinds CJ, Watson D 1996 Intensive care, 2nd edn. WB Saunders, London

Hodson C, Carroll S, Denehy L 1999 A survey of manual hyperinflation in Australian hospitals. Australian Journal of Physiotherapy 45(3): 185–193

Levick JR 1995 An introduction to cardiovascular physiology, 2nd edn. Butterworth-Heinemann, Oxford

Lindsay KW, Bone I, Callander R 1991 Neurology and neurosurgery illustrated, 2nd edn. Churchill Livingstone, Edinburgh

Marino P 1991 The ICU book. Lea and Febriger, Philadelphia

McCarren B, Chow CM 1998 Description of manual hyperinflation in intubated patients with atelectasis. Physiotherapy Theory and Practice 14: 199–210

Moxham J, Goldstone J (eds) 1994 Assisted ventilation, 2nd edn. British Medical Journal Books, London

Nunn JF 1993 Nunn's applied respiratory physiology, 4th edn. Butterworth-Heinemann, Oxford

Oh TE (ed) 1997 Intensive care manual, 4th edn. Butterworths, London

Shelly MP, Nightingale P 1999 ABC of intensive care: respiratory support. British Medical Journal 318: 1674–1677

Short A, Cumming A 1999 ABC of intensive care: renal support. British Medical Journal 319: 41–44.

Singer, M Little R 1999 ABC of intensive care: Cutting edge. British Medical Journal 319: 501–504

Singer M, Webb A 1997 Oxford handbook of critical care. Oxford University Press, Oxford

Smith G, Nielsen M 1999 ABC of intensive care: criteria for admission. British Medical Journal 318: 1544–1547

Wallace PGM, Ridley SA 1999 ABC of intensive care: transport of critically ill patients. British Medical Journal 319: 368–371

West JB 1992 Pulmonary pathophysiology, 4th edn. Williams and Wilkins, Baltimore

West JB 1995 Respiratory physiology, 5th edn. Williams and Wilkins, Baltimore

Winter B, Cohen S 1999 ABC of intensive care: withdrawal of treatment. British Medical Journal 319: 306–308

12

Surgery for adults

Sarah C Ridley
Amanda Heinl-Green

INTRODUCTION

Continued advances in minimal access surgery, combined with improved anaesthesia and pain management of the surgical patient, reflect the necessity for ongoing evaluation of physiotherapy practice in this field. Treatment should never be routine but in response to individual patient assessment and be based on the best clinical evidence available. Communication with members of the multidisciplinary team is essential in order to provide an efficient and effective service.

To avoid repetition, general physiotherapy management has been discussed and for individual surgical procedures the physiotherapy key points have been given additionally.

GENERAL ANAESTHESIA

The main objectives of a general anaesthetic (GA) are reversible loss of awareness and temporary blockade of gross responses to stimulation. During anaesthesia skeletal muscular contraction and autonomic responses such as increased heart rate, blood pressure and sweating are inhibited. A general anaesthetic may be divided into three main components coma, muscular relaxation and analgesia (Forrest et al 1995). Current anaesthetic agents enable proportional adjustment of each component to suit the patient and the procedure. The actual course of administering a GA may be divided into different stages.

Premedication

The premedicant drugs provide reduction in anxiety, pain relief, sedation and encouragement of amnesia. Other desired effects may be prevention of bradycardia, excess salivation and antiemesis. As the performance of day surgery increases and more patients are admitted close to the scheduled time of surgery, premedication is becoming less common.

Induction

The aim at this point is to start the anaesthetic process rapidly and pleasantly. This is usually achieved by intravenous injection of a short-acting coma-inducing drug such as propofol. Sometimes anaesthetic vapours may be inhaled to the same effect. Sevoflurane is the most commonly used agent for this as it has a pleasant smell and is not irritant to the airways. Anaphylaxis characterized by severe hypotension, hypoxia and bronchospasm is a rare but life-threatening reaction to parenterally administered drugs.

Maintenance

This follows induction and is the stage when surgery commences. A combination of inhaled anaesthetic (e.g. isoflurane, sevoflurane) and intravenous analgesics (e.g. morphine, fentanyl) may be given with muscle relaxants to enable controlled ventilation of the lungs. Total intravenous anaesthesia using an infusion of propofol, rather than an inhalation agent, is also becoming more popular. Muscle relaxants and analgesics are used as necessary in conjunction with propofol and may be given as infusions.

Reversal

The reversal of the effects of a GA is a short but potentially hazardous period. The concentration of the inhaled or intravenous anaesthetic will be reduced and drugs such as neostigmine are given to reverse the effect of muscle relaxants. Occasionally if a spontaneous respiratory rate has been re-established but is less than 6–8 breaths per minute, a narcotic antagonist may be given to reverse the respiratory depressant effect of the narcotic. Unfortunately this will also abolish the analgesic effect. Extubation is undertaken once the protective laryngeal reflexes have returned. The patient is normally positioned lying on their side (in the recovery position) to reduce the risk of aspiration and given supplemental oxygen, while the upper airway is maintained by jaw thrust, head tilt or an oropharyngeal airway.

Effects of general anaesthesia on respiratory function

Under GA the functional residual capacity (FRC) may be lowered by up to 30% at 24 hours postoperatively and remain reduced for several days. The reduction in FRC may be related to diaphragmatic dysfunction thought to be associated with increased abdominal tone (reflex muscle spasm) and/or a reflex reduction in phrenic nerve activity (Craig 1981). This reduction in lung volume and encroachment of the FRC on closing volume (CV) reduces lung compliance, increases airway resistance and may lead to atelectasis. Dependent lung collapse occurs within 15 minutes of anaesthetic induction and can last for up to 4 days postoperatively. Absorption atelectasis may also contribute to the development of postoperative pulmonary collapse. When the rate of gas leaving the alveolus, due to uptake in the blood, is greater than the rate of inspired gas entering it, absorption atelectasis may result. This process is facilitated when the airway leading to an area of lung is obstructed or collapsed (Joyce & Baker 1995).

There is also a reduction in lung recoil pressure, especially in overweight patients. Narcosis reduces the sensitivity of the respiratory centre and decreases the efficiency of the elimination of CO_2. A decrease in cardiac output potentially reduces pulmonary blood flow and alveolar perfusion, thus increasing physiological dead space. Ventilation/perfusion ($\dot{V}/\dot{Q}$) mismatch is accentuated by the patient being supine on the operating table, respiratory depression and reduced cardiac output.

Inhalation of dry, cold gas which bypasses the warming/humidification effect of the upper airways will increase mucus viscosity and a high inspired FiO$_2$ over a period of hours will slow down mucus velocity. Mucociliary clearance ceases altogether after 90 minutes of a GA (Lunn 1991).

The cough reflex is dampened centrally by sedation/opiates and peripherally by any abdominal/thoracic wounds. The resultant reduction in inspiratory and expiratory volumes makes it more difficult to generate pressure to detach mucus from the airways.

If infection ensues, this is primarily caused by *Streptococcus pneumoniae* or *Haemophilus influenzae.*

SPINAL ANAESTHESIA

During spinal anaesthesia a needle is inserted between the spinous processes of the lumbar vertebrae, passing through the ligamentum flavum, the epidural space and the dura-arachnoid and into the subarachnoid space (Fig. 12.1). The correct position of the needle can be confirmed by the escape of cerebrospinal fluid. The third and fourth lumbar vertebrae are normally selected as in adults the spinal cord has ended usually around the first lumbar vertebra (L1), thus reducing the risk of neurological complications. The spread of local anaesthetic solution, e.g. lidocaine (lignocaine) or bupivacaine, is determined by the dose, volume, puncture site and position of the patient. It will result in sensory, motor and sympathetic blockade of the specific nerve roots as they pass from the cord through the intervertebral foramen. Subarachnoid opiates may also be used to improve the quality of the sensorimotor blockade and to provide analgesia in the postoperative period. Adding vasoconstrictors such as epinephrine and phenylephrine may increase the duration of the blockade by up to 2 hours (Gaiser 1997). Disturbance of sympathetic outflow may result in hypotension and bradycardia (Lunn 1991).

Generally spinal anaesthesia is carried out for operations performed below the level of the

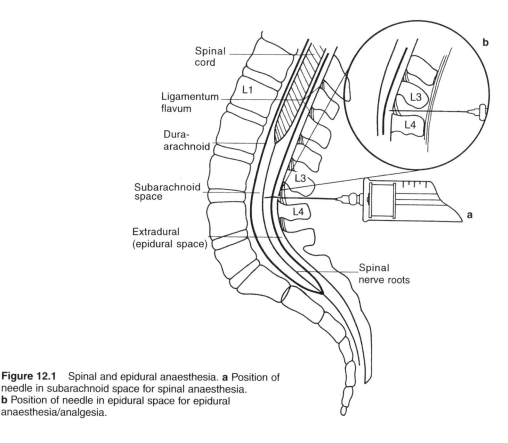

Figure 12.1 Spinal and epidural anaesthesia. **a** Position of needle in subarachnoid space for spinal anaesthesia.
b Position of needle in epidural space for epidural anaesthesia/analgesia.

umbilicus and is commonly used in joint replacement surgery. It is most suitable as an alternative to general anaesthesia for high-risk and elderly patients. Neurological complications are rare.

EPIDURAL ANAESTHESIA / ANALGESIA

This procedure involves a needle being inserted, at the appropriate level of the spinal column, into the epidural space; that is, passing through the ligamentum flavum but not the dura-arachnoid (Fig. 12.1). A band of anaesthesia will form depending on which nerve roots have been selected. Commonly this is done in the lumbar region but the epidural space can be approached from any level. The ideal block will provide a sensory block to the appropriate site but be narrow enough to reduce the risk of complications without causing motor blockade of the respiratory or lower limb muscles. Ideally the epidural catheter should be placed at the spinal level corresponding to the nerve roots supplying the proposed surgical incision; that is, at the appropriate dermatome level. The umbilicus is at the T10 dermatome level and the nipple line is at the T4 dermatome level. Epidurals for all upper abdominal and thoracic operations should ideally be performed at thoracic spinal rather than lumbar spinal level.

Regular testing is essential to prevent the block occurring above nipple level as this may lead to a reduction in cardiac output secondary to cardiac sympathetic blockade or motor blockade of the intercostal muscles, compromising respiratory function. An epidural catheter may potentially provide only a unilateral block so both sides of an incision should always be assessed. Epidural anaesthetic drugs delivered in lower concentrations and smaller volumes can provide analgesia and mild sympathetic blockade without significant motor block. This is due to motor fibres having a relatively larger diameter than pain and sympathetic fibres which makes them less penetrable by local anaesthetic.

If anaesthesia/analgesia is required for a period of hours or days following the operative procedure, a fine catheter is inserted over the needle as it is withdrawn. This enables repeated injections or continuous infusion of local anaesthetic, with or without the addition of an opioid. Current epidural protocols recommend very small doses of opioids to limit the opioid levels in the circulation (De Leon-Casasola et al 1994) and dilute mixtures of potent local anaesthetics such as bupivacaine or ropivacaine to reduce side effects such as motor block. Oxygenation, ability to cough and vital capacity are all improved with spinal or epidural analgesia compared with systemic narcotics (Gaiser 1997). It is suggested that epidural anaesthesia in abdominal surgery appears to decrease length of stay and pain experienced by patients postoperatively and results in a more rapid return of bowel function (Scott et al 1996).

A major advantage of an epidural compared to a spinal anaesthetic is that the dura is not punctured and that long-term analgesia/anaesthesia can be provided via a catheter which can safely be left in situ for a few days postoperatively.

Physiotherapy key points

- The patient may get up after a spinal anaesthetic once the effects have worn off. If, however, a post-dural puncture headache occurs secondary to leakage of cerebrospinal fluid, the patient is advised to lie flat until the symptoms have resolved. Post-dural puncture headaches most commonly occur after inadvertent dural puncture during the performance of an epidural block, but this is still very rare. It is due to the greater size of the epidural needle (usually 18 gauge) compared with a spinal needle (usually 26 gauge). The dural hole can be sealed with a clot, by injecting some of the patient's own blood into the space. This is referred to as an epidural blood patch and is effective in more than 95% of patients. Temporary back pain is the most common side effect (Gaiser 1997).
- In the recovery period after a spinal anaesthetic, patients will require care of their lower limbs due to temporary sensory and motor loss as well as monitoring of potential postural hypotension. This is another reason why

patients should not sit up until the spinal block has worn off.

- Respiratory depression can occur if opioids are being given via an epidural.
- A patient will experience pain if the epidural catheter becomes displaced or blocked or if a 'top-up' bolus of the anaesthetic/analgesic agent is required.
- Rarely, migration of an epidural catheter into the subarachnoid space combined with a substantial 'top up' could lead to an accidental spinal anaesthesia which would cause extensive bradycardia, hypotension and respiratory distress necessitating cardiopulmonary resuscitation.
- Close liaison with the medical and nursing staff and adherence to local guidelines are essential when considering the mobilization of a patient with an epidural in situ.

INTRAVENOUS REGIONAL ANAESTHESIA

This type of anaesthesia is used for simple limb surgery or manipulation of closed fractures. It involves the limb being injected with local anaesthetic while a tourniquet renders it ischaemic for the duration of the procedure.

Nerve block

This procedure involves injection of a local anaesthetic into the main nerve supplying the area under operation and is termed a nerve block. Examples of this technique include brachial plexus, intercostal nerve and ilio-inguinal blocks.

TOPICAL ANAESTHESIA

Local anaesthetic agents in the form of solutions or creams may be applied to the skin or mucosa and absorbed into the affected area. Lidocaine (lignocaine) is commonly used and may also be administered as a spray/gargle/gel or on soaked pieces of cotton wool. The effect is rapid and lasts approximately 30–60 minutes.

MANAGEMENT OF ACUTE POSTOPERATIVE PAIN
Effects of pain

It is essential that pain relief is managed well, especially over the immediate postoperative period when the patient may be spending more time in a bed or chair rather than walking around the ward. This is when patients are at greater risk of developing atelectasis and subsequent pulmonary infection. Acute pain is a complex process affected by the physiological reaction to injury or disease, as well as psychological and social factors. An individual's perception of pain may depend on their previous experience of pain as well as their current degree of control over their particular situation.

Pain following surgery may also indicate that a complication has occurred. The diagnosis of surgical complications should not be obscured by good pain control providing the patient's overall condition is assessed regularly (Attard et al 1992). If postoperative pain is not managed appropriately the following effects may occur:

- increased patient anxiety leading to fatigue and possible loss of confidence in the staff providing care
- increased heart rate and blood pressure resulting in increased myocardial oxygen consumption
- decreased movement therefore increased risk of deep venous thrombosis (DVT), pulmonary embolus (PE), breakdown of pressure areas and increased dependency on staff
- increased respiratory complications
- disturbance of sleep pattern.

Assessment of pain

Pain is a subjective experience and should be assessed by recording the patient's current perception of the pain using either a visual analogue scale or a verbal descriptor scale. Comparison of scores before and after administration of analgesics will provide essential information regarding the effectiveness of the pain relief. In some centres, as nausea and vomiting are common side effects of analgesia and potentially more distressing than the actual pain, they will also be assessed on a scale and be dealt with appropriately. A minimum of 1–4 hourly assessment of pain is recommended but should be tailored to meet the individual's needs.

Non-pharmacological methods

Emotions such as anxiety, fear and loss of autonomy are known to increase pain perception. Methods to reduce this include:

- provision of accurate information preoperatively regarding expected methods of pain relief and where the pain is most likely to occur
- advice on positioning, moving and wound support, etc.
- explanation of pain scales and the importance of reporting pain as early as possible
- awareness of side effects such as nausea and vomiting
- access to acupuncture and TENS as alternatives to medication
- techniques which promote relaxation such as self-hypnosis.

Drug therapy

Oral analgesia

As major surgery is often associated with gastrointestinal dysfunction resulting in variable drug absorption, oral analgesia is reserved for minor surgery or a few days after major surgery when the gut is working again and the pain is expected to be less acute.

Non-steroidal anti-inflammatory drugs (NSAIDs)

NSAIDs reduce inflammation at the site of injury as well as providing some central analgesic activity. They may be given orally, by intramuscular (IM) injection or rectally via a suppository. Side effects include gastric irritation, increased bronchospasm, decreased renal function and platelet dysfunction.

Opioids

This category is used to manage moderate to severe pain, especially of visceral origin. Side effects include nausea, vomiting, constipation, drowsiness and the possibility of upper airway obstruction during sleep, leading to hypoxaemia.

Despite these effects, opioids are the most commonly used postoperative analgesic, particularly over the first 3 days. Dosages required to relieve pain are very unpredictable and not necessarily linked to age, gender or body weight. They may be delivered orally, by IM injection or intravenous (IV) infusion. The aim of an IV infusion is to maintain constant plasma concentration of the opioid, therefore avoiding the peaks and troughs of intermittent regimens. It should be noted that analgesia should initially be established by bolus IV injection allowing the infusion to then maintain that level of pain relief. Additional subsequent boluses may be required depending on the patient's condition but the risk of respiratory depression is high and patients should be observed closely. Oxygen therapy is also advised during the period of infusion. It should be noted that the pump should always be placed at or below the level of the patient's heart and an anti-siphon valve incorporated into the system to avoid an inadvertent large bolus of opioid being delivered.

Patient-controlled analgesia (PCA)

The syringe containing the drug is put in a microprocessed controlled pump and connected to an intravenous cannula or IV infusion with a non-return valve. The pump is programmed to deliver a bolus dose and set with a minimum period between doses ('lockout' interval). Every time the patient presses the button on the control lead the preset dose is given unless the button is pressed during the 'lockout' period.

Each patient can administer as much or as little analgesia as they may need according to their pain and activity levels. This should be a safe technique if the patient is in control of the button, i.e. not staff or family members because as consumption increases, sleepiness should prevent self-administration continuing to the point of respiratory depression.

PCA may not be suitable for patients who are unable to comprehend the system or unable to operate the hand trigger, e.g. due to arthritis.

Nitrous oxide

Nitrous oxide (e.g. Entonox®) is a mixture of 50% oxygen and 50% nitrous oxide and provides good analgesia for severe pain of brief duration. Entonox® cylinder headsets have a demand valve which is patient activated on inspiration which should be administered 1 or 2 minutes before the painful procedure is carried out. As the mask is self-administered it will fall away from the face if the patient becomes too drowsy. Entonox® is contraindicated if:

- there is a low cardiac output because of peripheral vasodilatation
- a pneumothorax or subcutaneous emphysema is present as rapid diffusion of nitrous oxides impedes the absorption of air
- a patient requires more than 50% oxygen
- a patient is relying on his hypoxic drive to breathe.

If it is used in high dosages or over a protracted period of time it is associated with bone marrow suppression. As with any drug, Entonox® must be prescribed by a doctor prior to administration.

Entonox® can be particularly helpful during intermittent, relatively short episodes of pain such as removal of mediastinal drains, coughing with fractured ribs, repositioning a patient and contraction pains during labour. Occasionally it may be appropriate to deliver Entonox® through the ventilator circuit during manual hyperinflation or in conjunction with IPPB.

Side effects include nausea, euphoria (hence the lay term 'laughing gas'), tingling, numbness, light headedness and auditory disturbances. Cylinders are stored horizontally and it is good practice to invert the cylinder upside down approximately three times prior to use to ensure mixing of gases (BOC 1990).

INCISIONS AND SUTURES

Some common incisional sites are illustrated in Figure 12.2. These may vary according to the individual surgeon's preferences although they are designed to provide optimal exposure to the surgical area of interest.

Ideally, incisions are made along the lines of least tissue tension to enable prompt healing and a fine scar line. Transverse abdominal incisions cause less strain on the wound than vertical incisions (Garcia-Valdecasas et al 1988). Accurate suturing of the deeper layers of the wound facilitates the superficial skin layers coming together without tension and this allows apposition by adhesive tape or superficial sutures (e.g. silk or nylon). Deeper wound spaces that cannot be obliterated by suture should be drained to reduce the danger of exudate accumulation and possible consequent infection.

Absorbable sutures such as catgut or Dexon® are preferable for stitching deeper layers while stronger sutures are appropriate for those needed around joints and over the abdominal wall. Areas with a good blood supply such as the face and neck tend to heal quickly, possibly enabling suture removal at 3–5 days. In contrast, more peripheral areas such as the leg and foot may require sutures in situ for up to 14 days. Abdominal and chest wound sutures generally need 7–10 days prior to removal (Forrest et al 1995). Obesity increases the chance of infection, especially in traumatic or surgical wounds, presumed due to the relatively poor blood supply of large areas of subcutaneous adipose tissue.

A median sternotomy involves longitudinal division of the sternum and the aponeuroses of the pectoralis major muscle with all the thoracic muscles remaining intact. For this reason it is generally accepted that this incision is less painful than a thoracotomy or upper abdominal incision.

PREOPERATIVE PHYSIOTHERAPY MANAGEMENT

Appropriate patient selection

A number of factors should be taken into consideration when the physiotherapist is deciding

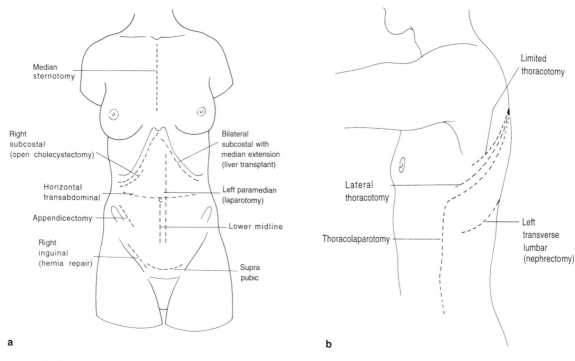

Figure 12.2   a and **b** Common surgical incisions.

which patients may be defined as 'high risk' and would benefit from input at this stage. Frameworks have been developed to identify patients at risk of developing postoperative pulmonary complications (Arozullah et al 2000, Brooks-Braun 1997).

Incisional site

Several studies have shown that upper abdominal and thoracic incisions lead to a high incidence of respiratory complications (Craig 1981, Ford et al 1983). This may result from a decrease in FRC, change in the ventilatory pattern to rapid shallow breathing and impaired oxygenation. This is not the case with lower abdominal surgery (Dureuil et al 1987) but it may be appropriate to assess the patient if they present with other significant risk factors.

Pre-existing respiratory problems

Infection. Upper respiratory tract infection may result in excessive mucus secretion and

reduction in mucociliary clearance. Lower respiratory tract infection may impair gas exchange, leading to possibilities of hypoxia secondary to pneumonia and exacerbation of infection. The immunocompromised patient is more susceptible to infection.

Restrictive defects. Lung fibrosis and pulmonary oedema can cause restrictive defects. Patients with kyphoscoliosis and ankylosing spondylitis are especially at risk after upper abdominal surgery since almost all tidal volume may be dependent on diaphragmatic movement. A large pleural effusion may compress lung tissue, thereby accentuating the reduced lung volume, and lead to an increase in airway resistance and closure following anaesthetic induction.

Obstructive defects. A deeper anaesthesia may be required in asthmatic patients due to bronchial hyperreactivity. An FEV_1 / FVC ratio of less than 35% is highly predictive of postoperative acute respiratory failure following thoracotomy (Brodsky 1995).

Obesity

Body mass index (BMI) is calculated by measuring a patient's weight in kilograms (kg) and then dividing by their height in metres (m) squared (kg/m^2). Generally there is a good correlation between BMI and body fat. A BMI of 18.5–24.9 is considered acceptable, 25.0–29.9 as overweight, 30.0–39.9 as obese and equal to or greater than 40.0 as morbidly obese (Garrow 1988).

Total lung compliance can be reduced to approximately one-third of the normal value due to the additional weight of the chest wall (Selsby & Jones 1993) and this leads to an increased work of breathing and O_2 consumption. FRC decreases and closing capacity increases, thereby predisposing to atelectasis. A 60% reduction in FRC is often observed at anaesthetic induction and this leads to an increased risk of basal atelectasis (Damia et al 1988). Hypoxaemia can be found at rest in obese patients, especially in the supine position where FRC is further reduced.

Age

Increasing age is associated with increasing closing volume and loss of elastic recoil. At approximately 65 years of age, small airways close during resting tidal volume in seated subjects. Even from the age of 44 years and upwards airway closure is observed in the supine position (Leblanc et al 1970). With increasing age, the respiratory muscles weaken and the rib cage stiffens, with a resultant decrease in excursion.

Smoking

Smoking results in small airway narrowing, increased mucus production, irritable airways, decreased mucus clearance and an elevated closing capacity. These factors predispose to a greater ventilation/perfusion ($\dot{V}/\dot{Q}$) shunt and impaired oxygenation during anaesthesia. Even short periods of abstinence from smoking (12–48 hours) are sufficient to decrease carboxyhaemoglobin (COHb) and nicotine levels and thus improve the work capacity of the myocardium (Anderson et al 1973). The patient's smoking history should be clarified as to whether they are a current or ex-smoker, including the time since last cigarette and total number of pack years accrued. Six weeks' cessation of smoking is required to reduce the volume of sputum produced by the patient but it takes several months for mucociliary clearance to return to normal (Egan & Wong 1992, Morgan & Nel 1996).

Patient motivation

Patients affected by impaired preoperative cognitive function, anxiety, depression, mental handicap or psychiatric disease may have a longer recovery period.

Nutritional status

Poor nutritional status has been shown to cause increased incidence of postoperative pneumonia. Impaired production of antibodies will also make these patients prone to infection. Protein and vitamin deficiencies can delay wound healing (Forrest et al 1995).

Functional status and intercurrent disease

Diseases such as multiple sclerosis, Parkinsonism and rheumatoid arthritis can increase the risk of complications through reduced mobility. Intercurrent disease, e.g. diabetes, leukaemia or haemophilia, should also be taken into consideration.

Alcohol and drug dependency

Potential problems with withdrawal symptoms and the possible need for high levels of anaesthesia/analgesia should be anticipated.

Preoperative physiotherapy assessment

Once the appropriate patients have been identified, further questioning may be necessary concerning the patient's smoking and respiratory history, including any relevant medications such as bronchodilators or steroids. It is important to establish the patient's exercise tolerance and to undertake a general examination of the musculoskeletal system. Examination of the chest (see Ch. 1) should also be carried out.

Teaching and information

Considering the amount of verbal information given to the patient at this stage, details should be brief and concise and ideally back-up written material should be provided. Preoperative explanation regarding the effects of surgery on respiratory function, the location of the wound, drips and drains may help to reduce pain and speed recovery after the operation (Auerbach & Kilmann 1977). Nelson (1996) reported that 75% of patients who participated in a preadmission education programme for patients undergoing cardiac surgery felt a resultant reduction in anxiety levels in response to the information that they received. The physiotherapist should also stress the importance of early mobilization (Mynster et al 1996), appropriate positioning while chair or bed bound, adequate pain control, regular thoracic expansion exercises and wound support during huffing or coughing if bronchial secretions are present. Close liaison with the nursing staff and provision of information leaflets will help to emphasize the importance of these activities to the patient. The use of video to convey preanaesthetic information may also be beneficial to increase recall (Done & Lee 1998).

Preoperative treatment

Occasionally a patient may need treatment to maximize pulmonary function in the preoperative stage because of, for example, a current chest infection or history of bronchiectasis. If major respiratory problems are anticipated postoperatively, a patient may benefit from instruction in the use of adjuncts such as intermittent positive pressure breathing (IPPB). In elective cases, advice from the surgeon on cessation of smoking and weight reduction should ideally be given weeks or months prior to admission.

POSTOPERATIVE PHYSIOTHERAPY MANAGEMENT

Generally the main aims in the postoperative phase are to promote the reinflation of areas of atelectasis and to maintain adequate ventilation, to assist in the removal of any excess bronchial secretions and to aid in the general positioning, bed mobility and early ambulation of the patient. Prevention of reduced joint movements or poor posture secondary to incisions or tubes, monitoring of adequate pain relief and appropriate oxygen therapy and humidification are also very important.

Physiotherapy techniques which help to achieve these aims include the following.

Early mobilization. With the development of laparoscopic surgery, improved anaesthetic and pain management, many patients are often able to mobilize independently from a very early stage postoperatively. Some patients will require assistance because of the presence of the various drips and drains and it is sometimes safer to have two people assisting for the first stand or walk because of the patient's general fatigue and the risk of postural hypotension. A graduated walking programme adapted to suit each patient should be encouraged with the introduction of stair climbing at an appropriate stage.

Manual handling teams can often be an excellent source of advice regarding current devices to assist standing and walking in highly dependent or obese patients. Suitable seating at a height appropriate to the individual can also improve patient independence, particularly for those patients who, following upper abdominal surgery (UAS), find it difficult to get up from sitting in a low chair to standing but are fully independent once up on their feet. The use of pressure-relieving devices should be considered for those patients who sit for long periods and are unable to easily shift their weight while seated.

Bed mobility / positioning. Advice on optimum and regular change of position while the patient is in bed is essential for patients in the early stages of recovery. Appropriate use of overhead 'monkey poles', rope ladders and cot sides can reduce the patient's reliance on staff to be 'mobile' if confined to bed. Simple advice on how to get in and out of bed without putting undue strain on the wound can also be of great value to the patient. Electronic beds which can adjust the patient automatically from lying to the seated position are available but expensive.

Thoracic expansion exercises. See p. 190. Patients who are unable to be frequently mobile in the ward and are at risk of developing atelectasis should be encouraged to carry out regular thoracic expansion exercises (TEE), e.g. 3 × 5 TEE every waking hour preferably with an end-inspiratory hold of a few seconds. Regular breathing exercises can also alert patients to the fact that their analgesia may be wearing off and that they need to inform a member of staff or self-administer the patient-controlled analgesia (PCA) system.

Incentive spirometry (IS) / intermittent positive pressure breathing (IPPB). These techniques are described in Chapter 6 and may be introduced for immobile patients who are unable to carry out thoracic expansion exercises or are ineffective at doing so and are showing signs of unresolved atelectasis.

Clearance of bronchial secretions. If sputum retention persists or difficulty in clearing secretions continues to be a problem, despite adequate analgesia and appropriate advice on thoracic expansion exercises, forced expiration technique (FET) and wound support, suction via the nasopharynx with or without a nasal airway or oral airway may be an option. If it is anticipated that this may be required more than once or twice, minitracheotomy should be considered.

POSTOPERATIVE COMPLICATIONS

The following section highlights some of the general complications following surgery.

Atelectasis and infection. The main postoperative respiratory problems are decreased lung volume leading to atelectasis and infection. Reports on the incidence of postoperative atelectasis vary from 20% to 69% (Dajczman et al 1991) and for pneumonia from 9% to 40% (Horowits et

al 1989). Any abdominal distension will tend to exacerbate these problems.

Wound complications. Infection rates vary depending on the type of operation, patient's condition and the ability of the surgeon. When managing clean wounds most centres have an infection rate of 2–4%. Complications such as dehiscence, incisional hernias and haematomas may raise the risk of infection to 5%. This rate would be even higher in traumatic or infected cases. In non-elective operations involving unprepared bowel or urinary tract infections the rate of wound complications can be as high as 50–60% (Moossa & Hart 1997).

Pulmonary oedema. Excessive administration of fluid in the early postoperative period may result in an increased workload for the heart and lungs and may lead to pulmonary oedema. This should be avoided by strict fluid balance monitoring, especially for patients with a history of cardiac disease.

Myocardial infarction. Evidence suggests that a recent myocardial infarction (MI) plays a major part in prediction of postoperative myocardial dysfunction and death (Mearns 1995). If there has been a history of MI within the last 3 months then there is a 20–30% chance of reinfarction. Perioperative MI has a mortality rate of up to 70% (Cavil 1999). The Goldman Cardiac Risk Index aims to predict the postoperative risk of cardiac complications after major non-cardiac surgery, with evidence of cardiac failure and recent MI being the most important factors (Goldman et al 1977).

Cardiovascular problems. Hypertension, ischaemic heart disease/angina, valvular heart disease, conduction defects and pacemakers may carry a risk to the patient. Cardiac dysrhythmias may be associated with hypotension.

Shock. Acute circulatory failure can be divided into three categories.

- *Hypovolaemic shock* is caused by a fall in circulating blood volume secondary to inadequate correction of perioperative fluid losses or continuing haemorrhage.
- *Cardiogenic shock* is usually caused by reduced cardiac output secondary to

myocardial ischaemia or infarction with left ventricular failure or arhythmias.

- *Septic shock* or septicaemia is defined as the proliferation of bacteria in the bloodstream and consequent circulatory collapse.

Deep venous thrombosis (DVT) / pulmonary embolus (PE). Low-dose heparin is commonly used in patients over 40 years of age undergoing a general anaesthetic. The risk of developing a thrombus is also increased by a history of smoking, immobility, malignancy, use of contraceptive pill and previous surgery, particularly pelvic or lower limb surgery. If a thrombosis develops in the calf veins there is a low risk of embolism. In this situation, ambulant patients are given thromboembolic deterrent (TED) stockings and encouraged to continue mobilizing. Immobile patients would be considered for systemic heparinization. If the site of thrombus is in the ileofemoral segment of the deep veins, the risk of embolism is high. These patients are anticoagulated and 48 hours of bedrest is advised with slight elevation of the foot of the bed. Clinical diagnosis of DVT is unreliable with only 50% of patients with evidence of DVT on venography showing any clinical signs. All patients who suffer a PE will require warfarin therapy for approximately 3–6 months. Fat embolization is occasionally seen and usually occurs following a long bone fracture. Amniotic fluid embolism is uncommon but may result in severe disseminated intravascular coagulation (DIC) secondary to extensive alteration of clotting function. Gas emboli occur due to introduction of gas into the circulation via the venous route. Laparoscopic procedures may result in embolization of insufflating gas.

Acute renal failure. Impairment of renal function results from inadequate perfusion of the kidneys due to hypovolaemia or sepsis. This usually presents as oliguria, defined as a urinary output of less than 0.5 ml per kg per hour which is the equivalent to 35 ml per hour for a patient weighing 70 kg.

Reduced gut motility. Paralytic ileus is characterized by reduced or absent bowel sounds and may result in considerable abdominal distension.

Gastric peristalsis usually returns 24–48 hours postoperatively and colonic activity after 48 hours.

Nausea and vomiting. Gastrointestinal upset is experienced in about one-third of patients undergoing surgery.

Aspiration pneumonitis is caused by aspiration of gastric contents which are normally sterile. Severe pneumonitis is associated with aspiration of greater than 25 ml of fluid with a pH value of less than 2.5 and can result in chemical burning of the airways. Very small food particles can cause intense inflammation if they reach as far as the distal airways. Larger food particles may obstruct more central airways leading to segmental or lobar collapse and possible hypoxic arrest if lodged in the larynx, trachea or main bronchi.

Aspiration pneumonia is usually a consequence of inhalation of contents from the oropharynx that may have a normal pH value but may contain bacteria. Patients who are unable to protect their upper airway are at high risk of aspiration. The onset of signs and symptoms often occurs gradually and may not be obvious if the patient is not being closely observed whilst eating or drinking. Input from a speech and language therapist may be appropriate to advise on management of this problem.

Postoperative psychosis and delirium. The incidence is approximately 0.2% in general surgical patients. Predisposing factors include age, alcohol and drug dependency, dementia and metabolic abnormalities (Moossa & Hart 1997).

Peripheral nerve injuries / pressure areas. Peripheral nerve injuries can be caused by stretching or compression of nerve trunks as a result of poor positioning of limbs on the operating table, which may be unavoidable. Incidence of recurring injuries should be investigated and may be alleviated by closer monitoring of pressure care or modification of positioning if possible, while the patient is in theatre and the recovery room. Injury to the skin and subcutaneous tissues may occur over bony prominences. The back of the head should not be forgotten when assessing for pressure areas.

Loss or chipping of teeth. Tooth fragments may be aspirated inadvertently into the respiratory tract.

Myalgia. Neck, chest and abdominal muscle pain may last up to one week if the muscle relaxant drug suxamethonium is given during anaesthesia.

THORACIC SURGERY

Intercostal chest drainage

Many thoracic surgical procedures and traumatic conditions require intercostal drainage. The main aim of intercostal chest drainage is to remove air and/or fluid from the pleural space in order to restore subatmospheric intrapleural pressure, enabling reexpansion of the deflated or compressed lung and to prevent the build-up of fluids, which may lead to the development of an empyema.

Chest tube

The chest tube should be clear, of adequate diameter (6–11 mm internal diameter in adults), with a radioopaque strip to outline the tube itself and the side holes should lie within the pleural space. Any connectors should also be clear to prevent blockage going undetected. Previously, apical tubes were positioned to drain air while basal drains were intended to drain fluid (Fig. 12.3). More recently, some surgeons prefer to place two apical drains which allow for the removal of air but also have a number of holes within the tube to allow for drainage of fluids as well.

Underwater seal drainage

To ensure that the air removed from the pleural space during expiration is prevented from reentering during inspiration, the drainage system must have an underwater seal. To achieve this the pleural drain is attached to a tight-fitting connector on the bottleneck (Fig. 12.4). This is connected to a rigid tube which is submerged about 2 cm below the surface level of the water, thus creating an underwater seal. The air is expelled against the

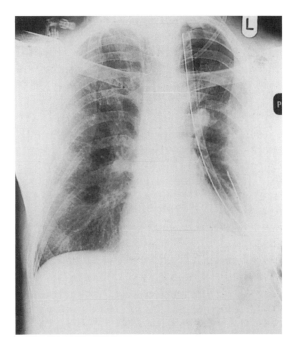

Figure 12.3 Chest radiograph showing apical and basal drains.

hydrostatic resistance of the water and out into the atmosphere via the vent. The vent is essential to avoid build-up of pressure within the container. It is important that the distal end of the underwater seal tube is always submerged but that the length of the tube below the water level is as short as possible whilst maintaining the seal as this reflects the work required to expel air or fluid from the pleural space. Fluids will drain by gravity and not spill back into the pleural space if, as recommended, the bottle is always kept below the level of the patient's chest.

Fluctuations in the level of the water column reflect the change in pleural pressure during breathing. In self-ventilating patients the intrapleural pressure becomes more negative during inspiration and the fluid column will rise. During expiration the intrapleural pressure is less negative, causing the fluid level to fall. If air is seen to bubble through the water it indicates a hole in the visceral pleura. If the air leak stops suddenly, kinking or blockage of the tube should be suspected. A more gradual cessation of bubbling usually means that the lung has fully re-expanded.

The simplest form of underwater seal drainage system consists of one bottle serving as both collection container and underwater seal drain for evacuation of fluid and air. This system is adequate if minimal drainage of fluid is expected. If a 'Y' connector is incorporated into this system, two separate intercostal drains may be attached to a single bottle (Fig. 12.4a). Alternatively two separate bottles may be used, enabling drainage of air and fluid (Fig. 12.4b). In a two-compartment system fluid is collected in the first container via the chest tube and air is bubbled through to a second container via a connecting tube where it can be vented to the atmosphere (Fig. 12.4c). The advantage of this system is that both containers have underwater seals, but the separate container for drainage of fluid only allows accurate monitoring of volume and expelled matter, e.g. pus, fibrin or blood clots. Integral sealed units without separate bottles are used in some institutions. Three- and four-compartment systems are also available.

Suction

Free drainage depends on gravity to expel air and fluid from the pleural space. In the presence of excess volume of fluid to be drained or a large air leak, suction may be applied to the vent tube at recommended pressures of between 5 and 20 cmH$_2$O. Greater pressures may be necessary for the management of a persistent air leak.

It is no longer advisable to intermittently compress and release the tubing, by gentle hand squeezing to dislodge any clots. 'Milking' or stripping of drains with rollers is thought to create high negative pressures, which could result in pulmonary trauma (Kam et al 1993).

Clamping

Clamping of tubes is generally avoided except:

- when the bottle needs to be temporarily lifted above the level of the patient's chest
- when the drainage container needs replacing
- when the drain has been inserted after a pneumonectomy

- when accidental disconnection of tubing or breakage of containers occurs
- when determining the absence of a pneumothorax on the chest radiograph prior to drain removal
- during chemical pleurodesis.

As there is a potential risk of a tension pneumothorax developing in the presence of a continuous air leak when the tubes are clamped, this procedure should be undertaken for very brief periods only.

It is essential that clamps are always readily available for any patient with an underwater seal drain in situ. In the situation where the intercostal drain is still within the patient's chest wall but has become disconnected or the bottle has broken, the tube should be clamped as close as possible to the patient's chest wall. The tubing should then be cleaned and reconnected or a new system applied as quickly as possible. If, however, the intercostal drain has become completely detached from the patient, he is requested to breathe out while at the same time pressure is applied to the wound at the end of expiration. While maintaining the pressure on the wound, the patient is encouraged to breathe normally while medical help is obtained.

Drain removal

Tubes that have been used solely to drain fluid will be removed once they drain 10–20 ml/hour or less. In the case of empyema where pus is being drained into a bag (open drainage), the length of the tube within the chest is gradually shortened, externally, by a few centimetres until the infection has resolved. Air drainage tubes are removed once the lung has fully reexpanded and the air leak has stopped. To avoid unnecessary reinsertion of a chest drain, the tube may be clamped for a period of 12–24 hours (functional removal) and a radiograph taken to confirm that the lung has not deflated prior to actually removing the drain. If a pneumothorax has reoccurred, the tube is simply unclamped for a further period of drainage. As the tube has nor-

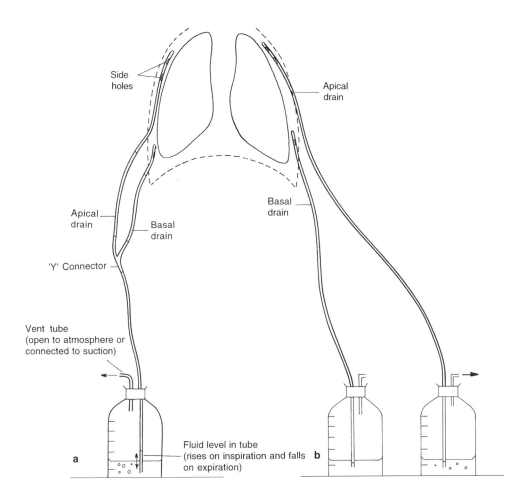

Side holes

Apical drain

Apical drain

Basal drain

Basal drain

'Y' Connector

Vent tube
(open to atmosphere or connected to suction)

a

Fluid level in tube
(rises on inspiration and falls on expiration)

b

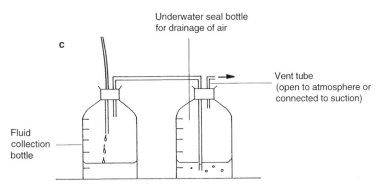

Underwater seal bottle for drainage of air

c

Vent tube
(open to atmosphere or connected to suction)

Fluid collection bottle

Figure 12.4 Underwater seal chest drainage. **a** Single bottle system allowing use of one bottle via a 'Y' connector to drain fluid and air. **b** Two separate bottles enabling drainage of air from the apical drain and fluid from the basal drain. **c** Two-compartment drainage system where two bottles are connected in series, the first collecting fluid and the second acting as the underwater seal drainage for air.

mally been sewn into position with a 'purse-string' suture, the patient is asked to breathe in deeply and hold at full inspiration as the tube is taken out and the sutures pulled together to avoid air escaping back into the pleural space. Adequate analgesia should be ensured for this procedure.

Physiotherapy key points

- Observation of changes in air leaks and drainage should be made before, during and after physiotherapy intervention.
- Care should be taken when handling patients so that the tubes are always visible, to avoid kinking, stretching or disconnection.
- Advice should be given on postural correction and upper limb exercises. Occasionally inappropriate taping of the drains with sleek tape around the chest wall can limit the patient's range of movement and should be addressed.
- Bottles should be at the side of a patient's bed and not hidden underneath, to avoid crushing of the container if the bed is inadvertently lowered too far.
- In the presence of an air leak, positive pressure techniques should be avoided if possible, as they may perpetuate the problem by maintaining the fistula. However, if gross atelectasis also persists then the application of positive airway therapy such as CPAP may aid reinflation of the lung and therefore lead to a reduction in the size of the pneumothorax.
- If suction is required to re-expand the lung then it is inadvisable to disconnect this to perform exercise. The suction tubing may be lengthened so that the patient is able to exercise at the side of the bed by walking on the spot, doing step-ups on a fixed single step or cycling on the spot, depending on age and clinical status.
- It must be stressed to the patient that the drains are held below the level of the chest and that clamps should be available at all times.
- Pain associated with the presence of chest drains should not be underestimated.

LUNG CARCINOMA

Guidelines have been developed regarding patients with lung cancer outlining specific criteria for fitness for surgery and operability (British Thoracic Society 2001).

Carcinoma of the lung occurs more frequently in the upper lobes than the lower lobes, with the middle lobe and lingula being least affected. It also affects the right more than the left lung (Sheilds 2000). The sites of tumours are classified as central if they are located in the main stem, lobar and segmental bronchi extending to the fifth generation. These tumours are firm, irregular-shaped masses of varying size and extra-bronchial spread can extend for a variable distance into the adjacent lung parenchyma. Secondary atelectasis and infection due to obstruction are common features. Peripheral tumours affect the bronchi past the fifth generation, the bronchioles and alveoli. These tumours are firm and irregular and may not be easily differentiated from surrounding lung tissue (Sheilds 2000).

Histological classification

Carcinoma of the lung is usually separated into the classifications of small cell lung carcinoma (SCLC) and non-small cell lung carcinoma (NSCLC).

SCLC

Small cell carcinomas account for 15–35% of all lung carcinomas. They are mostly found in the central area and are highly aggressive and malignant. They metastasize early and few patients are considered to be suitable surgical candidates. Radiotherapy and chemotherapy are the more common treatment options.

NSCLC

- *Squamous carcinoma tumours* constitute approximately 20–35% of all lung cancers (Sheilds 2000). These tumours are predominantly located in the central area, are often associated with distal collapse and consolidation and obstructive pneumonitis and are rarely seen in non-smokers. They grow relatively slowly and metastasize late.

- *Adenocarcinoma* accounts for 30–50% of all lung carcinomas (Sheilds 2000). This is most likely to present in peripheral lung regions. The growth of these tumours is intermediate between that of squamous and small cell types. These tumours metastasize early by means of the vascular and lymphatic systems.
- *Adenosquamous carcinomas* account for approximately 2.6–3.4% of lung carcinomas (Shimizu et al 1996). They are a mixture of adenocarcinoma and squamous cells, are predominantly peripheral and more commonly found in men (Shimizu et al 1996*)*. They metastasize early and have a worse prognosis than either squamous or adenocarcinoma in isolation.
- *Bronchioalveolar carcinomas* constitute 1.5–7% of all lung cancer; however, some groups do not view this as a separate entity but merely as a subset of adenocarcinoma. They rarely extend beyond the lung and lymph node metastases are uncommon (Daly et al 1991).
- *Undifferentiated large-cell carcinoma* accounts for 4.5–15% of all lung cancers (Sheilds 2000). These tumours are predominantly found in the lung periphery and metastasize early. Ninety percent of these patients are smokers and the prognosis is poorer than with other NSCLC.
- *Giant cell tumours* constitute less than 1% of all lung carcinomas and are said to be a variety of undifferentiated large cell carcinoma. The prognosis is extremely poor and most often they are rapidly fatal.

Metastasis of lung carcinoma

Metastatic spread of lung cancer may occur through the following mechanisms.

- Direct invasion of surrounding tissue. The sites are commonly the pleura, pulmonary vessels, chest wall, diaphragm, pericardium, heart, great vessels and spine.

- Lymphatic spread is common; approximately 50% of patients with NSCLC have mediastinal lymph node involvement at the time of presentation (Martini & Ginsberg 1990). The spread is usually ipsilateral. In general, the larger the primary, the greater the incidence of metastatic spread.
- Bloodborne metastases are common in patients with lung carcinoma. The organs affected are the brain, liver, lungs, skeletal system, adrenal glands, kidney and pancreas.

Physiotherapy key points

- When patients are admitted to hospital for pulmonary investigations they will often omit details from their medical history that they feel are irrelevant. Following discussion with a physiotherapist they often then disclose further information such as bone pain or joint problems, which they have not associated with their pulmonary condition. It is important that when a history is being taken the physiotherapist is alert to signs of potential metastatic spread which, if present, should be immediately reported to the medical staff for further investigation.
- Neurological metastases are often silent but can present secondary to raised intracranial pressure, e.g. headaches, nausea, blurred vision, diplopia and changes in levels of consciousness or mentation.
- Bone metastases commonly affect the spine, pelvis and femur and often present clinically as bone pain. Hypertrophic pulmonary osteoarthropathy also presents with bone pain due to proliferative periostitis affecting the distal ends of long bones. The most common bones affected are the tibia, radius, ulna and fibula but the humerus, femur, metacarpals and metatarsals may also be affected (Darling & Dresler 2000).
- As evaluation of tumours necessitates numerous invasive and non-invasive tests, it is important that prior to each visit the physiotherapist is up to date with all the test results as this may influence treatment.

Staging and investigations

Clinical staging classifications define the tumour size, location and the presence or absence of metastases and facilitate the decision as to which patients should be referred for surgery. The assessment, management and prognosis of the disease depend largely on the cell type and whether there has been metastatic spread. The TNM staging system (T = description of the primary tumour, N = extent of regional lymph node involvement and M = the absence or presence of metastases) identifies those patients who, following resection, will have improved survival compared with the natural history of the disease (Tisi 1985). This system has been modified to increase specificity and predictability of prognosis (Mountain 1997).

Non-surgical treatment of lung carcinoma

If surgery is not appropriate, alternative treatments include radiotherapy and chemotherapy. Endobronchial treatment also offers a variety of options for advanced lung tumours. Thermal resection with high-powered lasers (neodymium-yttrium-aluminium-garnet (Nd-YAG) and carbon dioxide) are used. In acute intrinsic obstruction of the airway, photodynamic therapy (PDT) with low-powered lasers is used to activate light-sensitive drugs which are preferentially retained by tumour cells. Fluorescence tumour detection uses certain drugs which will fluoresce if illuminated at the appropriate wavelength. Brachytherapy involves the implantation of radioactive isotopes (e.g. radioactive gold grains) into the tumour, which are then allowed to naturally decay. The patient has to be isolated for several days to avoid staff and other patients being affected by the radiation. Insertion of expanding metal or silastic stents may also relieve the pressure exerted on the airway by extrinsic tumours in the upper airway.

Currently patients selected for surgery may also be receiving simultaneous treatment with both chemotherapy and radiation. This impacts on their preoperative and postoperative state and they often suffer from malaise, fatigue, anaemia and thrombocytopenia and are more susceptible to nosocomial infection. It is important that all aspects of a patient's treatment programme are fully assessed prior to surgery in order that the appropriate physiotherapy treatments are tailored to individual needs.

LUNG SURGERY

In addition to lung surgery for carcinoma, localized bronchiectasis, sequestrated lobe and benign tumours may also be suitable for surgical intervention.

Thoracic incision

Access to the lung may be obtained through a full posterolateral thoracotomy, axillary (lateral) thoracotomy, limited thoracotomy (Fig. 12.2), median sternoscopy, transverse thoracosternotomy (clamshell) or thoracoscopy.

The *posterolateral* approach is now reserved for difficult cases where a wide area of access is required or for repeat thoracotomy where extensive adhesions are anticipated. This is the most painful of procedures involving muscular division of trapezius, latissimus dorsi, the lower portion of the rhomboids, serratus anterior, the intercostals and erector spinae. A rib retractor is used to spread the intercostal space. Whole or partial (2–4 cm) rib resection may be necessary to improve exposure of the lung, especially for repeat thoracotomies.

The *axillary thoracotomy*, sometimes referred to as the lateral thoracotomy, is primarily used for uncomplicated pulmonary operations. The only muscle group transected is the intercostals and it is therefore often referred to as a muscle-sparing thoracotomy. Upper lobe lesions are approached from the fourth intercostal space whereas middle and lower lobe lesions are approached from the fifth intercostal space. In a study by Kirby et al 1995 this approach was compared to videosassisted thoracoscopy (VATS) and no significant difference between length of hospital stay or postoperative pain experienced was identified between the two groups.

Median sternotomy is rarely used in thoracic surgery; however, it may be used for the removal of bilateral multiple tumours or for the treatment of bilateral spontaneous pneumothoraces and bilateral lung volume reduction surgery. The limitations of this incision are that it provides only limited access to the posterior hilar structures of the left lower lobe. Cosmetically for some patients, especially young women, the vertical incision is undesirable.

Transverse thoracosternotomy (clamshell) incision is primarily used for bilateral lung transplantation, but it is also an alternative for all the procedures listed under median sternotomy. The incision is made over the fourth or fifth intercostal space and the sternum is transected. The sternum may be reapproximated with Kirschner wires.

Thoracoscopy techniques have the advantages of offering minimal surgical trauma, are associated with less pain and respiratory embarrassment, a stronger cough and reduced recovery time in comparison to open thoracotomy (Mack et al 1992, Smith et al 1993a). It is an option for patients who are too severely compromised by their lung function to undergo open surgery. Diagnostic thoracoscopy may be carried out with a single direct-viewing thoracoscope but other techniques need video thoracoscopy (VATS) and simultaneous use of more than one port of access through trocars to manipulate instruments. The disadvantage of thoracoscopic surgery is that it may be difficult to locate a peripheral tumour and some surgeons feel that it does not provide enough access to fully manipulate the lung to feel for small metastases.

The following are some of the procedures performed under thoracoscopy.

- Pericardial window/pericardectomy for recurrent pericardial effusions
- Pleurectomy for recurrent pleural effusions
- Lung and mediastinal resection
- Resection of bullous emphysema

Lobectomy

This is the removal of an entire lobe. Generally two intercostal drains are placed in the pleural space at the time of operation to evacuate air and fluid/blood from the space (see Fig. 12.4). The drains may be attached to continuous suction to aid re-expansion of the remaining lung tissue. They usually remain until there is no air leak and less than 50 ml of fluid drains per 24 hours. Normally the hemidiaphragm on the affected side will rise slightly owing to the subsequent loss of lung volume. The remaining lung will reexpand and there will be a shift of the mediastinum to the ipsilateral side. The pleural space is usually obliterated in a few days to a week. In some patients there is a persistent air space, which can give rise to an empyema or bronchopleural fistula. If a pleural space is anticipated prior to surgery then some surgeons perform a muscle transplant to fill the gap. Alternatively, the phrenic nerve may be crushed, but this can give rise to an ineffective cough. Rarely an apical thoracoplasty may be performed to decrease the pleural space.

Sleeve resection

In this operation a section of the bronchus is removed, with or without a lobectomy, as a 'sleeve' and a primary bronchial reanastomosis is carried out to preserve the remaining lung tissue. The procedure is commonly carried out for tumours affecting the right upper lobe with spread into the right main bronchus.

Segmentectomy

Segmentectomy is the excision of one or more of the 10 bronchopulmonary segments. The subsequent loss of lung tissue is minimal and the procedure is therefore used in patients with limited pulmonary reserve or in those where resection of pulmonary metastases may provide a prolonged survival. An air leak may persist for several days, requiring an extended period of intercostal chest drainage and pleural exudate may be more marked.

Wedge resection

Patients with metastatic lesions often benefit from metastectomy using non-anatomical resections. Removing anatomical resections may lead to a removal of a significant amount of normal lung, which could restrict their pulmonary function and adversely affect quality of life. The approach may be a posterolateral incision, a median sternotomy, clamshell or VATS procedure. In-line staple devices are used to remove the lesions.

Physiotherapy key points

- The postoperative care of thoracic surgical patients is increasingly challenging, with the development of new technology and the treatment of increasingly elderly patients. More surgery is now performed on patients who are immunocompromised or in those patients who have previously received radiation and chemotherapy. The mortality of elective pulmonary and oesophageal resections remains 2–4 times higher than that of elective coronary artery bypass graft (CABG) (Ginsberg et al 1983). It should be remembered that extensive handling of the lung to exclude pulmonary metastases may lead to inflammation of the lung tissue.
- Preoperative assessment is vital. Most patients who present with lung carcinoma have a history of smoking and should be encouraged to cease smoking prior to surgery. Smoking cessation even for a few days decreases morbidity and improves ciliary clearance.
- Preoperative instructions, including breathing exercises, positioning and movement from bed to chair, should be practised before patients have to deal with the pain associated with a thoracotomy. High-risk patients in whom it is anticipated that non-invasive ventilation may be required after surgery should be shown the device, have the correct mask fitted and be familiar with its use prior to surgery in order to facilitate its application if required postoperatively.
- Thoracic surgery is painful so adequate analgesia must be given prior to treatment and titrated throughout the day to achieve optimal levels. A visual analogue scale, graded 1–10, may be useful for determining levels of pain.

- Liaison with the nursing staff is important as teamwork provides the most efficient use of time and causes the least amount of discomfort to the patient. For example, a physiotherapy exercise session can be tailored to include other activities the patient needs to perform, i.e. a walk to the bathroom, to the X-ray department or to get the patient out of bed in a chair ready for meal times.
- Breathing exercises should be started on the day of surgery.
- Early mobilization should be encouraged (Fig. 12.5). An airway clearance technique may be required if secretions are retained or when there are signs of atelectasis or lung collapse. Positioning to improve ventilation and perfusion (lying on the unaffected side) (Fig. 12.6) may be indicated. Adjuncts such as IPPB or CPAP may be considered, with caution, owing to the risk of perpetuating or increasing an air leak. Lower pressures should be used to minimize this effect.
- Adequate wound support for huffing and coughing should be taught. Assistance can be offered by placing one hand posteriorly below the thoracotomy incision and the other hand anteriorly to provide counter pressure.
- Damage to the recurrent laryngeal nerve can result in reduced effectiveness of coughing and lead to retention of secretions postoperatively. Huffing rather than coughing is better tolerated owing to the lower intrathoracic pressures generated. Nasopharyngeal suction or minitracheotomy may have to be considered if retained secretions become a persistent problem.
- Early mobilization on the first postoperative day progressing to stair climbing, often as soon as the third day postoperatively, should be encouraged. Exercise using a bicycle ergometer (Fig. 12.7) or a step may be appropriate for some patients with persistent air leaks where it is inappropriate to detach the drains from wall suction.
- Active/auto-assisted or resisted movements using proprioceptive neuromuscular facilitation techniques for the shoulder and shoulder girdle should be encouraged from the first

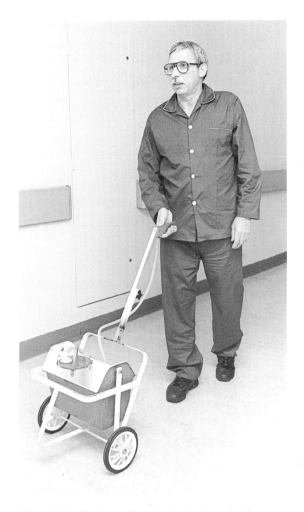

Figure 12.5 Walking with trolley for drainage bottles.

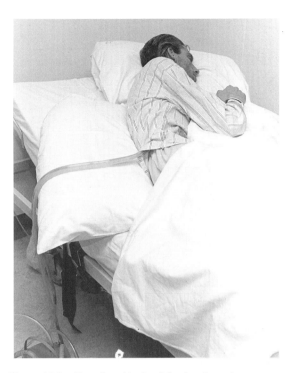

Figure 12.6 Use of positioning following thoracic surgery.

postoperative day. Postural correction is often needed as patients tend to side-flex the trunk toward the thoracotomy incision.

- Thoracic mobilizations, TENS or acupuncture may be beneficial for patients with persistent chest wall pain.
- Home advice to suit each patient regarding postural, shoulder and general mobility exercises should be given.

Pneumonectomy

This is the removal of a whole lung. Bronchial closure may be achieved by using either mechanical staples or sutures. Bloody fluid collects within the pneumonectomy space and the remaining air is progressively absorbed. The rate at which the fluid rises and the air is absorbed determines the position of the mediastinum. Some surgeons choose to insert a drain at the time of operation. The drain is usually in situ for 24 hours and is kept clamped except for 1–2 minutes every hour to allow a gradual build-up of fluid in the space, therefore maintaining an optimal mediastinal position. Usually after this 24-hour period, the air/fluid level in the space is at mid-hilar level. Monitoring of this position is aided by serial chest radiographs and palpation of the trachea to detect deviation. If the fluid accumulates too quickly the mediastinum will be pushed towards the unaffected lung, resulting in tracheal deviation and possible compression of the remaining lung. If a chest drain is not in situ, the mediastinal position may be altered by aspiration of air from the space until the pressure is negative in both phases of respiration.

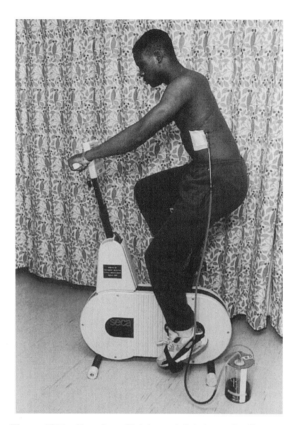

Figure 12.7 Exercise with intercostal drainage in situ.

Following a period of approximately 6 weeks the air will have been reabsorbed with subsequent loss of the fluid level and complete opacification of the hemithorax on chest radiograph. Over the following months organization of the pleural fluid takes place which may result in complete fibrosis. Consequently the pneumonectomy space contracts with progressive crowding of the intercostal spaces, elevation of the hemidiaphragm and possible mediastinal shift toward the side of surgery.

Physiotherapy key points

- The key points are similar to those described on p. 396. However, the pulmonary reserve of these patients is generally reduced to a greater extent and the mortality associated with pneumonectomy is higher.

- Post-pneumonectomy pulmonary oedema (PPO) has histopathological changes identical to acute respiratory distress syndrome (ARDS). The complication usually presents between 1 and 3 days postoperatively. The first clinical signs are tachypnoea, tachycardia and severe hypoxaemia refractory to supplemental oxygen. Later hypercapnia develops and a diffuse interstitial infiltrate is seen radiologically although this may lag behind clinical signs (Jordan et al 2000). It is important that the physiotherapist is alert to this serious complication and informs the medical staff immediately. Depending on the severity of the condition some of these patients may be supported with non-invasive positive airway devices. Usually, however, patients require intubation with the endotracheal tube selectively placed in the remaining bronchus to reduce any trauma to the bronchial stump of the resected lung.

- If tracheal deviation occurs, especially in the early postoperative period, the effectiveness of the cough mechanism may be reduced.

- Huffing rather than coughing is encouraged to minimize the increase in intrathoracic pressures created during clearance of secretions.

- If airway suctioning is necessary to clear secretions, either via the nasopharynx or a minitracheotomy, great care must be taken to avoid trauma to the bronchial stump, partcularly if the right lung has been removed, owing to the angle of the left and right main bronchi.

- Some surgeons may request avoidance of side lying in the first week postoperatively because if the patient lies on the non-thoracotomy side, the bronchial stump may become bathed in fluid. Others believe that if the suture line is secure the patient is not at risk and may lie on whichever side is more comfortable.

- The use of breathing control during activities such as stair climbing may increase exercise tolerance. Advice for energy conservation during activities of daily living may also be helpful.

Superior sulcus or Pancoast syndrome

The incidence is less than 5% of patients presenting with lung cancer (Mansour & Wanna 2000). Pancoast described the syndrome in 1932 which consists of pain usually in the shoulder, scapula or forearm and atrophy of the intrinsic muscles of the hand associated with a tumour in the superior sulcus and may also include Horner's syndrome. Symptoms are due to invasion of the brachial plexus, particularly the lower cords innervated by C7, C8 and T1, the intercostal nerves, chest wall and vertebral destruction. The tumour often invades the proximal ribs, intercostal muscles and vertebrae.

Upper airway stents

Insertion of expanding metal or silastic stents may relieve the pressure exerted on the airway by extrinsic tumours surrounding or invading the upper airway. These patients often have great difficulty clearing secretions, which tend to accumulate around the stent and can cause significant discomfort. The use of gravity-assisted positions with an airway clearance technique may encourage mucociliary clearance.

Bullectomy

Bullous emphysema is the presence of thin-walled air sacs under tension that impede expansion of surrounding lung tissue, causing compressive atelectasis. They may be single or multiple and can increase in size. A reduction in lung function may be a consequence of poor ventilation and perfusion in the presence of a large bulla. Only a few patients with bullous emphysema benefit from corrective surgery, the main aim of which is to ligate the bullae using a stapling device but removing the least possible amount of healthy lung tissue.

Pulmonary bullae can be classified into two groups based on the degree of structural changes of obstructive pulmonary disease in the non-bullous parenchyma (Deslauriers & Le Blanc 2000).

- Group 1: bullae associated with almost normal underlying parenchyma account for 20% of bullous disease.
- Group 2: bullae associated with diffuse emphysema account for 80% of bullous disease. This carries a 1–5% risk of surgical mortality (Deslauriers & Le Blanc 2000).

The indications for surgery are dyspnoea associated with a space-occupying lesion, which probably fills preferentially to more normal lung tissue. Surgery aims to restore the architecture and elasticity of the more normal tissue by removing the bullae. Other indications for removal, are troublesome pneumothoraces, haemoptysis, chest pain or infection.

Most bullectomies are performed through a standard posterolateral thoracotomy but with bilateral disease a median sternotomy or clamshell incision may be used. VATS is preferred by some surgeons, especially for patients who have a high risk of operative morbidity and mortality. Staples are used along the entire surface of the cysts and biological glues used to seal any remaining holes in order to reduce the risk of air leaks. Sometimes pleural tents are fashioned to reduce the pleural space if it is anticipated that the remaining lung will not expand sufficiently to occupy the space. Two chest drains are usually inserted and persistent air leaks are common.

Lung volume reduction surgery

The rationale for lung volume reduction surgery (LVRS) is the removal of non-functional distended air spaces, which are thought to be compromising the function of more normal lung parenchyma. Although the rationale for treatment is similar to that for bullectomy, the patient population is different. Patients undergoing LVRS have end-stage, severe emphysema refractory to medical management and consequently there is an increased level of surgical mortality. Surgery is performed via a median sternotomy or by VATS. Unlike bullectomy, which has a well-established role, this procedure has not been subjected to randomized controlled trials despite the fact that over 2000 LVRS cases have been reported.

Debate continues as to which precise patient population benefits most from this form of surgery and whether procedures should be carried out unilaterally in a staged procedure or bilaterally as a single operation. There is also controversy over whether laser ablation or a stapling device should be used. At most institutions pulmonary rehabilitation is performed prior to surgery, the aims being smoking cessation, improvement of aerobic capacity, improvement of respiratory muscle strength, strengthening of the upper limbs and improvement of thoracic mobility. During this time optimization of medical management, including a reduction in corticosteroids if possible, together with psychological preparation for surgery is undertaken.

As yet no randomized trial has been conducted to assess the value of pulmonary rehabilitation but improvements in quality of life have been reported (Debigare et al 1999). In a randomized controlled trial which compared pulmonary rehabilitation and surgery with pulmonary rehabilitation alone, a statistically significant improvement in FEV_1, shuttle walking distance and quality of life was reported in the surgical group (Geddes et al 2000). The rates of decline in lung function were similar in the two groups with an annual decrease of 100 ml in FEV_1. This indicates that surgery produced a one-time benefit but did not alter the natural progression of the underlying pulmonary disease and there was no significant difference in mortality between the groups. Although this was a small trial it highlights that LVRS remains a palliative procedure and that improvements need to be made in defining selection criteria.

Physiotherapy key points

Preoperatively
- Physiotherapy assessment is integral to improving patient selection and optimizing patient status prior to surgery. Shuttle walk tests or 6-minute walk tests are usually used in the preoperative assessment. A poor preoperative shuttle walk result (less than 150 m) has been shown to correlate with an increased mortality (Geddes et al 2000). It is therefore important that tests used for surgical selection are repeated just prior to surgery if a significant time period has elapsed between the date of assessment and date of surgery.
- Patients should also have serial sputum samples taken prior to surgery to identify pulmonary infection.
- Patients should be assisted with airway clearance if secretions are present.
- Pre- and post-bronchodilator lung function should be performed and inhaler technique checked.
- Patients should be familiarized with the breathing techniques and early rehabilitation exercises should also be carried out at this time.
- Preparation for non-invasive ventilation (NIV) is often advised as these are high-risk patients. Masks should be fitted and the machine shown to the patient prior to surgery. If it is required following surgery it needs to be applied without delay and it is of great benefit if the patient is familiar with and confident about its use. Very low pressures should be used preoperatively, as these patients are prone to pneumothoraces.

Postoperatively. Intensive physiotherapy is often required immediately postoperatively and for the first few days after surgery. The lack of pulmonary reserve in these patients means that even a small area of collapse or a slight increase in an air leak can lead to immediate respiratory embarrassment and imminent respiratory failure if not identified and treated immediately.

- Patients should be extubated as quickly as possible after surgery. If a prolonged period of ventilation is required a policy of low airway pressures with permissive hypercapnia and without positive end-expiratory pressure (PEEP) should be used. The postoperative arterial blood gases should be compared with the preoperative values, not with accepted normal values.

- The postoperative chest radiograph should be reviewed immediately to look for the presence of pneumothoraces.
- Drains are usually kept off suction but a brief period of suction may be required for the management of a pneumothorax. Great care must be taken with chest drains. These patients often have large air leaks and dislodgement or kinking of chest drains can quickly lead to lung collapse. If patients are on suction it is important that a step or cycle ergometer is available at the bedside so that they can exercise adequately.
- An airway clearance regimen should be started as soon as the patient is awake and repeated every 15–30 minutes on the day of surgery and the first postoperative day when the patient is awake. Over the proceeding days, as mobility is increased, the frequency of breathing exercises can usually be reduced.
- Patients should be sitting in a chair, to aid ventilation, as soon as they awaken. This may be with the endotracheal tube still in situ.
- Mobilization on the spot may also be started on the day of surgery.
- These patients have extremely limited pulmonary reserve and therefore treatments should be short and frequent throughout the day to prevent fatigue.
- Positive pressure, such as IPPB, CPAP or non-invasive ventilation, is avoided if possible as it may increase an air leak. However, there are times when these adjuncts are required for retained secretions, resistant airway collapse or to prevent reintubation in a patient who is sliding into respiratory failure. The indication should be discussed with the surgeon prior to application.
- There should be a low threshold for nasal suction or a minitracheostomy if these patients are having difficulty clearing secretions.
- Patients can start non-resistant arm, leg and thoracic mobility exercises on the first postoperative day. These are progressed until discharge and the exercise programme should be continued at home together with an outpatient rehabilitation programme.

PLEURAL SURGERY
Pleurectomy

Pleurectomy is an open procedure requiring thoracotomy where partial stripping of the parietal pleural layer enables the visceral pleura to stick to the subsequent raw surface of the chest wall. If at operation any blebs or bullae are identified these will be dealt with by oversewing, stapling, resection or ablation.

Pleurodesis

This entails the insufflation of a chemical irritant such as fibrin glue or iodized talc via a chest drain or thoracoscope. The latter technique has the advantage of allowing identification and treatment of any blebs or bullae. This procedure is painful and adequate analgesia must be provided.

Decortication

This may be necessary for patients presenting with chronic empyema. Rib resection is often required via a thoracotomy and with removal of the thickened pleurae, the previously restricted lung may reexpand. Any remaining pus must be drained.

Physiotherapy key points

- See p. 396.
- If these procedures are performed on young healthy patients, postoperative treatment should be directed accordingly such as running in the gym, fast cycling or fast stair climbing, to assist reinflation of the lung.

CHEST WALL SURGERY
Pectus excavatum

The primary defect results from the costal cartilages forming in a concave manner and therefore depressing the sternum. Most patients have few symptoms despite several studies showing that cardiac and respiratory function tends to be marginally below normal. On the whole, the primary indication for surgery is cosmesis because of psychological distress associated with altered body image (Sabiston 1990). Surgical correction involves a midline or transverse inframammary incision down to the periostium of the sternum. All cartilages are resected subperichondrially and the sternum repositioned. In adults internal fixation is carried out using retrosternal struts, plates or steel wires which can be removed during elective day surgery approximately 18 months later. The cartilages regenerate rapidly within several months, resulting in a firm anterior chest wall.

Physiotherapy key points

- These procedures can be very painful and adequate analgesia is required before treatment.
- Pulmonary atelectasis with fever may occur, therefore early mobilization is essential.
- Some surgeons restrict shoulder movements after surgery but if no restriction is applied early shoulder movemements should be encouraged.
- On discharge, patients are advised to avoid contact sports for several months or until the plate or wire, if in situ, has been removed.

Pectus carinatum

This is also commonly described as 'pigeon chest'. It is less common than pectus excavatum and is characterized by sternal protrusion caused by an upward curve of the 4th–5th costal cartilages. This usually results in reduced flexibility of the chest, impeding inspiratory expansion. The operative procedure is similar to that for pectus excavatum except that the sternum is manipulated into a normal position without the insertion of a plate or wire. Postoperative complications are rare.

Thoracoplasty

Thoracoplasty is the removal of ribs in order to collapse the underlying diseased lung. Originally the operation was devised as primary treatment for pulmonary tuberculosis prior to the availability of antituberculous chemotherapy. Nowadays it may be undertaken for treatment of bronchopulmonary fistulae and empyemas in patients who are immunosuppressed. This often applies to patients suffering from AIDS where tuberculosis and atypical mycobacterial infections do not respond well to chemotherapy and the patients are unable to withstand resectional surgery. The procedure will result in irreversible loss of lung function to the affected area. In the past the operation was staged and only 3–5 ribs would be resected at a time. Today the stages are often undertaken simultaneously.

Physiotherapy key points

- See p. 396.
- Postural reeducation is extremely important due to the high risk of deformity following this procedure. If the first rib and distal attachments of the scalene muscles have been removed, the head and neck are pulled over to the non-affected side. As the rhomboids have been cut, the shoulder on the affected side is raised and medially rotated. To counteract the head displacement, the trunk leans towards the affected side. Postural correction should be achieved in standing and maintained when walking. Early correction with the aid of a mirror will minimize the deformity, but the postural exercises may need to be continued by the patient for about 2 months.
- A firm pad should be applied if there is paradoxical movement of the chest wall.
- Shoulder girdle and arm movements should include depression of the shoulder girdle on the side of the thoracoplasty, retraction of the scapulae, bilateral full range movements and neck lateral lean towards the side of the operation.

SURGERY FOR THE DIAPHRAGM AND OESOPHAGUS

Diaphragm

Traumatic rupture of the diaphragm, more commonly the left hemidiaphragm, occurs because of injury to the chest or abdomen, for example following a road traffic accident (RTA) or from a penetrating wound. Herniation of visceral/abdominal contents into the thoracic cavity may not occur instantly and is therefore often misdiagnosed. The affected lung may collapse as a result, with mediastinal shift away from the rupture site. Repair of the diaphragm will be carried out via a thoracotomy with or without an abdominal incision.

Physiotherapy key points

- There is a risk of empyema developing if stomach contents have ruptured into the pleural space.
- Preoperative chest radiograph may reveal a fluid level secondary to stomach or bowel contents in the thoracic cavity.

Nissen fundoplication for hiatus hernia

This procedure corrects herniation of the stomach through the oesophageal hiatus in the diaphragm. Symptoms of gastric reflux and oesophagitis increase with stooping, straining, coughing and pregnancy. It is corrected via a thoracic or abdominal incision.

Oesophagectomy

Surgical correction involves two main incisions via a laparotomy and a thoracotomy with two small neck incisions posterior to sternomastoid. The resected portion of affected oesophagus may be replaced by a tube of stomach or colon, anastomosed to the oesophageal stump or pharynx if a total resection has been carried out. Resection of oesophageal carcinoma carries a high mortality rate and a 5-year survival rate of less than 5% (Forrest et al 1995).

Physiotherapy key points

- The head-down position is avoided to prevent gastric reflux, which could lead to pulmonary

infection secondary to aspiration and/or breakdown of the anastomosis.
- If dysphagia has been a problem preoperatively, patients are often malnourished and weak which can lengthen the recovery period.
- Extreme care must be taken if nasopharyngeal suction is indicated, as accidental entry of the catheter into the oesophagus may traumatize the anastomosis. Minitracheotomy may be a preferable option if retention of secretions is a problem.
- Restriction of particular neck movements, usually extension, to avoid possible tension on the anastomosis is requested by some surgeons.

Complications of thoracic surgery

Pain. Many complications after thoracic surgery arise due to poor pain control. It is vital that adequate analgesia is given prior to any physiotherapy sessions, but also throughout the day when the patient is performing exercises alone.

Bronchial secretions. The appropriate timing and selection of patients suitable for a minitracheotomy can help reduce the incidence of sputum retention. Patients should be encouraged to huff to move secretions and to cough to clear secretions from the central airways. Numerous bouts of coughing will increase pain and fatigue. Patients should be encouraged to keep up their fluid intake. Heated humidified oxygen should be used in patients with a high oxygen demand or in those who have retained secretions.

Pneumonia is a serious complication with a high mortality rate.

Acute lung injury (ALI)/acute respiratory distress syndrome (ARDS). Five percent of patients undergoing pneumonectomy or lobectomy will develop ALI which has an associated mortality of over 50%. In the worst cases it is indistinguishable from ARDS. There are many suggested triggers for ALI but it is thought that high oxygen concentrations associated with one-lung ventilation or ischaemia reperfusion may lead to a severe inflammatory process which in turn induces endothelial injury (Jordan et al 2000).

Atrial fibrillation is common with extensive resection in the elderly. Onset is usually 2–5 days postoperatively. If there is a compromise in cardiac output then the patient should not be mobilized and should continue with the airway clearance technique. If positive pressure adjuncts are required then haemodynamic monitoring should be performed to prevent any further decrease in cardiac output.

Myocardial infarction. Major surgery performed within 3 months of an acute myocardial infarction has been associated with a reinfarction rate of 30%. Postoperative myocardial infarctions are associated with higher rates of mortality than infarctions in general (Alexander & Anderson 2000).

Wound infection is a problem in approximately 10% of pulmonary resections. This percentage is reduced with the administration of prophylactic antibiotics at the time of anaesthetic induction.

Haemorrhage. Significant bleeding, usually involving the bronchial arteries occurs in 1–2% of patients. It is more likely after a pneumonectomy. Close monitoring of chest drains should be performed before, during and after treatment. If a patient has significant blood loss after surgery then physiotherapy treatment should be suspended until the bleeding has subsided and the medical staff should be informed.

Empyema. This complication of pus in the pleural space occasionally presents a few weeks following surgery. Often these patients have foul-smelling discharge from their wounds, which may cause significant embarrassment and requires very sensitive attention. Deodorizing sprays are available which can significantly assist with the management of this problem.

Bronchopleural fistula (BPF) is rare following a lobectomy but is seen more commonly after a pneumonectomy. If it occurs in the early postoperative period it is likely to be directly linked to the surgical closure of the stump. A classic sign on the chest radiograph is a drop in the fluid level in the pneumonectomy space and is usually associated with the patient coughing up loose brown liquid, i.e. space fluid, through the BPF. This fluid could potentially spill over into the healthy lung and therefore must be drained out

through an intercostal drain. Surgical repair of a chronic BPF fistula may be carried out by stump suturing with or without vascularized pedicle flaps of omentum (Sabanathan & Richardson 1994).

Surgical emphysema. The presence of air in the soft tissues is expected locally around wounds and will be absorbed over a few days. However, if surgical emphysema increases, review of intercostal chest drainage is necessary.

Recurrent laryngeal nerve damage. Palsy of the vocal cord may reduce the effectiveness of the cough mechanism and cause a weak or hoarse voice.

Dysfunction of the phrenic nerve. A persistently raised hemidiaphragm may indicate palsy or paralysis of the phrenic nerve. This may reduce the effectiveness of coughing.

Persistent air leaks and pneumothoraces. A persistent air leak often warrants the presence of a chest drain, which is a potential source of infection, is painful and can limit rehabilitation.

CHEST TRAUMA

There are many causes of chest trauma. The main areas of classification include stab/gunshot wounds, road traffic accidents (RTAs) or other accidents and blast injuries. One-third of patients hospitalized after RTAs have evidence of severe chest trauma (Besson & Saegesser 2000).

Gunshot wounds

If the wound arises from a low-velocity handgun, the damage to surrounding tissues is generally low. If, however, a high-velocity gun is used, this dissipates large amounts of damage to the surrounding tissues, which often require muscle and skin grafting to close the defect.

Simple rib fracture

Rib fractures are the most common thoracic injury and unless they are causing chest wall instability (flail) or are associated with major intrathoracic injury, the main aim is to relieve pain and to prevent pulmonary complications such as atelectasis and infection. Pain control is paramount and should not be overlooked, even with a single rib fracture, as this can produce respiratory complications, especially in the elderly.

Physiotherapy key points

- A great deal of injuring force is required to fracture the first rib, therefore visceral injury is likely to be present. Brachial plexus deficit, absent radial pulse, pulsating supraclavicular mass or widening of the superior mediastinum on radiograph should always be reported to medical staff.
- Intercostal nerve blocks can be a very effective form of pain management in this group of patients.
- Patients usually benefit greatly from early mobilization.
- Patients should be taught how to support the chest wall to facilitate an effective cough.
- Taping or restriction of the chest wall to reduce pain is not advised as this may lead to further respiratory complications. Other methods of pain relief should be considered.

Flail chest

A flail chest may be caused by multiple continuous, comminuted or segmented rib fractures resulting in paradoxical movement of the chest wall, i.e. the flail segment is 'sucked in' during inspiration and 'blown out' during expiration. This can also occur because of disruption of cartilaginous or ligamentous rib attachments. Although paradoxical movement may be marked, the main concern is often pulmonary contusion resulting in reduced lung compliance and atelectasis. If pain and respiratory fatigue are not addressed promptly, respiratory decompensation may ensue a few hours or days later. Epidural analgesia is universally useful in patients with multiple rib fractures (Wisner 1990).

Sternal fractures

Fractures of the sternum occur in approximately 4% of RTA patients (Otremski 1990). Generally these fractures are managed conservatively but if significant displacement has occurred they may require internal fixation. An associated pericardial contusion may also be present.

Scapula fractures

Scapula fractures are uncommon and arise due to a severe force of impact and are therefore usually associated with other injuries. Because of the high incidence of brachial plexus injuries a careful neurological assessment should be performed.

Physiotherapy key points

- Effective pain management is essential to maintain adequate ventilation and allow effective clearance of secretions.
- A cough pad may be supplied to ease the discomfort of coughing.
- Chest shaking and percussion are usually inappropriate, as patients will tend to 'splint' their chest in response to any increase in discomfort and delay of bone union may occur.
- Early mobilization is of great benefit.
- If patients have associated musculoskeletal injuries, especially affecting the shoulder joint, then they should be referred for outpatient rehabilitation.

Pulmonary contusion

Pulmonary contusion is a major component of chest trauma. Parenchymal damage consists of interstitial oedema and haemorrhage, which can result in obliteration of the alveolar space and large areas of consolidation. Hypoventilation and significant pulmonary shunting can occur. The contusion may present as unilateral or bilateral depending on the nature of the injury.

Pulmonary contusions are usually present on the initial chest radiograph. Other causes of an infiltrate such as an aspiration are often not present on the presenting radiograph but become evident a few hours later and are often confined by anatomical pulmonary segments. Contusions can also be misinterpreted as haematomas, although distinguishing features of the latter are that they tend to have defined margins. Chest radiographic findings of varying degrees of patchy consolidation may be very similar to that of ARDS and often co-exist. Close monitoring of fluid balance to avoid pulmonary oedema in lungs that may already have reduced compliance is essential.

Pneumothorax

A pneumothorax can be classed as open, tension or partial (Fig. 12.8).

Open pneumothorax

If an open chest wound is sufficiently large, intrapleural pressure will remain equal to atmospheric pressure and, with each breath, air will be sucked in and out of the chest wall, resulting in marked paroxysmal shift of the mediastinum with each respiratory effort. The subsequent hypoventilation and decreased cardiac output can be life threatening. In the emergency situation closure of the wound by any means should be attempted, followed by surgical closure and insertion of an intercostal drain.

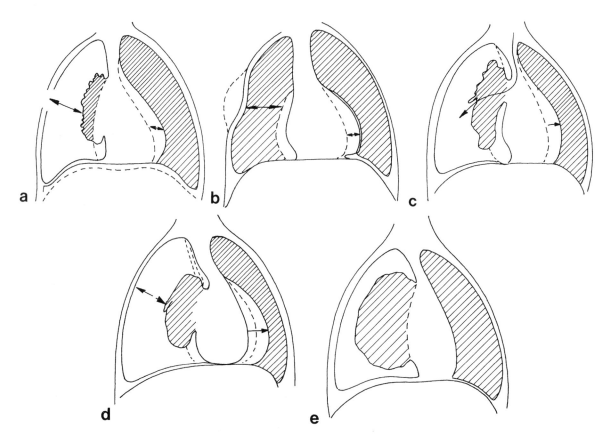

Figure 12.8 **a** Open pneumothorax secondary to chest trauma making respiration totally ineffective as air is sucked in and out of the open wound. **b** Flail chest secondary to multiple anterior and posterior rib fractures, resulting in chest wall instability. **c** Tension pneumothorax allowing air to enter the pleural space with each inspiratory breath. **d** Tension pneumothorax on expiration. The hole in the lung closes on expiration, resulting in a build-up of pressure in the pleural space with mediastinal shift. **e** Partial pneumothorax. Partial collapse of the lung away from the chest wall but not under tension.

Tension pneumothorax

Injury to the lung results in a continuing air leak which acts as a one-way valve, allowing air to progressively accumulate in the pleural space. This creates positive intrathoracic pressure leading to mediastinal shift and compression of the remaining lung and heart. These increasing pressures, if not corrected, can invert the diaphragm, cause subcutaneous emphysema, a decrease in cardiac output and ultimately a cardiorespiratory arrest. Signs and symptoms include surgical emphysema, absent breath sounds on the affected side, mediastinal shift and tracheal deviation to the opposite side, acute respiratory distress, tachycardia and hypotension. When an intercostal drain is inserted into the pleural space, the air is released under pressure.

Partial pneumothorax

This occurs with partial collapse of the lung away from the chest wall but is not 'under tension'. However, the pneumothorax may increase in size at any time and has the potential to develop into a tension pneumothorax.

Haemothorax

This involves accumulation of blood in the pleural space. Approximately 300–500 ml may be present before being evident on an erect chest radiograph. If a supine film is taken a haemothorax of up to 1000 ml may be missed. The source of bleeding may be attributed to the heart, aorta, intercostal arteries or internal mammary artery if a penetrating wound was the cause. It is often associated with a pneumothorax. Surgery to control bleeding will be considered if the immediate loss is greater than 1 litre or if the gradual loss is greater than 100 ml/hour for 4 hours or more (Hood 1990). If the blood has become clotted and cannot be cleared with an intercostal drain, thoracic evacuation of the pleural space will be necessary to avoid formation of a fibrothorax or empyema. This is usually performed as a VATS procedure 1–3 days post injury.

Chylothorax

The accumulation of chyle in the thorax occurs due to damage to the thoracic duct. Patients present with large amounts of chest drainage that is milky in colour when they are on an oral diet. Treatment consists of drainage of the chyle and total parenteral nutrition. If conservative management is unsuccessful, patients may benefit from a pleuroperitoneal shunt or ligation of the thoracic duct at the hiatus.

Tracheal injuries

These may take the form of a crushing injury to the larynx, a transverse tear or complete separation with retraction of the distal segment into the mediastinum. Main causes are RTAs and direct trauma to the neck. Resuturing will be carried out, with some patients requiring tracheostomy postoperatively.

Air embolism

Air embolism occurs in 4% of all major thoracic trauma cases following penetrating or blunt chest injury (Swanson & Trunkey 1989). These patients present with neurological signs, sudden cardiovascular collapse and froth in arterial blood samples. Emergency thoracotomy is required; the hilum of the affected lung is cross-clamped and the patient is placed in the Trendelenburg position, air is removed from the left ventricle and any lacerations in the lung oversewn. Occasionally a lobectomy or pneumonectomy is required (Swanson & Trunkey 1989).

Major bronchial injuries

These are normally caused by blunt trauma to either main bronchus resulting in circumferntial laceration with complete or partial separation. Lobar bronchi are less commonly affected. An incomplete laceration heals with stricture formation, resulting in recurrent collapse/infection leading to parenchymal destruction. A sleeve resection may be necessary (p. 395). In the case of complete laceration both ends of the severed bronchus granulate and heal. The distal bronchial tree fills with mucus and the affected lung collapses. Early surgery is required to carry out reanastomosis.

Cardiac and great vessel injury

This is usually secondary to a RTA where the steering wheel compresses the heart between the sternum and the vertebrae. As a result, myocardial contusion with or without tamponade commonly occurs. There is usually associated trauma to the anterior chest wall. Emergency thoracotomy is required to drain the blood from the pericardium. Cardiac tamponade is suspected if there is profound shock and low cardiac output. This is manifested by hypotension, tachycardia, elevated jugular venous pressure, poor urinary output and peripheral shutdown.

Thoracic aorta and branches

Injuries occur secondary to flexion or torsional forces. Aortic rupture results in immediate death unless a false aneurysm has formed in the periaortic tissue and pleura. In these cases immediate surgery is necessary but carries a high risk of fatal bleeding. For this reason patients are put on to partial bypass so that the aorta is cross-clamped, enabling an end-to-end anastomosis or Dacron patch to be performed.

CORONARY ARTERY DISEASE

Chronic myocardial ischaemia is one of the most frequent illnesses affecting the general population in the Western world. The primary pathophysiological process is an imbalance between myocardial oxygen supply and demand. This commonly arises from atherosclerotic coronary disease. The predominant clinical feature is usually chronic angina pectoris although some patients suffer from silent ischaemia. Despite effective medical therapy a significant number of these patients require coronary artery revascularization. The factors which determine revascularization are angina refractory to medical therapy and unfavourable coronary anatomy.

The two standard forms of revascularization are percutaneous coronary angioplasty (PTCA), with or without stents and coronary artery bypass grafts (CABG). CABG is usually performed if three or more coronary vessels are involved together with a reduction in left ventricular ejection fraction (LVEF), in the presence of a positive non-invasive stress test or if the left main stem is narrowed by more than 50%. In some patients with two-vessel disease of which one is the left anterior descending artery, CABG is also indicated. The beneficial effect of CABG on mortality compared to medical therapy has been conclusively demonstrated in several multicentre trials (Simons & Laham 1999).

The use of PTCA is based on the likelihood of a successful procedure and near-complete revascularization. PTCA is usually reserved for patients with one- or two-vessel disease. Advances in catheter and stent design have allowed multiple stent procedures to be performed in a single patient (Laham et al 1997). The drawback of PTCA and stenting is that 30% of patients suffer with in-stent restenosis within the first 6 months and require repeat procedures (Hoffman & Mintz 2000). A large multicentred study comparing the effectiveness of CABG to PTCA in 1205 patients with multivessel disease found CABG to be 14% more effective at reducing incidence of major cardiac and cerebrovascular events after one year, but there was a trend for the effectiveness of CABG to decrease with age. This was not evident in the stented group. The optimal treatment strategy may differ between age groups, with stenting being more effective in the older patient population (Disco 2000).

Despite the success of conventional medical and mechanical revascularization, a significant number of patients with ischaemic heart disease are not suitable candidates for PTCA or CABG or only incomplete revascularization is achieved with these techniques. This patient population is often referred to as 'no-option patients'.

There is therefore a need for alternative treatments in order to alleviate angina and improve myocardial function. Possible therapies which have been developed for these no-option patients are transmyocardial revascularization, angiogenesis and enhanced external counterpulsation (EECP).

Transmyocardial revascularization (TMR) and percutaneous myocardial revascularization (PMR)

A variety of techniques including needles, lasers and boring devices have been used to channel holes through the left ventricle in an attempt to emulate a reptilian circulation. The precise mechanism of action remains uncertain but suggested hypotheses include angiogenesis resulting from the release of growth factors and inflammatory mediators, perfusion through the channels and myocardial denervation resulting in a reduction in angina. The technique remains controversial. Early open studies suggested improvements in angina class and exercise tolerance but no improvement in objective measures of LVEF or myocardial perfusion.

Randomized controlled studies have been contradictory. One study, which followed 198 patients after TMR, found that compared to patients receiving medical therapy, TMR lead to a reduction in unstable angina episodes, improved myocardial perfusion and reduced hospitalizations (March 1999). However, a subsequent trial was unable to reproduce such significant improvements (Schofield et al 1999). The placebo effect associated with surgery may have contributed to the positive results demonstrated in the first study. The development of a percutaneous technique has enabled the inclusion of a control group, which is totally blinded to therapy. Phase II Biosense DIRECT trials in the United States and Europe are currently under way and will assist in determining whether this technique does in fact lead to myocardial revascularization.

Angiogenesis

Angiogenesis is the stimulation of blood vessel growth by a group of proteins known as angiogenic growth factors. The aim of this therapy is to produce a 'biological bypass' and to increase myocardial perfusion. There are a number of these proteins including vascular endothelial growth factor (VEGF), fibroblast growth factor (FGF) and master switch genes such as hypoxia-inducible factor (HIF-1α), which are capable of stimulating an upregulation of a number of growth factors and their receptors. The growth factors are thought to stimulate the extracellular matrix breakdown and proliferation and migration of endothelial and smooth muscle cells. This leads to the formation of endothelial tubes, which then have deposition of new matrix to stabilize the vessel and form a mature vessel. Again the mechanisms of action are complex and experimental microbiology is continually identifying new factors, receptors and inhibitors of angiogenesis.

Over the past few years a number of preclinical studies have demonstrated angiogenesis induced by growth factor therapy. These have been followed by a number of clinical studies. The administration of growth factors clinically has been via direct epicardial injection as an open approach (Losordo 1998), as an intravenous or intracoronary infusion (Henry et al 1998), as slow-release beads implanted into the myocardium as an adjunct to CABG (Laham 1999) or percutaneously via a cardiac catheter as endocardial injections. Preliminary efficacy data like those for TMR have reported improvements in exercise tolerance and angina class and quality of life. In the studies by Laham et al 1999 there were also improvements in target wall motion and perfusion demonstrated by magnetic resonance imaging (MRI). Most of these studies, however, have been open-blinded and have lacked a placebo group. Large double-blinded randomized controlled studies are currently under way in Europe and the United States to further define the role of therapeutic angiogenesis for advanced coronary artery disease.

Enhanced external counterpulsation (EECP)

EECP is a developing outpatient treatment for no-option patients. The mechanisms of action are similar to that of the intraaortic balloon pump

(IABP) in that it is designed to augment diastolic blood flow to the coronary arteries and reduce the left ventricular workload. This is achieved by three sets of external compressive cuffs which are applied to the patient's calves, lower and upper thighs. These are sequentially inflated and deflated with the timing of the cardiac cycle via the ECG. During diastole the cuffs are inflated sequentially from the calves to the upper thighs which 'milks' the venous return back to the heart. Theoretically, the increase in venous return should result in an increased cardiac output by the Frank Starling mechanism and increase coronary perfusion pressure. The cuffs are rapidly deflated just prior to the onset of systole, resulting in a rapid drop in diastolic pressure, which leads to unloading of the left ventricle and a reduction in myocardial workload.

Early experience in the USA showed anecdotal evidence of improvements in quality of life, exercise tolerance and reduction in episodes of angina. Subsequently, a multicentre placebo-controlled trial of 139 patients confirmed that EECP reduced angina and extended the time period to exercise-induced angina in patients with symptomatic coronary artery disease (Arora et al 1999). Although this is encouraging, further research is ongoing to validate the use of EECP for the treatment of end-stage myocardial ischaemia.

CARDIAC SURGERY

Owing to advancements over the years in anaesthetics, cardiopulmonary bypass and myocardial management, many patients undergoing heart surgery can now expect shorter operating times with fewer complications.

The commonest indications for adults undergoing heart surgery are coronary artery and valve disease. Surgery for correction of rhythm disorders, ventricular aneurysms and aortic coarctation will also be encountered. Advancements in surgical techniques now enable CABG to be performed without cardiopulmonary bypass and robotic minimally invasive surgery has now lead to CABG being performed through thoracoscopic ports. These techniques will be discussed later in 'Advances in cardiac surgery'.

Cardiopulmonary bypass

Open heart surgery is most commonly performed with cardiopulmonary bypass. This involves placing a cannula in the right atrium to drain blood away from the heart to a bypass machine where it is oxygenated and filtered before pumping it back into the systemic circulation, via another cannula, into the ascending aorta. Administration of cold cardioplegic solution and topical cooling will result in a hypothermic diastolic arrest, enabling the surgeon to operate on a non-beating, bloodless heart. The lungs are redundant during this procedure and are partially or totally collapsed. Oxygenation of the blood is carried out by the bypass machine. At the end of the operation, systemic rewarming is commenced until the heart reverts spontaneously or with the aid of direct current (D/C) conversion, to sinus rhythm.

Cardiopulmonary bypass causes derangements of intrinsic coagulation and fibrolytic systems. In some centres there has been renewed interest in carrying out cardiac surgery without the aid of cardiopulmonary bypass (Westaby 1995). If appropriate at the time of operation, temporary pacing wires will be attached to the ventricle or atrium and pericardial, mediastinal and pleural drains inserted as necessary. The sternum is closed with steel wires.

Coronary artery bypass grafting

The principal indications for CABG are angina pectoris and failed medical and/or previous surgical management. The preferred conduits for grafting are either reversed segments of the patient's own saphenous vein (SV), providing it is free from varicosities and deep vein thrombosis (DVT) or the internal mammary arteries (IMA) which have a much higher patency rate. At 10 years the patency rate for a SV graft is 40–60% compared to greater than 90% for an IMA graft (Lytle & Cosgrove 1992). The IMA graft appears especially suitable for grafting of the anterior descending coronary artery. However, owing to the delicate structure of the IMA, a longer operating time is required for mobilization of the vessel and a pleural drain is often required because the pleural space has been entered. Multiple arterial grafts are now more commonly performed utilizing both internal mammary arteries, the epigastric or radial arteries. There is generally an increased operative time associated with multiple arterial grafts but the rate of graft failure is slower than when vein grafts are used.

Generally 95% of patients undergoing CABG are either completely free from symptoms or greatly improved at 1 year following surgery. Approximately 90% of patients are alive at 5 years, 75% at 10 years and 60% at 15 years (European Coronary Surgery Study Group 1980). Video-assisted endoscopic techniques are beginning to be used in surgical correction of coronary or cardiac lesions and do not need cardiopulmonary bypass (Lin et al 1996).

Advances in cardiac surgery

Off-bypass CABG

Off-bypass CABG may provide a safer form of revascularization for high-risk patients because it avoids the side effects of cardiopulmonary bypass. The Medtronic Octopus System is a stabilizing device which has multiple suckers which attach to the epicardial surface of the heart. In 1997 three or more grafts were performed using this device on 24.6% of patients requiring CABG and by 1999, this had increased to 55.9%. Permanent stroke occurred in 0.6% of patients and operative mortality was 1% (Hart et al 2000). Octopus off-pump bypass was demonstrated in this study to be a safe procedure with increasing applicability. It is now possible to revascularize all territories with this technique.

Robotic endoscopic heart surgery

The introduction of voice-activated robotic endoscopic systems has enabled surgeons to perform CABG without the need for a sternotomy (Cichon et al 2000). This technique is only available in relatively few centres, but it appears to be able to achieve arterial revascularization with a significant reduction in surgical trauma.

Endoscopic robotic surgery has now been performed on the arrested as well as the beating heart (Boehm et al 1999). Clinical trials are ongoing.

Valvular heart disease

The commonest causes of diseased heart valves are childhood rheumatic fever, congenital abnormalities, endocarditis and collagen vascular disorders, e.g. Marfan's syndrome. The valves may become incompetent, leading to regurgitation or stenosis with or without calcification. Breathlessness, fatigue and cyanosis due to increased workload of the myocardium and lungs are the commonest symptoms. There is a high risk of sudden death associated with aortic stenosis even if the patient is free of symptoms.

Surgical management

Valvuloplasty. Balloon valvuloplasty entails a small balloon flotation catheter crossing the interatrial septum, enlarging the opening and then passing a larger balloon which is inflated through the orifice. This technique has virtually negated the need for open valvotomy via a thoracotomy.

Annuloplasty. This is the refashioning of the annulus which is part of the valve apparatus which may become calcified or dilated.

Open valvotomy. Requires cardiopulmonary bypass and the valve is incized under direct vision.

Valve replacement. Replacement valves may be classed as mechanical prostheses or bioprostheses (tissue valves). Mechanical valves are categorized into two major groups: the caged-ball, e.g. Starr–Edwards, which has a durability of up to 35 years; and the tilting disc, e.g. St Jude. Lifelong anticoagulation is required following insertion of a mechanical valve. Tissue valves were developed to overcome the risk of thromboembolism and may be divided into two groups, the first being porcine heterografts which are preserved in glutaraldehyde and mounted on a strut, e.g. Carpentier–Edwards. Anticoagulant therapy is still necessary in some cases. The second group are classed as homografts as they are harvested from human cadavers and placed in situ without the aid of a strut. A Ross procedure is sometimes performed for aortic valve replacement in which the individual's own pulmonary valve is transplanted to the aortic position and the pulmonary valve is replaced with a homograft.

Coarctation of the aorta

This is a localized thickening and infolding of the media of the aortic wall which causes obstruction to aortic flow at the site where, postnatally, the ductus undergoes obliteration. Resection of the narrowed portion is advized to avoid systemic hypertension and its inherent risks. An end-to-end anastomosis is normally carried out with occasional insertion of a Dacron graft.

Ventricular aneurysms

The aneurysm usually occurs as a result of transmural myocardial infarction, which leads to an area of ventricular scar tissue. Consequently the affected area is unable to contract effectively. Repair is carried out by resection or patching.

Surgical treatment of tachyarrhythmias

The aim of surgery is to excise, isolate or interrupt tissue in the heart responsible for triggering the tachycardia, while preserving or improving myocardial function. The appropriate layer of endocardium may be peeled off or cryoablation used to isolate areas of the ventricle that cannot be resected.

Postoperative management

Extubation within 3 hours of cardiac surgery is preferable in most non-complicated cases (Higgins 1992). Patients may remain in the recovery area for a few hours or on the ICU for up to 12–24 hours, depending on their cardiovascular status, before being transferred to the high-dependency area or postoperative ward.

Continuous monitoring of the patient's cardiac status is necessary until the patient is stable. See Chapter 9 for mechanical circulatory support devices.

Complications of cardiac surgery

Perioperative myocardial infarction can have major adverse effects on early and late prognosis.

Bleeding. Two to five percent of CABG patients are reopened for control of bleeding (Shainoff et al 1994). Cardiac tamponade occurs owing to haemorrhage into the pericardium causing pressure on the heart and prevention of filling during diastole. The clinical signs are tachycardia and hypotension. Cardiac arrest may result if the chest is not reopened to remove clots and stop the bleeding.

Hypertension is a problem in up to one-third of patients. The actual mechanism for this rise in blood pressure is unknown (Colvin & Kenny 1989). Hypertension is aggressively managed in the early postoperative period to reduce the stress on the newly anastomosed grafts.

Low cardiac output occurs secondary to hypovolaemia, myocardial stunning, heart failure or severe sepsis.

Arrhythmias can be induced by myocardial irritability secondary to surgery or because of electrolyte imbalances. Occasionally permanent rhythm problems arise, requiring pacing.

Atrial fibrillation presents in approximately 40% of patients within 2–3 days of surgery (Frost et al 1992). There is an increased risk of pulmonary embolism due to stasis of blood within the atrium. Atrial fibrillation can also compromise left ventricular filling, leading to a reduction in cardiac output.

Lower lobe collapse, particularly of the left lung, is present in the majority of patients, owing to the compression of the lower lobe during surgery and/or damage to the phrenic nerve through trauma or cold injury secondary to cardioplegia (Markand et al 1985).

Reduced lung volumes are thought to be attributable to alterations in rib cage mechanics.

Pulmonary infection can arise due to prolonged intubation, reduced mucociliary clearance and resistant atelectasis.

Pulmonary oedema may occur secondary to excessive fluid replacement to correct low volume states and also due to inflammatory mediated changes resulting from cardiopulmonary bypass.

Pleural effusions are particularly common after internal mammary artery grafts.

Pneumothorax/haemothorax is often a consequence of opening the chest wall and particularly after harvesting of the internal mammary artery.

Impairment of renal perfusion due to low cardiac output or vasoconstriction secondary to inotropic support may require temporary renal replacement therapy. Confusion may be clinically evident with electrolyte imbalances. The level of potassium should also be checked prior to treatment as abnormalities can give rise to significant arrhythmias.

Major wound complications such as mediastinitis and/or wound dehiscence affect 1% of patients (Loop et al 1990). After sternotomy the sternum may fail to unite necessitating rewiring. Dehiscence is more common after bilateral internal mammary grafts.

Intellectual dysfunction in the early postoperative period occurs in 75% of patients but major long-term problems are uncommon (Shaw et al 1986a). It is thought to be secondary to multiple emboli resulting in impaired cerebral perfusion induced by cardiopulmonary bypass. The risk is also greater with an increased time on cardiopulmonary bypass.

Stroke occurs in 1–5% percent of patients and is age related (Shaw et al 1986b). Significant aortic and carotid atherosclerotic disease are also risk factors.

Physiotherapy key points

- For management of physiotherapy problems on the intensive care unit, see Chapter 11. The guidelines for pre- and postoperative physiotherapy management are similar to those discussed for the general surgical patient (pp. 383–387) but the following points should be noted.
- The physiotherapist may find Box 12.1 useful in assessment of the postoperative cardiac surgical patient.

Box 12.1   Postoperative observations following cardiac surgery

Cardiovascular
- Heart rate – spontaneous or paced
- Arrhythmias – frequency and severity
- Blood pressure, central venous pressure
- Presence of left ventricular assist devices
- Cardiac output
- Urine output
- Presence of pacing wires, mediastinal drains
- Core to peripheral temperature
- Blood loss in past 24 hours
- Haemoglobin
- Electrolytes especially levels of potassium (K^+)

Respiratory
- Respiration – spontaneous or mechanical
- Ventilatory parameters – rate, mode, pressure, FiO_2
- Rate and depth of respiration
- Arterial blood gases and SaO_2
- Pleural drains, amount of fluid loss and presence of air leak
- Chest radiograph pre- and post drain removal
- Auscultation
- Bronchial secretions

Neurological
- Level of consciousness
- Signs of confusion
- Gross movement of all limbs
- Presence and severity of pain
- Electrolyte levels

Musculoskeletal
- Incisions
- Presence of a clicking sternum
- Swelling around vein or artery graft harvest sites
- Restrictions of movement or pain especially around the shoulder, thoracic spine and the lower limbs including graft sites

Pharmacology
- Sedation and paralysis
- Inotropic support
- Analgesia – frequency, type and strength

Miscellaneous
- Sleep deprivation
- Nausea and vomiting

- Patients who require IABP support are normally nursed supine. The IABP can be triggered either by the ECG trace or by cardiac pressures. It is advisable to change the trigger to 'pressures' if any techniques, e.g. movement/shakings/vibrations, disrupt the ECG signal, as interference with the IABP trigger can reduce the assistance the IABP gives to left ventricular function. If a side-lying position is indicated, due to lung pathology, at least three people should be used to perform the turn. The leg, which has the femoral sheath in situ, should be kept straight during the turn so that kinking of the IABP does not occur at the hip joint. Generally one person controls the leg, one the endotracheal tube and the other performs the turn. Patients can be nursed on either side as long as these principles are adhered to. Manual hyperinflation may further compromise a low cardiac output and if indicated should be carried out with caution and careful monitoring.

- Monitoring of blood pressure is essential to avoid excessive pressure on newly grafted vessels. The head-down position increases atrial pressure and is usually not indicated or tolerated by patients after cardiac surgery. Periods of unexplained hypertension may occur in patients following resection of aortic coarctation.
- It is important to give advice regarding positioning both during rest periods in bed and when sitting in a chair (Fig. 6.43).
- Reduced or bronchial breath sounds, especially in the left lower lobe, are a common finding and may persist even in an ambulant, apyrexial patient.
- In uncomplicated cases, early mobilization and supported huffing and coughing may be all that is necessary (Jenkins & Bourn 1992, Jenkins et al 1989).
- Stair climbing is introduced once the patient is cardiovascularly stable when walking for a reasonable distance on the flat. This generally occurs on the fourth or fifth day after surgery. However, with many patients being discharged as early as day 4 postoperatively, stair climbing may be started as early as 3 days postoperatively in appropriate cases.
- The use of CPAP may be indicated in persistent, problematic lung collapse. This can be combined with mobilizing on the spot. IPPB may be useful if retained secretions are a problem.
- Support of the sternal wound may be carried out by the patient using a pillow, 'cough-lock'

or towel to assist huffing and coughing. Particular attention should be paid to sternal support if a sternal click is heard or palpated. It should always be stressed that the 'cough-lock' should be tightened for coughing and any situations which may induce unwanted movement of the sternum, such as straining or getting in/out of bed and loosened in between use.

- Postural correction and gentle shoulder girdle exercises are encouraged. If shoulder joint stiffness is a problem then gentle, bilateral shoulder exercises are taught. For those patients with persistent chest wall pain of musculoskeletal origin, manual therapy techniques may help relieve symptoms (see Ch. 6).
- It is common for patients to feel depressed after the first few days following surgery or in the period following discharge from hospital. The patient should be reassured that this is a recognized feature of the recovery period.
- Prior to discharge the patient should be given advice regarding management of activities of daily living. A graduated, daily walking programme is generally advized but should be combined with rest periods of up to 1–2 hours each day. The distance walked should be increased at the patient's discretion, but it is hoped that the majority of patients should be able to manage 3–4 miles after 6 weeks (barring any complications and/or past medical history which would inhibit their progress). Common sense should prevail for those living in hilly areas and if possible, they should be driven to a flatter area to carry out the exercise programme. Patients themselves should not drive for at least 6 weeks to allow sternal healing. It is for this reason also that heavy work or lifting should be avoided for approximately 3 months. Sexual activity may be resumed as soon as the patient feels able; usually a good indication is being able to climb two flights of stairs. A passive position is recommended. Depending on the patient's occupation, the majority will return to work at around 3 months following surgery. Some centres offer cardiac rehabilitation but in the long term all patients who are able would benefit from

regular exercise such as swimming, walking and cycling. Advice/information on a general healthy lifestyle should also be made available to patients and their families.

MINIMAL ACCESS SURGERY

Over the last decade, there has been an increasing trend towards minimal access surgical procedures which aim to minimize the surgical trauma to the patient without compromising treatment efficacy and safety. This form of surgery is dependent on technology such as image display systems and specialized laparoscopic instruments as well as the skill of the operator. Laparoscopic surgery has been applied in both the diagnostic and therapeutic fields. Most abdominal procedures have been attempted using laparoscopic techniques and can be classified as:

- Group 1: established benefit to the extent of replacing open procedures such as cholecystectomy, anti-reflux surgery, nerve sections, splenectomy and adrenelectomy for non-malignant tumours
- Group 2: safe and probably beneficial but further research required, e.g. hernia repair, appendicectomy, segmental colonic resection for diverticular disease, distal pancreatic resection, oesophagectomy for oesophageal cancer and palliative bypass for inoperable cancer
- Group 3: currently under evaluation and not practised outside clinical trials. Such procedures include colonic cancer and laparoscopic liver resections
- Group 4: unsuitable with no benefit and associated high-risk factors, i.e. major resections, usually for cancer (Cuschieri & Houston 2000).

The technique is normally performed under general anaesthesia with a small incision made to insert a cannula to facilitate the introduction of carbon dioxide to create a pneumoperitoneum. A pressure of 10–12 mmHg is used in adults in order to ensure adequate lifting of the abdominal wall and facilitate exposure of organs. The peri-

toneal cavity may then be visualized through the laparoscope and a video camera allows the picture to be transmitted on to a monitor. Most procedures require additional portals (commonly 5–10 mm in diameter) for the passage of instruments, including diathermy devices and retractors.

The main advantage of this technique is a reduction in postoperative pain, possibly linked to decreased tissue handling and injury. Other benefits include fewer pulmonary complications and a shorter hospital stay with an earlier return to work compared with open procedures (Sawyers 1996). The disadvantages are the cost of training surgeons and the instrumentation, the increased duration of the operation and the possibility that the procedure may have to be converted to an open procedure if difficulties arise (Sawyers 1996). There are potential side effects to the creation of a positive pressure pneumoperitoneum secondary to carbon dioxide absorption, such as reduced cardiac output, hepatic, splanchnic and renal blood flow as well as increased preload, systemic and pulmonary vascular resistance. Gas embolism is a very rare but lethal complication.

Gasless laparoscopy is an option whereby an internal retracting device is placed through a small incision to lift the anterior abdominal wall (Smith et al 1993). Although this technique avoids the side effects of carbon dioxide and increased intraabdominal pressure, exposure is inadequate for many procedures. This situation can be improved if a low pressure (4–6 mmHg) of carbon dioxide insufflation is introduced.

The anticipated widespread introduction of minimal access surgery has been tempered by increased complication rates. The specific benefits of certain procedures continue to be evaluated in terms of efficacy and cost benefit. Master–slave manipulators are available in some centres and current models enable telepresence surgery which entails the surgeon operating via a console at a variable distance from the operating table. It is envisaged that this technique will be used for delicate microvascular surgery in the future (Cuschieri & Houston 2000).

The majority of patients undergoing laparo-scopic surgery do not require physiotherapy input as they are normally fully mobile from a very early stage postoperatively. However, if a patient presents with other high-risk factors or develops unexpected complications, physiotherapy treatment may be appropriate.

ADULT LIVER TRANSPLANTATION

Liver transplantation is indicated in irreversible (acute or chronic) end-stage liver disease which is unresponsive to conventional medical or surgical therapy and when life expectancy is judged to be less than 1 year. Quality of life should also be taken into consideration since this may become unacceptable due to a variety of associated symptoms, such as extreme disabling lethargy, progressive muscle wasting, intractable pruritis, recurrent oesophageal variceal bleeding, ascites and hepatic encephalopathy. Fulminant hepatic failure (FHF) is a less common but important indication for transplant and is defined as the development of hepatic encephalopathy within 8 weeks of the onset of symptoms in a patient without previous liver disease. In the United Kingdom, paracetamol overdose is the commonest cause of FHF (Mutimer 1994). Survival rates at 1 year for patients with benign disease undergoing elective transplant now exceed 90% in many centres with predicted 10-year survival rates of approximately 70% (Buckels 1997).

Orthotopic liver transplantation (OLT)

In this procedure the whole diseased liver is removed and replaced by a cadaveric liver in the same position. A bilateral subcostal incision with median extension to the xiphoid process is required. Many surgeons use venovenous bypass, where blood is diverted from the liver via the inferior vena cava and returned to the circulation via the axillary vein, thus ensuring portal and systemic decompression. The transplant procedure may last up to 10 hours during complex cases.

Recent advances in surgical procedures have enabled the splitting of the cadaveric liver, thus increasing the availability of donor organs. For an adult recipient a left lobe graft from a donor of the same weight will provide approximately 30–35% of standard liver volume, which is adequate to sustain liver function (Busuttil & Goss 1999). Though successful in children, the use of left lobe grafts is not without significant problems in adults. These are often related to the graft not being large enough for an adult recipient. As a result some centres are adopting the use of larger right lobe grafts in adult-to-adult living transplantation. It has been suggested that the future of these techniques may be self-limiting as only 15–20% of potential adult donors are suitable for the procedure (Belghuti & Durand 2000).

Following liver transplantation patients are routinely ventilated and admitted to the ICU. In uncomplicated cases, the patient may be extubated within 24 hours. In patients with FHF, signs of encephalopathy may be evident for several days following the procedure and there may often be a need for prolonged ventilation. Studies from the United Kingdom suggest that patients spend an average of 4 days in the ICU and a median total hospital stay of 43 days (Burroughs et al 1992).

Physiotherapy key points

- The majority of patients undergoing an elective procedure can be assessed during the preoperative work-up period. Guidelines are similar to those for any patient undergoing major upper abdominal surgery but the following points should also be noted.
- Patients with chronic end-stage liver disease can present with very poor mobility and exercise tolerance secondary to long-term malnourishment, progressive muscle wasting and excessive fatigue. Muscle wasting may be 'masked' by generalized oedema.
- Patients suffer from depression, often linked to poor quality of life and this should always be taken into consideration.
- Arterial hypoxaemia is relatively common in liver disease patients so pulse oximetry may be advisable when assessing exercise tolerance.
- Patients may be at high-risk of oesophageal variceal bleeding. If nasopharyngeal suction is

indicated, close liaison with medical staff and extreme caution are advised due to the risk of misplacement of the catheter and trauma resulting in a massive, life-threatening bleed.

- Postoperative pulmonary complications are common and may be secondary to the long anaesthetic times and a prolonged period of supine positioning during the procedure.
- The right phrenic nerve can be damaged during the procedure, leading to a raised right hemidiaphragm and lower lobe collapse.
- Ascites, if present, can result in reduced chest wall compliance and static and dynamic lung volumes.
- Reduced immunosuppression increases the risk of secondary infection.
- The majority of patients develop a right pleural effusion but less than one-third of these are clinically significant.
- Pressure on the common peroneal nerve is a relatively common event during and after surgery in the sicker patient and the temporary use of drop foot splints may be appropriate.
- Liver biopsies are carried out in the early postoperative period. Due to the risk of bleeding, patients usually undergo a period of bedrest for a few hours following the procedure. Physiotherapy should whenever possible be avoided during this time.
- In uncomplicated cases patients are often able to mobilize independently within a few days. However, some patients need a longer period of rehabilitation.

HEAD AND NECK SURGERY

Squamous cell carcinoma (SCC) of the head and neck is the fifth most common malignancy in males and the seventh most common in females worldwide (Parkin et al 1993). Tumours of the head and neck may involve the oral cavity oropharynx, larynx and hypopharynx.

The past decade has seen advances in microsurgical free tissue transfer techniques that have improved outcomes in pharyngo-oesophageal reconstruction.

Resection with primary closure may be adequate to clear some tumours. If, however, there has been metastatic spread to other tissues, a partial or radical neck dissection or the more extensive commando procedure may be indicated (Maran 1995).

When reconstructive surgery is necessary this may involve a variety of techniques.

- Split skin grafting.
- Musculocutaneous flaps using pectoralis major or, less commonly, trapezius and latissimus dorsi to provide single-stage reconstruction of pharyngo-oesophageal defects which can have disappointing long-term functional results.
- Radial forearm flaps which have thin, pliable skin ideal for restoration of the oral cavity and oropharynx and easily manipulated to form a tube to reconstruct the pharynx.
- Fibula free flaps which can provide up to 25 cm of vascularized bone for defects involving the mandible. Cutaneous portions of radial forearm and fibula flaps may also be used for sensory reinnervation through neural anastomoses.
- Rectus abdominis flaps are normally selected for reconstruction of skull base defects or during subtotal or total glossectomy.
- Organ transposition of the stomach or colon requires major upper abdominal and/or thoracic incisions. Vascularized free jejunal flaps are often used for defects of the lower pharyngeal space.

Surgery involving flaps which contain long vascular pedicles that reach the recipient vessels without requiring vein grafting contribute to the very low incidence of reconstructive complications (Blackwell 1999).

If the larynx has been removed this will result in loss of speech and a permanent tracheostomy. For patients undergoing surgery which does not entail a laryngectomy, a tracheostomy may still be required. This may only be a temporary measure to protect the airway from aspiration and compression from swelling in the surrounding structures in the early postoperative period.

Speech and language therapists will be involved with patients who have subsequent swallowing defects and those who require training in voice restoration. Oesophageal speech can be achieved by making a puncture in the tracheo-oesophageal wall and filling it with a unidirectional prosthesis that allows for diversion of pulmonary air into the oesophagus. By closing the tracheostoma manually, air is directed through the valve to an air chamber enclosed by soft tissue at the top of the oesophagus (pseudoglottis) which subsequently vibrates and acts as 'vocal folds'. Manual stoma closure can be impractical and unhygienic. New tracheostoma valves (TSV) being developed close the stoma by an inhalation of air which can allow the patient to speak for longer in one breath and improve the quality of speech. Another advantage of the new TSV is that it does not have to be removed from the stoma during coughing (Geertsema et al 1999).

The resultant quality of speech after pharyngo-laryngectomy surgery with free jejunal interposition reconstruction is significantly less intelligible than the voice produced by the majority of patients undergoing total laryngectomy (McAuliffe et al 2000). Alternatively speech may be facilitated by a laryngeal speech aid. The loss of speech and the possibility of severe facial disfigurement following some types of surgery can have devastating effects which need to be taken into consideration when caring for these patients.

Current research is indicating the feasibility of larynx-preserving techniques but further clinical trials are required (Lefebvre 2000).

Physiotherapy key points

- See Chapter 11 for tracheostomy management.
- In the early postoperative period following laryngectomy, fluid intake should be closely monitored until the patient's airways have become accustomed to the loss of upper airway humidification. Continuous, heated humidification via a tracheostomy mask should be provided.
- Patients requiring long-term or permanent tracheostomy should be taught general tracheostomy care, including airway suction. Family and carers should also be involved in teaching.

- Patients may be nursed in high sitting to minimize facial oedema following removal of lymph nodes, this problem being exacerbated in the case of bilateral neck dissection with bilateral removal of lymph nodes.
- If the patient has undergone extensive surgical resection respiratory complications are expected, especially if upper abdominal or thoracic incisions have been necessary. If indicated, incentive spirometers can be adapted for use by patients with a tracheostomy and/or laryngectomy (Tan 1995).
- Close liaison with the surgeon is essential where muscles have been resected or grafted as postural, neck and shoulder exercises may initially have to be avoided or modified to ensure that the graft is established and that the brachial plexus is not stretched. If the spinal accessory nerve has been affected following surgery, shoulder abduction may be reduced. The rhomboids and serratus muscles often compensate in the case of trapezius denervation. Patients may also have a restricted range of movement of the shoulder, even in the absence of nerve involvement. Rehabilitation of upper and lower limbs affected by the use of free tissue transfer techniques may be necessary. Commonly, partial weight bearing with a walking frame or elbow crutches is advized following a fibular or iliac graft.

VASCULAR SURGERY

The option to use minimally invasive endovascular treatment currently exists for the majority of common vascular surgical procedures (Dodds 1998).

Aortic aneurysm

An aneurysm occurs as a result of degeneration of the media and elastica lamina of the arterial wall of the aorta, leading to local dilatation. The majority of aneurysms occur in the abdominal aorta but can also affect the thoracic aorta. Patients who present as emergency cases with aneurysm rupture will be in hypovolaemic shock due to leakage or rupture of the aneurysm and require immediate surgical repair. The risk of rupture increases significantly with aneurysms which are 5 cm or more in size (Guirguis & Barber 1991).

Abdominal aortic aneurysm (AAA)

Approximately 95% of abdominal aortic aneurysms occur below the level of the renal arteries. Surgical repair therefore should not directly affect the blood supply to the kidneys or other viscera.

Open surgical repair of an abdominal aortic aneurysm involves a horizontal transabdominal or vertical incision, cross-clamping of the aorta above and below the affected area, resection of the thrombi and insertion of Dacron tubing to bridge the resection. Alternatively, a 'trouser' bifurcation graft may be anastomosed distally to the iliac and femoral arteries. Transfemoral, endovascular repair of AAA using endoluminal stents attached to prosthetic grafts has been proven to be feasible and avoids the need for extensive abdominal incisions, minimizes aortic clamp time and facilitates surgery under local anaesthesia (Chuter et al 1993, Parodi et al 1991). Further studies are required to test the long-term outcomes regarding the durability of this procedure.

Thoracic aortic aneurysm (TAA)

Thoracic aortic aneurysms are less common than infrarenal aneurysms. Some patients with an AAA will also have thoracic extension of the aneurysm. Thoracoabdominal aneurysms may be classified into four types:

- Type I – aneurysm affecting the descending thoracic and proximal abdominal aorta
- Type II – aneurysm affecting all of the descending and abdominal aorta
- Type III – aneurysm affecting the distal thoracic and all of the abdominal aorta
- Type IV – aneurysm affecting the upper aorta from which the visceral arteries arise.

If a thoracic aortic aneurysm is being repaired an aortic valve replacement may also be necessary at the time of operation. Cardiac problems may be evident from aortic valve stretching or compression of the pulmonary artery or right ventricle. Dissecting ascending thoracic aneurysms may result in upper limb ischaemia. Descending aneurysms can lead to lower limb ischaemia or paralysis, acute renal failure if the renal arteries are affected and possible bowel ischaemia where the mesenteric arteries are involved.

Physiotherapy key points

- The majority of patients presenting with AAA are over 70 years old with varying degrees of arteriosclerosis. Decreased mobility and exercise tolerance is often a problem both pre- and postoperatively.
- Early mobilization, within the patient's capabilities, is important to avoid respiratory complications.
- TAA may cause stretching of the recurrent laryngeal or phrenic nerve and, less commonly, vertebral body erosions leading to back pain or spinal nerve compression. Pre- and postoperative management should include close monitoring for early detection of neurological complications.

SURGERY IN THE ELDERLY

It has been estimated that 50% of people currently aged 65 years and over will undergo some form of surgery in their remaining lifetime (Davenport 1986). Elderly patients who present without previous medical problems have low postoperative morbidity and mortality rates.

The elderly surgical patient has reduced autonomic responses so perioperative blood loss or fluid overload are poorly tolerated. Acute confusional state is more common with advancing age and may be secondary to infection, hypoxia, major organ failure or alcohol withdrawal or may be drug induced. Older patients are also more sensitive to narcotic analgesia and temperature control mechanisms are less effective. Elective surgical procedures in this patient group carry a 2–7 times lower mortality rate when compared to emergency procedures (Seymour et al 1992).

Elderly women with osteoporosis are the commonest group of patients to suffer from fractured neck of femur. Surgical treatment should be immediate and involve internal fixation of the femur, allowing early mobilization and thus reducing the risk of postoperative respiratory complications. Sepsis and pulmonary embolus after major orthopaedic surgery is one of the main causes of death in the elderly population. Although early mobilization alone is insufficient to prevent postoperative thromboembolism, the advantages regarding bone density, neuromuscular and respiratory function, skin integrity, increased independence and sense of well-being are invaluable (Devas et al 1992).

Acknowledgements

In memory of Anna Carey. Sarah Ridley is grateful to Dr John McClure and the postoperative pain group of the Royal Infirmary of Edinburgh NHS Trust regarding the section on pain management which is based on their 1995 second edition of *Guidelines for the management of postoperative pain* and would also like to thank the following people for all their support and advice: David Lindsay, Professor Garden, Dr Swan, Dr Sim, Dr McClure, Professor Ruckley, Mr Campanella, Mr Purves, Ian Lennox, Morag McNaughton and all the staff at the physiotherapy department of the Royal Infirmary of Edinburgh, Lothian University Hospitals NHS Trust.

REFERENCES

Alexander JC and Anderson RW 2000 Preoperative cardiac evaluation of the thoracic surgical patient and management of perioperative cardiac events. In: Sheilds TW, LoCicero III J, Ponn R, Lippincott B (eds) General thoracic surgery, 5th edn. Williams and Wilkins, Philadelphia, pp 305–312

Anderson EW, Andleman RJ, Strauch JM et al 1973 Effect of low carbon monoxide exposure on onset and duration of angina pectoris. Annals of Internal Medicine 79: 46–50

Arora RR, Chou TM, Jain D et al 1999 The multicenter study of enhanced external counterpulsation (MUST-EECP): effects of EECP on exercise-induced myocardial ischaemia and anginal episodes. Journal of the American College of Cardiology 33: 1833–1840

Arozullah AM, Daley J, Henderson WG et al 2000 Multifactorial risk index for predicting postoperative respiratory failure in men after non cardiac surgery. Annals of Surgery 232: 242–253

Attard AR, Corlett MJ, Kidner NJ et al 1992 Safety of early pain relief for acute abdominal pain. British Medical Journal 305: 554–556

Auerbach SM, Kilmann PR 1977 Crisis intervention: a review of outcome research. Psychological Bulletin 84: 1189–1217

Belghuti J, Durand F 2000 Living donor liver transplantation present and future. British Journal of Surgery 87: 1441–1443

Besson FD, Saegesser JR 2000 Blunt and penetrating injuries of the chest wall, pleura and lungs. In: Sheilds TW, LoCicero III J, Ponn R, Lippincolt B (eds) General thoracic surgery, 5th edn. Williams and Wilkins, Philadelphia, pp 815–831

Blackwell KE 1999 Unsurpassed reliability of free flaps for head and neck reconstruction. Archives of Otolaryngology Head and Neck Surgery 125: 295–299

Boehm DH, Reichenspurner H, Gulbins H et al 1999 Early experience with robotic technology for coronary artery surgery. Annals of Thoracic Surgery 68: 1542–1546

British Oxygen Company 1990 Entonox fact sheet. Boc, Guildford, Surrey

British Thoracic Society and Society of Cardiothoracic Surgeons of Great Britain and Ireland Working Party 2001 Guidelines on the selection of patients with lung cancer for surgery. Thorax 56: 89–108

Brodsky JB 1995 Anaesthesia for thoracic surgery. In: Healy TEJ, Cohen PJ (eds) Wylie and Churchill-Davidson's a practice of anaesthesia, 6th edn. Edward Arnold, London, p 1148

Brooks-Braun JA 1997 Predictors of postoperative pulmonary complications. Chest 111: 564–571

Buckels JAC 1997 Liver transplantation. In: Carter DC, Garden OJ, Patterson-Brown S (eds) A companion to specialist surgical practice transplantation surgery. WB Saunders, London, p 165

Burroughs AK, Blake J, Thorne S et al 1992 Comparative hospital costs of liver transplantation and the treatment of complications of cirrhosis: a prospective study. European Journal of Gastroenterology and Hepatology 4: 123–128

Busuttil RW, Goss JA 1999 Split liver transplantation. Annals of Surgery 229: 313–321

Cavil G 1999 Pre-operative management. In: Pinnock C, Lin T, Smith T (eds) Fundamentals of anesthesia Greenwich Medical Media, London, p 31

Chuter TAM, Green RM, Ouriel K et al 1993 Transfemoral endovascular aortic graft replacement. Journal of Vascular Surgery 18: 185–197

Cichon R, Kappert U, Schneider J et al 2000 Robotic-enhanced arterial revascularisation for multivessel coronary artery disease. Annals of Thoracic Surgery 70: 1060–1062

Colvin JR, Kenny GNC 1989 Automatic control of arterial pressure after cardiac surgery. Anaesthesia 44: 37–41

Craig DB 1981 Post-operative recovery of pulmonary function. Anaesthesia and Analgesia 60: 46–52

Cuschieri A, Houston G 2000 Minimal access therapy. In: Cuschieri A, Steele RJ, Moossa A (eds) Essential surgical practice, vol 1, 4th edn. Butterworth Heinemann, Oxford, p 504

Dajczman E, Gordon A, Kreisman H et al 1991 Longterm post thoracotomy pain. Chest 99: 270–274

Daly RC, Trastek VF, Pairolero PC et al 1991 Bronchoalveolar cell carcinoma: factors affecting survival. Annals of Thoracic Surgery 51: 368–377

Darling G, Dresler C M 2000 Clinical presentation of lung cancer. In: Sheilds TW, LoCicero III J, Ponn R, Lippincott B (eds) General thoracic surgery, 5th edn Williams and Wilkins, Philadelphia, pp 1269–1282

Damia G, Mascheroni D, Croci M et al 1988 Peri-operative changes in functional residual capacity in morbidly obese patients. British Journal of Anaesthesia 60: 574–578

Davenport HT 1986 Anaesthesia in the elderly. Heinemann, London

Debigare R, Maltais F, Whihom F et al 1999 Feasibility and efficacy of home exercise training in emphysema before lung volume reduction. Journal of Cardiopulmonary Rehabilitation 19: 235–241

De Leon-Casasola OA, Parker B, Lema MJ et al 1994 Post-operative epidural bupiviacaine-morphine therapy. Experience with 4227 surgical patients. Anesthesiology 81: 368–375

Deslauriers J, Le Blanc 2000 Bullous and bleb diseases, emphysema of the lung and lung volume reduction operations. In: Sheilds TW, LoCicero III J, Ponn R, Lippincolt B (eds) General thoracic surgery, 5th edn Williams and Wilkins, Philadelphia, pp 1001–1038

Devas M, Plumpton FS, Seymour DG 1992 Orthopaedics. In: Crosby DL, Rees GAD, Seymour DG (eds) The ageing surgical patient: anesthetic, operative and medical management. John Wiley, Chichester.

Disco CM 2000 Comparison of effectiveness and cost effectiveness of CABG versus percutaneous intervention in patients with multi-vessel disease assessed by age. European Heart Journal 21: 478

Dodds SR 1998 Recent advances in the management of arterial disease. In: Johnson CD, Taylor I (eds) Recent advances in surgery. Churchill Livingstone, Edinburgh, p 147

Done ML, Lee A 1998 The use of a video to convey pre-anesthetic information to patients undergoing ambulatory surgery. Anesthesia and Analgesia 87: 531–536

Dureuil B, Cantineau JP, Desmonts JM 1987 Effects of upper and lower abdominal surgery on diaphragmatic function. British Journal of Anaesthesia 59: 1230–1235

Egan TD, Wong KC 1992 Perioperative smoking cessation and anesthesia: a review. Journal of Clinical Anesthesia 4: 63–72

European Coronary Surgery Study Group 1980 Prospective randomized study of coronary artery bypass surgery in stable angina pectoris. Lancet 2: 491–495

Ford GT, Whitelaw WA, Rosenal TW et al 1983 Diaphragm function after upper abdominal surgery in humans. American Review of Respiratory Disease 127: 431–436

Forrest APM, Carter DC, Macleod IB 1995 Principles and practice of surgery, 3rd edn. Churchill Livingstone, Edinburgh

Frost L, Molgaard H, Christiansen EH et al 1992 Atrial fibrillation and flutter after coronary artery bypass surgery: epidemiology, risk factors and preventative trials. International Journal of Cardiology 36: 253–261

Gaiser RR 1997 Spinal, epidural and caudal anesthesia. In: Longnecker E, Murphy FL (eds) Introduction to anesthesia, 9th edn. WB Saunders, Philadelphia, p 222

Garcia-Valdecasas JC, Almenara R, Carbrer C et al 1988 Subcostal incision versus midline laparotomy in gallstone surgery: a prospective and randomized trial. British Journal of Surgery 75: 473–475

Garrow JS 1988 Measurement of energy stores. In: Obesity and related diseases. Churchill Livingstone, Edinburgh

Geddes D, Davies M, Koyamo H et al 2000 Effect of lung volume reduction surgery in patients with severe emphysema. New England Journal of Medicine 343: 239–245

Geertsema AA, Cornelis WB, Harm KS et al 1999 Design and test of a new tracheostoma valve based on inhalation. Archives of Otolaryngology Head and Neck Surgery 125: 622–626

Ginsberg RJ, Hill LD, Eagan RT et al 1983 Modern 30 day operative mortality for surgical resection in lung cancer. Journal of Thoracic and Cardiovascular Surgery 86: 654–658

Goldman L, Caldera DL, Nussbaum SR et al 1977 Multifactorial index of cardiac risk in non cardiac surgical procedures. New England Journal of Medicine 297: 845–850

Guirguis EM, Barber GG 1991 The natural history of abdominal aortic aneurysms. American Journal of Surgery 162: 481–483

Hart JC, Spooner TH, Pym J et al 2000 A review of 1,582 consecutive Octopus off-pump coronary bypass patients. Annals of Thoracic Surgery 70: 1017–1020

Henry T, Rocha-Singh K, Isner JM et al 1998 Results of intracoronary recombinant human vascular endothelial growth factor (rh VEGF) administration trial. Journal of American College of Cardiology 31: 65A

Higgins TL 1992 Pro: early endotracheal extubation is preferable to late extubation in patients following coronary artery surgery. Journal of Cardiothoracic and Vascular Anesthesia 6: 488–493

Hood RM 1990 Trauma to the chest. In: Sabiston DC, Spencer FC (eds) Surgery of the chest, 5th edn. WB Saunders, Philadelphia, ch 14

Hoffman RM, Mintz GS 2000 Coronary in-stent restenosis predictors, treatment and prevention. European Heart Journal 21: 1739–1749

Horowits MD, Ancalmo N, Ochsner JL 1989 Thoracotomy through auscultatory triangle. Annals of Thoracic Surgery 47: 782–783

Jenkins S, Bourn J 1992 Post-operative respiratory physiotherapy. Indications for treatment. Physiotherapy 78: 80–85

Jenkins SC, Soutar SA, Loukota JM et al 1989 Physiotherapy after coronary artery surgery: are breathing exercises necessary? Thorax 44: 634–639

Jordan S, Mitchell JA, Quinlan GJ et al 2000 The pathogenesis of lung injury following pulmonary resection. European Respiratory Journal 15: 790–799

Joyce CJ, Baker AB 1995 What is the role of absorption atelectasis in the genesis of perioperative pulmonary collapse? Anaesthesia and Intensive Care 23: 691–696

Kam AC, O'Brien M, Kam PCA 1993 Pleural drainage systems. Anaesthesia 48: 154–161

Kirby TJ, Mack MJ, Landreneau RJ et al 1995 Lobectomy video-assisted thoracic surgery versus muscle-sparing thoracotomy. A randomized controlled trial. Journal of Thoracic and Cardiovascular Surgery 109: 997–1001

Laham RJ 1999 Local perivascular delivery of basic fibroblast growth factor in patients undergoing coronary bypass surgery: results of phase l randomized, double blind, placebo-controlled trial. Circulation 100: 1865–1871

Laham RJ, Ho KK, Bairn DS et al 1997 Multi-vessel Palmaz-Schatz stenting: early results and one-year outcome. Journal of the American College of Cardiology 30: 180–185

Leblanc P, Ruff F, Milic-Emili J 1970 Effects of age and body position on 'airway closure' in man. Journal of Applied Physiology 28: 448–451

Lefebvre JL 2000 What is the role of primary surgery in the treatment of laryngeal and hypopharyngeal cancer? Archives of Otolaryngology Head and Neck Surgery 126: 285–288

Lin PJ, Chang CH, Chu JJ et al 1996 Video-assisted mitral valve operations. Annals of Thoracic Surgery 61: 1781–1787

Loop FD, Lytle BW, Cosgrove DM et al 1990 Sternal wound complications after isolated coronary bypass grafting: early and late mortality, morbidity and cost of care. Annals of Thoracic Surgery 49: 179–186

Losordo DW 1998 Gene therapy for myocardial angiogenesis: initial clinical results with direct myocardial injection of ph VEGF-165 as sole therapy for myocardial ischaemia. Circulation 98: 2800–2804

Lunn JN 1991 Lecture notes on anaesthetics. Blackwell Science, Oxford.

Lytle BW, Cosgrove DM 1992 Coronary artery bypass surgery. Current Problems in Surgery 29: 733–807

Mack MJ, Aronoff RJ, Acuff TE et al 1992 Present role of thoracoscopy in the diagnosis and treatment of diseases of the chest. Annals of Thoracic Surgery 54: 403–408

Mansour KA, Wanna FS 2000 Extended resection of bronchial carcinoma in the superior pulmonary sulcus. In: Sheilds TW, LoCicero III J, Ponn R, Lippincott B (eds) General thoracic surgery, 5th edn. Williams and Wilkins, Philadelphia, p 467

Maran AGD 1995 Head and neck surgery. In: Cuschieri A, Giles GR, Moossa AR (eds) Essential surgical practice, 3rd edn. Butterworth-Heinemann, Oxford, p 1656

March RJ 1999 Transmyocardial laser revascularization with the CO2 laser: one year results of the randomized controlled trial. Seminars in Thoracic and Cardiovascular Surgery 11: 12–18

Markand ON, Moorthy SS, Mahomed Y et al 1985 Post operative phrenic nerve palsy in patients with open-heart surgery. Annals of Thoracic Surgery 39: 68–73

Martini N, Ginsberg RJ 1990 Surgical approach to non-small cell lung cancer stage 111a. Hematology and Oncology Clinics of North America 6: 1121

McAuliffe MJ, Ward EC, Bassett L et al 2000 Functional speech outcomes after laryngectomy and pharyngolaryngectomy. Archives of Otolaryngology Head and Neck Surgery 126: 705–709

Mearns AJ 1995 Tumours of the lung. In: Cuschieri A, Giles GR, Moossa AR (eds) Essential surgical practice, 3rd edn. Butterworth-Heinemann, Oxford, p 794

Moossa AR, Hart ME 1997 Surgical complications. In: Sabiston DC (ed) Textbook of surgery. The biological basis of modern surgical practice. WB Saunders, Philadelphia

Morgan M, Nel MR 1996 Smoking and anaesthesia revisited. Anaesthesia 51: 309–311

Mountain CF 1997 Revision in the international system for staging lung cancer. Chest 111: 1710–1717

Mutimer D 1994 Fulminant and subacute hepatic failure. In: Neuberger J, Lucey M (eds) Liver transplantation: practice and management. BMJ Books, London, p 76

Mynster T, Jensen LM, Kehlet H et al 1996 The effect of posture on late post-operative oxygenation. Anaesthesia 51: 225–227

Nelson S 1996 Pre-admission education for patients undergoing cardiac surgery. British Journal of Nursing 5: 335–340

Otremski I 1990 Fracture of the sternum in motor vehicle accidents and its association with mediastinal injury. Injury 21: 81–83

Parkin DM, Pisani P, Ferlay J et al 1993 Estimates of the worldwide incidence of 18 major cancers in 1985. International Journal of Cancer 54: 594–606

Parodi JC, Palmaz JC, Barone HD 1991 Transfemoral intraluminal graft implantation for abdominal aortic aneurysms. Annals of Vascular Surgery 5: 491–499

Sabanathan S, Richardson J 1994 Management of post pneumonectomy bronchopleural fistulae. A review. Journal of Cardiovascular Surgery 35: 449–457

Sabiston DC 1990 Disorders of the sternum and the thoracic wall. In: Sabiston DC, Spencer FC (eds) Surgery of the chest, 5th edn. WB Saunders, Philadelphia

Sawyers JL 1996 Current status of conventional (open) cholecystectomy versus laparoscopic cholecystectomy. Annals of Surgery 223: 1–3

Schofield PM, Shatpes LD, Coine N et al 1999 Transmyocardial laser revascularisation in patients with refractory angina: a randomized controlled trial. Lancet 353: 519–524

Scott AM, Starling JR, Ruscher AE et al 1996 Thoracic versus lumbar epidural anesthesia's effect on pain control and ileus resolution after restorative proctocolectomy. Surgery 120: 688–697

Selsby DS, Jones JG 1993 Respiratory function and the safety of anaesthesia. In: Taylor TH, Major E (eds) Hazards and complications of anaesthesia, 2nd edn. Churchill Livingstone, Edinburgh

Seymour DG, Rees GAD, Crosby DL 1992 Introduction and general principles. In: The ageing surgical patient: anaesthetic, operative and medical management. John Wiley, Chichester

Shainoff JR, Estafanous FG, Yared JP et al 1994 Low factor X111A levels are associated with increased blood loss after coronary artery bypass grafting. Journal of Thoracic and Cardiovascular Surgery 108: 437–445

Shaw PJ, Bates D, Cartridge NE et al 1986a Early intellectual dysfunction following coronary bypass surgery. Quarterly Journal of Medicine 58: 59–68

Shaw PJ, Bates D, Cartridge NE et al 1986b Neurological complications of coronary artery bypass graft surgery. British Medical Journal 293: 165–167

Sheilds TW 2000 Pathology of carcinoma of the lung. In: Sheilds TW, LoCicero III J, Ponn R, Lippincott B (eds) General thoracic surgery, 5th edn. Williams and Wilkins, Philadelphia, pp 1249–1268

Shimizu J, Makoto O, Yoshinobu H et al 1996 A clinicopathological study of resected cases of adenosquamous carcinoma of the lung. Chest 109: 989–994

Simons M, Laham RJ 1999 Chronic myocardial ischaemia: contemporary management strategies. Drugs of Today 35: 667–684

Smith R S, Fry W R, Edmund K M T et al 1993 Gasless laparoscopy and conventional instruments: the next phase of minimally invasive surgery. Archives of Surgery 128: 1102–1107

Smith RS, Fry WR, Tsoi EKM et al 1993a Preliminary report on videothoracoscopy in the evaluation and treatment of thoracic injury. American Journal of Surgery 166: 690–693

Swanson J, Trunkey DD 1989 Trauma to the chest wall, pleura and thoracic viscera. In: Sheilds TW (ed) General thoracic surgery, 3rd edn. Lea and Febiger, Philadelphia

Tan AK 1995 Incentive spirometry for tracheostomy and laryngectomy patients. Journal of Otolaryngology 24: 292–294

Tisi GM 1985 Neoplastic diseases. In: Bordon RA, Moser KM (eds) Manual of clinical problems in pulmonary medicine, 2nd edn. Little, Brown, Boston, p 411

Westaby S 1995 Coronary surgery without cardiopulmonary bypass. British Heart Journal 73: 203–205

Wisner DH 1990 A stepwise logistic regression analysis of factors affecting morbidity and mortality after thoracic trauma: effects of epidural analgesia. Journal of Trauma 30: 799–804

13

Paediatrics

S Ammani Prasad   Eleanor Main

INTRODUCTION

Anatomical and physiological differences between adults and children mean that the care of children with respiratory disorders can differ significantly. Additional criteria need to be used for assessing and treating children, who should at all times be handled with care and respect.

Fear of the unknown is more acute in children than in adults and information about treatment should be explained carefully in a way that is appropriate for their age. Physiotherapy treatments are easier and more pleasant when children are cooperative and compliant. Cooperation can often be obtained by persuasion, distraction with games, television, cassette tapes or reading books suited to the child's age and interest. It may be helpful in some situations to reward good behaviour or bravery with balloons or stickers, but occasionally children do refuse treatment (either because they simply do not want it or perhaps due to fear). However, if the benefits of treatment are considered to outweigh the risks, treatment must be given after thorough and careful explanation.

It is essential to include parents, relatives and carers as part of the care team. Parents should always have a full explanation of why treatment is required and how it is to be carried out. Parents are able to refuse physiotherapy treatment for their child but this rarely occurs in practice. Parents of sick children are extremely vulnerable to stress and should at all times be handled with tact and understanding. Parental stress may manifest in different ways, including hysteria, apparent lack of concern or anger. Some parents are so distressed that they are unable to stay with or visit their sick child and may need special help to cope with their feelings of fear and panic.

Parents benefit from the physiotherapist's support when they are required to carry out physiotherapy treatment themselves at home. When children and parents are intensively involved in treatment sessions, such as may occur in chronic illness, e.g. cystic fibrosis, siblings may often feel left out. It is therefore important to include them in some way, perhaps even in helping with treatment.

Children's awareness of the implications of illness and treatment develop as they grow older. Explanations that are suitable for younger children will need to be expanded as the child grows older and begins to understand how his body works. Teenagers, particularly, have a more sophisticated understanding and may be beginning to think about the future and the impact of illness on school and social life, as well as body image. Although they may often object to being told what to do, careful handling and education should be used to encourage them to develop some responsibility for their treatment.

Physiotherapists treating children with acute or chronic respiratory problems must be aware of the psychological problems affecting the child and parents and adapt their approach accordingly.

DEVELOPMENT OF THE LUNGS

The development of the lung can be divided into four stages (Inselman & Mellins 1981).

- Embryonic period (weeks 3–5)
- Pseudoglandular period (weeks 6–16)
- Canalicular period (weeks 17–24)
- Alveolar sac period (week 24–term)

Embryonic period (weeks 3–5)

The lung bud starts as an endodermal outgrowth of fetal foregut. The single tube thus formed soon branches into two, forming the major bronchi. By cell division, the process of growth continues until, at the end of this period, the major lung branches are formed.

Pseudoglandular period (weeks 6–16)

During this period the airways grow by dichotomous branching so that by week 16 all generations of the airway from trachea to terminal bronchioles (i.e. the preacinus) are formed. During this period the pulmonary circulation also develops, cartilage and lymphatic formation occur and cilia appear (week 10 onwards) (Langman 1977).

Canalicular period (weeks 17–24)

The respiratory bronchioles, alveolar ducts and alveoli (i.e. the acinus) start to develop during this time, simultaneously with the lung capillaries, thus preparing the lungs for their future role in gas exchange (Hislop & Reid, 1974). The air-blood barrier first appears at week 19 and towards the end of this period surfactant synthesis begins.

Terminal sac period (week 24–term)

Development of the pulmonary circulation continues and the respiratory bronchioles subdivide to form air spaces. Two different cell types (types I and II pneumocytes) line the air spaces. Type–I pneumocytes flatten and elongate to cover the majority of the surface area of the saccular air spaces. Type–II cells only occupy approximately 2% of the surface and are responsible for surfactant synthesis and storage (Greenough 1996a). Surfactant is a phospholipid, which stabilizes surface tension in the alveolus and prevents alveolar collapse on expiration. Small quantities of surfactant are present at weeks 23–24 of gestation and the amount present gradually increases until a surge at about week 30. Birth itself and the onset of respiration stimulate surfactant production.

Towards the end of the terminal sac period, the air spaces have developed into primitive multilocular alveoli. After birth, alveoli increase in size and number. The average number of alveoli in the newborn is 150 million. By the age of 3–4 years, the adult number of 300–400 million alveoli has been reached, but alveolar growth continues until about 8 years of age (Hislop et al 1986).

ANATOMICAL AND PHYSIOLOGICAL DIFFERENCES BETWEEN CHILDREN AND ADULTS

Anatomical differences

- Differences in upper airway anatomy allow infants to feed and breathe simultaneously up to approximately 3–4 months of age. Until this time infants are preferential nose breathers, therefore any nasal blockage can lead to increased work of breathing and spells of apnoea (Rodenstein et al 1987).
- The lymphatic tissue (adenoids and tonsils) may be enlarged in the infant and the tongue is also relatively large. These factors may contribute to upper airway obstruction.
- The smaller diameter airways of infants, particularly those born preterm, offer very high resistance to airflow and any mucosal oedema will significantly increase the work of breathing.
- Bronchial wall structure is different in infants. Cartilage is less firm and there are proportion-
ately more mucous glands. Both these factors predispose to airway obstruction and collapse (Reid 1984).
- There are fewer alveoli in young children and, therefore, less surface area for gaseous exchange (Reid 1984).
- The collateral ventilatory channels between alveoli, respiratory bronchioles and terminal bronchioles are poorly developed until 2–3 years of age, predisposing towards alveolar collapse.
- Infants' ribs are horizontally positioned (Fig. 13.1), so there is no 'bucket handle' movement of respiration. In addition, weak intercostal muscles mean that the infant is more reliant on the diaphragm for respiration. Adult rib configuration develops as the child adopts a more upright posture when gravity pulls the anterior ribs downwards (Openshaw et al 1984).
- The horizontal angle of insertion of the diaphragm combined with the compliant cartilaginous rib cage of the infant mean less efficient ventilation and distortion of chest wall shape on inspiration (Muller & Bryan 1979).

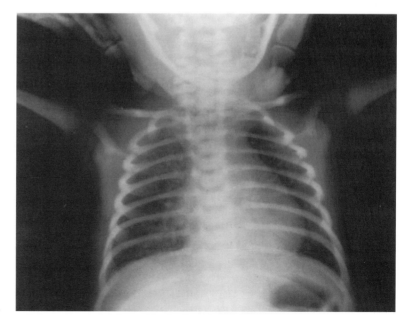

Figure 13.1 Normal chest radiograph.

- The heart and other organs, e.g. thymus, are relatively large in infants and therefore there is relatively less space for lung tissue.

Physiological differences

- The lungs of infants are less compliant than those of older children and adults, particularly in preterm infants (< 37 weeks' gestation) where there may also be a lack of surfactant.
- Neonates, especially those born preterm, have irregular breathing patterns which may lead to apnoea. Although short spells of apnoea are considered normal, longer periods and those which require stimulation to restart breathing will need investigation.
- Anatomical differences in rib cage configuration do not allow the infant to increase lung volume to the same extent as an adult (Konno & Mead 1967). Therefore when in respiratory difficulties, the infant must increase respiratory rate rather than depth to maintain minute volume.
- Neonates may sleep for up to 20 hours a day and 80% of this time may be in active (rapid eye movement, REM) sleep compared with 20% in adults. During active sleep there is a decrease in postural tone, causing a drop in functional residual capacity, and thereby increasing the work of breathing (Muller & Bryan 1979).
- The diaphragm in the adult is composed of approximately 50% of fatigue-resistant type I muscle fibres whereas the neonate has only 25% and preterm infants may have as little as 10%. Therefore there is an increased susceptibility to fatigue of the diaphragm (Muller & Bryan 1979).
- Children have a higher resting metabolic rate with a greater oxygen demand. Any increase in demand can cause hypoxia more rapidly than in adults. Hypoxia in infants causes bradycardia (less than 100 bpm), rather than tachycardia as in adults.
- Infants and children preferentially ventilate the uppermost lung regions, rather than dependent lung regions as in the adult (Davies et al 1985), although the pattern of perfusion is

similar (Bhuyan et al 1989). This difference may persist as late as the second decade of life. In acutely ill children with unilateral lung disease, oxygenation may be optimized by placing the good lung uppermost.
- In the small infant the closing volume exceeds the functional residual capacity. In dependent regions airway closure may occur even during normal tidal breathing.

RESPIRATORY ASSESSMENT OF THE INFANT AND CHILD

Careful assessment is essential to identify problems requiring physiotherapy intervention. Many aspects of assessment will be the same as in adults, but specific differences are listed below.

Medical notes

Information can be extracted from the medical notes relating to present and past medical history. When assessing a neonate, history of pregnancy, labour and delivery are relevant as well as gestational age and weight. In addition, the Apgar score at birth should be noted. This score relates to heart rate, respiratory effort, muscle tone, reflex irritability and colour and gives an indication of the degree of asphyxiation suffered by the infant at birth.

Discussion with the relevant carers

Discussion with medical staff, nursing staff and the parent/carer is essential to obtain correct information about recent changes. In chronically ill children who require home physiotherapy, liaison with the primary healthcare team is essential.

When assessing the hospitalized child, information should be obtained about:

- the stability of the child's condition over the last few hours
- how well the infant tolerates handling. Does the infant become rapidly hypoxic or bradycardic? How long does he take to recover from the handling episode?

- whether the child is fed via the oral, nasogastric or intravenous route and the timing of the last feed
- whether the child is sufficiently rested to tolerate a physiotherapy treatment.

Observation charts and investigations

- Pyrexia may indicate a possible respiratory infection. The core-to-peripheral temperature gradient should be noted, particularly in the critically ill patient.
- Tachycardia can be due to sepsis or shock. It may also be caused by inadequate levels of sedation or analgesia. In preterm infants, bradycardias may be due to many causes, including retention of secretions.
- Apnoeic spells in the infant may indicate respiratory distress, sepsis or presence of secretions in the upper or lower respiratory tract.
- The trend of arterial gases and their relationship to oxygen saturation and transcutaneous oxygen should be noted together with the degree and type of respiratory support.
- Results of investigations and other relevant observations should be referred to as appropriate.

Examination

Examination of the older child is similar to that of the adult (Ch. 1). The following specific factors should be considered in younger children.

Clinical signs

Clinical signs of respiratory distress are listed in Box 13.1.

Recession occurs when high negative intrathoracic pressure during inspiration pulls the soft, compliant chest wall inward. It may be sternal, subcostal or intercostal. Mild recession may be normal in preterm infants but in older infants is a sign of increased respiratory effort.

Nasal flaring is a dilatation of the nostrils by the dilatores naris muscles and is a sign of respiratory distress in the infant. It may be a primitive response attempting to decrease airway resistance.

Box 13.1 Clinical signs of respiratory distress

Respiratory
- Recession
  - intercostal
  - subcostal
  - sternal
- Nasal flaring
- Tachypnoea
- Expiratory grunting
- Stridor
- Cyanosis
- Abnormal breath sounds

Cardiac
- Tachycardia/bradycardia
- Hypertension/hypotension

Other/general
- Neck extension
- Head bobbing
- Pallor
- Reluctance to feed
- Irritability/restlessness
- Altered conscious level
- Headache

Tachypnoea (respiratory rate greater than 60 breaths/min) may indicate respiratory distress in infants. Normal values are listed in Table 13.1.

Grunting occurs when an infant expires against a partially closed glottis. This is an automatic response which increases functional residual capacity in an attempt to improve ventilation.

Stridor is heard in the presence of a narrowing of the upper trachea and/or larynx. This may be due to collapse of the floppy tracheal wall, inflammation or an inhaled foreign body. It is most commonly heard during inspiration, but in cases of severe narrowing it may be heard during both inspiration and expiration.

Cyanosis refers to the bluish colour of the skin and mucus membranes caused by hypoxaemia.

Table 13.1 Normal values

Age group	Heart rate mean (range) (beats/min)	Respiratory rate – range (breaths/min)	Blood pressure systolic/diastolic (mmHg)
Preterm	150 (100–200)	40–60	39–59 / 16–36
Newborn	140 (80–200)	30–50	50–70 / 25–45
< 2 years	130 (100–190)	20–40	87–105 / 53–66
> 2 years	80 (60–140)	20–40	95–105 / 53–66
> 6 years	75 (60–90)	15–30	97–112 / 57–71

In infants and young children it is an unreliable sign of respiratory distress as it depends on the relative amount and type of haemoglobin in the blood and the adequacy of the peripheral circulation. For the first 3–4 weeks of life, the newborn infant has an increased amount of fetal haemoglobin which has a higher affinity for oxygen than adult haemoglobin. The result is a shift of the oxygen saturation curve to the left in infants.

Auscultation of the infant and young child is sometimes complicated by the easy transmission of sounds. In the infant who is ventilated, referred sounds such as water in the ventilator tubing may be transmitted to the chest. In the older child, secretions in the nose or throat may lead to referred sounds in both lung fields. Wheezing in the younger child or infant may be due to bronchospasm but could also be due to retained secretions partially occluding smaller airways. It is sometimes very difficult to hear breath sounds in the spontaneously breathing preterm infant.

Cardiac manifestations of respiratory distress include an initial tachycardia and possible increase in systemic blood pressure. This changes with worsening hypoxia to bradycardia and hypotension.

Neck extension in an infant with respiratory distress may represent an attempt to reduce airway resistance.

Head bobbing occurs when infants attempt to use the sternocleidomastoid and the scalene muscles as accessory muscles of respiration. It is seen because the relatively weak neck extensors of infants are unable to stabilize the head.

Pallor is commonly seen in infants with respiratory distress and may be a sign of hypoxaemia or other problems, including anaemia.

Reluctance to feed is often associated with respiratory distress and infants may need to take frequent pauses from sucking when tachypnoeic.

Alterations in levels of consciousness should be noted. A reduction in activity may be due to neurological deficit or as a result of opiate analgesia but may also be due to hypoxia. It may be accompanied by an inability to feed or cry. Irritability and restlessness may also be indicative of a hypoxic state.

Other relevant observations

The behaviour of a child can often give important clues about their respiratory status. Agitation or irritability may be a sign of hypoxia, while the child in severe respiratory distress may be withdrawn and lie completely still.

It is important to note muscle tone in the infant or child with respiratory distress. A hypotonic child may have increased difficulty with breathing, coughing and expectorating, while hypertonia may also be associated with difficulty in clearing secretions.

Abdominal distension can cause or exacerbate respiratory distress, because the diaphragm is placed at a mechanical disadvantage. In infants this is of greater concern as the diaphragm is the primary muscle of respiration.

PHYSIOTHERAPY TECHNIQUES IN INFANTS AND CHILDREN

Most physiotherapy techniques used in adults can be applied in children and the same contraindications apply. Treatment should never be performed routinely as it may have potentially detrimental effects (Horiuchi et al 1997, Krause & Hoehn 2000, Stiller 2000). Ideally treatment should occur before feeds or adequate time allowed following a feed to avoid problems associated with vomiting and aspiration.

Technological advances in recent years have meant that modern ventilators often incorporate pressure and flow sensors which allow continuous monitoring and calculation of tidal breathing parameters or respiratory mechanics from which an assessment of respiratory function can be made (MacNaughton & Evans 1999). It is imperative that physiotherapists familiarize themselves with these devices, the interpretation of data generated from them and their limitations in the clinical environment. There is great potential for such equipment to provide objective feedback about efficacy and tolerance of treatments in individual patients and to provide excellent tools for systematic evaluation of physiotherapy treatment in mechanically ventilated infants.

Chest percussion

Chest percussion (sometimes referred to as chest clapping) using the hand, fingers or a facemask is generally well tolerated and widely used in children. Percussion using one hand is used in small children and babies (Fig. 13.2a). In neonates and preterm infants 'tenting' (using the first three or four fingers of one hand with slight elevation of the middle finger; or the use of a soft plastic cup–shaped object such as a facemask may be more appropriate (Fig. 13.2b) (Tudehope & Bagley 1980).

Vibrations and shaking

The chest wall is very compliant in infants and young children. Vibrations can be applied effectively when the respiratory rate is normal or near normal (30–40 breaths/min). If infants are breathing very rapidly, e.g. more than 60 breaths/min, the expiratory phase is so short that vibrations are more difficult to perform.

Precautions for chest percussion and vibratory techniques

- In children with dietary deficiencies, liver disease, bone mineral deficiency (e.g. rickets) or coagulopathies manual techniques should be applied with caution.
- Manual techniques may not be appropriate in extremely premature infants and specific issues related to this group of patients are discussed on page 441.
- Chest percussion has been reported to cause an increase in bronchospasm in adults with chronic lung disease (Campbell et al 1975), (Wollmer et al 1985). Premedication with bronchodilator therapy may reduce this effect but in severe cases percussion should be avoided.

Postural drainage (gravity-assisted positioning)

Gravity-assisted positions can be used in children to assist clearance of bronchial secretions. The

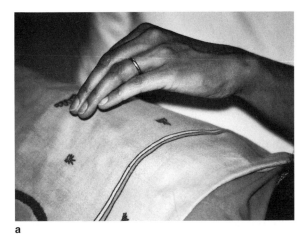

a

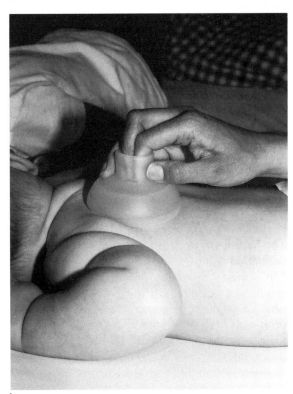

b

Figure 13.2 **a** Single-handed percussion. **b** Percussion with face mask.

upper lobes, particularly the right side, are more frequently affected by respiratory problems and appropriate gravity-assisted positioning may be helpful. A head-down tip should be avoided in children with raised intracranial pressure and in preterm infants who are at risk of periventricular haemorrhage. This position should also be avoided in the presence of abdominal distension as this places the diaphragm at a further mechanical disadvantage. Care should be taken in infants with a history of reflux although the effect of head-down tipping on gastro-oesophageal reflux remains unclear (Taylor & Threlfall 1997). Some evidence suggests that it may aggravate reflux and potentially cause aspiration (Button 1999, Button et al 1997, Demont et al 1991) while other reports suggest little or no effect on reflux (Phillips 1996). Reflux may affect approximately 80% of preterm infants (Newell et al 1989).

Positioning

Positioning may be used to optimize respiratory function. The supine position has been shown to be the least beneficial, while prone positioning has been shown to improve respiratory function (Dean 1985), decrease gastro-oesophageal reflux (Blumenthal & Lealman 1982) and reduce energy expenditure (Brackbill et al 1973). It is often used in closely monitored infants with respiratory problems in a hospital setting, but parents should be advised against using this position when babies are sleeping unattended because of its association with sudden infant death (Southall & Samuels 1992).

Patterns of regional ventilation in infants differ significantly from adults (Davies et al 1985), with ventilation in infants and small children being preferentially distributed to the uppermost regions of the lungs. In acutely ill children with unilateral lung disease, care should be taken if positioning the child with the affected lung uppermost as this may cause rapid deterioration of respiratory status. Spontaneously breathing newborn infants are better oxygenated when tilted slightly head up (Thoresen et al 1988) and show a drop in PaO_2 if placed flat or tilted head down.

Manual ventilation

Manual lung inflation involves disconnection of the patient from mechanical ventilation to provide temporary manual ventilation. The same contraindications apply for children and adults (Chs 6 & 11). However, special consideration should be applied in preterm infants whose lung tissue is easily damaged by high inflation pressures and in children with hyperinflated lungs (e.g. asthma and bronchiolitis) in whom there is a greater risk of pneumothorax. For infants 500 ml bags should be used and 1 litre bags for older children. They may be valved or open-ended so that expulsion of excess pressure is controlled by the operator's fingers. A manometer should be placed in the circuit whenever possible to monitor the inflation pressures (Fig. 13.3). As a general guideline, manual ventilation pressures during physiotherapy should not exceed $10 \text{ cmH}_2\text{O}$ above the ventilator pressure. In order to prevent airway collapse, some positive end-expiratory pressure (PEEP) should be maintained in the bag. Self-inflating bags are used in some units. The flow rate of gas is adjusted according to the size of the child: 4 l/min for infants increasing to 8 l/min for children.

In paediatric patients manual ventilation is used to achieve the following:

- *Hyperinflation* – a long inspiration with an inspiratory pause followed by rapid release of the bag. The aim of this technique is to recruit lung units by improving collateral ventilation and increasing lung volume. Following hyperinflation a high expiratory flow may assist in mobilizing secretions towards central airways. Some studies support the use of hyperinflation for improving compliance and ventilation/perfusion matching, while others dispute its efficacy (Bartlett et al 1973, Clement & Hubsch 1968, Windsor et al 1972). Controversy exists regarding the safety and effectiveness of manual lung hyperinflation in intubated patients. The volumes, pressures and FiO_2 are not controlled and there are inherent dangers of barotrauma (Brandstater & Muallem 1969, Gattinoni et al. 1993). Novak et al (1987) were unable to demonstrate improvement in gas exchange or pulmonary compliance following hyperinflation for 15–30 seconds. In patients with compromised

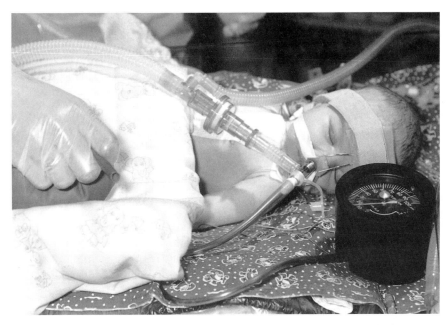

Figure 13.3 Manual hyperinflation in small child showing pressure gauge in circuit.

cardiac output the long inspiratory phase with pause may be contraindicated.

- *Hyperventilation* – in order to reduce CO_2 in patients with head injury so that physiotherapy can be safely undertaken. CO_2 should not be allowed to drop too low as this may lead to excessive reduction in cerebral blood flow. In those with a large cardiac shunt, hyperventilation may be contraindicated.
- *Hyperoxygenation* – may be used prior to suction in order to reduce suction-induced hypoxia or pulmonary hypertension. Stone & Turner (1989) critically reviewed research on the efficacy of ventilator versus the manual hyperinflation in delivering hyperoxygenation or hyperinflation breaths before, during and/or after endotracheal suctioning. Findings were that hyperoxygenation or hyperinflation breaths at 100% O_2 delivered via the ventilator were either superior or equivalent to manually delivered breaths in preventing suction-induced hypoxaemia, but delivery of manual hyperinflation breaths resulted in increased airway pressure and increased haemodynamic consequences (Stone 1990). In the presence of pulmonary hypertension, it is generally not

advisable to use a FiO_2 of 1.0 during manual hyperinflation as this may further increase blood flow to the lungs.

Breathing exercises

Laughing and crying are very effective means of lung expansion in infants. It is possible to encourage children to deep breathe from about 2 years of age by using games such as bubbles, paper windmills or incentive spirometers, although the efficacy of these treatments is unproven. As children get older, they are able to play a more active role in their treatment and appropriate airway clearance techniques can be introduced.

Coughing

Children from about 18 months of age often mimic coughing if asked to do so, but it is often very difficult to persuade an acutely ill child to cough and expectorate.

Positioning or activity may mobilize secretions and stimulate a cough reflex. Secretions will usually be swallowed as the ability to expectorate is not usually developed before 3–4 years of age. Tracheal compression can some-times be used to stimulate a cough in children who are unable to cough on request. Gentle pressure is briefly applied to the trachea below the thyroid cartilage which causes apposition of the soft and pliant tracheal walls, stimulating the cough reflex. This technique must be used with care in small infants as they can become bradycardic. If cough is ineffective and there are copious secretions, airway suction may be necessary.

Airway suction

Airway suction is discussed in Chapters 6 and 11. Suction techniques may be either naso- or oropharyngeal or endotracheal, depending on whether there is an artificial airway in situ. Adverse effects have frequently been reported and include hypoxaemia, mechanical trauma, apnoea, bronchospasm, pneumothorax, atelectasis, cardiac arrhythmias and even death on rare occasions (Clark et al 1990, Clarke et al 1999, Czarnik et al 1991, Kerem et al 1990, Shah et al 1992, Singer et al 1994, Stone & Turner 1989, Wood 1998).

Methods for reducing complications associated with suction include the following:

- Preoxygenation prior to suction using ventilator or manually delivered breaths with a higher FiO_2 (Chulay & Graeber 1988, Goodnough 1985). Preoxygenation with ventilator breaths has been recommended in preference to disconnection and manual hyperinflation because of the reduced risk of barotrauma, loss of PEEP and FiO_2 (Glass et al 1993, McCabe & Smeltzer 1993, Stone et al 1991). Particular care should be taken in preterm infants to avoid hyperoxia as this is associated with retinopathy of prematurity (Roberton 1996).
- Suctioning via a port adapter or closed suction systems in patients who require maintenance of PEEP and/or positive pressure ventilation during suction (Harshbarger et al 1992).
- Infants are at particular risk of infection, so care should be taken to avoid crossinfection.

- High vacuum pressures have been associated with mechanical trauma of the tracheal mucous membranes (Kleiber et al 1988). Suction pressures should therefore be as low as possible, without compromising the efficacy of secretion clearance.
- When suctioning artificial airways the external diameter of the catheter should not exceed 50% of the internal diameter of the airway (Imle & Klemic 1989). Most commonly used catheters are 6 and 8 French gauge (FG). Size 5 FG and below are usually ineffective in removing thick secretions. Size 10 FG and above should be reserved for use with older children.
- Saline instillation into the tracheal tube of ventilated patients aims to loosen thick or sticky secretions to facilitate easy removal with suction, although evidence for the practice is variable. Some suggest that saline instillation at best is not effective and at worst is harmful (Blackwood 1999, Hagler & Traver 1994, Kinloch 1999, McKelvie 1998), while others suggest it is well tolerated even in infants and may be helpful in removing secretions adherent to the chest wall (Shorten et al 1991). Other mucolytics (n-acetylcysteine) in aliquots of 0.5–5 ml may be used to enhance secretion clearance. Larger quantities of irrigants are sometimes used as part of bronchoalveolar lavage procedures.
- Pneumothorax due to direct perforation of a segmental bronchus by a suction catheter has been reported in intubated preterm infants (Vaughan et al 1978). Graduated catheters with centimetre markings are available to gauge how far the catheter has been passed.
- The non-intubated child requiring nasopharyngeal suction should be firmly restrained. The child should be positioned in side lying to avoid potential aspiration of gastric contents (Fig. 13.4). Constant reassurance should be given throughout the procedure. Supplemental oxygenation and resuscitation equipment should be available.
- Particular care should be taken with nasopharyngeal suction of neonates as reflex bradycardia and apnoea can occur.

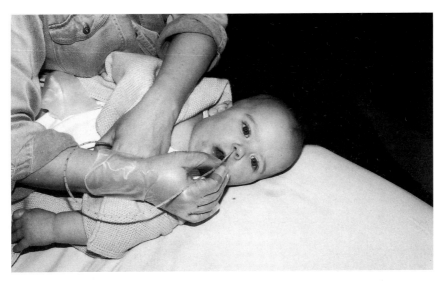

Figure 13.4 Nasopharyngeal suction.

● Nasopharyngeal suction should be avoided if the child has stridor or has recently been extubated as it may precipitate laryngospasm.

Passive movements

Passive movements and two-joint muscle stretches should be given regularly to older children in intensive care, although they are at less risk of developing joint stiffness than adults. Care should be taken when handling children and infants who are hypotonic in order to avoid soft tissue damage. Preterm infants are hypotonic and require minimal handling, so passive movements are not usually indicated.

MANAGEMENT OF THE ACUTELY ILL INFANT OR CHILD

Respiratory failure in acutely ill infants and children may result from many different medical problems. In the neonate the most common causes are prematurity, respiratory distress syndrome, asphyxia and aspiration pneumonia. Under 2 years of age bronchopneumonia, bronchiolitis, status asthmaticus, croup, foreign body inhalation and congenital heart anomalies are more common aetiologies. In chil-

dren over 2 years asthma, central nervous system infection (e.g. meningitis) and trauma are more frequent.

Equipment used in neonatal and paediatric intensive care

Physiotherapists working in an intensive care unit should be familiar with equipment used on that unit (Fig. 13.5). They should be able to respond when a problem is indicated by the monitors and be able to ascertain whether the problem is patient or equipment related.

Incubators and radiant warmers

Infants, especially preterm babies, may have difficulty maintaining their temperature and are therefore nursed in incubators or under radiant warmers.

Incubators are enclosed units of transparent material with portholes in the sides for access. They can be warmed and humidified air or oxygen can be delivered to the infant inside. The temperature inside an incubator is maintained in the thermoneutral range which is the environmental temperature at which oxygen consumption is minimal in the presence of a normal body

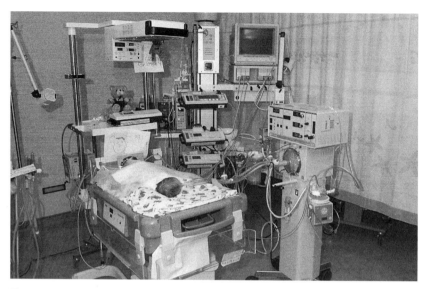

Figure 13.5 Equipment used in a paediatric intensive care unit. Figure shows an infant undergoing high-frequency oscillatory ventilation.

temperature. This will vary according to the patient's gestation and weight.

A radiant warmer is an open-topped unit with a radiant heating device above it. It allows free access to the infant but there is more convective heat loss and insensible fluid loss than with an incubator.

Phototherapy unit

These units consist of white or blue lamps which emit light of wavelength 400–500 nm. Light of these wavelengths oxidizes unconjugated bilirubin into harmless derivatives and so is very important in the treatment of jaundice in neonates. Infants receiving phototherapy have to be nursed naked, which can cause problems of temperature control. There is also increased insensible fluid loss and a theoretical risk of eye damage, so eye shields are placed on the infant.

Electrocardiogram (ECG), respiratory and blood pressure monitors

These are similar to the monitors used on adults (Ch. 4), although normal values vary according to age (Table 13.1).

Pulse oximetry

Pulse oximetry is a tool which non-invasively measures arterial oxyhaemoglobin (Ch. 4), giving a percentage value for oxygen saturation (SaO_2). The relative inaccuracy of these machines (i.e. their unreliability in reflecting arterial oxygenation) means that they cannot be used as the only method of monitoring oxygen in the critically ill infant. They are, however, useful in terms of monitoring trends of change in arterial oxygenation in acutely ill infants and children.

Transcutaneous oxygen monitors

Most neonatal units use transcutaneous oxygen monitors to give an indication of oxygenation. These monitors provide a non-invasive means of measuring the partial pressure of oxygen (PaO_2) in arterialized capillaries through the skin. Transcutaneous oxygen (TcO_2) monitors have electrodes which are heated and placed on an area of thin skin, e.g. the abdomen. The heating produces a superficial erythema so that the PaO_2 in the dilated capillaries can be assessed by the machine and displayed on a visual monitor. Normal values are 8–12 kPa (60–90 mmHg). Accuracy is checked by regular comparison with arterial blood gases.

Electrodes need to be moved to a different position every 4 hours in order to prevent burning. In order to remain accurate, the electrodes need careful positioning and calibration.

Carbon dioxide monitoring

When necessary it is possible to monitor CO_2 levels either transcutaneously or using infra-red end-tidal monitoring from the expiratory breath.

Respiratory support

Humidification of therapeutic gases

Humidification of inspired gases is essential for infants and children as narrow- bore endotracheal tubes (ETT) and small calibre airways can easily be blocked by thick secretions. Children requiring ventilation usually have a heated humidifier as part of the ventilator circuit. The amount of humidity received by the child is dependent upon the temperature of the humidifier, ambient room and/or incubator temperature, gas flow rate, level of water in the humidifier chamber, the length of ventilator tubing and the position of the temperature probe in the ventilator circuit (Tarnow-Mordi et al 1989). The optimum temperature of the inspired gas is unknown, but temperatures greater than 36.5°C have been shown to reduce the incidence of chronic lung disease in infants weighing less than 1500 grams (Tarnow-Mordi et al 1989).

Oxygen

Supplemental oxygen therapy for the treatment or prevention of hypoxia may be administered by several means and is discussed in detail in Chapter 6. However, the potentially adverse effects of excessive oxygen administration in premature infants or infants with high pulmonary blood flow will be discussed later in this chapter.

Carbon dioxide

Carbon dioxide is rarely used as a therapeutic gas but may be helpful in reducing pulmonary blood flow, for example in infants with large intracardiac shunts at risk of pulmonary hypertension.

Nitric oxide

Nitric oxide gas (NO) has a potent pulmonary vasodilatory effect and can be delivered directly to the lungs via the ventilator circuit for the effective relief of pulmonary hypertension in infants and children. Very small doses are used to reduce pulmonary arterial pressures, while systemic blood pressure is not affected (doses larger than 80 parts per million can be toxic) (Cheifetz 2000, Haddad et al 2000, Kinsella & Abman 2000).

Head box and nasal cannulae

Oxygen can be delivered directly into an incubator via an inlet but such delivery rarely exceeds an FiO_2 of 0.4. Head box oxygen delivery via a clear plastic box placed over an infant's head (Fig. 13.6) is a very effective means of delivering supplemental oxygen and FiO_2 levels of up to 0.95 can be effectively achieved. If used with small infants, the humidification of inspired gas should be warmed. Other means of O_2 delivery include the use of a nasopharyngeal catheter inserted 4–6 cm or paediatric nasal cannulae which can achieve an FiO_2 of 0.5 with a flow of 6 l/min. Older children are much more able to tolerate a facemask or nasal cannulae.

Continuous positive airway pressure (CPAP) and bilevel positive airway pressure (BiPAP)

Continuous positive airway pressure (CPAP) or bilevel positive airway pressure (BiPAP) (Ch. 9) may be used as a first-line treatment in infants and children requiring respiratory support or as part of the process of weaning from full ventilation. CPAP or BiPAP may be applied via an endotracheal tube or, in non-intubated infants, via a facemask or nasal prong.

Negative extrathoracic pressure ventilation

Negative extrathoracic pressure ventilation (NEPV) was first used in the treatment of children

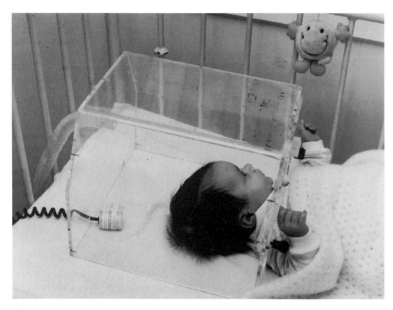

Figure 13.6 Humidified oxygen delivered via a head box.

with respiratory failure due to poliomyelitis. It is now most commonly used in patients with respiratory failure due to myopathy or other neuromuscular disorders and can be applied via a rigid thoracic jacket such as the Hayek jacket or cuirass shell.

Endotracheal intubation and mechanical ventilation

Details of paediatric mechanical support are described in Chapter 9.

Indications for endotracheal intubation are:

- maintenance of a patient's airway
- protection of the airway in states of altered consciousness
- facilitation of pulmonary toilet
- for mechanical ventilation due to inadequate spontaneous ventilation.

Tubes may be nasal or oral (Fig. 13.7). Historically infants and young children were preferentially intubated with uncuffed tubes to reduce the risk of damage to the tracheal mucosa and subsequent stenosis (Deakers et al 1994, Khine et al 1997). Although it was considered desirable

to have a small tracheal tube leak to prevent mucosal damage, there are considerable disadvantages to having moderate to large tracheal tube leaks in terms of inconsistent delivery of ventilation (Main et al 1999, Kuo et al 1996) and inaccurate monitoring of respiratory mechanics.

A variety of mechanical ventilators are used in neonatal and paediatric practice. Pressure-limited ventilators avoid excessive inflating pressures and reduce the risk of barotrauma. Time cycling allows the ratio of the inspiration to expiration to be controlled. Continuous flow of gas around the circuit will allow the infant to breathe spontaneously between ventilator breaths.

Volume-cycled (pressure-limited) ventilators deliver a preset tidal volume and are thus effective in situations where respiratory compliance is low and resistance is high. However, this can result in the delivery of excessively high inflation pressures which increase the risk of intrathoracic air leak and barotrauma. In the presence of tracheal tube leak, more of the delivered tidal volume will be lost with volume-controlled ventilation than with pressure preset ventilation (Watt & Fraser 1994).

The use of PEEP is standard when mechanically ventilating infants and children to prevent

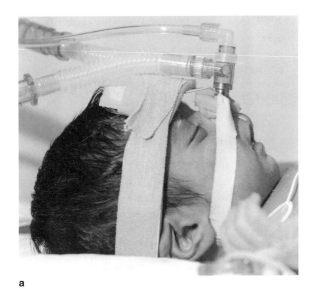

a

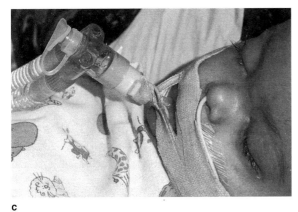

c

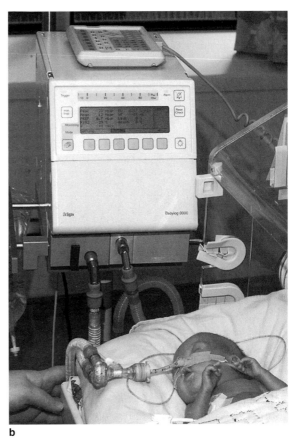

b

Figure 13.7 **a** & **b** Nasal intubation. **c** Oral intubation.

airway closure at end expiration as closing volume is much closer to FRC.

High-frequency ventilation employs small tidal volumes and high respiratory rates (1–15 Hz) to achieve adequate ventilation and has been shown to be safe and effective in the treatment of respiratory failure in paediatric practice (Arnold 1996).

Extracorporeal membrane oxygenation

Extracorporeal membrane oxygenation (ECMO) involves cardiopulmonary bypass to provide support for the heart and lungs or lungs alone when patients have severe but potentially reversible cardiac or respiratory failure (Ch. 9).

It has been reported to be beneficial in both neonates and children with acute lung injury and respiratory failure (Pearson et al 1993, UK Collaborative ECMO Trial Group 1996).

Liquid ventilation

Liquid breathing has been proposed as a means of improving gas exchange in infants with acute respiratory failure since the 1970s. It has been suggested that the use of partial liquid ventilation can improve ventilation/perfusion mismatch by promoting a more even distribution of pulmonary blood flow and improving compliance through the elimination of the gas–liquid interface. The ability to lower surface tension directed the initial clinical focus on neonatal therapy in the treatment of premature lung disease. The first clinical trial of perfluorochemical ventilation was performed in neonates in 1989 and additional trials have been performed since, which conclude that liquid ventilation appears to be safe, improve lung function and recruit lung volume. The results of such trials are encouraging, but randomized trials have yet to be completed (Arnold 1999, Bartlett 1999, Davies 1999, Greenspan et al 2000).

Complications of ventilatory support

- Pneumothorax may be caused by many factors including high peak inspiratory pressures, high positive end-expiratory pressure and long inflation times or by the infant actively expiring against the ventilator's inspiration (Greenough et al 1983). A tension pneumothorax will cause a sudden deterioration and will require immediate insertion of an intercostal drain. Small pneumothoraces may not require drainage. Pneumothoraces occur commonly in preterm infants with immature lungs or in association with congenital bullae. A predisposing factor is the hyperinflation of alveoli occurring in conditions such as meconium aspiration and respiratory distress syndrome (RDS).
- Pulmonary interstitial emphysema (PIE) occurs when gas leaks out of an alveolus, tracks along the cardiovascular bundle and remains trapped, forming interstitial gas pockets. PIE is most common in preterm infants; the incidence is inversely proportional to gestational age. Fast-rate, low-pressure ventilation with a long expiratory time has been helpful in reducing air trapping. In severe cases, where ventilation is becoming difficult, needle scarification of the lung surface may be helpful. Unresolved PIE may require surgical resection in severe cases.
- Subglottic stenosis occurs in some infants following prolonged intubation and leads to upper airway obstruction. It should be avoidable by attention to tracheal tube placement and fixation and care with suction (Albert

1995). Acquired neonatal tracheobronchial stenosis (particularly in preterm infants) has a poor outcome. Stridor is often present and may respond to adrenaline via a nebulizer. In more severe cases a tracheostomy may be necessary until the airway has increased sufficiently in size to allow adequate ventilation. Some patients will also require surgical laryngo-tracheoplasty before successful decannulation of the tracheostomy can be achieved. More recently, primary repair of subglottic stenosis with laryngotracheal reconstruction has been successfully developed.

- Retinopathy of prematurity is a condition of preterm infants seen when the capillaries in the retina proliferate, leading to haemorrhage, fibrosis and scarring. In the most severe form, this may result in permanent visual impairment. The cause is unknown, but periods of hyperoxia (exact length of time unknown) with a PaO_2 of above 12 kPa are thought to be a major predisposing factor (Roberton 1996). Careful oxygen monitoring, preferably using an arterial catheter, is essential to attempt to prevent this condition.
- Chronic lung disease (CLD) is defined as a requirement for ventilatory support at one month of age. Infants with the severest form who have specific radiographic changes are said to have bronchopulmonary dysplasia (BPD). CLD is discussed further later in this chapter.

NEONATAL INTENSIVE CARE

The reasons for admission to a neonatal intensive care unit (NICU) include the following.

- *Preterm delivery*: defined as less than 37 completed weeks of gestation (full term is 38–42 weeks). Preterm infants who require admission to a NICU are usually less than 32 weeks of gestation with a birth weight less than 2500 g. Some infants are born as early as 23 weeks gestation and weigh as little as 450 g. Causes of preterm birth include antepartum haemorrhage, cervical incompetence, multiple pregnancies or infection. There is also an association with deprived socioeconomic circumstances and in some cases the cause of preterm delivery is unknown.

- *Low birth weight:* often due to prematurity but more mature infants may also be of low birth weight due to intrauterine growth retardation. Causes include placental dysfunction, smoking and intrauterine infection, e.g. rubella.
- *Perinatal problems:* such as birth asphyxia or meconium aspiration.
- *Congenital abnormalities* include congenital heart disease and diaphragmatic hernia.

Prophylactic ventilation is often started from birth in infants <1000 g. Other indications for ventilation are: deteriorating blood gases (hypoxaemia or hypercapnia) despite a high FiO_2, recurrent or major apnoea, major surgery pre- or postoperatively for congenital anomalies.

Preterm low birth-weight infants have been shown to be better oxygenated with fast rates of ventilation (60–150 breaths/min) using time-cycled, pressure-limited devices (Greenough et al 1987). This seems to allow the infant to synchronize with the ventilator and thus reduce the occurrence of pneumothoraces. If synchrony cannot be achieved, it is necessary to use paralysing agents when ventilating these infants (Greenough et al 1984).

Weaning from ventilation in infants and small children is achieved by initial reduction of the inspiratory pressures and the inspired oxygen concentration. Intermittent mandatory ventilation (IMV) can then be used, followed by CPAP. Extubation is usually performed from CPAP via the endotracheal tube (ETT), but some infants require a period of support on CPAP via a nasopharyngeal airway (nasal prong) prior to unsupported spontaneous breathing. The weaning process in older infants is similar to that in adults.

Patient-triggered ventilation has been shown to assist weaning from conventional ventilation in some infants during the acute stage of respiratory distress syndrome (RDS) (Greenough & Pool 1988). It is not as useful in very preterm low birth-weight infants whose respiratory efforts are often inadequate and inconsistent. Modified neonatal ventilators that respond quickly to small changes in airflow are needed in these infants.

General problems of infants in the NICU

- Preterm and critically ill neonates tolerate handling poorly and should therefore be handled as little as possible. Physiotherapy and suction should only be carried out when indicated and careful assessment is essential prior to intervention.
- An association between chest physiotherapy and brain lesions, termed encephaloclastic porencephaly, in extremely preterm infants was reported by Harding et al in 1998. This study involved a retrospective analysis of 454 infants with birth weights less than 1500 g delivered between 24 and 27 weeks' gestation. Affected subjects received 2-3 times as many chest physiotherapy treatments as did the control group but the group also had more prolonged and severe episodes of hypotension in the first week than controls and were less likely to have had a cephalic presentation at delivery. The lesions were considered to be caused by impact of the brain with the skull during shaking movements, which could occur during chest physiotherapy with percussion (Harding et al 1998). Since this publication, however, several authors have disputed the association between encephaloclastic porencephaly and chest physiotherapy (Beby et al 1998, Gray et al 1999, Vincon 1999). The significant methodological errors in this work have been highlighted and it is possible that these lesions occurred only in the sickest infants and the fact that they had more chest physiotherapy may be a reflection of their degree of illness (Gray et al 1999). No cases of encephaloclastic porencephaly were reported over the same 3-year period, despite similar criteria for initiation of chest physiotherapy, in two separate studies (Beby et al 1998, Gray et al 1999). Although an association between chest physiotherapy and encephaloclastic porencephaly seems unlikely, it highlights the need

for very careful assessment of these preterm infants and a judicious approach to treatment. If chest physiotherapy is indicated and chest percussion thought appropriate, the baby should be kept in a stable position, with the head well supported, and vital signs carefully monitored throughout treatment.

- The preterm infant is particularly vulnerable to infection. The most important means of preventing and reducing cross-infection is by meticulous attention to hygiene by both staff and visitors. The skin is very thin and easily damaged and manual techniques should be applied with care.

- Physiological jaundice is common in the normal full-term infant owing to the breakdown of fetal haemoglobin causing a raised level of unconjugated bilirubin in the blood. It usually begins 2 days after birth and disappears by days 7–10. High levels of unconjugated bilirubin may diffuse into the basal ganglia and lead to a condition called kernicterus, characterized by athetoid cerebral palsy, deafness and mental retardation. Preterm infants are particularly prone to developing jaundice and run an increased risk of subsequent kernicterus. Serum bilirubin levels are closely monitored and treatment, if required, consists of phototherapy or in severe cases exchange transfusion. In this procedure, small amounts of blood are replaced by donor blood until twice the infant's blood volume has been exchanged.

- Pulmonary haemorrhage, defined as acute intrapulmonary bleeding, may be a life-threatening event. It is relatively uncommon but can occur after surfactant therapy. Physiotherapy is contraindicated, although regular suctioning may be required to keep the airway clear. When fresh blood is no longer being aspirated, physiotherapy techniques may assist removal of residual blood. Prognosis is often poor.

- Infants who have been resuscitated and require immediate admission to a NICU shortly after birth will not have had the chance for physical contact with their parents. Incubators and other equipment may be a further barrier to contact. Parents should be encouraged to give physical comfort to their infant by stroking and cuddling when possible.

- Nutrition: adequate calorie intake and weight gain are important in preterm and low birthweight infants to avoid hypoglycaemia, persistent jaundice and delayed recovery from RDS. Feeding should be started as soon as possible either enterally, in those who can tolerate it, or intravenously. Preterm infants have poor sucking, gag and cough reflexes so will be fed nasogastrically until these develop. Continuous infusion of milk may be preferable to bolus feeds which can increase respiratory distress, regurgitation and aspiration because of abdominal distension. Feeds are often better tolerated when the infant is lying in the prone position. Orogastric tubes may be used rather than nasogastric ones in order to avoid blockage of the nostril in spontaneously breathing infants with respiratory distress.

- Temperature control: preterm and low birthweight infants have difficulty in maintaining their body temperature because they have a large surface area relative to their body mass. They also have a smaller proportion of brown fat in comparison with full-term infants and easily lose heat through the skin by evaporation and radiation. Hypothermia can cause acidosis, hypoglycaemia, increased oxygen consumption and decreased surfactant production. Infants should therefore be kept in a thermoneutral environment (incubators or under radiant warmers) to maintain body temperature. Heat shields are used to reduce radiant heat loss and the ambient room temperature is kept high at 27–28°C. A core temperature of less than 36.5°C in preterm infants indicates that non-essential handling should be delayed until the infant's temperature has risen.

Respiratory distress

Respiratory distress syndrome (RDS) is a common complication of preterm infants, primarily caused by lack of surfactant. Steroids are usually administered to women in preterm labour in order to enhance lung maturation

(Crowley 1995). The more preterm the infant, the higher the incidence of RDS and symptoms develop within 4 hours of delivery with sternal and costal recession, grunting and tachypnoea. The chest radiograph shows a 'ground-glass' appearance due to lung collapse. Preterm infants, however, may be electively intubated and ventilated at birth before they develop these classic signs.

Treatment includes supplemental oxygen to avoid hypoxia, which may hinder surfactant production. Depending on severity, infants may require head box humidified oxygen, CPAP or full ventilatory support.

Pulmonary surfactant production usually begins 36–48 hours after birth, regardless of gestational age. The more mature infant will start to recover at this time. Very preterm infants who have other problems compounding their respiratory distress or infants who have developed complications of treatment may require ventilatory support for much longer.

During the last decade there have been many trials investigating the use of surfactant therapy to try to prevent or ameliorate RDS (Clements & Avery 1998, Morley 1997). Natural or artificial surfactant in fluid form is introduced into the endotracheal tube prophylactically or after signs of RDS have appeared. These trials have shown a reduction in mortality in very preterm infants given surfactant therapy.

As lung collapse in RDS is primarily caused by lack of surfactant, physiotherapy is not required for this condition. Secretions may become a problem after the infant has been intubated for more than 48 hours, owing to irritation of the tracheal mucosa by the endotracheal tube. These secretions may be cleared easily by suction alone. Physiotherapy may be indicated when suction is not adequately clearing secretions.

Respiratory distress in the preterm infant can also be caused by pneumonia. Organisms causing pneumonia may be bacterial, viral or fungal and may be acquired before, during or after birth. The most serious bacterial cause is group B *Streptococcus*. The presenting features of this pneumonia are similar to RDS with an indistinguishable chest radiograph. Group B streptococcal pneumonia can be rapidly fatal unless antibiotic therapy is started early. For this reason all infants presenting with respiratory distress are given antibiotics.

Periventricular haemorrhage and periventricular leucomalacia

Periventricular haemorrhage (PVH) is a major cause of mortality and morbidity in very preterm and low birth-weight infants. The incidence is inversely proportional to birth weight, occurring most frequently and severely in the smallest and least mature infant. The haemorrhages arise from the capillaries in the floor of the lateral ventricles and may occur spontaneously, but are most often associated with fluctuations in cerebral blood flow caused by apnoea, changes in blood pressure, carbon dioxide or oxygen concentrations.

There are four grades of severity.

- Grade I – bleeding into the floor of the ventricle
- Grade II – bleeding into the ventricle (intraventricular haemorrhage (IVH))
- Grade III – IVH with dilatation of the ventricle
- Grade IV – IVH and bleeding into the cerebral cortex causing areas of ischaemia

Grades I and II may be asymptomatic and chances of recovery are good. Grades III and IV are likely to cause residual problems such as hydrocephalus or neurological deficit. Severe grade IV haemorrhage may result in the death of the infant.

Prevention of PVH is directed towards minimal handling of 'at-risk' infants and avoidance of hypoxic and hypotensive episodes.

Periventricular leucomalacia (PVL) may occur on its own or associated with PVH. Ischaemia of cerebral tissue adjacent to the ventricles causes formation of cystic lesions. There is an association with neurological problems, particularly diplegia.

Regular cerebral ultrasound scanning is used to monitor the presence and progression of PVH and PVL.

Perinatal problems

Birth asphyxia

Birth asphyxia occurs in approximately 10% of births and if severe, may necessitate admission to the NICU. Careful monitoring will be required as these infants may develop cardiac failure, neurological damage or renal failure. Some may have fits and will need to have anticonvulsant therapy. As these infants are often very irritable, handling should be kept to a minimum.

Meconium aspiration

Meconium aspiration usually occurs in full-term infants who become hypoxic due to a prolonged and difficult labour. Hypoxia causes the infant to pass meconium into the amniotic fluid and to make gasping movements, thereby drawing meconium into the pharynx.

If the mother's liquor is meconium stained, a paediatrician should suction the infant's airway as soon as the head is delivered to prevent aspiration when the first breath is taken. Once delivered, the infant may require intubation for further suction. The irritant properties of meconium can cause a chemical pneumonitis and predispose to bacterial infection, especially *Escherichia coli*. A severely affected infant may require ECMO and/or assisted ventilation, although ventilation is often difficult because of the risk of pneumothorax due to gas trapping.

Physiotherapy. Physiotherapy is very important when meconium aspiration has occurred in order to remove the extremely thick and tenacious green secretions. Treatment consists of gravity-assisted positioning, as tolerated, with chest percussion and should be carried out as soon as possible after aspiration has occurred, preferably within 1 hour. Physiotherapy is often well tolerated soon after aspiration and in these cases removal of meconium plugs may allow the infant to be better ventilated. However, if severe pneumonitis develops these babies are often very sick, tolerate handling poorly and should be treated with caution.

CARDIAC INTENSIVE CARE

Congenital heart disease and cardiac surgery

Congenital heart disease is the most common congenital anomaly with an incidence of 8 per 1000 live births (Hoffman & Christianson 1978). Only about one-third of these will require surgical intervention, with the rest either resolving spontaneously or being haemodynamically insignificant. Major congenital cardiac defects can often be detected antenatally by ultrasound examination, while more minor defects may not be detected until the postnatal period. Diagnosis is usually confirmed by echocardiography. Postnatally most cardiac defects are amenable to surgery and overall mortality has fallen to less than 5% in the best units (Elliott & Hussey 1995). Early complete repair is attempted whenever possible, with the majority of operations being performed in the first year of life.

Management of congenital heart defects must involve agreement between cardiologist, surgeon, family and the child, if he or she is old enough. Each aspect of the child's care is an integrated process requiring the skills of a multidisciplinary team before, during and after surgery. The normal anatomy of the heart is shown in Figure 13.8.

Palliative procedures

When a primary repair is not possible, palliative or staging procedures will provide temporary or extended relief of symptoms. They are usually indicated to deal with excessive pulmonary blood flow, inadequate pulmonary blood flow or inadequate mixing between oxygenated and deoxygenated blood in the heart.

Pulmonary artery band. The pulmonary artery band is designed to restrict excessive blood flow to the lungs by reducing the diameter of the pulmonary artery with a constricting tape. A child with excessive pulmonary blood flow (ventricular and atrioventricular septal defects or truncus arteriosus) may present with poor feeding, heart failure, tachypnoea and, if uncorrected, pulmonary hypertension. If a corrective procedure is

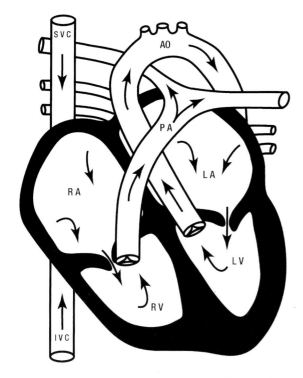

Figure 13.8 Anatomy of the normal heart: AO, aorta; PA, pulmonary artery; SVC, superior vena cava; IVC, inferior vena cava; RA, right atrium; LA, left atrium; RV, right ventricle; LV, left ventricle.

not possible pulmonary artery banding may be performed via left thoracotomy, to protect the lungs from the progression of pulmonary vascular disease. The pulmonary artery pressure is reduced to approximately one-third of the systemic pressure.

The modified Blalock–Taussig shunt. The modified Blalock–Taussig shunt (MBTS) is the most common palliative procedure used to improve pulmonary blood flow by connecting the subclavian artery and the pulmonary artery via thoracotomy. Inadequate pulmonary blood flow will result in poorly oxygenated blood and central cyanosis (e.g. tetralogy of Fallot, pulmonary or tricuspid atresia). If primary repair is not possible, the MBTS temporarily improves pulmonary perfusion, thereby significantly improving oxygen saturation (80–85%). The shunt (polytetrafluoroethylene conduit) is usually ligated at the time of definitive repair.

Septostomy. In defects such as transposition of the great arteries where there is inadequate mixing of oxygenated and deoxygenated blood within the heart, the foramen ovale may be enlarged using either a balloon atrial septostomy in neonates or surgically in older children via a Blalock–Hanlon septectomy.

Corrective surgery: closed procedures

Patent ductus arteriosus. The ductus arteriosus is the fetal vascular connection between the main pulmonary trunk and the aorta (usually distal to the origin of the left subclavian artery), which normally closes soon after birth. If it remains open, excessive blood shunts from the aorta to the lungs causing pulmonary oedema and, in the long term, pulmonary vascular disease. Symptoms may be mild or severe, depending on the magnitude of the left-to-right shunt. This defect occurs very commonly in premature infants and may cause difficulty weaning from ventilation or congestive cardiac failure.

In some circumstances (for instance, neonates with transposition of the great arteries) it is desirable to delay closure of the ductus arteriosus and this may be achieved by the administration of prostaglandin.

It may be possible to induce closure of the duct in preterm infants with indomethacin. Surgical correction involves left thoracotomy and ligation using silk ligature or a liga clip. In older infants closure may be achieved via cardiac catheterization using a double umbrella device.

Coarctation of the aorta. This is a congenital narrowing of the aorta. It usually occurs proximal to the junction of the ductus arteriosus and distal to the left subclavian artery origin. Neonatal presentation with symptoms of congestive heart failure requires early surgical repair. This is usually performed by resection of the stenosis and end-to-end anastomosis. If the aortic arch is hypoplastic a more extensive procedure, aortic arch angioplasty, is necessary. Repair of simple coarctation carries almost zero mortality. For severe forms of coarctation such as interrupted aortic arch (where upper and lower aortic arches are separated) the mortality rate is higher. Paraplegia is an extremely rare complication specific to correction of this defect (Brewer et al 1972) and may be associated with longer cross-clamping times.

Vascular ring. This defect is caused when malformations of the aorta or pulmonary artery compress the trachea, oesophagus or both (examples include double aortic arch, abnormally positioned innominate artery or abnormal course of the left pulmonary artery crossing behind the trachea). Symptoms include stridor, respiratory difficulties, repeated chest infections or feeding problems. Surgical decompression of the vascular ring will often improve symptoms but tracheal stenosis or malacia are frequently associated with vascular rings and may require further surgery to repair or replace the stenotic area.

Physiotherapy. Manual hyperinflation following tracheal repair may be associated with greater risk of pneumothorax, since the tracheal anastomosis is not initially airtight. In addition, the tracheal anastomosis is often distal to the tracheal tube and suction procedures should avoid traumatizing the site.

Corrective surgery: open procedures

Open procedures require cardiopulmonary bypass, modified for children in terms of size, flow rate, perfusion, temperature and drugs (Elliott & Hussey 1995).

Atrial septal defect (ASD). Atrial septal defect is one of the most common congenital cardiac anomalies, characterized by a hole in the atrial septum that separates the left and right atria. Types of ASD include ostium primum defects, also referred to as partial atrioventricular septal defects (AVSD), discussed below and ostium secundum defects due to failure of fusion of the two atrial septa and patency of the foramen ovale. Ostium secundum ASD is often associated with one or more of the superior pulmonary veins draining into the superior vena cava.

Children with ASD are generally asymptomatic and diagnosis is usually made after a murmur is detected at routine examination. If undiagnosed, slow development of symptoms may occur with rising pulmonary artery pressure and pulmonary vascular disease. If pulmonary vascular disease becomes severe and pulmonary hypertension is irreversible, then corrective surgery is not possible and heart-lung transplantation is the only palliative option. Because of the severe late consequences of pulmonary hypertension, repair is usually undertaken before the age of 5 years via median sternotomy or right anterior thoracotomy. The septal defect is usually closed by direct suture, pericardial or synthetic patch. Umbrella or balloon devices have also successfully been used to close small, round defects via cardiac catheterization.

Ventricular septal defect (VSD) Ventricular septal defects are the most common congenital cardiac lesions, defined by a hole in the septum that separates left and right ventricles. VSDs are often found in conjunction with other cardiac defects and the clinical presentation will depend on the size of the VSD and the presence or absence of other cardiac anomalies. Infants may present with congestive cardiac failure, recurrent chest infections and failure to thrive. More than half of all VSDs close spontaneously and do not require surgery (Elliott & Hussey 1995). However, as with ASDs, undiagnosed larger defects can lead ultimately to severe irreversible pulmonary hypertension.

VSDs (Fig. 13.9) are defined according to their position in either the perimembranous inlet, the trabecular portion or the muscular outlet of the ventricular septum. Primary repair is usually performed using synthetic or bovine pericardial patches via median sternotomy, with the cardiac approach varying according to the position of the defect. Conduction disturbances are common following surgery.

Although operative mortality approaches zero for isolated septal defects, multiple VSDs or 'Swiss cheese' defects carry a higher risk (De Leval 1994a).

Atrioventicular septal defect (AVSD). Incomplete development of the inferior atrial septum, superior ventricular septum and atrioventricular valves results in a spectrum of anomalies termed atrioventricular septal defects. Symptoms vary in severity according to the magnitude and direction of the shunt and the extent of the ASD, VSD, valve incompetence or combination of these. They may

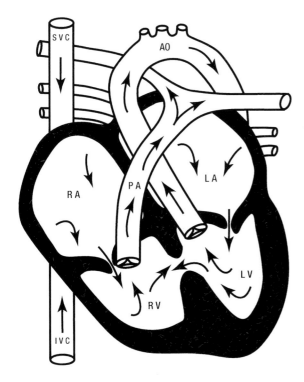

Figure 13.9 Ventricular septal defect, showing mixing of blood between the left and right ventricle: AO, aorta; PA, pulmonary artery; SVC, superior vena cava; IVC, inferior vena cava; RA, right atrium; LA, left atrium; RV, right ventricle; LV, left ventricle.

be associated with other cardiac defects (transposition of the great arteries, tetralogy of Fallot) and are also strongly associated with chromosomal abnormalities such as Down's syndrome. Some patients may be asymptomatic despite high pulmonary vascular resistance, but a high left-to-right shunt causes dyspnoea, recurrent chest infection and congestive cardiac failure.

Partial AVSD refers to an ostium primum type of ASD above the mitral and tricuspid valves which are displaced into the ventricles and may be incompetent. The development of pulmonary vascular disease is uncommon.

Complete AVSD is distinguished by a single six-leafed atrioventricular valve between the right and left atrioventricular chambers and continuous with the ASD above and VSD below. Over 50% of infants with this defect will die within the first year of life because of pulmonary vascular disease if left untreated. The remaining children will almost all have died within 5 years.

Both types of AVSD are repaired with patches on cardiopulmonary bypass via a median sternotomy. Hospital mortality is usually less than 10% but may be greater in patients with major associated anomalies. Early complete repair is preferred so that irreversible development of pulmonary vascular disease may be avoided but conduction problems and valve incompetence are relatively common postoperatively.

Tetralogy of Fallot. The four components of Fallot's tetralogy are classically described as a large VSD, right ventricular (infundibular) outflow obstruction, right ventricular hypertrophy and an overriding aorta (Fig. 13.10).

Inadequate blood flow to the pulmonary circulation and preferential flow of deoxygenated blood to the aorta may cause cyanosis, but severity of symptoms will depend on the degree of

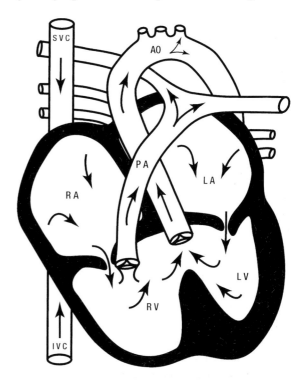

Figure 13.10 Tetralogy of Fallot, showing VSD, right ventricular hypertrophy, aorta overriding both ventricles and stenosis of the pulmonary artery: AO, aorta; PA, pulmonary artery; SVC, superior vena cava; IVC, inferior vena cava; RA, right atrium; LA, left atrium; RV, right ventricle; LV, left ventricle.

obstructed pulmonary blood flow. The majority of infants are pink at birth but become progressively cyanosed as they grow. Periodic spasm of the infundibulum prevents blood flow to the lungs and may cause 'spelling' episodes in which infants become irritable. Continued crying leads to increasing cyanosis and eventual loss of consciousness. The spasm then relaxes and the child gradually recovers. These episodes are dangerous and may lead to death or cerebral anoxia. Older undiagnosed children may intuitively squat following exercise, which reduces blood flow to and from the lower extremities in an effort to compensate for the large oxygen debt accrued during physical activity. In the presence of cyanosis, this behaviour may suggest diagnosis of this defect.

Some controversy exists about whether it is better to do primary repair or palliative shunt with repair when the child is older. Corrective surgery will involve closure of the VSD, resection of the hypertrophied infundibulum and reconstruction of the pulmonary arteries. Long-term results are good with actuarial survival of 93% at 15 years and good quality of life (Castenda 1994).

Pulmonary atresia. The infant with pulmonary atresia may be cyanosed at birth and this may become rapidly worse as the ductus arteriosus closes. Palliation in the form of a modified Blalock–Taussig shunt is the immediate treatment of choice so that adequate blood supply to the lungs can be established. Prostaglandins may be used to delay closure of the ductus arteriosus until surgery. This defect can occur with a VSD, in which case the right ventricle may be hypertrophied or hypoplastic and the pulmonary valve atretic. Sometimes the coronary arteries are supplied with desaturated blood from the right ventricle and major aortopulmonary collateral arteries (MAPCAs) often develop to augment pulmonary blood flow. The technique used for definitive surgical repair is variable depending on the size of the right ventricle. In the absence of right ventricular hypoplasia and coronary artery abnormalities, mortality is very low.

Transposition of the great arteries (TGA) This defect is characterized by the aorta originating from the right ventricle and the pulmonary

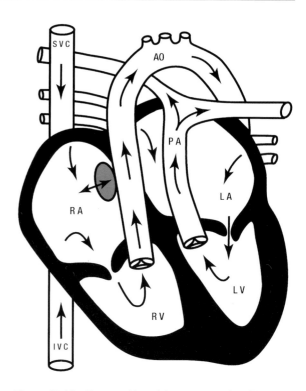

Figure 13.11 Transposition of the great arteries. Shaded area shows either position of a patent foramen ovale or site of balloon septostomy allowing some mixing of oxygenated and deoxygenated blood between the systemic and pulmonary circulations: AO, aorta; PA, pulmonary artery; SVC, superior vena cava; IVC, inferior vena cava; RA, right atrium; LA, left atrium; RV, right ventricle; LV, left ventricle.

artery from the left (Fig. 13.11). Oxygenated pulmonary blood recirculates through the lungs without reaching the body and deoxygenated blood recirculates through the body without reaching the lungs. The two closed circulations would quickly lead to death but there is usually a degree of mixing through the PDA and, if present, associated anomalies such as ASD or VSD. Babies therefore present soon after birth with cyanosis and immediate treatment aims to keep the ductus arteriosus open with prostaglandins until surgery. This can be followed by cardiac catheterization and balloon atrial septostomy if necessary.

The arterial switch operation has been performed with good results since 1985 and is the preferred option for simple TGA or for TGA with VSD. It is generally performed in the first 2–3 weeks of life, while the pulmonary vascular resistance is high and the left ventricle is 'trained' to receive the systemic workload. The aorta and pulmonary arteries (above the level of the coronary vessels) are transected and transferred to their correct anatomical positions. The coronary arteries are also transferred to their appropriate positions. Operative mortality is low (< 2%) and long-term results appear to be far superior to the earlier Mustard or Senning operations which redirected blood flow via intra–atrial tunnels (Jordan & Scott 1989).

Interrupted aortic arch. This rare condition is characterized by a discontinuous aortic arch and will result in death within the first month if left untreated. The most common site for interruption is distal to the left carotid artery. A VSD is almost always present, as is a PDA through which blood flows to the distal aorta. Soon after birth, when the ductus arteriosus begins to close, the pulmonary vascular resistance increases and severe congestive cardiac failure develops. Early surgical repair is the treatment of choice but is technically difficult and the postoperative course is often prolonged.

Total anomalous pulmonary venous connection (TAPVC). This anomaly is rare and involves two or more pulmonary veins connecting to either the vena cava or the right atrium. The reduced left atrial pressure keeps the foramen ovale open post–natally and mixed arterial and venous blood is transported systemically. Thus symptoms in the first few days of life will include congestive cardiac failure and cyanosis. There are often associated cardiac anomalies and surgical repair will depend on the nature of these, if present.

Truncus arteriosus. Truncus arteriosus is characterized by a single arterial trunk arising from both ventricles and from which the aorta and pulmonary arteries originate via a single semi–lunar valve. A VSD permits flow up the common trunk. Congestive cardiac failure and irreversible pulmonary vascular disease rapidly develop in early infancy and untreated infants rarely survive beyond their first year. Surgical treatment involves separating the pulmonary arteries from the truncal artery and connecting them via a conduit to the right atrium. The VSD

is closed to divert the left ventricular flow up the aorta.

Cardiac valve abnormalities

Aortic stenosis. Obstruction to left ventricular outflow may occur in isolation or in combination with other cardiac defects. They may be found at valvular, subvalvular, supravalvular or combined levels. Critical stenoses present neonatally with congestive cardiac failure and reduced peripheral pulses and require immediate intervention. Relief of aortic stenosis may be obtained with aortic valvotomy, aortic valve replacement, homograft insertion or balloon dilatation. However, mortality is high (10%) and reoperation common (Elliott & Hussey 1995). Aortic stenosis may not cause problems until adulthood although by then, a degree of left ventricular hypertrophy may have developed.

Pulmonary stenosis. The neonate with pulmonary stenosis may become progressively more cyanosed as the PDA closes and this may be reversed or delayed by the use of prostaglandins to keep the PDA patent. Management is similar to that of pulmonary atresia, with surgery dependent on the nature and extent, if any, of associated cardiac anomalies. Homograft valve replacement may be required at a later stage. Less critical pulmonary stenosis may present later in life with breathlessness on exertion and fatigue.

Tricuspid valve. Tricuspid valve disease is rare in childhood but is seen in Epstein's anomaly. Patients present with severe cardiac failure, cyanosis and dysrhythmia. Neonatal surgery carries a high mortality and a palliative approach with a later Fontan procedure may be preferred (De Leval 1994b). In the older child it is possible to perform a more complex repair of the anomaly.

Mitral valve. Mitral valve problems present either as stenosis or incompetence, usually associated with other cardiac anomalies. Repair is the preferred option though replacement may be the only option. Early replacement is associated with a high mortality (20%) (Carpenter 1994).

Hypoplastic left heart syndrome. This defect is defined by aortic valve stenosis or atresia associated with severe left ventricular hypoplasia.

Early mortality in untreated patients is high. The systemic blood flow derives almost entirely from the right ventricle through the ductus arteriosus and depending on the size of it, peripheral pulses may be normal, reduced or absent. Immediate management involves keeping the ductus arteriosus open with prostaglandins. Surgical management options include early heart-lung transplantation or staged surgical interventions which aim to turn the left ventricle into the systemic circulation pump while venous return passively enters the pulmonary circulation (Norwood, Fontan, bi-directional Glenn shunts and total caval pulmonary connection procedures are examples of this type of surgery) (Norwood & Jacobs 1994). Success of these types of surgery depends on the lungs being free of pulmonary vascular disease.

Physiotherapy management

In addition to the altered pulmonary dynamics and respiratory insufficiency seen after general anaesthesia, open heart surgery with cardiopulmonary bypass leads to further changes in respiratory function. Loss of perfusion and diminished surfactant production lead to poor compliance postoperatively. In addition, the lungs may be compressed intraoperatively, contributing to atelectasis. Pain due to the incision and presence of intercostal drains may cause splinting of the chest wall and reduced excursion.

Preoperative assessment

Preoperative assessment of both respiratory function and motor development is important. Any preoperative neurological problems or developmental delay should be documented and appropriate management plans formulated. The assessment of respiratory status provides an opportunity to evaluate postoperative risks and occasionally it may be necessary to administer treatment preoperatively. The value of meeting the child and family preoperatively is to explain carefully the postoperative process and procedures, in order to prepare them and relieve some of the anxiety of the unknown.

Postoperative management

Thorough assessment prior to any physiotherapy intervention is essential in these patients who may be significantly haemodynamically compromised. Heart rate is an important component in determining cardiac output in infants whose ventricles are less responsive to filling pressure changes. Bradycardia can significantly compromise cardiac output and in infants is easily induced by hypoxia. Adequate pain relief must be ensured and in the immediate postoperative period continuous infusion is the method of choice. In the older child patient-controlled systems can be used.

Treatment should only be performed when the child is stable and never following any potentially destabilizing manoeuvres. Continuous observation of heart rate, blood pressure, pulmonary artery pressure and oxygen saturation should guide the progression of treatment. Treatment techniques have been discussed earlier but a few specific points should be noted.

- As soon as the child is relatively stable it is usually feasible to use the side-lying position, with care not to kink or disrupt lines, wires or infusions, particularly neck lines, which may impede the delivery of inotropic agents. Hussey et al (1996) demonstrated a greater fall in oxygen saturation in children post-cardiac surgery who were turned as part of their physiotherapy treatment. More frequent but shorter episodes of treatment, performed only in situ or allowing for sufficient time lapse between turning and continuing with treatment, should be considered in the unstable child.
- Percussion and vibrations should be avoided if postoperative bleeding is persistent or excessive. Manual hyperinflation may be indicated to enhance secretion clearance and has been shown to have a negligible effect on oxygen saturation when used as part of a chest physiotherapy regimen for children post-cardiac surgery (Hussey et al 1996). However, care should be taken when cardiac output is low as the increase in intrathoracic pressure may decrease venous return, lowering the cardiac output further and leading to a fall in arterial oxygenation. Higher intrathoracic pressure

may also decrease pulmonary blood flow and should be avoided in children with low pulmonary flow anomalies (e.g. tetralogy of Fallot, pulmonary atresia). In duct-dependent children manual hyperinflation with 100% oxygen should be avoided as the response of the specialized ductal tissue to oxygen is constriction and closure.

Specific considerations

Pulmonary hypertensive crises. This phenomenon is described as an acute elevation of the pulmonary artery (PA) pressure (owing to contraction of the arteriolar musculature) which restricts flow through the lungs. It is associated with a fall in left atrial pressure and a dramatic fall in cardiac output. PA pressure may approach or even exceed systemic pressure. It is seen in the presence of hypertrophic reactive arteriolar muscle in the lungs and is therefore common in those patients who have had significant left-to-right shunts (VSD, AVSD, truncus arteriosus). The partial pressures of blood O_2 and CO_2 relative to each other will determine the ratio of systemic–pulmonary blood flow. Low O_2 and high CO_2 will increase pulmonary vascular resistance and reduce pulmonary blood flow. High O_2 and low CO_2 cause an increase in pulmonary blood flow.

Pulmonary hypertensive crisis is a critical, life-threatening event and prevention is the key to its management. Airway suction and chest physiotherapy have the potential both for precipitating a hypertensive crisis (by creating an imbalance in the pulmonary–systemic flow ratio) and for correcting an imbalance (caused by excess secretions). Treatment should be undertaken with great caution, inspired oxygen should be increased during chest physiotherapy and treatment times kept to a minimum. Particular attention should be paid to oxygen saturation and the PA pressure in relation to systemic blood pressure.

Delayed sternal closure. Occasionally postoperative closure of the sternum is impeded by pulmonary, myocardial or chest wall oedema (due either to prolonged bypass times or particularly complicated intracardiac repairs). If sternal closure is likely to constrict cardiopul-

monary function, closure may be delayed for days or even weeks. During this period children are paralysed, sedated and are preferentially nursed in supine. They are therefore at much greater risk of pulmonary complications. However, if stable and if the sternum is stented (to keep its edges separate), the child can with care be quarter turned into a side-lying position. Manual hyperinflation is usually well tolerated and gentle posterior and posterolateral vibrations can be applied. When the sternum is finally closed there is often a fall in respiratory function which may be important in terms of timing physiotherapy treatments (Main et al 2000).

Phrenic nerve damage. Damage to the phrenic nerve is a well-documented complication of paediatric cardiac surgery (Main 1995). It occurs most commonly where dissection is required close to the mediastinal vessels and pericardium with which its course is closely associated. The result may be an inability to wean from mechanical ventilation or severe respiratory compromise once extubated. Paradoxical movement during inspiration may compress the ipsilateral lung and cause mediastinal shift to the contralateral side, causing a further loss in lung volume. Physiotherapy intervention will depend on clinical symptoms but it is important that the patient is positioned head up to relieve the pressure from the abdominal viscera and reduce the work of breathing. It is sometimes necessary to surgically plicate the affected diaphragm.

GENERAL PAEDIATRIC INTENSIVE CARE

Patients with a wide variety of medical and surgical diagnoses are admitted to general paediatric intensive care units. The intensive care management of severe acute asthma and bronchiolitis is discussed in Chapter 9. Physiotherapy management is discussed later in the section on respiratory disease in childhood.

Trauma

Accidents are the most common cause of child death after the first year of life and 50% are road traffic accidents. Children who have been severely injured may require intensive care and mechanical ventilation, particularly after head injury.

Head injury

In the acutely head- injured child the primary injury refers to the damage sustained during trauma caused by bleeding, contusion or neuronal shearing. Secondary injury is due to the resultant complicating events. These may be intracranial factors such as bleeding, swelling, seizures and raised intracranial pressure (ICP) or systemic factors such as hypoxia, hypercarbia, hyper- or hypotension, hyper- or hypoglycaemia and fever. In the United Kingdom, 90–95% of injuries are managed without the need for neurosurgical intervention (Jennett & Macmillan 1981). When required, for example in the presence of an acute subdural bleed, surgical evaluation should be facilitated immediately.

The most common presentation of acute, severe head injury in children is with coma. Clinical scores, such as the paediatric modifications of the Glasgow Coma Scale (GCS) (Teasdale & Jennett 1974), allow bedside assessment of neurological function and the degree of impairment of consciousness in children. Such scores are designed to allow early identification of pathology when it is still potentially reversible by medical or surgical intervention.

Coma in children may present after a longer interval than in adults. Continued extradural bleeding following a relatively minor injury may lead to a deteriorating level of consciousness. Cerebral oedema may be focal or generalized; the latter may result in an increase in intracranial pressure and cause a more rapid deterioration.

Raised intracranial pressure

Raised intracranial pressure (ICP) represents an increase in the volume of the intracranial contents. In addition to trauma, it can be caused by space-occupying lesions or encephalopathy. The normal value of ICP is below 15 mmHg. The cerebral perfusion pressure (CPP) is the driving pressure for cerebral perfusion and is defined as the difference between mean arterial blood pressure and ICP. It is a crucial parameter which lies within the range of 50–70 mmHg. A variety of methods to monitor ICP can be used including intraventricular catheters, subdural or subarachnoid monitors and cerebral intraparenchymal catheters. While considered the 'gold standard' measurement, intraventricular catheters carry a risk of secondary infection.

Once the child is stabilized, medical management aims to avoid or minimize secondary brain injury. Factors which may precipitate a rise in ICP resulting in a potential fall in CPP should be avoided. The management of children with acute head injury has been extensively reviewed (Tasker 2001) and some of the strategies for management are discussed below.

- *Hyperventilation*: intubation and mechanical hyperventilation have been widely used to reduce ICP. It is suggested that hyperventilation may be detrimental as hypocapnia may induce cerebral ischaemia, but it is generally felt that it may be necessary for short periods during acute deterioration or when intracranial hypertension is unresponsive to other therapy.
- *Diuretics*: osmotic agents such as mannitol have been widely used to increase serum osmolality and reduce cerebral oedema. Renal function should be closely monitored, as renal dysfunction is a side effect of this therapy. Other agents, termed loop diuretics, such as furosemide (frusemide) have also been used for reducing cerebral swelling and this agent acts synergistically with mannitol.
- *Barbiturates*: in children barbiturate agents such as phenobarbitone and thiopentone are effective in managing raised ICP. The induction of barbiturate coma as a means of protecting the brain post injury has, however, not been shown to be of benefit clinically.
- *Hypothermia*: moderate hypothermia is used in some centres to reduce the cerebral metabolic rate and trials are currently being undertaken to evaluate the beneficial effects of this therapy. Most centres currently aim to keep the child normothermic, as fever leads to an

increase in cerebral blood flow and a consequent rise in ICP.

Physiotherapy

Immobility, impaired cough, depression of the respiratory centre and pulmonary dysfunction due to anaesthetic and paralysing agents predispose these patients to pulmonary complications. The frequency of pneumonia in severely head-injured patients requiring prolonged mechanical ventilation has been reported to be as high as 70% (Demling & Riessen 1993).

Safe and effective treatment should be based on careful assessment and judicious use of appropriate physiotherapy techniques (Prasad & Tasker 1995). The use of bolus doses of analgesics and sedatives or, in more unstable cases, thiopentone prior to intervention can help reduce acute swings in ICP. Length of treatment time is an important factor, with longer treatment more likely to produce larger elevations of ICP. Sustained increases in ICP during cumulative interventions should be avoided by allowing a return to baseline values between procedures.

Careful monitoring of CPP during treatment is essential and treatment should be withheld or abandoned if levels fall below 50 mmHg.

A head-down position is generally contraindicated and any change in position should maintain the head midline in relation to body position. A 30° head-up tilt has been shown to significantly reduce ICP in the majority of patients (Feldman et al 1992). Chest clapping may be better tolerated than vibrations and manual hyperinflation may be used with careful monitoring (Prasad & Tasker 1995). Endotracheal suctioning may have severe prolonged effects on ICP (Rudy et al 1986) and great care must be taken to avoid hypoxia. A protocol for physiotherapy management is shown in Figure 13.12.

Passive movements to maintain joint mobility may be felt necessary and it has been shown that these can be undertaken without detrimental effect on ICP in adults, provided that Valsalva-like manoeuvres are avoided (Brimioulle et al 1997).

SURGERY IN INFANTS AND CHILDREN

The effects of surgery, anaesthesia and immobility are the same in infants and children as in adults (Ch. 12). Owing to the anatomical and physiological differences, however, the potential for respiratory complications may be greater. Infants and children undergoing major surgery should therefore be regularly assessed by a physiotherapist.

Preoperative management

In some hospitals preoperative visits and handbooks are available which help to reduce some of the fear of being in hospital. Except in emergency situations, children and their parents should be seen by a physiotherapist preoperatively. Explanation of postoperative procedures should be given at a level appropriate to the child's understanding. Overloading the child with information which he does not understand only increases preoperative stress and anxiety. It is important that parents are fully aware of the need for postoperative physiotherapy intervention. Parents can play an important role in encouraging postoperative mobility.

Assessment by the physiotherapist should include respiratory function and motor development. If indicated, older children may be taught an airway clearance technique. Incentive spirometry can be useful in children, especially those techniques specifically designed for their use, for example the 'Coach' incentive spirometer which has a spaceship which moves upwards on inspiration.

When a child has preexisting pulmonary disease, for example cystic fibrosis, he may need to be admitted some time before surgery to clear his chest as effectively as possible. Some children may require physiotherapy and suction in the anaesthetic room following intubation and before entering the operating theatre.

Postoperative management

Children and infants should be regularly reviewed and treated as required. Effective pain

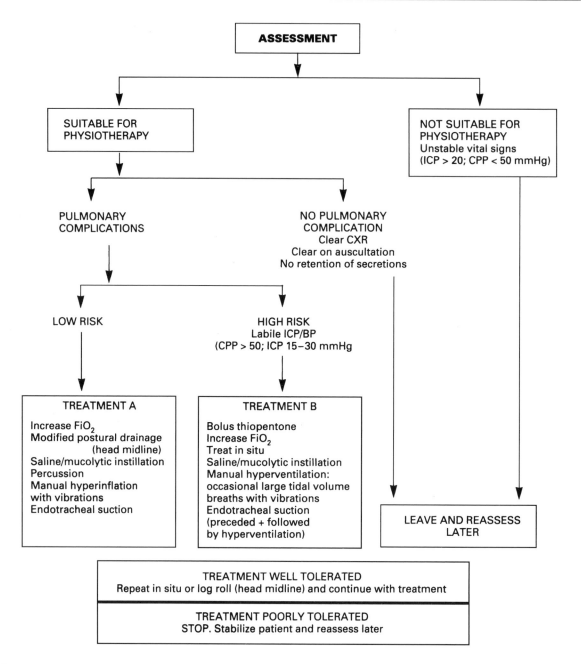

Figure 13.12 Flow diagram of an approach to chest physiotherapy in children with raised intracranial pressure. (Reproduced with permission from Prasad & Tasker 1990.)

relief is essential for children postoperatively prior to any intervention. It may be difficult to assess the severity of pain, as crying may be due to other causes. Lack of crying does not necessar- ily indicate lack of pain as children in pain are often totally withdrawn and immobile. Infants in pain may be tachycardic and tachypnoeic. Many children who have a fear of needles will deny pain in order to avoid injections. Infusions of analgesia are often used following major surgery for effective and continuous pain relief.

Treatment is directed towards early mobilization. When in bed, children should be comfortably positioned in alternate side lying or sitting upright and the 'slumped posture' should be avoided. As soon as possible children should be sat out of bed and walking encouraged when appropriate. Drips, drains and catheters can all be carried to allow early ambulation. Attention to posture is important, particularly following thoracotomy when shoulder exercises to the affected side are also essential.

If sputum retention is a problem postoperatively, airway clearance techniques may be required. A child often prefers not to have his wound supported or to support his own wound when coughing. At all times firm but sympathetic and gentle handling is important to avoid undue distress.

Congenital diaphragmatic hernia

Diaphragmatic herniation occurs when abnormal fetal development of the diaphragm weakens the muscular barrier and abdominal contents (most commonly stomach or small bowel) are displaced into the thoracic cavity, posteriorly, on the left side. The incidence is approximately 1 in 3000 births (Morin et al 1994). The abnormality may be diagnosed antenatally by ultrasound or postnatally in significant defects when the infant presents with neonatal respiratory distress. A chest radiograph will show abdominal viscera in the thoracic cavity. Unless the herniation has occurred late in pregnancy, which is very unusual, there will be associated pulmonary hypoplasia on the affected side as the abdominal viscera occupy the space normally available for the growing lung. The contralateral lung is also smaller than expected because of compression due to mediastinal shift during fetal development. There are also commonly other associated anomalies such as persistent foetal circulation and abnormalities of the pulmonary vasculature.

The infant with diaphragmatic hernia is often very unwell, particularly as the bowel in the

chest distends with air and further compresses the lungs, and requires immediate gastric decompression with simultaneous intubation and ventilation. Surgery is not carried out until the infant's condition is fully stabilized and extracorporeal membrane oxygenation may sometimes be required to support the infant until surgery is possible. Surgical correction is via a laparotomy. The abdominal viscera are carefully returned to the abdominal cavity and the defect in the diaphragm is closed.

Postoperatively, the infant may require ventilation for some time, depending on the amount of pulmonary hypoplasia. Prognosis is variable and mortality for isolated hernias is about 45% (Wenstrom et al 1991).

Physiotherapy. Physiotherapy may be indicated postoperatively if retention of secretions is a problem. Manual hyperinflation techniques should not generate excess pressures within hypoplastic lungs.

Other congenital anomalies of the lung

Congenital conditions of the lung such as lobar emphysema, lung cysts and adenomata are very rare. They may be diagnosed by ultrasound antenatally or by chest radiography postnatally. Treatment may involve surgical resection (lobectomy) if the condition is severe, but in some cases the lesions appear to resolve spontaneously in infancy.

Acquired lobar emphysema and lung cysts are more common as complications of respiratory distress syndrome and its treatment. Most of these cases will resolve with medical management though some do require resection.

Physiotherapy. Physiotherapy may be indicated postoperatively if there is sputum retention, but manual hyperinflation is contraindicated if cysts are present.

Oesophageal atresia and tracheo-oesophageal fistula

There are five recognized types of this anomaly. In the most common variety the oesophagus ends in a blind proximal pouch and there is a fistula between the trachea and the lower section of the oesophagus. About 10% of affected infants have oesophageal atresia with a tracheal fistula. The incidence is approximately 1 in 3000 births (Depaepe et al 1993).

The infant presents postnatally with episodes of choking, coughing and respiratory distress due to an inability to swallow saliva or feeds and consequent aspiration into the larynx or trachea. It is often difficult to pass a nasogastric tube, which on chest radiograph appears curled in the upper oesophagus.

Surgical correction is usually attempted as soon as possible and involves division of the fistula and anastomosis of the ends of the oesophagus. Some anastomoses may have to be performed under tension and the infant has to be electively ventilated and paralysed with the neck kept in flexion postoperatively. In a few cases, where the gap between the two ends of the oesophagus is too large, primary anastomosis is not possible and a feeding gastrostomy is performed. Oesophageal anastomosis or replacement by colonic, jejunal or gastric interposition is delayed until a later date.

Physiotherapy. If recurrent or continuous aspiration occurs before corrective surgery, physiotherapy (in the head-up position) may be indicated to clear excess secretions or treat lung collapse due to reflux of gastric contents. Preoperatively the airway is often kept clear by continuous suction of the upper pouch and the infant should be nursed head up to prevent reflux of gastric contents through the fistula.

Postoperatively, head-down postural drainage is contraindicated and patients are often nursed in the head-up position for the first few days, to reduce the risk of reflux. Care must be taken not to extend the neck, especially in patients with a tight oesophageal anastomosis. Naso- or oropharyngeal suction should not in general exceed the external distance between the nasal cavity and the ear. This distance is effective at producing cough and inadvertent damage to the oesophageal anastomosis is avoided.

Gastroschisis and exomphalos (omphalocele)

These conditions are relatively rare abdominal wall defects, occurring in approximately 1 in 5000 births (Baird & MacDonald 1982). Affected infants often have other major associated anomalies. Gastroschisis refers to an anterior abdominal wall defect through which the small and large bowel and sometimes the liver herniate. In exomphalos a membranous sac encloses the hernial contents. The defect is usually diagnosed antenatally by ultrasound.

Immediately after birth, the abdominal contents are covered to prevent heat and fluid loss until corrective surgery can be undertaken. In most cases primary repair is possible but where the defect is large a staged procedure is required.

Postoperatively the infant may require ventilation as the tightly packed, rigid abdomen causes respiratory embarrassment and compromises venous return. Where a staged procedure is necessary prolonged ventilation may be required. Some infants have impaired antenatal lung growth and a proportion continue to have abnormal lung function during infancy.

Physiotherapy. These infants are particularly at risk from retention of secretions and lobar collapse due to the distended abdomen and predominantly supine nursing position (with the abdominal contents suspended above the abdomen). If treatment is required, techniques which increase intrathoracic pressure and consequently intra-abdominal pressure, such as vibrations, should be used cautiously and manual hyperinflation is contraindicated. Postoperative respiratory compromise, if related to increased abdominal pressure, is unlikely to respond to physiotherapy. A slightly head-up position may relieve the thorax of some of the weight of the abdominal contents and reduce the work of breathing.

Transplantation surgery in children

The problems of cardiac, lung and heart-lung transplant surgery in children are similar to those in adults, and are discussed in detail in Chapter 16.

Liver transplantation

Liver transplantation is used for chronic end-stage liver disease and fulminant hepatic failure. Shortage of paediatric donors means that more and more grafts are reductions of adult livers. In some situations one donor liver can be used for two patients.

Postoperative complications include bleeding and splinting of the right side of the diaphragm. Patients invariably develop a pleural effusion which is usually right sided but may be bilateral.

Acute rejection is common 5–7 days post-transplant. Some patients develop chronic rejection and require retransplantation (Salt et al 1992).

Physiotherapy. Physiotherapists may have the opportunity to assess these patients preoperatively but often patients with fulminant hepatic failure are operated on as an emergency or are too ill to be seen preoperatively.

Postoperatively, the risk of bleeding in some patients means that handling is kept to a minimum. Patients are assessed regularly and treated as appropriate.

Following extubation, ambulation is encouraged as soon as possible. Large pleural effusions coupled with ascites mean patients are often very breathless and unable to mobilize.

RESPIRATORY DISEASE IN CHILDHOOD

Respiratory disease in childhood is very common. Most of the illnesses are mild; only a small proportion are more serious, involving the lower respiratory tract. The highest morbidity and mortality from lower respiratory tract disease occur in the first year of life. Respiratory disease is more common in children: from a poor socio-economic background, with a family history of respiratory disease; from an urban rather than country environment; with a school-age sibling or with a mother who smokes.

Respiratory disease is more severe in infants with congenital heart or lung abnormalities, immunodeficiency, cystic fibrosis or chronic lung disease.

Asthma

The prevalence rates of asthma vary considerably regionally and have been reported to be between 1.6% and 36.8% with the highest rates in America, Australasia and the United Kingdom. Much lower rates are reported in prevalence studies from Africa and Asia. Prevalence also varies considerably within countries regionally. Atopic (allergic) disease in general has increased over the past few decades and possible explanations for this rise include outdoor pollution, social deprivation/socioeconomic status, dietary factors and passive smoking (particularly maternal smoking during pregnancy). There has also been a significant increase in the number of children admitted to hospital with asthma, although this rise seems to have levelled out over the past few years (Ninan & Russel 2000).

Pathology

The main problem in asthma is a chronic inflammatory process within the airway resulting in recurrent episodes of wheezing, breathlessness and cough. There is an increased responsiveness of the smooth muscle in the bronchial wall to various stimuli. Hypertrophy of the mucus glands may lead to mucus plugging. These changes cause variable airway obstruction, which may become chronic and severe.

Aetiology

Children are more likely to develop asthma if parents or close relatives are asthmatic or atopic. There is an important link between atopy and bronchial hyperreactivity, and children with asthma often have other atopic features such as eczema, food allergy, hay fever or urticaria. Exposure to specific allergens such as house dust mite, pollen and animal dander can precipitate bronchospasm and wheeze. Exercise, particularly running, can precipitate an acute attack (exercise-induced asthma (EIA)), as can emotional upset or upper respiratory tract infections.

Management

The mainstay of asthma treatment is drug therapy. There are agreed guidelines on how asthma should be managed on a regular basis and during attacks (British Thoracic Society et al 1997, Rachelefsky & Warner 1993). Bronchodilator preparations are used to decrease bronchospasm and the most potent antiinflammatory agents are corticosteroids. The use of continuous oral steroids for prophylaxis is unusual nowadays, though more severely affected children may require them intermittently during exacerbations. Administration of corticosteroids by the inhaled route is safer and results in fewer systemic effects. Their early use is indicated when there is insufficient response to initial treatment with bronchodilators and a trial of sodium cromoglicate. It is important when using inhaled corticosteroids in children that growth is carefully monitored.

Bronchodilators may be given orally in children under the age of 2 years, but administration via this route is thought to be less effective and is generally no longer recommended. Inhalation of asthma medications provides topical effective therapy, which usually requires smaller doses and has fewer systemic effects. However, the method of drug delivery is very important and has been extensively reviewed (O'Callaghan 2000). The choice of device depends both on the drug to be delivered and the patient, particularly in relation to age.

Metered dose inhalers (MDI) can be manually or breath actuated and contain a mixture of propellant and drug which is emitted at a high velocity. Breath-actuated devices require an inspiratory flow of at least 30 l/min to trigger the device and there is very little published work on the efficacy of these in young children. With manual devices it is necessary to coordinate actuation of the device with inspiration. This makes them inherently difficult to use in young children unless given via a valved spacer device (Volumatic®, AeroChamber® or Nebuhaler®). These allow the infant or child to breathe (via mask or mouthpiece) from a reservoir of drug within a chamber. This also reduces the amount of drug impacting on the oropharynx and the potential for systemic absorption via the alimentary tract.

The mask of the spacer is held gently over the nose and mouth with the device held upright, at an angle greater than 45° to ensure the valve is open. The drug can then drift down through the open valve to be inhaled (Fig. 13.13a). As infants can exhibit paradoxical bronchoconstriction following inhaled bronchodilators, it is recommended that the first dose be given in controlled circumstances, for example in a hospital or clinic (O'Callaghan et al 1986, 1989). From the age of 2 years, the spacer device can be used conventionally with the MDI (Fig. 13.13b,c). Five tidal volume breaths are needed to inhale each dose of the drug (Gleeson & Price 1988). The click of the valve opening will be heard with each breath. It should be noted that different spacer devices have been shown to deliver varying drug doses (Barry & O'Callaghan 1996). Accumulation of static charge on the surfaces of the spacer attracts drug particles and can reduce the output. It is therefore advised that before the first use and at monthly intervals the spacer is washed in detergent and allowed to dry without rinsing or wiping (Drug and Therapeutics Bulletin 2000).

Dry powder inhalers do not use a propellant action but instead the drug is dispersed and delivered by inspiratory effort. Orophayngeal deposition is, however, quite high and therefore even older patients who require higher doses of inhaled corticosteroids should use metered dose inhalers with spacer devices in preference. The most commonly used dry powder inhalers are the Turbohaler® and Accuhaler®. From approximately 5 years of age, a child's inspiratory flow rate is usually fast enough to use a powdered device.

Nebulizers in the home setting are now being used much less in asthma. In severe cases or during exacerbations it may, however, be necessary to deliver bronchodilators and steroids via a nebulizer. It is preferable to use a mouthpiece (if the child is able) so as to avoid drug deposition on the face. Children with an acute severe attack usually display signs of respiratory distress, but wheezing may not necessarily be present. When airway obstruction in the presence of hyperinflation is severe, the airflow may be so low that

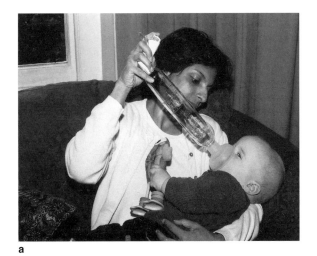

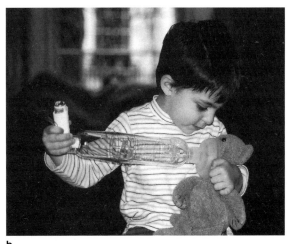

a

b

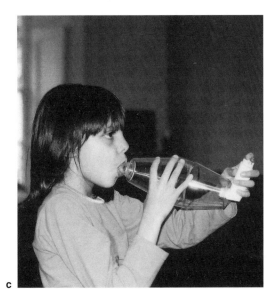

c

Figure 13.13   Administration of bronchodilator by spacer device to (**a**) an infant, (**b**) a teddy bear – to familiarize a young child with the device, and (**c**) a young child.

wheezing is not heard. Admission to hospital may be necessary and it is important to note that if nebulized bronchodilator therapy is given during an acute attack it should be oxygen driven to avoid hypoxaemia (Inwald et al 2001).

Newer breath-activated devices such as the Halolite® (Medic-Aid Ltd, UK) deliver pulses of drug during early inspiration only and may prove to be more efficient than the current conventional devices.

Physiotherapy. A crucial part of the management of asthma is education of the child and parents about the condition and its treatment. Often much of this is undertaken by the primary care team. The role of specialist nurses has also increased greatly in this field although physiotherapists are still involved in teaching children how to take their medication.

Physiotherapists should also be able to advise on exercise which is important in the asthmatic child to maintain general fitness. Where EIA is a problem (Godfrey 1983), bronchodilators should be taken before beginning exercise. Swimming is the activity least likely to cause EIA. Some physiotherapists organize swimming and exercise classes especially designed for asthmatic children. These classes include instruction in drug therapy, progressive exercise programmes to increase exercise tolerance, posture awareness and breathing control to help cope with breathlessness during an acute attack. Peak expiratory flow is monitored regularly to judge the effectiveness of treatment. Other than physical improvement, classes are also important psychologically, particularly for those with more severe asthma as these children are often afraid to exercise and lack confidence. Older children who do not have access to such classes should have the opportunity to consult a physiotherapist, if necessary, for education in breathing control and posture awareness.

Improvements in aerobic capacity after exercise programmes have been documented in asthmatic patients (Bingol Karakoc et al 2000, Matsumoto et al 1999, Neder et al 1999), but there is no clear evidence to suggest that exercise training can influence the dose of medication required or improve asthma control in some other way (Carrol & Sly 1999). Systematic reviews of the use of breathing exercises have also not been conclusive as to the efficacy of this form of intervention in asthma (Ernst 2000, Holloway & Ram 2000).

The child with acute asthma may need to be admitted to hospital and in severe cases may require mechanical ventilation (Ch. 9). Often the situation will resolve with careful medical management and appropriate respiratory support. Physiotherapy intervention is not always necessary. However if problems arise, due to mucus plugging or retained secretions, chest physiotherapy may be of benefit. It is essential that bronchospasm is adequately controlled before physiotherapy techniques are started. Treatment

should proceed cautiously and if bronchospasm increases it should be discontinued.

Although there is no routine indication for chest physiotherapy in asthma (Hondras et al 2000), children with persistent areas of lung collapse following an acute attack may respond well to an appropriate airway clearance technique. Parents may need to continue physiotherapy at home if bronchial hypersecretion persists.

Bronchiolitis

Bronchiolitis caused by human respiratory syncytial virus (RSV) is the most common severe lower respiratory tract disease in infancy. It occurs most frequently in the winter months. The cause is viral with RSV being the main agent in more than 70% of cases. As many as 1–2% of infants may require hospital management for RSV infection (Hodge & Chetcuti 2000) but other causes include parainfluenza, influenza and adenoviruses.

Pathology

Bronchiolar inflammation occurs with necrosis and destruction of cilia and epithelial cells, leading to obstruction of the small airways. Ventilation/perfusion mismatch cause hypoxia and hypercapnia.

Clinical features

The initial presenting symptoms are coryzal, such as the common cold. The infant develops a dry irritating cough and has difficulty in feeding. As the disease progresses, the infant becomes tachypnoeic and wheezy with signs of respiratory distress. The chest radiograph shows hyperinflation and patchy areas of collapse or pneumonic consolidation. Widespread inspiratory crepitations and expiratory wheezes can be heard on auscultation.

Management

Management of this condition is mainly supportive. The infant is given humidified oxygen via a head box as required. In those with severe respiratory distress blood gas monitoring and even ventilatory support may be necessary. Intensive care management of the infant with acute bronchiolitis is discussed in Chapter 9.

Most infants have difficulty with feeding due to respiratory distress. Milder cases may tolerate small, frequent nasogastric feeds, although the nasogastric tube causes obstruction of one nostril and may itself significantly increase the work of breathing. For this reason some centres prefer to use orogastric tubes. Small-volume feeds lessen the risk of vomiting and aspiration. More severely affected infants may require intravenous nutrition.

Antibiotics are not required as the cause of the illness is viral, although they are often used if there is suspicion of secondary bacterial infection. The risk of this is increased if the infant is ventilated and many centres would use intravenous antibiotics for those requiring mechanical ventilation.

Bronchodilators may be used in cases with severe wheeze, but effective response is variable and unreliable.

Ribavirin is an antiviral agent, which has been shown to be effective in reducing severity and duration of the disease (Barry et al 1986). It is delivered as an aerosol by a small particle aerosol generator for long periods (> 3–5 days). The drug is expensive and its efficacy remains controversial. Concerns regarding efficacy, the complicated mode of delivery and high cost have led to its clinical use being limited to those infants with pre-existing cardiac or pulmonary problems, immunodeficiency or severe respiratory failure.

Passive immunization with intravenous human immune globulin or intramuscular humanized monoclonal antibody given monthly during the bronchiolitis season has been investigated in high-risk infants but is very expensive and mixed results have been reported (Pringle 2000).

Physiotherapy. Physiotherapy is not indicated in the acute stage of bronchiolitis when the infant has signs of respiratory distress. Studies which have examined the efficacy of physiotherapy intervention compared to no treatment in these patients have not shown any benefit in terms of the course of the disease (Niclolas et al 1999, Webb et al 1985). The ventilated infant with bronchiolitis needs careful assessment and physiotherapy techniques should only be applied when sputum retention or mucus plugging is a problem.

Pertussis

Pertussis, commonly called 'whooping cough', is caused by the organism *Bordetella pertussis*. It occurs in epidemics every 3–4 years and is largely preventable by immunization. Following adverse publicity about side-effects in the 1970s, the uptake of immunization was greatly reduced, leading to an increased incidence of the disease.

Pertussis is particularly dangerous in infants less than 6 months of age and in children with other pulmonary problems, for example asthma and chronic lung disease.

Clinical features

The disease starts with coryza lasting 7–10 days during which the child is most infectious. The cough then becomes paroxysmal and can be provoked by crying, feeding or any other disturbance. It is particularly bad at night. The spasms of coughing may cause hypoxia and apnoea, especially in infants, and may lead to further problems such as convulsions, intracranial bleeding and encephalopathy.

At the end of the coughing spasm, the inspiratory whoop may occur followed by vomiting. Some very thick, tenacious sputum may be expectorated. This phase of paroxysmal coughing may last for 6–8 weeks and is exhausting for the child and parents. The Chinese call pertussis the '100-day cough'.

Bronchopneumonia is the most common complication, particularly in infants and may be due to the disease itself or to secondary bacterial infection with *Staphylococcus*, *Haemophilus* or *Pneumococcus*. The chest radiograph in severe cases shows hyperinflation and patchy areas of collapse and consolidation.

Management

Most children with pertussis will be managed at home. Infants and children with pneumonia may need admission to hospital. Treatment is supportive. Minimal handling in a quiet environment is essential for the infant with pertussis in order to reduce disturbance, which may precipitate coughing. Nutritional and fluid support should be given throughout the stage of paroxysmal coughing. Antibiotics do not affect the course of the disease but erythromycin may reduce infectivity and may also be given prophylactically to close contacts.

A small number of cases, particularly infants who have had frequent apnoeic attacks or hypoxic convulsions, will need intensive care and artificial ventilation.

Physiotherapy. Any physiotherapy manoeuvre during the acute phase can precipitate the paroxysmal cough with its complications. Treatment is therefore contraindicated in children during this stage.

If the child or infant requires ventilation, physiotherapy is very important to remove the extremely tenacious secretions, which easily block large and small airways and endotracheal tubes. The paroxysmal cough is not a problem when the child is paralysed in order to be ventilated.

When the stage of paroxysmal coughing is over, there may occasionally be persistent lobar collapse. This lung pathology often responds to an appropriate airway clearance technique. Parents can be taught how to treat the child at home.

Pneumonia

The most common cause of pneumonia in the neonate is *Staphylococcus*, in the infant RSV or *Mycoplasma*, and in the child *Mycoplasma*, *Streptococcus* or *Haemophilus influenzae*. Staphylococcal pneumonia can be an indication of underlying lung disease, for example cystic fibrosis.

Clinical features

Presenting signs are pyrexia, dry cough, tachypnoea and sometimes recession of the ribs and sternum. The chest radiograph shows areas of consolidation. Chest signs are often minimal compared with the degree of illness. Children with underlying pulmonary disease are particularly at risk from pneumonia.

Management

Treatment is supportive with adequate fluid intake and humidified oxygen, if required. In younger children it is impossible to distinguish between viral and bacterial pneumonia and broad-spectrum antibiotics are usually given.

Physiotherapy. In many cases of pneumonia there is consolidation of lung tissue with no excess secretions and there is no evidence that physiotherapy is of benefit (Stiller 2000). Where sputum retention is a problem, appropriate gravity-assisted positions with clapping, and in the older child breathing techniques, can be used. Copious amounts of sputum may be cleared in one treatment following which the pyrexia may settle and the child will feel better. Reassessment of the child is often necessary as retention of secretions may become a problem as the pneumonia resolves.

Acute laryngotracheobronchitis (croup)

Croup is a common problem occurring between the ages of 6 months and 4 years. The illness is usually viral and produces acute inflammation and oedema of the airway.

Clinical features

The presenting symptoms are coryzal and later the symptoms include a harsh barking cough and hoarse voice. There may be fever. Stridor, initially inspiratory only, is much worse at night and may become inspiratory and expiratory. Signs of respiratory obstruction are seen and the severely affected child may develop respiratory failure. The acute stage of respiratory obstruction may only last 1–2 days but the stridor and cough may continue for 7–10 days. Some children have recurrent bouts of croup.

Management

Mild cases can be managed at home. Extra humidity is often given, for example by sitting with the child in a warm steamy bathroom, but there is no objective evidence of benefit from this treatment.

More severely affected infants will be admitted to hospital and given humidified oxygen if hypoxic or distressed. Treatment is supportive but with minimal handling as any disturbance that upsets the child will increase the laryngeal obstruction. Nebulized adrenaline may be given with careful observation, in case of rebound and an acute collapse, and has been shown to provide short-term relief but is probably not useful in the long term. Antibiotics are not usually required unless there is some specific evidence of bacterial cause, for example purulent secretions. Glucocorticoids (dexamethasone and budesonide) have rapid beneficial effects on symptoms and have been shown to decrease the length of time of hospital admission (Ausejo et al 2000).

Very few children with croup who are admitted to hospital go on to require intubation in order to maintain the airway due to severe respiratory obstruction. A few of these, particularly infants, may also require some additional form of respiratory support, e.g. IPPV or CPAP.

Physiotherapy. Physiotherapy is contraindicated in the non-intubated child with croup. Treatment may be required when the child is intubated if sputum cannot be cleared by suction alone.

Acute epiglottitis

Epiglottitis is caused by *Haemophilus influenzae* but is now rarely seen due to the introduction of the Hib (*Haemophilus influenzae*) vaccine. It is, however, a very dangerous condition which occurs between the ages of 1 and 7 years.

Clinical features

The onset is sudden, with a severe sore throat and high temperature. Stridor and dysphagia develop rapidly, the child is unable to swallow saliva and dribbles. The neck is held extended in an attempt to open the airway. Acute and possibly fatal obstruction of the airway can develop.

Management

The child with suspected epiglottitis should not be disturbed in any way. No attempt should be made to examine the throat as this may precipitate obstruction. Usual management is intubation with a nasotracheal tube. In extreme circumstances tracheostomy may be necessary but should only be required for 3–4 days following which there is usually complete recovery.

Physiotherapy. Physiotherapy techniques may be required in the intubated child if secretions cannot be removed by suction alone.

Chronic lung disease

Over the past few decades there has been a steady improvement in the survival of very preterm infants with birth weights of less than 1500g. Chronic respiratory morbidity is common in these infants; those who have abnormalities on chest radiograph and are chronically oxygen dependent are said to have chronic lung disease (CLD) and those with a more severe form are described as having bronchopulmonary dysplasia. The incidence of CLD varies between 4% and 40% according to the initial respiratory illness, birth weight and gestational age at delivery (Greenough 1996b). It is more common in preterm infants who have had acute RDS requiring oxygen and ventilatory support. High peak pressures in positive pressure ventilation cause barotrauma and high inspired oxygen concentrations cause an acute inflammatory response leading to local tissue damage. Other precipitating factors are fluid overload, persistent ductus arteriosus (PDA), pulmonary interstitial emphysema (PIE) and infection.

The infant with CLD shows an increased oxygen requirement and carbon dioxide retention and has decreased lung compliance with increased airway resistance. Tachypnoea and persistent sternal and costal recession are usually present. The condition may be progressive, requiring more ventilatory support and eventually leading to respiratory and cardiac failure.

Radiographic appearances can vary but include alternating areas of collapse and hyperinflation, widespread fibrosis and scarring of the lung with compensatory emphysema.

Treatment consists of appropriate respiratory support, which may include mechanical ventilation or added oxygen via a head box or nasal cannulae. Good nutrition is essential and the infant may require fluid restriction and diuretics. Some infants respond to bronchodilators and steroids. Antibiotics may be required as these infants are prone to recurrent chest infections. The prognosis is variable. Mortality may be as high as 40% in severe cases. CLD is associated with lung function abnormalities during the preschool years. These may remain detectable even in adolescents who required chronic oxygen supplementation after premature birth even though they may not have respiratory symptoms (Kennedy 1999). Those who survive are often small and underweight, have lung function abnormalities, recurrent upper and lower respiratory tract infections, wheezing and gastric reflux (Greenough 1996b, 2000). Some children may require oxygen for several years and are therefore managed at home if the family is able to cope with home oxygen therapy. The long-term prognosis for those who survive the first 2 years is good.

Physiotherapy. Infants with CLD are particularly prone to chest infections and physiotherapy may be indicated if secretion retention is a problem. However, these infants often have severe wheeze and airway collapse and some physiotherapy techniques may not be appropriate. Careful assessment is important before any intervention. If wheezing is not too severe, careful treatment may be possible following bronchodilator therapy, providing the infant has a good response (O'Callaghan et al 1986, 1989). Modified gravity-assisted positions with chest percussion may be useful in infants and nasopharyngeal suction may be required. In older children an appropriate airway clearance technique should be used either during episodes of infection or if retained secretions are a persistent problem. Children, particularly infants, in whom supplemental oxygen is delivered via nasal cannulae often have a problem with thick, dry nasal secretions and may need humidification. Humidifiers which bubble oxygen through cold water counteract the absolute dryness of the oxygen to some extent but are unlikely to be effective in loosening secretions. If necessary, the infant should have nasal cannulae while awake during the day to allow social interaction, but should have humidified oxygen via a head box for long periods of sleep. Normal saline or a mucolytic via a nebulizer may be helpful and sometimes saline nose drops are used, but these have a limited effect.

Inhaled foreign body

Aspiration of a foreign body into the respiratory tract can occur at all ages, but is most common between the ages of 1 and 3 years. All types of foodstuffs may be aspirated, for example peanuts, pieces of fruit and vegetables, as well as small plastic or metal toys.

Objects are most commonly aspirated into the right main bronchus. The left main bronchus and trachea are the next most common, and smaller objects may be inhaled into right middle and lower lobe bronchi or occasionally into the left lower lobe bronchus.

When aspiration has been witnessed by parents or carers, the child should be taken immediately to hospital. On examination there may be wheeze and some signs of respiratory distress. Breath sounds may be reduced over the affected lung. The chest radiograph taken on expiration may show gas trapping in the area distal to the blockage.

In some cases the aspiration is not witnessed and the acute changes just described may be assumed to be the onset of a respiratory infection. The bronchial wall becomes oedematous, especially if the inhaled object is vegetable matter. Total obstruction of the bronchus gradually occurs and secondary pneumonic changes develop in the area distal to the obstruction. After a few days the child may become unwell with a persistent cough. The longer the obstruction remains, the more permanent the lung damage, eventually leading to bronchiectasis (Dinwiddie 1997). An inhaled foreign body should be suspected in a child with a pneumonia which does not respond to conventional treatment.

Management

All children who have aspirated a foreign body into the airway should have an urgent rigid bronchoscopy for removal of the foreign body. If symptoms persist, a repeat bronchoscopy may be necessary to ensure complete removal. Rarely bronchoscopic removal may fail and thoracotomy may be required.

Physiotherapy. Physiotherapy is not indicated to attempt to remove the object before bronchoscopy. Usually physiotherapy is ineffective as the object is firmly wedged in the bronchus. However if the object is dislodged by physiotherapy manoeuvres, it may travel up the bronchial tree and obstruct the trachea, leading to respiratory arrest.

Following bronchoscopy, gravity-assisted positioning and chest clapping may be necessary to clear excess secretions, particularly if the object has been aspirated for some time and secondary bacterial infection has occurred.

Primary ciliary dyskinesia

Primary ciliary dyskinesia (PCD) is a rare, inherited (autosomal recessive) condition in which cilial motility is severely reduced because of structural defects within the cilia.

Disorders of ciliary structure or function result in recurrent sinusitis and bronchiectasis due to decreased clearance of secretions (Cowan et al 2001). Males are often infertile because of reduced cilial motility of the sperm tails. A classic triad of sinusitis, bronchiectasis and dextrocardia is known as Kartagener's syndrome, but only about 50% of patients with ciliary dyskinesia present with this picture. Cilia can be examined for motility using nasal epithelial brushings.

Infants with this condition may present in the neonatal period with pneumonia, but many children present later with chronic upper and lower respiratory tract infection. This condition is not curable, so treatment is directed towards preventing infection and chronic lung damage. Appropriate antibiotic therapy is required during periods of infection. Children usually require daily physiotherapy to clear bronchial secretions. An individualized programme of airway clearance should be formulated using an appropriate airway clearance technique (Ch. 6). There has been very little work published on chest physiotherapy in this condition, but it has been suggested that airway clearance techniques may play a relevant role (Gremmo & Guenza 1999) (see also Ch. 20).

Cystic fibrosis

Cystic fibrosis (CF) is the most common inherited condition in Caucasians, occurring in about 1 in 2500 births. The major clinical and diagnostic features result from abnormalities of the exocrine glands, the most important areas affected being the respiratory and digestive tracts. Twelve percent of children present at birth with meconium ileus, where thickened meconium causes blockage of the colon and ileum. The infant presents in the first day of life with abdominal distension, vomiting and failure to pass meconium. The obstruction can often be conservatively managed but occasionally laparotomy may be required. Other modes of presentation include recurrent chest infections and/or failure to thrive. Diagnosis of CF is confirmed with a sweat test and blood sampling for genotype.

Physiotherapy. Physiotherapy is usually implemented from the time of diagnosis in an attempt to prevent progressive lung damage caused by persistent airway inflammation and infection. Cystic fibrosis is fully described in Chapter 20.

Acknowledgement

The authors would like to thank Annette Parker for her contributions which have been retained from 'Paediatrics' in the second edition of *Physiotherapy for respiratory and cardiac problems*.

REFERENCES

Albert D 1995 Management of suspected tracheobronchial stenosis in ventilated neonates. Archives of Disease in Childhood 72: 1–2

Arnold JH 1996 High frequency oscillatory ventilation: theory and practice in paediatric patients. Paediatric Anaesthesia 6: 437–441

Arnold JH 1999 Partial liquid breathing: more questions than answers. Critical Care Medicine 27: 2058–2060

Ausejo M, Saenz A, Pham B et al 2000 Glucocorticosteroids for croup (Cochrane Review). In: The Cochrane Library, Issue 4. Update Software, Oxford

Baird PA, MacDonald EC 1982 An epidemiologic study of congenital malformations of the anterior abdominal wall in more than half a million consecutive live births. American Journal of Human Genetics 34: 517–521

Barry P, O'Callaghan C 1996 Inhalational drug delivery from seven different spacer devices. Thorax 51: 835–840

Barry W, Cockburn F, Cornall R, Price JF, Sutherland G, Vardag A 1986 Ribavirin aerosol for acute bronchiolitis. Archives of Disease in Childhood 61: 593–597

Bartlett RH 1999 Liquid ventilation: background and clinical trials. Pediatric.Pulmonology 18: 182–183

Bartlett RH, Gazzaniga AB Geraghty, TR 1973 Respiratory manoeuvres to prevent postoperative pulmonary complications. A critical review. *JAMA* 224: 1017–1021

Beby PJ, Henderson-Smart DJ, Lacey JL, Rieger I 1998 Short and long term neurological outcomes following neonatal chest physiotherapy. Journal of Paediatric Child Health 34: 60–62

Bhuyan U, Peters AM, Gordon I, Helms P 1989 Effect of posture on the distribution of pulmonary ventilation and perfusion in children and adults. Thorax 44: 480–484

Bingol Karakoc G, Yilmaz M, Sur S, Ufuk Altintas D, Sarpel T, Guneter Kendirli S 2000 The effects of daily pulmonary rehabilitation program at home on childhood asthma. Allergology Immunopathology (Madr) 28: 12–14

Blackwood B 1999 Normal saline instillation with endotracheal suctioning: primum non nocere (first do no harm). Journal of Advanced Nursing 29: 928–934

Blumenthal I, Lealman GT 1982 Effects of posture on gastro-oesophageal reflux in the newborn. Archives of Disease in Childhood 57: 555–556

Brackbill Y, Douthitt T C, West H 1973 Psychophysiological effects in the neonate of prone versus supine placement. Journal of Pediatrics 82: 82–83

Brandstater B, Muallem M 1969 Atelectasis following tracheal suction in infants. Anesthesiology 31: 468–473

Brewer LA, Fosburg RG, Mulder GA, Verska JJ 1972 Spinal cord complications following surgery for coarctation of the aorta–a study of 66 cases. Journal of Thoracic and Cardiovascular Surgery 64: 368

Brimioulle S, Moraine JJ, Norrenberg K, Kahn RJ 1997 Effect of positioning and exercise on intracranial pressure in a neurosurgical intensive care unit. Physical Therapy 77: 1682–1689

British Thoracic Society et al 1997 The British guidelines on asthma management. Thorax 52(suppl 1): S1–S21

Button BM (1999) Postural drainage techniques and gastro-oesophageal reflux in infants with cystic fibrosis [letter]. European Respiratory Journal 14: 1456–1457

Button BM, Heine RG, Catto-Smith AG, Phelan PD, Olinsky A 1997 Postural drainage and gastro-oesophageal reflux in infants with cystic fibrosis. Archives of Disease in Childhood 76: 148–150

Campbell AH, O'Connell JM, Wilson F 1975 The effect of chest physiotherapy upon the FEV1 in chronic bronchitis. Medical Journal of Australia 1: 33–35

Carpenter A 1994 Congenital malformation of the mitral valve. In: Stark J, De Leval M (eds) Surgery for congenital heart defects, 2nd edn. WB Saunders, Philadelphia, pp 599–614

Carrol N, Sly P 1999 Exercise training as an adjunct to asthma management. Thorax 54: 190–191

Castenda AR 1994 Tetralogy of Fallot. In: Stark J, De Leval M (eds) Surgery for congenital heart defects, 2nd edn. WB Saunders, Philadelphia, pp 405–416

Cheifetz IM 2000 Inhaled nitric oxide: plenty of data, no consensus. Critical Care Medicine 28: 902–903

Chulay M, Graeber GM 1988 Efficacy of a hyperinflation and hyperoxygenation suctioning intervention. Heart and Lung 17: 15–22

Clark AP, Winslow EH, Tyler DO, White KM 1990 Effects of endotracheal suctioning on mixed venous oxygen saturation and heart rate in critically ill adults. Heart and Lung 19: 552–557

Clarke RC, Kelly BE, Convery PN, Fee JP 1999 Ventilatory characteristics in mechanically ventilated patients during manual hyperventilation for chest physiotherapy. Anaesthesia 54: 936–940

Clement AJ, Hubsch SK 1968 Chest physiotherapy by the 'bag squeezing' method: a guide to technique. Physiotherapy 54: 355–359

Clements JA, Avery ME 1998 Lung surfactant and neonatal respiratory distress syndrome. American Journal of Respiratory and Critical Care Medicine 157: S59-S66

Cowan MJ, Gladwin MT, Shelhamer JH 2001 Disorders of ciliary motility. American Journal of Medical Science 321: 3–10

Crowley P 1995 Update on the antenatal steroid meta-analysis. American Journal of Obstetrics and Gynecology 173: 322–335

Czarnik RE, Stone KS, Everhart CJ, Preusser BA 1991 Differential effects of continuous versus intermittent suction on tracheal tissue. Heart and Lung 20: 144–151

Davies H, Kitchman R, Gordon G, Helms P 1985 Regional ventilation in infancy. Reversal of the adult pattern. New England Journal of Medicine 313: 1627–1628

Davies M 1999 Liquid ventilation. Journal of Paediatrics and Child Health 35: 434–437

De Leval M 1994a Ventricular septal defects. In: Stark J, De Leval M (eds) Surgery for congenital heart defects, 2nd edn. WB Saunders, Philadelphia, pp 355–371

De Leval M 1994b Tricuspid valve. In: Stark J, De Leval M (eds) Surgery for congenital heart defects, 2nd edn. W B Saunders, Philadelphia, ch 23, pp 453–466

Deakers TW, Reynolds G, Stretton M, Newth CJ 1994 Cuffed endotracheal tubes in pediatric intensive care. Journal of Pediatrics 125: 57–62

Dean E 1985 Effect of body position on pulmonary function. Physical Therapy 65: 613–618

Demling RH, Riessen R 1993 Respiratory failure after cerebral injury. Critical Care Medicine 1: 440–446

Demont B, Escarrou P, Vincon C, Cambas CH, Grisan A, Odievre M 1991 Effects of respiratory physical therapy and nasopharyngeal suction on gastrooesophageal reflux in infants less than one year of age with or without abnormal reflux. Archives Francaises de Pediatrie (Paris) 48: 621–625

Depaepe A, Dolk A, Lechat M F 1993 The epidemiology of tracheo-oesophageal fistula and oesophageal atresia in Europe. Archives of Disease in Childhood 68: 743–748

Dinwiddie R 1997 Aspiration syndromes. In: The diagnosis and management of paediatric respiratory disease, 2nd edn. Churchill Livingstone, New York, pp 247–260

Drug and Therapeutics Bulletin 2000 Inhaler devices for asthma. Drugs and Therapeutics Bulletin 38(2): 914

Elliott M, Hussey J 1995 Paediatric cardiac surgery. In: Prasad SA, Hussey J (eds) Paediatric respiratory care. Chapman and Hall, London, pp 122–141

Ernst E 2000 Breathing techniques–adjunctive treatment modalities for asthma? A systematic review. European Respiratory Journal 15: 969–972

Feldman Z, Kanter MJ, Robertson CS et al 1992 Effect of head elevation on intracranial pressure and cerebral blood flow in head injured patients. Journal of Neurosurgery 59: 206–211

Gattinoni L, Pesenti A, Bombino M, Pelosi P, Brazzi L 1993 Role of extracorporeal circulation in adult respiratory distress syndrome management. New Horizons 1: 603–612

Glass C, Grap MJ, Corley MC, Wallace D 1993 Nurses' ability to achieve hyperinflation and hyperoxygenation with a manual resuscitation bag during endotracheal suctioning. Heart and Lung 22: 158–165

Gleeson JG, Price JF 1988 Nebuhaler technique. British Journal of Diseases of the Chest 82: 172–174

Godfrey S 1983 Exercise induced asthma. Archives of Disease in Childhood 52: 1–2

Goodnough SK. 1985 The effects of oxygen and hyperinflation on arterial oxygen tension after endotracheal suctioning. Heart and Lung 14: 11–17

Gray PH, Flenady VJ, Blackwell L 1999 Potential risks of chest physiotherapy in preterm infants. Journal of Pediatrics 135: 131

Greenough A 1996a Lung maturation. In: Greenough A, Roberton NRC, Milner A (eds) Neonatal respiratory disorders. Arnold, London, pp 13–26

Greenough A 1996b Chronic lung disease. In: Greenough A, Roberton NRC, Milner A (eds) Neonatal respiratory disorders. Arnold, London, pp 393–425

Greenough A 2000 Measuring respiratory outcome. Seminars in Neonatology 5: 119–126

Greenough A, Pool J 1988 Neonatal patient triggered ventilation. Archives of Disease in Childhood 63: 394–397

Greenough A, Morley CJ, Davis JA 1983 The interaction of the preterm infants spontaneous respiration with ventilation. Journal of Pediatrics 103: 769–773

Greenough A, Morley CJ, Wood S, Davies JA 1984 Pancuronium prevents pneumothoraces in ventilated premature infants who actively expire against positive pressure inflation. Lancet i: 1–3

Greenough A, Pool J, Greenall F, Morley C J, Gamsu H 1987 Comparison of different rates of artificial ventilation in preterm neonates with respiratory distress syndrome. Acta Paediatrica Scandinavica 76: 706–712

Greenspan JS, Wolfson MR, Shaffer TH 2000 Liquid ventilation. Seminars in Perinatology 24: 396–405

Gremmo ML, Guenza MC 1999 Positive expiratory pressure in the physiotherapeutic management of primary ciliary dyskinesia in the paediatric age. Monaldi Archives of Chest Disease 54: 255–257

Haddad E, Lowson SM, Johns RA, Rich GF 2000 Use of inhaled nitric oxide perioperatively and in intensive care patients. Anesthesiology 92: 1821–1825

Hagler DA, Traver GA 1994 Endotracheal saline and suction catheters: sources of lower airway contamination. American Journal of Critical Care 3: 444–447

Harding JE, Miles FK, Becroft DM, Allen BC, Knight DB 1998 Chest physiotherapy may be associated with brain damage in extremely premature infants. Journal of Pediatrics 132: 440–444

Harshbarger SA, Hoffman LA, Zullo TG, Pinsky MR 1992 Effects of a closed tracheal suction system on ventilatory and cardiovascular parameters. American Journal of Critical Care 1: 57–61

Hislop A, Reid L 1974 Development of the acinus in the human lung. Thorax 29: 90–94

Hislop A, Wigglesworth JS, Desai R 1986 Alveolar development in the human fetus and infant. Early Human Development 13: 1–11

Hodge D, Chetcuti PAJ 2000 RSV: management of the acute episode. Paediatric Respiratory Reviews 1: 215–220

Hoffman JI, Christianson R 1978 Congenital heart disease in a cohort of 19502 births with long term follow up. American Journal of Cardiology 42: 641–646

Holloway E, Ram FSF 2000 Breathing exercises for asthma (Cochrane Review). In: The Cochrane Library, 4. Update Software, Oxford

Hondras MA, Linde K, Jones AP 2000 Manual therapy for asthma (Cochrane Review). In: The Cochrane Library, 4. Update Software, Oxford Oxford

Horiuchi K, Jordan D, Cohen D, Kemper MC, Weissman C 1997 Insights into the increased oxygen demand during chest physiotherapy. Critical Care Medicine 25: 1347–1351

Hussey J, Hayward L, Andrews M, Macrae D, Elliott M 1996 Chest physiotherapy following paediatric cardiac surgery: the influence of mode of treatment on oxygen saturation and haemodynamic stability. Physiotherapy Theory and Practice 12: 77–85

Imle PC, Klemic N 1989 Methods of airway clearance: coughing and suctioning. In: Mackenzie CF, Imle PC, Ciesla N (eds) Chest physiotherapy in the intensive care unit. Williams and Wilkins, Baltimore, pp 153–187

Inselman LS, Mellins RB 1981 Growth and development of the lung. Journal of Pediatrics 98: 1–15

Inwald D, Roland M, Kuitert L, McKenzie S, Petros A 2001 Oxygen for all in acute severe asthma. British Medical Journal 27: 722–729

Jennet B, Macmillan R 1981 Epidemiology of head injury. British Medical Journal 282: 101–104

Jordan SC, Scott O 1989 Cyanotic lesions with increased pulmonary blood flow. In: Jordan SC, Scott O (eds) Heart disease in paediatrics, 3rd edn. Butterworths, London, pp 170–185

Kennedy JD 1999 Lung function outcome in children of premature birth. Journal of Paediatrics and Child Health 35: 516–521

Kerem E, Yatsiv I, Goitein KJ 1990 Effect of endotracheal suctioning on arterial blood gases in children. Intensive Care Medicine 16: 95–99

Khine HH, Corddry DH, Kettrick RG et al 1997 Comparison of cuffed and uncuffed endotracheal tubes in young children during general anesthesia. Anesthesiology 86: 627–631

Kinloch D 1999 Instillation of normal saline during endotracheal suctioning: effects on mixed venous oxygen saturation. American Journal of Critical Care 8: 231–240

Kinsella JP, Abman SH 2000 Clinical approach to inhaled nitric oxide therapy in the newborn with hypoxemia. Journal of Pediatrics 136: 717–726

Kleiber C, Krutzfield N, Rose EF 1988 Acute histologic changes in the tracheobronchial tree associated with different suction catheter insertion techniques. Heart and Lung 17: 10–14

Konno K, Mead J 1967 Measurement of the separate volume changes of rib cage and abdomen during breathing. Journal of Applied Physiology 22: 407–422

Krause MF, Hoehn T 2000 Chest physiotherapy in mechanically ventilated children: a review. Critical Care Medicine 28: 1648–1651

Kuo CY, Gerhardt T, Bolivar J, Claure N, Bancalari E 1996 Effect of leak around the endotracheal tube on measurements of pulmonary compliance and resistance during mechanical ventilation: a lung model study. Pediatric Pulmonology 22: 35–43

Langman J 1977 Medical embryology, Williams and Wilkins, Baltimore

MacNaughton PD, Evans TW 1999 Pulmonary function in the intensive care unit. In: Hughes JMB, Pride NB eds Lung function tests: physiological principles and clinical applications. London, WB Saunders, London, pp 185–199

Main E 1995 Phrenic nerve latency testing: assessing post operative diaphragmatic function in infants. MSc thesis, University of London

Main E, Castle R, Stocks J, James IG, Hatch DJ 1999 Respiratory function in the PICU: How much tracheal tube leak is permissible? European Respiratory Journal 14: 155s–155s

Main E, Elliott MJ, Schindler M, Stocks J 2001 Effect of delayed sternal closure after cardiac surgery on respiratory function in ventilated infants. Critical Care Medicine 29(9): 1798–1802

Matsumoto I, Araki H, Tsuda K et al 1999 Effects of swimming training on aerobic capacity and exercise induced bronchoconstriction in children with bronchial asthma. Thorax 54: 196–201

McCabe SM, Smeltzer SC 1993 Comparison of tidal volumes obtained by one-handed and two-handed ventilation techniques. American Journal of Critical Care 2: 467–473

McKelvie S 1998 Endotracheal suctioning. Nursing Critical Care 3: 244–248

Morin L, Crombleholme TM, D'Alton ME 1994 Prenatal diagnosis and management of fetal thoracic lesions. Seminars in Perinatology 18: 228–253

Morley CJ 1997 Systematic review of prophylactic vs rescue surfactant. Archives of Disease in Childhood 77: F70-F74

Muller NL, Bryan AC 1979 Chest wall mechanics and respiratory muscles in infants. Pediatric Clinics of North America 26(3): 503–516

Neder JA, Nery LE, Silva AC, Cabral ALB, Fernandes ALG 1999 Short term effects of aerobic training in the clinical management of moderate to severe asthma in children. Thorax 54: 202–206

Newell SJ, Booth W, Morgan ME, Durbin GM, McNeish AS 1989 Gastro oesophageal reflux in preterm infants. Archives of Disease in Childhood 64: 780–786

Niclolas KJ, Dhouibe MO, Marchall TG, Edmunds AT, Grant MB 1999 Physiotherapy in patients with bronchiolitis. Physiotherapy 85(12): 669–674

Ninan TK, Russel G 2000 The changing picture of childhood asthma. Paediatric Respiratory Reviews 1: 71–78

Norwood WI, Jacobs ML 1994 Hypoplastic left heart syndrome. In: Stark J, De Leval M (eds) Surgery for congenital heart defects, 2nd edn. WB Saunders, Philadelphia, pp 587–598

Novak RA, Shumake L, Snyder JV, Pinsky, MR 1987 Do periodic hyperinflations improve gas exchange in patients with hypoxemic respiratory failure? Critical Care Medicine 15: 1081–1085

O'Callaghan C 2000 How to choose delivery devices for asthma. Archives of Disease in Childhood 82: 185–191

O'Callaghan C, Milner A, Swarbrick A 1986 Paradoxical deterioration in lung function after nebulized salbutamol in wheezy infants. Lancet ii: 1424–1425

O'Callaghan C, Milner A, Swarbrick A 1989 Paradoxical bronchospasm in wheezing infants after nebulized preservative-free iso-osmolar ipratropium bromide. British Medical Journal 299: 1433–1434

Openshaw P, Edwards S, Helms P 1984 Changes in rib cage geometry during childhood. Thorax 39: 624–627

Pearson GA, Grant J, Field D, Sosnowski A, Firmin RK 1993 Extracorporeal life support in paediatrics. Archives of Disease in Childhood 68: 94

Phillips G 1996 To tip or not to tip? Physiotherapy Research International 1(1): 1–6

Prasad SA, Tasker RC 1990 Guidelines for physiotherapy management of critically ill children with acutely raised intracranial pressure. Physiotherapy 76(4): 248–250

Prasad SA, Tasker RC 1995 Neurological intensive care. In: Prasad SA, Hussey J (eds) Paediatric respiratory care. Chapman and Hall, London, pp 142–149

Pringle CR 2000 Prevention of bronchiolitis. Paediatric Respiratory Reviews 1: 228–234

Rachelefsky GS, Warner JO 1993 International consensus on the management of pediatric asthma: a summary statement. Pediatric Pulmonology 15: 125–127

Reid L 1984 Lung growth in health and disease. British Journal of Diseases of the Chest 78: 113–132

Roberton NRC 1996 Intensive care. In: Greenough A, Roberton NRC, Milner A (eds) Neonatal respiratory disorders. Arnold, London, pp 174–195

Rodenstein DO, Kahn A, Blum D, Stanescu DC 1987 Nasal occlusion during sleep in normal and near miss for sudden death syndrome in infants. Bulletin European Physiopathologie Respiratoire 23: 223–226

Rudy EB, Baun M, Stone K, Turner B 1986 The relationship between endotracheal suctioning and changes in intracranial pressure: a review of the literature. Heart and Lung 15: 488–494

Salt A, Noble-Jameson G, Barnes ND et al 1992 Liver transplantation in 100 children: Cambridge and King's College Hospital series. British Medical Journal 304: 416–421

Shah AR, Kurth CD, Gwiazdowski SG, Chance B, Delivoria-Papadopoulos M 1992 Fluctuations in cerebral oxygenation and blood volume during endotracheal suctioning in premature infants Journal of Pediatrics 120: 769–774

Shorten DR, Byrne PJ Jones, RL 1991 Infant responses to saline instillations and endotracheal suctioning. Journal of Obstetric, Gynecological and Neonatal Nursing 20: 464–469

Singer M, Vermaat J, Hall G, Latter G, Patel M 1994 Hemodynamic effects of manual hyperinflation in critically ill mechanically ventilated patients. Chest 106: 1182–1187

Southall DP, Samuels MP 1992 Reducing risks in the sudden infant death syndrome. British Medical Journal 304: 260–265

Stiller K 2000 Physiotherapy in intensive care: towards an evidence-based practice. Chest 118: 1801–1813

Stone KS 1990 Ventilator versus manual resuscitation bag as the method for delivering hyperoxygenation before endotracheal suctioning. AACN: Clinical Issues in Critical Care Nursing 1: 289–299

Stone KS, Turner B 1989 Endotracheal suctioning. Annual Review of Nursing Research 7: 27–49

Stone KS, Talaganis SA, Preusser B, Gonyon DS 1991 Effect of lung hyperinflation and endotracheal suctioning on heart rate and rhythm in patients after coronary artery bypass graft surgery. Heart and Lung 20: 443–450

Tarnow-Mordi WO, Reid E, Griffiths P, Wilkinson AR 1989 Low inspired gas temperature and respiratory complications in very low birthweight infants. Journal of Pediatrics 114: 438–442

Tasker RC 2001 Neurocritical care and traumatic brain injury. Indian Journal of Paediatrics 68: 257–266

Taylor CJ, Threlfall D 1997 Postural drainage techniques and gastro-oesophageal reflux in cystic fibrosis. Lancet 349: 1567–1568

Teasdale G, Jennett B 1974 Assessment of coma and impaired consciousness: a practical scale. Lancet 2: 81–84

Thoresen M, Cavan F, Whitelaw A 1988 Effect of tilting on oxygenation in newborn infants. Archives of Disease in Childhood 63: 315–317

Tudehope DI, Bagley C 1980 Techniques of physiotherapy in intubated babies with RDS. Australian Paediatric Journal 16: 226–228

UK Collaborative ECMO Trial Group 1996 UK collaborative randomised trial of neonatal extracorporeal membrane oxygenation. Lancet 348: 75–81

Vaughan RS, Menke JA, Giacoia GP 1978 Pneumothorax: a complication of endotracheal suctioning. Journal of Pediatrics 92: 633–634

Vincon C 1999 Potential risks of chest physiotherapy in preterm infants. Journal of Pediatrics 135: 131–132

Watt JW, Fraser MH 1994 The effect of insufflation leaks upon ventilation. A quantified comparison of ventilators. Anaesthesia 49: 320–323

Webb MSC, Martin JA, Cartlidge PHT, Ng YK, Wright NA 1985 Chest physiotherapy in acute bronchiolitis. Archives of Disease in Childhood 6: 1078–1079

Wenstrom KD, Weiner CP, Hanson JW 1991 A five-year statewide experience with congenital diaphragmatic hernia. American Journal of Obstetrics and Gynecology 165: 838–842

Windsor HM, Harrison GA, Nicholson TJ 1972 "Bag squeezing": a physiotherapeutic technique. Medical Journal of Australia 2: 829–832

Wollmer P, Ursing K, Midgren B, Eriksson L 1985 Inefficiency of chest percussion in the physical therapy of chronic bronchitis. European Journal of Respiratory Disease 66: 233–239

Wood CJ 1998 Endotracheal suctioning: a literature review. Intensive Critical Care Nursing 14: 124–136

FURTHER READING

Dinwiddie R 1997 Diagnosis and management of paediatric respiratory disease, 2nd edn. Churchill Livingstone, New York

Prasad SA, Hussey J 1995 Paediatric respiratory care. Chapman and Hall, London

14

Pulmonary rehabilitation: a multidisciplinary intervention

Rachel Garrod   Jadwiga Wedzicha

INTRODUCTION

Physical training for patients with respiratory disease is not a new concept; as long ago as 1895 exercise was recognized to be beneficial in the management of respiratory disorders. The identification of dyspnoea as a major disabling symptom of chronic obstructive pulmonary disease (COPD) led Charles Dennison (Casaburi & Petty 1993) to introduce a programme of physical exercise and chest wall expansion termed 'Exercise for Pulmonary Invalids'. Later, research began investigating the effect of positioning and breathing exercises on dyspnoea and exercise tolerance (Barach 1955) and in 1966 a study aimed at evaluating the benefit of a programme of 'comprehensive and rehabilitative care' was undertaken (Petty et al 1969).

In 1994, at a National Institute of Health pulmonary rehabilitation workshop, a working definition was decided upon (National Institute of Health 1994):

Pulmonary rehabilitation is a multidisciplinary continuum of services directed to persons with pulmonary disease and their families, usually by an interdisciplinary team of specialists, with the goal of achieving and maintaining the individual's maximum level of independence and functioning in the community.

Pulmonary rehabilitation is a multidisciplinary intervention that is predominantly concerned with issues of disability. The physiotherapist has played an important role in the management of patients with respiratory disease for many years. Techniques aimed at reducing the work of breathing and improving disability have been an integral part of the physiotherapist's management. Effective positioning (O'Neill & McCarthy 1983), mobilization, relaxed breathing and techniques to aid the removal of secretions are recognized treatment interventions for these patients (Hough 1996).

Physiotherapists have traditionally been active in the education of patients with respiratory disease. The aim is to promote healthy attitudes and recognition of the benefits of exercise in the management of a variety of conditions. Pulmonary rehabilitation is an holistic approach to the treatment of patients and their families with respiratory disease and as such requires the participation of a large number of health professionals. Physiotherapists may supervise and deliver the exercise programme whilst specialist input is provided from occupational therapy, nursing, dietetics, social work and psychology. All patients should be assessed prior to entry in order to optimize medical therapy and nutritional status. Assessment for portable oxygen may be appropriate at this time although the response to oxygen may alter as a result of physical training, suggesting a need for reassessment (Fig. 14.1) (Garrod et al 2000a).

RATIONALE FOR REHABILITATION IN OBSTRUCTIVE DISEASE

The predominant symptom reported by patients with respiratory disease is dyspnoea. It has been well documented that dyspnoea is associated with anxiety and fear (Devito 1990, O' Donnell 1994, Smoller et al 1996) and it is not surprising that this 'dyspnoea spiral' is itself a cause of further disability. One model proposes that:

It is the individual's fear of and misinterpretation of the physical sensations associated with dyspnoea, hyperventilation, or other symptoms that are thought to be crucial in producing panic attacks. (Clark 1986)

Over a decade ago it was found that subjects who had experience of loaded breathing during exercise reported less breathlessness in further tests compared with subjects who had no prior experience (Wilson & Jones 1990). This suggests that the perception of dyspnoea can be influenced by training modalities and cognitive behavioural interventions.

Patients who suffer dyspnoea report significant limitations during daily life and reductions in exercise tolerance. One study has reported high levels of disability in patients with COPD, with 50% of patients studied requiring assistance with

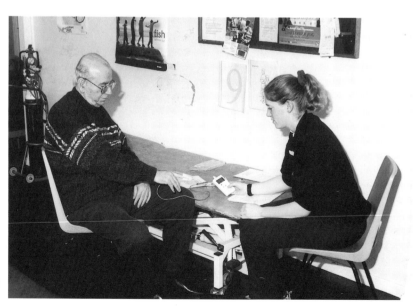

Figure 14.1 Assessment of oxygen saturation using a pulse oximeter.

household chores (Garrod et al 2000b). Almost all the patients investigated reported some degree of breathlessness during washing and dressing. Exercise limitation may be attributable to both the illness itself and to pre-existing levels of cardiovascular fitness. Furthermore, physical deconditioning substantially contributes to a reduction in mobility, with 60% of patients with COPD citing leg fatigue as a factor limiting walking distance (Killian et al 1992) . Moreover, leg fatigue is experienced at lower work intensities in COPD patients compared with normal subjects (Killian et al 1992). Debate persists concerning the nature of peripheral muscle weakness in COPD; is weakness caused by metabolic abnormality or as a result of inactivity?

Whittom and co-workers from Canada (1998) have identified differences in the fibre distribution of the quadriceps muscles of patients with COPD compared with normal age-matched subjects. There was a marked decrease in type I fibres (associated with endurance) and in type IIb fibres (associated with maximum strength). Correspondingly, this study reported a reduction in the cross-sectional area of the peripheral muscles as measured by computerized tomography (CT). This suggests that the quadriceps muscle is significantly weaker and more prone to fatigue in patients with COPD compared with normal subjects. However, this is not reflective of a generalized myopathy since there is evidence of an increase in endurance fibres of the accessory muscles of respiration, in response to increased demand (American Thoracic Society & European Respiratory Society 1999).

Bernard and colleagues (1998) have identified an association between the degree of airflow obstruction and the strength of the quadriceps. Strength may be reduced as a result of inactivity or conversely as an effect of worsening inflammatory processes.

Patients with COPD are exposed to a number of factors that may contribute to peripheral muscle dysfunction. The recent American Thoracic Society statement describes in further detail the deleterious effects of chronic hypoxia and hypercapnia, corticosteroid damage and nutritional defects (American Thoracic Society & European

Respiratory Society 1999). Indeed, COPD is recognized as a disease with systemic effects; the peripheral muscles may be further impaired by systemic inflammatory agents contributing to cytokine production and a picture of cachexia similar to that seen in patients with cancer.

Studies have, however, shown that the peripheral muscles in COPD respond to training in a similar manner to muscles in healthy individuals (Casaburi et al 1991). This suggests that the contractile mechanism of the peripheral muscles in patients with COPD remains intact and muscle strength can be modified with an appropriate programme (Bernard et al 1999, Maltais et al 1997, Simpson et al 1992).

Thus it is important to remember that the peripheral muscles of patients with COPD are responsive to training but that other factors will also contribute to weakness, namely nutritional status, hypoxia and hypercapnia, inflammatory mediators and circulating hormones. These further developments in our understanding of the causes of myopathy in COPD reinforce the need for a thorough multidisciplinary assessment and intervention.

The aims of pulmonary rehabilitation are to:

- reduce dyspnoea
- increase muscle endurance (peripheral and respiratory)
- improve muscle strength (peripheral and respiratory)
- ensure long-term commitment to exercise
- help allay fear and anxiety
- increase knowledge of lung condition and promote self-management.

EXERCISE PRESCRIPTION

Exercise training for patients with respiratory disease follows the same principles as those applied in healthy subjects. Training effects depend on three things: frequency of training, duration of the training programme and intensity of the programme. The response achieved depends upon which muscles are involved and the training regimen adopted, for strength or endurance.

- How often? Daily/×2 week/×3 week
- How long ? 4 weeks/8 weeks/ 12 weeks
- Length of sessions? 40–60 minutes
- Time of day? Afternoons/mornings
- Exercise? Resisted/unloaded training/aerobic/walking
- Intensity? Limited by dyspnoea (Borg 1982) /by $\dot{V}O_2$ peak
- Regimen? Endurance/maximal
- Assessment? Physiological/functional

A variety of training regimens have been employed in the management of patients with COPD, all with generally good results. Some authors advocate high-intensity aerobic training (Casaburi et al 1991) while others support the view that training should focus on endurance and strength (Clark et al 1996). Most programmes incorporate an element of walking. One group of workers use outdoor circuit walking as the main component of their training (Singh et al 1998), while others base training on the principle of high-repetition contractions and cycle ergometry (Clark et al 1996, Wedzicha et al 1998).

A recent study has compared interval training with continuous training in COPD patients (Coppoolse et al 1999); although no significant difference was found between the groups there was a trend towards greater oxidative adaptive changes with continuous training compared with interval training. The numbers in this study were small, suggesting that a significant finding may have been obscured by low power.

Weight training may be a useful addition to pulmonary rehabilitation programmes. Simpson and co-workers (1992) demonstrated a significant increase in muscle strength after a randomized trial of weight lifting, as did Bernard et al (1999) who also reported an increase in muscle mass. However, in both of these studies there was no additional effect of strength training on maximal exercise capacity or walking distance. These studies reinforce the need for specific functional training.

Debate persists concerning the relative merits of endurance versus strength training, though to a certain extent the type of training will vary according to the needs of the individual. Patients who report weakness or fatigue as a cause of exercise limitation may benefit most from strength training, while patients in whom dyspnoea is a predominant cause of exercise intolerance may benefit most from endurance training. To date, no study has evaluated the response to a training programme prescribed on the basis of reported symptoms, although most authors recognize the value of individualized training regimens.

Assessment of training intensity

A further element of exercise prescription concerns the intensity of exercise. A number of earlier studies into pulmonary rehabilitation showed methodological flaws concerning the description of exercise intensity. Before considering appropriate levels of intensity it is necessary to revisit relevant assessment tools. Two common methods of prescribing intensity are used; symptom-limited exercise prescription and physiological testing derived from maximal oxygen consumption (or related measures). In the first method patients are instructed to exercise to a prescribed symptom level, for example 'moderately or somewhat short of breath' on the Borg breathlessness score (Horowitz et al 1996). Although this provides an effective training stimulus for most patients, problems may occur when patients demonstrate very high levels of dyspnoea, thus limiting the intensity of training. Dyspnoea is very much a subjective perception, meaning that fear and anxiety at the start of a programme may heighten scores, so if using this method it may be necessary to reassess the dyspnoea levels midway through the programme and target a higher training level.

Calculating the exercise intensity from maximum oxygen consumption ($\dot{V}O_2$max) is probably more reliable and is easily performed using cycle ergometry or derived from an associated measure such as the shuttle walk test (Singh et al 1994). However, it is worth remembering that for patients with COPD a true $\dot{V}O_2$max may be unattainable due to ventilatory limitations (Singh et al 1994). An effective compromise is to determine the initial exercise prescription at 70–80% of the derived $\dot{V}O_2$max and then use breathlessness scores to monitor the training and adjust accordingly.

Intensity of training

Casaburi and colleagues (1991) demonstrated greater physiological and cardiovascular benefits in patients who exercise at higher intensities when compared with patients exercising for a longer duration but at a lower intensity. The same group later showed that supervised training programmes were more effective than lower intensity self-monitored training (Puente-Maestu et al 2000). These authors recommend training intensities of up to 80% of maximal oxygen consumption to achieve the greatest effects. However, a cautionary note concerns the relative severity of the patients under investigation. Patients in the study by Casaburi and colleagues showed moderate airflow obstruction and were fairly young (mean age 49 years).

In contrast, Roomi and co-workers (1996), investigating patients over 70 years of age, used self-prescribed dyspnoea levels to limit exercise. In this study patients continued exercising until they perceived themselves to be 'moderately breathless' using the Borg breathlessness score (Borg 1982). The authors demonstrated significant improvements in exercise tolerance after this programme. This approach was confirmed in a further trial of older COPD patients who were instructed to exercise until moderately to severely short of breath (Wedzicha et al 1998). Here significant improvements were seen in patients with a mean age of 68 years.

A pragmatic approach needs to be taken when prescribing the intensity of physical training for patients with obstructive disease, particularly when more severe airflow obstruction is present. Kearon and colleagues (1991) investigated the relationship between work performed and dyspnoea in patients with COPD. They observed two important findings: first, that prolonged respiratory activity increased ventilation and accordingly dyspnoea, and second, that dyspnoea was more affected by increases in exercise intensity than by increments in the duration of exercise. Thus lower intensity training of longer endurance may be more appropriate for patients with more severe ventilatory limitation.

It may be necessary to adopt different strategies for patients with differing airflow obstruction. One approach that may be useful when considering the type of programme is a classification of severity according to predicted values of forced expiratory volume in one second (FEV_1) (Table 14.1).

PHYSIOLOGICAL TRAINING RESPONSES

Physiological training effects differ according to the training regimen. The first aspect of training that occurs is a learning effect or improved neuromuscular coordination. This is not associated with physiological training effects per se, but may result in improved gait efficiency and increased stride length after a programme involving repeated walks (McGavin et al 1977).

Training results in fundamental recognized benefits to the individual. The effects may be classified under three headings:

- improved mechanical efficiency
- cardiovascular
- muscle changes.

Table 14.1 Suggested training programme according to severity of disease

Severity of disease	Type of training
Mild (FEV_1 < 60% predicted)	High-intensity aerobic training, with resistive training
Moderate (FEV_1 40 – 59% predicted)	Moderate intensity aerobic, with or without weight lifting
Severe (FEV_1 < 40% predicted)	Low intensity, high repetition of large muscles, unresisted/resisted work

Improved mechanical efficiency

Much of the improvement in exercise tolerance after pulmonary rehabilitation is likely to be a result of improvements in mechanical efficiency (O'Donnell 1994). Measures that may suggest an improvement in efficiency include stride length and gait coordination. McGavin and co-workers (1977) showed improvements in exercise tolerance after a programme of low-intensity exercise provided at home for 12 weeks. There was a modest increase of approximately 8% in walking distance which was probably attributable to improvements in mechanical efficiency rather than cardiovascular changes per se. Similarly, a group of patients housebound because of dyspnoea showed some improvement in exercise tolerance after a home programme, although this was not significant when compared to a control group (Wedzicha et al 1998). Another programme of home exercise, continued over a period of 1 year, showed larger changes, suggesting that where exercise intensity is low a longer period of time may be needed to achieve true physiological training effects (Sinclair & Ingram 1980).

Cardiovascular

Cardiovascular adaptations to training that one might expect to see in a normal subject after training include a reduction in the heart rate after training for a given level of work, reductions in minute ventilation, a lowering of the onset of lactic acidosis and a lower maximum oxygen uptake ($\dot{V}O_2$max) for a given work rate. Numerous studies show evidence of these changes in patients with COPD, with both moderate and severe obstruction (Casaburi et al 1991, Griffiths et al 2000, Ries et al 1995).

Muscle changes

It is necessary to reiterate the fact that changes will depend upon the type of training performed. Endurance exercise consisting of submaximal sustained efforts results in the transformation of type IIb fibres to type IIa, increasing their oxidative capacity. Type I fibres increase in size and number and the concentration of mitochondrial

enzymes is greater after training (Maltais et al 1996). Strength training is predominantly associated with an increase in size of muscle cells and number of myofibrils. Most importantly, muscle capillaries and myoglobin levels within a trained muscle are higher after training, thus improving the transport of oxygen to exercising muscles. The result of this is an improvement in oxygen uptake and the ability to maintain aerobic muscle metabolism for a prolonged period.

MEASUREMENT OF EXERCISE TOLERANCE

Evidence-based guidelines indicate that patients undergoing a period of rehabilitative training show improvements in exercise tolerance without evidence of adverse complications (ACCP/AACVPR 1997). Exercise training is a key component in pulmonary rehabilitation and all patients should perform a standardized test of exercise capacity before and after training. Laboratory tests measuring maximal oxygen consumption ($\dot{V}O_2$max), heart rate, workload, arterial oxygenation and blood lactate levels remain the gold standard in exercise testing and are appropriate in patients with COPD (Pelange et al 1994). Assessment of exercise tolerance is required in order to set targets of training intensity, assess the benefit of rehabilitation programmes, motivate patients to continue with training regimens and characterize initial disability.

However, where resources are limited, 'field tests' (tests of exercise tolerance applied in the clinical setting rather than the laboratory) may be performed, although these tests may be more susceptible to bias. Moreover, laboratory tests may offer limited information, particularly in patients with severe disease where work capacity is very reduced, resulting in an inability to reach ventilatory threshold levels (Midorikawa et al 1997). Indeed, the functional ability of patients will not necessarily reflect the true daily activities performed by them. Field tests may be considered superior to laboratory measurements due to simplicity and functional appropriateness, but the effects of motivation and the lack of physiological correlates remain disadvantages.

The 12-minute walking distance

The 12-minute walking distance test (12MWD) is a simple field test measuring the distance walked over 12 minutes. However, it is susceptible to practice effects and requires a number of practice walks (McGavin et al 1978). Moreover, this test lacks standardization and is dependent upon patient motivation.

The 12MWD was used in early rehabilitation trials (Cockcroft et al 1981, McGavin et al 1977, Sinclair & Ingram 1980) whilst Strijbos and colleagues (1996) used an adapted version, the 4-minute walking distance, and Wijkstra et al (1996) used the 6-minute walking distance (6MWD). Such variability makes comparison of trials difficult.

Furthermore, statistically significant changes need to be interpreted in the light of clinically significant changes: 'how big is big?' (Guyatt et al 1991). The threshold of clinical differences is a measured value which equates to a level of change at which the patient perceives either an improvement in symptoms or a deterioration. Redelmeir et al (1997) have identified the clinical threshold of the 6MWD as an increase or decrease of 54 metres after an intervention. Many results of rehabilitation trials in COPD patients fall short of this threshold (Cambach et al 1997, Wijkstra et al 1996).

The shuttle walking test

A 'field walking' test that is less susceptible to motivation is the shuttle walking test (SWT) (Singh et al 1992). This test is externally paced, enhancing standardization, does not include patient stops and correlates to $\dot{V}O_2$max (Singh et al 1994). The SWT demonstrates validity with other measures of exercise tolerance and is reliable on test-retest, requiring only one practice walk (Singh et al 1992). It has been shown to be a sensitive measure of change after rehabilitation in patients with severe COPD (Wedzicha et al 1998). A further test from this group measures endurance in a standardized manner (Revill et al 1999). A review article by Ambrosino (1999) states that the information obtainable with the

Table 14.2 Comparison of the shuttle walking test and the 12-minute walking distance

SWT	12MWD
Standardized	Open to variability
Facility to extrapolate $\dot{V}O_2$max from results	Evidence of validity and weak association with $\dot{V}O_2$max
Externally paced	Susceptible to patient motivation
Requires one practice walk	Requires three practice walks
Maximal test	Submaximal timed test
Requires tape and recorder	Requires no equipment
No clinical threshold identified	Clinical threshold identified (6MWD)

shuttle test may be considered of greater value than other unpaced walking tests. Field tests are an appropriate measure of exercise capacity in these patients and, although limiting with respect to mechanisms of improvement, combined with other functional assessments they help to provide a practical evaluation of pulmonary rehabilitation (Table 14.2).

PRACTICAL ASPECTS OF TRAINING

As with all physical training programmes, there are practical aspects to the provision of the service. One of the first issues to consider is the location of the programme or the setting. Rehabilitation programmes have shown favourable results in most settings, from cost-intensive inpatient programmes (Goldstein et al 1994) to more simple home-based programmes.

Location

There are arguments in favour of rehabilitation in a number of settings, from the hospital inpatient setting to the outpatient, home or community setting. The advantage of home programmes relates to improved compliance and prolonged benefits with an additional focus on functional and meaningful activities (Strijbos et al 1996). The disadvantages relate to the lack of peer group support (Wedzicha et al 1998) and the potentially limited space for mobilization. Individual supervision is required and patients

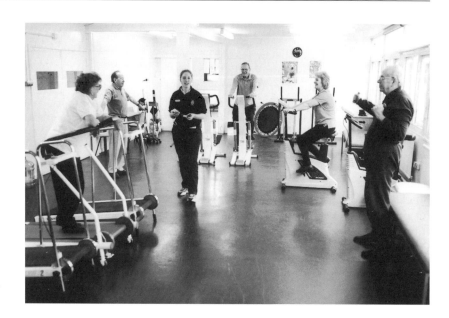

Figure 14.2 A pulmonary rehabilitation group provides peer support.

may need input for a longer period of time than compared with outpatient programmes (Fig. 14.2) (Sinclair & Ingram 1980). The pros and cons of pulmonary rehabilitation at home are reviewed (Garrod 1998) and summarized in Table 14.3.

Other avenues are being explored, from community care settings (Cambach et al 1997) to primary care interventions in local surgeries and sports centres, but further trials will be needed to evaluate the role of rehabilitation in primary care. Recent advances in 'exercise on prescription' schemes run in conjunction with local sports facilities and general practitioner surgeries point towards greater community involvement and better use of private sector resources. Future developments look likely to make greater use of community facilities. Physiotherapists are ideally placed to lead the way with referrals and support and training of local members.

The most appropriate location for pulmonary rehabilitation should be determined by the needs of the patient. Patients with severe COPD and exercise hypoxaemia must be assessed at a specialist centre with a view to oxygen requirements and monitoring during exercise. However, patients with mild to moderate disease may perform all aspects of training in the community, only requiring initial supervision from a physiotherapist. The role of the physiotherapist will expand to include education and support of exercise practitioners, relatives of patients and a wider perspective of health promotion.

Equipment

Equipment requirements for pulmonary rehabilitation are simple: a mat for floor exercises, dumbbells or hand weights and space to perform

Table 14.3 The pros and cons of pulmonary rehabilitation at home (adapted from Garrod 1998)

Pros	Cons
Encourages lifestyle changes	Practical constraints, i.e. space
May help further address ADL	May make multidisciplinary approach more difficult to manage
Greater accessibility for patients	Requires supervision (at least weekly?) – related to intensity
Individual supervision enables cognitive and behavioural approach to exercise	Requires a longer duration to achieve maximal changes
Cost-effective management of severe COPD?	Lacks group support
	Less cost effective than outpatient rehabilitation for moderate COPD?

aerobic training. As mentioned previously, functional exercise programmes are of the utmost importance to the success of pulmonary rehabilitation. Simple exercises aid clarity, and practical measures to include exercise in daily life may aid long-term compliance. Moreover, for older patients with COPD exercise must be seen as 'appropriate'; for patients with less severe disease swimming, bike riding, golfing, bowling and walking are all appropriate forms of exercise.

The type of equipment needed will depend primarily on the type of training to be performed and local financial resources. Where endurance training is the main objective equipment such as cycle ergometry (Fig. 14.3a) and a treadmill may be helpful. However, walking practice and blocks to simulate stair climbing (Fig. 14.3b) will have

more functional applicability. In order to achieve long-term benefits patients must be able to continue exercising effectively after the programme has ended. For strength training a multigym may be ideal but simple hand and ankle weights will also be sufficient. It is important to note the necessity of training both the upper and lower limbs (Lake et al 1990, Sivori et al 1998) and the use of breathing control throughout exercise.

Breathing control is defined as 'gentle breathing using the lower chest with relaxation of the upper chest and shoulders; it is performed at normal tidal volume, at a natural rate and expiration should not be forced' (Partridge et al 1989). Patients should be encouraged to breathe slowly and naturally. Appropriate terminology may help instruction, with words such as 'let the air

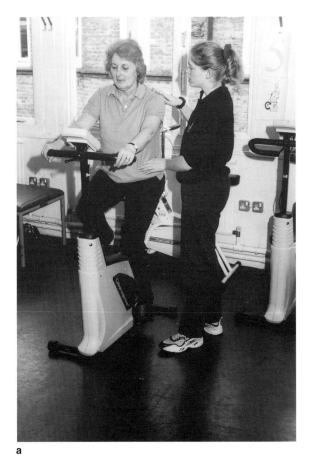

a

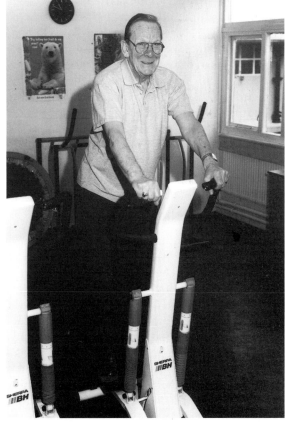

b

Figure 14.3 **a** Cycle ergometry. **b** Stepping machine.

flow in' rather than 'breathe in' which implies that a forced breath in is required. Effective positioning can reduce the work of breathing (O'Neill & McCarthy 1983) and should be utilized during exercise. Patients may use the 'lean forward position' in standing, against walls or equipment or in sitting (Bott 1997). Breathing control can be used during stair climbing (inhale, climb up one step; exhale, climb up two steps) to reinforce a rhythmical breathing pattern and minimize breath holding during activities. Although there is little empirical evidence for the value of these techniques, anecdotal and physiological evidence supports their continuing use (Sharp et al 1980). Breathing control during exercise remains a subject worthy of investigation.

When training the upper limbs it is important to consider the principles of positioning during exercise. Exercise endurance is less during unsupported upper limb activities than compared with supported upper limb work (Astrand et al 1968), especially when the arms are elevated above the head such as in 'reaching' or 'arching the arms'. Stabilization of the accessory muscles only occurs during movements where the shoulder girdle is fixed. These principles can be utilized during training. Unsupported upper limb work may achieve greater desensitization of dyspnoea, whilst strength training will be best performed with the upper limbs supported in order to minimise dyspnoea and maximize repetitions.

Cognitive training

Fear and anxiety influence the breathing pattern. Many patients fear exercise, which further exacerbates dyspnoea. The underlying philosophy of pulmonary rehabilitation states implicitly that exercise is beneficial. During the programme the therapist attempts to help the patient to replace negative thought processes with positive ones. Teaching patients to perceive breathlessness as a positive effect of 'good' exercise rather than a negative effect of their health enhances training effects (Atkins et al 1984). This philosophy must, of course, extend to relatives and demands the education and involvement of the families of those with respiratory disease.

Safety issues in rehabilitation

Many elderly people perceive exercise at 'their age' to be dangerous (O'Brien Cousins & Keating 1995). Issues of safety are obviously compounded in older people with respiratory disease and considerable reassurance may be required concerning safety. The issues of safety are somewhat unknown in the field of pulmonary rehabilitation. Although full exercise testing with ECG heart monitoring is recommended as routine for patients with COPD (American Thoracic Society 1999), a maximal incremental cycle ergometry test is unrealistic for many patients with severe disease. Even unloaded cycling can be exhausting for these patients, while adding incremental loads can cause distressing dyspnoea, ultimately preventing further exercise and disheartening the patient.

Most programmes exclude patients with unstable angina. For most patients, a field walking test with pulse oximetry and heart rate monitoring will identify oxygen needs and enable prescription of exercise intensity. In the hospital setting resuscitation equipment and oxygen should be readily available and the personnel involved trained in the use of equipment. However, a more pragmatic approach is required in the community setting where patients may be exercising at home or in local centres. There is evidence that patients with COPD demonstrate arterial desaturation during routine activities but the long-term effects of temporary falls in arterial saturation are unknown and warrant further investigation (Schenkel et al 1996). Patients with COPD often demonstrate ventilatory limitation or report fatigue before there is significant cardiovascular stress. However, this will not be the same for all groups of patients with respiratory disease and further research is required in this area. In the authors' experience the only complications of exercise in these patients have been related to minor musculoskeletal injuries.

Supplemental oxygen during exercise training

There are relatively few studies evaluating the benefit of supplemental oxygen during training programmes in COPD. A study by Zack & Pelange (1985) showed an improvement in exercise tolerance after a 12-week outpatient training programme in which all patients trained while breathing oxygen. However, the study was not controlled and it is not known whether additional benefits resulted from the use of supplemental oxygen. One randomized study investigated the role of oxygen in patients with severe COPD and exercise desaturation (Garrod et al 2000a). This showed an improvement in dyspnoea after rehabilitation that was greater in the patients who trained with oxygen compared with those who did not. However, in accordance with an earlier study (Rooyakers et al 1997), there were no differences in the changes in exercise tolerance between the two groups. This implies that although additional oxygen may augment desensitization to dyspnoea, it does little to enhance changes in exercise tolerance.

Supplemental oxygen has a greater effect on submaximal exercise, improving endurance rather than intensity (Bradley et al 1978). Casaburi and colleagues (1991) have shown that higher intensities of exercise result in greater physiological changes after training. The small increases in exercise tolerance due to oxygen may do little to enhance training effects when considered as part of comprehensive pulmonary rehabilitation programmes. It is likely that if there is an additional benefit of oxygen during pulmonary rehabilitation, a randomized trial would require a large sample of patients to identify the difference and these studies have yet to be completed.

More research is required concerning the cardiovascular complications and implications of exercise. At the present time it is prudent to advise that patients who are on long-term oxygen therapy (LTOT) should exercise with supplemental oxygen. The routine use of oxygen during pulmonary rehabilitation has clinical implications. Instruction to exercise with supplemental oxygen during rehabilitation for patients not already prescribed LTOT or ambulatory oxygen relays a confused message. This will adversely affect adherence to both the rehabilitation programme and the use of oxygen. Patients with exercise desaturation, but without resting daytime hypoxaemia, should have their saturation levels monitored throughout training and where a clear benefit is shown, they should train with oxygen and be provided with ambulatory oxygen for home use.

TRAINING IN ACTIVITIES OF DAILY LIVING

The importance of training in management of activities of daily living (ADL) has been outlined as the cornerstone of rehabilitation (Walsh 1986). ADL training includes conservation of energy achieved through practical approaches to daily problems such as the use of high stools at the sink, breathing re-education during exertion and exercises mimicking functional activities such as reaching and stair climbing. An apparent paradox arises when considering energy conservation in the light of the philosophy of exercise training for these patients. On the one hand patients are instructed to train and work hard; on the other hand, they are taught to minimise energy and reduce the effort involved. Of course, the aim is to maximize the patient's exercise programme whilst improving his functional ability.

Without an integrated multidisciplinary approach, throughout all aspects of the rehabilitation programme, messages can be misleading. It is tempting to compartmentalize the team's roles during rehabilitation but it is imperative that this does not occur. The team should be seen to present a united front, with members involved in all aspects of the programme. To some extent a blurring of roles is inevitable during a package of care such as pulmonary rehabilitation. With good teamwork and cooperation, this will maximize the benefits of treatment for the patient, with poor teamwork and communication it will result in mixed messages, repetition and ineffective management.

Assessment of activities of daily living

At present the assessment of daily activities remains poorly evaluated in COPD. However, there have been significant advances in the development of assessment tools in the last decade. Lareau and co-workers (1994) developed a 70-item ADL assessment tool employed as a measure of outcome after pulmonary rehabilitation. The tool was modified to form a shorter questionnaire of 40 items and has been successful in identifying improvements in daily activities after pulmonary rehabilitation (Lareau et al 1998). More recent developments concern the validation of a short, 15-item questionnaire, the London Chest Activity of Daily Living Scale (Garrod et al 2000b) (Table 14.4). Significant improvements in dyspnoea during ADL were documented after pulmonary rehabilitation and the change in ADL was associated with change in exercise tolerance (Garrod et al 2000a,c). Improvement in ADL provides a recognizable measure of the benefit of pulmonary rehabilitation to the individual. Further research is required to identify thresholds of clinical relevance in the patient population.

Assessment of health-related quality of life

A broad definition of quality of life includes factors that healthcare may not directly affect (though there may be indirect effects on health). Such factors include financial status, housing, employment and social support. Health-related quality of life (HRQoL) instruments can vary from disease specific questionnaires, which measure a single item such as dyspnoea or numerous items, to generic measures intended for use in any disease. Generic questionnaires were originally designed to define the health of populations and not to measure therapeutic efficiency. They are considered to be useful for comparing different populations of patients. Disease specific questionnaires were designed especially to detect and quantify health gain following treatment (Table 14.5).

HRQoL instruments have been useful in assessing benefits of pulmonary rehabilitation programmes. There have been numerous reports of improvements in exercise tolerance and health status after such programmes (Garrod et al 2000a, c, Griffiths et al 2000, Wedzicha et al 1998).

In a study from the Netherlands (Wijkstra et al 1994), HRQoL was measured using the disease specific Chronic Respiratory Questionnaire (CRQ) which measures four aspects of HRQoL: dyspnoea, mastery, emotion and fatigue (Guyatt et al 1987). Another commonly used questionnaire, the St George's Respiratory Questionnaire (SGRQ) (Jones et al 1991), has recently provided strong evidence of a change in health status after rehabilitation (Griffiths et al 2000). The clinical threshold for the CRQ has been identified as requiring a change of at least 0.5 points per item (Jaeshchke et al 1989) while a change of 4 points or more in the total score of the SGRQ is required to achieve a clinical effect (Griffiths et al 2000). An empirical comparison of the SGRQ and the CRQ showed strong similarities between the questionnaires in terms of validity and reliability, suggesting that either would be an appropriate measurement tool (Rutten-van Mölken et al 1999).

Assessment of dyspnoea

Repeated trials of rehabilitation have shown improvement in dyspnoea using validated measures (Goldstein et al 1994, Reardon et al 1994, Ries et al 1995). In 1997 a meta-analysis by Lacasse and colleagues concluded that training resulted in significant relief of dyspnoea. Dyspnoea can be measured in a variety of ways, graded scales such as the Baseline and Transition Dyspnoea Index (BDI) (Mahler et al 1984) and the Medical Research Council (MRC) Breathlessness Score (Fletcher 1960) are examples.

The MRC Breathlessness Score, which is self-administered, grades dyspnoea during walking according to five levels, with grade 5 representing patients who consider themselves to be housebound due to breathlessness. It is a valid and reliable questionnaire which has been found to be useful in stratification of patients prior to entry to pulmonary rehabilitation (Bestall et al 1999). However, the problem with such scales concerns the wide variation of disability evident between the grades which, although improving the reliability of the questionnaire, reduces its sensitivity (Jones 1992).

Table 14.4 The London Chest Activity of Daily Living Scale

THE LONDON CHEST ACTIVITY OF DAILY LIVING SCALE

NAME ....

DATE OF BIRTH ....

DO YOU LIVE ALONE?   YES ☐   NO ☐

Please tell us how breathless you have been during the last few days whilst doing the following activities.

SELF-CARE						
Drying	0	1	2	3	4	5
Dressing upper body	0	1	2	3	4	5
Putting shoes / socks on	0	1	2	3	4	5
Washing hair	0	1	2	3	4	5
DOMESTIC						
Make beds	0	1	2	3	4	5
Change sheet	0	1	2	3	4	5
Wash windows / curtains	0	1	2	3	4	5
Clean / dusting	0	1	2	3	4	5
Wash up	0	1	2	3	4	5
Vacuuming / sweeping	0	1	2	3	4	5
PHYSICAL						
Walking up stairs	0	1	2	3	4	5
Bending	0	1	2	3	4	5
LEISURE						
Walking in home	0	1	2	3	4	5
Going out socially	0	1	2	3	4	5
Talking	0	1	2	3	4	5

How much does your breathing affect you in your normal activities of daily living?
A lot ☐   A little ☐   Not at all ☐

The London Chest Activity of Daily Living Scale (score sheet)

Please read carefully and circle the relevant number next to each activity.
This questionnaire is designed to find out whether there are activities that you can no longer do because of your breathlessness and how breathless the things that you still do make you. All answers are confidential.

If you do not do an activity because it is not relevant, or you have never done it, please answer:
0 – Wouldn't do anyway

If an activity is easy for you, please answer:
1 – Do not get breathless

If the activity makes you a bit breathless, please answer:
2 – I get moderately breathless

If the activity makes you very breathless, please answer:
3 – I get very breathless

If you have stopped doing this **because of your breathlessness** and *have no one else to do it for you*, please answer:
4 – I can't do this anymore.

If someone else does this for you, or helps you, BECAUSE you are too breathless, e.g. The home help does your shopping, please answer:
5 – I need someone else to do this.

Other scales used to measure dyspnoea include the Borg Scale of Perceived Dyspnoea (Borg 1982), the dyspnoea component of the CRQ (Guyatt et al 1987), the UCSD shortness of breath questionnaire (Eakin et al 1998) and the visual analogue scale (VAS) (Aitken 1969).

Table 14.5 Examples of disease specific and generic health-related quality of life tools

Disease specific	Generic
Chronic Respiratory Disease Questionnaire (CRQ)	Sickness Impact Profile (SIP)
St George's Respiratory Disease Questionnaire (SGRQ)	MOS Short-Form 36 (SF36)
Breathing Problems Questionnaire (BPQ)	Quality of Well-Being Scale(QWB)
Oxygen Cost Diagram (OCD)	Nottingham Health Profile (NHP)

Assessment tools enable the therapist to reflect on practice, provide insight into the mechanisms of improvement and therefore aid development of programmes and allow the patient the opportunity to monitor progress in meaningful terms. The choice of assessment tool remains predominantly that of the investigator whilst remembering the basic principles of validity, reliability and sensitivity.

DO ALL PATIENTS BENEFIT?

This is a contentious question and to some extent remains unanswered in the field of pulmonary rehabilitation. It is probably fair to say that all patients have the potential to gain some benefit, albeit modest in some cases. As yet, it has not been possible to establish specific predictive factors. ZuWallack and co-workers (1991), investigating 50 COPD patients after rehabilitation, were unable to show a relationship between improvements and age, gender, pulmonary function or initial walking distance. However, they did show that patients with the greatest ventilatory reserve at baseline had the greatest improvement in walking distance after training. Likewise, Moser and colleagues (1980) reported that patients who achieved the highest levels of maximal exercise showed the greatest postcourse improvements. As yet unpublished data show a negative correlation between carbon dioxide tension and change in exercise tolerance, suggesting that patients with chronic respiratory failure show smaller improvements.

In contrast to these findings a retrospective analysis of 33 patients (including seven with asthma) after rehabilitation found that improvements after training tended to be greater in those patients with the lowest initial performance (Niederman et al 1991). However, findings from retrospective studies must be viewed with caution. Indeed, the authors also identified a positive relationship between FEV_1 and submaximal endurance, suggesting that those patients with the greatest FEV_1 at baseline were able to tolerate the most exercise.

One study stratified patients into two groups, according to ability to reach anaerobic threshold, and showed similar functional improvements after training (Punzal et al 1991). However, even the more severe patients in this study had a baseline FEV_1 of greater than 1 litre.

More recent research also concludes that physiological changes are unrelated to initial impairment (Vogiatzis et al 1999). These authors also performed a retrospective analysis after rehabilitation and showed no relationship between baseline percent predicted FEV_1 and change in exercise tolerance. However, the sensitivity of FEV_1 as a stratification tool may be questioned. Randomized studies are required in groups of patients with differing severity of disease and disability before it can be confidently concluded that all patients respond similarly.

Midorikawa and co-workers (1997) investigated whether the ventilatory (anaerobic) threshold could be reached in 25 patients with severe COPD. Their findings showed that in 56% of the patients the ventilatory threshold was undetectable. They concluded that rapidly developing dyspnoea in some patients may preclude high-intensity training. Thus, in a subgroup of patients with greater dyspnoea, low-intensity training may lead to functional improvements attributable to greater mechanical efficiency following training (O'Donnell 1994). For the majority of patients pulmonary rehabilitation programmes will show a beneficial effect in terms of exercise performance and quality of life. However, for severe patients, strategies aimed at minimizing dyspnoea during exercise may yield greater benefits (O'Donnell 1994). Functional assessment including activities of daily living, walking distance and health status are more appropriate outcome measures in severe COPD than physiological testing.

Smoking status

There is no evidence that continued smoking reduces the response to pulmonary rehabilitation. There has been much debate concerning whether patients who refuse to stop smoking should be eligible for pulmonary rehabilitation. However, it has been our experience that for many smokers, the combined positive influence of pulmonary rehabilitation and the effect of peer pressure has indeed helped a number of patients to stop smoking. Until trials show positively that the benefit of training is reduced in current smokers, we would recommend that smokers be supported throughout pulmonary rehabilitation programmes and offered appropriate smoking cessation help (Kawane 1997).

EDUCATION AS PART OF REHABILITATION

There are few trials specifically evaluating the benefit of education programmes as part of pulmonary rehabilitation. Education programmes are often provided as control groups on the grounds that they have little effect on exercise tolerance (Ries et al 1995, Wedzicha et al 1998). Education alone appears to do little to reduce the sensation of dyspnoea (Hunter & Hall 1989), improve quality of life (Gallefoss et al 1999, Ries et al 1995) or exercise tolerance (Wedzicha et al 1998). Moreover, a review by Folgering and co-workers (1994) suggests that education programmes in COPD patients show ambiguous results and compare poorly with asthmatic patient education on the grounds of cost effectiveness.

However, appropriate assessment of health education requires evaluation of benefits on patient knowledge, therapeutic compliance, cost effectiveness and dyspnoea. In an article by Mackay in 1996, COPD patients displayed improved knowledge and understanding after receiving dietary advice at home. However, no follow-up assessment was made of change in eating habits. A review of patient education by Mazzuca (1982)

states that although general education may have little benefit 'behaviour (regimen orientated) instruction has therapeutic value'. Regimen orientated instruction includes interactive sessions such as medical management with instruction on inhaler technique, teaching relaxation techniques, practical demonstrations of energy conservation techniques and stress management.

Psychosocial education

A meta-analysis of psychoeducational components of COPD management has shown a significant beneficial effect of behavioural education on inhaler use and a small non-significant effect on healthcare utilization (Devine & Pearcy 1996). Previous studies have shown reductions in dyspnoea after training in relaxation skills (Renfroe 1988) and coping strategies (Sassi-Dambron et al 1995). Moreover, Eiser and colleagues (1997) have shown improvements in exercise tolerance after group psychotherapy.

In another study investigating psychosocial interventions, a combined behavioural and cognitive approach to exercise in COPD patients achieved greater improvements in walking distance than single interventions alone (Atkins et al 1984). Behaviour-orientated approaches to pulmonary rehabilitation such as goal setting may improve compliance and task performance (Locke et al 1981). Education programmes must be task orientated, specific to the population and provided in a manner that is accessible to the patient. Analysis of the effects of education should focus on patient knowledge and its translation into reductions in hospitalization, prompt identification of problems and improved self-management. An educational programme combined with physical training optimizes functional ability as well as self-mastery.

RESPIRATORY MUSCLE TRAINING

Many workers have focused on specific training for the respiratory muscles, hypothesizing that increased respiratory muscle strength will translate into increased exercise tolerance via a reduction in dyspnoea (Belman et al 1994). By improving the strength or endurance of the diaphragm, greater inspiratory loads may be tolerated, thereby prolonging exercise tolerance. The diaphragm is a skeletal muscle consisting of type I and type II fibres with a slight predominance of type I. Strength training results in an increased number of fibres and increased inspiratory pressures. Trials have shown evidence of this in patients with COPD (Belman & Shadmehr 1988, Harver et al 1989). However, results have been variable (Belman et al 1986, Chen et al 1985, Guyatt et al 1992).

More recent studies have evaluated the role of respiratory muscle training in conjunction with general body training and once again have achieved variable results. Wanke and co-workers (1994) showed an additional effect of respiratory muscle training in COPD patients compared with cycle endurance alone. In contrast, Berry et al (1996) and more recently Larson and co-workers (1999) showed no significant additive effects of respiratory muscle training compared with general training alone.

Differences in the results may exist because of different training schedules, differing duration and intensity of programmes. Goldstein (1993) reports that in many studies no attempt to control breathing pattern was made and measurements of endurance were often unreliable.

A review by Reid & Samrai (1995) notes that training intensity is often below that required to achieve physiological effects and that changes in breathing pattern during training alter the resistance provided. In addition, the type of training regimen alters the response. A meta-analysis of respiratory muscle training studies has shown that the effects of treatment on respiratory muscle strength and endurance are small when looking across all studies (Smith et al 1992). Furthermore, there is little evidence of benefit on functional outcomes and health status. Future work in respiratory muscle training must ensure standardization of breathing frequency and pattern with training regimens of sufficient intensity to achieve a training effect.

Few workers have investigated the role of the expiratory muscles during exercise, although training these muscles may help prevent dynamic hyperinflation in some patients. This may prove a fruitful area for research.

ADJUNCTS TO REHABILITATION

There are adjuncts other than respiratory muscle training and oxygen that have been incorporated into pulmonary rehabilitation programmes. Recent authors have investigated the role of anabolic hormone therapy in the management of COPD. It has been hypothesized that hormone therapy may enhance muscle changes after rehabilitation. However, one early study has shown no significant effect of added growth hormone on exercise tolerance or muscle strength (Burdet et al 1997). Other authors have demonstrated a significant relationship between exercise tolerance and nutritional status, indicating that malnourishment is a poor prognostic factor irrespective of airflow obstruction (Schols et al 1991).

One interesting study evaluated the effect of acupressure practised daily in conjunction with a 6-week exercise programme (Maa et al 1997). The study was randomized with the control group receiving 'sham' acupressure. There were significant benefits of acupressure on dyspnoea although these were not reflected in differences in exercise tolerance. Unfortunately, the study was single blinded and the investigator, who met with the patients weekly to reinforce 'sham' or 'real' acupressure, was aware of the randomization. A repeat of this study with a double-blind design would be recommended.

Two randomized controlled trials have investigated the addition of non-invasive positive pressure ventilation (NPPV) administered during exercise and have shown similar, positive results (Bianchi et al 1998, Keilty et al 1994). Keilty and colleagues (1994) showed that inspiratory pressure support during treadmill walking was associated with a significant increase in walking distance and reduction in dyspnoea. Similarly, the use of proportional assist ventilation during cycle training produced a significant increase in cycling compared with sham ventilation (Bianchi et al 1998). Changes in exercise tolerance were associated with changes in dyspnoea.

The use of non-invasive ventilation (NIV) during exercise enhances performance and improves dyspnoea, probably as a result of the unloading of the respiratory muscles. However, there are practical difficulties to providing ventilation during a training session, limiting the type of exercise and questioning the adherence to exercise. A recent randomized controlled trial has evaluated the role of domiciliary NIV provided overnight in conjunction with a comprehensive exercise programme for patients with severe COPD (Garrod et al 2000c). The results of this study show significant improvements in exercise tolerance and quality of life after training in conjunction with NIV, when compared with exercise training alone. Additionally, only the group treated with NIV showed a significant improvement in inspiratory muscle strength at the end of the rehabilitation programme. Improvement in exercise tolerance may have resulted from overnight relief of low-level fatigue of respiratory muscles caused during exhaustive exercise. However, criticisms of this work concern the relatively short period of time spent using the ventilators (mean 2.5 hours) and the lack of placebo ventilation.

Although for most patients, this additional aid will be unnecessary, for those patients severely disabled by dyspnoea this treatment may enable them to exercise at sufficient intensity to achieve an effective training response. Patients with cystic fibrosis or emphysema, awaiting lung transplantation, or those recently discharged from intensive care with significant ventilatory limitation may be suitable candidates for additional support. The role of exercise in patients with respiratory disease will be wider than its present application. It is our role to ensure that we maximize the function of all patients where possible, using relevant adjuncts.

LONG-TERM EFFECTS OF PULMONARY REHABILITATION – IS BENEFIT MAINTAINED?

Many studies have assessed the short-term benefits of pulmonary rehabilitation. These studies have shown that patients can gain significant benefits in exercise capacity, health status and dyspnoea immediately after a rehabilitation programme. However, full assessment of pulmonary rehabilitation requires an evaluation of the long-term benefits of such programmes.

Vale et al (1993) assessed the maintenance of improvements in exercise tolerance and health status approximately 1 year after training. They compared two groups of patients; the first group had participated in a structured follow-up programme whereas the second group had no follow-up programme. Both groups showed a decline in measured parameters with no significant difference evident between the groups. The authors suggested that follow-up programmes were of little benefit and that other strategies are required to prolong effects. However, caution is recommended in the interpretation of these findings as no control group (those who did not receive rehabilitation) was included.

Health status improvements are still evident at 12 months after rehabilitation (Griffiths et al 2000) and Wijkstra and colleagues (1995) demonstrated that improvements were greater in patients who received monthly follow-up sessions for up to 18 months. They assessed three types of maintenance programme; group 1 received no follow-up, group 2 received weekly follow-up sessions and group 3 received monthly follow-up sessions. Results revealed that the group receiving monthly follow-up sessions had significantly maintained their improvements, in health status over and above that of the other two groups. This would suggest that while patients may require some assistance to maintain improvement, too much may be counter productive. The aim of pulmonary rehabilitation is to achieve the highest level of independent functioning and too much support may prevent the patient from attaining an adequate level of independence. However, these results suffer from low sample numbers and may not be replicated in a larger study.

One of the most extensive follow-up studies was carried out by Ries et al (1995). This group reported on a 6-year follow-up with monthly reinforcement programmes. They showed that improvements in exercise tolerance, dyspnoea and daily activity declined between 6 and 12 months. However, improvements in self-efficacy and perceived breathlessness were maintained for up to 24 months.

More recently Griffiths and colleagues (2000) have reported on follow-up data 1 year after a pulmonary rehabilitation programme. They collected data on hospital admissions and consultations as well as health status and exercise tolerance. The results showed a significant effect of rehabilitation on the number of days spent in hospital 1 year post rehabilitation. However, there was no evidence of a significant difference in the number of hospital admissions between the treatment and control groups. This suggests that physical training may have an effect on the recovery phase of exacerbations rather than altering the number of exacerbations experienced.

CONCLUSION

Pulmonary rehabilitation is an effective therapy. There is evidence to support the following.

● Improvement in exercise tolerance

● Improvement in the sensation of dyspnoea
● Improvement in the ability to perform routine activities of daily living
● Improvement in health-related quality of life
● Improvement in muscle strength and mass
● Reductions in number of days spent in hospital

Evidence is emerging which suggests that pulmonary rehabilitation is a cost-effective intervention (Griffiths et al 2000) and there is recent indication that pulmonary rehabilitation may improve mortality (Senjyu et al 1999).

With the bulk of evidence in favour of pulmonary rehabilitation it must be considered an important therapeutic intervention for these patients, particularly, in the light of many therapeutic treatments routinely provided for which there is significantly less evidence to support efficacy. Cost and resources will remain difficult obstacles to overcome but pulmonary rehabilitation is a relatively low-budget intervention. A multidisciplinary combined approach will spread the workload and ensure that we offer the most effective, proven treatments to our patients.

REFERENCES

ACCP/AACVPR 1997 Pulmonary rehabilitation guidelines panel. Pulmonary rehabilitation. Joint ACCP/AACVPR Evidence-based guidelines. Chest 112: 1363–1396

Aitken RB 1969 A growing edge of measurement of feelings. Procedings of the Royal Society of Medicine, 62: 989–993

Ambrosino N 1999 Field tests in pulmonary disease. Thorax 54: 191–193

American Thoracic Society 1999 Pulmonary rehabilitation: an official statement. American Journal of Respiratory and Critical Care Medicine 159: 1666–1682

American Thoracic Society and European Respiratory Society 1999 Skeletal muscle dysfunction in chronic obstructive pulmonary disease. American Journal of Respiratory and Critical Care Medicine 159 (4): S1-S40

Astrand I, Guharay A, Wahren J 1968 Circulatory responses to arm exercise with different arm positions. Journal of Applied Physiology 25: 528–532

Atkins CJ, Kaplan RM Timms RM, et al 1984 Behavioural exercise programmes in the management of chronic obstructive pulmonary disease. Journal of Consulting and Clinical Psychology 52 (4): 591–603

Barach AL 1955 Breathing exercises in pulmonary emphysema and allied chronic respiratory disease. Archives of Physical Medicine and Rehabilitation 36: 379–390

Belman MJ, Shadmehr R 1988 Targeted resistive muscle training in COPD. Journal of Applied Physiology 65: 2726 –2735

Belman MJ, Thomas S, Lewis M 1986 Resistive breathing training in patients with chronic obstructive pulmonary disease. Chest 90: 662-669.

Belman MJ, Botnick WC, Nathan SD et al 1994 Ventilatory load characteristics during ventilatory muscle training. American Journal of Respiratory and Critical Care Medicine 149 (4): 925–929

Bernard S, Leblanc P, Whittom F et al 1998 Peripheral muscle weakness in patients with chronic obstructive pulmonary disease. American Journal of Respiratory and Critical Care Medicine 158: 629–634

Bernard S, Whittom F, Leblanc P et al 1999 Aerobic and strength training in patients with chronic obstructive pulmonary disease. American Journal of Respiratory and Critical Care Medicine 159: 896– 901

Berry M, Norman A, Sevensky S et al 1996 Inspiratory muscle training and whole body reconditioning in COPD. American Journal of Respiratory and Critical Care Medicine 153: 1812–1816

Bestall JC, Paul EA, Garrod R et al 1999 Usefulness of the Medical Research Council (MRC) dyspnoea scale as a measure of disability in patients with COPD. Thorax 54: 581–586

Bianchi L, Foglio K, Pagani M et al 1998 Effects of proportional assist ventilation on exercise tolerance in COPD patients with chronic hypercapnia. European Respiratory Journal 11: 422–4277

Borg C 1982 Psychophysical basis of perceived exertion. Medicine and Science in Sports Exercise 14: 377–381

Bott J 1997 Physiotherapy. In: Singh SJ, Morgan MDL (eds) Practical pulmonary rehabilitation. Chapman and Hall, London, pp 156–176

Bradley BL, Garner AE, Billiu D et al 1978 Oxygen-assisted exercise in chronic obstructive lung disease. American Review of Respiratory Disease 118: 239–243

Burdet L, Muralt B, Schutz Y et al 1997 Administration of growth hormone to underweight patients with chronic obstructive pulmonary disease. A prospective randomized, controlled study. American Journal of Respiratory and Critical Care Medicine 156: 1800–1806

Cambach W, Chadwick-Straver RVM, Wagenaar RC et al 1997 The effects of a community based pulmonary rehabilitation programme on exercise tolerance and quality of life: a randomised controlled trial. European Respiratory Journal 10: 104–113

Casaburi R, Petty TL 1993 Principles and practice of pulmonary rehabilitation. WB Saunders, Philadelphia, p 2

Casaburi R, Patessio A, Ioli F et al 1991 Reductions in exercise lactic acidosis and ventilation as a result of exercise training in patients with obstructive lung disease. American Review of Respiratory Disease 143: 9–18

Chen H, Dukes R, Martin B 1985 Inspiratory resistance training in patients with COPD. American Review of Respiratory Disease 131: 251–255

Clark CJ, Cochrane L, Mackay E 1996 Low intensity peripheral muscle conditioning improves exercise tolerance and breathlessness in COPD. European Respiratory Journal 9(12): 2590–2596

Clark DM 1986 A cognitive approach to panic. Behaviour Research and Therapy 24: 461–470

Cockcroft AE, Saunders MJ, berry G 1981 Randomised controlled trial of rehabilitation in chronic respiratory disability. Thorax 36: 200–203

Coppoolse R, Schols A, Baarends E et al 1999 Interval versus continuous training in patients with severe COPD: a randomized controlled trial. European Respiratory Journal 14: 258–263

Devine E, Pearcy J 1996 Meta-analysis of the effect of psycho-educational care in adults with COPD. Patient Education and Counselling 29 (2): 167–178

Devito AJ 1990 Dyspnoea during hospitalisations for acute phase of illness as recalled by patients with COPD. Heart and Lung 19: 186–191

Eakin E, Resnikoff P, Prewitt L et al 1998 Validation of a new dyspnoea measure: The UCSD shortness of breath questionnaire. Chest 113: 619–624

Eiser N, West C, Evans S et al 1997 Effects of psychotherapy in moderately severe COPD: a pilot study. European Respiratory Journal 10 (7): 1581–1584

Fletcher CM 1960 Standardised questionnaire on respiratory symptoms: a statement prepared and approved by the MRC committee on the aetiology of chronic bronchitis (MRC Breathlessness Score). British Medical Journal 2: 1665

Folgering H, Rooyakkers J, Herwaarden C 1994 Education and cost benefit ratios in pulmonary patients. Monaldi Archives of Chest Disease 49: (2) 166–168

Gallefoss F, Bakke PS, Kjaersgaard P 1999 Quality of life assessment after patient education in a randomised controlled study on asthma and chronic obstructive pulmonary disease. American Journal of Respiratory and Critical Care Medicine 159: 812–817

Garrod R 1998 Pulmonary rehabilitation: the pros and cons of rehabilitation at home. Physiotherapy 84(12): 603–607

Garrod R, Paul EA, Wedzicha JA 2000a Supplemental oxygen during pulmonary rehabilitation in patients with COPD and exercise hypoxaemia. Thorax 55: 539–543

Garrod R, Bestall J, Wedzicha JA et al 2000b Development and validation of a standardised measure of activity of daily living in patients with COPD: the London Chest Activity of Daily Living Scale (LCADL). Respiratory Medicine 94 (6): 589–596

Garrod R, Mikelsons C, Paul EA, Wedzicha JA 2000c Randomized controlled trial of domiciliary noninvasive positive pressure ventilation and physical training in severe chronic obstructive pulmonary disease. American Journal of Respiratory and Critical Care Medicine 162 (41): 1335–1341

Goldstein R 1993 Ventilatory muscle training. Thorax 48: 1025 –1033

Goldstein RS, Gort EH, Stubbing D et al 1994 Randomised controlled trial of respiratory rehabilitation. Lancet 344: 1394–1397

Griffiths TL, Burr ML, Campbell IA et al 2000 Results at 1 year of out-patient multidisciplinary pulmonary rehabilitation: a randomised controlled trial. Lancet 355: 362–368

Guyatt GH, Townsend M, Berman L et al 1987 A measure of quality of life for clinical trials in chronic lung disease. Thorax 42: 773–778

Guyatt GH, Feeny D, Patrick D 1991 Issues in quality of life measurement in clinical trials. Controlled Clinical Trials 81S–90S

Guyatt GH, Keller J, Singer J et al 1992 Controlled trial of respiratory muscle training in chronic airflow limitation. Thorax 47: 598–602

Harver A, Mahler D, Daubenspeck J 1989 Targeted inspiratory muscle training improves respiratory muscle function and dyspnoea in patients with COPD. Annals of Internal Medicine 111 (2): 117–124

Horowitz MB, Littenberg B, Mahler DA 1996 Dyspnoea ratings for prescribing exercise intensity in patients with COPD. Chest 109(5): 1169–1175

Hough A 1996 Physiotherapy in Respiratory Care (2nd edn) Stanley Thornes, Cheltenham

Hunter S, Hall S 1989 The effect of an educational support programme on dyspnoea and the emotional status of COPD clients. Rehabilitation Nursing Journal 14 (4): 200–202

Jaeshchke R, Singer J, Guyatt GH 1989 Measurement of health status. Ascertaining the minimal clinically important difference. Controlled Clinical Trials 10 (4): 407–415

Jones PW 1992 Measurement of health in asthma and chronic obstructive airways disease. Pharmaceutical Medicine 6: 13–22

Jones PW, Quirk FH, Baveystock CM 1991 The St George's Respiratory Questionnaire (SGRQ). Respiratory Medicine 85 (suppl B): 25–31

Kawane H 1997 Smoking cessation in comprehensive pulmonary rehabilitation. Lancet 349: 285

Kearon MC, Summers E, Jones N et al 1991 Effort and dyspnoea during work of varying intensity and duration. European Respiratory Journal 4: 917– 925

Keilty S, Ponte J, Fleming T et al 1994 Effect of inspiratory pressure support on exercise tolerance and breathlessness in patients with severe stable COPD. Thorax 49: 990–994

Killian KJ, Leblanc P, Martin DH et al 1992 Exercise capacity and ventilatory, circulatory, and symptom limitation in patients with chronic airflow limitation. American Review of Respiratory Disease 146: 935–940

Lacasse Y, Guyatt GH, Goldstein RS 1997 The components of a respiratory rehabilitation programme. Chest 111: 1077–1088

Lake F, Henderson K, Briffa T et al 1990 Upper limb and lower limb exercise training in patients with chronic airflow obstruction. Chest 97: 1077–1082

Lareau SC, Carrieri-Kohlmon V, Janson-Bjerklie S et al 1994 Development of the Pulmonary Functional Status and Dyspnea Questionnaire (PFSDQ). Heart and Lung 23 (3): 242–250

Lareau SC, Meek PM, Roos PJ 1998 Development and testing of the modified version of the Pulmonary Functional Status and Dyspnea Questionnaire (PFSDQ-M). Heart and Lung 27 (3): 159–168

Larson J, Kim J, Sharp T et al 1999 Inspiratory muscle training with a pressure threshold breathing device in patients with COPD. American Review of Respiratory Disease 138: 689–96

Locke E, Shaw K, Sari L et al 1981 Goal setting and task performance 1969–1980. Psychological Bulletin 90(1): 125–152

Maa SH, Gauthier D, Turner M 1997 Acupressure as an adjunct to a pulmonary rehabilitation programme. Journal of Cardiopulmonary Rehabilitation 17 (4): 268–276

Mackay L 1996 Health education and COPD rehabilitation: a study. Nursing Standard 10 (40): 34 –3 9

Mahler DA, Weinberg DH, Wells CK et al 1984 The measurement of dyspnea; contents, inter-observer agreement and physiologic correlates of two new clinical indexes. Chest 85: 751–758

Maltais F, Leblanc P, Simard C et al 1996 Skeletal muscle adaptation to endurance training in patients with COPD. American Journal of Critical Care Medicine 154: 442–447

Maltais F, Leblanc P, Jobin J et al 1997 Intensity of training and physiologic adaptation with COPD. American Journal of Respiratory and Critical Care Medicine 155: 555–561

Mazzuca S 1982 Does patient education in chronic disease have therapeutic value? Journal of Chronic Diseases 35 (7): 521– 529

McGavin CR, Gupta SP, Lloyd EL et al 1977 Physical rehabilitation for the chronic bronchitic: results of a controlled trial of exercises in the home. Thorax 32: 307–311

McGavin CR, Artvinili M, Naoe H et al 1978 Dyspnoea, disability and distance walked – comparison of estimates of exercise performance in respiratory disease. British Medical Journal 2: 241–243

Midorikawa J, Hida W, Taguchi O et al 1997 Lack of ventilatory threshold in patients with COPD. Respiration 64: 76–80

Moser KM, Bokinsky GE, Savage RT et al 1980 Results of a comprehensive rehabilitation programme; physiologic and functional effects on patients with COPD. Archives of Internal Medicine 140: 1596–1601

National Institute of Health 1994 Pulmonary rehabilitation research. National Institute of Health workshop summary. American Review of Respiratory Disease 49: 825–893

Niederman MS, Clemente PH, Fein AM et al 1991 Benefits of a multidisciplinary pulmonary rehabilitation program – improvements are independent of lung function. Chest 99: 798–804

O'Brien Cousins S, Keating N 1995 Life cycle patterns of physical activity among sedentary and older women. Journal of Ageing and Physical Activity 3: 340– 359

O'Donnell D 1994 Breathlessness in patients with chronic airflow limitation. Chest 106: 905–912

O'Neill S, McCarthy DS 1983 Postural relief of dyspnoea in severe chronic airflow limitation. Thorax 38: 595–600

Partridge C, Pryor J, Webber B 1989 Characteristics of the forced expiration technique. Physiotherapy 73 (3): 193–194

Pelange P, Carlone S, Forte S et al 1994 Cardiopulmonary exercise testing in the evaluation of patients with ventilatory vs circulatory causes of reduced exercise tolerance. Chest 105: 1122–1126

Petty TL, Nett LM, Finnigan MM et al 1969 A comprehensive care program for chronic airways obstruction; methods and preliminary evaluation of spirometric and functional improvement. Annals of Internal Medicine 70: 1109–1120

Puente-Maestu L, Sanz M, Sanz P et al 2000 Comparison of effects of supervised versus self-monitored training programmes in patients with chronic obstructive pulmonary disease. European Respiratory Journal 15 (3): 517–525

Punzal PA, Ries AL, Kaplan RM et al 1991 Maximum intensity training in patients with COPD. Chest 100: 618–623

Reardon J, Awad E, Normandin E et al 1994 The effect of comprehensive outpatient pulmonary rehabilitation on dyspnea. Chest 105: 1046–1052

Redelmeir D, Bayoumi A, Goldstein R et al 1997 Interpreting small differences in functional status: the Six Minute Walk test in chronic lung disease patients. American Journal of Respiratory and Critical Care Medicine. 155 (4): 1278–1282

Reid W, Samrai B 1995 Respiratory muscle training for patients with COPD. Physical Therapy 75(11): 70–79

Renfroe K 1988 Effect of progressive relaxation on dyspnoea and state anxiety in patients with COPD. Heart and Lung 17: 408–413

Revill SM, Morgan MDL, Singh SJ et al 1999 The endurance shuttle walk: a new field test for the assessment of endurance capacity in chronic obstructive pulmonary disease. Thorax 54: 213–220

Ries AL, Kaplan RM, Limberg TM et al 1995 Effects of pulmonary rehabilitation on physiologic and psychosocial outcomes in COPD. Annals of Internal Medicine 122: (11): 823–831

Roomi J, Johnson MM, Waters K et al 1996 Respiratory rehabilitation, exercise capacity and quality of life in chronic airways disease in old age. Age and Ageing 25: 12–16

Rooyakers JM, Dekhuijzen PNR, Van Herwaarden CLA et al 1997 Training with supplemental oxygen in patients with COPD and hypoxaemia at peak exercise. European Respiratory Journal 10: 1278–1284

Rutten-van Mölken M, Roos B, Van Noord JA 1999 An empirical comparison of the St George's Respiratory Questionnaire (SGRQ) and the Chronic Respiratory Disease Questionnaire (CRQ) in a clinical trial setting. Thorax 54 (11): 995–1003

Sassi-Dambron DE, Eakin EG, Ries AL et al 1995 Treatment of dyspnea in COPD. A controlled clinical trial of dyspnea management strategies. Chest 107: 724–729

Schenkel NS, Muralt BB, Fitting JW 1996 Oxygen saturation during daily activities in chronic obstructive pulmonary disease. European Respiratory Journal 9: 2584–2589

Schols A, Mostert R, Soeters P et al 1991 Body composition and exercise performance in patients with chronic obstructive pulmonary disease. Thorax 46 (10): 695–699

Senjyu H, Moji K, Takemoto T et al 1999 Effects of pulmonary rehabilitation on the survival of emphysema patients receiving long-term oxygen therapy. Physiotherapy 85 (5): 251–258

Sharp JT, Drutz WS, Moisan T et al 1980 Postural relief of dyspnoea in severe COPD. American Review of Respiratory Disease 122: 201–211

Simpson K, Killian K, McCartney N et al 1992 Randomised controlled trial of weightlifting exercise in patients with chronic airflow limitation. Thorax 47: 70–75

Sinclair DJM, Ingram CG 1980 Controlled trial of supervised exercise training in chronic bronchitis. British Medical Journal 280: 519–521

Singh SJ, Morgan MDL, Scott S et al 1992 Development of a shuttle walking test of disability in patients with chronic airways obstruction. Thorax 47: 1019–1024

Singh SJ, Morgan MDL, Hardman AE et al 1994 Comparison of oxygen uptake during a conventional treadmill test and the shuttle walk test in chronic airflow limitation. European Respiratory Journal 7: 2016–2020

Singh SJ, Smith DL, Hyland ME et al 1998 A short outpatient pulmonary rehabilitation programme: immediate and longer-term effects on exercise performance and quality of life. Respiratory Medicine 92(9): 1146–1154

Sivori M, Rhodius E, Kaplan P et al 1998 Exercise training in chronic obstructive pulmonary disease. Comparative study of aerobic training of lower limbs vs combination with upper limbs. Medicina 58 (6): 712–727

Smith K, Cook D, Guyatt G et al 1992 Respiratory muscle training in chronic airflow limitation: a meta-analysis. American Review of Respiratory Disease 145: 533–539

Smoller JW, Pollack MH, Otto MW et al 1996 Panic anxiety, dyspnoea and respiratory disease. Theoretical and clinical implications. American Journal of Respiratory and Critical Care Medicine 154: 6–17

Strijbos JH, Postma DS, Van Altena R et al 1996 A comparison between an outpatient hospital based pulmonary rehabilitation program and a home care pulmonary rehabilitation program in patients with COPD. Chest 109: 366–372

Vale F, Reardon J, ZuWallack R 1993 The long term benefits of outpatient pulmonary rehabilitation on exercise endurance and quality of life. Chest 103:42–45

Vogiatzis I, Williamson AF, Miles J et al 1999 Physiologic responses to moderate exercise workloads in a pulmonary rehabilitation program in patients with varying degrees of airflow obstruction. Chest 116 (5): 1200–1207

Walsh R 1986 Occupational therapy as part of a pulmonary rehabilitation programme. Occupational Therapy and Health Care 3: 65 -77

Wanke TH, Formanek D, Lahrmann H et al 1994 Effects of combined inspiratory muscle and cycle ergometer training on exercise performance in patient with COPD. European Respiratory Journal 7: 2205–2211

Wedzicha JA, Bestall JC, Garrod R et al 1998 Randomised controlled trial of pulmonary rehabilitation in severe chronic obstructive pulmonary disease patients, stratified with the MRC scale. European Respiratory Journal 12: 363–369

Whittom F, Jobin J, Simard PM et al 1998 Histochemical and morphological characteristics of the vastus lateralis muscle in patients with chronic obstructive pulmonary disease. Medicine and Science in Sports and Exercise 30(10): 1467–1474

Wijkstra PJ, Van Altena R, Kraan J et al 1994 Quality of life in patients with COPD improves after rehabilitation at home. European Respiratory Journal 7: 269–273

Wijkstra PJ, Ten Vergert EM, Van Altena R et al 1995 Long term effects of rehabilitation at home on quality of life and exercise tolerance in patients with chronic obstructive pulmonary disease. Thorax 50: 824–828

Wijkstra PJ, Mark TW, Kraan J et al 1996 Long term effects of home rehabilitation on physical performance in chronic obstructive pulmonary disease. American Journal of Respiratory and Critical Care Medicine 153: 1234–1241

Wilson R, Jones PW 1990 Influence of prior ventilatory experience on the estimation of breathlessness during exercise. Clinical Science 78: 149–153

Zack MB, Pelange AV 1985 Oxygen supplemented exercise of ventilatory and nonventilatory muscles in pulmonary rehabilitation. Chest 88 (5): 669– 675

ZuWallack RL, Patel K, Readon J et al 1991 Predictors of improvement in the 12 minute walking distance following a 6 week outpatient pulmonary rehabilitation programme. Chest 99 (4): 805–808

15

Cardiac rehabilitation

*Ann Taylor   Jenny Bell
Fiona Lough*

INTRODUCTION

Cardiac rehabilitation is a widely accepted form of management for patients with cardiac disease. It attempts to enable patients to regain full physical, psychological and social status and to promote and undertake secondary prevention for optimum long-term prognosis. It should be an integral part of both acute care and long-term follow-up. There is large variation in the format and organization of rehabilitation programmes both within and between countries, but programmes traditionally encompass a period of exercise training, education sessions, psychosocial support and advice/counselling for both the patient and their family. In the UK a National Service Framework has been written to provide guidance on the management of people with coronary heart disease (National Service Framework, 2000). One of the standards of recommended care is the provision of a multidisciplinary programme of secondary prevention and cardiac rehabilitation. The emphasis of the chapter is on exercise training, as this is the area in which most physiotherapists are involved within a comprehensive rehabilitation programme. To facilitate access to the information the chapter is divided into three parts and includes an overview of the research evidence, a discussion of exercise prescription and exercise programmes and concludes with issues related to the delivery of cardiac rehabilitation.

RESEARCH EVIDENCE

Both providers and recipients of cardiac rehabilitation are able to benefit from an extensive base of research, making this an area of informed evidence-based practice. With a plethora of research information it is tempting to consider that the case for rehabilitation programmes is beyond question, but the findings of studies need to be placed in context within the period when they were performed, the type of programme offered and the recipients. The period between the 1960s and 1980s witnessed a flurry of research activity involving patients recovering from a myocardial infarction (MI), reflecting the evolution of rehabilitation programmes. At that time the management of those patients bore little resemblance to that of the present day. Thrombolysis and the pharmacological control of secondary complications was not available. Additionally, several weeks of enforced inactivity was the norm, resulting in patients with low levels of exercise tolerance entering rehabilitation programmes. Consequently these programmes tended to focus on exercise rehabilitation in contrast to the multifaceted comprehensive programmes offered today. Therefore the evaluation of a single intervention is now of limited benefit, as the sum of the programme may be greater than its individual parts. The combination of these factors means that most of the early studies related to cardiac rehabilitation are only of historical interest and have limited relevance to the present population of patients. Patients with most forms of heart disease may now be found participating in rehabilitation programmes, including those who were previously considered to be 'high risk'. With increased levels of infarction survival, there may be an increase in the number of the latter group who may develop secondary cardiological complications. Hence the patients now involved in cardiac rehabilitation form a heterogeneous group in terms of clinical features and exercise tolerance compared to those of the past.

A continuing problem with many studies is that they do not reflect clinical practice, with exercise prescription often based on laboratory measurements unavailable to clinicians, an idealistic training programme and highly selected patients. An important deficit in most studies is the lack of female and elderly patients, as they generally involve men under the age of 65 years. Consequently the evidence for cardiac rehabilit-

ation is incomplete and we need to evaluate its benefits in areas of deficient information and continue to evaluate its effects with changes in the management of patients with heart disease and use current findings as a basis for clinical practice.

Exercise training

The previous large improvements in physiological measures following exercise training were to be expected due to the patient's poor entry status (Certo 1985, Detry et al 1971, Paterson et al 1979, Rousseau et al 1974, Thompson 1988). Patients who are now recovering from a MI have a different physiological baseline due to changes in management and different expectations compared with their predecessors (DeBusk 1992, Franklin et al 1992). Consequently patients generally show more modest improvements compared with 20 years ago. This has implications for the objectives of cardiac rehabilitation programmes and not all patients may require formal rehabilitation, with some gaining similar benefits by alternative means, e.g. home-based programmes (Ades et al 2000, Bar et al 1992, Chua & Lipkin 1993, DeBusk et al 1985, Haskell 1994a, Lewin et al 1992, Lindsay et al 1991, Sparks et al 1993). As most patients recovering from an uncomplicated MI now quickly regain their premorbid level of exercise tolerance it has been suggested that the emphasis of programmes for this group should focus on secondary prevention, rather than restoration of physical activity (DeBusk 1992, Gohlke & Gohlke-Barwolf 1998, Gordon & Haskell 1997, Thompson & De Bono 1999, Verges et al 1998). Exercise training, as part of a comprehensive programme, has a role in achieving this aim (Brubaker et al 2000, Jolliffe & Taylor 1998, Niebauer et al 1997). Some studies have suggested patients who have recently experienced an anterior MI, and therefore have poor left ventricular function, should delay participating in exercise programmes because of the possible detrimental effect of remodelling on the myocardium (Jugdutt et al 1988, Kloner & Kloner 1983). However, recent studies involving more appropriate forms of exercise have demonstrated that exercise does not contribute to the onset of remodelling (Cannistra et al 1999, DuBach et al

1997, Giannuzzi et al 1993, Myers et al 2000) and may improve cardiac perfusion (Linxue et al 1999).

While most studies demonstrate the benefits of encouraging patients to perform regular exercise after a MI, they also illustrate the diversity of exercise regimens offered within a rehabilitation programme. Patients in the early stages of recovery are thought to derive similar physiological and psychosocial benefits from a low-intensity aerobic exercise programme compared with one of higher intensity (Blumenthal et al 1988, Goble et al 1991, Worcester et al 1993). Utilization of a low-intensity programme would facilitate both compliance and safety. Until recently programmes tended to exclude resistance exercises, but some studies have suggested these aid return to full function without patients incurring any detrimental effects (Adams et al 1999, Beniamini et al 1999, McCartney 1998). There is also some evidence to suggest that participation in a high-frequency training programme confers greater improvement in quality of life than performing exercise less frequently, with younger patients deriving most benefit (Nieuwland et al 2000). The studies that have focused on elderly patients following a MI indicate that participation in rehabilitation programmes confers similar benefits to those seen in middle-aged patients (Ades 1999, Lavie & Milani 1997, McGee 1999, Stahle et al 1999).

The duration of the period of exercise training may be influenced by the objectives of the programme. Aspects of both physiological and psychosocial recovery after a MI are thought to occur at different rates (Joughin et al 1999, Morrin et al 2000) and achievement of secondary prevention requires a prolonged period of exercise training (Brubaker et al 2000, Niebauer et al 1997). Patients may need support to adopt behavioural changes to optimize compliance and long-term adherence. There is a general paucity of information on how long any changes persist once the rehabilitation programme or training period is completed, with few studies including long-term follow-up measures (Dugmore et al 1999, Van Dixhoorn & Duivenvoorden 1999). Both Oldridge et al (1988) and O'Connor et al (1989) have suggested that a period of exercise training decreases mortality in patients after a MI, but the conclusions of these meta-analysis may no longer be relevant due to the changes in management of this group of patients and the reviews have been criticized (Gohlke & Gohlke-Barwolf 1998, Jolliffe et al 2000a, NHS 1998, West 1995). However, a recent systematic review of exercise-based rehabilitation (Jolliffe et al 2000a) continues to support the beneficial effect of exercise training in reducing mortality in middle-aged men after a MI.

Although patients with chronic heart failure are now included in many exercise programmes, they still form a disproportionately small population of participants. This is despite a growing collection of recent studies indicating that these patients derive both physiological and psychosocial benefits from modest periods of exercise training (Belardinelli et al 1999, Coats 1999, Dziekan et al 1998, Hambrecht et al 2000, Keteyian et al 1996, McKelvie et al 1995, Meyer et al 1996, Taylor 1999, Wielenga et al 1997). The exercise programmes that achieved these effects were varied in organization and patients were generally class II and III of the New York Health Association classification system for chronic heart failure (Squires 1998). There is some evidence to suggest that patients with ischaemic chronic heart failure show less improvement in aerobic function than patients whose origin is dilated cardiomyopathy (Keteyian et al 1996, Yokoyama et al 1994). At present there is no information available concerning the effect of regular exercise on mortality, but any gains are quickly lost on cessation of exercise training (Coats et al 1992, Taylor 1997).

Education and psychosocial support

When comprehensive rehabilitation programmes are offered it is difficult to determine whether all the components are contributing to the attainment of the objectives or whether one component is more influential than another (Thompson & De Bono 1999). Programmes that have only offered educational or psychosocial interventions to patients recovering from a MI have generally been found to have minimal benefit or only lower some risk factors in the short-term, with any gains being short-lived and not influencing morbidity or mortality (Dusseldorp et al 1999, NHS 1998, Sivarajan et al 1983, Stern et al 1983, Taylor 1997). In contrast, some studies have shown that the inclusion of psychosocial interventions within a comprehensive programme does reduce mortality and morbidity, suggesting a beneficial additive effect (Linden et al 1996, Van Dixhoorn & Duivenvoorden 1999).

While mortality and morbidity are easy endpoints to measure, patients may consider return to normal function to be a better reflection of a successful recovery. Improvements in quality of life after attending rehabilitation programmes have received less attention than changes in the patient's physiological state, although the two are interrelated. This may be due in part to the difficulty in measuring these areas. Whilst there are many valid and reliable measures for changes in physiological status, this is not the situation when monitoring changes in the psychosocial domain. Many different outcome measures have been utilized, which makes comparisons between studies difficult (Fitzpatrick et al 1992, Gorkin et al 1993, Langosch 1988, Mayou & Bryant 1993, Wiklund & Welin 1992). Questionnaires have been widely used to measure quality of life and health status and they may be generic, e.g. Short form-36 (SF-36) (Ware et al 1994), which allows comparison with other disease states, or disease specific, e.g. quality of life after myocardial infarction. Studies which have used generic questionnaires have generally been unable to detect any benefit from attending rehabilitation programmes (Burgess et al 1987, Morrin et al 2000, Ott et al 1983), whilst those utilizing disease-specific questionnaires have usually found only short-term benefits (Oldridge et al 1991). These findings may reflect methodological issues, as the ability of previously established measurement tools to detect change in this area is now being challenged (McGee et al 1999, Ni et al 2000, Smith et al 2000, Taylor et al 1998).

Prediction models and cost effectiveness

In order to optimize finite resources, the ability to predict which patients would derive the greatest benefit from a period of formal cardiac rehabilitation would be desirable. However, this task is fraught with difficulty and a robust prediction model is not yet available (Shepherd et al 1998, Van Dixhoorn et al 1990). Programmes vary in organization, duration, intensity of exercise training, frequency and stage within the patient's disease process: all these factors interact to influence the response of the patient. Similarly the diversity of the programmes also makes it difficult to generalize on the cost effectiveness of cardiac rehabilitation (Ades et al 1997, Oldridge 1998, Taylor & Kirby 1997). In many cases the latter is also hampered by the absence of an appropriate audit tool, although this is evolving within the United Kingdom (Thompson et al 1997), and the lack of formal evaluation of the effectiveness of individual rehabilitation programmes. Reduction in the utilization of health services as a result of cardiac rehabilitation programmes may enable a net saving to be identified after several years have elapsed.

RATIONALE AND IMPLEMENTATION OF A CARDIAC REHABILITATION PROGRAMME

Cardiac rehabilitation (CR) should meet the emotional, educational and physical needs of patients and their families in the acute hospital phase, through outpatient care and long-term follow-up in the community. Rehabilitation should be an integral part of cardiological management with common goals to:

- decrease cardiac morbidity and relieve symptoms
- promote risk modification and secondary prevention
- decrease anxiety and increase knowledge and self-confidence
- increase fitness and resume normal activities.

Cardiological management involves assessment, risk stratification, diagnostic testing, drug therapy and revascularization interventions (e.g. angioplasty and coronary artery bypass grafting). The rehabilitation package should encompass psychosocial and activity management, providing:

- reassurance, support and information
- risk factor modification and an appropriate behavioural change programme

- assessment and risk stratification
- exercise prescription and an individualized activity programme.

Optimum shared patient care involves close collaboration between cardiology and rehabilitation professionals, e.g. before prescribing, when modifying treatment in symptomatic patients or implementing exercise prescription the 'risk' of further cardiac events (risk stratification) must be determined.

Cardiac rehabilitation provision spans four phases of care (BACR 1995).

- Phase I – in-hospital period (average 5–7 days)
- Phase II – immediate post-discharge/ convalescence stage (2–6 weeks)
- Phase III – supervised outpatient programme (6–12 weeks)
- Phase IV – long-term maintenance programme in the community

The aims and duration of each phase may vary in accordance with the needs of individual patients and local resources. Dividing the care package into four phases with a flexible timescale enables patients to 'travel' between phases as circumstances, need and progress dictate; for example, more complex patients with recurrent unstable episodes who require further cardiological treatment will not proceed as quickly as an uncomplicated patient following a small myocardial infarction.

In spite of common service aims, considerable variation still exists in the timing, content, style and delivery of CR programmes, e.g. hospital group setting versus home based; exercise training only without education and psychosocial components; programmes limited to 4–6 weeks versus provision for up to 1 year. However, there is now consensus on clinical guidelines, 'models' of service delivery and audit tools which should enable more widespread use of recommended protocols and outcome measures, leading to an increase in the standardization and effectiveness of cardiac rehabilitation services (AACVPR 1999, BACR 1995).

In the following sections the rationale for and implementation of a cardiac rehabilitation exercise programme are reviewed. First, programme implementation is considered in terms of:

- to whom it should be available
- by whom it should be delivered.

Second, the benefits of exercise training and principles of exercise prescription are described.

Finally the implementation of an exercise programme across the four phases of rehabilitation is described together with special exercise considerations for specific groups within the general coronary heart disease (CHD) population.

To whom should cardiac rehabilitation be available?

CR should be offered to all cardiac patients who would benefit. Traditionally programmes have been targeted at post-MI and coronary artery bypass graft patients with limited and variable service provision for patients with angina, chronic heart failure, following angioplasty or those who have undergone cardiac transplantation. Uptake of service is often poor amongst women, multi-pathology patients, ethnic groups and the elderly. Therefore issues relating to access, distance, timing and flexibility of cardiac rehabilitation programmes are very important considerations when trying to optimize service provision for such under-represented groups.

By whom should cardiac rehabilitation be delivered?

The challenge of delivering a broad spectrum of care requires the combined skills and close collaboration of a multidisciplinary team of professionals. The team should be led by a cardiologist and include nursing, physiotherapy, dietetics, occupational therapy, pharmacy and psychology staff with specialist training in cardiology and rehabilitation. Additional input may be required from social services and vocational guidance staff. Continuation of care in the community includes the primary healthcare team, principally GP and practice nurse, Phase IV exercise instructor and possibly attendance at a cardiac patient support group. Long-term risk factor monitoring/management, coupled with a regular activity programme, is promoted at Phase IV to reinforce the need for ongoing secondary prevention.

Physiotherapists posess core skills in the assessment and rehabilitation management of multi-pathology patients and in the delivery of health education and exercise advice (Jolliffe et al 2000b). Consequently, the role of the physiotherapist within the team should focus on exercise prescription, training and education in Phases I–III. Exercise prescription should not, however, be addressed in isolation by one professional. Modification of prescription may need to be discussed with medical and nursing colleagues, not only when there is a change in clinical status but also in response to the patient's changing psychological status, e.g. fear, negative attitude to exercise, inappropriate activity goals. Activity management requires teamwork with other professionals who are aware of concurrent medical and psychosocial issues. There should also be full discussion and agreement of activity goals with the patient and family and liaison with Phase IV community instructors who will be continuing the long-term exercise prescription.

WHAT ARE THE BENEFITS OF EXERCISE TRAINING?

Improved exercise capacity

The development of cardiovascular endurance is the primary objective for CHD patients. Endurance training, defined as any activity which uses large muscle groups, can be sustained for a prolonged period and is rhythmic and aerobic in nature, results in an increase in maximal oxygen uptake ($\dot{V}O_2$max), i.e the highest rate of oxygen consumption attainable during maximal exercise. Maximal oxygen uptake is limited centrally by cardiac output (CO = HR (heart rate) x SV (stroke volume)) and by peripheral factors, in particular by the capacity of skeletal muscle to extract oxygen from the blood (arteriovenous oxygen difference (a-vO_2diff)). Consequently an increase in $\dot{V}O_2$max depends upon the potential for inducing central and/or peripheral adaptations.

Central changes

In healthy individuals, endurance training results in a significant increase in maximal cardiac output. Maximum heart rate does not alter with training and so the increase in CO must arise from a training-induced increase in maximal SV. This is achieved primarily through:

● increased left ventricular mass and chamber size
● increased total blood volume
● reduced total peripheral resistance at maximal exercise.

Peripheral changes

Training-induced changes within skeletal muscle which contribute to increased extraction and utilization of oxygen include:

● increased number and size of mitochondria
● increased oxidative enzyme activity
● increased capillarization
● increased myoglobin.

In cardiac patients, the increase in $\dot{V}O_2$max is attributed predominantly to peripheral adaptation. Central changes are associated with prolonged periods of high-intensity training and, although in selected patients central changes have been provoked (Ehsani et al 1986, Schuler et al 1992), the high intensity of the training regimen would be inappropriate for the heterogeneous group of patients accepted into typical cardiac rehabilitation programmes.

Consequences of increase in maximal oxygen uptake

The significance of an increase in $\dot{V}O_2$max for cardiac patients is not that it permits a higher level of maximal effort (as this is rarely demanded in everyday life) but that repeated submaximal activities of daily living constitute a smaller percentage of the increased maximal capacity and therefore impose relatively less physiological stress. This is reflected in a reduction in heart rate (attributed to both increased vagal tone and reduced sympathetic outflow), blood pressure and plasma catecholamine concentrations at rest and at submaximal workloads. Since myocardial oxygen consumption ($M\dot{V}O_2$) is determined by heart rate and systolic blood pressure (referred to as rate pressure product (RPP) or double product) a reduction in either or both delays the onset of ischaemia and lessens the potential for arrhythmias. A further benefit of the training-induced bradycardia is that, at any reference submaximal workload, the period of diastole is extended and since 80% of coronary blood flow occurs during the relaxation phase of the cardiac cycle, myocardial perfusion is significantly enhanced.

Risk factor modification

In cardiac patients exercise may have an important secondary prevention role (Haskell 1994b). The 'acute' effects of each bout of exercise in healthy people include:

● a raised post-exercise metabolic rate
● changes in lipoprotein metabolism with consequent increased synthesis of high-density lipoprotein (HDL)
● improved insulin sensitivity
● decreased blood pressure.

These effects all relate to local changes in the previously exercised muscle and are evident even after light to moderate exercise, suggesting that a general increase in physical activity is likely to make a significant contribution to the patient's continued well-being.

Principles of exercise prescription

When developing an individual training regimen, several factors (often referred to as the FITT principles) must be considered.

● Frequency   **F**
● Intensity   **I**
● Duration/time   **T**
● Mode/type   **T**

Prescribing and monitoring intensity

This issue is critical because vigorous activity carries a greatly increased risk of precipitating adverse events such as myocardial infarction or arrhythmias (Willich et al 1993). Frequent, moderate-intensity exercise is recommended for CHD patients since it will optimize benefits without increasing the risk of adverse events (Dafoe & Huston 1997). For individuals with very diminished functional capacity, several short bouts (as little as 5–10 minutes) throughout the day may be advisable. There are a number of established methods for prescribing and monitoring intensity which may be used separately or in combination with one another.

Use of heart rate. Ideally, training heart rate is based on information derived from a maximal or symptom-limited exercise electrocardiogram (ECG) test. Where a maximal test has been achieved, training heart rate should be set at 60–75% of maximal heart rate. If the test was symptom limited, training intensity should be set at 10–20 beats per minute (bpm) below the heart rate at which symptoms were apparent and the patient's heart rate should be monitored throughout exercise. ECG test information is, however, not always available to health professionals. In the absence of test data or if, for diagnostic purposes, a patient performs the exercise test 'off medication', other methods for establishing appropriate training intensity have to be used.

Age-adjusted predicted maximal rates can be used (220 bpm minus age in years is one formula) and the training heart rate set at 60–75% of the predicted maximum; this is equivalent to 40–65% $\dot{V}O_2$max. However, the standard deviation (SD) for maximal heart rate during exercise is ± 10 bpm and some individuals will, therefore, have an actual maximum heart rate 20 bpm higher or lower (2 SD above or below the population mean) than that predicted. An alternative approach is to prescribe training at 60–75% of heart rate reserve (HRR), i.e. the difference between resting and maximal heart rate. This approach is convenient since it is known that 60–75% of heart rate reserve is equivalent to 60–75% of $\dot{V}O_2$max. An example of the calculation is shown below for an individual with a resting heart rate of 60 bpm and maximal heart rate of 180 bpm.

$180 - 60 = 120$ (heart rate reserve – HRR)

Training heart rate = 60–75% of heart rate reserve + resting heart rate (RHR)

$120 \times 0.60 = 72 + 60$ (RHR) = 132 bpm (60%)

$120 \times 0.75 = 90 + 60$ (RHR) = 150 bpm (75%)

NB. The formula is intended for use with known maximal heart rates. In the absence of these data, the substitution of age-adjusted predicted maxima introduces the same potential for error as previously mentioned. Consequently, any prescription which is based on predicted maximal heart rates should be used in conjunction with a rating of perceived exertion scale (RPE).

Since the relationship between exercise intensity and the percent of maximal heart rate is preserved in patients on beta-blockers, the above formula can be adopted for calculating a training heart rate for this group but the maximal or peak heart rate must be established from an exercise test performed on medication.

Use of rating of perceived exertion Cardiorespiratory and metabolic variables are strongly related to rating of perceived exertion which is accepted as a valid and reproducible indicator of the intensity of steady-state exercise. On the 15-point Borg scale (Table 15.1) a rating of 12–13 (equivalent to 3–4 on the Borg CR10 scale (Table 15.2)) corresponds to approximately 60% of heart rate reserve or $\dot{V}O_2$max and a rating of 15 corresponds to 75% of either.

Use of metabolic equivalent values (METs). Exercise may also be regulated by choice of activities according to their known MET (metabolic equivalent) values (for which tables are available in most exercise physiology texts). If an individual assesses walking at 3 miles per hour (mph) as 12–13 on the Borg RPE scale (corresponding to 60% of $\dot{V}O_2$max), then activities of comparable MET value can be prescribed in the knowledge that they will present an appropriate training stimulus. Knowledge of MET values is also important in

Table 15.1 15-Grade Borg scale for rating perceived exertion, reproduced with permission

6	No exertion at all
7	
8	Extremely light
9	Very light
10	
11	Light
12	
13	Somewhat hard
14	
15	Hard (heavy)
16	
17	Very hard
18	
19	Extremely hard
20	Maximal exertion

Table 15.2 The Borg CR10 scale for rating perceived exertion, reproduced with permission

0	Nothing at all	No "1"
0,3		
0,5	Extremely weak	Just noticeable
0,7		
1	Very weak	
1,5		
2	Weak	Light
2,5		
3	Moderate	
4		
5	Strong	Heavy
6		
7	Very strong	
8		
9		
10	Extremely strong	"Strongest 1"
11		
⌇		
●	**Absolute maximum**	Highest possible

Patient instructions: This is a scale for rating perceived exertion. Perceived exertion is the overall effort or distress of your body during exercise. The number 0 (6 if using the 15-grade scale) represents no perceived exertion or leg discomfort and 10 (20 if using the 15-grade scale) represents the greatest amount of exertion that you have ever experienced. At various times during the exercise you will be asked to select a number that indicates your rating of perceived exertion at the time. Do you have any questions?

terms of excluding those activities which might pose a risk to certain individuals. Skipping (8–12 METs) or freestyle swimming (9–10 METs), for example, would be entirely inappropriate for someone with a peak capacity of 7 METs.

Some activities have a wide range of MET values, while others are relatively constant between individuals, mainly because they permit little variation in individual execution, e.g. there is very little difference in the way individuals walk or cycle. In contrast, there can be great variation in the way 'free-moving' activities such as dancing, skipping or rebounding on a mini-trampoline are executed. Because precise control of the exercise prescription, in a cardiac population, is necessary (particularly in early recovery post-event and for stable angina patients) activities which can be maintained at prescribed workloads and which permit uniform modification, e.g. altering the speed of walking or jogging or the resistance on a cycle ergometer, are preferred to those which are not amenable to standardized prescription.

Regardless of the objective method used for monitoring intensity, it is important to observe individuals for signs of excessive breathlessness, loss of quality of movement, unusual pallor or excessive sweating, all of which are inappropriate responses to moderate levels of exertion. Indications for ceasing exercise and contraindications to initiating exercise are included in the section on programme implementation.

Training modes

The inclusion of a variety of training modes within the individual prescription or the class format will minimize the incidence of overuse injuries, maximize peripheral adaptation (as, for example, when activities which require a contribution from both upper and lower body musculature are included) and increase patient motivation and adherence.

It is well documented that coronary artery disease (CAD) patients who expend about 250–300 kcal per session and 1000–1500 kcal per week in additional physical activity will improve their aerobic capacity by 15–30% over a 4–6-month period (Balady et al 1994). There appears to be a continuous gradient in the benefits conferred and there is evidence that a minimum of 1600 kcal per week may halt the progression of CAD whereas atherosclerotic regression may be achieved with a weekly energy expenditure of about 2200 kcal (Hambrecht et al 1994). Within the recommended ranges of frequency, intensity and time (or duration) of training, similar conditioning effects can be expected from any programme which realizes comparable weekly energy expenditure. Consequently the FITT components may be adjusted to provide an optimal prescription for individuals of varying cardiovascular and general medical status.

The exercise programme

Warm-up. Preparation for activity in older adults and especially in the cardiac population must be more gradual than for apparently healthy individuals. Fifteen minutes devoted to the warm-up component is recommended (Bell 2001). Low-impact, dynamic movements which use large muscle groups and which take all major joint complexes through their normal range of motion should be incorporated. A gradual increase in the size and range of movements performed will delay the onset of ischaemia by allowing adequate time for coronary blood flow to increase in response to the greater myocardial demand. Gradual increments in myocardial workload will also lessen the risk of arrhythmias which can be a consequence of abrupt increases in demand and concomitant elevated sympathetic activity. As a guideline individuals should be within 20 bpm of their prescribed training heart rate at the end of the warm-up or, if RPE is used in place of heart rate monitoring, a rating no higher than 3 on the Borg CR10 scale or 10–11 on the original scale (Borg 1982).

Although evidence of the benefit is not equivocal, preparing for exercise has traditionally included static stretches which are performed after the pulse raising and mobility phase. Because static stretches are used, the need to maintain pulse rate and body temperature during this time must be addressed.

Cardiovascular conditioning. The type of activity used for conditioning may adopt a continuous or interval approach. Continuous training, as the name implies, involves uninterrupted activity usually performed at a constant submaximal intensity. Its advantage is the ease with which intensity may be prescribed and monitored. Walking, jogging, cycling, rowing, bench stepping and swimming all lend themselves to a continuous approach. Interval training entails bouts of relatively intense work separated by periods of rest or less intense activity. Its main advantage is that, especially for debilitated patients, the total volume of work accomplished is generally greater than when exercise is continuous; consequently the stimulus to physiological change is greater. In an older cardiac population, the transition from one activity to another also provides a time for social interaction and support which probably aids long-term compliance.

In clinically supervised programmes, interval-style circuit training is the favoured format for rehabilitation classes (Fig. 15.1). Participants spend a fixed time (ranging from 30 seconds to 2 minutes) at 'cardiovascular (CV) stations' and either rest or perform a lower intensity activity before moving on to the next CV station. The lower intensity or 'active recovery' stations are usually designed to increase the endurance of specific muscle groups, e.g. triceps, pectorals, trapezius, used in activities of daily living.

Individualization of the cardiovascular component of the programme is achieved through variation in:

- the duration at each CV station*
- the intensity (by changing the resistance or the speed or range of movement)*
- the period of rest between stations
- the overall duration of conditioning.

* In general the duration of activity is extended before increasing the intensity.

Exercises involving a recumbent position are discouraged because:

- some older participants have difficulty in getting up and down
- following vigorous activity, the increase in venous return on lying down enhances preload and thereby myocardial workload

which increases the risk of arrhythmias and angina in some individuals
- there is an increased risk of orthostatic hypotension.

It is therefore recommended that any recumbent work (e.g. for the abdominals or erector spinae) should be performed after completion of the circuit and a cool-down period.

Resistance training. Traditionally, training to increase the strength (as opposed to endurance) of specific muscle groups was considered to be inappropriate for individuals with established heart disease. This was because resistance training is associated with an increase in arterial blood pressure which increases myocardial workload. Some early studies suggested that the isometric component caused reduced ejection fraction, left ventricle wall motion abnormalities and increased incidence of arrhythmias. Further studies (Squires et al 1991, Williams 1994) have generally reported that cardiovascular and haemodynamic responses to resistance training in CHD patients and in normal subjects are similar and, because of increased diastolic pressure, may even enhance myocardial perfusion. However, in the UK, it is rare to incorporate strength training into clinically supervised programmes unless it is indicated for vocational reasons.

In the absence of further research, guidelines remain relatively conservative; two sets of 8–10 exercises involving the major muscle groups, performed a minimum of twice per week, is generally recommended but the American College of Sports Medicine (1994) advocates a single set of up to 10–12 exercises using 10–12 repetitions which can be performed 'comfortably'. This is based on evidence that strength gains derived from one set are very similar to those reported when several are performed and adherence to programmes which are less time consuming is increased.

Contraindications for resistance training are:

- abnormal haemodynamic responses with exercise
- ischaemic changes during graded exercise testing
- poor left ventricular function
- uncontrolled hypertension or arrhythmias
- exercise capacity less than 6 METs.

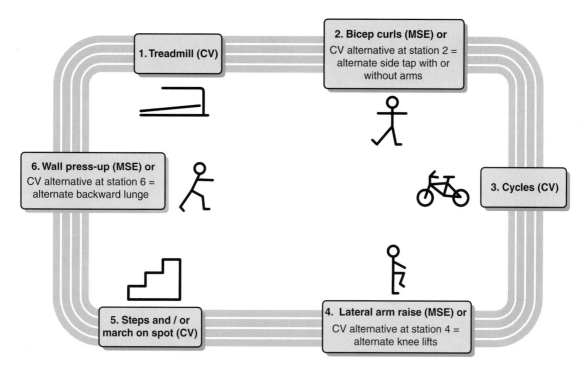

CV= Cardiovascular work. MSE= muscular strength and endurance work

Figure 15.1 An example of interval-style circuit training suitable for a phase III cardiac rehabilitation exercise programme.

Class Management
Patients spend 2 minutes on stations 1, 3 and 5. At stations 2, 4 and 6, 1 minute is spent on the MSE work followed by 1 minute walking round the outside of the circuit. The patient's attention needs to be drawn to the start of each 2 minute activity period and (for the benefit of those at the even MSE stations) when the 1st minute has passed. One full circuit constitutes 12 minutes and 2 circuits, 24 minutes.

Individualization and Progression
The emphasis should be on improving cardiovascular endurance and greater duration of cardiovascular work may be achieved by individuals (as and when appropriate) being encouraged to adopt some of the CV alternatives at even station numbers. The intensity of the cardiovascular component may also be progressed at CV stations.
station 1   via speed and / or gradient of the treadmill
station 3   via resistance setting of the cycle
station 5   via progression from 2 minutes marching on spot to 1 minute of stepping & 1 minute marching and finally to
              2 minutes stepping. To any of these armwork may be added. The height of the step may also be increased.
Progression on the alternative CV stations is achieved at:
station 2   via increased range of movement and / or lifting arms up to shoulder level as alternate legs go out to side
station 4   via increased range of movement and / or lifting arms up between each knee lift
station 6   via increased range of movement and / or lifting arms in front as alternate legs are extended back.

The intensity of the MSE component may be progressed by introducing dumbells or resistance bands or, in the case of station 6, taking the feet further from the wall or introducing backward extension of the arm at the elbow (tricep 'kick-back') using a dumbell.

Determining appropriate workloads using fixed equipment
Although individuals will vary considerably in the amount of cardiovascular work they can achieve it is suggested that for:
– the treadmill – a walking speed of 2.5–3.0 miles per hour (mph) or 4.0–4.8 kilometres per hour (kph) is prescribed with the gradient altered to elicit a heart rate response within the target training heart rate range
– the cycle – 50–55 revolutions per minutes (rpm) is prescribed with the resistance altered to elicit a heart rate response within the target heart rate range
– the steps – a stepping speed to between 18 and 24 cycles per minute is prescribed (1 cycle – 4 footfalls i.e. up, up, down down) and the step height altered to elicit a heart rate response within the target training heart rate range

The circuit when completed twice provides a minimum of 12 minutes CV work and a maximum of 24 minutes (if all CV alternatives at even numbered stations are used).

Cool-down component. A period of 10 minutes is recommended for cool-down at the end of the cardiovascular component. This is because:

- there is an increased risk of hypotension in this group. For some this is a specific side effect of their medication. In addition, there is an age-related slowing of baroreceptor responsiveness which increases the risk of venous pooling following sustained exercise
- in older adults heart rates take longer to return to pre-exercise rates
- raised sympathetic activity during vigorous exercise increases the risk of arrhythmias during the immediate period following cessation of exercise.

The cool-down should incorporate movements of diminishing intensity and passive stretching of the major muscle groups used during the conditioning phase.

Patient observation for up to 30 minutes after the exercise session is recommended. Many programmes follow the exercise session with an education or relaxation component which affords the opportunity for extended observation and supervision of participants.

Progression. The duration, frequency or intensity of training can be increased in order to maintain the training stimulus. Ideally serial exercise testing will form the basis on which the prescription is modified in order to ensure that it provokes physiological adaptation. In the absence of exercise testing, heart rate monitoring and rating of perceived exertion, at reference workloads, may be used to establish the appropriateness of increasing any of the three variables, either singly or in combination with one another. The way in which exercise prescription is progressed and the rate at which it is progressed will be highly variable between individuals with CHD and will be a function of many factors including age, severity of disease, motivation, dual pathology and compliance.

The exercise ECG test

In the cardiology setting an exercise ECG using an incremental protocol is the most common method for determining cardiac perfusion and function. Its major applications are:

- diagnosis – to identify patients with CHD and the severity of their disease
- prognosis – to identify high , moderate and low-risk patients
- evaluation – to establish the effectiveness of a selected intervention
- measurement of functional capacity – on which advice about activities of daily living and a formal exercise prescription may be based
- measurement of acute exercise responses including blood pressure, heart rate, ventilatory responses and detection of exercise-induced arrhythmias.

Numerous exercise protocols have been developed which utilize a variety of different exercise modes but in the United Kingdom, an incremental treadmill protocol is the traditional test mode. Prior to acceptance into a Phase III programme, usually 2–6 weeks post MI, a symptom-limited test (i.e. the patient continues until signs or symptoms which necessitate test termination are evident) is customary; the Bruce protocol is the most common. Sub-maximal tests which use a predetermined endpoint such as an age-predicted maximum heart rate are usual before discharge. The modified Bruce protocol is the most commonly used since it introduces two preliminary, less strenuous stages (Table 15.3).

Table 15.3 Commonly used treadmill exercise protocols (adapted from Bruce 1973)

Stage		Speed (mph)	Grade %	Duration (Mins)	METs
Modified Bruce	Full Bruce				
1	–	1.7	0	3	1.7
2	–	1.7	5	3	2.9
3	1	1.7	10	3	4.7
4	2	2.5	12	3	7.1
5	3	3.4	14	3	10.2
6	4	4.2	16	3	13.5
7	5	5.0	18	3	17.3
8	6	5.5	20	3	24.6
9	7	6.0	22	3	28.4

Criteria for terminating an exercise test include:

- horizontal or down-sloping ST segment depression greater than 2 mm, indicating ischaemia
- marked drop in systolic blood pressure (> 20 mmHg) indicating poor left ventricular function or severe coronary disease
- serious arrhythmias, e.g. ventricular tachycardia
- patient fatigue and/or excessive breathlessness at low workloads which may simply indicate poor functional capacity but may also be suggestive of serious problems such as heart failure.

In general an exercise ECG test is considered to be negative if haemodynamic responses to the increasing workload are normal and the patient satisfactorily completes a workload equivalent to the second stage of the full Bruce protocol (7 METs). The test is considered positive if the patient is symptomatic at low workloads, if there are significant ECG changes or there is an inappropriate heart rate/blood pressure response to the incremental workload.

PROGRAMME IMPLEMENTATION

Phase I: in-hospital activity component

Graduated mobilization of cardiac patients following acute MI or coronary artery bypass graft (CABG) is initiated by nursing or physiotherapy staff on acute units as part of overall patient care. Activities in the first 24–48 hours are usually restricted to breathing exercises, simple arm/leg range of movement exercises and limited self-care activities. Sitting out of bed, short walks and progressive self-care including showering and dressing are gradually included over the next 2–3 days, depending on cardiac status. Although the physiotherapist may be involved in the earlier stages with a multi-pathology patient, their customary role is to supervise the patient's individual mobilization plan, e.g. pre-discharge walk or stair assessments in order to monitor exercise intensity, symptoms and/or limitations. By discharge, all patients should be conversant with the signs and symptoms of

excessive exertion and be able to rate level of effort using, for example, the Borg scale or a similar locally developed scale. Both the patient and family should be advised on how to manage chest pain and encouraged to keep symptom and activity diaries to discuss with staff at follow-up appointments.

A home exercise programme with guidance on convalescence activities over the first 6 weeks and written advice on specific 'do and don't activities' should be provided. Emphasis is on walking and resumption of light household tasks as the main means of gradually increasing functional capacity. A sample walking schedule suggesting distance/speed ratios and progressions should also be incorporated. There are a number of sources of professionally produced written material if none is available locally.

Although exercise prescription is always dependent on individual clinical status, symptoms and medical history, the following FITT criteria may be used as general guidelines at discharge.

- **Frequency**   2–3 times daily
- **Intensity**   Resting HR + 20 bpm post MI (arbitrary target)
  Resting HR + 30 bpm post CABG (arbitrary target)
  RPE <11 (6–20 Borg scale) or to individual tolerance, i.e. symptom limited by excess breathlessness/angina/fatigue at or below these suggested targets
- **Timing**   5–20 mins; intermittent bouts of activity <5 min interspersed with rest periods – overall duration of activity progressed to about 20 min
- **Type**   Sitting/standing functional activities; range of movement exercises; walking

Phase II: immediate post-discharge convalescence activity phase

This home-based period may typically last from 2 to 6 weeks depending on local protocols and resources as well as the patient's fitness to attend the supervised outpatient programme. The immediate post-discharge phase is a time of high anxiety for patients and families and unfortunately rehabilitation services vary considerably from either no or limited contact to regular phone follow-up and home visiting arrangements. A home programme for MI patients in the form of a workbook, the Heart Manual (Lewin et al 1992), is used in some areas either as the complete rehabilitation package or more usually as an interim measure or adjunct to a Phase III programme. Contact from rehabilitation staff at this stage provides the opportunity to answer questions, reinforce daily walking and home exercises as appropriate, discuss symptom and activity diaries. It also facilitates the review of risk factor modification goals and achievements and preparation for the transition to Phase III. Depending on the duration of Phase II, uncomplicated post-MI and CABG patients may have increased the duration and frequency of activities and be achieving up to 30 minutes of walking once or twice daily.

Phase III: supervised outpatient exercise programme

Comprehensive Phase III rehabilitation is composed of safe, incremental progression of physical activity, risk factor modification and health education to address secondary prevention and psychosocial support through counselling and stress management. The onset and duration of Phase III programmes vary considerably and are usually dependent on local resources. They are usually delivered in a group setting and include patients at different stages in their recovery. Programmes may start any time from 3 to 8 weeks post-event and last for up to 6–12 weeks. They are often hospital based but there are also rehabilitation centres in the community.

Exercise component: assessment and risk stratification. The transition between low-level convalescence activity and a more progressive exercise prescription should be preceded by detailed assessment and risk stratification (CSP 1999). Local referral protocols should include appropriate screening and consent from a hospital physician or cardiologist prior to commencing exercise. The following information should be available:

● the site and size of the infarct or operation details for surgical patients
● current cardiac status and any complications
● risk stratification outcome following an exercise ECG
● current medication
● progress since discharge – symptoms, activity level, psychological status
● relevant previous medical history (e.g. musculoskeletal problems, respiratory or neurological conditions)
● CHD risk factors.

Prognosis and clinical risk stratification, i.e. determining the relative risk of future cardiac events and complications, should be carried out for all cardiac patients at the earliest possible stage. Mortality is highest in the first 4 weeks post MI with 1-year rates cited at 10–15% and 5% annually thereafter. The criteria published by AACVPR (1999) (Table 15.4) stratify patients into low- , medium- or high-risk groups depending on their current cardiac status including cardiac damage, complications and associated signs and symptoms. Patients who have had more than one MI, an anterior rather than inferior infarction, large increases in cardiac enzymes and a low ejection fraction consistent with impaired left ventricular function and complications such as serious arrhythmias, left ventricular failure or cardiogenic shock are at greater risk of complications and future cardiac events. The main risk to cardiac patients attending an exercise programme is ventricular fibrillation. Key factors to consider when 'predicting' risk from clinical evidence and exercise ECG assessment are the patients who have suffered extensive cardiac damage, have residual ischaemia and demonstrate ventricular arrhythmias on exercise.

A patient with a significantly positive exercise ECG test would be considered to be in a poorer prognostic category, at higher risk of cardiac events, requiring further cardiological investigation and consequently only able to undertake a very cautious rehabilitation exercise programme. If HR and BP responses to the exercise test are

Table 15.4 Stratification for risk of event (not specific solely to exercise). Reprinted by permission, from AACPVR 1999 Guidelines for Cardiac Rehabilitation and Secondary Prevention Programs edited by the AACPVR (Champaign, 1L: Human Kinetics Table 4.2 p45).

Lowest risk	Moderate risk	Highest risk
• No significant LV dysfunction (EF >50%) • No resting or exercise-induced complex dysrhythmias • Uncomplicated MI; CABG; angioplasty, atherectomy or stent; – absence of CHF or signs/symptoms indicating post-event ischaemia • Normal haemodynamics with exercise or recovery • Asymptomatic including absence of angina with exertion or recovery • Functional capacity ≥7.0 METS* • Absence of clinical depression **Lowest risk classification is assumed when each of the risk factors in the category is present.**	• Moderately impaired left ventricular function (EF = 40–49%) • Signs/symptoms including angina at moderate levels of exercise (5–6.9 METs) or in recovery **Moderate risk is assumed for patients who do not meet the classification of either highest risk or lowest risk.**	• Decreased LV function (EF <40%) • Survivor of cardiac arrest or sudden death • Complex ventricular dysrhythmia at rest or with exercise • MI or cardiac surgery complicated by cardio-genic shock, CHF and/or signs/symptoms of post-procedure ischaemia • Abnormal haemodynamics with exercise (especially flat or decreasing systolic blood pressure or chronotropic incompetence with increasing workload) • Signs/symptoms including angina pectoris at low levels of exercise (<5.0 METS) or in recovery • Functional capacity <5.0 METS* • Clinically significant depression **Highest risk classification is assumed with the presence of any one of the risk factors included in this category.**

*NOTE: If measured functional capacity is not available, this variable is not considered in the risk stratification process. Abbreviations: LV, left ventricular; EF, ejection fraction; MI, myocardial infarction; CABG, coronary artery bypass graft; CHF, chronic heart failure

satisfactory then limits for exercise prescription may be determined by onset of other symptoms, e.g. breathlessness or fatigue, and very importantly by evidence of ischaemia, with or without the presence of angina (silent ischaemia). Peak exercise prescription should always be set at least 10 bpm below the ischaemia threshold (AACVPR Guidelines 1999). When assessing and setting exercise heart rates, further consideration must also be given to the impact of medication, e.g. the blunting effect of beta-blockers (Table 15.5).

Patient safety when exercising is the main consideration for rehabilitation professionals. This involves not only initial risk stratification and assessment at entry to Phase III to establish the exercise prescription but also ongoing clinical assessment prior to each exercise session. It is recommended that patients should not exercise if they are generally unwell, symptomatic or clinically unstable on arrival, e.g. if they present with:

• fever and acute systemic illness
• unresolved/unstable angina
• resting blood pressure (BP) systolic >200 mmHg and diastolic >110 mmHg
• significant unexplained drop in blood pressure
• tachycardia >100 bpm
• new or recurrent symptoms of breathlessness, palpitations, dizziness
• swelling of ankles or significant lethargy.

If any of these signs or symptoms are present the patient should be seen by their general prac-

Table 15.5 A guide to medication (from BACR 2000, reproduced with permission)

Medication	Used for	Possible side effects	Relevance to exercise
Beta-blockers Atenolol (Tenormin) Propranolol (Inderal) Metoprolol (Lopresor) Sotalol (Beta-cardone) Bisoprolol (Monocor)* Carvedilol (Eucardic)*	Hypertension Angina Tachycardia/arrhythmias Migraine prevention Panic attacks Heart failure*	Slow pulse Hypotension Tiredness, lethargy Dizziness Airway constriction Cold fingers/toes Impotence Nightmares	Suppressed heart rate response Rate of perceived exertion (RPE) more appropriate than heart rate to monitor intensity Risk of postural hypotension with floor exercises
Alpha-blockers Prazosin (Hypovase) Doxazosin (Cardura) Indoramin (Baratol)	Hypertension not controlled by other drugs	Postural hypotension Headache	
Nitrates GTN spray or tablets Isosorbide dinitrate (Isordil) Isosorbide mononitrate (Imdur/Ismo)	Angina – relief and prevention Heart failure	Facial flushing Headache Dizziness Nausea Postural hypotension	Possible postural hypotension especially when used with beta-blockers Rest after using GTN in case of drop in blood pressure Can increase exercise tolerance by preventing angina and increasing ischaemic threshold
Calcium channel blockers Nifedipine (Adalat) Felodipine (Plendil) Nicardipine (Cardene) Amlodipine (Istin) Diltiazem (Tildiem) Verapamil (Cordilox)	Hypertension Angina Control arrhythmias	Facial flushing Palpitations Pounding headaches Mild ankle swelling Constipation	Possible reduced heart rate response to exercise (verapamil & diltiazem only)
Potassium channel activators Nicorandil (Ikorel)	Angina	Dizziness Headache Hypotension Tachycardia	Possible hypotension or tachycardia
ACE inhibitors Trandolapril (Gopten, Odrik) Penindopril (Coversyl) Captopril (Capoten) Enalapril (Innovace) Lisinopril (Zestril Carace) Fosinopril (Staril) Ramipril (Tritace)	Hypertension Heart failure Post-myocardial infarction for LV function	Dry annoying cough Hypotension Skin rash Metallic taste Angio-oedema of lips and tongue Reduced kidney function	Possible increased exercise capacity due to treatment of heart failure
Angiotensin receptor antagonists Losartan (Cozaar) Valsartan (Diovan)	Hypertension	Fatigue Hypotension Taste disturbance Skin rash	None known
Diuretics Frusemide (Lasix) Bumetanide (Burinex) Amiloride (Midamor) Triamterene (Dytac) Spironolactone (Aldactone)	Acute heart failure Mild heart failure – short term Hypertension	Loss of potassium with some types Tiredness Muscle weakness/cramps Loss of appetite	Dehydration effects – keep encouraging fluids in hot weather

continued

Table 15.5 *(continued)*

Medication	Used for	Possible side effects	Relevance to exercise
Bendrofluazide Hydrochlorothiazide (Hydrosaluric) Moduretic Frumil Burinex A. Metaolazone (Metenix)		Ventricular arrhythmias Gout Diabetes Impotence Raised cholesterol and triglycerides	Aching legs may affect exercise capability
Bile acid binders Cholestyramine (Questran)	Reduce LDL cholesterol	Unpalatable and causes gastrointestinal problems Raised triglycerides	
Fibrates Bezafibrate (Bezalip) Clofibrate (Atromid-S) Fenofibrate (Lipantil) Gemfibrozil (Lopid)	Reduce triglycerides and LDL cholesterol Increase HDL cholesterol	Gallstones Rash Gastrointestinal upset Acute pain in calf or thigh muscle if kidney function impaired	Aching legs otherwise no exercise considerations
Statins Simvastatin (Zocor) Pravastatin (Lipostat) Fluvastatin (Lescol) Atorvastatin (Lipitor) Cerivastatin (Lipostay)	Potent at reducing LDL cholesterol Moderately reduce triglycerides and increase HDL cholesterol	Well tolerated Gastrointestinal upset	
Antiarrhythmics Digoxin (Lanoxin)	Supraventricular tachycardia Atrial fibrillation Heart failure (limited use)	Nausea/loss of appetite Vomiting Fatigue Slow pulse	Possible slower heart rate response
Amiodarone (Cordarone)	Mainly atrial fibrillation or flutter	Photosensitivity Nightglare Metallic taste Nightmares	Possible reduced exercise capacity
Flecainide (Tambocor)	Ventricular tachycardia	Dizziness Visual disturbances	

titioner and/or cardiologist. Home activity and exercise goals should be adjusted appropriately and they should be reviewed by rehabilitation staff before re-commencing the gym session.

Safe delivery of exercise also depends on:

- staff with appropriate skills and training – to lead and supervise exercise
- appropriate staff:patient ratio – to ensure safe monitoring/management of patients (recommended ratio 1:5; inclusion of higher risk patients would require a higher ratio)
- monitoring of patient HR/BP, symptoms, pacing and coordination during exercise;

surveillance of patients in immediate post-exercise period (for up to 30 minutes)
- all staff competent and regularly updated in basic life support and preferably one professional with advanced life support training
- local policy for emergency situation, e.g. cardiac arrest, access to staff/emergency equipment, regular practice of emergency drill
- induction and education of each patient, i.e. aims of programme, circuit design/use of equipment, safety/self-monitoring/pacing of exercise, exercise goals, home exercise/activity log book

- equipment maintenance and suitable venue – adequate space, temperature (65–72°F, 18–22°C), ventilation, humidity (65%).

There is a perception that exercise training for cardiac patients is dangerous but if the above safety issues are implemented, available data suggest that cardiac rehabilitation programmes result in very few complications and the incidence of death is one per 1.3 million exercise hours (Van Camp & Peterson 1986).

The FITT principles for Phase III and particular considerations for CHD patients are well covered in a number of specialist texts but may be summarized as follows.

- Frequency   1–2 times per week at a rehabilitation class and 1–2 times per week home exercise circuit Other days at home: walk/leisure activities
- Intensity   60–75% maximal HR (calculated from an exercise ECG or derived from an agreed formula) 12–13 RPE (Borg scale) or 3–4 RPE (Borg CR10 scale) 40–60% of $\dot{V}O_2$peak
- Time   20–30 minutes conditioning period exclusive of warm-up (15–20 minutes) and cool-down (10 minutes)
- Type   Aerobic/endurance training involving large muscle groups in dynamic movement.

When applying these FITT principles to cardiac patients close attention should be paid to the following points to ensure safe and effective training.

- Extended warm-up of 15–20 minutes reduces the potential for ischaemia and arrhythmias; aim for intensity within 20 bpm of training HR zone (adjust if beta-blocker medication/blunted HR response).
- Extended cool-down of 10 minutes reduces post-exercise hypotension and arrhythmias arising from elevated sympathetic activity.

- Increase frequency and duration of exercise before intensity.
- Ensure moderate intensity workload to reduce risk of arrhythmias.
- If combining cardiovascular activities and muscle strength endurance work in a multiple-station circuit training approach:
  - progress intensity by increasing: duration of circuit/stations; speed/range of movement; resistance; or by decreasing recovery/rest intervals between exercises
  - caution with strength training (low resistance/high repetitions)
  - avoid Valsalva manoeuvres
  - avoid abrupt posture shifts, e.g. upright work to recumbent position and recumbent to upright
  - avoid excessive use of arm/upper body exercise relative to leg work as armwork (at a given workload) results in a higher systolic and diastolic BP than when the same work is performed by a larger muscle mass such as the legs.
- Observe for 30 minutes post-exercise.

The Phase III exercise instructor must also be aware that many of the patients joining the exercise class may be fearful, anxious, cavalier or aggressive in response to the situation. Many will be alarmed and daunted at the prospect of taking part in a formal exercise class, perhaps for the first time in their lives. The importance of creating a safe, welcoming, supportive, positive, non-intimidating environment to encourage patients (and perhaps their partners) to participate in an enjoyable and effective exercise session cannot be overemphasized. The skill of the instructor is to combine the science of exercise prescription with the art of persuading and engaging patients through Phase III and into a long-term commitment to an active lifestyle to achieve the optimum secondary prevention. Ensure patients and their families have a good understanding of how the body works and responds to exercise by including educational issues such as:

- listen to your body – signs and symptoms of exertion
- warm-up and cool-down advice

- caution with isometric activities
- relative haemodynamic responses to armwork versus legwork
- environmental issues, e.g. heat/dehydration; cold/circulation constriction
- avoiding exercise after a heavy meal, i.e. potential cardiovascular stress due to the conflicting demands of additional circulation directed to digestive system and exercising muscles
- avoiding exercise with systemic illness and when fatigued.

Special considerations

Chronic heart failure. In patients with chronic heart failure (CHF), activity levels are limited by breathlessness and muscle fatigue. In the past, heart failure was considered an absolute contraindication to participation in the exercise component of cardiac rehabilitation but current recommendations exclude only decompensated patients. BACR guidelines (BACR 1995) recommend that the patient must be comfortable at rest and be able to exercise for 5 minutes at twice their resting energy expenditure (2 METs). A left ventricular ejection fraction of 20% or less is compatible with participation and patients can usefully take part when on a cardiac transplantation list as long as they are stable.

In heart failure patients, the benefits conferred by exercise training are thought to be predominantly due to peripheral adaptations and only a few studies have found changes in cardiac output. Benefits demonstrated include:

- increased exercise duration
- increased peak oxygen uptake
- decreased resting heart rate
- decreased heart rate at reference submaximal workloads
- delayed onset of anaerobic metabolism
- decreased breathlessness.

It has been suggested that patients with ischaemic CHF show less improvement in oxygen uptake than those with idiopathic dilated cardiomyopathy and further evaluation is needed to determine optimal training regimens and to investigate the influence of different aetiologies. In the meantime current exercise recommendations, based on AACVPR Guidelines (1999), are similar to those for other cardiac patients and include:

- education of patients: about recognition of signs and symptoms, e.g. extreme fatigue, weakness, shortness of breath, dyspnoea on exertion, orthopnoea, oedema and weight gain. Extended warm-up and cool-down are essential
- interval training: 1–6 minutes of activity at 40–60% of functional capacity or 11–13 RPE followed by rest
- light resistance training
- progression: should be achieved by increasing duration before intensity
- weight bearing: to improve ability to perform activities of daily living
- monitoring exercising blood pressure: a drop or failure to rise can be an indication of impending failure
- use of dyspnoea scales as well as RPE
- rigorous monitoring: patients are at high risk for ventricular arrhythmias.

Considerations for prescribing exercise for special groups within the CHD population are summarized in Table 15.6.

Transition of patients to long-term community-based exercise provision

Three criteria have been specified by the Massachusetts Association for Cardiovascular and Pulmonary Rehabilitation (BACR 1995) as goals in order to achieve transfer from Phase III to Phase IV. These are useful general objectives by which to assess CHD patients and determine whether they should indeed progress from the closely supervised environment of Phase III into a Phase IV programme.

- Significant improvement in functional capacity.
- Psychological adaptation to chronic disease.
- The foundation of behavioural and lifestyle changes required for continued risk factor modification.

Table 15.6 Considerations for prescribing exercise for special groups within the CHD population

	Management	Precautions/safety
Diabetes	• Diabetes must be stable • Monitor blood sugar before and after exercise • When new to exercise stay with other people in case of adverse incidents • Autonomic neuropathy may alter HR or BP responses • Peripheral neuropathy may cause sensory loss, impaired balance and coordination • Footwear and foot care are important as healing is slow	• Insulin may need to be reduced on exercise days • Insulin uptake may be increased if injected into exercising limb • Carry medical information about condition • Have rapid acting glucose source available • Late evening exercise is inadvisable • 'Silent' ischaemia is more common in diabetics than in non-diabetics
Hypertension	• Classification for clinical intervention: For those not at high risk of CHD: SBP >160 mmHg, DBP >90 mmHg Individuals with CHD/CVD: SBP >140 mmHg, DBP >85 mmHg Individuals with diabetes: SBP >130 mmHg, DBP >80 mmHg • Use FITT principles but adopt lower end of range of training intensity • Adopt lower resistance/higher repetitions for resistance work	• Contraindication to exercise in CHD & CVD patients – SBP >180 mmHg, DBP >100 mmHg • Medication may lead to hypotension – ensure extended active recovery post-exercise with feet constantly moving to aid venous return • Avoid Valsalva manoeuvre • Avoid high-intensity armwork and overgripping of equipment, e.g. cycle handlebars
Peripheral vascular disease	• Promote daily walking and other weight-bearing exercise • Increase duration before intensity • Interval work may be better tolerated than continuous • Non-weight bearing exercise, e.g. cycling can be used to ensure adequate CV dose when pain is severe and will improve compliance	• Cold weather leading to vasoconstriction may exacerbate problem – encourage warm-up, e.g. slow walking gradually increasing to normal pace • Reassure/support patient to exercise through discomfort and teach PVD scale of discomfort • PVD sufferers are more at risk of CHD – monitor for angina
Ageing population	• FITT principles apply for CV training but at lower end of 60–75% HRmax until ability is established • Extended gradual warm-up and cool-down is required • Promote strength work for major muscle groups: 2–3 of 8–12 repetitions at 40–60% of 1 repetition max. × 2 per week • Include flexibilty and general mobility work within the programme	• Avoid exercise in extremes of temperature • Consider hydration especially if diuretics have been prescribed • Avoid using a partner for support or in resistance work • Instructions must be especially clear/precise/unhurried and should be enhanced by good visual demonstration • Avoid exercises which will aggravate urinary incontinence

Abbreviations: HR, heart rate; BP, blood pressure; CHD, coronary heart disease; CVD, cardiovascular disease; SBP, systolic blood pressure; DBP, diastolic blood pressure; PVD, peripheral vascular disease; CV, cardiovascular

More specific objectives may be related to the level of risk stratification and may include the patient demonstrating the ability to:

- exercise safely and effectively, according to an individual exercise prescription
- monitor own heart rate or use scale of perceived exertion effectively
- recognize warning signs and symptoms and take appropriate action (e.g. stop/reduce exercise level, take glyceryl trinitrate)

- identify specific goals for long-term maintenance of lifestyle change and risk factor reduction, relating to own personal history
- ability to identify goals relating to psychological interventions and plan necessary support.

Rehabilitation staff must be satisfied that the patient meets these criteria before discharge to the care of general practitioner and Phase IV instructor; in particular that the patient should be medically and psychologically stable and adjusted to the cardiac event. A functional capacity of approximately 5 METs, i.e. equivalent to a walking speed of about 4 mph, is recommended as the basis for Phase IV exercise prescription.

In the period following assessment the cardiac rehabilitation team should negotiate a long-term management plan with the patient. Issues may include the following.

- Who will monitor risk factors (i.e. smoking, blood pressure, cholesterol and diabetes) – their general practitioner, the practice nurse, the hospital?
- Would regular follow-up be required, e.g. annually? Patients with signs of residual ischaemia should have a treadmill test every 1–3 years.
- Further assessment may be required in patients with signs of residual ischaemia, e.g. treadmill tests. Some 'stable' patients may be on a routine angiogram waiting list. Results of the investigation and possible implications for management and exercise prescription should be reported.

- Where does the patient (and hopefully his/her partner) plan to exercise regularly and how will they keep the momentum going? Fifty percent of patients are likely to drop out of any exercise programme after 6 months (Dishman 1988). This is an important issue.
- Does the patient wish to join a local coronary support club?

A discharge communication with the patient's general practitioner summarizing achievements and future plans regarding follow-up should be written before the patient moves on to Phase IV. Either a similar version of this discharge summary or the recommended BACR Information Sheet, for transition between Phases III and IV, should be completed and given to the patient so that he/she may take this information to the proposed Phase IV instructor.

CONCLUSION

Cardiac rehabilitation is beneficial for many patients but, as with all interventions, it needs to be offered to patients who would benefit and its effectiveness needs to be reassessed with changes in management.

REFERENCES

AACVPR 1999 Guidelines for cardiac rehabilitation and secondary prevention programs, 3rd edn. Human Kinetics, Champaign, Illinois
Adams KJ, Barnard KL, Swank AM, Mann E, Kushnick MR, Denny DM 1999 Combined high-intensity strength and aerobic training in diverse phase II cardiac rehabilitation cardiac patients. Journal of Cardiopulmonary Rehabilitation 19: 209–215
Ades PA 1999 Cardiac rehabilitation in older coronary patients. Journal of the American Geriatrics Society 47: 98–105
Ades PA, Pashkow FJ, Nestor JR 1997 Cost-effectiveness of cardiac rehabilitation after MI. Journal of Cardiopulmonary Rehabilitation 17: 222–231
Ades PA, Pashkow FJ, Fletcher G, Pina IL, Zohman LR, Nestor JR 2000 A controlled trial of cardiac rehabilitation in the home setting using electrocardiographic and voice transtelephonic monitoring. American Heart Journal 139: 535–548
American College of Sports Medicine 1994 Position stand – exercise for patients with coronary artery disease. Medicine in Science and Sports Exercise 26: 1–4
BACR 1995 Guidelines for cardiac rehabilitation Blackwell Science, Oxford

BACR 2000 Phase IV exercise instructor manual, 2nd edn. British Association for Cardiac Rehabilitation, London
Balady GJ, Fletcher BJ, Froelicher ES et al 1994 Cardiac rehabilitation programs. A statement for healthcare professionals from the American Heart Association. Circulation 90: 1602–1610
Bar FW, Hoppener P, Diederiks J et al 1992 Cardiac rehabilitation contributes to the restoration of leisure and social activities after myocardial infarction. Journal of Cardiopulmonary Rehabilitation 12: 117–125
Belardinelli R, Georgiou D, Cianci G, Purcaro A 1999 Randomized, controlled trial of long-term moderate exercise training in chronic heart failure: effects on functional capacity, quality of life and clinical outcomes. Circulation 99: 1173–1182
Bell J 2001 Delivering an exercise prescription for patients with coronary artery disease. In: Young A, Harries M (eds) Physical activity for patients: an exercise prescription. Royal College of Physicians, London
Beniamini Y, Rubenstein JJ, Faigenbaum AD, Lichtenstein AH, Crim MC 1999 High-intensity strength training of patients enrolled in an outpatient cardiac rehabilitation program. Journal of Cardiopulmonary Rehabilitation 19: 8–17

Blumenthal JA, Rejeski WJ, Walsh-Riddle M et al 1988 Comparison of high and low-intensity exercise training early after acute myocardial infarction. American Journal of Cardiology 61: 26–30

Borg GA 1982 Psychophysical bases of perceived exertion. Medicine and Science in Sports and Exercise 14: 276–280

Brubaker PH, Rejeski WJ, Smith MJ, Sevensky KH, Lamb KA, Sotile WM 2000 A home-based maintenance exercise program after centre-based cardiac rehabilitation: effects on blood lipids, body composition and functional capacity. Journal of Cardiopulmonary Rehabilitation 20: 50–56

Bruce RA 1973 Principles in exercise testing. In: Naughton JP, Heuerstein HK (eds) Exercise testing and exercise training in coronary heart disease. Academic Press, New York

Burgess AW, Lerner DJ, D'Agostino RB, Vokonas PS, Hartman CR, Gaccione P 1987 A randomised controlled trial of cardiac rehabilitation. Social Science and Medicine 24: 359–370

Cannistra LB, Davidoff R, Picard MH, Balady GJ 1999 Moderate-high intensity exercise training after myocardial infarction: effect on left ventricular remodeling. Journal of Cardiopulmonary Rehabilitation 19: 373–380

Certo CM 1985 History of cardiac rehabilitation. Physical Therapy 65: 1793–1795

Chua TP, Lipkin DP 1993 Cardiac rehabilitation should be available to all who would benefit. British Medical Journal 306: 731–732

Coats AJ 1999 Exercise training for heart failure: coming of age. Circulation 99: 1138–1140

Coats AJ, Adamopoulos S, Radaelli A et al 1992 Controlled trial of physical training in chronic heart failure: exercise performance, haemodynamics, ventilation and autonomic function. Circulation 85: 2119–2131

CSP 1999 Standards for the exercise component of Phase III cardiac rehabilitation. Chartered Society of Physiotherapy, London

Dafoe W, Huston P 1997 Current trends in cardiac rehabilitation. Canadian Medical Association Journal 156: 527–532

DeBusk RF 1992 Why is cardiac rehabilitation not widely used? Western Journal of Medicine 156: 206–208

DeBusk RF, Haskell WL, Miller NH et al 1985 Medically directed at-home rehabilitation soon after clinically uncomplicated acute myocardial infarction: a new model for patient care. American Journal of Cardiology 55: 251–257

Detry JM, Rousseau M, Vandenbroucke G, Kusumi F, Brasseur LA, Bruce RA 1971 Increased arteriovenous oxygen difference after physical training in coronary heart disease. Circulation 44: 109–118

Dishman RH (ed) 1998 Exercise adherence: its impact on public health. Human Kinetics, Champaign, Illinois

DuBach P, Myers J, Dziekan G et al 1997 Effect of exercise training on myocardial remodeling in patients with reduced left ventricular function after myocardial infarction. Circulation 95: 2060–2067

Dugmore LD, Tipson RJ, Phillips MH et al 1999 Changes in cardiorespiratory fitness, psychological wellbeing, quality of life, and vocational status following a 12 month cardiac exercise rehabilitation programme. Heart 81: 359–366

Dusseldorp E, Van Eldren T, Maes S, Mealman J, Kraaij V 1999 A meta-analysis of psychoeducational programs for coronary heart disease patients. Health Psychology 18: 506–519

Dziekan G, Myers J, Goebbels U et al 1998 Effects of exercise training on limb blood flow in patients with reduced ventricular function. American Heart Journal 136: 22–30

Ehsani AA, Biello DR, Schultz J, Sobel BE, Holloszy JO 1986 Improvement of left ventricular contractile function in patients with coronary artery disease. Circulation 74: 350–388

Fitzpatrick R, Fletcher A, Gore S, Jones D, Spiegelhalter D, Cox D 1992 Quality of life measures in health care: applications and issues in assessment. British Medical Journal 305: 1074–1077

Franklin BA, Gordon S, Timmis GC 1992 Amount of exercise necessary for the patient with coronary artery disease. American Journal of Cardiology 69: 1426–1432

Giannuzzi I, Tavazzi L, Temporelli PL et al for EAMI 1993 Long term physical training and left ventricular remodeling after anterior myocardial infarction: results of the Exercise in Anterior MI (EAMI) trial. Journal of the American College of Cardiology 22: 1821–1829

Goble AJ, Hare DL, MacDonald PS, Oliver RG, Reid MA, Worcester MC 1991 Effect of early programmes of high and low intensity exercise on physical performance after transmural acute myocardial infarction. British Heart Journal 65: 126–131

Gohlke H, Gohlke-Barwolf C 1998 Cardiac rehabilitation. European Heart Journal 19: 1004–1010

Gordon NF, Haskell WL 1997 Comprehensive cardiovascular disease risk reduction in a cardiac rehabilitation setting. American Journal of Cardiology 80 (8B): 69H–73H

Gorkin L, Norvell NK, Rosen RL et al 1993 Assessment of quality of life as observed from the baseline data of the Studies of Left Ventricular Dysfunction (SOLVD) trial quality-of-life substudy. American Journal of Cardiology 71: 1069–1073

Hambrecht R, Niebauer J, Marburger C et al 1994 Various intensities of leisure time physical activity in patients with coronary athersclotic lesions. Journal of Cardiopulmonary Rehabilitation 14: 167–168

Hambrecht R, Gielen S, Linke A et al 2000 Effects of exercise training on left ventricular function and peripheral resistance in patients with chronic heart failure. Journal of the American Medical Association 23: 3095–3101

Haskell WL 1994a The efficacy and safety of exercise programs in cardiac rehabilitation. Medicine and Science in Sports and Exercise 26: 815–823

Haskell WL 1994b Health consequences of physical activity: understanding and challenges regarding dose-response. Medicine and Science in Sports and Exercise 26: 649–660

Jolliffe JA, Taylor R 1998 Physical activity and cardiac rehabilitation: a critical view of the literature. Coronary Health Care 2: 179–186

Jolliffe JA, Rees K, Taylor RS, Thompson D, Oldridge N, Ebrahim S 2000a Exercise-based rehabilitation for coronary heart disease (Cochrane review). In: The Cochrane Library, Issue 4. Update Software, Oxford

Jolliffe J, Taylor R, Ebrahim S 2000b A report on the clinical and cost effectiveness of physiotherapy in cardiac rehabilitation. Chartered Society of Physiotherapy, London

Joughin HM, Digenio AG, Daly L, Kgare E 1999 Physiological benefits of a prolonged moderate-intensity endurance training programme in patients with coronary artery disease. South African Medical Journal 89: 545–550

Jugdutt BI, Michorowski BL, Kappagoda CT 1988 Exercise training after anterior Q wave myocardial infarction: importance of regional left ventricular function and topography. Journal of the American College of Cardiology 12: 362–372

Keteyian SJ, Levine AB, Brawner CA et al 1996 Exercise training in patients with heart failure. A randomized, controlled trial. Annals of Internal Medicine 124: 1051–1057

Kloner RA, Kloner JA 1983 The effect of early exercise on myocardial infarct scar formation. American Heart Journal 106 (5, partt 1): 1009–1013

Langosch W 1988 Psychological effects of training in coronary patients: a critical review of the literature. European Heart Journal 9 (suppl M) (10): 37–42

Lavie CJ, Milani RV 1997 Benefits of cardiac rehabilitation and exercise training in elderly women. American Journal of Cardiology 79: 664–666

Lewin B, Robertson IH, Cay EL, Irving JB 1992 Effects of self-help post-myocardial infarction rehabilitation on psychological adjustment and use of health services. Lancet 339: 1036–1040

Linden W, Stossel C, Maurice J 1996 Psychosocial interventions for patients with coronary artery disease: a meta-analysis. Archives of Internal Medicine 156: 745–752

Lindsay C, Jennrich JA, Biemolt M 1991 Programmed instruction booklet for cardiac rehabilitation teaching. Heart and Lung 20: 648–653

Linxue L, Nohara R, Makita S et al 1999 Effect of long-term exercise training on regional myocardial perfusion changes in patients with coronary artery disease. Japanese Circulation Journal 63: 73–78

Mayou R, Bryant B 1993 Quality of life in cardiovascular disease. British Heart Journal 69: 460–466

McCartney N 1998 Role of resistance training in heart disease. Medicine and Science in Sports and Exercise 30 (suppl 10): S396–402

McGee HM 1999 Psychosocial issues for cardiac rehabilitation with older individuals. Coronary Artery Disease 10: 47–51

McGee HM, Hevey D, Horgan JH 1999 Psychosocial outcome assessments for use in cardiac rehabilitation service evaluation: a 10-year systematic review. Social Science and Medicine 48: 1373–1393

McKelvie RS, Teo KK, McCartney N, Humen D, Montague T, Yusuf S 1995 Effects of exercise training in patients with congestive heart failure: a critical review. Journal of the American College of Cardiology 25: 789–796

Meyer K, Schwaibold M, Westbrook P et al 1996 Effects of short term exercise training and activity restriction on functional capacity in patients with severe chronic congestive heart failure. American Journal of Cardiology 78: 1017–1022

Morrin L, Black S, Reid R 2000 Impact of duration in a cardiac rehabilitation programme on coronary risk profile and health related quality of life outcomes. Journal of Cardiopulmonary Rehabilitation 20: 115–121

Myers J, Goebbels U, Dzeikan G et al 2000 Exercise training and myocardial remodeling in patients with reduced ventricular function: one-year follow-up with magnetic resonance imaging. American Heart Journal 139: 252–261

NHS Centre for Reviews and Dissemination 1998 Effective healthcare bulletin: cardiac rehabilitation. University of York

National Service Framework 2000 Coronary Heart Disease. Modern Standards and Service Models. http://www.doh.gov.uk/nsf/coronary.htm

Ni H, Toy W, Burgess D, Wise K, Nauman DJ, Crispell K, Hershberger RE 2000 Comparative responsiveness of Short-form 12 and Minnesota Living with Heart Failure Questionnaire in patients with heart failure. Journal of Cardiac Failure 6: 83–91

Niebauer J, Hambrecht R, Valich T et al 1997 Attenuated progression of coronary artery disease after 6 years of multifactoral risk intervention. Circulation 96: 2534–2541

Nieuwland W, Berkhuysen MA, Van Veldhuisen DJ et al 2000 Differential effects of high-frequency versus low-frequency exercise training in rehabilitation of patients with coronary artery disease. Journal of the American College of Cardiology, 36: 202–207

O'Connor GT, Buring JE, Yusuf S et al 1989 An overview of randomised trials of rehabilitation with exercise after myocardial infarction. Circulation 80: 234–244

Oldridge NB 1998 Comprehensive cardiac rehabilitation: is it cost-effective? European Heart Journal 19 (suppl O: 42–50

Oldridge NB, Guyatt GH, Fischer ME, Rimm AA 1988 Cardiac rehabilitation after myocardial infarction. Combined experience of randomized clinical trials. Journal of the American Medical Association 260: 945–950

Oldridge NB, Guyatt GH, Jones N et al 1991 Effects on quality of life with comprehensive rehabilitation after acute myocardial infarction. American Journal of Cardiology 67: 1084–1089

Ott CR, Sivarajan ES, Newton KM, Almes MJ, Bruce RA, Bergner M, Gilson BS 1983 A controlled randomised study of early cardiac rehabilitation: the Sickness Impact Profile as an assessment tool. Heart and Lung 12: 162–170

Paterson DH, Shepherd RJ, Cunningham D, Jones NL, Andrew G 1979 Effects of physical training on cardiovascular function following myocardial infarction. Journal of Applied Physiology 47: 482–489

Rousseau MF, Degre S, Messin R, Brasseur LA, Denolin H, Detry J-MR 1974 Haemodynamic effects of early physical training after acute myocardial infarction: comparison with a control untrained group. European Journal of Cardiology 2: 39–45

Schuler G, Hambrecht R, Schlierf G et al 1992 Regular physical exercise and low-fat diet. Effects on progression of coronary artery disease. Circulation 86: 1–11

Shepherd RJ, Kavanagh T, Mertens DJ 1998 On the prediction of physiological and psychological responses to aerobic training in patients with stable congestive heart failure. Journal of Cardiopulmonary Rehabilitation 18: 45–51

Sivarajan ES, Newton KM, Almes MJ, Kempe TM, Mansfield LW, Bruce RA 1983 Limited effects of out-patient teaching and counselling after myocardial infarction: a controlled study. Heart and Lung 12: 65–73

Smith HJ, Taylor R, Mitchell A 2000 A comparison of four quality of life instruments in cardiac patients: SF-36, QLI, QLMI and SEIQoL. Heart 84: 390–394

Sparks KE, Shaw DK, Eddy D, Hanigosky P, Vantrese J 1993 Alternatives for cardiac rehabilitation patients unable to return to a hospital-based program. Heart and Lung 22: 298–303

Squires RW 1998 Exercise prescription for the high-risk cardiac patient. Human Kinetics, Champaign, Illunois, p 37

Squires RW, Muri AJ, Anderson LJ, Allison TG, Miller TD, Gau GT 1991 Weight training during phase II (early outpatient) cardiac rehabilitation: heart rate and blood pressure responses. Journal of Cardiac Rehabilitation 11: 360–364

Stahle A, Mattsson E, Ryden L, Unden A, Nordlander R 1999 Improved physical fitness and quality of life following training of elderly patients after acute coronary events. A 1 year follow-up randomized controlled study. European Heart Journal 20: 1475–1484

Stern MJ, Gorman PA, Kaslow L 1983 The group counselling v exercise therapy study. A controlled intervention with subjects following myocardial infarction. Archives of Internal Medicine 143: 1719–1725

Taylor AE 1997 Cardiac rehabilitation – do exercise programmes make a difference? Journal of Coronary Health Care 1: 193–199

Taylor AE 1999 The effects of exercise training on patients with chronic heart failure. Physical Therapy Review 4: 195–202

Taylor R, Kirby BJK 1997 The evidence base for the cost effectiveness of cardiac rehabilitation. Heart 78: 5–6

Taylor R, Kirby B, Burdon D, Caves R 1998 The assessment of recovery in patients after myocardial infarction using three generic quality-of-life measures. Journal of Cardiopulmonary Rehabilitation 18: 139–144

Thompson DR, De Bono DP 1999 How valuable is cardiac rehabilitation and who should get it? Heart, 82: 545–546

Thompson DR, Bowman GS, De Bono DP, Hopkins A 1997 Cardiac rehabilitation: guidelines and audit standards. Royal College of Physicians, London

Thompson PD 1988 The benefits and risks of exercise training in patients with chronic coronary artery disease. Journal of the American Medical Association 259: 1537–1540

Van Camp SP, Peterson RA 1986 Cardiovascular complications of outpatient cardiac rehabilitation programmes. Journal of the American Medical Association 256: 1160–1163

van Dixhoorn JJ, Duivenvoorden HJ 1999 Effect of relaxation therapy on cardiac events after myocardial infarction: a 5-year follow-up study. Journal of Cardiopulmonary Rehabilitation 19: 178–185

van Dixhoorn JJ, Duivenvoorden HJ, Pool J 1990 Success and failure of exercise training after myocardial infarction: is the outcome predictable? Journal of the American College of Cardiology 15: 974–982

Verges BL, Patois-Verges B, Cohen M, Casillas JM 1998 Comprehensive cardiac rehabilitation improves the control of dyslipidemia in secondary prevention. Journal of Cardiopulmonary Rehabilitation 18: 408–415

Ware JE, Kosinski M, Keller SD 1994 SF-36 physical and mental health summary scales: a user manual. The Health Institute, New England Medical Center, Boston, Massachusetts

West R 1995 Evaluation of rehabilitation programmes. In: Jones D, West R (eds) Cardiac rehabilitation. BMJ Books, London, pp 192–194

Wielenga RP, Coats AJS, Willem WL, Huisveld IA 1997 The role of exercise training in chronic heart failure. Heart 78: 431–436

Wiklund I, Welin C 1992 A comparison of different psychological questionnaires in patients with myocardial infarction. Scandinavian Journal of Rehabilitation Medicine 24: 195–202

Williams MA 1994 Exercise testing and training in the elderly cardiac patient. Current issues in cardiac rehabilitation series. Human Kinetics, Champaign, Illinois

Willich SN, Lewis M, Lowel H, Arntz JR, Schubert F, Schroder R 1993 Physical exertion as a trigger of acute myocardial infarction. New England Journal of Medicine 329: 1684–1690

Worcester MC, Hare DL, Oliver RG, Reid MA, Goble AJ 1993 Early programmes of high and low intensity exercise and quality of life after acute myocardial infarction. British Medical Journal 307: 1244–1247

Yokoyama H, Sato H, Hori M Takeda H, Kamada T 1994 A characteristic change in ventilation mode during exertional dyspnea in patients with chronic heart failure. Chest 106: 1007–1013

16

Cardiopulmonary transplantation

Catherine E Bray

INTRODUCTION

Cardiopulmonary transplantation is now a recognized treatment for end-stage cardiac and pulmonary disease in adults and paediatrics. The first human adult cardiac transplant was performed in 1967 by Dr Christian Barnard, although work on this procedure had started much earlier. Paediatric transplantation was first carried out in 1967 by Kantrowitz but it was not until December 1980 that it was felt to be a therapeutic option.

This may be a reflection of the disappointment following the initial enthusiasm about transplant surgery, mainly due to problems associated with acute rejection. It was not until the advent of cyclosporin A in 1980 (Borel 1980) as the principal immunosuppressant that cardiopulmonary transplant became an accepted therapeutic option. This new therapy then saw the first long-term survivors of heart – lung (Reitz 1982), single lung (Cooper et al 1987) and double lung (Patterson et al 1988) transplantation.

With a more stable immunosuppressant regimen of cyclosporin, azathioprine and prednisolone in place, over 300 centres worldwide took up cardiopulmonary transplantation. Through to 1999 more than 69 000 thoracic organs have been transplanted (Hosenpud et al 2000).

In children cardiac transplantation is undertaken when the heart is in terminal failure and no other treatment options are available (e.g. end-stage acquired or viral myopathy). Outcome is worst in patients who are transplanted at less than 1 year of age, with a 3-year survival of 60%.

In children over 6 years of age, 3-year survival exceeds 70% (Hosenpud et al 1996). Coronary artery disease is not uncommon as a result of chronic immunosuppression. More children require lung or heart-lung transplantation than cardiac transplantation alone. However, fewer donors are available with lungs suitable for transplantation. Most children (two-thirds) requiring lung or heart – lung transplantation have cystic fibrosis (CF) (and usually the choice of procedure is limited by the availability of donor organs). Other indications include Eisenmenger's complex, fibrosing alveolitis and interstitial pneumonitis. The 5-year survival for this group of patients is below 50% (Hosenpud et al 1996). Outcome post transplantation for children with CF seems to be similar for both a younger and older age group, with survival at 3 years for children below 10 years of age recently reported as 41% and 46% for older children (Balfour-Lynn et al 1997). The development of obliterative bronchiolitis seems to be the major obstacle to long-term success in this field.

In adults the primary indication for cardiac transplantation today is for the relief of severe symptoms in individuals with severe heart failure (Stevenson 1996). Cardiopulmonary and pulmonary transplantation is increasingly utilized for patients with end-stage pulmonary disease, which may or may not be associated with cor pulmonale. The indications for the various forms of cardiopulmonary transplantation are outlined in Table 16.1. Survival following heart transplant is 81% at 1 year and 37% at 12 years and heart-lung transplant is 63% at 1 year and 23% at 12 years. The 5-year survival for adult recipients is as follows: heart 65%, heart-lung 40%, single lung 45% and double lung 50% (Hosenpud et al 2000).

ASSESSMENT

The assessment of potential recipients is usually carried out by a multidisciplinary team. This process involves both a clinical and psychological assessment, which includes:

- severity of cardiac and/or pulmonary dysfunction
- identification of contraindications
- immunological status (ABO group, human leucocyte antigen (HLA)), tissue typing (usually retrospectively)
- previous exposure to potentially complicating infection: cytomegalovirus (CMV), toxoplasmosis, hepatitis B, hepatitis C, methicillin-resistant Staphylococcus aureus (MRSA), Epstein–Barr virus (EBV) and HIV
- nutritional status
- psychological status (Keogh et al 1991).

Once accepted for the active waiting list (Table 16.2), transplantation can occur at any time. Timing to transplant is variable, with more hearts being available than lungs. Potential recipients are reviewed regularly.

Table 16.1 Indications for cardiopulmonary transplantation

Heart transplantation	Heart-lung transplantation	Single lung transplantation	Double/bilateral sequential single lung transplantation
End-stage heart failure as a result of: • post-viral cardiomyopathy • ischaemic cardiomyopathy • idiopathic cardiomyopathy Disabling angina with inoperable coronary artery disease	Pulmonary vascular disease, e.g. primary pulmonary hypertension Eisenmenger's syndrome pulmonary parenchymal disease (with non-reversible cardiac dysfunction), e.g. bronchiectasis, cystic fibrosis, sarcoidosis, fibrosing alveolitis, chronic airflow limitation	End stage fibrotic lung disease, e.g. pulmonary fibrosis, occupational lung disease, sarcoidosis, chronic airflow limitation	An alternative to heart-lung transplantation for patients with satisfactory right ventricular function and bilateral pulmonary sepsis, e.g. bronchiectasis, cystic fibrosis, chronic airflow limitation

Table 16.2 Contraindications to transplantation (procedure-specific exclusion criteria)

General	Heart	Heart-lung	Single/double/bilateral sequential single lung
Absolute exclusion			
Irreversible renal dysfunction (except in combined heart-kidney transplantation) Irreversible hepatic dysfunction Active malignancy Immunodeficiency Alcohol/drug abuse Morbid obesity	Raised transpulmonary gradient (>15 mmHg) and/or pulmonary vascular resistance (>4 mmHg) (Patients who are excluded may be reconsidered for heterotopic heart or heart-lung transplantation)		Right ventricular ejection fraction <25% (Patients who are excluded may be reconsidered for heart-lung transplantation) Systemic corticosteroids
Relative exclusion			
Active systemic infection Recent pulmonary infarction Insulin-dependent diabetes mellitus Peripheral or cerebrovascular disorders Psychological instability		Systemic corticosteroids (retard healing, especially tracheal or bronchial anastomosis) Previous extensive pleural surgery Malnutrition Immobility Cachexia	Previous extensive pleural surgery Malnutrition Immobility Cachexia

THE TRANSPLANTATION PROCESS

Donors

Potential donors are individuals who have been declared dead for a variety of reasons, the most common being a head injury or injuries sustained from a road traffic accident, which has not compromised the heart and lungs. The donor selection criteria are outlined in Table 16.3.

The basics of donor recipient matching are:

- blood group
- size – donor weight and height
- age
- cause of death
- inotropic requirement
- blood gases in 100% and 30% oxygen for lung transplant
- length of time ventilated
- infection
- past medical history.

Table 16.3 Donor selection criteria

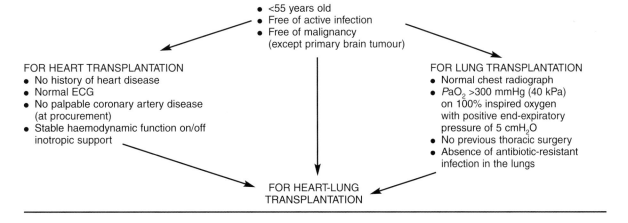

- <55 years old
- Free of active infection
- Free of malignancy (except primary brain tumour)

FOR HEART TRANSPLANTATION
- No history of heart disease
- Normal ECG
- No palpable coronary artery disease (at procurement)
- Stable haemodynamic function on/off inotropic support

FOR LUNG TRANSPLANTATION
- Normal chest radiograph
- PaO_2 >300 mmHg (40 kPa) on 100% inspired oxygen with positive end-expiratory pressure of 5 cmH_2O
- No previous thoracic surgery
- Absence of antibiotic-resistant infection in the lungs

FOR HEART-LUNG TRANSPLANTATION

In paediatrics for patients under 6 months of age, there is a possibility of ABO mismatch. A further problem in paediatric transplant is that of the availability of organs of a suitable size for the recipient.

It is normal practice to seek consent from the next of kin before the donor is referred to the transplant coordinator, who will then offer the organs on to the respective recipient centre. Most donors today are multiorgan donors and this means that many retrieval teams are involved in the retrieval of various organs. The donor will need to be given expert medical and nursing care to maximise its potential as an organ donor. This can place an immense emotional pressure on both the donor family and the staff caring for the donor. For cardiopulmonary retrieval teams, timing of retrieval is important. Most cardiac teams would look for an ischaemic time of under 4 hours, from the time of cross-clamping the aorta to reperfusing the organ. This indicates how important coordinating the retrieval is.

To improve donor availability recipients who receive heart-lung blocks (mainly patients with cystic fibrosis) are asked to donate their hearts to a cardiac patient (the domino procedure). Cardiac patients can sometimes take organs from donors up to three times their body weight, whereas pulmonary donors are matched by donor/recipient weight, height and dimensions of the thoracic cavity.

In the early days of transplantation it was necessary for the donor to be transported to the transplant centre. Today hearts, heart-lung blocks, lungs and other transplantable organs/tissues are utilized via distant procurement and preservation procedures.

Operative procedures

Heart transplantation (HTx)

Orthotopic transplantation. Preparation of the heart (and heart-lung) transplant recipient is similar to that for any patient undergoing cardiac surgery (anaesthesia, median sternotomy and cardiopulmonary bypass). When the donor heart is present in the recipient theatre and has passed

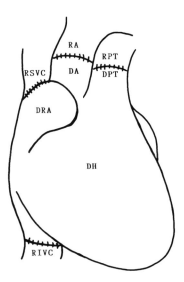

Fig. 16.1 Orthotopic technique: the donor heart following implantation: DH, donor heart; RPT, recipient pulmonary trunk; DPT, donor pulmonary trunk; RA, recipient aorta; DA, donor aorta; RSVC, recipient superior vena cava; DRA, donor right atrium; RIVC, recipient inferior vena cava.

a final inspection, the recipient heart is removed, by incising the atria, pulmonary artery and aorta (leaving the posterior walls of both atria, including the sinoatrial (SA) node). The donor heart is sutured in place, the anastomoses joining recipient and donor atria, the pulmonary arteries and finally the aortas (Keogh et al 1986) (Fig. 16.1).

Heterotopic transplantation. Heterotopic transplantation is a less commonly used procedure than orthotopic transplantation. In this 'piggy-back' procedure the recipient heart is left in place and the donor heart (connected to the recipient's in parallel by anastomoses made between the two hearts at the atria, pulmonary arteries and aortas) is positioned in the right chest. Both hearts contribute to the cardiac output (Weber 1990).

Heart-lung transplantation (HLTx)

The heart and lungs are excised separately, allowing identification and protection of the phrenic, recurrent laryngeal and vagus nerves, a most critical part of the procedure. The heart is removed, leaving the posterior wall of the right atrium. The left and then right lungs are removed

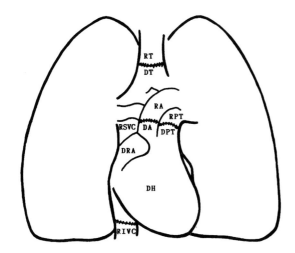

Fig. 16.2   The donor heart-lung block following implantation: DH, donor heart; RPT, recipient pulmonary trunk; DPT, donor pulmonary trunk; RA, recipient aorta; DA, donor aorta; RSVC, recipient superior vena cava; DRA, donor right atrium; RIVC, recipient inferior vena cava; RT, recipient trachea; DT, donor trachea.

(following stapling of the bronchi, to minimize the risk of contaminating the area) and the trachea is divided above the bifurcation. The donor heart-lung block is implanted, starting with the tracheal, then the atrial and aortic anastomoses. Ventilation is established (ensuring the patency of the airway anastomosis) and the heart resuscitated (Jamieson et al 1984) (Fig. 16.2).

Lung transplantation

Single lung transplantation (SLTx). The procedure commences as a lateral thoracotomy. The recipient's lung is removed and the donor lung positioned in the chest. Cuffs on the left atrium of the donor and recipient heart are joined. The pulmonary artery anastomosis is completed and circulation is restored to the lung, allowing for inspection of the arterial and atrial anastomoses. The bronchial anastomosis is performed and ventilation is resumed (Cooper et al 1987, Gaissert & Palterson 1996, Weill et al 1999). Cardiopulmonary bypass is made available for the procedure but is rarely needed.

Double lung transplantation (DLTx)/bilateral sequential single lung transplantation (BSSLTx). The early experiences of DLTx involved the implantation 'en bloc' of both lungs via a median sternotomy, utilizing an omental wrap to secure the tracheal anastomosis (Patterson et al 1988). In an effort to avoid the high incidence of airway complications associated with the original procedure, the technique of BSSLTx via anterolateral, bilateral thoracotomies with transverse sternotomy is now preferred. The procedure of direct revascularization of the bronchial arteries with the internal mammary artery is sometimes used to promote healing (Madden et al 1992). The donor procedure for double lung transplantation allows for the separate excision of the heart, facilitating the utilization of donor organs (Kaiser et al 1991).

Other lung techniques. The scarcity of organs available for transplantation has led to the development of the split-lung technique (Couetil 1996) and living donor lobar lung transplantation (Abecassis et al 2000, Starnes et al 1999). These techniques have been carried out in limited numbers only and raise many recipient-specific issues. Living donor transplantation also raises donor-specific issues, none more important than the risk posed to the two living donors who are needed for each recipient procedure.

Postoperative care

The intensive care area and ward management of the cardiopulmonary transplant patient is similar to that for any patient having undergone cardiac or thoracic surgery. The major differences include drug therapy and the intensive and comprehensive monitoring necessary because of the potential for rejection and infection. The degree and duration of protective isolation of recipients vary considerably between centres. Some units protectively isolate recipients in laminar airflow rooms, while others only require thorough hand washing before contact with the patient (Cooper & Lidsky 1996, Daly & McGregor 1996).

Patients can be discharged from the hospital to home (if within reasonable access to the unit) or to the hospital accommodation as early as 4 days postoperatively. Patients continue to be closely monitored on an outpatient basis, usually for the first 3 months postoperatively. Regular follow-up continues until most patients can be reviewed on a 6–12-monthly basis. All patients are well informed of the signs or symptoms with which they must contact their carer centre.

Rejection of the transplanted organs

The same immune response that protects the body against foreign chemicals and organisms is also responsible for graft (transplanted organ) rejection. The presence of the transplanted organs triggers the immune system to respond; that is, to reject them. Both humoral (B lymphocyte mediated) and cellular (T lymphocyte mediated) immune responses may be involved in graft rejection. Rejection may occur at any time following transplantation, but the risk is greatest in the first 3 months post transplantation (Du Toil et al 1996, Weber 1990).

Acute rejection

Acute rejection occurs within the first 3 months after transplantation. Most recipients can anticipate two or more episodes of this cell-mediated immune response. The patient may be asymptomatic despite a definitive biopsy diagnosis.

In heart recipients it may be associated with malaise, shortness of breath, peripheral oedema, low-grade fever, nausea, vomiting, a voltage drop on ECG and/or an atrial arrhythmia (Keogh et al 1986). Endomyocardial biopsy (using a bioptome, passed down the right internal jugular vein and sampling tissue from the right ventricle) is currently the only objective way to diagnose rejection. Biopsies are performed routinely on a regular basis for the first year following transplantation and then only if indicated symptomatically.

A clinical diagnosis of acute lung rejection is usually made from a combination of findings such as low-grade fever, shortness of breath, increasing infiltrates on chest radiograph, deteriorating gas exchange and lung function, the exclusion of infection and rapid symptomatic improvement with augmented immunosuppression (Lawrence 1990, Tyndall & Cooper 1996) (Fig. 16.3).

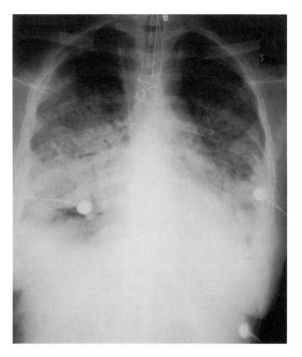

Fig. 16.3 A chest radiograph showing acute pulmonary rejection in a heart-lung recipient.

To establish a diagnosis of lung rejection and to identify infection, transbronchial lung biopsy may be utilized. There are, however, intrinsic difficulties in obtaining adequate tissue samples and performing the procedure on critically ill patients. Transbronchial lung biopsies are carried out on a regular basis and when symptoms necessitate.

Chronic graft dysfunction

Chronic graft dysfunction occurs over months to years. In the transplanted heart it is characterized by diffuse and rapidly progressing coronary artery disease (CAD) manifesting in myocardial infarction, congestive heart failure or sudden cardiac death. CAD is postulated to be the result of chronic undetected rejection. It is a major factor limiting long-term survival and is seen in approximately 40% of patients 5 years following transplant (Squires 1990). Periodic coronary angiography is utilized for the diagnosis and monitoring of this process.

Obliterative bronchiolitis (OB), associated with lung transplantation, involves an inflammatory process in the small airways which leads to the obstruction and destruction of pulmonary bronchioles (Kriett & Jamieson 1996) (Fig. 16.4). It is suggested that OB is the result of 'late' rejection and may be advanced (or even triggered) by respiratory infection. It is one of the major factors influencing long-term survival of heart-lung and lung recipients. Its successful management requires the close monitoring of pulmonary function and aggressive, early immunosuppression augmentation (Theodore et al 1990) as well as aggressive surveillance and treatment of infection.

Immunosuppression

Immunosuppressive therapy is necessary for the rest of the recipient's life. Most maintenance immunosuppressive regimens utilize a combination of two or three drugs. By combining a number of drugs the doses of each can be adjusted to reduce associated side effects (Tyndall & Cooper 1996) (Table 16.4).

Infection

Infection continues to be a complicating and life-threatening feature of transplantation, especially in the first 3 months following the surgery. High-dose immunosuppressive therapy allows for the

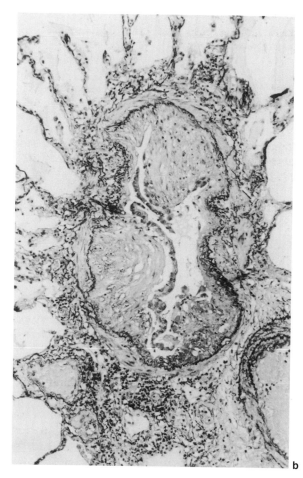

a

b

Fig. 16.4 **a** A normal bronchiole lined by ciliated, columnar epithelium deep to which there is a thin layer of smooth muscle. **b** Obliterative bronchiolitis: nodules of submucosal fibrous tissue have developed, elevating the lining mucosa and substantially occluding the lumen.

Table 16.4 Immunosuppression

Drug	Effect	Side effects
Maintenance immunosuppression		
Cyclosporin (CsA) or cyclosporin-neoral (CsA-neoral)	T cell suppressor, lesser B cell effect CsA together with a surfactant, developed to reduce the erratic absorption of CsA	Nephrotoxicity, hepatic dysfunction, hirsutism, tremor, hypertension, susceptibility to malignant neoplasms
or Tacrolimus (FK506): used as an alternative to CsA for refractory/steroid-resistant rejection or CsA intolerance	Suppresses T-cell mediated immunity, some B cell effect Immunosuppressive activity up to 100 times more potent than CsA	Hypertension, diabetes, nephrotoxicity, increased risk of malignancy, neurotoxicity
with Azathioprine	Decreases the body's ability to generate T cells	Bone marrow suppression, hepatic dysfunction, nausea, anorexia
and Corticosteroid: many centres now attempt to withdraw corticosteroid treatment after the 'acute' rejection risk period	Decreases antibody production and depresses the maturation of T cells	Sodium and fluid retention, hypokalaemia, hyperglycaemia, gastrointestinal ulceration, osteoporosis, skin fragility, increased appetite, mood changes
Anti rejection therapy		
Corticosteroid (methylprednisolone)	Reverses acute rejection as above	As above
Antithymocyte globulin (ATG)	T cell cytolytic (may be used as prevention therapy)	Fever, rigors, neutropenia, 'serum' sickness
OKT3	Blocks generation and function of T cells (T cell cytolytic) For cardiac recipients rather than lung	Acute pulmonary oedema, fever, rigors, headache and tremor
Mycophenolate mofetil	Inhibits T and B cell proliferation by blocking DNA replication Use as an alternative to azathioprine	Diarrhoea, bone marrow suppression, opportunistic infection (especially invasive CMV)
Methotrexate/cyclophosphamide	Cytotoxic to T and B lymphocytes	Bone marrow suppression, hepatic and renal toxicity

growth of opportunistic organisms (Rubin 1994) (Table 16.5).

SPECIAL CONSIDERATIONS FOR THE PHYSIOTHERAPIST

The key to a successful cardiopulmonary transplant programme is a well-informed, communicative, multidisciplinary team. With medical and nursing staff, social worker, pharmacist and dietitian the physiotherapist is vitally involved in the monitoring and education of the recipients, throughout each phase of the transplantation process. To do so effectively, the physiotherapist needs a strong knowledge base, particularly focused on the features of transplantation that will strongly influence the recipient's ability to participate in rehabilitation and, later, to resume employment and leisure activities. Physiotherapy specialization in this field, with continuity of care from assessment to postoperative rehabilitation, offers significant advantages in patient confidence, education and compliance.

Denervation of the heart / lungs

At rest. Most heart and heart-lung block recipients will have a higher than normal resting heart rate: they lack the inhibitory vagal influence. The lungs of heart-lung and lung recipients are denervated distal to the tracheal/bronchial anastomosis. As a result, the recipient's ability to cough spontaneously in response to secretions accumulating distal to the anastomosis is impaired.

Exercise. Denervation of the heart, in particular, has significant implications for the exercising

Table 16.5 Common infections seen in heart or lung transplant recipients

Infection	Common manifestation	Management (infection can be rapid and fatal. Investigation and treatment must be aggressive and expeditious (Chaparro et al 1997))
Bacterial		
Especially postoperative days 0–14 Gram-negative organisms: *Pseudomonas, Klebsiella* and *Haemophilus influenzae* After 2 weeks, as above and Gram-positive organisms: *Staphylococcus aureus*	Respiratory involvement; bronchial and/or lobar pneumonias	Specific antibiotic therapy
CF recipients are frequently colonized with *Pseudomonas* Where there is resistance to antibiotic agents, morbidity is higher		CF recipients with *Burkholderia cepacia* may be excluded from transplant as some units have experience high morbidity and mortality, especially in the early postoperative period
Patients who develop OB are frequently colonized with *P. aeruginosa*		
Viral		
Cytomegalovirus (primary or reactivation infection), especially subacute phase	Systemic, gastrointestinal inclusion/ulceration, penumonitis (especially lung and heart-lung recipients)	Ganciclovir (intravenous twice daily, 10–14 days; prophylaxis, inravenous, 3 times weekly for donor–recipient CMV mismatch)
Herpes (simplex and zoster)	Usual manifestations	Acyclovir
Epstein–Barr virus (primary or reactivation infection)	Lymphoma	Acyclovir
Fungal		
Candida	Oral, oesophageal	Nystatin, fluconazole, amphotericin B
Aspergillus	Respiratory, cerebral	Amphotericin B, itraconazole
Protozoal		
Pneumocystic carinii	Respiratory	Bactrim (treatment and prophylaxis)
Toxoplasma gondii	Systemic	As above
Mycobacterial infections		
Tuberculosis Atypical mycobacteria	As in other immunosuppressed populations, principally respiratory involvement. Limited information on incidence and outcomes	Specific antibiotic treatment, even in the absence of clinical disease

of heart and heart-lung recipients. In the normally innervated heart it is changes in heart rate, not stroke volume, which account for the increase in cardiac output in response to dynamic exercise. There is substantial evidence that the denervated heart also increases its cardiac output in response to exercise. It does so early in the activity by increasing its stroke volume (based on the Frank–Starling mechanism). The heart rate of the recipient rises more gradually than that of a normal individual following the commencement of exercise, does not reach a similar peak and slows more gradually once exercise is stopped. This pattern of heart rate response is primarily the result of changing levels of circulating catecholamines, which play an increasingly important role in increasing cardiac output at high workloads.

It is important to note that, although the transplanted heart does demonstrate compensatory exercise responses, the peak intensity of exercise and the duration of activity may be lower than that of normal individuals. If these limitations are present, it has been suggested that it may be the result of the donor heart having undergone an ischaemic period and reperfusion, myocyte necrosis as a result of acute rejection episodes, undetected or chronic rejection and/or diffuse CAD (Bussieres et al 1995, Horak 1990, Lampert et al 1998, Scott et al 1995, Squires 1990).

Denervation also prevents the transmission of pain from any ischaemic area of myocardium (Weber 1990). Although partial reinnervation occurs in some recipients, the majority of patients will not experience anginal symptoms and should be advised against unsupervised exercise at high intensities for long periods. This is especially important if angiography indicates the presence of CAD (Hosenpud 1999, Kavanagh 1996).

Immunosuppression

It is important that physiotherapists working with transplant recipients are mindful of the effects of immunosuppressive drug therapy, particularly corticosteroids, on the musculoskeletal system. The overall exercise capability of many transplant recipients is limited by peripheral musculoskeletal factors (Kavanagh et al 1988). Drug-related myopathy and prolonged periods of inactivity, pre- and postoperatively, may be responsible for these limitations. Cyclosporin is nephrotoxic and via its vasopressor effect contributes to significant hypertension in the majority of patients (Scott et al 1995).

The contribution of corticosteroids to the process of osteoporosis must also be acknowledged, particularly for those patients whose preoperative management (at any stage) has involved the prolonged use of steroid therapy. Special care when exercising and immediate and thorough investigation of reports of pain (especially back and hip pain) are essential for these patients (Aris et al 1996, Negri et al 1999).

When prescribing exercise and advising patients on resuming sporting activities, both physiotherapist and patient must be mindful of the inhibiting influence of steroid therapy on healing.

Other drug therapies

Hyperlipidaemia is a common problem amongst recipients and has been associated with both steroid and cyclosporin use. Antilipaemic agents such as the statin group (which are frequently utilized in the transplant population) have been associated with myositis which may lead to rhabdomyolysis (Reaven & Witztum 1988). Cyclosporin may induce changes to antilipaemic drug metabolism and add to the risk of myositis in the transplant recipient (Kobashigawa et al 1995).

Infection / rejection

When a recipient is diagnosed as being in severe rejection (and provided that his cardiac rhythm and oxygen saturation are stable) his activity should be limited to walking at a slow, comfortable pace. The rehabilitation programme is recommenced when the antirejection therapy is being reduced and the patient is asymptomatic.

In instances of minimal and moderate rejection or infection, exercise is continued according to the patient's presentation and symptoms. For acute-phase lung and heart-lung recipients it is of paramount importance to monitor oxygen saturation regularly at rest and throughout any exercise activities, even when they report no symptoms, but acute rejection has been confirmed by transbronchial biopsy. Again, monitoring of the patient's heart rate, rhythm and blood pressure is of importance.

PHYSIOTHERAPY MANAGEMENT

Physiotherapy has always played an important part in cardiopulmonary transplantation. The number of centres carrying out these procedures has expanded over recent years and so has the role of the physiotherapist within these units. Physiotherapy is now an integral part of all stages of the patient's management at assessment, preoperatively and at both the acute and rehabilitation phases of postoperative care.

Assessment

All patients referred for formal assessment should be seen by the physiotherapist. The assessment of potential heart transplant recipients focuses on:

- previous and current activity levels, including a measure of exercise tolerance (e.g. 6-minute walk, shuttle test or step test) (Aurora et al 2001, Cahalin 1996, Lipkin et al 1986, Singh et al 1992, Steele 1994).
- musculoskeletal condition such as: muscle bulk and strength (including limb girth strength measures), flexibility and preexisting joint and postural difficulties
- respiratory history and function.

At this interview/assessment the physiotherapist may provide advice on dividing fatiguing activities of daily living (ADL) into more easily managed subtasks and outline a programme of stretches and exercises to maintain/improve mobility, strength and muscle bulk. Previously, heart failure was a contraindication to involvement in a cardiac rehabilitation programme. There is an increasing body of research demonstrating that the negative effects of long-term cardiac failure on skeletal muscle contribute significantly to the poor quality of life experienced by sufferers (Clark et al 1996, Keteyian et al 1997). Appropriately prescribed exercise can have lasting benefits without placing the patient at risk (Coats 1993, Demopoulos et al 1997).

All potential heart-lung and lung transplant recipients accepted for formal assessment are seen by the physiotherapist who assesses the patient's:

- activity/exercise tolerance/oximetry
- muscle range and strength (upper limb, trunk, quadriceps, etc.)
- cervical and thoracic spine posture and mobility
- breathing pattern (at rest and while exercising)

- previous musculoskeletal injuries/current musculoskeletal problems (such as osteoporosis), including sources of acute and chronic pain and their management
- current strategies for maintaining respiratory status such as management of acute shortness of breath and monitoring/clearing airway secretions.

The findings are then reviewed with those of other team members in considering if the patient is an appropriate candidate for transplantation. Patient compliance with both medical management and activity is an important issue for all team members.

Preoperative care

The principal goal for the physiotherapist in the preoperative period is that shared by all the transplant team: to maintain, improve and/or slow the decline of the potential recipient's physical and functional capacity. The preoperative contact is also an opportunity to:

- establish a good rapport between patient and physiotherapist
- provide each potential recipient with a thorough understanding of his role in transplantation
- assist the patient to use his time constructively to improve his quality of life while awaiting transplant.

Children's activity levels are assessed and advice given regarding exercise and the importance of maintaining physical fitness preoperatively. Many adult patients awaiting heart and lung transplants are included in a conditioning rehabilitation programme (CRP). Patients living close to the hospital attend the gymnasium once or twice a week and continue elements of the programme in a home routine. Patients who regularly attend other hospitals for ongoing outpatient treatment should be supervised by their local physiotherapist in a modified form of the conditioning programme. Patients who live beyond the reach of regular hospital attendance should be worked through a home conditioning programme, managed and reviewed at clinic visits.

The CRP involves five treatment/training components:

- patient education
- 'aerobic/endurance' training
- specific muscle strength training
- thoracic mobility techniques
- relaxation and stress management techniques.

Each of the five components specifically addresses one or more previously identified problems and involves a number of techniques (Table 16.6). The patient's heart rate and rhythm, blood pressure, oxygen saturation and rating of perceived exertion are checked before and as indicated, during the gymnasium activities. Supplementary oxygen is used as appropriate.

The ongoing monitoring of all potential recipients is the responsibility of each team member who regularly reviews the patient. Each patient's walk or shuttle test, weight and muscle bulk and strength should be reassessed regularly (every 4–6 weeks would seem to be ideal) and the results recorded and compared over time (Cahalin 1996). If significant deterioration in the potential recipient's functional status and/or physical condition is noted, an intervention strategy involving one or a number of intensive therapies may be employed in an effort to optimize the patient's condition or 'bridge to transplant'. In particular cases of increasing hypercapnic respiratory failure or left ventricular failure, the application of a form of non-invasive ventilation (following diagnostic and prescriptive sleep studies) may be of benefit. CPAP, BIPAP or nasal positive pressure ventilation during rest and sleep periods is frequently utilized in adults pre-transplant to provide ventilatory support, reducing respiratory muscle energy expenditure and ventricular strain, and can result in a reduction of symptoms and some

Table 16.6 A conditioning rehabilitation programme for potential heart-lung and lung recipients

Problem(s) addressed	Management / techniques
Component 1: Patient education	
Poor quality of life while awaiting transplantation	ADL advice
	Alternative strategies for recreational time
	Instruct family in massage and relaxation techniques
Fear of intubation/ventilation	Explanation of surgical and intensive care procedures
	Visit to intensive care unit
	Talk with (selected) recipients
Poor awareness of patterns of breathing	Review of chest anatomy, muscles of breathing, normal and abnormal breathing patterns
	Practice in 'isolating'/focusing on specific muscles and patterns of breathing
Component 2: Endurance training	
Poor endurance	Treadmill and bicycle ergometer programmes (intermittent work/rest periods)
	Home walking programme
Component 3: Specific muscle training	
Muscle weakness	Upper limb/trunk programme
	Abdominal programme
	Quadriceps programme
	Home weight programme
Component 4: Thoracic mobility techniques	
Preoperative musculoskeletal discomfort and postoperative pain	Soft tissue techniques
	Joint mobilization for cervical, thoracic, costal and sternal articulations
Component 5: Relaxation and stress management	
Preoperative respiratory crisis management and postoperative pain management	Relaxation techniques

participation in preoperative rehabilitation (Carrey et al 1990).

Potential recipients' nutritional status must be constantly monitored. Nutritional supplements and easy-to-consume foods are utilized in the care of respiratory failure patients, particularly those with cystic fibrosis. Nocturnal nasogastric or gastrostomy feeding may also be utilized for deteriorating, cachexic patients (Poindexter 1991, Schwartz 1989,).

Patients with a chronic respiratory problem will need to continue an appropriate airway clearance regimen. This should be reviewed regularly and modified as necessary.

Increasingly, ventricular assist devices are being utilized to sustain adult patients awaiting heart transplant. These devices vary considerably with respect to the degree of mobility they afford the patient. Some require the patient to be maintained on complete bedrest whilst others allow the patient to ambulate or be managed on an outpatient basis. The obvious benefit of the ambulatory devices is that they allow the physical condition of the patient to be preserved or improved while waiting for transplant. For some cardiac failure patients (particularly older individuals or those who weigh more than 85 kilograms) left or biventricular assist devices are now utilized as an alternative to transplantation (Frazier 1993, Hill et al 1993).

Postoperative care

Acute care

Following transplant, the team's focus shifts to optimizing function, both of the graft organ and the recipient.

The physiotherapist's role in the acute phase is to employ techniques that will facilitate oxygen transport without causing undue stress on a systemic physiology, which may take months to 'normalize' following prolonged cardiac insufficiency and/or hypoxaemia and deconditioning (Dean 1997, Manning et al 1999). Occasionally a recipient may require prolonged ventilatory support. As with other intensive care patients, all physiotherapy interventions must be assessment based and individualized for each patient. Recipients who struggle to maintain an adequate cardiac output and/or oxygen level may be managed (amongst other therapies) on inhaled nitric oxide (Troncy et al 1997). The gas, which is titrated into the inspiratory oxygen/air mix, has a potent pulmonary vasodilatory effect and may assist in decreasing the load on the right heart and improving oxygenation. If assessment indicates a need for assisted secretion clearance, the technique chosen must not disrupt the titrated percentage of inspired nitric oxide. Changes in patient position should be trialled in stages, as with any critically ill patient, to ensure that the position change has no negative effect on cardiac output, blood and airway pressures or oxygen saturation. In heart-lung and lung recipients the need for prolonged intensive care, especially ventilatory assistance, may be a preservation-reperfusion injury to the lung or lungs (Daly & McGregor 1996). In children the anastomosis may be distal to the end of the endotracheal tube and therefore suction should be performed with the greatest care. In the immediate postoperative period the anastomosis may not be 'air tight' and care should be taken when performing manual hyperinflation to ensure that excessive pressures are not delivered.

The physiotherapist may be involved in weaning patients from mechanical ventilation and establishing energy cost-efficient patterns of breathing. Well-supported positioning, utilization of the stimulation of hands-on instruction alternated with shoulder and cervical soft tissue techniques can bring about a change in respiratory pattern and rate and positively affect arterial blood gases and haemodynamics. These techniques are especially effective when the physiotherapist–patient relationship has been well established in the preoperative period. In some instances it is also appropriate to encourage the patient to utilize the relaxation method he chose and practised in the preoperative conditioning programme. Non-invasive ventilatory support may be useful in assisting patients who have experienced difficulties in weaning and extubation or, in instances of postextubation hypoxaemia, hypercapnia and/or fatigue, particularly in lung recipients who required support preoperatively.

For the majority of patients, postoperative physiotherapy is started after extubation, which is usually 3–12 hours following transfer to the intensive care area from theatre. Thorough and comprehensive monitoring and reassessment of the patient by every health professional involved in the acute care are of paramount importance to both the individual patient and the ongoing quality assurance of the programme as a whole. It is essential that the physiotherapist assesses and reassesses the patient at each treatment, remembering the vulnerability of the transplant recipient to infection and rejection. Subjective and objective assessment findings must be reviewed along with the latest microbiology results, arterial blood gases, chest radiograph, lung function measurements and oxygen saturation at rest and while changing position or mobilizing.

Following through from preoperative physiotherapy care, the emphasis of physiotherapy postoperatively is on active, functional movement and strengthening and patient education. The techniques utilized, frequency and duration of treatments in the early postoperative days are dependent upon the patient's presentation, needs and progress. Experience suggests that frequent, brief treatments are the most effective during this period. From the first postoperative treatment, patients are taught to monitor themselves with their therapist and to utilize respiratory techniques not as a compulsory 'drill' but according to clinical measures. Most patients quickly become proficient in using a huff to assess the presence of upper airway secretions and their oximetry monitor to provide feedback on the effectiveness of their pattern of breathing.

If patients are hypoventilating, thoracic expansion exercises combined with breathing control (in conjunction with augmented analgesia) in different positions, e.g. sitting and standing, may be beneficial. Current intensive care beds allow even patients who are limited to bed (such as those requiring significant ionotropic support) to be treated in a foot-down, high sitting position, offloading abdominal and postoperative drain pressure from the lower segments of the lungs. Frequent, well-supported, effective huffing and

coughing, in a variety of positions, is of paramount importance for lung recipients because of their inability to cough spontaneously in response to secretions accumulating distal to the airway anastomosis. If sputum retention becomes a problem for a recipient, inhalation therapy and an appropriate airway clearance technique should be considered.

Bronchoscopy is utilized to check on the airway anastomosis but can be used more frequently for bronchial toilet if accumulating secretions compromise the patient. Physiotherapy before and during a bronchoscopy may assist clearance by mobilizing sputum to the central airways for suction.

In keeping with the increased emphasis on progressive rehabilitation rather than differentiating respiratory physiotherapy and exercise therapy, many centres now allow patients to be sat out of bed (depending on their cardiovascular stability) as early as the day of surgery. Patients usually start mobilizing from bed to chair on day 1. Recipients (especially the very debilitated patients) may commence a light weight programme as early as day 3, depending on their wound pain and stability (using weights of 1–1.5 kg).

Patients may be transferred to the ward as early as day 2 postoperatively. At this stage, patients are usually seen three or four times daily. Once able to mobilize from the bed area, patients are commenced on stair walking and gentle bicycle ergometer work. Usually on day 4 or 5, soft tissue (Chaitow 1988), joint mobilization (Maitland 1986) and/or thoracic stretching techniques are commenced as indicated. These have proven particularly valuable with the SLTx and BSSLTx recipients whose primary pain following removal of the now routine epidural infusion appears to be associated with the articulations and muscle groups that have been stressed during surgery.

In children, following extubation and removal of inotropic support an individually tailored graduated programme of rehabilitation can be instituted both to enable the child to regain confidence in his/her ability and to achieve a good level of fitness. Bicycle ergometry is useful in the early stages and motivation may be enhanced by using charts to provide a measure of improvement in function. Chest physiotherapy is only required in the presence of infection and retained secretions.

Rehabilitation

The primary goals in the rehabilitation phase after transplantation are to:

- improve the patient's physical condition (posture, strength and endurance)
- improve the patient's confidence in becoming involved in a full range of activities of daily living and appropriate exercise activities
- nurture realistic expectations for employment, sport and leisure activities
- promote independence in maintaining and monitoring their physical condition.

Gymnasium-based rehabilitation

When the patients are allowed to mobilize from the ward area, they should commence a gymnasium-based rehabilitation programme. This may begin as early as day 3 postoperatively. Each patient's programme is tailored to suit his current physical status and is oriented toward his specific goals for employment and recreational pursuits. Even the most debilitated patient is included in the gymnasium programme and his support person/s are also encouraged to attend and become involved in supervising and encouraging exercise activities and in extending the patient's off-ward activities to include walking out of doors and eating 'out'.

Inpatients attend the gymnasium once or twice daily. Outpatients are encouraged to attend the gymnasium 3–5 times weekly, depending upon their condition and distance from the hospital, for a period of 8–12 weeks.

Each patient's gymnasium programme is based on varying times and intensities of work in a number of activities. The activities are introduced gradually according to the patient's physical condition, wound/musculoskeletal discomfort and level of confidence. Table 16.7 outlines the activities/equipment used, their primary purpose(s) and the varying duration of activities through which patients are progressed (Kjaer et al 1999, Lampert et al 1998, Quittan et al 1999).

In our experience, the most effective way to determine the appropriate intensity of an activity has been to exercise according to a scale of perceived exertion such as the Borg scale (Borg 1970, Pandolf 1983). Activities are introduced at an intensity such that the patient's subjective description of his level of exertion is 'very light' or 'light'. The intensity is subsequently progressed to levels of exertion described as 'somewhat hard' and 'hard'. The same scale of exertion used in this rehabilitation phase is also used in the preoperative conditioning programme and the patient's home-based, maintenance work. By the time a patient is ready for discharge from the immediate supervision of the gymnasium environment, he is well practised in judging and progressing activity intensity and is encouraged to apply this scaling to his recreational activities and workplace tasks.

Thorough supervision/monitoring of recipients before and while participating in gymnasium activities is of the utmost importance, especially in the early weeks of rehabilitation, while patients are unfamiliar with 'reading' the symptoms often associated with infection/rejection episodes. Prior to commencing their gym activities, patients are asked to comment on their ability to cope with

Table 16.7 Gymnasium activities utilized in the post-transplant rehabilitation programme

Activity	Purpose	Time/repetitions
Treadmill/bicycle ergometer	Warm-up	12 minutes
Bicycle ergometer/treadmill	Endurance/aerobic fitness	5–40 minutes
Weights	Quadriceps strengthening Upper limb and shoulder girdle strengthening Glutei and lower limb strengthening	1–10 kg, 10–30 repetitions

activities of daily living and walking and how it compares with their performance in the previous days. Patients are checked for any change in weight, lung function tests (for heart–lung and lung recipients this includes twice-daily self-monitoring of FEV_1 and FVC), blood pressure, heart rate and rhythm and resting oxygen saturation. Heart rate and blood pressure (and oxygen saturation for heart–lung and lung recipients) are monitored throughout the gymnasium session. Any uncharacteristic changes in the above parameters are noted, as is any decline in a patient's ability to cope comfortably with an activity that previously has been well within his ability. Medical staff in the outpatients' clinic are notified and the patient is reviewed and investigated accordingly.

Patient participation in and progression through a rehabilitation programme needs to be flexible and readily modified and 'back tracked' to accommodate the sometimes unpredictable nature of the recipient's postoperative course. There will be occasions when patients are unable to exercise:

- immediately following cardiac or transbronchial biopsy (or other 'minor' procedures/investigations)
- when symptoms and/or a biopsy are indicative of a significant rejection or infection episode.

When exercise can be resumed, it will need to be at a lesser intensity than when the patient last participated in the activities and, as always, progressed considering the recipient's presenting condition. This is particularly important if the patient has just completed a course of intravenous steroid therapy and has noted symptoms of peripheral myopathy.

At 3–4 weeks postoperatively, abdominal and lower back strengthening exercises are added to the work-out. These exercises and upper limb weight work are outlined in each patient's maintenance programme, which is based on a once-a-day aerobic activity of the patient's choice, whether it be walking, cycling, swimming, running or a combination of these. Specific stretching/strengthening programmes are also outlined for patients returning to physically demanding employment and sporting activities (Derman et al 1996).

As the number of long-term transplant survivors increases it is apparent that physiotherapy intervention may be needed for some individuals many years after their actual procedure. Some recipients require ongoing assistance with acute and chronic musculoskeletal problems while others may periodically need specific programmes for weight loss or simply guidelines for recommencing exercise after neglecting their fitness for a time. The quality of life experienced by many recipients can be excellent. Experience suggests that those who regularly exercise, particularly focusing on both cardiovascular and weight- bearing activities, can be safely involved in most recreational and employment pursuits.

CONCLUSION

Physiotherapy is an integral part of the management of the cardiopulmonary transplant recipient. The role of the physiotherapist has expanded considerably in the last decade and the future looks equally exciting. There are many avenues of research in the area of thoracic organ replacement. Permanent cardiac replacement with a mechanical device is an experimental reality and although xenotransplantation to date has been of limited success, research continues. Promising experimentation in biological augmentation of the failing myocardium (such as cardiomyoplasty and culturing cardiomyocytes) is well under way in a number of centres worldwide (Cooper & Liosky 1996).

The greatest challenge facing cardiopulmonary transplant programmes continues to be the limited number of donor organs available for the ever-expanding potential recipient waiting list. Limited donor numbers have necessitated the development of transplant alternatives in the management of respiratory and cardiac failure and the expertise gained in maintaining potential recipients has allowed many transplant centres to develop special cardiac and respiratory failure programmes. The development and rapidly increasing utilization of lung volume reduction surgery in the management of emphysema and pulmonary endarterectomy in the treatment of pulmonary hypertension have taken some pressure off transplant waiting lists. Physiotherapy has much to offer these patients also and it is essential that the therapist be actively involved in the cardiopulmonary transplant programme.

Acknowledgements

For the paediatric contribution I acknowledge the input from Pauline Whitmore, Clinical Nurse Specialist, Great Ormond Street Hospital, London.

I would like to acknowledge the assistance of Ms Samantha Edwards, Ms Susan Colley, Mr Matthew Tallis and Ms Kirsty Krieg (physiotherapists) in the preparation of this chapter and thank the Heart and Lung Transplant Team, St Vincent's Hospital, Sydney, Australia, for their continued encouragement to develop physiotherapy in this challenging area.

REFERENCES

Abecassis M, Adams M, Adams P, et al 2000 Consensus statement on the live organ donor. JAMA 284(22): 2919–2926

Aris R, Neuringer I, Weiner M, Egan T, Ontjes D 1996 Severe osteoporosis before and after lung transplantation. Chest 109(5): 1176–1183

Aurora P, Prasad SA, Balfour-Lynn IM, Slade G, Whitehead B, Dinwiddie R 2001 Exercise tolerance in children with cystic fibrosis undergoing lung transplantation assessment. European Respiratory Journal 18: 293–297

Balfour-Lynn IM, Martin I, Whitehead BF, Rees PG, Elliot MJ, De Leval MR 1997 Heart-lung transplantation for patients under 10 with cystic fibrosis. Archives of Disease in Childhood 76: 1–3

Borel JF 1980 Immunosuppressive properties of cyclosporin A (CY-A). Transplantation Proceedings 12: 233

Borg G 1970 Perceived exertion as an indicator of somatic stress. Scandinavian Journal of Rehabilitation Medicine 2(3): 92–98

Bussieres L, Pflugfelder P, Menkis A, Novick R, McKenzie F, Taylor A, Kostuk W 1995 Basis for aerobic impairment in patients after heart transplantation. Journal of Heart and Lung Transplantation 14(6): 1073–1080

Cahalin L 1996 Preoperative and postoperative conditioning for lung transplantation and volume-reduction surgery. Critical Care Nursing Clinics 8(3): 305–322

Carrey Z, Gottfried S, Levy R 1990 Ventilatory muscle support in respiratory failure with nasal positive pressure ventilation. Chest 97: 150–158

Chaitow L 1988 Soft-tissue manipulation: a practitioner's guide to the diagnosis and treatment of soft tissue dysfunction and reflex activity. Healing Arts Press, New York

Chaparro C, Kesten S 1997 Infections in lung transplant recipients. Clinics in Chest Medicine 18(2): 339–351

Clark A, Poole-Wilson P, Coats A 1996 Exercise limitation in chronic heart failure: central role of the periphery. Journal of the American College of Cardiology 28(5): 1092–1102

Coats A 1993 Exercise rehabilitation in heart failure. Journal of the American College of Cardiology 22(4): 172A–177A

Cooper D, Lidsky N 1996 Immediate postoperative care and potential complications. In: Cooper D, Miller L, Patterson G (eds) The transplantation and replacement of thoracic organs, 2nd edn. Kluwer Academic , Dordrecht

Cooper J, Pearson F, Patterson G, Todd T, Glinsberg R, Goldberg M, DeMajo W 1987 Technique of successful lung transplantation in humans. Journal of Thoracic and Cardiovascular Surgery 93: 173–181

Couetil J 1996 The split-lung technique for lobar transplantation. In: Cooper D, Miller L, Patterson G (eds) The transplantation and replacement of thoracic organs, 2nd edn. Kluwer Academic, Dordrecht

Daly R, McGregor C 1996 Postoperative management of the single lung transplant patient In: Cooper D, Miller L, Patterson G (eds) The transplantation and replacement of the thoracic organs, 2nd edn. Kluwer Academic , Dordrecht

Dean E 1997 Oxygen transport deficits in systemic disease and implications for physical therapy. Physical Therapy 77(2): 187–202

Demopoulos L, Bijou R, Fergus I, Jones M, Strom J, LeJemtel T 1997 Exercise training in patients with severe congestive heart failure: enhancing peak aerobic capacity while minimising the increase in ventricular wall stress. Journal of the American College of Cardiology 29(3): 597–603

Derman E, Derman K, Noakes T 1996 Exercise rehabilitation of cardiac transplant recipients. In: Cooper D, Miller L, Patterson G (eds) The transplantation and replacement of thoracic organs, 2nd edn. Kluwer Academic, Dordrecht

Du Toil E, Oudshoorn M, Smith D 1996 Pretransplant immunological considerations. In: Cooper D, Miller L, Patterson G (eds) The transplantation and replacement of thoracic organs, 2nd edn. Kluwer Academic, Dordrecht

Frazier O 1993 Long-term ventricular support with the HeartMate in patients undergoing bridge-to-transplant operations. In: Ott R, Gutfinger D, Gazzaniga A (eds) Cardiac surgery: state of the art reviews, vol 7. Hanley and Belfus, Philadelphia, pp 353–362

Gaissert H, Patterson G 1996 Surgical techniques of single and bilateral lung transplantation. In: Cooper D, Miller L, Patterson G (eds) The transplantation and replacement of thoracic organs, 2nd edn. Kluwer Academic , Dordrecht

Hill J, Farrar D, Topic N 1993 The Thoratec experience in bridge to cardiac transplantation. In: Ott R, Gutfinger D, Gazzaniga A (eds) Cardiac surgery: state of the art reviews, vol 7. Hanley and Belfus, Philadelphia, pp 317–326

Horak A 1990 Physiology and pharmacology of the transplanted heart. In: Cooper D, Novitzky D (eds) The transplantation and replacement of thoracic organs. Kluwer, Lancaster Hosenpud J 1999 Coronary artery disease after heart transplantation. American Heart Journal 138(5 Pt 2): 469–472

Hosenpud J, Novick RJ, Bennett LE, Keck BM, Fiol B, Daily OP 1996 The registry of the International Society for Heart and Lung Transplantation: thirteenth official report. Journal of Heart and Lung Transplantation 15: 655–674

Hosenpud J 1999 Coronary artery disease after heart transplantation. American Heart Journal 138(5 Pt 2): 469–472

Hosenpud J, Bennett L, Keck B, Boucek M, Novick J 2000 The registry of the International Society for Heart and Lung Transplantation: seventeenth official report Journal of Heart and Lung Transplantation 19(10): 909–931

Jamieson S, Stinson E, Oyer P, Baldwin J, Shumway N 1984 Operative technique for heart–lung transplantation. Journal of Thoracic and Cardiovascular Surgery 87: 930–935

Kaiser L, Pasque M, Trulock E, Low D, Dresler C, Cooper J 1991 Bilateral sequential lung transplantation: the procedure of choice for double-lung replacement. Annals of Thoracic Surgery 52: 438–446

Kavanagh T 1996 Physical training in heart transplant recipients. Journal of Cardiovascular Risk 3: 154–159

Kavanagh T, Yacoub M, Mertens D, Kennedy J, Campbell R, Sawyer P 1988 Cardiorespiratory responses to exercise training after orthotopic cardiac transplantation. Circulation 77(1): 162–171

Keogh A, Baron D, Spratt P, Esmore D, Chang V 1986 Cardiac transplantation in Australia. Australian Family Physician 15(11): 1474–1481

Keogh A, Macdonald P, Chang V et al 1991 Seven years of heart transplantation in Australia – the St Vincent's Hospital experience. On the Pulse III(2): 2–7

Keteyian S, Brawnwe C, Schairer J 1997 Exercise testing and training of patients with heart failure due to left ventricular systolic dysfunction. Journal of Cardiopulmonary Rehabilitation 17: 19–28

Kjaer M, Beyer N, Secher N 1999 Exercise and organ transplantation. Scandinavian Journal of Medicine and Sports Science 9(1): 1–14

Kobashigawa J, Katznelson S, Laks H 1995 Effect of pravastatin on outcomes after cardiac transplantation. New England Journal of Medicine 333: 621–626

Kriett J, Jamieson S 1996 Diagnosis and management of bronchiolitis obliterans. In: Cooper D, Miller L, Patterson G (eds) The transplantation and replacement of thoracic organs, 2nd edn. Kluwer Academic, Dordrecht.

Lampert E, Mettauer B, Hoppeler H, Charloux A Charpentier A, Lonsdorfer J 1998 Skeletal muscle response to short endurance training in heart transplant recipients. Journal of the American College of Cardiology 32(2): 420–426

Lawrence E 1990 Diagnosis and management of lung allograft rejection In: Grossman R, Maurer J (eds) Clinics in chest medicine, vol 2 WB Saunders, Philadelphia, pp 269–278

Lipkin D, Scriven A, Crake T, Poole-Wilson P 1986 Six minute walk test for assessing exercise capacity in chronic heart failure. British Medical Journal 292: 653–655

Madden B, Hodson M, Tsang V, Radley-Smith R, Khaghani A, Yacoub M 1992 Intermediate-term results of heart–lung transplantation for cystic fibrosis. Lancet 339: 1583–1587

Maitland G 1986 Vertebral manipulation. Butterworths, London

Manning F, Dean E, Ross J, Abboud R 1999 Effects of side lying on lung function in older individuals. Physical Therapy 79(5): 456–466

Negri A, Plantalech L, Russp Picasso M, Otero A, Sarli M 1999 Post-transplantation osteoporosis. Medicina (B Aires) 59(6): 777–786

Pandolf K 1983 Advances in the study and application of perceived exertion. Exercise, Sports Science Review 11: 118–158

Patterson G, Cooper J, Goldman B et al 1988 Technique of successful clinical double-lung transplantation. Annals of Thoracic Surgery 43: 626–633

Poindexter S 1991 Nutrition in a heart transplant program. (Abstract) American Dietetic Association. San Fransisco

Quittan M, Sturm B, Wiesinger G, Fialka-Moser V, Pacher R, Rodler S 1999 Skeletal muscle strength following orthotopic heart transplantation. Wiener Klinische Wochenschrift 111(12): 476–483

Reaven P, Witztum J 1988 Lovastatin, nicotinic acid and rhabdomyolysis. Annals of Internal Medicine 109: 597–603

Reitz B 1982 Heart and lung transplantation. Heart Transplantation 1(1): 80–81

Rubin R 1994 Infections in the organ transplant recipient. In: Rubin R, Young L (eds) Clinical approach to infection in the compromised host, 3rd edn Plenum Press, New York

Schwartz D 1989 Respiratory disease and mechanical ventilation. In: Skipper A (ed) Dietitian's handbook of enteral and parenteral nutrition. Aspen, Rockville, MD

Scott C, Dark J, McComb J 1995 Evolution of the chronotropic response to exercise after cardiac transplantation. American Journal of Cardiology 76: 1292–1296

Singh S, Morgan M, Scott S, Walters D, Hardman A 1992 Development of a shuttle walking test of disability in patients with chronic airway obstruction. Thorax 47(12): 1019–1024

Squires R 1990 Cardiac rehabilitation issues for heart transplantation patients. Journal of Cardiopulmonary Rehabilitation 10: 159–168

Starnes VA, Woo MS, MacLaughlin EF et al 1999 Comparison of outcome between living donor and cadaveric lung transplantation in children. Annals of Thoracic Surgery 68(6): 2279–2283; discussion 2283–2284

Steele B 1994 The six-minute walk. American Association of Cardiovascular and Pulmonary Rehabilitation procedings, 9th annual meeting, Portland, Oregan, 383–388

Stevenson L 1996 Selection and management of the potential candidate for cardiac transplantation. In: Cooper D, Miller L, Patterson G (eds) The transplantation and replacement of thoracic organs, 2nd edn. Kluwer Academic, Dordrecht

Theodore J, Starnes V, Lewiston N 1990 Obliterative bronchiolitis. In: Grossman R, Maurer J (eds) Clinics in chest medicine, vol 2 WB Saunders, Philadelphia, pp 309–321

Troncy E, Francoeur M, Blaise G 1997 Inhaled nitric oxide: clinical applications, indications, and toxicology. Canadian Journal of Anaesthesia 44(9): 973–988

Tyndall K, Cooper D 1996 Maintenance immunosuppressive drug therapy and potential major complications. In: Cooper D, Miller L, Patterson G (eds) The transplantation and replacement of thoracic organs, 2nd edn. Kluwer Academic, Dordrecht

Weber B 1990 Cardiac surgery and heart transplantation. In: Hudak C, Gallo B, Benz J (eds) Critical care nursing: a holistic approach, 5th edn. JB Lippincott, Philadelphia

Weill D, Hodges F, Olmos J, Zamora M 1999 Acute native lung hyperinflation is not associated with poor outcome following single lung transplant for emphysema. Journal of Heart and Lung Transplantation 18(11): 1080–1087

FURTHER READING

American Association of Cardiovascular and Pulmonary Rehabilitation 1999 Guidelines for cardiac rehabilitation and secondary prevention programs, 3rd edn. Human Kinetics, Champaign, Illinois

Cooper D, Miller L, Patterson G (eds) 1996 The transplantation and replacement of thoracic organs, 2nd edn. Kluwer Academic, Dordrecht

Grossman R, Maurer J (eds) 1990 Clinics in chest medicine: pulmonary considerations in transplantation. WB Saunders, Philadelphia

Kavanagh T, Yacoub M, Mertens D, Campbell R, Sawyer P 1989 Exercise rehabilitation after heterotopic cardiac transplantation. Journal of Cardiopulmonary Rehabilitation 9: 303–310

Keteyian S, Ehrman J, Fedel F, Rhoads K 1990. Heart rate-perceived exertion relationship during exercise in orthotopic heart transplant patients. Journal of Cardiopulmonary Rehabilitation 10: 287–293

Paul L, Solez K (eds) 1996 Organ transplantation: long-term results. Marcel Dekker, New York

Solez K, Racusen L, Billingham M (eds) 1996 Solid organ transplant: rejection mechanisms, pathology and diagnosis. Marcel Dekker, New York

Squires R, Allison T, Miller, Gau G 1991 Cardiopulmonary exercise testing after unilateral lung transplantation: a case report. Journal of Cardiopulmonary Rehabilitation 11: 192–196

Vibekk P 1991 Chest mobilisation and respiratory function. In: Pryor J (ed) Respiratory care. Churchill Livingstone, Edinburgh

17

Spinal cord injury

Trudy Ward   Kathryn Harris

INTRODUCTION

The prognosis for the patient sustaining spinal cord injury was poor until the latter part of the 20th century. An unknown Egyptian physician of 2500BC describing spinal cord injury in the Edwin Smith Papyrus wrote: 'An ailment not to be treated' (Grundy & Swain 1996). This view continued until the work of Guttmann and others encouraged development of special centres throughout the world and saw the problems associated with spinal cord injury at last being addressed, although the mortality from tetraplegia until the 1960s remained at 35% (Grundy & Swain 1996). Improvements in administering care at the time of the accident, technological advances in diagnosis and in management have contributed to a continuing fall in mortality and morbidity rates over recent years. In a 50-year study in the United Kingdom Frankel et al (1998) found that 92.3% of spinal cord injuries survived, the primary cause of death being attributed to respiratory complications. Another study has shown a projected mean life expectancy of 84% of normal for paraplegia and 70% for tetraplegia (Yeo et al 1998). DeVivo et al (1999) reported on mortality of patients who were admitted to one of the 'Model spinal cord injury system' hospitals in the USA. Patients admitted to such a centre between 1993 and 1998 were found to be 67% less likely to die than those admitted to the system between 1973 and 1977. There are no comparative figures for patients treated outside this system model but the assumption is that mortality is higher.

The respiratory care of patients with spinal cord injury is examined in this chapter. It should, however, be remembered that the total management of patients requires a holistic, multidisciplinary approach, preferably in a spinal cord injuries unit, to ensure effective rehabilitation.

MECHANICS OF RESPIRATION AND THE EFFECT OF SPINAL CORD INJURY

Normal respiration

An understanding of normal respiratory mechanics is needed to appreciate the effect a spinal cord injury will have. Fig. 17.1 lists the muscles of respiration and their level of innervation.

The contraction and downward movement of the diaphragm and contraction of the intercostal muscles cause normal inspiration by generation of negative intrapleural and subsequent negative intrathoracic pressure (Lucke 1998). The intercostal muscles also work to stabilize the rib cage against the tendency for paradoxical inward movement caused by the negative intrathoracic pressure during inspiration.

Expiration is normally a passive process except during a forceful manoeuvre such as coughing or sneezing. This force is generated mainly by the abdominal muscles assisted by the intercostals at large lung volumes (De Troyer & Heilporn 1980).

Respiratory complications are a major cause of death in the early stages of spinal injury (Lanig & Peterson 2000, Van Buren et al 1994), and those at the highest risk are:

- tetraplegic patients
- patients with associated injuries such as rib fractures or chest trauma
- patients who have preexisting lung disease.

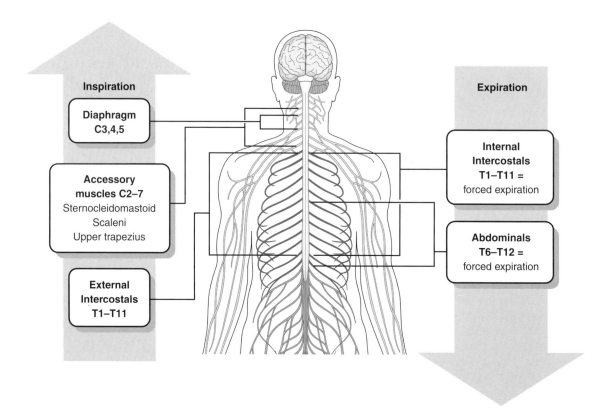

Fig. 17.1 Spinal innervation of the respiratory muscles.

Effects of spinal cord injury

Following a spinal cord injury the muscles below and, not uncommonly, at the level of the injury are paralysed. The higher the level of injury, the greater the effect on respiration (Linn et al 2000). To gain a more precise picture of the muscles affected, the physiotherapist should refer to the level of innervation of the respiratory muscles and relate this to the neurological level of injury.

Tetraplegic patients (i.e. those with an injury affecting T1 or above) will have lost the use of their intercostal muscles which has a profound effect on respiratory function. Depending on the level of their injury, they may only have part of their diaphragm spared to provide them with all of their respiratory effort (Cohn 1993).

Paradoxical breathing

Tetraplegic patients injured at or below C4 will have partial or total innervation of the diaphragm and some accessory muscles of respiration and hence can be totally independent of mechanical ventilation. However, in the initial spinal shock stage, tetraplegic patients will have paralysis of their intercostal muscles which, when flaccid, cause disruption to the mechanics of respiration. The usual splinting function of the intercostal muscles is lost and the negative intrathoracic pressure during inspiration causes paradoxical inward depression of the ribs (Lucke 1998, Menter et al 1997) (Fig. 17.2). This may lead to microatelectasis and an increase in the work of breathing (Fishburn et al 1990). With time the tendons, ligaments and joints of the rib cage stiffen owing to decreased active movement. This, together with spasticity of the intercostals, will provide some compensation for the loss of active control of these muscles and stabilize the rib cage, so that paradoxical breathing lessens (Axen et al 1985, Mansel & Norman 1990).

Cough

The ability to produce an effective cough is severely impaired in patients with cervical or high thoracic spinal cord injury (Roth et al 1997,

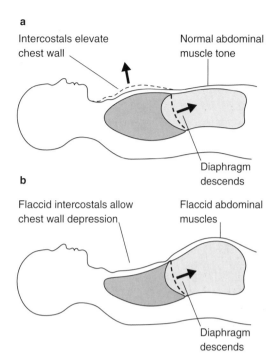

Fig. 17.2 Paradoxical breathing in tetraplegia.

Wang et al 1997). This is most marked when the intercostals are flaccid and the rib cage is at its most mobile. Patients who have loss of innervation to the abdominal muscles and the internal intercostals lose the ability to produce a forced expiration (Gouden 1997). De Troyer & Estenne (1991) have shown that patients with injuries at C5–8 can utilize the clavicular portion of pectoralis major to generate an expulsive force, although the extent to which this is functional is not clear. Linn et al (2000) found that in a group of patients with high tetraplegia (above C5) loss of peak expiratory flow rate was greater than 50% predicted. An effective cough for these patients requires external compression to produce the necessary large intrathoracic pressures; assisted coughing is discussed later.

The effect of position

In the normal subject, mechanisms exist to ensure that adequate ventilation is maintained in all positions. In the supine position, contraction of the diaphragm displaces the abdominal contents without significantly expanding the rib cage, as the abdomen is more compliant than the rib cage. In standing, abdominal tone increases to support the abdominal contents, thereby decreasing abdominal wall compliance. Contraction of the diaphragm, intercostal and accessory muscles causes greater rib cage expansion, resulting in an increase in vital capacity in standing of about 5% (Chen et al 1990).

Positional changes will, however, affect the respiratory function of the tetraplegic patient. In supine, the weight of the abdominal contents forces the diaphragm to a higher resting level so that contraction produces greater excursion of the diaphragm. In sitting or standing, the weight of the unsupported abdominal contents increases the demand on the diaphragm which now rests in a lower and flatter position (Chen et al 1990, Lucke 1998), decreasing effectiveness and restricting available excursion for creating negative intrapleural pressure (Fig. 17.3). Chen et al (1990) recorded a 14% drop in predicted vital

capacity in the tetraplegic patient on changing position from supine to sitting or standing. Conversely, vital capacity of a tetraplegic patient rises by 6% when the bed is tipped 15° head down from supine (Bromley 1998). Linn et al (2000) showed a statistically significant decrease in FVC in the erect position as compared to supine. It is therefore important with these patients not to assume that their respiratory ability will be sufficient in all positions.

Abdominal binders have been used on patients with high spinal cord injury for many years, both to minimize the effect of postural hypotension and aid respiration (Goldman et al 1986, McCool 1986, Scott et al 1993). Their effect is achieved by providing support to the abdominal contents, decreasing the compliance of the abdominal wall and thereby allowing the diaphragm to assume a more normal resting position in the upright posture (Alvarez et al 1981). Goldman et al (1986) investigated the effect of abdominal binders on breathing in tetraplegic patients and concluded that in the supine position there was no change but when sitting there was a trend for improvement in lung volumes. This may help the patient considerably during the early stages of mobilization.

RESPIRATORY ASSESSMENT

Accurate assessment and regular review of the respiratory status are vital. Initial assessment must be carried out as soon as possible to establish a baseline against which future deterioration or improvement can be monitored. The assessment procedure is discussed in Chapter 1 but in patients with spinal cord injury, the following details should be considered.

1. Motor and sensory neurological examination, relating this to the respiratory muscle innervation and hence likely function (Roth et al 1997).
2. Associated injuries – rib fractures and flail segments are particularly likely in the patient with thoracic spinal injury and these may require modification of treatment techniques. Patients involved in diving accidents may

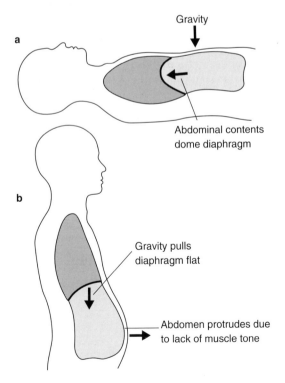

Fig. 17.3 The effect of position on diaphragm function in tetraplegia **a** lying; **b** sitting or standing.

present with the additional respiratory complications of water aspiration. The presence of intraabdominal trauma or complications such as paralytic ileus, acute gastric dilatation or gastrointestinal bleeding will also require modification of the techniques used by the physiotherapist, especially in assisted coughing.

3. Associated lung trauma – common injuries include pneumothorax, haemothorax and pulmonary contusion.
4. Preexisting lung disease – problems such as asthma or chronic airflow limitation may exist and should be treated as indicated.
5. Presence of ventilatory support.
6. Psychological state – major psychological adjustment is required by the patient with spinal cord injury, not only to the injury itself but also to the necessary treatment procedures. Sensory deprivation may cause loss of orientation, made worse by enforced immobilization and restricted visual input. Anxiety and interrupted sleep patterns caused by frequent turns and other procedures can result in increased patient confusion and fatigue. These factors will all affect respiratory function and must be considered by the physiotherapist to enable the most effective and appropriate planning of respiratory treatment.
7. Results of the chest radiograph and arterial blood gases, if available.
8. Altered levels of consciousness.
9. Respiratory rate at rest – with normal diaphragm activity the rate remains regular at 12–16 breaths/min. In the presence of a weak or fatiguing diaphragm the rate will increase (Alvarez et al 1981).
10. Assessment of breathing pattern to establish the degree of paradoxical movement or presence of unequal movement of the chest wall.
11. Assessment of diaphragm function, by inspection or palpation of the upper abdomen.
12. Assessment of cough to ascertain effectiveness.
13. Measurement of vital capacity – repeated measurements of vital capacity provide an indication of trends developing in respiratory function and should be recorded in all the positions in which the patient may be nursed to detect postural variations (Lucke 1998). This will be especially pronounced in the presence of unilateral phrenic nerve damage. Values will vary depending on the level of injury. Lucke (1998) reports observed initial vital capacities of 24% of predicted normal value in mid-cervical injuries and 31% in lower cervical injuries; this can rise to 50% after spinal shock has resolved. Vital capacity may fall over the first few days post injury owing to factors such as muscle or patient fatigue, respiratory complications or cord oedema which result in a rise in neurological level (Alderson 1999). Improvement is usually seen as oedema resolves and respiratory function stabilizes (Axen et al 1985, Ledsome & Sharp 1981). Vital capacity values of less than 15 ml per kilo of body weight may, in conjunction with clinical assessment, indicate the need for ventilation (Thomas & Paulson 1994).
14. Auscultation of the chest to detect areas of lung collapse, pleural effusion or secretions.

PHYSIOTHERAPY TECHNIQUES

Respiratory management of the patient with spinal cord injury requires the application of the same principles as other respiratory problems; the skills used are discussed in Chapters 5 and 6. The goals of treatment include:

- clearance of secretions from the lungs
- improvement in breath sounds
- increase in lung volumes
- strengthening of the available muscles of respiration
- improvement of pulmonary and rib cage compliance
- education of the patient and their carer.

Treatment may be prophylactic or directed to treat specific problems.

Prophylactic treatment

This will include breathing exercises, modified postural drainage by regular turning and assisted coughing.

Breathing exercises to encourage maximal inspiration must be established at an early stage, but the therapist should be aware of the implications of lack of sensation of the chest wall. Exercises are directed to improve lateral basal and apical chest wall expansion and diaphragmatic excursion, but care must be taken to avoid tiring the diaphragm. Patients with intercostal paralysis, however, are usually unable to perform localized breathing exercises.

Respiratory muscle training. Many authors have reported on the use of respiratory muscle training for tetraplegia but there is a lack of randomized controlled trials, which makes the findings of the often small studies difficult to apply to the general patient group. Stiller & Huff (1999) could not recommend routine use of respiratory muscle training for tetraplegic patients (see also p. 187).

There have been some recent favourable findings; Liaw et al (2000) found that resistive inspiratory muscle training in tetraplegic patients who were between 30 days and 6 months of injury improved ventilatory function but noted that the patients needed to be highly motivated to gain benefit. Uijl et al (1999) reported on nine tetraplegic patients who underwent target flow endurance training and showed enhanced endurance capacity and an increase in aerobic exercise performance.

Incentive spirometry enables respiratory training with immediate visual feedback to reinforce success. However, caution is needed in providing these patients with such a device as a balance is needed between maintaining and improving lung volumes and respiratory muscle fatigue.

Intermittent positive pressure breathing (IPPB) and non-invasive positive ventilation (NIV) can be used in conjunction with other methods of treatment, particularly assisted coughing; see below. Work by Rose et al (1987) concluded that solely increasing lung volumes had no major effect on lung function in stable tetraplegics. IPPB may be useful to aid the clearance of secretions by increasing inspiratory volume in patients with sputum retention and lung collapse (p. 209). The introduction of ventilators for NIV has overcome some of the limitations of IPPB machines such as lack of choice of interface and requirement for pressurized gas (Bott et al 1992). NIV is useful to initiate at an early stage before the onset of fatigue to enable the patient to get used to the machine (Tromans et al 1998) and if the patient does tire then the system can be used to provide assistance for up to 24 hours if required. This has been shown to be an effective way of preventing intubation and ventilation in acute spinal cord injury (Tromans et al 1998).

Unfortunately, in the case of acute spinal cord injury the psychological impact is devastating. Acceptance of a facemask or nosemask by the patient is often poor when they are also dealing with profound sensory deprivation from immobility and sensory loss. Kannan (1999) acknowledges that patient comfort and mental status can be reasons for failure of NIV and in clinical experience this can often be the case.

Glossopharyngeal breathing is another technique that can be used to increase lung volumes and assist secretion clearance (p. 206) in the high tetraplegic. Vital capacity may be increased by as much as 1000 ml (Alvarez et al 1981). Bach refers to the technique for augmenting inspired volume for patients with neuromuscular disorders to the extent where they can achieve a vital capacity of up to 1.7 litres (Bach 1993, Bach & McDermott 1990, Bach et al 1993). Pryor (1999) suggests glossopharyngeal breathing is a useful technique for increasing cough effectiveness in tetraplegia. In the high tetraplegic patient dependent on mechanical ventilation, other important benefits of learning GPB are to give security in case of ventilator failure and independence from the ventilator for periods of time (p. 209).

Assisted coughing

Assisted coughing is a vital inclusion in any respiratory programme. Patients may be able to clear sputum from small to large airways, but will need assistance to produce an effective cough for expectoration. Assistance is provided by the application of a compressive force directed inwards and upwards against the thorax to create a push against the diaphragm, thus replacing the work of the abdominal and internal intercostal muscles. Pressure on the abdominal wall alone must be avoided. The sound of the resultant cough is the best indicator of the force required, but care must be taken to avoid movement of any fracture. Pressure directed down through the abdomen must be avoided, especially in the acute patient, due to the possibility of associated abdominal injury or paralytic ileus. Care should also be taken in the presence of rib fractures or other chest injuries and therapists should position their hands away from the problem area to perform an assisted cough.

Bromley (1998) describes various methods of achieving assisted cough. More recently, the literature describes various other methods of assisting cough, which centre on the use of electrical stimulation (Stanic et al 2000). Assisted coughing remains one of the most important techniques for airway clearance in the patient with an acute spinal cord injury. The technique needs to be rel-

atively forceful and for this reason it is advisable for the therapist to lower the bed to gain the most advantageous position from which to perform the technique. However, great care must be taken not to allow any weights used for cervical traction to touch the floor.

The spinal stability of the patient must be carefully considered and for the patient with an unstable cervical spine, a shoulder hold should be used to counter any movement of the fracture site. The methods which may be used in the supine patient requiring a shoulder hold are illustrated in Fig. 17.4.

If one person is assisting the cough, hands should be placed so that one rests on the near side of the thorax and the other on the opposite side of the thorax, with the forearm resting across the lower ribs (Fig. 17.4a). As the patient attempts to cough the physiotherapist pushes inwards and

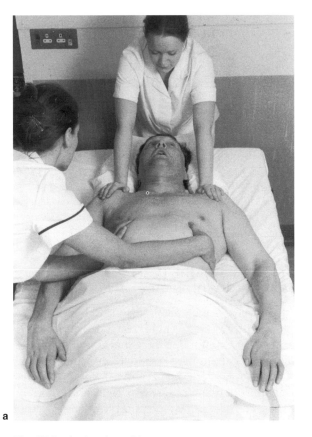

a

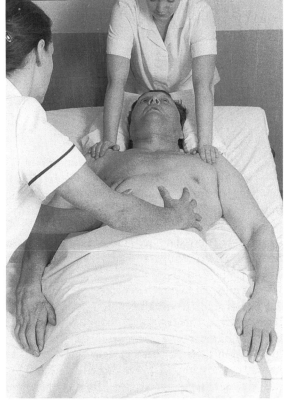

b

Fig. 17.4   Assisted coughing.

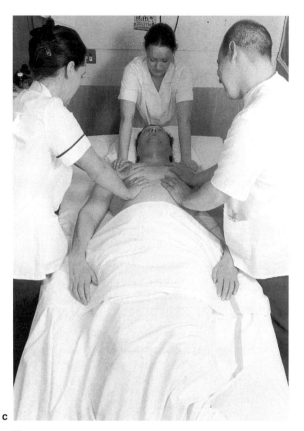

c

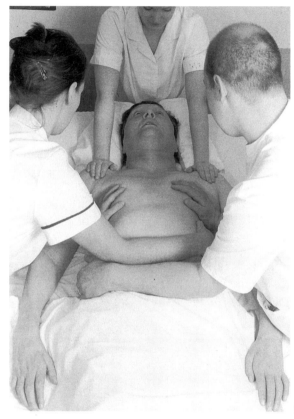

d

Fig. 17.4 Assisted coughing. *Continued*

upwards with the forearm and stabilizes the thorax with the hands.

Alternatively, the hands are positioned bilaterally over the lower thorax (Fig. 17.4b) and, with elbows extended, the physiotherapist pushes inwards and upwards evenly through both arms.

In the case of the patient with a large thorax or having particularly tenacious sputum, two people may be required to produce an effective cough (Fig. 17.4c,d).

Care must be taken to synchronize the applied compressive force with the expiratory effort of the patient. Once the cough is completed, pressure must be lifted momentarily from the lower ribs, thus enabling the patient to use his diaphragm to initiate the next breath. In the presence of paralytic ileus or internal injury, extreme care must be taken during assisted coughing to avoid the application of pressure over the abdomen. Patients should

be encouraged to cough 3–4 times per day, with nursing staff involvement in this process. If possible, patients should be taught self-assisted coughing when in a wheelchair and relatives should learn how to assist the patient to cough in both lying and sitting.

Treatment of the patient with respiratory problems

In the presence of respiratory problems such as retained secretions or lung collapse, sputum clearance is of paramount importance and vigorous, aggressive treatment is often needed. Physiotherapy treatment plans will be determined by ongoing assessment. Unless contraindicated by other complications, postural drainage, either with an electric turning bed or manual turn into supported side lying, should be used as appropriate. Great care must be taken to maintain spinal alignment and cervical traction throughout treatment. The effect of positioning on lung ventilation and perfusion must be considered (Ch. 5). Patients should never be left unsupervised during postural drainage in case of sudden sputum mobilization, which could cause the patient to choke unless it is cleared by assisted coughing. Treatment may consist of the active cycle of breathing techniques (Pryor 1999), vibration, shaking and chest clapping as necessary, followed by assisted coughing. 'Little and often' is the general rule as patients will tire quickly, but treatment must be effective, using two physiotherapists if necessary. Where possible, treatment should link in with planned turn times to allow some rest between various procedures. American authors recommend use of the mechanical exsufflator which has been used to great effect for many years in the USA (Bach 1993, Bach et al 1993, Tzeng & Bach 2000).

Nasopharyngeal suction may be used as a last resort if clearance by assisted cough alone is insufficient, but great care must be taken as pharyngeal suction can cause stimulation of the parasympathetic nervous system via the vagus nerve, resulting in bradycardia and even cardiac arrest. Hyperoxygenation of the patient with 100% oxygen prior to treatment will help minimize this possibility (Wicks & Menter 1986). Atropine or an equivalent drug should be available for administration intravenously should profound bradycardia occur, which can be defined as a heart rate of less than 50 with a continuing downward trend.

Occasionally, bronchoscopy using a fibreoptic bronchoscope may be necessary to treat cases of unresolving lung or lobar collapse.

Care of the ventilated patient

Mechanical ventilation of the patient with spinal cord injury may be necessary in the following circumstances:

- injury to the upper cervical spine C1–3, resulting in paralysis of the diaphragm
- deterioration in respiratory function as a result of oedema or bleeding within the

spinal canal causing the neurological level to rise, so affecting the diaphragm. Patients are most at risk during the first 72 hours
- respiratory muscle fatigue. The use of non-invasive ventilation, e.g. a bilevel positive pressure device, may be helpful in providing ventilatory assistance without the need for full ventilation (Tromans et al 1998) (Ch. 10). Tracheostomy may be beneficial in reducing the dead space by up to 50% (Bromley 1998)
- associated chest or head injuries, which require management by elective ventilation.

Insertion of a minitracheostomy may be considered for patients with problems purely of retained secretions (Gupta et al 1989).

Physiotherapy goals for treatment of the ventilated patient are the same as those for the non-ventilated patient. Treatment will include modified postural drainage, vibration and shaking with manual hyperinflation followed by suction to remove secretions. As previously stated, hyperoxygenation may be needed to prevent overstimulation of the vagus nerve resulting in bradycardia. Other methods for minimizing this are to use a suction catheter that is no more than half the diameter of the tracheostomy tube and to be as gentle and brief as possible (Carroll 1994, Dean 1997, Glass & Grap 1995). Frequency of treatment will be determined by assessment of the respiratory condition but should not exceed 15–20 minutes (Bromley 1998). Patients requiring ventilation due to complications from spinal cord injury are often not sedated and a system of communication must be established before physiotherapy is started.

Ventilation and weaning considerations

Early intervention with a non-invasive ventilatory technique may avoid progression of respiratory failure and the need for sedation, intubation and full mechanical ventilation (Tromans et al 1998). Where ventilation is necessary, weaning will typically progress from IPPV to pressure support and then, in the neurologically intact patient, CPAP is often used. However, in patients with hypercapnic respiratory failure as is seen in spinal cord injury CPAP is not indicated, as it cannot influence tidal volume or respiratory rate and hence does not lower carbon dioxide (Keilty & Bott 1992) . Bilevel positive pressure may be of use during the weaning period, as it assists both expiration and inspiration. Some of these machines have a very sensitive flow trigger which decreases the work of breathing.

There are other associated injuries and complications, which may affect the results.

Weaning from the ventilator should start as soon as the patient's condition permits and is best performed with the patient supine, allowing the most effective diaphragm function (Chen et al 1990, Mansel & Norman 1990). Weaning must take into account the possibility that the patient's respiratory muscles will have atrophied if ventilation has been prolonged. Cohn (1993) suggests that weaning should be thought of as a conditioning process for the diaphragm and also warns that fatigue of the muscle should be avoided. The goal must therefore be to achieve spontaneous breathing for short periods several times a day to avoid fatigue. A study by Peterson et al (1994) compared weaning onto a T-piece for progressive periods of time with the synchronised intermittent mandatory ventilation (SIMV) mode of ventilation, the latter being used frequently in the neurologically intact patient (Cull & Inwood 1999). Compared to SIMV, the T-piece group was almost twice as likely to wean successfully from the ventilator. Tromans et al (1998) reported on the use of BiPAP for weaning 15 patients from ventilation. They reported success in 13 out of 15 patients who weaned in an average of 32 days using a gradual decrease in pressure. Menter et al (1997) quote average weaning times for 74 spinal cord injured patients to be 36 days using progressive T-piece weaning. Peterson et al (1999) report on the use of high tidal volumes to ventilate tetraplegic patients in association with T-piece weaning and conclude that tidal volumes of more than 20 ml per kilo of body weight were most successful. McKinley (1996) reports on the case of an initially ventilator-dependent tetraplegic patient with a C3–4 lesion who was successfully weaned

from a ventilator after 5 years. Other authors support the view that weaning can be prolonged and can take months, if not years (Fromm et al 1999, Oo et al 1999).

Whichever technique is used, regular recording of vital capacity, oxygen saturation and respiratory rate are minimal requirements to effectively monitor the patient's progress (Menter et al 1997). If end-tidal carbon dioxide can be monitored it is very useful and less traumatic than arterial blood gas sampling if no arterial access is in situ (Cull & Inwood 1999). However, arterial blood gases are the gold standard and if the patient is unable to sustain his vital capacity, arterial carbon dioxide is likely to be rising and weaning should not be progressed until it has stabilized.

For the patient on long-term ventilation, a battery-driven ventilator may be attached to the wheelchair to enable mobility (Fig. 17.5). With increasing numbers surviving the initial injury due to greater public awareness of resuscitation skills, home ventilation is now becoming more common, enabling these patient to undergo rehabilitation and go home (Alderson 1999, Carter 1993). Planning, education and support must be provided for all involved to achieve successful integration of the patient and his family back into the community.

The ethical dilemmas surrounding the ventilation of the high tetraplegic patient have challenged, and will continue to challenge, medical practice (Gupta et al 1989, Maynard & Muth 1987). Only the ventilated tetraplegic knows what it is like to be a ventilated tetraplegic and only his carer knows what it is like to care for him. In one review of 21 patients who had required artificial ventilation (Gupta et al 1989), 18 stated that they would prefer a further period of continuous ventilation to being allowed to die. Sixteen of the 21 nearest caring relatives indicated that they were glad that their relative had been kept alive by ventilation. The study concluded that patients with spinal cord injury should be ventilated, provided that total emotional, educational and physical support could be given and maintained to all involved. This would seem to be most important.

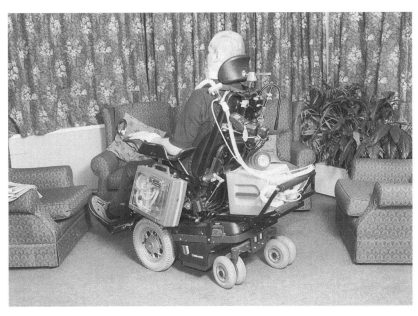

Fig. 17.5 Ventilated patient in a wheelchair.

In a case study, Maynard & Muth (1987) reveal how one individual's request to cease life-supporting ventilation was met. They suggest that 'if rehabilitation is defined as achieving optimal quality of life for people with severe disability then quality must be defined by the disabled individual'. An individual's perception of what constitutes acceptable quality of life will change over time (Purtilo 1986) and this poses the question of the feasibility of involvement of the newly injured patient and relatives in the decision regarding ventilation, unable as they are to appreciate the global implications of tetraplegia. However, the patient and his family must be kept fully informed and their views taken into account before any decisions are made (Gardner et al 1985).

Diaphragmatic pacing. A paralysed diaphragm can be electronically stimulated if the phrenic nerve is intact and the cell bodies of C3, C4, C5 at the spinal cord are viable. The technique was first developed by Dr Glenn in the 1960s (Carter 1993). Electrodes may be placed to stimulate the phrenic nerve in either the neck or thorax and are connected to a receiver embedded in the skin of the anterior chest wall. Stimulation is achieved by means of a radio transmitter placed over the receiver. Extensive postoperative training is necessary to increase diaphragmatic endurance and teach the patient, his family and carers the necessary skills and understanding of the device. For some patients, phrenic nerve pacing will provide an alternative to the ventilator, but the ventilator will remain an emergency back-up. For others, pacing provides selective periods of freedom from mechanical ventilation, enabling easier wheelchair mobility, speech, less noise from the ventilator, less need for carer input and improved psychological status (DiMarco 1999).

CONCLUSION

Greater understanding of the problems of the spinal cord-injured patient has led to continuing improvements in morbidity and mortality rates. Respiratory complications can now be managed more effectively as understanding of the problems facing these patients improves. Physiotherapists have, and will continue to have, much to offer in the respiratory care of the patient with spinal cord injury.

REFERENCES

Alderson JD 1999 Spinal cord injuries. Care of the Critically Ill 15 (2): 48–52

Alvarez S, Peterson M, Lunsford B 1981 Respiratory treatment of the adult patient with spinal cord injury. Physical Therapy 61(12): 1737–1745

Axen K, Pineda H, Shunfenthal I, Haas F 1985 Diaphragmatic function following cervical cord injury: neurally mediated improvement. Archives of Physical Medicine and Rehabilitation 66: 219–222

Bach JR 1993 Mechanical insufflation-exsufflation: comparison of peak expiratory flows with manually assisted and unassisted coughing techniques. Chest 104: 1553–1562

Bach JR, McDermott IG 1990 Strapless oral-nasal interface for positive-pressure ventilation. Archives of Physical Medicine and Rehabilitation 71 (11): 910–913

Bach JR, Smith WH, Michaels J, Saporito L, Alba AS, Pan J 1993 Airway secretion clearance by mechanical exsufflation for poliomyelitis ventilator-assisted individuals. Archives of Physical Medicine and Rehabilitation 74 (2): 170–177

Bott J, Keilty SJ, Noone L 1992 Intermittent positive pressure breathing – a dying art? Physiotherapy 78 (9): 656–660

Bromley I 1998 Tetraplegia and paraplegia. A guide for physiotherapists, 5th edn. Churchill Livingstone, Edinburgh

Carroll P 1994 Safe suctioning. Registered Nurse. 57 (5): 32–36

Carter RE,. 1993. Experience with ventilator dependent patients. Paraplegia 31: 150–153.

Chen C, Lien I, Wu M 1990 Respiratory function in patients with spinal cord injuries: effects of posture. Paraplegia 28: 81–86

Cohn JR 1993 Pulmonary management of the patient with spinal cord injury. Trauma Quarterly 9(2): 65–71

Cull C, Inwood H 1999 Weaning patients from mechanical ventilation. Professional Nurse 14 (8): 535–538

De Troyer A, Estenne M 1991 Review article: the expiratory muscles in tetraplegia. Paraplegia 29: 359–363

De Troyer A, Heilporn A 1980 Respiratory mechanics in quadriplegia. The respiratory function of the intercostal muscles. American Review of Respiratory Disease 122: 591–600

Dean B 1997 Evidence-based suction management in accident and emergency: a vital component of airway care. Accident and Emergency Nursing 5: 92–97

DeVivo MJ, Stuart Kraus PHJ, Lammertse DP 1999 Recent trends in mortality and causes of death among persons with spinal cord injury. Archives of Physical Medicine and Rehabilitation 80: 1411–1419

DiMarco AF 1999 Diaphragm pacing in patients with spinal cord injury. Topics in Spinal Cord Injury Rehabilitation 5(1): 6–20

Fishburn MJ, Marino RJ, Ditunno JF 1990 Atelectasis and pneumonia in acute spinal cord injury. Archives of Physical Medicine and Rehabilitation 71: 197–200

Frankel HL, Coll JR, Charlifue SW et al 1998 Long term survival in spinal cord injury: a fifty year investigation. Spinal Cord 36 (12): 868–869

Fromm B, Hundt G, Gerner HJ et al 1999 Management of respiratory problems unique to high tetraplegia. Spinal Cord 37: 239–244

Gardner B, Theocleous F, Watt J, Krishnan K 1985 Ventilation or dignified death for patients with high tetraplegia. British Medical Journal 291: 1620–1622

Glass CA, Grap MJ 1995 Ten tips for safer suctioning. American Journal of Nursing 5: 51–53

Goldman J, Rose L, Williams S, Silver J, Denison D 1986 Effect of abdominal binders on breathing in tetraplegic patients. Thorax 41: 940–945

Gouden P 1997 Static respiratory pressures in patients with post-traumatic tetraplegia. Spinal Cord 35: 43–47

Grundy D, Swain A 1996 ABC of spinal cord injury, 3rd edn. BMJ Books, London

Gupta A, McClelland M, Evans A, El Masri W 1989 Minitracheostomy in the early respiratory management of patients with spinal cord injury. Paraplegia 27: 269–277

Kannan S 1999 Practical issues in non-invasive positive pressure ventilation. Care of the Critically Ill 15 (3): 76–79

Keilty SEJ, Bott J 1992 Continuous positive airways pressure. Physiotherapy 78 (2): 90–92

Lanig IS, Peterson WP 2000 The respiratory system in spinal cord injury. Physical Medicine and Rehabilitation Clinics of North America 11 (1): 29–43

Ledsome J, Sharp J 1981 Pulmonary function in acute cervical cord injury. American Review of Respiratory Disease 124: 41–44

Liaw MY, Lin MC, Cheng PT, Wong MKA, Tang FT 2000 Resistive inspiratory muscle training: its effectiveness in patients with acute complete cervical cord injury. Archives of Physical Medicine and Rehabilitation 81: 752–756

Linn WM, Adkins RH, Gong H, Waters RL 2000 Pulmonary function in chronic spinal cord injury: a cross-sectional survey of 222 Southern California adult outpatients. Archives of Physical Medicine and Rehabilitation 81: 757–763

Lucke KT 1998 Pulmonary management following acute SCI. Journal of Neuroscience Nursing 30 (2): 91–103

Mansel J, Norman J 1990 Respiratory complications and management of spinal cord injuries. Chest 97(6): 1446–1452

Maynard F, Muth A 1987 The choice to end life as a ventilator dependent quadriplegia. Archives of Physical and Medical Rehabilitation 68: 862–864

McCool FD, Pichurko BM, Slutsky AS, Sarkarati M, Rossier A, Brown R 1986 Changes in lung volume and rib configuration with abdominal binding in quadriplegia. Journal of Applied Physiology 60 (4): 1198–1202

McKinley WO 1996 Late return of diaphragm function in a ventilator–dependent patient with a high tetraplegia: case report, and interactive review. Spinal Cord 34: 626–629

Menter RR, Bach JR, Brown DJ, Gutteridge G, Watt J 1997 A review of the respiratory management of a patient with high level tetraplegia. Spinal Cord 35: 805–808

Oo T, Watt J, Soni BM, Sett PK 1999 Delayed diaphragm recovery in 12 patients after high cervical spinal cord injury. A retrospective review of the diaphragm status of 107 patients ventilated after acute spinal cord injury. Spinal Cord 37: 117–122

Peterson W, Charlifue MA, Gerhart A, Whiteneck G 1994 Two methods of weaning persons with quadriplegia from mechanical ventilators. Paraplegia 32: 98–103

Peterson W, Barbalata L, Brooks CA, Gerhart KA, Mellick DC, Whiteneck GG 1999 The effect of tidal volumes on the time to wean persons with high tetraplegia from ventilators. Spinal Cord 37: 284–288

Pryor JA 1999 Physiotherapy for airway clearance in adults. European Respiratory Journal 14 (6): 1418–1424

Purtilo R 1986 Ethical issues in the treatment of chronic ventilator dependent patients. Archives of Physical and Medical Rehabilitation 67: 718–721

Rose L, Geary M, Jackson J, Morgan M 1987 The effect of lung volume expansion in tetraplegia. Physiotherapy Practice 3: 163–167

Roth EJ, Lu A, Primack S, Oken J, Nussbaum S, Berkowitz M, Powley S 1997 Ventilatory function in cervical and high thoracic spinal cord injury. American Journal of Physical Medicine & Rehabilitation 76 (4): 262–267

Scott MD, Frost F, Supinski G, Gonzalez M 1993 The effect of body position and abdominal binders in chronic tetraplegic subjects more than 15 years post injury. Journal of the American Paraplegia Society 16 (2): 117

Stanic U, Kandare F, Jaeger R, Sorli J 2000 Functional electrical stimulation of abdominal muscles to augment tidal volume in spinal cord injury. IEEE Transactions on Rehabilitation Engineering 8 (1): 30–34

Stiller K, Huff N 1999 Respiratory muscle training for tetraplegic patients: a literature review. Australian Journal of Physiotherapy 45: 291–299

Thomas E, Paulson SS 1994 Protocol for weaning the SCI patient. SCI Nursing 11 (2): 42–45

Tromans AM, Mecci M, Barrett FH, Ward TA, Grundy DJ 1998 The use of the BiPAP biphasic positive airway pressure system in acute spinal cord injury. Spinal Cord 36: 481–484

Tzeng AC, Bach JR 2000 Prevention of pulmonary morbidity for patients with neuromuscular disease. Chest 118 (5): 1390–1396

Uijl SG, Houtman S, Folgering HTM, Hopman MTE 1999 Training of the respiratory muscles in individuals with tetraplegia. Spinal Cord 37: 575–579

Van Buren R, Lemons MD, Franklin C, Wagner MD Jr 1994 Respiratory complications after cervical spinal cord injury. Spine 19 (20): 2315–2320

Wang AY, Jaeger RJ, Yarkony GM, Turba RM 1997 Cough in spinal cord injured patients: the relationship between motor level and peak expiratory flow. Spinal Cord 35: 299–302

Wicks A, Menter R 1986 Long-term outlook in quadriplegic patients with initial ventilator dependency. Chest 3: 406–410

Yeo JD, Walsh J, Rutkowski S, Soden R, Craven M, Middleton J 1998 Mortality following spinal cord injury. Spinal Cord 36: 329–336

18

Care of the dying patient

Wendy Burford   Stephen J Barton
Mandy Bryon

INTRODUCTION

Palliative care is the essence of care for many people with respiratory conditions because so many of these diseases are disabling and incurable.

The palliative care approach aims to promote both physical and psychosocial well being. It is a vital and integral part of all clinical practice, whatever the illness or its stage, informed by a knowledge and practice of palliative care principles. The key principles underpinning palliative care which should be practised by all health care professionals in primary care, hospital and other settings comprise:

• focus on quality of life which includes good symptom control
• whole-person approach taking into account the person's past life experience and current situation
• care which encompasses both the dying person and those who matter to that person
• respect for patient autonomy and choice (e.g. over place of death, treatment options)
• emphasis on open and sensitive communication, which extends to patients, informal carers and professional colleagues. (National Council for Hospice and Specialist Palliative Care Services 1995).

It is to be emphasized that it is the disease itself which is terminal and not the patient; because the disease is in the terminal phase this does not mean the withdrawal of appropriate treatment. In 1992 the Standing Medical Advisory Committee and Standard Nursing and Midwifery Advisory Committee recommended that all patients requiring palliative care services should have access to them and that they should be developed as for patients with terminal cancer. To maintain contact with the patient, by a short visit, when it is no longer appropriate to continue active interventions is important to the patient, carer and physiotherapist.

Throughout the disease process it is important to maintain an holistic approach; the physical symptoms are often glaringly obvious but other components are often forgotten by the professionals. Good symptom control takes into account the physical, social, psychological and spiritual aspects affecting both the patient and those caring for him (Fig. 18.1).

PSYCHOLOGICAL FACTORS

The psychological factors of the disease process reverberate around the patient, relatives and the staff involved. For both the patient and the carer the grieving process begins with the diagnosis of a life-threatening condition. The patient anticipates lack of function and the thought of leaving the family: 'How will they cope without me?'. The family tree (Fig. 18.2) can be used to show who is important to the patient and if they have faced a significant loss before.

It is important to recognize that an understanding of the psychological aspects of dying is as important as the understanding of the physiological changes that are occurring within the dying patient.

When a patient and the family have been given the diagnosis of a terminal illness and learn that the emphasis of treatment will now be aimed at palliative care and the effective control of symptoms, to allow for quality of life instead of a cure, the grieving process begins.

Effective care of the dying patient lies in the ability of the different members of the healthcare team to understand the problems faced by each individual patient and family and then to initiate the appropriate actions.

The stages of the grieving process have been described (Worden 1982) and these apply both to the individual facing up to their own inevitable death and to the loved ones who are bereaved. It is now known, however, that there is not a set

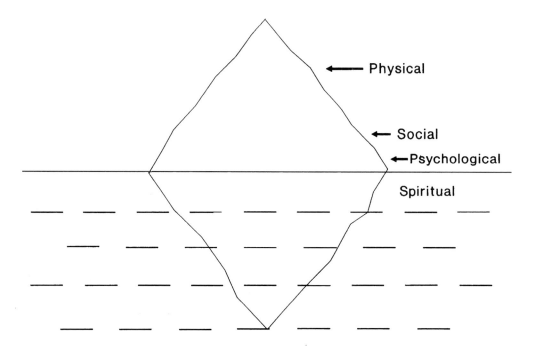

Fig. 18.1 An 'iceberg' demonstrates how healthcare professionals perceive the physical, social, psychological and spiritual needs of patients.

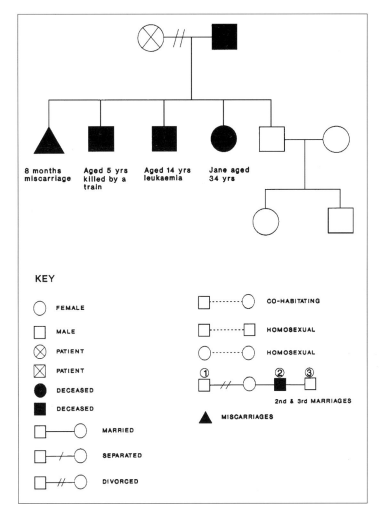

Fig. 18.2   A family tree.

grieving process that a person goes through. Instead, the stages are best viewed as a list of possible emotions to do with death and dying. It is likely that some of these emotions will be experienced in any order and, for the bereaved individuals, intermittently for a considerable length of time after the loss.

The list of 'stages' has been found useful for the professional in recognizing or anticipating what dying or bereaved people may be going through. Additionally, it is often useful to be able to reassure the bereaved that their reactions are normal and expected. For this reason the conven-

tional stages of the grief process are described as follows (see Fig. 18.3).

Denial

After the initial shock that the patient has a terminal illness, the denial phase begins. 'There must be some mistake', 'They don't really mean me' or 'They must have someone else's results'. This behaviour continues in the hope that if it is denied long enough the illness will eventually go away or the result will change. It is a coping mechanism used to protect the individual from

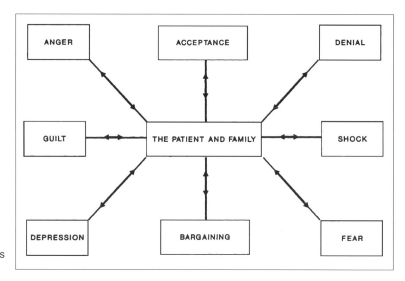

Fig. 18.3 The psychological components of terminal care.

something unpleasant. It is hard to accept the news of a terminal disease if one has a sense of well-being and one's physical condition is not yet compromised by symptoms. For example, some newly diagnosed lung cancer patients present to their general practitioners with a cough that is not resolving or responding to conventional antibiotic therapy. The chest radiograph shows a mass and subsequent fibreoptic bronchoscopy confirms that there is a tumour present. Cytology confirms small cell (oat cell) lung cancer. It is even harder for patients to accept that without treatment their life expectancy is approximately 3 months and with treatment probably between 12 and 18 months, especially if they are still able to lead a near-normal lifestyle.

Shock

No matter how much preparation is given before confirmation of bad news, it can still surprise and shock when given. The two most common reactions seen in hospital are the hysterical and inconsolable or the numbing and emotionless response. Of these two responses the hysterical reaction is often the easier to deal with, once the patient and family are through the initial stage. Working with them, it is possible to build up a relationship of mutual trust and respect and to help them come to terms with the future and what it may hold.

With the latter response, it may be impossible to help patients until they have let down the barriers that they are using to protect themselves. It will inevitably be a long process trying to win the patient's and relatives' confidence and so helping them face up to the future.

Anger

Anger may be felt by many people during the terminal phases of a person's life, varying from the patient to the immediate members of the family. Their reactions will be as diverse as their reasons for trying to understand what is happening.

The patient or relatives may initially become angry with the doctor or nurse when informed of the diagnosis and although this anger is directed at them, it should not be taken personally. It is usually an automatic response when given information that one cannot cope with. It may also be an aspect of some people's coping ability that they have to retaliate when faced with a situation that is alien to them. Often patients become angry and frustrated as the illness progresses, owing to a loss of their physical ability and independence, becoming more dependent on the carer either in the home or in hospital. It is therefore very important that both the patient and carer should be involved in all decisions made with regard to medical and nursing management which helps to maintain their autonomy.

The family may become angry and highly critical of the treatment and care being offered to their loved one. This anger may be a result of their own feelings of guilt and inadequacy and inability to cope with the fact that their partner is actually going to die and leave them alone and it is this fear that is presenting itself as anger.

Many parents when faced with the death of their child will initially respond with anger – anger at God for allowing this to happen, anger at the medical profession for not doing enough to help and anger at each other for allowing this to happen by not caring enough.

Guilt

Guilt is an emotion common to all involved in the life of a terminally ill patient. The patients themselves may feel a sense of guilt for becoming a burden on their family. The burden may be physical because they are no longer able to look after themselves or it may be financial, especially if they are the main breadwinner of the family. They may have feelings of guilt that they will eventually be leaving their partner to cope alone after they have gone.

The carers will often feel guilty if they are unable to cope with the patient in the community and hospital admission is required. They often see this as letting their loved one down. There may also be feelings of guilt on the part of the family that they are being left behind and will have to cope.

Depression

Depression is the emotion that everyone expects to see at some time in someone faced with the prospect of dying. Depression can present in different forms and has many components that need to be considered. These vary from feelings of melancholia and somatic complaints to feelings of deep despair and suicidal tendencies.

The more common symptoms are changes in behaviour, with the person becoming withdrawn, having reduced concentration, loss of interest and increased irritability; for example,

laughter and the noise of children are no longer welcomed with a tolerant smile but arouse irritation and frustration. There may be changes in the sleep pattern which consist of early morning waking rather than difficulty in getting off to sleep. This can lead to insomnia which is highly resistant to hypnotics and, although the answer lies in treatment of the underlying depression, the patient and the family cannot see this and often demand more powerful drugs.

Changes in appetite are commonly associated with depression and in mild cases compulsive eating may be witnessed. Generally appetite is diminished and weight loss is more common and in severe cases it can be dramatic.

Somatic complaints are multiple and include the common tension symptoms, such as pain in the head, back and neck. The tension can manifest itself locally or can be very generalized.

Fear

Fear is a natural component of terminal care and the uncertainty that people face. It may only be a temporary feeling or it can remain with the patient and family until the end. Usually this feeling can be overcome by a little thought on the part of the doctor and the nurse. Quite often a simple explanation of any procedures that are about to be performed will suffice to reassure the patient and carer. Honest and realistic answers to any of their questions will help reassure the patient and reinforce what is happening and what to expect.

Bargaining

Bargaining is a mental process that many people will experience when faced with a terminal disease; for example, the patient with lung cancer who promises to give up smoking if it will buy more time. This process is often associated with feelings of guilt and will be faced by both the patient and the family.

Acceptance

Acceptance is the coming to terms with the grieving or bereavement process; it is the resolution of one's emotions or the resolving of conflicts. It is only when this phase is reached that patients can be at peace with themselves, accepting and preparing for a death with dignity. To allow for this to happen, all components have to be equal and when this equilibrium between physical symptoms and psychological state is balanced, then a peaceful death can follow. Acceptance of the death may never be reached by some bereaved people. For some there is more likely to be an adaptation to life without loved ones. The periods of time between feelings of acute distress get longer and there is the reassuring knowledge from experience that despair will resolve to something more manageable. Adaptation can be said to have been reached when the bereaved person can participate in daily activities with enjoyment. Many bereaved individuals report, however, that feelings of loss and longing recur intermittently for many years.

PHYSICAL FACTORS

Respiratory conditions which physiotherapists may see in the terminal care stage include lung cancer, cystic fibrosis, emphysema and cryptogenic fibrosing alveolitis. The period between the time of diagnosis of a terminal condition and the stage of terminal care varies from years to several weeks. Most patients with cystic fibrosis will have lived with the knowledge that their life expectancy is limited, but for patients with lung cancer the diagnosis will probably be a shock to them and to their families.

There are different types of lung cancer and these include squamous cell carcinoma, adenocarcinoma, large cell and small cell carcinoma. Half of the lung cancers arise peripherally but the others are situated more centrally, proximal to a segmental bronchus and are less often resectable. The cell type will be identified by histological or cytological investigation and will influence the treatment the patient will receive. Of all cases presenting, only about 25% are suitable for surgery. The majority of patients who develop lung cancer have a relatively poor prognosis (Mountain 1986). The median survival time after diagnosis is less than 4 months and about 80% of patients die within 1 year (NHS Executive 1998).

Psychologically, patients who are found to have an inoperable tumour may find it difficult to accept that no 'active' treatment is offered whilst they remain asymptomatic. Radiotherapy in the treatment of lung cancer is primarily palliative but is reserved for the control of symptoms; that is, haemoptysis, bone pain or nerve pain, superior vena caval obstruction, breathlessness (intraluminal radiotherapy), dysphagia, cough, spinal cord compression, lymphangitis and cerebral metastases. It may be possible to relieve the patient's symptoms of breathlessness and stridor by the use of laser treatment if the tumour is visible and accessible through bronchoscopy. With small cell (oat cell) carcinoma there is usually evidence of disease elsewhere in the body at the time of diagnosis which therefore excludes surgery. The overall prognosis is very poor but the tumour does respond for a time to chemotherapy and/or radiotherapy.

Symptom control in lung cancer

Pain

Pain is the symptom most feared by both the patient and carer and once a diagnosis of cancer is made physical pain is the symptom which they all anticipate, although one-third of patients with cancer do not experience any physical pain (Twycross & Lack 1990).

Pain is influenced by physical, social, psychological and spiritual attitudes. Pain is whatever the patient says it is. It is individual and is affected by the patient's previous experience of pain and there are racial and cultural differences. Patients often fear the process of dying rather than death itself and it is important to emphasize that measures can be taken to control physical pain in the majority of patients.

Analgesics should be given on a regular basis; there is no place for 'as required' analgesia in the situation of chronic pain. The aim is to ensure that the patient is pain free and this can only be achieved by the regular administration of drugs, often in combination. Pain should be assessed regularly and adjustments made to the analgesia.

It is important to gain patients' trust and confidence and to restore their sense of worth, well-being and self-esteem, thereby enabling them to feel more relaxed. Some patients find this by utilizing complementary therapies, for example aromatherapy, reflexology, gentle massage and relaxation techniques (possibly including a relaxation tape). Time spent with patients allaying their fears will often enable a reduction in the amount of analgesia required.

Bone pain. This is usually the result of metastatic deposits (which may present as a pathological fracture and may require surgery). Radiotherapy as a single treatment is often very beneficial for bone pain. A non-steroidal antiinflammatory agent combined with an opiate drug may control the pain. Bone pain related to hypercalcaemia may respond when a bisphosphonate is administered (Bower & Coombes 1993).

Nerve pain. This is caused by the invasion or destruction of nerve fibres, for example by superior sulcus tumours (Pancoast tumour). These tumours grow in the apex of the lung and invade the brachial plexus. Mesotheliomas are tumours usually occurring in patients who have had exposure to asbestos. They grow in the pleura and cause intractable chest wall nerve pain.

Nerve pain can be difficult to control and is often opiate resistant. Drugs which may be helpful are tricyclic agents, anticonvulsants, corticosteroids and local anaesthetic congener drugs such as flecainide. Nerve blocks may be attempted and transcutaneous electrical nerve stimulation may bring some relief to this type of pain.

Liver pain. This is caused by metastases invading the liver capsule. This pain responds to corticosteroids.

Headaches. These may be caused by raised intracranial pressure from cerebral metastases. Corticosteroids and cranial irradiation will relieve this symptom.

Muscle spasm. This may be experienced following convulsions if the patient has cerebral metastases. Muscle relaxants (benzodiazepines) may be administered.

Drugs for the control of chronic pain must be given regularly (Fig. 18.4):

● mild analgesics (non-opioid) – aspirin, other non-steroidal anti-inflammatory drugs (NSAIDs), paracetamol

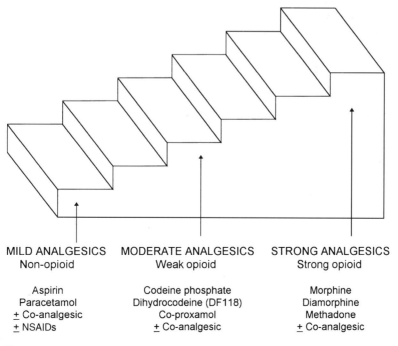

MILD ANALGESICS	MODERATE ANALGESICS	STRONG ANALGESICS
Non-opioid	Weak opioid	Strong opioid
Aspirin	Codeine phosphate	Morphine
Paracetamol	Dihydrocodeine (DF118)	Diamorphine
± Co-analgesic	Co-proxamol	Methadone
± NSAIDs	± Co-analgesic	± Co-analgesic

Fig. 18.4 The analgesic ladder.

- moderate analgesics (weak opioid) – codeine phosphate, dihydrocodeine (DF 118), co-proxamol
- strong analgesics (strong opioid) – morphine, diamorphine, methadone.

At all levels co-analgesics may be used for specific symptoms. There is no minimum or maximum amount of opiate which can be given. The advent of the syringe driver, which delivers a controlled regular amount of drug, has made it possible for many patients with terminal illness to be nursed at home until their death.

Other types of analgesia to be considered include fentanyl (Durogesic®) transdermal patches. For patients whose pain is non-morphine receptive, methadone, oxycodone and hydromorphone may be used as an alternative.

Nausea

Nausea may be a side effect of chemotherapy or a result of the administration of opiates. It may also be caused by severe constipation, electrolyte imbalance or a raised intracranial pressure. Some patients obtain relief of nausea from antiemetic drugs and steroids. Dexamethasone may help to reduce a raised intracranial pressure. (Cold fizzy drinks, e.g. ginger ale, may be tolerated by the nauseated patient.)

Breathlessness

Positioning the patient plays a very important part and the high side lying position can be of great assistance to the breathless patient (see Fig. 6.12, p. 183). Many patients prefer sitting upright in an armchair and may wish to sleep in the armchair at night. Some find resting on a pillow across a small table helpful (see Fig. 6.16, p. 186).

Oxygen therapy may be necessary for patients with coexisting respiratory or cardiac conditions and patients with lymphangitis carcinomatosis or stridor or if they are continuously dyspnoeic. However, for many patients with lung cancer oxygen therapy is usually of no value, except psychologically for the patient with terminal malignant disease, and sets up yet another physical barrier between patients and their family/carer.

Occasionally when a tumour is causing tracheal obstruction, heliox, a mixture of helium (79%) and oxygen (21%), is used to relieve respiratory distress (p. 226).

Opiate drugs can be helpful in the relief of breathlessness and may be administered either orally or by subcutaneous infusion. An anxiolytic may be of use, for example diazepam. Nebulized morphine has been shown to relieve breathlessness in some patients with severe chronic lung disease (Young et al 1989).

Superior vena caval obstruction

Superior vena caval obstruction is caused by the spread of a tumour into the mediastinum or by enlarged lymph nodes. Pressure on the superior vena cava leads to oedema in the face, neck and arms. The patient may complain of difficulty breathing, headaches and feeling faint when he bends down. Stridor may be present.

Urgent treatment is necessary and radiotherapy is probably the most effective except for patients with small cell carcinoma who usually respond to chemotherapy. Opiate and corticosteroid drugs may alleviate breathlessness. The head of the bed may be raised in an attempt to reduce the facial oedema during the night.

It may be possible in severe cases of superior vena caval obstruction, following other symptomatic treatment to insert a stent providing there is no evidence of clotting. This will relieve the pressure and dramatically improve the symptoms.

Death rattle

This noise is produced by the movement of secretions in the hypopharynx in association with the inspiratory and expiratory phases of respiration. This is heard in patients who are too weak to expectorate. Repositioning the patient is often effective in reducing the sound, which helps both patient and family. Oropharyngeal suction is unpleasant for the patient, particularly if conscious, and is usually ineffective. Hyoscine may be given by subcutaneous injection. If the patient is unconscious and the syringe driver is being used, the administration of hyoscine subcutaneously is the treatment of choice and can be combined with diamorphine.

Glycopyrronium can be used as an alternative if the patient fails to respond to hyoscine.

Physiotherapy

The physiotherapist may have been involved with the patient throughout his illness and there will be a stage when most physical treatment techniques are inappropriate, but it is important that the physiotherapist maintains contact with both the patient and the family during the terminal stages. Positioning the patient for comfort and relief of breathlessness and assisting the patient to clear a plug of sputum may be beneficial. Even if the physiotherapist feels she is achieving very little, the patient would feel abandoned if her visits stopped.

SOCIAL FACTORS

Social factors affect the total well-being of the patient. The patient may be concerned about his inability to work and the financial implications which may affect the whole family. This can cause depression and it is important that the patient is aware of the social benefits to which he is entitled. Industrial claims can be instigated if it is an industry-related disease, for example mesothelioma. A social worker should be available and good communication among the multiprofessional team will lead to more effective treatment.

The patient may fear rejection by family, friends and colleagues and this may lead to social isolation. As the disease progresses the patient experiences a loss of libido and those who have received cytotoxic chemotherapy become sterile. This has implications for family life.

The control of symptoms enables a more socially acceptable lifestyle. Family and friends should be included in the decision making and care of the patient both at home and during hospitalization. This helps the carers to cope when death occurs.

SPIRITUAL CARE

To help a patient attain or maintain peace of mind it is important to be aware that the patient's personal value system may have been shaken as a result of the illness. 'It may be that the person's concept of God or his understanding of the spiritual dimensions of his life are stunted; that religious ceremonies are neither meaningful, nor supportive, nor a source of strength to him' (Kitson 1985).

Sensitive listening may enable the patient to express his fears, hopes and conflicts. The lack of a firm commitment to a religion does not mean that the patient does not have spiritual requirements. Religious practices should be observed and patients and families are usually happy to explain practices which are unfamiliar to members of the multiprofessional team of carers. Ministers and religious leaders should be available.

RESPONDING TO THE DYING PATIENT AND HIS RELATIVES

It is important to be natural and to spend time with the dying patient. You do not have to talk all the time, but give the patient an opportunity to express his fears and anxieties. Patients often ask questions which are uncomfortable to answer.

Having discussed the diagnosis and prognosis with the patient and their relatives it is essential that their wishes regarding their cardiopulmonary resuscitation status is established.

Am I going to die? The patient will put this question to the person he trusts and an honest reply is being sought. The response 'Do you think you are?' gives the patient the chance to vocalize his fears and opens up an opportunity for you to say 'Yes, but I don't know when' and to ask him if he is afraid. Many patients say that they are not afraid of death but of the process of dying.

When am I going to die? This is always difficult because we cannot predict the answer. We can say 'Yes, you are very sick but we do not know when you are going to die'.

All questions should be handled very sensitively. Sit with the patient and do not rush away. It is not appropriate to tell patients not to worry but listen to their fears and anxieties. You cannot say that you know how they are feeling because we all have individual ways of coping.

Tell the nurse who is looking after the patient about the type of questions you have been asked. Return to the patient later in the day as this will allow him to ask you more questions if he wishes and shows that you are offering him support at a difficult time.

How am I going to die? This is a question frequently asked by dying patients. Always be honest. Ask the patient how he feels he might die. This allows him to express his fears. Many breathless patients lie awake at night, afraid to go to sleep in case they do not wake up. It is often the fear of dying alone, without anyone noticing, that keeps them awake. During the day there are people around. Breathless patients need reassurance that they are not going to suffocate and that drugs can be given to relieve symptoms.

If good symptom control is maintained the patient should die quite peacefully.

The dying child

Communicating with a dying child about their death is a daunting task for professionals and the family. Unfortunately, this often means that a child dies without having had the opportunity to express their fears or receive emotional comfort. Patients and other family members report being plagued by regrets following the child's death because they didn't say something important. The management of the terminal phase of childhood illness has a dramatic effect on the psychological recovery of the family following the death (Whittam 1993). Though it is a difficult time, the family should have the opportunity for support and, importantly, the dying child should have the option of speaking to someone about their experience.

Parents frequently report their fears that if their child knows they are dying then they will give up hope. However, most children know what is happening and keep silent because they don't want to upset their parents. There is often a mutual avoidance of the subject (Bluebond-Langer 1978). When parents and other family members have been helped to speak to their children they often find this gives them a role and lessens their feelings of helplessness. Speaking to a child about your understanding of death and dying is not very different to the way you would speak to an adult; the approach and questions are the same although the words the child uses may be simpler. Some children may have a naïve view of what is happening or may refer to heaven and angels; before any of this is challenged, it is essential to speak to the parents and respect their views and wishes.

How to approach relatives before and after a death

The relatives should be kept informed of the patient's deteriorating condition and should be encouraged to participate in the care of the patient as much as they wish. In stressful situations we all behave differently and it is important to allow relatives to express their worries and fears. Many adults have never seen anyone die except on films or television where death is often portrayed as being frightening.

The staff should explain to the relatives how they think a patient will die, that the breathing will get slower and eventually stop. Following the patient's death the relatives should have the opportunity to stay with the patient until they feel ready to leave.

It is important to acknowledge what has happened. This may be verbally by saying how sorry you are to hear of the patient's death. Non-verbal communication can be very comforting. A gentle touch on the arm can convey more than a list of platitudes.

The actual death of a loved one, no matter how prepared or how expected, is always traumatic. There is a powerful physical and emotional reaction which can last for days and relatives often panic that they will never recover. Reassuring support is required and often just a presence. It is useful to remember that there is very little that can be said that is helpful and simple platitudes should be avoided. There are some self-help publications which can also be used to guide staff input, e.g. *Dying, death and bereavement* (Cystic Fibrosis Trust 2000).

There are a few common reactions in this 'acute' phase immediately following the death. First, many relatives spend hours trying to think of something that could have been done to avoid the death. This is a result of the shock and disbelief which occur following bereavement. Some relatives need to spend time with staff discussing the medical management and sometimes this develops into a need to find someone to blame. It is important that this is taken seriously and the relatives should not feel patronized, but they can be helped to see that probably nothing could have been done differently.

Second, there is a variation in the ways that mothers and fathers grieve (Schwab 1996). Mothers tend to experience a wider range of emotions than fathers and frequently flit between emotional states. Fathers, however, tend to have one stable emotional reaction but find it more difficult than mothers to express their feelings so consequently become more isolated. This gender differential should be recognized by staff as family members may accuse each other of failing to be supportive when in fact they were mismatched in their emotional reactions at the time.

Finally, all families eventually learn to live with their loss. They will never get over it and that should not be their aim. Relatives can instead be helped to live with their memories, to highlight the positives about the life of their loved one.

Support for staff

Staff need the opportunity to talk through the problems they are experiencing when working with the dying patient. This helps the individual to cope with their feelings and physiotherapists should be sensitive to these needs. It is particularly difficult when patients are young or in the same age group as the professional.

Many dilemmas have arisen for staff working with patients who are terminally ill but awaiting transplantation. When the patient's physical condition is deteriorating, what would normally be considered appropriate management may be withheld in anticipation of donor organs becoming available.

It is important that the patient is able to live until he dies. 'We cannot judge a biography by its length, by the number of pages in it; we must judge by the richness of the contents... Sometimes the "unfinisheds" are among the most beautiful symphonies' (Frankl 1964).

REFERENCES

Bluebond-Langer M 1978 Mutual pretence: causes and consequences. In: The private lives of dying children. Guilford, Princeton, pp 210–230.

Bower M, Coombes RC 1993 Endocrine and metabolic complications of advanced cancer. In: Doyle D, Hanks GWC, MacDonald N (eds) Oxford textbook of palliative medicine. Oxford University Press, Oxford, p 449

Cystic Fibrosis Trust 2000 Dying, death and bereavement: help for all the family when someone is dying or dies from cystic fibrosis. Cystic Fibrosis Trust, Bromley

Frankl V 1964 Man's search for meaning. Hodder and Stoughton, London

Kitson A 1985 Spiritual care in chronic illness. In: McGilloway O, Myco F (eds) Nursing and spiritual care. Harper and Row, London, p 145

Mountain CF 1986 A new international staging system for lung cancer. Chest 89: 225S–233S

National Council for Hospice and Specialist Palliative Care Services 1995 Specialist palliative care, a statement of definitions. Occasional Paper 8, section 4.3, NCHSPCS, London, p 6

NHS Executive 1998 Improving outcomes in lung cancer. Department of Health, London, p 11

Schwab R 1996 Gender differences in parental grief. Death Studies 20: 103–113

Standing Medical Advisory Committee and Standing Nursing and Midwifery Advisory Committee Joint Report 1992 The principles and provision of palliative care. HMSO, London, p 27

Twycross R, Lack S 1990 Therapeutics in terminal cancer, 2nd edn. Churchill Livingstone, Edinburgh, p 11

Whittam EH 1993 Terminal care of the dying child, Psychosocial implications of care. Cancer 71: 3450–3462

Worden WJ 1982 Grief counseling and grief therapy. Cambridge University Press, Cambridge

Young I, Daviskas E, Keena VA 1989 Effect of low dose nebulised morphine on exercise endurance in patients with chronic lung disease. Thorax 44: 387–390

FURTHER READING

Buckman R 1988 I don't know what to say. Papermac, London

Doyle D, Hanks GWC, MacDonald N (eds) 1993 Oxford textbook of palliative medicine. Oxford University Press, Oxford

Hoogstraten B, Addis BJ, Hansen H et al (eds) 1988 Lung tumours. Springer-Verlag, Berlin

Kübler Ross E 1970 On death and dying. Macmillan, New York

Lugton J 1987 Communicating with dying people and their relatives. Austen Cornish/Lisa Sainsbury Foundation, London

McGilloway O, Myco F (eds) 1985 Nursing and spiritual care. Harper and Row, London

Murray Parkes C 1986 Bereavement studies of grief in adult life, 2nd edn. Penguin, Harmondsworth

Souhami R, Tobias J 1986 Cancer and its management. Blackwell Science, Oxford

19

Hyperventilation

Diana M Innocenti

INTRODUCTION

Hyperventilation is a 'physiological response to abnormally increased respiratory "drive" which can be caused by a wide range of organic, psychiatric and physiological disorders, or a combination of these' (Gardner & Bass 1989). It is a state of breathing in excess of metabolic requirements resulting in a lowering of the alveolar partial pressure of carbon dioxide ($PACO_2$), the arterial partial pressure of carbon dioxide ($PaCO_2$) and respiratory alkalosis. 'Hyperventilation', in its strictly physiological sense, is synonymous with 'hypocapnia'.

Acute hyperventilation is a normal physiological response to stress and may result in self-regulating paraesthesia, dizziness and palpitations and, in extreme cases, tetany. The disorder of chronic hyperventilation is a condition characterized by the spontaneous occurrence of multiple and often alarming somatic symptoms associated with anxiety. In 1937 Kerr et al described a group of patients who, in addition to their anxious tensional state, presented with 'a variety of symptoms referable to many structures in the body; and in whom hyperventilation precipitates and maintains a state of hyperirritability'. In the table of the laboratory work they coined the term 'hyperventilation syndrome' (Kerr et al 1937). A syndrome is, by definition, identified by its combination of symptoms and is therefore not able to be contained within a single diagnostic measurement. The difficulty regarding the understanding of the various mechanisms producing the symptoms, of finding a definitive form of diagnostic test and agreeing a more appropriate name for this disorder, has created some discussion in the recent literature (Gardner 2000, Hornsveld et al 1996, Howell 1997, Malmberg et al 2000, Troosters et al 1999). Meanwhile, this more subtle form of chronically disturbed breathing, referred to as the hyperventilation syndrome (HVS), can be recognized clinically as a constellation of continuous or intermittent symptoms and physiological changes with or without recognizable provocative stresses (Magarian 1982) or known aetiology.

The diagnosis was not uncommon in the past (Baker 1934, Wood 1941) but in the present technological era, hyperventilation in its various chronic recurrent forms often tends to go unrecognized and the diverse symptoms are labelled as functional. Even though it has been shown that severe chronic hyperventilation with profound hypocapnia can be present in the absence of psychiatric, respiratory or other organic abnormalities (Bass & Gardner 1985), patients may attend a succession of clinics, presenting with increasingly disturbing symptoms, and yet receive little help. The new anxiety aroused by the situation increases the hyperventilation–anxiety spiral which is already in operation. The spiral may be perpetuated by physiological and/or psychological causes, setting up conditioned reflexes of new and incorrect habitual patterns of breathing and a re-setting, or loss of fine tuning, of the respiratory centre's trigger mechanisms (Fig. 19.1).

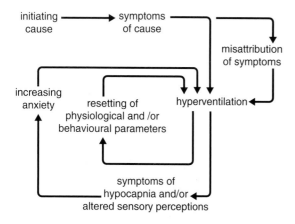

Fig. 19.1 Factors contributing to the hyperventilation–anxiety spiral.

Today, hyperventilation is more likely to be recognized in association with panic disorders or phobic states because of its causal, consequential or perpetuating relationships (Cowley & Roy-Byrne 1987). Patients presenting with panic disorder or anxiety have been shown to have lower resting levels of carbon dioxide than normal (van den Hout et al,1992) and may demonstrate a greater basilar artery sensitivity in response to hyperventilation than normal (Ball & Shekhar 1997).

SIGNS AND SYMPTOMS

The vast array of commonly reported signs and symptoms can be loosely grouped as they affect different systems (Table 19.1). Some patients present with a constant resting level of hypocapnia and others present with resting levels of carbon dioxide within the normal range. Both groups feel generally unwell and experience 'attacks' featuring a galaxy of symptoms which appear to occur sometimes with no apparent reason. Further hypocapnia may or may not be recorded at these times.

Hypocapnia induces vascular constriction, resulting in decreased blood flow, and as a response to the Bohr effect there is also inhibition of transfer of oxygen from haemoglobin in the circulating blood to the tissue cells. Hypocapnia produces a characteristic range of symptoms and most cerebral, peripheral and cardiac symptoms probably occur as a consequence. Fluctuations in $PaCO_2$ can have a destabilizing effect on the autonomic system resulting in a sympathetic dominance (Freeman & Nixon 1985). The patients are often in a state of arousal. It has been shown that the mean urinary excretion of adrenaline in a group of hyperventilators was three times as high as in a group of normals (Folgering et al 1983). The respiratory alkalosis associated with hyperventilation causes a lowering of calcium ions in the plasma, which precipitates hyperirritability of motor and sensory axons (Macefield & Burke 1991). Altered patterns of breathing can cause musculoskeletal dysfunction with subsequent chest pain, which may be due to intercostal muscle tension, spasm or fatigue,

Table 19.1 Commonly reported signs and symptoms can be loosely grouped into systems

System	Signs and symptoms
Cardiovascular	Palpitation Chest pain (pseudoangina) Peripheral vasoconstriction
Gastrointestinal	Dysphagia Dyspepsia Epigastric pain Diarrhoea
General	Exhaustion Lethargy Weakness Headache Sleep disturbance Excessive sweating Disturbance of concentration and memory
Musculoskeletal	Muscle pains Tremors Involuntary contractions Cramps Tetany (rarely)
Neurological	Paraesthesiae Lack of coordination Dizziness Disturbance of vision and hearing Syncope (rarely)
Respiratory	Breathlessness Difficulty in taking a satisfying breath Excessive sighing Chest pain Bronchospasm
Psychological	Anxiety Panic attacks Phobic states 'Depersonalization'

costochondritis, costosternal or costovertebral joint pain.

Chest pain and the sensation of dyspnoea could be due to the altered sensory responses in the cerebral cortex. It has been suggested that hyperventilation increases circulating histamine, which may be the cause of the high incidence of allergies reported, and that as the cerebral symptoms of hypoglycaemia are similar to those of hypocarbia, the cerebral effects of hyperventilation are highlighted at times of low blood sugar (Lum 1994). In some patients the symptoms seem to precede the event of hypocapnia rather than be a consequence (Hornsveld et al 1996). If symptoms in some patients are not generated by hypocapnia, what other mechanisms could be the cause? Are the symptoms a direct consequence of the disordered movements of overbreathing and their abnormal sensory feedback? Which sensory, motor or behavioural mechanisms could be involved?

CAUSES OF HYPERVENTILATION

There are many circumstances that may stimulate a hyperventilatory response (Box 19.1). Other than HVS being the primary cause of the patient's symptoms, it is not uncommon for chronic hyperventilation to coexist with other conditions and to be a sustaining factor within the complex interaction of a number of physiological, organic and psychological disorders (Gardner 1994). Before embarking on a treatment programme, it is necessary to ensure that the patient has been suitably investigated in order to diagnose any underlying treatable disease or disorder and to recognize any other possible coexisting factors.

Box 19.1 Some causes of hyperventilation

Drugs	Drug ingestion (causing acidosis or respiratory dyskinesia) Alcohol Caffeine Nicotine
Organic disorder	Anaemia Asthma Chronic severe pain Central nervous system disorders Diabetes mellitus Pneumonia Pulmonary embolus Pulmonary oedema (LVF) Recurrent laryngeal nerve paralysis Vestibular disorder
Physiological	Altitude Pyrexia Pregnancy Luteal phase of the menstrual cycle
Psychiatric	Anxiety Depression
Psychological	Anxiety Panic disorders Phobic states

DIAGNOSTIC TESTS

There are no generally accepted measurable diagnostic criteria and it is probably not possible to devise a satisfactory or conclusive diagnostic test for HVS because of the multifactorial effects and complex systemic interactions. Various tests have been described but time has shown that none should be used alone. Each test can be useful when used with other information.

The voluntary hyperventilation provocation test (HVPT)

The voluntary hyperventilation provocation test (HVPT) (Hardonk & Beumer 1979) records end-tidal $PACO_2$ and all symptoms provoked during the test. Using end-tidal $PACO_2$ recordings, the patient is requested to hyperventilate for 3 minutes. If the $PACO_2$ falls by at least 1.33 kPa (10 mmHg) and the rate of recovery is less than two-thirds of the former resting level after 3 minutes, the result is recorded as a positive diagnosis of a hyperventilation syndrome. However, as about a quarter of 'normals' also show this phenomenon, the test in this form is losing favour as an instrument for diagnosis if used alone. Immediately after the voluntary hyperventilation the patient is asked to compare any symptoms provoked during the test with recognized complaints. When two major symptoms are reproduced the HVPT is considered positive. Generally, tingling of fingers and dizziness are not included because these symptoms occur in 'normal' subjects. Sometimes provoked symptoms are new experiences and not related to the patient's complaints. Caution should be exercised on using this test if the patient complains of cardiac symptoms or pseudoangina.

The Nijmegen questionnaire

This was first drawn up as a list of 16 complaints (Box 19.2), chosen by a team of specialists from different disciplines, from 45 clinically relevant symptoms related to hyperventilation syndromes (van Doorn et al 1982). The complaints fall into three categories or dimensions, corresponding with the classic triad of breathing disruption, paraesthesiae and central nervous system effects. The list does not include fatigue or behavioural disturbances. Patients score on a five-point scale from 0–4 (0 = never, 1 = rare, 2 = sometimes, 3 = often, 4 = very often) against each of the 16 listed symptoms and a score over 23 is recognized as positive.

The questionnaire can be useful for physiotherapists to record symptoms and, if used at regular intervals, it could record the changing status in relation to treatment and a final score at discharge could be used as a semi-objective outcome measure. The efficacy of the questionnaire was investigated by comparing patients who hyperventilate with persons who do not. It showed a high ability to differentiate between the two groups (van Dixhoorn & Duivenvoorden 1985) and, although not conclusive, it was recognized that the questionnaire was suitable to be used as a screening instrument in diagnosing HVS when used with additional information. A correlation has been shown between positively rated Nijmegen questionnaire results (score of 24 or more) and positive HVPT results (recognition of at least two major symptoms) (Vansteenkiste et al 1991).

The 'Think test' (Nixon & Freeman 1988)

This provides a patient-specific stimulation which can have an advantage over unspecific

---

Box 19.2 Nijmegen questionnaire: the list of 16 symptoms

- Chest pain
- Feeling tense
- Blurred vision
- Dizzy spells
- Feeling confused
- Faster or deeper breathing
- Short of breath
- Tight feelings in the chest
- Bloated feeling in the stomach
- Tingling fingers
- Unable to breathe deeply
- Stiff fingers or arms
- Tight feelings round the mouth
- Cold hands or feet
- Heart racing (palpitations)
- Feelings of anxiety

challenges in testing for episodic hypocapnia. Approximately 3 minutes after a period of forced voluntary hyperventilation the patient is invited to close the eyes and to think about the circumstances, feelings and sensations surrounding or initiating the experience of symptoms. A fall in $PaCO_2$ greater than 1.33 kPa (10 mmHg) is considered to be significant.

Ambulatory monitoring of transcutaneous $PaCO_2$ ($P_{Tc}CO_2$)
(Pilsbury & Hibbert 1987)

The patient is attached to the transcutaneous monitor and instructed on how to press the 'event button' and in the use of a diary. The 'event button' marks the recording tape and the diary entry records the type of symptoms, severity of symptoms (on a visual analogue scale 0–8), type of activity or non-activity and the extent of the physical exertion (visual analogue scale 0–8).

Breath-holding time

This is a semi-objective measure which generally shows a direct relationship between the maximum breath-holding time and the resting $PaCO_2$ (short breath-holding time is usually associated with a low or unstable resting $PaCO_2$). Breath-holding time tends to increase as the breathing pattern becomes more regular and the $PaCO_2$ rises. If breath-holding time is recorded at regular intervals it could be used as a semi-objective outcome measure.

CONTROL OF BREATHING

Normally breathing takes place without thought or sensation and is controlled by a very complex physiological and psychological feedback system. It is only when breathing becomes disordered in anatomical or physiological parameters that it impinges on the consciousness.

Breathing control (Fig. 19.2) is centred on the rhythm generator and pneumotaxic centre in the medulla and pons. Carbon dioxide and oxygen chemoreceptors, mechanoreceptors in the muscles, joints and lung tissue, emotion,

temperature and vestibular influences all moderate this breathing centre in the brain stem. This sensory feedback may be filtered through and integrated by the reticular formation and limbic autonomic system or be transmitted directly to the breathing centre. Behavioural and voluntary stimuli from the cerebral cortex also feed back to the breathing centre and, in addition, can influence the respiratory muscles directly by bypassing the reflex pathways. Adaptation of any of the components of these neuro-pathways of respiration can influence or concentrate disordered responses, breathing patterns and carbon dioxide levels, resulting in what appears to be a re-setting of the respiratory centre's triggering mechanisms and new conditioned patterns of breathing.

Why are some people more prone to respond to physiological, organic, psychological or environmental stimuli with grossly altered breathing patterns? Why do some people appear to have hypersensitive respiratory control mechanisms? One hypothesis is that the sensitivity of the respiratory centres is personality linked (Clark & Cochrane 1970) and related to mood-state and disposition. Another related hypothesis is that there is an underlying biological and often inherited vulnerability leading to a hypersensitive central nervous 'alarm system'. This is triggered inappropriately, causing the 'fight and flight' response (Cowley & Roy-Byrne 1987).

PATTERNS OF BREATHING

Normal breathing patterns at rest involve an active inspiratory phase and a passive expiratory phase at approximately 8–14 breaths per minute. Naturally, air is drawn in through the nose where it is warmed, moistened and the flow controlled before entering the airways. The body movement is predominantly a gentle swelling of the abdomen on inspiration which reflects the descent of the diaphragm and which returns to rest on expiration. Thoracic movement is minimal at rest and increases on exercise. Rate, size and place of movement change with posture, varying stimuli, disease or dysfunction.

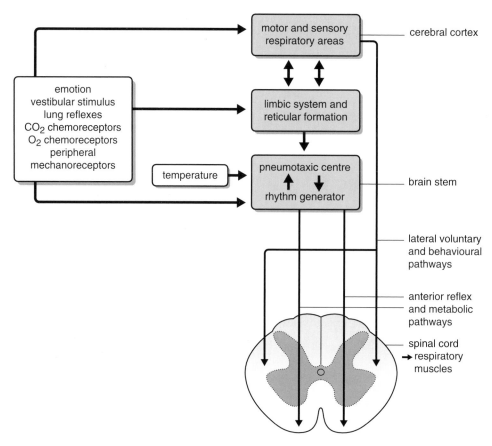

Fig. 19.2 Major pathways involved in the control of breathing.

The breathing patterns related to the chronic hyperventilation syndromes (or idiopathic symptomatic hyperventilation) vary widely from gross upper thoracic movement with sternomastoid action at a rate of 50 breaths/min to a near-normal rate and volume and minimal upper thoracic movement. The degree of lower thoracic movement and abdominal movement also varies from almost nil to normal.

The respiratory rate and volume may be extremely irregular and the pattern interspersed with sighs (Fig. 19.3). At the other extreme, once habitual hypocapnia has been established, it may only require an occasional deep sigh to maintain the new low levels of carbon dioxide and the general breathing pattern may appear normal.

The breathing patterns vary with each patient and within the daily experience of each patient. The only constant feature in HVS is that the patient's breathing appears to respond inappropriately to the changing metabolic and emotional requirements of daily living and that symptoms generally vary throughout the day for no apparent reason. Often there are 'good days' and 'bad

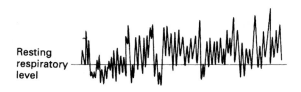

Fig. 19.3 Diagrammatic representation of an irregular pattern taken from a spirometry trace.

days'. There does not seem to be a strict correlation between the abnormality of the breathing pattern, the depression of $PaCO_2$ and the severity and type of symptoms.

TREATMENT

We have seen that there appear to be various groups of patients with symptoms related to hyperventilation. Patients presenting for physiotherapy tend to fall into three main groups.

1. Hyperventilation syndrome (HVS) in the absence of psychiatric, respiratory or other organic abnormalities – generally there is low or fluctuating $PaCO_2$.
2. Chronic hyperventilation with associated physical symptoms, presenting with panic or phobic states or other psychological disturbance. There may or may not be a low resting $PaCO_2$.
3. Chronic hyperventilation presenting as a conditioned physiological or behavioural pattern related to other organic conditions. Generally when the underlying condition is resolved the hyperventilating component is also resolved. However, in some instances the disordered breathing pattern needs to be addressed and treated in order to help resolve the lingering symptoms of any long-standing problems. In some conditions involving the vestibular system and recurrent laryngeal nerve palsy, breathing pattern reeducation and control should be part of the overall long-term plan. It has been shown that hyperventilation during phonation is one of the causes of fatigue in patients with vocal chord disorders (Miyazaki et al 1999). Inability to close the vocal chords to maintain sufficient subglottal pressure for speech appears to result in disrupted breathing patterns in order to compensate for excessive breath loss on vocalization. Hyperventilation appears to be a common occurrence with patients suffering with vestibular lesions and work has shown the relationship between the vestibular and respiratory pathways in the brainstem (Yates & Miller 1998).

The sooner a hyperventilating component is recognized and treated, the less likely it is that the situation will escalate. Where there is related disorder then an interdisciplinary approach is often helpful (psychiatric, counselling, behavioural or speech therapy or vestibular rehabilitation).

Whether hyperventilation is the primary or secondary factor, an improvement of subjective symptoms, exercise tolerance, general fitness and quality of life can be gained by reeducating the breathing pattern with the subsequent reordering of the patient's responses to the internal and external environment.

Reeducation of the breathing pattern for all groups will follow similar lines, involving a conscious control of nose breathing, place of movement, rate, volume and regularity of the breathing cycle. If the $PaCO_2$ is low or labile, the programme will be devised to help to raise and stabilize the resting level. If low $PaCO_2$ is not an issue, attention will remain with making the pattern slow and regular. If the $PaCO_2$ is raised as a result, it can only be an added benefit. A predominantly relaxed, passive abdominal movement (reflecting the movement of the diaphragm) is preferred and movement directed away from the upper thorax. This abdominal pattern of movement may in turn help to induce physical and mental relaxation. Relaxation is often aided by a regular, slow pattern of breathing. It may be necessary with some patients to practise a relevant relaxation technique before, during or after the breathing control. The long-term goal is to reestablish a more normal and slower pattern of movement and to decrease ventilation sufficiently to raise the resting $PaCO_2$ by a small measure.

In the short term, until the new pattern of breathing becomes the natural, constant, unconscious, spontaneous method of breathing, the patient is likely to continue to experience episodes of symptoms. These symptoms may be related to certain recognizable situations, stresses or exercise. The patient needs to learn to control the breathing pattern at these times and/or take 'first aid' measures of breath holding or rebreathing expired carbon dioxide. In time, with reassurance and perseverance, it should be possible to control the pattern of breathing and any intermittent dropping of $PaCO_2$ by identifying the provoking situations and practising precautionary measures.

Treatment sessions usually take approximately 1 hour. Outpatients should attend weekly at first. As the patient progresses the sessions become less frequent. Some patients need only two or three sessions others 12 or 14 spaced out over 12 or 18 months. At the time of discharge it is important for the patient to know where to telephone in an emergency for advice and review if necessary. Inpatients will probably be treated daily at first. Sessions will be given less frequently as soon as possible, to allow the patient more responsibility to practise alone.

ASSESSMENT

The assessment should include:

- history
- signs and symptoms
- personality
- physical examination.

History

It is helpful to ask open-ended questions to elicit when the patient was first aware of symptoms and the response to them. The first awareness may have been an acute 'attack', for instance driving home on the motorway on a Friday night after a stressful week and experiencing dizziness, tingling in the limbs and central chest pain. The response to this could be that of believing it to be a heart attack. This would be very understandable, especially if a member of the family had recently died of coronary disease. The anxiety would stimulate the respiratory rate further and the symptoms would increase, possibly to the point of admission to the nearest A&E department. Misrepresentation of the symptoms of an acute short-term episode of stress may cause a single natural response to be transformed into a pattern of inappropriate responses thereafter.

Signs and symptoms may not present so dramatically. Commonly symptoms may be traced back to a history of glandular fever or a long viral illness or fever, bereavement, failed expectations, change of lifestyle or job or house, family breakdown, frightening experience or prolonged emotional pressures or conflicts. A definitive triggerpoint may not be found and the first experience of the disorder be related to an array of stimuli or events which happened together or in close succession. History of chronic pain should be noted as this may be the underlying cause (Glyn et al 1981). Hypermobility syndrome may have an effect on the ventilation because of abnormally compliant lungs and hypermobility of the thoracovertebral joints.

Family history. Any similar symptoms, allergy, anxiety, cardiac or respiratory disease experienced by other members of the family should be elicited. Not uncommonly, the habit of overbreathing can be traced back to family illness patterns or relationships.

Childhood history. History of premature birth, oxygen therapy or artificial ventilation immediately after birth are incidents which are increasingly reported. It is also helpful to record childhood general health, including any tonsil or adenoid problems, physical ability, exercise tolerance and some idea of the quality of the relationships at school.

Signs and symptoms

There may be difficulty in describing the symptoms, as many of them are not usually within our experience. The symptoms generally occur when the brain is trying to function in a hypoxic condition, causing difficulty in perception, retention and recall of phenomena. The symptoms should be recorded, listed and numbered in relation to severity, occurrence and concern. The degree to which a symptom is incapacitating could rate 0–10 on a *disability scale* and the degree to which a symptom is fear provoking could rate 0–10 on a *distress scale*, while the frequency of occurrence of the symptom could also be rated 0–10. These records will give a guide to progress and ultimately give a semi-objective outcome measure.

Assessment of personality

A detailed analysis of the personality is neither possible nor necessary in this setting. However, a simple assessment may be made by noticing the posture, facial expression, demeanour of the hands, manner in which the history is given and the patient's emotional responses and reactions to the situations related in the history. One patient may be overtly obsessive and perfectionist and obviously reacting against the uncertainties of life, whilst another may be superficially tranquil, masking the underlying burden of troubles and emotions which are being carried. These may come spilling out at any time during the sessions.

Physical examination

It may not be appropriate to make a physical examination if pertinent information is given in the referral. When examination is deemed necessary and with the chest unclothed, note should be made of:

- the shape of the chest (including any physical deformity)
- the findings from auscultation.

The pattern of breathing can be assessed with the patient dressed. The place of movement, size, regularity and rate of breathing should be recorded and whether the patient breathes through the nose or mouth. The physiotherapist should have a watch with a second hand available to record the breathing rate per minute. It will be helpful to make a record of the number of breaths per minute at each visit and ultimately this record can be used as an outcome measure. The patient should not be informed at this stage of the rate per minute, as the reeducation of the pattern will take place at the level of the individual breath or phase of breath and a knowledge of the greater timescale can be damaging.

Treatment plan

The treatment plan will be agreed after discussion of symptoms and findings. The transfer of oxygen and carbon dioxide should be described in lay terms and related to the patient's manner of moving air. Once patients are able to connect their symptoms to the manner of breathing and not to some life-threatening disease, they are usually only too delighted to make a firm commitment to learn more about the manner of breathing and its control and to take responsibility for the home treatment programme. They happily recognize that it is possible to help themselves and to gain a degree of mastery over symptoms and the environment.

Treatment is not a matter of learning 'breathing exercises', but of learning how to alter the manner of breathing.

The treatment plan in the short term (to control symptoms) and in the long term (spontaneously to maintain a corrected pattern of breathing) should be described and agreed. Agreement should also be sought to look constructively at the activities of the day and to try to identify possible factors influencing the onset of symptoms. A fitness programme may be discussed at this stage but it should not be introduced until later in the plan when there is some semblance of breathing control.

Breathing education

The most comfortable position for learning breathing awareness is lying with suitable support. Most people with chronic hyperventilation do not have respiratory disease and therefore can lie flat without distress. The suggested position is supported with one or two pillows under the head and a pillow under the knees. The knee pillow helps to prevent tension in the abdominal muscles and thus enables a natural passive abdominal movement during the respiratory cycle. For patients who find that this position is uncomfortable or if it precipitates breathlessness or a feeling of vulnerability, another position should be found. Sitting with adequate support is usually acceptable to most people.

The first step of breathing awareness is the recognition of the relationship of body movements to the flow of air while breathing. Sensory input and body awareness is increased if the patient rests both hands on the abdomen. The physiotherapist lightly covers them with her hands. This light contact helps to bond the physiotherapist – patient relationship and allows the physiotherapist to feel, as well as observe, the movements related to the breathing cycle.

Again, a simple description of respiration is given, relating the flow of air in and out to the chest, diaphragmatic and abdominal movements. If the patient is a mouth breather time should be spent describing the purpose of breathing through the nose and practising nose breathing. Tuition and discussion should continue in this position until the physiotherapist is satisfied that the patient has grasped a basic and simple anatomical and physiological understanding. Generally the patient will become more relaxed as the interaction distracts from excess self-awareness.

Having had the breathing described, the patient is asked to close the eyes and try to feel and sense what is happening with regard to the breathing. It may be necessary for the physiotherapist to relate what is happening.

Care must be taken not to direct the pattern but merely to describe:

'You are now breathing in… and now you are breathing out'

'Your abdomen is swelling… and now your abdomen is falling back to rest'.

At this early stage it is helpful for the patient to establish the relationship between the air movement and the associated body movement and to recognize that as the air moves 'in' the body moves 'out' and vice versa. As soon as one becomes conscious of one's breathing there is a natural feeling of discomfort. Breathing is naturally reflex and subconscious but has a voluntary pathway. When breathing is brought into the consciousness, as it has to be for reeducation, there is a discomfort which has to be recognized and accepted and yet at the same time disregarded. Reeducation has to take place within this forum.

The patient is then asked to focus on the 'in breath' and notice when and how it starts and finishes. This 'quiet attentiveness' is then transferred to the 'out breath' and note taken of the beginning and end of this phase. Particular attention should be given to the end of the phase to recognize when the breath gently stops. The spontaneous rest point is identified as the natural rest point in the breathing cycle and the patient is helped to feel it as a place of relaxation, a place of balance, not a place of tension. It may be helpful to practise general relaxation into this place of 'no movement'. Most patients can accept this experience and begin to recognize it as a welcome rest.

In order to recognize the full breathing capacity it is helpful to stop the breath at the upper point of the tidal volume and then to request a continuation of inspiration until full inflation is achieved. In this way it is possible to experience the inspiratory capacity. Similarly, the expiratory reserve can be experienced by breath holding at the bottom of the tidal volume and then exhaling entirely by using all the expiratory muscles. Having practised these two manoeuvres, the patient will also realize that the relaxed tidal volume is relatively easy compared with the muscle work needed above and below the tidal flows. Patients may be able to use this information to perceive a change in their breathing pattern before symptoms occur. The learned corrective steps could then be made before full-blown symptoms take hold.

Breathing pattern re-education

The initial education and breathing awareness training is followed by reeducation of the components that have been identified as being disordered. These components are:

- tidal volume
- flow rate
- regularity
- place of movement.

The new breathing cycle may be of two or three phases, depending on the patient's body preference. The two-phase cycle would consist of a gentle inspiration followed by a slower expiration. In a three-phase cycle the natural rest point at the end of expiration is inserted and/or extended. A gentle inspiration is followed by an easy (passive) expiration which naturally changes into the rest period, which is comfortably extended until the next inspiration is gently initiated. Care has to be taken not to extend this rest to the point where a gasping inspiration is stimulated.

Method

By this stage the patient and physiotherapist will be aware of the size, speed and rhythm of the breathing pattern. The physiotherapist will describe these components and clarify with the patient what changes need to be made. Breathing is a very personal activity and the new pattern should not be imposed by another from the outside. The changes have to be made by the patient from within, guided carefully by the physiotherapist. A change of volume, speed of flow, regularity and place of movement may be required. One component, a combination or all of these may be involved. The new pattern will be remade with the least possible interference.

As many patients who hyperventilate have a predominantly thoracic movement, this needs to be changed to a gentle passive movement of the abdominal wall. Some patients find it extremely difficult to obtain any abdominal movement and it may be necessary to spend several treatment sessions using different word combinations and images until a more relaxed abdominal movement is achieved. Large or forced movements must be discouraged. Any increase in ventilation will increase or precipitate symptoms. In general, most patients manage to recognize what is needed to change from a thoracic 'in and up' pattern to an abdominal 'in and down' pattern. Special care also needs to be taken in order not to increase the volume if the flow is slowed, nor to increase the flow rate if the volume is decreased. A new pattern is introduced by gradual and patient work. It will be very individual. Guidance should be given breath by breath and phase by phase, relating which movement is good and which incorrect, thus reinforcing correct patterns of volume, movement and rest, which will of course be smaller and slower and more regular.

This decrease in body movement and ventilation may cause the patient an uncomfortable sensation akin to suffocation. This sensation is probably due to altered responses from the stretch reflexes in muscles, joints and lung tissue and from the rising $PaCO_2$. The patient is helped to accept this sensation of unease or discomfort as the sensation is described, discussed and understood.

It is necessary to experience this sensation at a minimal level while practising the corrected pattern. It should be barely perceptible and acceptable. Changes should not be so great that they create an unacceptably strong sensation, as the new pattern would not be physiologically sustainable and it would stimulate a sense of anxiety. By maintaining the controlled pattern for as long as possible, the new movement pattern will be reinforced and the respiratory centre reprogrammed to trigger inspiration at a higher level of carbon dioxide. The reprogramming is similar to that which occurs in patients with ventilatory insufficiency in chronic obstructive disease. An imperceptible increase in $PaCO_2$ over a period of time appears to condition the respiratory centre to accept higher levels before triggering inspiration.

If the desire to breathe becomes too great to contain, simple swallowing may ease the discomfort. If this is not sufficient, a slow, controlled deep breath may be taken. To compensate for moving this large volume of air, a longer period of time must be used. It is helpful to hold the breath after expiration, if it is possible, for a count of five or six (2–3 seconds). In a normal subject the $PaCO_2$ drops as the result of a deep breath and takes 3–4 minutes to return to normal if no compensatory measures are taken. Patients need to learn of this phenomenon and to use the knowledge positively by compensating for deep breathing or sighing by breath holding (preferably at the point of expiration) for a count of five or six. It is helpful to practise this slow deep breath, with the small breath hold on expiration, to ensure that it is not excessive.

Once a pattern has been found that fulfils the change criteria and suits the patient, it needs to be reinforced in the patient's mind. Some are able to recognize the pattern without external help; others find it difficult to recognize the timescale required. The correction in time may be helped by the physiotherapist guiding, by counting monotonously, the timespan of the phases of each breath. The possibilities are many and individual. They may vary from *in out in out in …* to a slower more natural pattern of *in and out two three and rest and in and out two three …* (Fig. 19.4). The use of a tape recorder, to capture the timing of the pattern during a treatment session, may help the patient to practise more effectively at home. The chosen new pattern of breathing may be the ideal to control the symptoms and enable the patient to feel better. However, it is sometimes necessary to move forward more slowly and, having achieved a very small step, to make further corrective changes until a curative pattern can be accepted.

The patient will need to learn control of the breathing pattern in sitting, standing, walking and during and after exercise. Recent work appears to offer evidence to support this practice. Malmberg et al (2000) reported that when changing body posture from supine to standing, patients with HVS increase their pulmonary ventilation in excess of metabolic needs greater than healthy controls. The work of Yates (1998) and his colleagues has shown an important relationship between vestibular stimulation and respiratory control. It may be necessary to practise changing positions and exercising during treatment sessions. Natural breathlessness will occur on exercise and should be recognized and accepted as normal. Some patients may feel better on exercise, as the body's metabolic needs rise to equilibrate with the respiratory physiology. Others may overbreathe on exercise; this will be recognized by an increase in, or occurrence of, symptoms. Appropriate control measures will need to be introduced and practised. If the natural breathlessness does not subside within an acceptable timespan after exercise, help may be given with control by changing one component of the breathing cycle at a time. First slow the rate, then decrease the volume, then slow the rate, etc., until control is achieved.

Compensatory procedures in the short term

If the patient falls back into the old habit (irregularity, deep breaths or frequent sighs) it may precipitate symptoms. Coughing or laughing may also precipitate symptoms. One first-aid measure is a conscious compensation for the movement of a large volume of air by gentle breath holding. This is so planned that a natural size of breath is subsequently possible. Intermittent breath holding is a useful manoeuvre to practise throughout the day. It should not be anticipated by a deep breath; rather, the breathing cycle is stopped anywhere in the cycle for a count of two or three or such time that does not provoke a large following inspiration. It can be practised and linked to simple everyday activities (like walking through a doorway) until it becomes a conditioned reflex. The hypothesis of this manoeuvre is to raise the $PaCO_2$ minimally and regularly to help to lessen the falling of carbon dioxide to symptomatic levels as a result of overbreathing and slow recovery times.

Planned rebreathing

It has been recorded that paper bag rebreathing may carry the hazard of hypoxia (Callaham 1989). However, poorly programmed rebreathing in acute hyperventilators who may have undiagnosed cardiac or respiratory conditions should not rule out the careful, controlled use of rebreathing

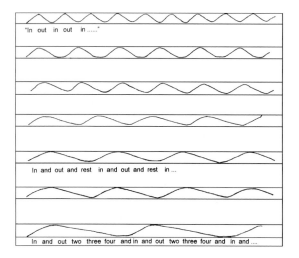

Fig. 19.4 Some suggested breathing patterns demonstrating a regular small tidal volume with various flow rates and rest periods.

therapy for chronic hyperventilators. There is a small group of people who cannot control the breathing pattern when it is most needed. There may be many reasons for this. One possibility is that the low $PaCO_2$ has an effect on memory programming and recall. If the $PaCO_2$ can be raised by rebreathing, the patient becomes more clear headed and can then remember the breathing control programme.

At times of acute distress or inability to control the disordered breathing, a bag of 25 cm × 30 cm minimum may be used as a rebreathing apparatus. The bag must be shaken out so that it is full of room air. The open end of the bag is placed loosely over the nose and mouth, allowing free passage of air between face and bag. The patient should breathe freely within the bag. Rebreathing of the expired gases takes place, thus raising the $PaCO_2$. After approximately 6–8 breaths, the bag should be removed from the face and shaken out to refill it with fresh room air. The procedure should continue with regular shaking of the bag until the acute presenting symptoms subside or until the patient is capable of controlling the breathing pattern effectively. For safety reasons the rebreathing bag must only be used in the sitting or standing position and never in lying. Should the patient lose consciousness, the bag would fall away from the face and not remain in situ, with the risk of asphyxia. Cupped hands held over the nose and mouth form another suitable and less obvious rebreathing procedure.

Rebreathing only raises the $PaCO_2$ during the procedure and, if the breathing pattern is not changed, the $PaCO_2$ would fall back when rebreathing ceased. The purpose of the procedure is to raise the carbon dioxide sufficiently to enable conscious control of the breathing pattern.

An ordinary oxygen mask with large holes, as used for inhalation therapy, may be used for patients who are unable to control the breathing sufficiently at certain times or who, as a result of hyperventilation, are housebound and unable to do household and personal routines. The facemask may be worn for the duration of the task. The $PaCO_2$ is artificially raised by the rebreathing function of the mask. The vent holes are left open so that room air can be drawn in to maintain sufficient oxygen concentration.

A facemask may be the short-term therapy of choice for patients who are terminally ill and hyperventilate with anxiety.

It is unwise to use bags or masks too freely as some patients can become dependent on the aid and never learn to reorder the breathing cycle. They should only be used when the patient's personality and situation are understood and when all other avenues have been investigated.

Speech

Many patients report that speaking and singing stimulate the symptoms. Normal conversational speech occurs at the upper end of expiratory tidal flows and there is a delicate interplay between breathing and speaking. Complex coordination of the respiratory muscles is required to produce the necessary subglottal pressures and the intricate manipulations needed to produce and maintain sound.

So often the old pattern of speech is very fast, as the patient endeavours to say as much as possible on one breath, before snatching at the next. Speech requires longer controlled expirations and shorter, faster inspirations than resting breathing. These inspirations need to be taken at suitable points in the sentence in order to maintain fluency and intelligibility. The aim is to articulate each word more slowly, to say fewer words on each breath and to try not to move down into the expiratory reserve volume. The new patterns of breathing required to incorporate these requirements need to be found and carried out. It is usually helpful if the physiotherapist works with the patient, who practises reading aloud while listening carefully to the new pattern of speech. This process helps to reeducate the breathing control and the sensory feedback loop.

Home programme

Therapy is directed towards reeducating the breathing pattern, not to breathing exercises. Practice sessions should be as many and for as long as possible. By using a practical approach, an acceptable programme must be worked out by the physiotherapist and the patient. At first it may only be possible to practise for 5 minutes a day, but three or four sessions of 20–30 minutes each is obviously more beneficial. Many patients find that as their lifestyle changes, more time can be made available for breathing control and relaxation sessions.

It is good to start the day with a period of conscious control of breathing. It is suggested that 10–15 minutes is spent in practice before rising in the morning. Travelling by bus or train is time well spent in conscious breathing control and relaxation. Car drivers can constructively use the time while waiting at traffic lights. Coffee, lunch and tea breaks could afford a few minutes of practice. Some people prefer to remember to practise breathing control for a few minutes each hour, on the hour, during the day. Fifteen or 20 minutes should be put aside when returning home from work or shopping to relax and practise breathing control. It is worth spending this time after a working day to allow the body to equilibrate. The evening can be more enjoyable when not fighting symptoms. The last period of practice can be done having retired to bed using the favourite sleeping position.

Compensatory breath holding, intermittent breath holding and general physical and mental relaxation should become part of the normal day. People who have experienced HVS are probably always at risk, even after the presenting episode has been resolved. It would be judicious always to remember to practise breathing control before aggravating situations such as flying, travelling to a high altitude, heat, hot baths and periods of prolonged excitement, stress or risk.

Exercise and fitness programmes

As a result of the disordered breathing pattern, many patients have been unable to exercise and have become unfit, thus compounding the problem. Guidance in a slowly graded exercise scheme can be helpful. It may need to start with very simple movements two or three times only. The progression must be carefully graded and to err on the slow side is preferable to advancing too quickly. Impatience for progress may cause decline rather than improvement. Swimming is an excellent form of free exercise, which encompasses general movement synchronized with breathing.

Group therapy

Some centres arrange self-help groups for exercise, relaxation and discussion. These sessions can be beneficial after an individual pattern of breathing control has been mastered and the patient is progressing with control in exercise. At a later stage, fitness training can be carried out in a group, although it should never be competitive. Each person should be following an individual programme.

These group sessions must be monitored carefully to ensure that they are not used for 'swapping symptoms'. With careful guidance they can help to give confidence and enhance the patient's ability to return to a more active life.

HYPERVENTILATION AND ASTHMA

The relationship between hyperventilation and asthma is ambiguous. Hyperventilation appears to be one factor in acute asthma, either in cause or effect, and panic or anxiety could exacerbate the symptoms of asthma by their propensity to stimulate hyperventilation. Recent work has suggested that chest discomfort and dyspnoea in children, precipitated by exercise, can be associated with hypocapnia from hyperventilation, rather than be a true exercise induced asthma (Hammo & Weinberger 1999).

Osborne et al (2000) have demonstrated that decreased airflow in a group of mild asthmatic patients, was related to a low $PaCO_2$ and end-tidal PCO_2 in association with hyperresponsive airways, rather than to airway obstruction or mucosal inflammation. Thus, in some people with mild asthma, hypocapnia may be responsible for an increase in their smooth muscle contractility.

Based on the understanding that the pattern of breathing and the central control mechanisms can be changed (Grossman et al 1985), a programme of breathing reeducation based on the individual's mode of breathing behaviour could be a helpful part of the total care management plan for the condition of asthma. The ability to recognize the onset of problems, to identify the breathing disorder and then, in association with the appropriate use of medication, to regulate the manner of breathing could not only decrease the anxiety involved but also make a positive input to the actual process of ventilation. The breathing reeducation would aim to lead the gasping-in and squeezing-out breaths into a smoother pattern and, on inspiration, to encourage a gentle swelling of the abdominal wall and relaxation of the accessory muscles of respiration. It would be directed towards controlling the pace and raising the respiratory level of each breath, in such a way that the airflow is kept as laminar as possible and the airways are not compressed excessively on expiration. The control of air movement through the nose should help to prevent any unnecessary irritation of the airways, as when cold, fast-moving air is drawn in through the mouth.

Recently, the Buteyko breathing technique of 'reducing the depth and frequency of respiration' and of breath holding is being introduced in the West, as a treatment for asthma. It appears to be based on a similar understanding of the need to upregulate the $PaCO_2$ levels. The regimen of breathing exercises seems to be of a fairly fixed formula which is taught in a group (Bowler et al 1998) and modified on an individual basis.

CONCLUSION

Patience and perseverance of physiotherapist and patient are necessary for the long-term reeducation of the breathing pattern, which aims at decreasing the rate and slowly increasing the resting $PaCO_2$ to more normal levels. Each patient's respiratory system is very particular and each physiotherapist will learn new nuances of breathing patterns and new ways of helping to reeducate the system from each patient. The treatment programmes can never be exactly the same, nor should they be imposed rigidly. Each patient needs to be guided to find their own particular corrected breathing arrangement, which fulfils the basic physiological principles. This chosen pattern should eventually become the new, unconscious, habitual method of breathing. This chapter is related mainly to the description of this method of reeducating this manner of breathing. It does not discuss methods of associated relaxation techniques, which may need to be part of the treatment.

Chronic habitual hyperventilators are often gifted and interesting people who are generally highly motivated and compliant with treatment. A high proportion of sufferers are helped by a systematic, individual treatment programme and by an intelligent and sympathetic approach to the syndrome. The condition is a challenging one for the physiotherapist and the patient's improvement is pleasing.

At discharge the outcome could be measured by:

- Nijmegen questionnaire
- breath-holding time
- disability/distress records
- respiratory rate
- breathing pattern, measured by spirography or Respi-vest if these services are available.

Breathing is a very complex system, which is affected by many stimuli and appears to have effects other than the exchange of gases (van Dixhoorn 1996). Some patients' symptoms may be attributed to various dysfunctional aspects within the inherent mechanisms of the afferent and efferent responses of the breathing system, other than the variable or low levels of $PaCO_2$. Many phenomena are not yet understood and there are many areas inviting research. Work is currently in progress in a few centres, which is offering a greater understanding of the physiological sensitivities and complexities and the interplay of feedback loops in the breathing system, in relation to individual responses to life events.

The effects of reeducation of the breathing pattern merit further study and the field is wide open for physiotherapists to research.

REFERENCES

Baker DM 1934 Sighing respiration as a symptom. Lancet 1: 174–177

Ball S, Shekhar A 1997 Basilar artery response to hyperventilation in panic disorder. American Journal of Psychiatry 154(11): 1603–1604

Bass C, Gardner WN 1985 Respiratory and psychiatric abnormalities in chronic symptomatic hyperventilation. British Medical Journal 290: 1387–1390

Bowler SD, Green A, Mitchell CA 1998 Buteyko breathing techniques in asthma: a blinded randomized controlled trial. Alternative Medicine 169: 575–578

Callaham M 1989 Hypoxic hazards of traditional paper bag rebreathing in hyperventilating patients. American Emergency Medicine 18(b): 622–628

Clark TJH, Cochrane GN 1970 Effect of personality on alveolar ventilation in patients with chronic airways obstruction. British Medical Journal 1: 273–275

Cowley DS, Roy-Byrne PP 1987 Hyperventilation and panic disorder.American Journal of Medicine 83: 929–937

Folgering H, Ruttern H, Rouman Y 1983 Beta–blockade in the hyperventilation syndrome. A retrospective assessment of symptoms and complaints. Respiration 44 (1): 19–25

Freeman LJ, Nixon PGF 1985 Chest pain and the hyperventilation syndrome: some etiological considerations. Postgraduate Medical Journal 61: 957–961

Gardner WN 1994 Diagnosis and organic causes of symptomatic hyperventilation. In: Timmons BH, Ley R (eds) Behavioural and psychological approaches to breathing disorders. Plenum Press, New York, p 111

Gardner W 2000 Orthostatic increase of respiratory gas exchange in hyperventilation syndrome. Thorax 55: 257–259

Gardner WN, Bass C 1989 Hyperventilation in clinical practice. British Journal of Hospital Medicine 41(1): 73–81

Glyn C , Lloyd JW, Folkard S 1981 Ventilatory responses to intractable pain. Pain 11(2): 201–211

Grossman P, De Swart JCG, Defares PB 1985 A controlled study of a breathing therapy for treatment of hyperventilation syndrome. Journal of Psychosomatic Research 29(1): 49–58

Hammo AH, Weinberger MM 1999 Exercise-induced hyperventilation: a pseudoasthma syndrome. Annals of Allergy, Asthma and Immunology 82(6): 574–578

Hardonk HJ, Beumer HM 1979 Hyperventilation syndrome. In: Vinken PJ, Bruyn GW (eds) The handbook of clinical neurology. North Holland, Amsterdam, pp 309–360

Hornsveld HK, Garssen B, Fiedeldij Dop MJC, Van Spiegel PI, De Haes JCJM 1996 Double blind placebo-controlled study of the hyperventilation provocation test and the validity of the hyperventilation syndrome. Lancet 348: 154–158

Howell JBL 1997 The hyperventilation syndrome: a syndrome under threat? Thorax 52(3): S30-S34

Kerr WJ, Dalton JW, Gliebe PA 1937 Some physical phenomena associated with the anxiety states and their relation to hyperventilation. Annals of Internal Medicine 11: 961–992

Lum LC 1994 Hyperventilation syndromes: physiological considerations in clinical management. In: Timmons BH, Ley R (eds) Behavioural and psychological approaches to breathing disorders. Plenum Press, New York, pp 118, 120

Macefield G, Burke D 1991 Parasthesia and tetany induced by voluntary hyperventilation. Brain 114: 527–540

Magarian GJ 1982 Hyperventilation syndromes: infrequently recognized common expressions of anxiety and stress. Medicine 61(4): 219–236

Malmberg LP, Tamminen K, Sovijarvi ARA 2000 Orthostatic increase of respiratory gas exchange in hyperventilation syndrome. Thorax 55: 295–301

Miyazaki H, Yamashita H, Masuda T, Yamamoto T, Komiyama S 1999 Transcutaneous PCO2 monitoring in the evaluation of hyperventilation of patients with recurrent nerve paralysis. European Archives of Oto-Rhyno-Laryngology 256 (1) : S47–S50

Nixon PGF, Freeman LJ 1988 The 'think test': a further technique to elicit hyperventilation. Journal of the Royal Society of Medicine 81: 277–279

Osborne CA, O'Connor BJ, Lewis A, Kanabar V, Gardner WN 2000 Hyperventilation and asymptomatic chronic asthma. Thorax 55: 1016–1022

Pilsbury D, Hibbert GA 1987 An ambulatory system for long term continuous monitoring of transcutaneous PCO_2. Clinical Respiratory Physiology 23: 9 – 13

Troosters T, Verstraete A, Ramon K, Schepers R, Gosselink R, Decramer M, Van De Woestijne K P 1999 Physical performance of patients with numerous psychosomatic complaints suggestive of hyperventilation. European Respiratory Journal 14: 1314–1319

van den Hout MA, Hoekstra R, Arntz A et al 1992 Hyperventilation is not diagnostically specific to panic patients. Psychosomatic Medicine 54(2): 182–191.

van Dixhoorn J 1996 Hyperventilation and dysfunctional breathing. A presentation at the Third Annual Meeting of the International Society for the Advancement of Respiratory Psychophysiology (ISARP), University of Nijmegen

van Dixhoorn J, Duivenvoorden HJ 1985 Efficacy of Nijmegen questionnaire in recognition of the hyperventilation syndrome. Journal of Psychosomatic Research 29(2): 199–206

van Doorn P, Colla P, Folgering H 1982 Control of end-tidal PCO_2 in the hyperventilation syndrome: effects of biofeedback and breathing instructions compared. Bulletin Europeen de Physiopathologie Respiratoire 18: 829–836

Vansteenkiste J, Rochette M, Demedts M 1991 Diagnostic tests of hyperventilation syndrome. European Respiratory Journal 4: 393–399

Wood P 1941 Da Costa's syndrome (or effort syndrome). British Medical Journal 1: 767–772, 805–811, 845–851

Yates BJ 1998 Vestibular autonomic regulation: overview and conclusions of a recent workshop at the university of Pittsburg. Journal of Vestibular Research 8 (1): 1–5

Yates BJ, Miller AD 1998 Physiological evidence that the vestibular system participates in autonomic and respiratory control. Journal of Vestibular Research 8 (1): 17–25

FURTHER READING

Bradley D 1998 Hyperventilation syndrome – breathing pattern disorders, 3rd edition. Kyle Cathie, London

Lum LC 1976 The syndrome of chronic hyperventilation. In: Hill O (ed) Modern trends in psychosomatic medicine. Butterworths, London, pp 196–230

Tenny SM, Lamb TW 1965 Physiological consequences of hypoventilation and hyperventilation. In: Handbook of physiology. American Physiological Society, Bethesda, MD, pp 979–1003

Timmons BH, Ley R 1994 (eds) Behavioural and psychological approaches to breathing disorders. Plenum Press, New York

20

Bronchiectasis, primary ciliary dyskinesia and cystic fibrosis

Mary E Dodd   A Kevin Webb

BRONCHIECTASIS

'Bronchiectasis' is the term used for chronic dilatation of one or more bronchi (Cole 1995), which leads to impaired drainage of bronchial secretions. These secretions often become chronically infected, producing a persistent host inflammatory response. The combination of infection and a chronic inflammatory host response results in a progressive destructive lung disease. Depending upon the aetiology, bronchiectasis can affect specific lobes or both lungs.

The incidence and prevalence of bronchiectasis are unknown. Chest radiography is less sensitive than computed tomography (CT), which is the gold standard in the detection of bronchiectasis, but population screening using CT is not justified. With the decline in childhood tuberculosis, measles and whooping cough there is an impression that bronchiectasis is less prevalent. However, treatment of bronchiectasis has improved and it is important to try and establish the exact cause. Diagnosing the cause may define a specific approach to treatment and provide a prognosis as in the case of cystic fibrosis. A recent survey of the causative factors of bronchiectasis identified that 29% of cases were post infectious, 8% due to an immune defect and 7% due to allergic bronchopulmonary aspergillosis (ABPA) but for 53% of patients no cause was found (Pasteur et al 2000). A list of the common causes of bronchiectasis is set out in Table 20.1.

Delivery of care for complex diseases requires experience, expertise and teamwork. This maxim applies to lung cancer, transplantation

Table 20.1 Commoner causes of bronchiectasis

Post-infective	Tuberculosis
	Measles
	Whooping cough
Mucociliary clearance defects	Cystic fibrosis
	Primary ciliary dyskinesia
	Young's syndrome
Immune defects	Immunoglobulin deficiency
	Cellular defects
Allergic bronchopulmonary aspergillosis	
Localized bronchial obstruction	Foreign body
	Benign tumour
	External compression
Gastric aspiration	

and interstitial lung disease and it may improve the outcome for patients with bronchiectasis if they were cared for by a specialist multidisciplinary team in a similar way that patients with cystic fibrosis have benefited.

Clinical features

The range of disease expression may vary from patients who are totally asymptomatic to those who have severe disease with a cough productive of large amounts of purulent sputum which is sometimes bloodstained. The latter require treatment of high intensity with frequent hospital attendance. Severe exacerbations may be accompanied by chest pain, breathlessness and fevers. Patients with inherited diseases such as cystic fibrosis and primary ciliary dyskinesia will often have accompanying sinus disease with nasal blockage, a purulent discharge and facial pain.

Clinical signs are non-specific. On auscultation there may be localized or widespread inspiratory and expiratory crackles with occasional wheezing. Clubbing is infrequent except with severe disease and cystic fibrosis.

Diagnosis and investigations

- *Assessment* using subjective and objective findings, as discussed in Chapter 1.
- *The chest radiograph* may be normal or there may be signs of thickened bronchial walls (tramlining), crowding of vessels with loss of

volume and cyst-like shadows with fluid levels. The chest radiograph on its own is an insensitive test, detecting less than 50% of patients with bronchiectasis (Currie et al 1987).
- *High-resolution CT* is the imaging method of choice as a diagnostic tool in bronchiectasis. It has a high specificity, greater than 90% (Smith & Flower 1996).
- *Sputum specimens* for examination and culture to identify the micro-organisms and their sensitivity to antibiotics. The most common bacteria found in bronchiectatic sputum are *Haemophilus influenzae* (70%), *Streptococcus pneumoniae* and *Pseudomonas aeruginosa*. The latter is found in patients with diffuse bronchiectasis and associated with accelerated lung disease (Evans et al 1996). Patients infected with *Ps. aeruginosa* require a higher intensity of treatment.
- *Bronchoscopy* should be considered if a foreign body or tumour is suspected.
- *Lung function tests* are used to assess severity of airflow obstruction and airways reversibility.
- *Serum immunoglobulins* will detect patients with hypogammaglobulinaemia.
- The diagnosis of ABPA is difficult. The routine investigations should include: skin prick tests, eosinophil count, Aspergillus precipitins, total IgE levels with specific IgG and IgE levels to *Aspergillus*. Plain radiography may show fleeting shadows responsive to steroids. CT scanning may show the typical proximal bronchiectasis.
- *Gene mutation analysis*. This should be performed on all cases of idiopathic bronchiectasis to exclude some of the more benign mutations of cystic fibrosis (Pasteur et al 2000).
- *Nasomucociliary clearance test* and microscopic examination of the cilia to exclude cilial defects.

Medical management

Progression of bronchiectasis is related to poor clearance of infected secretions. Physiotherapy (see below) is probably the most important component of long-term treatment. Antibiotics are fundamental to treating infective exacerbations and controlling the severity of bronchiectasis. The choice of antibiotic will be determined by the frequency and sensitivity of micro-organisms grown in sputum culture. The route and frequency of delivery will be decided by the severity of the disease. Antibiotics can be given orally, nebulized and intravenously. Getting the best results from antibiotic usage will depend upon the skill and experience of the team looking after the patient.

Indications for antibiotics

Oral antibiotics can be given as prophylaxis, for occasional infective exacerbations or continuously for repeated severe infections. Viral infections can produce a bacterial infective exacerbation which will often require a course of prophylactic oral antibiotics. Patients with severe disease and persistent purulent sputum who repeatedly relapse following a short course of antibiotics can be maintained on long-term oral antibiotics. Those commonly used are the penicillins and more recently the macrolides.

Nebulized antibiotics are indicated for patients with severe bronchiectasis whose disease is progressive and difficult to control (Currie 1997). Nebulized antibiotics can delay persistent infection with *Ps. aeruginosa* in patients with cystic fibrosis if instituted at the time of first colonization (Valerius et al 1991). Although there are no clinical trials, this practice should be used in bronchiectasis since acquisition of *Ps. aeruginosa* is associated with greater morbidity (Evans et al 1996). Randomized controlled trials using nebulized antibiotics for bronchiectatic patients chronically infected with *Ps. aeruginosa* have shown a reduction in sputum density of *Ps. aeruginosa* (Barker et al 2000) and a lessening of disease severity (Oriols et al 1999).

Intravenous antibiotics are used for severe disease, patients who fail to respond to oral antibiotics and those chronically infected with *Ps. aeruginosa*.

Other treatment measures

Influenza vaccination should be given annually to all bronchiectatic patients unless there is a medical contraindication.

Topical medication may be indicated for chronic mucopurulent rhinosinusitis and the recommended technique for inhaled topical deposition of drugs is the head-down and forward position to encourage entry of the drops to the ethmoid and maxillary sinuses (Wilson et al 1987).

Where there is an immunoglobulin deficiency, replacement therapy should be given in an attempt to prevent further lung damage.

Surgical resection should only be considered if the bronchiectasis is localized but there are no randomized controlled trials to compare surgical versus conservative treatment in the decision-making process (Corless & Warburton 2000). In very severe widespread bronchiectasis with respiratory failure, lung transplantation may be considered.

The inhalation of recombinant human deoxyribonuclease (rhDNase) does not appear to improve ciliary transportability, spirometry, dyspnoea or quality of life in patients with bronchiectasis not associated with cystic fibrosis (Wills et al 1996).

Inhaled steroids have been evaluated, with a trend to improving some respiratory parameters, but larger studies are needed (Kolbe & Wells 2000). A subset of bronchiectatic patients respond to bronchodilators and all patients should be tested for a response (Hassan et al 1999).

Physiotherapy management

Physiotherapy may help in the treatment of patients' problems of excess bronchial secretions, breathlessness, reduced exercise tolerance and chest wall pain of musculoskeletal origin.

Excess bronchial secretions

It is important that the patient understands the pathology of the condition and the reasons for treatment. Clinically, effective physiotherapy should reduce the episodes of superimposed infection and may help to minimize further lung damage.

An airway clearance technique, for example the active cycle of breathing techniques (ACBT) (p. 190), should be introduced and self-treatment encouraged. Each patient should be assessed to determine the positions which may increase the efficiency of secretion clearance and a CT scan, if available, would facilitate this.

Clinical experience suggests that a minimum of 10 minutes in any one productive position will be necessary and the endpoint of treatment must be recognized by self-assessment. The sitting position may be adequate for patients with minimal secretions. The horizontal position may be a more acceptable and comfortable alternative to the head-down tipped position and has been shown to be equally effective in patients who expectorate >20 g of sputum per day (Cecins et al 1999).

There may be concern in those patients who present with gastrooesophageal reflux that postural drainage will exacerbate the problem. Chen et al (1998) have shown that there was no difference in the duration or frequency of symptoms in the various drainage positions. There are other techniques which may be used to facilitate airway clearance and may be of use in bronchiectasis. These are discussed in Chapter 6.

Regular daily treatment is essential but the frequency will vary among individuals and should be increased during episodes of superimposed infection. For many patients treatment once a day is sufficient. Some patients find their chest is 'dry' at the beginning of the day. The timing of treatment should take into consideration both the time of day that the chest is most productive and the patient's lifestyle. Compliance/adherence may also be increased by agreeing a suitable home programme with the patient.

Patients using gravity-assisted positions for the lower and middle zones may find a full-length postural drainage frame (Fig. 20.1) comfortable and convenient for treatment. Elderly or frail patients may require assistance from a relative or carer who should be carefully instructed by a physiotherapist.

It is important that the physiotherapy techniques and positions for treatment are reassessed at intervals. Currie et al (1986) recommended regular review. Most patients should be reassessed within 3 months of initial instruction and at least annually thereafter.

Acute exacerbation of infection. Patients may be admitted to hospital with an acute exacerbation of their chest infection. The patient will probably be expectorating an increased amount of more purulent sputum, may be febrile, dehydrated and breathless. Haemoptysis is not uncommon and pleuritic chest pain may be present. The most severely affected may present with respiratory failure.

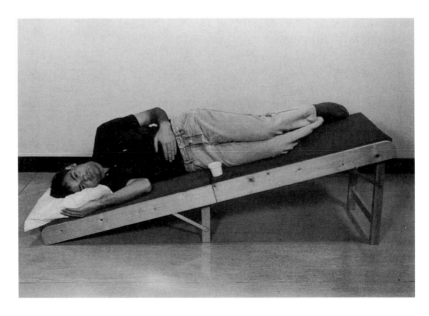

Fig. 20.1 Postural drainage frame.

It is likely that mechanical adjuncts will be required in addition to an airway clearance technique to assist the clearance of excess bronchial secretions. A nebulized bronchodilator and/or humidification (Conway et al 1992) before treatment may help in the mobilization of tenacious secretions.

Intermittent positive pressure breathing (IPPB) may help both in the clearance of secretions and in relief of the work of breathing. Patients who, many years ago, received the more radical treatment of resection of more than one lobe will probably have very poor respiratory reserve by the time they reach middle age. A superimposed infection in these patients may precipitate respiratory failure. Modified positioning, for example side lying or high side lying, combined with IPPB may be an effective form of treatment in minimizing the effort of clearing secretions (p. 209). Non-invasive ventilation may be indicated in acute respiratory failure although the outcome is less successful in the presence of excess bronchial secretions (Ch. 10).

Following resection of lung tissue the anatomy of the bronchial tree may alter and the traditional positions for drainage of segments of the remaining lobes may be unsuitable or in appropriate. The physiotherapist should try varying positions until the optimal ones are found.

The presence of blood streaking in the sputum is not a contraindication to physiotherapy and treatment should be continued. If there is frank haemoptysis physiotherapy should be temporarily discontinued but resumed as soon as the sputum is only mildly bloodstained to avoid retention of old blood and mucus. Before discharge from hospital it is important that the patient is able to take the responsibility for his treatment and is confident with the positions and techniques required to continue regularly at home. If a bronchodilator has been prescribed, this should be taken before treatment and a few patients with bronchiectasis may also be prescribed nebulized antibiotic drugs which should be inhaled after clearance of secretions. A breath-enhanced nebulizer or adaptive aerosol delivery (AAD) device is recommended for delivery of antibiotics (Ch. 6). If a patient is on the waiting list for lung transplantation, a preoperative rehabilitation programme should be established and postoperative treatment would be as outlined in Chapter 6.

Breathlessness

Some patients with bronchiectasis also demonstrate a degree of bronchospasm and will benefit from the inhalation of a bronchodilator before physiotherapy to clear secretions. Instruction in the use of an appropriate device for drug delivery is important.

A minority of patients with bronchiectasis complain of breathlessness and for these patients rest positions to relieve breathlessness and breathing control while walking and stair climbing should be included in the treatment programme (Ch. 6, Figs 6.18, 6.19)

Reduced exercise tolerance

Exercise should be encouraged to improve general physical fitness. It will also assist the mobilization of bronchial secretions. Patients with severe bronchiectasis may benefit from a group pulmonary rehabilitation programme (Ch. 14).

Chest wall pain of musculoskeletal origin

See p. 273–277

Evaluation of physiotherapy

Effective treatment can be recognized by a decrease in the quantity and purulence of sputum, absence of fever, improvements in spirometry, a reduction in breathlessness, an increase in exercise tolerance, more energy and a reduction or absence of chest wall pain. Improvements in oxygen saturation and blood gas tensions may also be apparent.

PRIMARY CILIARY DYSKINESIA

Primary ciliary dyskinesia (PCD) is an autosomal recessive disorder with an incidence of between

1 in 15 000 and 1 in 30 000 (Cole 1995) and an expected prevalence of 3000 cases in the UK. Currently genetic testing is not available for carrier screening or prenatal diagnosis, which may explain why late diagnosis is a feature of the disease and many cases are under diagnosed. This can be inferred from the relatively few cases known to the UK primary ciliary dyskinesia support group (Bush et al 1998).

PCD is characterized by abnormal structure of the cilia, normal structure but with abnormal function, or absence of the cilia. This results in recurrent infections in the nose, ears, sinuses and lungs. Fertility may be affected, both in the female because the fallopian tubes are lined with cilia and in the male due to reduced sperm motility. In 50% of cases, PCD is associated with dextrocardia or situs inversus. Kartagener described a syndrome of bronchiectasis, sinusitis and situs inversus in 1933. Later it was recognized that there was also a ciliary abnormality and this could occur without situs inversus. Cilia defects were described first in spermatazoa and later in nasal and bronchial cilia and the term 'immotile cilia syndrome' was applied to this group of conditions. With the discovery of a range of cilial defects, with variation in beat frequency and ultrastructure and the recognition that not all abnormal cilia are immotile, the term primary ciliary dyskinesia was adopted (Greenstone et al 1988).

The age of presentation can vary from the newborn to 51 years (Turner et al 1981). Chronic sputum production and nasal symptoms are the main presenting symptoms but this can vary from pneumonia and rhinitis in the newborn, 'asthma' with a productive cough, chronic and severe secretory otitis media, with associated hearing problems and severe oesophageal reflux in the older child and the problems of infertility and ectopic pregnancy in the adult. Specific investigations which would clarify the diagnosis of PCD include the nasal mucociliary clearance test, i.e. the saccharin test (Stanley et al 1984), photometric determination of ciliary beat frequency (Rutland & Cole 1980) and electron micrographic analysis. DNA testing should be undertaken to exclude the diagnosis of cystic fibrosis. Exhaled and nasal nitric oxide is very low in PCD (Karadag et al 1997) but increased in bronchiectasis and asthma. Although the measurement is not recommended as a diagnostic test, if levels are low in a patient with bronchiectasis then the diagnosis of PCD should be excluded.

Medical management

Early diagnosis is essential and the medical treatment is centred around the prevention of lung damage and bronchiectasis with aggressive use of antibiotics and daily chest physiotherapy. Intravenous treatment may be necessary for unresponsive infections and long-term nebulized antibiotics should be considered for patients colonized with *Ps. aeruginosa*. In childhood, careful regular assessment and monitoring of hearing should indicate the requirement for hearing aids or grommet insertion due to the build-up of fluid in the middle ear. Hearing aids are considered preferable because grommets may cause additional discharge. Hearing loss is temporary and resolves spontaneously later in childhood.

Recent studies have focused on the influence of drugs on cough clearance (Houtmeyers et al 1999, Noone et al 1999). In PCD airway clearance is dependent on cough, but an increased amount of secretion is necessary to ensure effective clearance with coughing. Aerolized uridine-5'-triphosphate has been shown to improve whole lung clearance during cough after a single dose when compared to 0.12% saline (Noone et al 1999). Further trials of this drug are required to determine the clinical significance of long-term administration. Two case reports have suggested benefit from inhalation of rhDNase in the acute situation (Desai et al 1995, ten Berge et al 1999). However, its use has not been validated in PCD in a controlled trial. Inhaled β_2 agonists are frequently prescribed in PCD for their effect on bronchodilation, mucociliary transport and thinning of secretions (Rubin 1988). Regular use in asthma may be associated with increased bronchial responsiveness and decreased airway calibre. Koh et al (2000) have shown that no such adverse effects or decrease in lung function were seen in PCD over a 6 week period. Severe gastro-oesophageal reflux, which can compromise airway clearance, is a problem for some patients and requires appropriate management with a proton pump inhibitor.

Referral for assisted conception may be necessary for both males and females who are infertile or subfertile. Psychosocial support will include help with benefits, liaison with schools about infections and possible deafness and counselling may be appropriate to cope with the problem of infertility. Care is centred around daily home chest clearance and the control of infection by the general practitioner. Periodic review in a specialist centre by a multidisciplinary team with expertise in respiratory disorders is recommended.

Physiotherapy management

Daily physiotherapy, if introduced at the time of diagnosis, becomes a way of life for the child. It is important that parents detect signs of infection early: a child may be lethargic, 'off colour' and feel abnormally hot. Physiotherapy should be increased during infective episodes and parents must understand that effective treatment is not achieved by antibiotics alone.

Due to the cilial defect, secretions are most likely to collect in the dependent areas: the lower lobes and often the middle lobe and lingula. The middle lobe which may be situated on the left side, owing to situs inversus, is more commonly affected than the lingula. The goal of treatment should be to assist clearance of secretions from the dependent parts of the lungs using an effective airway clearance technique. Even when the chest sounds dry and non-productive, parents should probably be shown drainage positions for the middle lobe (Fig. 20.2), lingula and lateral segments of the lower lobes. Children should be encouraged to blow their noses regularly.

Huffing games and airway clearance devices can usually be introduced at an early age and by 8 or 9 years the child can begin to do some of the treatment himself, gradually becoming independent. It has been suggested that the PEP mask may be a useful technique, based on the theoretical benefits of peripheral mobilization of secretions, and can be used at any age, including neonates (Gremmo & Guenza 1999). Some patients may require nebulized antibiotics and inhaled Beta-2 agonists for their beneficial effect on mucociliary clearance. Beta-2 agonists should be inhaled before and antibiotics after chest clearance. Exercise, which increases bronchodilation to a greater extent than Beta-2 agonists (Philips et al 1996), should be encouraged from the time of diagnosis and its importance emphasized to parents and patients (Fig. 20.3). Even with grommets in place children can enjoy swimming (Pringle 1992).

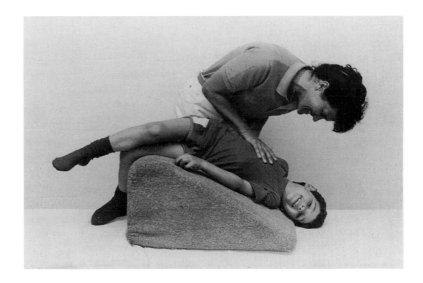

Fig. 20.2 Assisted treatment for the right middle lobe.

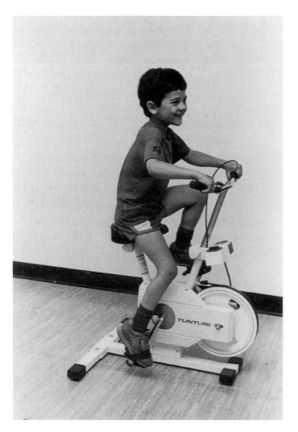

Fig. 20.3 Exercise on a stationary bicycle.

Very occasionally, nasopharyngeal suction may be indicated in the infant when it is impossible to clear nasal and bronchial secretions by any other means.

Regular assessment of techniques, remotivation of the patient and support for the parents are important aspects of physiotherapy. It is probable that chronic lung damage will be minimized if physiotherapy is continued on a regular basis.

Evaluation of physiotherapy

In the young patient with PCD, effective treatment in the stable condition may be recognized by the presence of only minimal coughing on exertion. During an infective episode signs and symptoms of effective treatment include a reduction in shortness of breath, coughing, wheeze and fever if either or both had been present.

In addition, in the older patient, a constant volume of sputum would be expectorated while stable and during an infective episode, the volume of expectorated sputum should lessen with effective treatment.

CYSTIC FIBROSIS

Cystic fibrosis (CF) is the most frequent cause of suppurative lung disease in caucasian children and young adults and is characterized by chronic pulmonary disease, pancreatic insufficiency and increased concentrations of electrolytes in the sweat (Høiby & Koch 1990).

Cystic fibrosis is an autosomal recessive condition most commonly found in Caucasian populations with a carrier rate of 1 in 25 and the disease occurring in approximately 1 in 2500 live births (Dodge et al 1993). Carriers of the genetic defect show no signs of cystic fibrosis but if both parents carry the abnormal gene each child born has a 1 in 4 chance of inheriting the condition. When the condition was first described by Anderson (1938) life expectancy was less than 2 years but with increased recognition of the disease, especially in its milder forms, and improved treatment the median age of survival is currently approximately 31 years (Shale 1997a). Cohort survival graphs indicate an improvement in survival with time in the UK in all age groups (Dodge et al 1993). If the trend for improved survival continues it is likely that many of the patients born in the 1990s will live well into their 50s (Lewis 1997 personal communication).

Prior to the identification of the gene in 1989, a diagnosis of cystic fibrosis was made using the sweat test which measures the amount of sodium in the sweat (Di Sant'Agnese & Davis 1979).

The basic defect for CF lies on chromosome 7 and was identified in 1989 (Rommens et al 1989). Genes are made from the chemical deoxyribonucleic acid (DNA) and some pieces of DNA code for protein. The faulty gene in CF codes for the transmembrane conductance regulator (CFTR). The abnormality in this protein leads to changes in ion transport (McBride 1990) which produce changes in the nature of the mucous and serous secretions produced by the exocrine glands, cells of the respiratory system and digestive tract.

Ion transport in human airways is dominated by the absorption of sodium ions from the mucosal surface (Alton et al 1992) and this is associated with the movement of water into the epithelial cells. It is also thought that chloride ions pass from the epithelial cells into the airway lumen, taking water with them. The balance between the movement of sodium and chloride probably determines the volume and composition of the airway surface liquid and may affect mucociliary clearance (Alton et al 1992).

In cystic fibrosis there is a reduction in chloride secretion from the epithelial cells of the respiratory mucosa. This results in excess absorption of sodium and increased movement of fluid from the lumen of the airway into the cells, reducing the airway surface liquid (mucous layer), increasing the viscosity of mucus and impairing mucociliary clearance.

The lungs are structurally normal at birth (Reid & De Haller 1967), but studies have demonstrated evidence of inflammation and infection in infants and children with CF (Birrer et al 1994, Khan et al 1995) and in asymptomatic adults with normal lung function (Konstan et al 1994). Infection stimulates further mucus secretion and a generalized obstructive, suppurative cycle becomes established. Repeated infections result in a neutrophil bronchiolitis. The neutrophils are ineffective at eliminating the microorganisms which chronically infect the small airways. They break down, releasing numerous peptides, and in particular neutrophil elastase, which destroy lung tissue. The consequences are a destructive progressive suppurative bronchiectasis. The cycle of infection and inflammation impairs ciliary function and reduces mucus clearance.

As the suppurative bronchiectasis progresses, chronic hypoxia leads to pulmonary hypertension. The majority of patients die from respiratory failure when they no longer respond to medical treatment or if transplant organs fail to become available.

Diagnosis and presentation

Screening may be undertaken if there is a known family history of CF (Super et al 1994). Recently national neonatal screening has been approved. Long-term outcome may be influenced by early diagnosis (Ranieri et al 1994). Currently, the majority of patients are diagnosed early in life with symptoms related to either the respiratory or gastrointestinal systems.

In the neonate, meconium ileus is the most common presenting feature, occurring in about 10–15% of cases (Park & Grand 1981). Signs of intestinal obstruction may occur within 48 hours of birth. The infant fails to pass meconium after birth because the bowel is obstructed by sticky inspissated intestinal contents, but in milder cases there may only be a delay in the passage of meconium. A blood test for genotyping to clarify the diagnosis should be performed in infants with meconium ileus, as this condition can occur in infants who do not have CF.

Another presenting sign in infants and young children is a voracious appetite and failure to thrive due to pancreatic malabsorption. Abnormalities in ion transport in the pancreas lead to inflammation and later to fibrosis of the acinar portion of the gland and to hyposecretion of the major digestive enzymes secreted by the pancreas. The presenting symptom is steatorrhoea with the passage of characteristically fatty and offensive stools. Pancreatic steatorrhoea is often accompanied by abdominal discomfort and distension. The majority of patients (85%) are pancreatic insufficient (Davidson 2000). The remaining 15% usually have better nutrition and pulmonary function.

Additional signs and symptoms

The complication of diabetes mellitus in the older patient results from progressive fibrosis damaging the endocrine cells which produce insulin. The onset of diabetes, if not detected and treated promptly, can result in a decline in the patient's clinical condition (Lanng et al 1992). The basic defect affects the hepatobiliary system which can result in a biliary cirrhosis. Patients with severe disease can develop portal hypertension. The main complication is bleeding from gastric or oesophageal varices.

Distal intestinal obstruction syndrome (DIOS) is small bowel obstruction occurring in children and adults and is similar to that seen in neonates presenting with meconium ileus. Often the cause is poor compliance with pancreatic supplements. It presents as small bowel obstruction with abdominal distension and discomfort, vomiting and reduced or absent bowel signs. Diagnosis is confirmed by the classic radiographic appearances of small bowel obstruction.

Puberty may be delayed for both male and female patients. Most women with cystic fibrosis have normal or near-normal fertility. Improving survival has resulted in an increasing number of the female population having children. Outcome of pregnancy is improved if pulmonary function is greater than 60% predicted (Edenborough et al 1995).

Most males are infertile because of developmental defects of the vas deferens, which is either absent or blocked, but they can produce sperm. Improved technology, whereby sperm can be aspirated from either the testis or epididymal sac in conjunction with intracytoplasmic sperm injection (ICSI), has resulted in CF biological fathers (Phillipson et al 2000).

Approximately one-third of adult patients with CF develop rheumatic symptoms (Bourke et al 1987). The two most common forms are an episodic and recurrent arthritis and hypertrophic pulmonary osteoarthropathy. They are characterized by joint pain, tenderness, swelling and limitation of movement, usually symmetrical and affecting particularly the knees, ankles and wrists (Johnson & Knox 1994). More important has been the recent recognition of the high prevalence of low bone mineral density in children and adults (Bachrach et al 1994, Bhudmkanok et al 1996, Haworth et al 1999) which leads to a high incidence of fractures. Rib fractures can result in considerable pain, sputum retention and morbidity.

The respiratory signs and symptoms vary. The majority of older children and adults have a cough productive of sputum with varying degrees of purulence. Chest pain is common and may be musculoskeletal or pleuritic. Breathlessness may be associated with infective exacerbations and increasing disease severity. Pneumothorax should be considered if there is an acute onset of breathlessness and pain. As

breathlessness increases appetite may fall and weight loss is common.

Haemoptysis is common and usually mild, although episodes of frank haemoptysis may occur. Most patients develop finger clubbing which is associated with more severe disease.

Auscultation is often unrewarding when compared with the severity of radiological disease. Coarse crackles are often heard over the upper lobes. A pleural rub may be heard in association with infective exacerbations. The respiratory pathogens most commonly isolated in sputum are *Pseudomonas aeruginosa* (61%), *Staphylococcus aureus* (28.3%), *Haemophilus influenzae* (8.9%) and *Burkholderia cepacia* (3.2%) (FitzSimmons 1993). Infection with *B. cepacia* is often associated with accelerated pulmonary disease and a worse prognosis (Muhdi et al 1996).

The chest radiograph is often normal at birth but early changes include bronchial wall thickening, initially in the upper zones. As the disease progresses, hyperinflation may be noticeable with ill-defined nodular shadows, numerous ring and parallel line shadows indicating bronchial wall thickening and bronchiectasis (Fig. 2.21, p. 51).

Some patients develop nasal polyps; these may grow rapidly and are frequently recurrent. They may be related to chronic sinus infection.

Pulmonary function tests initially show signs of airways obstruction, but with advanced disease a restrictive pattern may be superimposed on the obstructive defect and a diffusion abnormality will also become apparent.

Pulmonary function measurements (FEV_1, PaO_2, $PaCO_2$) have been shown to be predictors of mortality (Kerem et al 1992). As the disease progresses ventilation/perfusion imbalance occurs, leading to hypoxaemia and pulmonary hypertension. Carbon dioxide retention occurs in patients with severe disease.

Asthma is as common in patients with CF as it is among the normal population. Many patients with CF have a positive skin test to *Aspergillus fumigatus*. This is often seen in the sputum of patients but ABPA is less common, occurring in approximately 11% of patients (Brueton et al 1980, Nelson et al 1979). ABPA is recognized by recurrent wheezing, deteriorating chest symptoms, fleeting fluffy shadows on the chest radiograph and elevated IgE levels which are specifically raised to *Aspergillus*. Diagnosis is sometimes difficult radiologically because the chest radiograph in cystic fibrosis is abnormal.

Medical management

Paediatric and adult patients with CF should receive care from a specialist CF centre. Pulmonary function and nutrition, the two main prognostic indicators for survival, are better when care is delivered from paediatric and adult CF centres (Mahadeva et al 1998). Models for shared care between the CF centre and the district hospital at the paediatric level have worked extremely well for many years but this process is not commonly practised at the adult level. Most specialist units have a system of annual review whereby a comprehensive battery of tests is undertaken annually by the patient.

Cystic fibrosis is an extremely complex disease. Care is best delivered by a multidisciplinary team composed of doctors, physiotherapists, dietitians, nurses, social workers, psychologists and other disciplines who will complement each other in their individual areas of expertise. The patient should also be closely involved in choice of care and self-care at home.

Morbidity and mortality are primarily related to chronic progressive respiratory infection. Therefore the mainstay of treatment is oral, nebulized and intravenous antibiotics. Long-term oral anti-staphylococcal antibiotics are given in the early years to treat *Staphylococcus aureus* which is often the main micro-organism causing chronic infection. Subsequently patients become chronically infected with *Ps. aeruginosa* which increases treatment requirements and morbidity. The practice of starting nebulized and oral antibiotics at time of first culture of *Ps. aeruginosa* has been shown to be effective in eradicating and delaying persistent infection (Valerius et al 1991).

Intravenous antibiotics are frequently used for acute infective exacerbations but opinions differ as to the regular or symptomatic use of intravenous antibiotics (Elborn et al 2000). Treatment usually needs to continue for at least 14 days and

can be evaluated by monitoring respiratory function, sputum quantity, body weight, blood gases and blood inflammatory markers such as C-reactive protein (Hodson 1996).

Nebulized antibiotics (Webb & Dodd 1997) have been shown to be effective in the treatment of chronic *Ps. aeruginosa* infection (Mukhopadhyay et al 1996, Touw et al 1995). Antibiotics are usually inhaled twice daily and should follow airway clearance.

Patients needing frequent or prolonged antipseudomonal treatment, who have poor venous access, may require implantable intravenous access devices. These devices can maintain continuity of antibiotic infusions and quality of life for the patient undertaking treatment at home (Shale 1997b, Stead et al 1987).

Segregation of patients colonized with *Burkholderia cepacia* from other patients with cystic fibrosis limits the spread of the organism by social contact (Govan et al 1993, LiPuma et al 1990, Muhdi et al 1996). Health professionals must pay particular attention to hygiene and thorough hand washing between patients (Cystic Fibrosis Trust 1999). More recently there has been concern regarding the emergence of transmissible strains of *Ps. aeruginosa*. Some clinics now practise segregation by microbiological status (Cystic Fibrosis Trust 2001).

Contamination of nebulizers is common and patients must be given instruction in the cleaning and care of nebulizer equipment. To minimize contamination, cleaning and drying of this equipment after use are essential (Hutchinson et al 1996).

Some patients benefit from the inhalation of bronchodilator drugs. Steroids may be indicated if asthma or ABPA complicates cystic fibrosis. The use and value of inhaled steroids to treat the inflammatory component of airflow obstruction in the long-term management of cystic fibrosis are still under review with prospective controlled trials.

As a consequence of lung infection there are large quantities of DNA from the breakdown of inflammatory cells, e.g. neutrophils. The inhalation of rhDNase acts on the DNA in the purulent lung secretions (Range & Knox 1995). It has been shown to improve lung function (Shah et al 1996), reduce viscoelasticity of the mucus (Shah et al 1996) and decrease exacerbations of bronchopulmonary infection (Fuchs et al 1994). Occasionally alteration in voice and episodes of pharyngitis may be experienced, but these are usually minor and transient (Hodson & Shah 1995).

Hypertonic saline inhaled before physiotherapy may also assist in clearance of secretions (Eng et al 1996, Robinson et al 1996). There is little evidence to support the use of other mucolytic agents such as acetylcysteine (Parvolex). Some mucolytic agents may induce bronchoconstriction and a bronchial challenge (pp. 219–220) should be undertaken at the time of the first inhalation.

In CF a high energy intake is needed as a result of malabsorption and the increased metabolic requirements during infection. The dietary energy intake should exceed the normal daily recommendation to sustain and maintain adequate weight, muscle bulk and function (Poole 1995). Supplements of fat-soluble vitamins and vitamin K are usually necessary in addition to pancreatic enzymes which should be taken with all meals and snacks.

When nasal obstruction by polyps is incomplete a corticosteroid nasal spray may be tried. Complete obstruction is unusual and polypectomy may be indicated.

Haemoptysis will usually stop spontaneously but if bleeding is severe and prolonged, embolization of the bronchial artery to the affected lobe would be considered (Cohen 1992, Fairfax et al 1980). The current use of short courses of oral or intravenous tranexamic acid for moderate haemoptyses is effective.

Pneumothorax can occur spontaneously in the older patient. Small pneumothoraces may resolve without treatment, but most pneumothoraces require the insertion of an intercostal drain. Surgical intervention is required for large non-resolving leaks. Video-assisted thorascopic surgery (VATS) may be used to avoid a thoracotomy.

Heart-lung and double lung transplantation (Ch. 16, p. 520) have been successfully carried out in patients with end-stage lung disease but there is a critical shortage of donor organs. Non-invasive ventilation may be life saving and indi-

cated for patients developing severe respiratory failure to bridge the waiting time to transplantation (Hodson et al 1991).

If medical treatment has failed and the patient is distressed palliative care must be expertly employed so the patient dies comfortably and with dignity. It is important not to withhold such care even if the patient is listed for transplantation.

Home treatment

In many countries the emphasis on treatment is moving from hospital to home. The benefits for patients of treatment at home include less disruption to school, work and family life while avoiding the isolation from friends and family that hospitalization incurs.

For the newly diagnosed or newly referred patient, a home visit by a member of the specialist team (usually the clinical nurse specialist) provides an opportunity for advice, education and support for the patient and family, as necessary. Domiciliary physiotherapy services are sometimes available and can provide the opportunity for discussion and demonstration of physiotherapy techniques in the home, an opportunity for a more effective assessment of the necessity and appropriateness of equipment and the possibility of specialist physiotherapy during terminal care. There is also evidence of improved compliance with treatment and a reduction in the stress of coping with the disease (Rogers & Goodchild 1996).

Many patients awaiting heart-lung transplantation can be cared for at home with a clinical nurse specialist visiting to provide assessment and to identify the needs for changes in treatment to maintain optimal health status. It may be appropriate for a patient to either receive a course of intravenous antibiotics at home or to continue a course started in hospital. This has been facilitated by developments in technology: for example, the small, portable, prefilled antibiotic infusion devices (Bramwell et al 1995).

The future

Cystic fibrosis is a complex disease. An enormous amount of effort is being expended to improve standards of care (De Boeck 2000), provide guidelines for antibiotic treatment (Cystic Fibrosis Trust 2000, Doring et al 2000) and evidence based upon controlled trials for different aspects of treatment (Cheng et al 2000). More patients (but not enough) are being transplanted and survival figures are improving with greater experience (Vizza et al 2000). The physicians and scientists are continuously evaluating current care (Davis et al 1996) and searching for new therapies to improve quality of life and long-term survival (Rubin 1998).

Gene therapy aims to correct the basic defect. The gene is transferred in a 'carrier'. Liposomes and adenovirus have been used, but difficulties have been experienced. The adenovirus can stimulate an inflammatory response and the liposome is not as efficient as a 'carrier' (Du Bois 1995). Theoretically the transfer of sufficient normal copies of the CFTR gene to sufficient numbers of affected cells should result in the production of enough normal protein to reduce the clinical manifestations of cystic fibrosis (Stern & Geddes 1994). There is considerable research in progress which may lead to effective gene therapy in the future.

Physiotherapy management

Advances in the medical management of cystic fibrosis have increased the expectation of survival into the fifth decade of life (Elborn et al 1991). As the science of the basic defect is translated into a greater understanding of the pathophysiology of the disease and novel complications of an ageing population emerge, the physiotherapist's role is continually challenged. The management encompasses the treatment from birth through childhood and adolescence into adulthood and parenting. It is adapted through changing lifestyles, disease severity and the changes of the acute exacerbation and stable state of the disease. Physiotherapy requires detailed accurate assessment and treatment tailored to the individual as lifestyle and disease severity change. In parallel with the advances in the medical management, the role of the physiotherapist has expanded from the clearance of

bronchial secretions to include the assessment of exercise capacity and the prescription of safe and effective exercise programmes, assessment and education of inhalation therapy and in the later stages of the disease the use of oxygen therapy and non-invasive ventilation (NIV). More recently the problems of musculoskeletal pain, low bone mineral density and urinary incontinence have emerged. The physiotherapist's treatment is confounded by the many complications of this multisystem disease, e.g. diabetes, distal intestinal obstruction syndrome and arthropathy. Improved survival is also attributed to the enormous burden of self-care imposed on patients. To enhance adherence to this treatment regimen it is crucial that the physiotherapist works with the patient and their family/carers to encourage an effective but realistic treatment plan balanced with their wishes to lead a normal life.

Excess bronchial secretions

The removal of bronchial secretions remains the mainstay of physiotherapy management as bronchial infection and respiratory failure continue to be the major causes of morbidity and mortality. Currently airway clearance is recommended from the time of diagnosis. The debate of its value for the asymptomatic infant continues. However, there is evidence of inflammation and infection at this stage of the disease (Armstrong et al 1995, Khan et al 1995, Konstan et al 1994) and the concern of withdrawing a well-established treatment raises ethical issues when considering a randomized controlled trial. Most paediatricians recommend introducing physiotherapy at this time in an attempt to delay the destructive process of infection and fibrosis. If physiotherapy becomes an accepted part of life, compliance may be better than if it (physiotherapy) is introduced at a later stage. A close bonding usually develops between the parents and the child. It is important that both parents are involved and that the siblings are included in the care of the affected child so that they do not feel left out.

Traditionally, in the infant, treatment has comprised the use of gravity-assisted positions and chest clapping. In the absence of specific radiological signs, drainage of the apical segments of the upper lobes is included as the infant will spend much of his time lying down. The position is sitting upright on the parent's lap with the head and shoulders supported (see Fig. 6.31). Other recommended positions are alternate side lying and prone in a head-down position and supine flat. When the child begins to sit and stand the apical segments can be omitted from treatment, but it is then important to include the anterior segments of the upper lobes. Although the cause is unknown, the upper lobes are frequently the most severely affected (Tomashefski et al 1986). If an infant or child has specific radiological signs, treatment may need to be more frequent and, if tolerated, of slightly longer duration. Treatment is usually advised before feeds and for 10–15 minutes twice a day.

Infants with cystic fibrosis have a higher incidence of gastro-oesophageal reflux (GOR), but there is conflicting evidence as to whether this is exacerbated by the head-down tipped position (Button et al 1997, Phillips 1996, Taylor & Threlfall 1997). Gravitational effects in the tipped position lead to a lowering of intraabdominal pressure and an increase in intrathoracic pressure. This, together with an increase in diaphragmatic activity, may enhance the competence of the oesophageal sphincter (Sindel et al 1989). When an increase in GOR has been confirmed anti-reflux medication should be prescribed and the effect of positioning must be assessed.

Although this traditional form of treatment is still practised widely, many centres internationally are now using alternative methods of treatment in infants and small children, e.g. PEP, physical activity and other airway clearance techniques, and the value of routine treatment in asymptomatic infants is under discussion.

Even at a young age treatment should be fun. The young child can be bounced up and down on his parent's knees and another exercise that is fun for the family is 'wheelbarrows' (Fig. 20.4). Laughing will also stimulate coughing and the mini-trampoline can be introduced (Fig. 20.5). From the age of 2 years the child can be encouraged to actively participate in breathing tech-

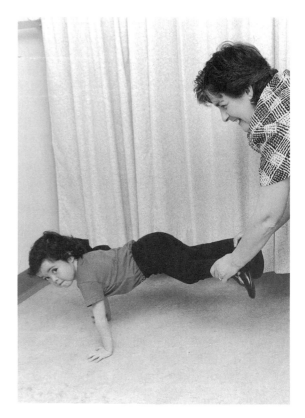

Fig. 20.4 'Wheelbarrows'.

niques in the form of play. The whole family can be involved in these games.

Infants and small children swallow their bronchial secretions, but as soon as possible expectoration should be encouraged. Nasopharyngeal suction should only be used if it is essential to obtain a sputum specimen or if the infant is distressed by the secretions. Learning to blow the nose is important to keep the upper airways clear.

From as early an age as possible children should be encouraged to play a more active role in their treatment. With increased cooperation the child can be introduced to various airway clearance techniques and become independent with treatment (Table 20.2).

Infected bronchial secretions are responsible for many complications in the airways and lung tissue (Fig. 20.6). Obstruction occurs initially in the small airways, with repeated infections and hypersecretion resulting in damage to the airway

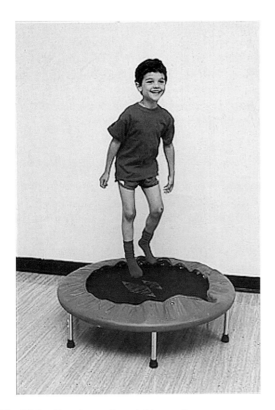

Fig. 20.5 Exercise on the mini-trampoline.

Table 20.2 Airway clearance techniques

Active cycle of breathing techniques (ACBT)
Autogenic drainage (AD)
Modified autogenic drainage (M AD)
Exercise
High-frequency chest wall oscillation (HFCWO)
Intrapulmonary percussive ventilation (IPV)
Oscillating positive expiratory pressure:
   Flutter®
   R-C Cornet®
Positive expiratory pressure (PEP):
   PEP
   High PEP
Postural drainage and percussion

wall, central airway instability and hyperreactivity. Infected secretions in cystic fibrosis are dehydrated, hyperadhesive and hyperviscoelastic. Studies of the techniques have attempted to identify characteristics to address some of the problems of the airway and secretions. The presenting pathological problem should be considered

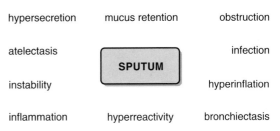

Fig. 20.6 The pathophysiological consequences of sputum.

when choosing an airway clearance technique (Lapin 2000).

In order to achieve effective treatment, secretions have to be mobilized and removed without causing an increase in airway obstruction or fatigue. Mobilization may be achieved by improving collateral ventilation and allowing air to get behind obstructive secretions (e.g. the thoracic expansion exercises of ACBT and positive expiratory pressure of PEP), the concept of interdependence (p. 190) (e.g. the thoracic expansion exercises of ACBT) and breath holding to improve ventilatory asynchrony (e.g. the thoracic expansion exercises of ACBT and autogenic drainage).

Theoretically, altering the rheological properties of sputum may improve clearance. High-frequency chest wall oscillation (HFCWO) and oscillating PEP, e.g. Flutter® and R-C Cornet®, have been shown to decrease the viscoelasticity of secretions (App et al 1998, Scherer et al 1998). The oscillatory movements which occur with forced expiratory manoeuvres (Freitag et al 1989) and the relationship of reduced viscosity with increasing shear forces (Lapin 2000) explain the mechanism of huffing.

The removal of secretions is enhanced by increasing expiratory airflow. Manoeuvres which cause airway compression by increasing intrathoracic pressure will increase expiratory flow in proportion to the degree of compression (van der Schans 1997). However, in the presence of bronchial wall instability expiratory airflow is reduced when intrathoracic pressures are high (Zach et al 1985). Huffing generates less intrathoracic pressure than coughing (Langlands 1967) and it has been suggested that it is as effective as coughing for mucociliary clearance (Hasani et al 1994). Autogenic drainage prevents airway collapse by maximizing airflow at different lung volumes and avoiding high-pressure peaks (Schöni 1989). By altering the intrathoracic pressure and the lung volume at which the expiratory manoeuvre is performed, the physiotherapist can tailor the point of compression to the area of obstruction without causing airway collapse.

Exercise offers an important contribution to sputum expectoration (Baldwin et al 1994, Sahl et al 1989), but in the majority of patients it should be complementary and not exclusive (Bilton et al 1992). Patients perceive exercise differently to other forms of treatment (Abbott et al 1996) and some prefer this method of airway clearance. It is important for the physiotherapist to be sensitive to the patients' beliefs (Carr et al 1996) but encourage formal airway clearance during an acute exacerbation when the patient is unable to exercise at their normal level.

The frequency and duration of treatment will vary. When secretions are minimal, treatment once a day may be sufficient but additionally some form of exercise should be encouraged. Many patients will require treatment two or three times a day, but the programme should be realistic and allow for other normal activities. If a session is required in the middle of the day, this can probably be done in a sitting position at school, college or work.

Currently there is no evidence to suggest that any technique is superior. Trials are confounded by small numbers, inconsistency of techniques and no control population (Prasad & Main 1998). To date the majority of trials have been short term and undertaken mainly in adults. A meta-analysis of chest physiotherapy suggested that chest clearance produced significantly greater sputum expectoration than no treatment and the addition of exercise further improved lung function (Thomas et al 1995). However, a systematic review was not able to demonstrate a benefit for treatment compared with no treatment, although short-term studies indicate that there may be deterioration in lung function during periods without treatment (van der Schans et al 2000).

Some techniques can be time consuming to perform, difficult to learn and may be position dependent. Others involve equipment which requires meticulous cleaning. The choice of technique should be individualized to suit the patient's age, lifestyle and disease severity and be acceptable to patient and carer.

Maintenance / increase in exercise tolerance

The value of exercise in the management of CF is now well established. Short-term studies of exercise training programmes in cystic fibrosis have been shown to have considerable therapeutic benefit and the majority of patients wish to include exercise in their routine self-care (Webb & Dodd 2000). Studies have shown improved exercise tolerance (Andreasson et al 1987, Edlund et al 1986, Freeman et al 1993), ventilatory muscle endurance (Keens et al 1977), cardiorespiratory fitness (Orenstein et al 1981), muscle bulk and body image (Strauss et al 1987), decreased breathlessness (O'Neill et al 1987) and improved quality of life (de Jong et al 1997). More recently, two randomized controlled trials of home exercise programmes have demonstrated the long-term value of exercise (Moorcroft et al 2000, Schneiderman-Walker et al 2000). Early studies demonstrated that patients with mild to moderate disease ($FEV_1 \geq 55\%$ predicted) could exercise to the same level as their peers, but those with more severe disease ($FEV_1 < 55\%$ predicted) would require individualized recommendations and supervised exercise programmes (Cropp 1982). Everyone can exercise and no patient should be excluded because of disease severity (Webb & Dodd 2000).

Assessment of exercise capacity

The patient's baseline exercise capacity should be assessed, when the patient is clinically stable, to determine their level of fitness and limitations. The results will give guidance for effective and safe exercise recommendations. The test will provide a baseline measure for further testing to monitor improvement or change in any values and evaluate an intervention. Assessment should

Table 20.3 Types of exercise test

Endurance exercise	Progressive maximal • Treadmill • Cycle ergometer • Modified shuttle walk Sub maximal • Treadmill • Cycle ergometer • Step test
Peak power output	Wingate protocol
Strength	Isokinetic dynamometer Isometric dynamometer Maximal weight which can be lifted comfortably (1RM)

Table 20.4 Measurements and equipment required for assessing exercise capacity

Measurements	Equipment
Peak work capacity	• Bicycle – resistance • Treadmill – speed and incline • Walking – speed and distance
Peak heart rate	• Cardiac monitor • Pulse meter • Fingers
Oxygen saturation	• Pulse oximeter
Spirometry (pre- and post-exercise)	• Spirometer
Perceived breathlessness	• Borg or VAS scores • 15-count breathlessness score
Perceived muscular fatigue	• Borg or VAS scores
Respiratory rate	• Count or 'on-line'
Ventilation ($\dot{V}_E$, V_T, TiTOT,RR) Oxygen uptake CO_2 output End-tidal CO_2	• On-line system
Blood lactate	• Lactate analyser or blood to laboratory
PaO_2 and $PaCO_2$	• Arterial line

consider the choice of protocol, the type of test and the measurements required. The choice of protocol (Table 20.3) depends on the information required, the facilities available and the patient's clinical condition. It may be desirable to determine a functional level of exercise in preference to peak performance (Jones 1988).

Space may be limited and a cycle ergometer may therefore be more appropriate than the modified shuttle test (Bradley et al 1999). The patient may be too breathless to perform a maximal test and some tests may be too difficult for children to perform. The step test may be a validated alternative to measure functional exercise capacity (Balfour-Lynn et al 1998). The measurements and equipment required are outlined in Table 20.4. The standard measures of work capacity (distance walked, wattage), pulse, oxygen saturation and a subjective measure of breathlessness and muscle fatigue are sufficient for routine assessment (Fig. 20.7). More sophisticated measures give additional information but are not necessary for routine use. Safety precautions during testing should include personnel trained in resuscitation; oxygen and appropriate drugs for resuscitation should be immediately available in the exercise department. From the results of the test the physiotherapist can recommend a level of exercise to provide an appropriate training effect which is safe. It is a useful complement to an exercise test to establish the pattern of habitual activity. Some patients are unwilling to participate in formal exercise programmes but are happy to increase everyday activity.

Exercise programmes

Exercise is limited by the symptoms of breathlessness or muscle fatigue. The aim of an exercise programme is to improve exercise performance, make a given level of exercise more comfortable and increase the activities of daily living. It is important to establish the goals of an exercise programme for the individual patient, which may be different for carer and patient (Table 20.5). Exercise programmes must be tailored to the individual, based on disease severity, level of fitness and patient preference.

Types of exercise

An exercise programme should combine endurance and strength-training exercises for upper and lower body.

● Endurance exercise aims to improve the capacity to endure more exercise without discomfort, e.g. swimming, running, cycling, skipping, aerobic classes, step aerobics, trampolines

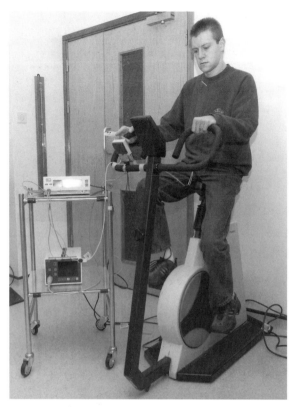

Fig. 20.7 Assessing exercise capacity with cycle ergometry and pulse oximetry monitoring.

Table 20.5 The differing aims of exercise programmes for the patient and carer

Aims of carer	Aims of patient
• ↑ Maximal exercise performance, endurance and strength	• Healthy lifestyle
• ↓ Breathlessness	• Enjoyment and social interaction
• ↑ Nutritional status	• Improved body image
• ↑ Quality of life	• Improved stamina for socializing
• ↓ Respiratory tract infections	• Improved fitness for a sporting activity
• Preserve lung function	• A replacement for chest clearance
• ? Decrease mortality	

(Edlund et al 1986, Orenstein et al 1981, Sahl et al 1989) (Fig. 20.8).

• Strength training aims to increase muscle mass and strength, e.g. weights and sprint training (Strauss et al 1987) (Fig. 20.9).
• Interval training may be useful for those patients unable to sustain long periods of

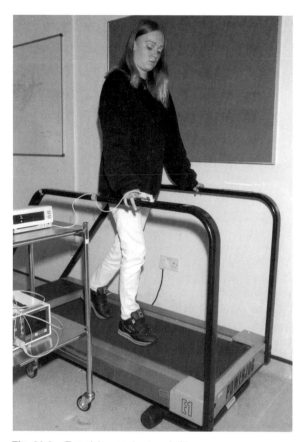

Fig. 20.8 Exercising on the treadmill.

exercise. Short bursts of exercise at higher rates will enhance a training response. It may be of benefit for those patients with prolonged periods of desaturation.
• The evidence for inspiratory muscle training is conflicting (Asher et al 1982, Sawyer & Clayton 1993) and to date has shown no advantage over general upper body muscle training (Keens et al 1977).
• There are no studies to date evaluating the benefits of a lifestyle change. Parents of children and adolescents with CF are less positive about the benefits of exercise than the parents of healthy children (Boas et al 1999). It is important to establish from the time of diagnosis the importance of the contribution of exercise to a healthy lifestyle and to encourage participation of the whole family. There is a decline in physical activity in late adolescence (Britto et al

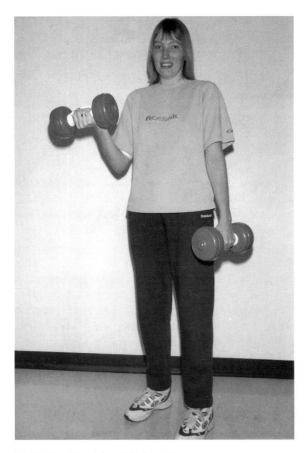

Fig. 20.9 Exercising with dumbells.

2000). Careful consideration and encouragement should be given to this age group at this time. Contact by the physiotherapist with local gym and sports facilities can often lead to reduced rates for exercise sessions.

Intensity, duration and frequency

Endurance exercise. An effective exercise programme should make reasonable demands on the patient's physical capacity and be progressive. The intensity can be derived from the results of the exercise test. Various recommendations have been suggested:

- 50% of peak work capacity is below the anaerobic threshold for most patients and represents a functional level of activity (Marcotte et al 1986)

- 50–60% $\dot{V}O_2$peak is necessary to improve physical fitness (Astrand & Rodahl 1977) and the patient's capability is related to the percentage of their individual $\dot{V}O_2$peak
- 70–85% of the measured maximum heart rate is sufficient to achieve a training effect (Orenstein et al 1981)
- 'breathlessness without distress' for those patients with severe disease who are limited by ventilatory mechanics (Godfrey & Mearns 1971).

Exercise should begin at the chosen intensity for a period of time sufficient to cause breathlessness or muscle fatigue without undue stress and progress to 20–30 minutes 3–4 days a week. Progression for the patient who is limited by breathlessness will be at a slower rate than the unfit patient who is limited by muscular fatigue.

Strength training. This should begin with a weight that can be lifted comfortably 10–15 times and progressed by increasing the repetitions to 20–30 and then by increasing the weight. The intensity should be sufficient to leave the patient 'pleasantly tired without soreness'. The duration and frequency can progress to 15–30 minutes on alternate days. It is important to ensure correct positioning, correct technique and coordination of breathing for each exercise. A warm-up, stretching exercises and cool-down should be incorporated into each session to avoid injury. A more aerobic programme would include low weights and high repetitions whereas high weights and low repetitions constitute an anaerobic programme.

Strength training in children should be approached with care. Growing bones are sensitive to repetitive loading and the epiphysial plate is susceptible to injury before full growth is complete. Overstrenuous resistance training is as dangerous for children as it is for adults and joints should not be subjected to repetitive stress. As with adults, exercises should be carefully planned and well performed in a correct position.

Precautions

There are no absolute precautions but exercise should cease temporarily for the following medical problems: abdominal obstruction, an acute bronchopulmonary exacerbation associated with fever, transient arthralgia and arthritis, pneumothorax, persistent haemoptysis and surgery, including a caesarian section. Exercise-induced bronchoconstriction is rare in CF and can be controlled with pre-exercise bronchodilators. Patients undertaking exercise in hot climates should be well hydrated and advised to take salt tablets (Bar-Or et al 1992). Exercise for the diabetic patient should be encouraged (see below). Certain sporting activities carry a medical risk (Webb & Dodd 1999). Contact sports, bungee jumping and parachute jumping are not advised for those patients with diagnosed osteoporosis, portal hypertension and significant enlargement of the spleen and liver. Scuba diving could be hazardous for patients with air trapping and sinus disease. In the hypoxic patient, exercise at altitude poses a potential risk (Speechley-Dick et al 1992). Careful advice should be given to patients contemplating skiing and any fierce aerobic and anaerobic exercise at altitude.

Exercising the patient with advancing disease

There is no evidence that carefully tailored and supervised exercise is harmful in these patients and they should not be excluded from a training programme. For patients with severe disease and those awaiting transplantation deconditioning rapidly occurs. Maintaining mobility is crucial and strength and endurance exercises should be encouraged (Webb et al 1996). A maximal exercise test will define the limits of breathlessness and muscle fatigue and exercise programmes should be planned with these in mind. Positions for breathing control (Ch. 6, p. 182) should be introduced to alleviate exertion breathlessness and increase mobility.

Studies have reported the benefits of oxygen supplementation for patients with severe disease (Heijerman et al 1992, Marcus et al 1992). Oxygen may be required to ease the symptom of breathlessness and increase exercise performance. Many patients are reluctant to use oxygen for activity, especially outdoors. Considerable benefits are achieved using oxygen before and after exercise for recovery. Small oxygen cylinders can be used discreetly by patients to enable them to travel and socialize in the community. During exercise and periods of recovery, inspiratory flow rates increase, so the oxygen prescription and delivery device should be adjusted to relieve exercise-induced breathlessness. Patients mouth breathe during exercise and periods of breathlessness and a fixed concentration mask at low concentration and high flows may provide greater relief than nasal cannulae (Dodd et al 1998). The oxygen flow should be titrated to a level of comfort which provides a SpO_2 >90% (Heijerman et al 1992). For patients who are dependent on non-invasive ventilation, exercise should also be performed using the equipment (Webb et al 1996). This can take the form of weight training in sitting and step-ups in standing or walking on a treadmill (Fig. 20.10). Careful assessment with attention to respiratory rate and perceived breathlessness and exertion can provide a comfortable level of exercise without undue breathlessness, with or without oxygen to maintain mobility and quality of life.

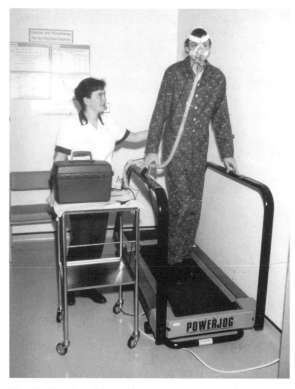

Fig. 20.10 Exercising with non-invasive ventilation. (Reproduced with permission from Webb et al 1996.)

Inhalation of drugs

Patients are prescribed an ever-increasing number of drugs delivered by inhalation. Delivery is potentially maximized by matching the patient's inspiratory flow rate and drug characteristics to the delivery device. Inhalers are more convenient and less time consuming than nebulizers but some drugs can only be delivered by the nebulized route.

Bronchodilators

Bronchodilators are prescribed to relieve obstruction and careful evaluation by reversibility testing and subjective benefit will determine the response and the merits of the inhaled or nebulized route for the individual patient. Beta-adrenergic drugs increase cilial action, improve mucociliary clearance (Wood et al 1975) and may be of benefit before chest clearance (Kuhn & Nahata 1985). During an acute exacerbation, when secretions are excessive and the obstruction is increased, the nebulized route is recommended (Conway & Watson 1997). Inhalers are available in a range of doses. It is preferable and less time consuming for the patient to be prescribed a higher dose than to increase the number of puffs of a lower dose.

The value of long-acting beta-2 agonists has been described (Bargon et al 1997) but the role of inhaled corticosteroids is as yet inconclusive (Bisgaard et al 1997, Balfour-Lynn et al 1997). Serial PEFR measurements may identify objective benefit. CF patients often show a dip in PEFR and report symptoms of tightness in the early evening. One can speculate that this is because drugs are metabolized faster in patients with CF so that the benefits of long-acting drugs are shortened. It is important to select a device which is both acceptable to the individual patient and matches their inspiratory flow rate. Generally CF patients have high inspiratory flow rates. There are various teaching devices to assess patient technique and suitability for the required flow rate of the device, but careful consideration must be given to the risk of cross-infection in this patient group. Some commercially prescribed devices require specific inspiratory flow rates for effective deposition. The Accuhaler® (GlaxoSmithKline) is a dry powder inhaler which is less dependent on inspiratory flow (Hill & Slater 1998). It is less confusing for the patient if the same device is prescribed for all drugs. It is sometimes possible to combine two types of drug in one device, e.g Seretide® (GlaxoSmithKline). The physiotherapist should always be mindful of the treatment burden on CF patients.

Mucolytic agents

Inhalation of hypertonic saline by an ultrasonic nebulizer has been shown to improve lung function and perceived effectiveness of chest physiotherapy over a 2-week period (Eng et al 1996) and to improve mucociliary clearance after one inhalation (Robinson & Anderson 1996). In both of these studies the positive effects were significantly increased when compared to 0.9% saline. Hypertonic saline may induce bronchoconstriction (Rodwell et al 1996). A test dose should be given, with recordings of PEFR or FEV_1 before and 5 minutes after inhalation, to identify any increase in airflow obstruction. Pre-treatment with a bronchodilator would be recommended for those patients at risk (Suri et al 2000a).

The optimal drug effect of rhDNase is different for each individual and can vary from 30 minutes to several hours. It is recommended initially that inhalation should be performed before early evening to avoid coughing during sleeping hours and 30 minutes to 2 hours before chest clearance (Conway & Watson 1997). Some patients who have difficulty clearing sputum in the morning gain considerable benefit from inhalation of rhDNase at night, without coughing during sleeping hours. Treatment regimens should therefore be individualized and frequently assessed as the disease changes. When the optimum time has been determined, inhalation in relation to chest clearance can be recommended. RhDNase should not be mixed with other drugs as it requires isotonic conditions and a neutral pH for maximal activity. If nebulized antibiotics or inhaled steroids are part of the treatment regimen, the pH of these solutions is acidic and may denature the protein (Ramsey & Dorkin 1994). At least 30 minutes should separate antibiotic and rhDNase inhalation (Conway & Watson 1997). A sidestream nebulizer (Medic Aid, Bognor Regis, West Sussex) has been recommended for inhalation (Shah et al 1997). The nebulizer chamber used for rhDNase should not be used for any other drug. RhDNase should be stored at 0–4°C and should be removed from the refrigerator and brought to room temperature (approximately 15 minutes) before inhalation to avoid bronchoconstriction.

Mucolytic agents, for example acetylcysteine (Parvolex), are said to reduce mucus viscosity.

Antibiotics

Aerosol antibiotics should be inhaled after secretions have been cleared. Studies have shown that bronchoconstriction may be induced (Chua et al 1990, Maddison et al 1994, Nikolaizik et al 1996). A test dose should be performed when the patient is clinically stable to detect any increase in airflow obstruction. Spirometry should be performed before, immediately and up to 30 minutes post inhalation (Webb & Dodd 1997). Bronchoconstriction may be prevented by altering the tonicity of the solution to iso- or hypotonic (Dodd et al 1997). The long-term effects of repeated bronchoconstriction are unknown and it is now recommended that the inhalation of antibiotics should be preceded by an inhaled bronchodilator (Chua et al 1990, Webb & Dodd 1997).

The details of inhaling several drugs can be complex. It is crucial that the patient is given verbal and written instructions of how to use (including the cleaning and maintenance of any equipment), when to use and the order of use in relation to chest clearance and other drugs. An individualized timetable should be agreed, taking into account social and work commitments. Assessment and techniques should frequently be reviewed as the disease progresses.

Acute bronchopulmonary infection

Increased cough and sputum production with a fall in spirometry, decreased exercise tolerance, weight loss, lack of energy and increased breathlessness are the usual signs and symptoms of an acute exacerbation. Fever and chest pain are additional symptoms. It is likely that the duration and frequency of airway clearance should be increased and, if necessary, assistance given with manual techniques. Periods of breathing control may need to be lengthened to avoid fatigue and the treatment should be discontinued before the patient feels exhausted. Positions for treatment may need to be modified to reduce breathlessness. During periods of rest the positions of high side lying and forward lean sitting may facilitate contraction of the diaphragm, by altering the length–tension status (Sharp et al 1980), and ease the work of breathing. There are such wide variations in pathology, signs and symptoms that for the inexperienced physiotherapist it is very difficult to know when to discontinue a treatment session. As a guide, a treatment session may range from about 20 to 45 minutes.

Various adjuncts may be required to improve the effectiveness of treatment. The relief of airway obstruction should be maximized. Regular nebulized bronchodilators are recommended (Conway & Watson 1997) and benefits have been reported following the use of intravenous terbutaline (Finnegan et al 1992) or aminophylline (Hodson 2000). There is no evidence that inhaling bland aerosols, e.g. normal saline, is effective in improving the rheological properties of mucus, increasing ciliary clearance or increasing mucus transport in CF (Wanner & Rao 1980). Inhalation of hypertonic saline and rhDnase has been shown to be effective (Fuchs et al 1994). Although rhDNase is recognized to be the treatment of choice (Suri et al 2000b) there is individual variability and both drugs are worthy of consideration.

IPPB may be indicated for the tiring breathless patient who is having difficulty clearing secretions because of compromised ventilatory mechanics. Careful consideration must be given in patients who have had a previous pneumothorax.

Supplemental oxygen, during airway clearance, is advised if the PaO_2 is below 8.0 kPa (60 mmHg) or SpO_2 is below 92%. Theoretically improving hypoxia will decrease respiratory rate and improve tidal volume, hence promoting a more effective treatment. Airway clearance techniques may be better tolerated and breathlessness reduced with the use of supplemental oxygen. The high total gas flows of low-concentration Venturi masks may be more acceptable and provide greater relief than nasal cannulae for recovery from coughing (Dodd et al 1998).

Oxygen therapy for respiratory failure

CF patients have a supra-normal drive to breathe, with an increased ventilatory response to increasing hypoxia resulting in a lower than usual PCO_2. Inspiratory time is increased, which further increases the work of breathing. Patients are therefore unlikely to chronically retain carbon dioxide but at a PaO_2 below 50 mmHg, ventilation decreases and respiratory failure easily ensues (Bureau et al 1981) (presumably due to muscle fatigue in the presence of an increasing respiratory drive). CF patients have high inspiratory flow rates and the normal recommended flow rates of fixed-concentration masks may be insufficient to meet that demand. It is important to increase the normal recommended flow rate to meet the peak inspiratory flow rate, i.e. a 24% mask may require settings of 2–4 litres or more and a 28% mask 4–6 litres or more. Failure to increase the flow rate will result in a decreased oxygen concentration and increased work of breathing. For the severely breathless patient requiring >28% concentration, oxygen delivery by a high-flow generator at low concentrations of oxygen (32%) may be necessary (Dodd et al 1998) (Fig. 20.11).

CF patients hypoventilate at night with a significant increase in $PaCO_2$ (Spier et al 1984). The ventilatory response to hypercapnia is blunted in CF and although the long-term consequences of increasing hypercapnia are unclear one can speculate that ventilatory drive and CO_2 sensitivity may be blunted (Gozal 1997). A fixed-concentration mask should be considered for the safe delivery of oxygen at night time but NIV may be required for those patients with increasing levels of $PaCO_2$ in response to oxygen. CF patients may not be hypercapnic during the day but may retain carbon dioxide at night and may therefore respond differently to supplemental oxygen administered at night than during the day. An accurate prescription will be necessary for night time, exercise and at rest with details of delivery device, concentration and flow rate.

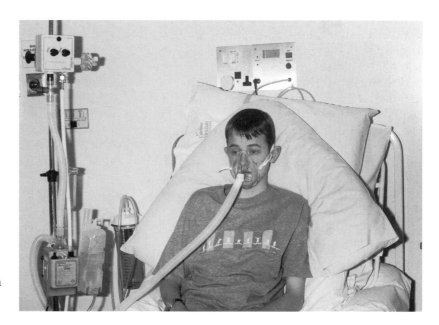

Fig. 20.11   Oxygen delivered by a high-flow generator (Vital Signs, Brighton, Sussex).

NIV has reported benefits for patients who are listed for transplantation (Hodson et al 1991, Hill et al 1998) and for the stable hypercapnic patient at home (Piper et al 1992). The physiotherapist may be involved with introducing the patient to the ventilator and adjusting the settings to meet the patient's comfort and give adequate oxygenation. For some patients NIV may be continued during airway clearance with appropriate adjustment to the settings, but for others airway clearance alone or in conjunction with IPPB is just as effective. The development of a pneumothorax in patients who are dependent on NIV causes a medical management dilemma. If a patent intercostal tube is in situ, NIV can be delivered safely with a pressure preset ventilator. Each patient will require supervised and individualized management with the risks of mechanical ventilation being balanced against the potential benefits (Haworth et al 2000).

Humidification of oxygen

It is recommended that oxygen should be humidified in CF, due to the basic defect in the airway. It is suggested that water vapour humidity is preferable to nebulised humidity for maintenance of PaO_2 (Kuo et al 1991). Oxygen delivered by nasal cannulae can be humidified with a bubble through water vapour humidifier to a maximum flow of 6 litres. A heated humidifier (e.g. Aerodyne, Kendall, Basingstoke, Hampshire; Fisher & Paykel, Maidenhead, Berkshire) is necessary to humidify the large volumes of gas delivered by 24% and 28% concentration masks and a high-flow generator because the time interval for moisture transfer decreases as flow rate increases above 20 l/min (p. 224). The large volumes of air delivered by NIV may cause drying of secretions and require humidification by a heated water vapour source (HC 100 Sullivan). This may increase the problem of breakdown of the skin on the bridge of the nose and in those patients, humidification may have to be reserved for the acute exacerbation. In the terminal stage of the disease when secretions are very tenacious it may be necessary to humidify the oxygen delivered to the nasal mask with a bubble-through humidifier.

Domiciliary oxygen

Transferring oxygen into the community can be a challenge (Dodd et al 1998). Oxygen concentrators are usually prescribed for night-time use. The driving pressure is much lower than that of a cylinder and although adequate for use with nasal cannulae and NIV, there may be difficulties with the use of venturi masks. Cylinders and 24% or 28% venturi masks are recommended for relief of breathlessness, but domiciliary flow heads are limited to 2 or 4 litres. A multiflow head can be supplied by the CF centre for those patients who require higher flow rates. Liquid oxygen is the ideal system for CF patients and allows mobility outside the home. It is not prescribable and funding may be required.

Complications of cystic fibrosis

Advanced cystic fibrosis

The late stages of the disease are characterized by repeated exacerbations, often with continuous intravenous antibiotics and increased hospitalization, respiratory failure and reduced mobility. It is essential to maximize the reversal of airway obstruction with airway clearance techniques, nebulized and intravenous bronchodilators and steroids. Sputum viscosity is reduced with rhDNase and intravenous fluids. Shortness of breath is decreased with humidified oxygen, careful positioning and relaxation techniques. Type I respiratory failure requires meticulous evaluation at rest and during mobility for the requirements of oxygen. Hypercapnic respiratory failure may be reversed with NIV. Mobility is crucial for patients who are listed for transplantation (p. 527) and to maintain quality of life. Some patients have difficulty coming to terms with their loss of independence and input from a clinical psychologist experienced in the treatment of cystic fibrosis may prove beneficial.

Despite optimal medical and physiotherapeutic care the terminal stage of the disease will ensue. It is inappropriate to withdraw support in the terminal stages even though physiotherapy may no longer be effective. Assistance can be given with positioning the breathless patient in high side lying or sitting leaning forward to make him as comfortable as possible. Occasionally IPPB can be used to assist the clearance of secretions from the upper airways, but care must be taken to use it only as a part of physiotherapy treatment and not as a form of pseudoventilation. Nasotracheal suction is not indicated as it would serve no useful purpose at this stage. Morphine or one of its derivatives will help to relieve anxiety and breathlessness.

Allergic bronchopulmonary aspergillosis

Tenacious mucus plugs, often brown in colour, and wheezing are the common presenting symptoms of allergic bronchopulmonary aspergillosis (ABPA). Airway obstruction is increased and there is a marked reduction in lung function. The mucus plugging can lead to lobar or segmental collapse and subsequent bronchiectasis (Alfaham & Goodchild 1996). Treatment should include nebulized bronchodilators and airway clearance techniques, adapted to minimize airway obstruction. IPPB may be indicated. Exercise tolerance may be reduced (Simmonds et al 1990) and programmes may need to be modified.

Arthropathy and joint pain

CF-related arthropathy can present as hypertrophic pulmonary osteoarthropathy (HPOA) or periodic arthritis (Koch & Lanng 2000). HPOA is related to pulmonary disease and presents most frequently in adults. Episodes of transient arthritis appear to be unrelated to pulmonary disease. HPOA is characterized by pain, swelling and warmth of the involved area and occasionally small joint effusions. Arthritis can be associated with fever and vasculitis. Active physiotherapy is not generally indicated. Joints should be rested and gentle mobilization encouraged within the limits of the symptoms. The medical management for a pulmonary exacerbation may lead to a resolution of symptoms (Rush et al 1986) and CF arthritis usually resolves spontaneously (Turner et al 1997).

Cystic fibrosis-related diabetes

The specific changes in glucose metabolism in CF are well described (Koch & Lanng 2000). The incidence increases with age and it is suggested that survival is reduced in this group. Hyperglycaemia causes polyuria which leads to dehydration and a possible increase in sputum viscosity. Expectoration is difficult and lung function declines. The physiotherapist should be alert to the results of blood glucose monitoring (BM) in the analysis of chest symptoms and formulation of a treatment plan. It is essential that the medical management includes control of blood sugar and rehydration with intravenous fluids. When diabetes is difficult to control attention should be directed to the application of airway clearance techniques which reduce viscosity and the consideration of rhDNase.

Insulin requirements will change with exercise. Exercise can sometimes improve overall blood glucose control by reducing insulin requirements. When diabetes is well controlled, exercise may induce hypoglycaemia. The balance of insulin requirement and carbohydrate intake should be discussed with the CF dietitian and physician and individualized for both normal activity and exercise programmes. It is important to maintain exercise during admission to hospital because reduced activity will result in an increase in BM values. If the diabetes is labile during an acute exacerbation a pre-exercise BM is advisable in addition to close liaison with the dietitian.

Distal intestinal obstruction syndrome

This complication describes intestinal obstruction occurring after the neonatal period (Davidson 2000). It is characterized by abdominal pain, distension, vomiting, palpable faecal masses and partial or complete intestinal obstruction. Urgent medical management includes intravenous rehydration, gastrograffin and possibly a balanced electrolyte solution. The symptoms of immobility, pain, decreased FRC and dehydration compromise the clearance of secretions. It is important for airway clearance to continue but techniques should be modified until the problem resolves. Mobilization is encouraged and may help bowel movement. For patients with a persistent problem, a lower body exercise programme may be useful.

Gastro-oesophageal reflux

This is well recognized in CF with a higher incidence in infants. The cause and effect of physiotherapy positioning for this group are controversial. Treatment is directed at medical management with the use of prokinetic agents and/or gastric suppressants, thickening of feeds and appropriate positioning. The adult is often unaware that gastro-oesophageal reflux is a complication of CF and the symptoms may be underreported. It is often initially recognized by the physiotherapist during airway clearance.

Haemoptysis

Blood streaking of sputum frequently occurs, especially at the time of an acute exacerbation. It is appropriate to continue with the normal airway clearance regimen and to reassure the patient. Frank haemoptysis can be considered moderate at <250 ml or severe at >250 ml (Hodson 1994) and it is important to establish the volume expectorated over 24 hours to determine the treatment plan. (Table 20.6). It is important to continue with chest clearance to remove the blood and infected secretions (Hodson 1994). Management is aimed at clearing secretions without increasing the bleeding. Noting the activity and position at the time of haemoptysis will provide a clue to the cause and influence management. The weakened artery may rupture due to increasing heart rate or increasing the flow of blood when the area of lung supplied by the artery is dependent (the bronchial arteries lie posteriorly). If the patient can establish the location of the bleed, it is advisable to avoid chest clearance with the affected lobe dependent (Bilton et al 1990).

When haemoptysis is severe the location of the bleeding should be dependent to avoid asphyxiation (Jones & Davis 1990). When the bleeding has subsided chest clearance can be resumed. Bronchoscopy will locate the bleeding for those patients with persistent haemoptysis and the management usually requires embolization (King et al 1989). Chest clearance can resume after the procedure in consultation with the radiologist. Implantable venous access devices, which require flushing with an anticoagulant to maintain patency, may increase the risk of haemoptysis during intravenous therapy. If this occurs, the use of normal saline for flushing may lead to cessation of bleeding.

Liver disease

Liver disease usually presents as biliary cirrhosis, but fatty infiltration is a recognized feature. Hepatosplenomegaly and portal hypertension ensue with the development of oesophageal varices and potentially life-threatening haematemesis (Westaby 2000). Liver transplantation is an increasing feature of adult CF care. An enlarged liver and spleen will compromise respiratory mechanics and cause breathlessness. Careful consideration should be given to positioning during airway clearance. Airway clearance should be discontinued during acute haemorrhage. Careful exercise advice is recommended. See exercise section p. 597.

Low bone mineral density

Osteopenia and osteoporosis are recognized complications of CF in both children and adults (Bachrach et al 1994, Bhudmkanok et al 1996).

Table 20.6 The treatment of haemoptysis

Mild Streaking	• Normal airway clearance regimen
Moderate < 250 ml	• Careful positioning • Thoracic expansion exercises • Gentle huffing to low lung volume • Minimize coughing. Airway clearance techniques should minimize increases in intrathoracic pressure • Exercise advice (avoid sudden increases in heart rate)
Severe > 250 ml **Embolization**	• Oxygen / humidification • When the bleeding has subsided resume treatment as for moderate • Chest clearance can resume after the procedure in consultation with the radiologist

The correlates of low bone mineral density include poor absorption of vitamins, minerals and protein from the gut, oral steroids, inactivity, increased cytokines from infection and hypogonadism (Haworth et al 1999). The problem is one of reduced bone accretion in childhood and early and increased rate of bone reabsorpbtion in adult life. Lack of physical activity is a known correlate and weight-bearing exercises should be encouraged from an early age. There is an increased risk of rib fractures (Bachrach et al 1994) and for patients with severe osteoporosis any manual techniques associated with airway clearance would be contraindicated (Chartered Society of Physiotherapy 1999).

Musculoskeletal dysfunction

Patients with CF develop alterations in chest wall mechanics and spinal deformities due to progressive lung disease, malnutrition and poor bone mineralization (Tattersall et al 2000). This leads to poor posture and often musculoskeletal pain. Postural adjustments may correct kyphosis and lordosis but the value of postural therapy needs further evaluation in CF. Manual therapy techniques may increase thoracic mobility (p. 161) and may improve lung function (Vibekk 1991). Flexibility and postural exercises should be introduced in childhood as part of an exercise regimen.

Pneumothorax

In CF a pneumothorax usually occurs in patients with advanced disease and chronic Pseudomonas infection (Penketh et al 1982). It is associated with increased mortality and may be an independent indicator of prognosis. A pneumothorax may occur due to rupture of a subpleural bleb through the visceral pleura or, rarely, as a result of misplacement of a central line. The physiotherapist will be alerted to the problem by a sudden increase in breathlessness and shoulder tip pain.

The aim of physiotherapy management is to clear secretions and aid re-expansion of the collapsed lung and prevent infection in the re-expanding lung (Table 20.7). It is usual for prophylactic intravenous antibiotics to be given at this time because chest clearance and mobility are compromised. When the pneumothorax is small (<20% of lung volume) treatment is conservative and chest clearance should continue with the aim of clearing secretions without increasing the size of the pneumothorax. Techniques which increase intrathoracic pressure and paroxysmal coughing should therefore be avoided and positive pressure devices should be used with caution. Mobility is encouraged but exercise programmes should temporarily cease. An increase in symptoms may be an indication that the pneumothorax has increased in size. This should be immediately reported and an urgent chest X-ray requested.

Table 20.7 The treatment of a pneumothorax

Small (up to 20% of lung volume)	Chest clearance techniques are aimed at clearing secretions without increasing the size of the pneumothorax. ↑ Intrathoracic pressure should be minimized. • Position the patient with affected side uppermost • Thoracic expansion exercises and 'hold' • Gentle huffing • Minimize coughing • Exercise advice
Large (with intercostal drain)	Treatment is aimed at clearing secretions of all lung areas with adequate pain relief. • Thoracic expansion exercises and 'hold' • Huffing • Coughing • Exercise advice • Care with moving and handling. Drainage bottle should always be lower than the patient
Removal of intercostal drain	• Treatment as for small pneumothorax • Care is taken in the short term to prevent any reoccurrence of the resolving pneumothorax
Unresolved	VATS or thoracotomy

Larger pneumothoraces will require an intercostal drain and if persistent, a video assisted thorascopic surgery (VATS) procedure is the preferred treatment. In the light of lung transplantation, pleurodesis should be avoided. Whilst the drain is in situ airway clearance techniques are reintroduced as indicated at assessment with appropriate analgesia. Mobilization and gentle exercise are encouraged. When the intercostal tube is removed, care should be exercised with chest clearance in the short term to prevent any reoccurrence of the resolving pneumothorax. Normal activities are advised but strenuous exercise and lifting are not recommended. Patients should be cautioned about driving and air travel is contraindicated for 6 weeks (British Thoracic Society 2000). Following surgery airway clearance should be restarted as soon as possible with adequate analgesia.

Pregnancy

Improved survival has resulted in more females reaching reproductive age. Pregnancy is well tolerated by patients with an FEV_1 >60% predicted but associated with increased maternal and fetal complications in those with an FEV_1 <60% predicted (Edenborough et al 1995). As pregnancy can stress the pulmonary, nutritional and cardiovascular reserves of the CF patient, knowledge of the normal changes (Elkus & Popovich 1992, Weinberger et al 1980) and their implications in CF (Kotloff et al 1992) is useful (Table 20.8). Airway clearance techniques should continue throughout pregnancy and be modified as pregnancy progresses with consideration of the degree of breathlessness and discomfort. Breathlessness commonly occurs in the first and second trimesters and may be normal. Careful monitoring of the vital capacity is essential to identify the onset of an acute exacerbation. Elevation of the diaphragm reduces functional residual capacity and causes early airway closure. Attention should be paid to clearance of the lung bases to prevent the possibility of trapped secretions.

Gentle exercise during pregnancy should be encouraged and established aerobic programmes can continue. Non-weight bearing exercises, e.g. swimming and cycling, have less energy cost than weight-bearing exercises (Kotloff et al 1992).

Table 20.8 The normal changes of pregnancy and the implications for patients with cystic fibrosis

Normal changes	Implications in cystic fibrosis
Thoracic cage • 4 cm elevation of diaphragm with ↓ abdominal tone • ↑ AP and transverse diameter due to laxity of ligaments • Normal pressures of respiratory muscles	• Normal excursion of the diaphragm
Cardiovascular • ↑ Cardiac output by 30–40% • ↑ Blood volume by 50%	• In the presence of cor pulmonale and pulmonary hypertension the risk of cardiovascular collapse is greater due to the inability to cope with the increased circulating blood volume, particularly during and immediately following delivery
Hormones (peak in the 3rd trimester) • ↑ Oestrogen results in hypersecretion and mucosal oedema of airways • ↑ Progesterone = ↑ respiratory drive, ↑ minute ventilation resulting in chronic hyperventilation by ↑ TV • ↑ PaO_2 ↓$PaCO_2$ • ↓ Bronchomotor tone • Threefold ↑ in cortisol level and prostaglandins	• Potential ↑ airway obstruction • Breathlessness most commonly occurs in the 1st and 2nd trimesters and may be normal • Careful monitoring of vital capacity determines the cause, i.e. normal mechanism of pregnancy or ↑ disease severity • Instability of airways may be increased • This may improve airways obstruction
Lung volumes • ↓ ERV ↓ RV ↓ FRC (due to diaphragmatic displacement) • Normal VC ↓ TLC	• ↓ FRC results in early airway closure at lung bases and possible retention of secretions • Hypoxaemia may result from ventilation perfusion mismatch

Weight training should not be introduced during pregnancy but an established programme should be modified and discussed with the medical team. The importance of pelvic floor exercises should be stressed at the beginning of pregnancy and reinforced at each clinic visit. Leakage of urine is a problem for many women (Orr et al 2001) and pregnancy will further stress the pelvic floor. Abdominal supports are available for patients who suffer lower back pain or sacroiliac strain, in combination with postural advice and gentle exercise. Gastro-oesophageal reflux may present for the first time. Medication will relieve symptoms and prevent potential aspiration.

Following the birth, chest clearance begins immediately and physiotherapy may be required while the patient is in the delivery room. It is important to liaise with the midwife and medical team to ensure that pain relief is adequate. Sputum production may increase as the diaphragm descends and ventilation to the lower lobes improves. Postural drainage can resume as soon as the mother feels comfortable. Pelvic floor exercises should continue and foot and leg exercises are introduced while the mother is immobile. Mobility begins as soon as the mother feels comfortable. The return to physical activity depends on prenatal fitness, maternal health during pregnancy and progress during the postnatal period. It is usual to begin with gentle forms of exercise such as walking and build up to low-impact aerobics. Returning to an established programme will depend on the discomfort of the women's abdomen and perineum; every mother will require individualized advice. In the postnatal period pelvic floor exercises should continue for at least 12 weeks, but many mothers give up after the postnatal check-up at 6 weeks.

Surgery

The incidence of the complications of CF requiring surgery is increasing as survival improves (Weeks & Buckland 1995). For the different surgical procedures, refer to Chapter 12. Adequate intravenous hydration is recommended from the time the patient is 'nil by mouth'.

Transplantation

The physiotherapist should be involved both before and after heart-lung or lung transplantation. Before transplantation the patient's exercise ability will be very limited, but an exercise programme should be undertaken to optimize muscle strength and cardiovascular function. Postoperatively an extensive rehabilitation programme is essential to gain maximum benefit and improved quality of life (Ch. 16, p. 533).

Following heart-lung or double lung transplantation the lungs are denervated below the tracheal anastomosis with loss of all pulmonary innervation except postganglionic efferent nerves (Hathaway et al 1991). With the loss of the cough reflex and impaired mucociliary clearance, early recognition of signs of a chest infection is particularly important to minimize granulation tissue formation in the region of the large airway anastomoses and pooling of secretions in the transplanted lung, which may lead to bronchiectasis (Madden & Hodson 1995). It is therefore often recommended that a short session of physiotherapy for airway clearance be continued on a daily basis and increased as necessary during periods of chest infection.

Urinary incontinence

Leakage of urine is recognized as an emerging problem in females with CF (Hilal et al 1999, Cornaccia et al 2001, Orr et al 2001) with a prevalence of 55–68% and the age of onset as early as 10 years. Expiratory manoeuvres are the major cause for the majority of women and leakage affects the ability to perform spirometry and chest clearance. In CF the cause may be multifactorial: lifelong chest clearance, a weak pelvic floor due to poor nutrition and raised intraabdominal pressure. Further studies are required to determine the mechanisms before treatment is recommended for CF females who are already burdened with daily self-care. Patients are embarrassed and are rarely forthcoming about the problem; a sensitive and open approach with early recognition of symptoms needs to be developed to evaluate this distressing problem.

Infection control

The physiotherapist should have knowledge of the respiratory pathogen harboured by the patient, the risk of transmission and the potential for cross-infection. Infection control policies specific to cystic fibrosis should be in place and attention paid to the risk of cross-infection between patients and from physiotherapy equipment. All physiotherapy treatment sessions should be with individual patients.

Evaluation of physiotherapy

Sputum weight

In clinical practice sputum weight or volume is a useful outcome measure of airway clearance in the stable state. It provides a baseline measure of the normal sputum production for the individual. Ideally, with appropriate airway clearance and medical management, sputum will be expectorated only during periods of chest clearance. Any increase, either during treatment or out of treatment, is a possible indication of an acute exacerbation. Total daily sputum weight during an acute exacerbation is less informative but, together with lung function, will determine if the problem is one of increased infection or sputum retention (Table 20.9). During an admission for an acute exacerbation it is the physiotherapist's goal to reduce sputum expectoration to periods of airway clearance. Measures of treatment and out-of-treatment sputum weight will provide this information and indicate to the less adherent patient the value of airway clearance techniques.

Lung function

Spirometry provides a measure of the degree of airway obstruction. It is the gold standard of measurement which influences medical management and monitors long-term progression. PEFR is less useful in the long term; as disease progresses central airway instability results in an increase in PEFR, with a decrease in FEV_1. However, PEFR is a useful measure of any change in obstruction following a short-term intervention, e.g. airway clearance technique, introduction of inhaled drugs and changes in treatment during an acute exacerbation. It also identifies diurnal variation. Daily peak flow recordings may be of value during an acute exacerbation. The expiratory flow volume curve identifies the location of any flow limitation throughout expiration from TLC to RV. This will vary from the early detection of small airway limitation to large airway collapse and gives the physiotherapist an invaluable insight into the problems of airway clearance. The manoeuvre is performed with an open glottis and therefore mimics a huff from TLC to RV. In the long term, measurements of small airway function (FEF_{25} and FEF_{75}) are not comparable due to changes in TLC and RV and should therefore be interpreted with caution.

The physiotherapist should be mindful of the many confounding factors that affect sputum weight and lung function, e.g. raised blood glucose levels, the hours of use of NIV, while the rate and volume of overnight feeding can compromise the diaphragm and influence early morning breathlessness. The normal observations of temperature pulse and respiration are vital routine measurements of assessment.

Arterial / capillary blood gases

Serial measurements of PaO_2 and $PaCO_2$ monitor decreases in oxygen tension and ensuing hypercapnia. $PaCO_2$ levels inform the physiotherapist of ventilatory drive and the work of breathing.

Table 20.9 The value of spirometry and sputum weight during an acute exacerbation

Outcome		Analysis	Action
↑ FEV_1	↓ Sputum weight	Treatment goal	Continue present treatment
↑ FEV_1	↑ Sputum weight	↑ Ventilation	↑ Airway clearance
↓ FEV_1	↑ Sputum weight	↑ Infection	↑ Airway clearance
			Review antibiotics
↓ FEV_1	↓ Sputum weight	Sputum retention	Review airway clearance techniques

Pulse oximetry gives a quick measure of oxygen saturation but should not be used to prescribe oxygen.

Subjective measures

Visual analogue scales (VAS) and Borg scores (p. 115) provide important subjective measures of breathlessness, chest tightness, muscle fatigue and pain. More recently the 15-count breathlessness score has been developed for use in children (Prasad et al 2000). Other useful measures include health status/quality of life questionnaires (Congleton et al 1997, Gee et al 2000, Orenstein et al 1989, Shepherd et al 1992) and activities of daily living.

Adherence

The daily timetable of self-care can be an enormous burden for the patient and carer who are trying to balance treatment with family, work and social commitments. This can be particularly difficult for the adolescent and young adult and studies show a decline in adherence with increasing age (Gudas et al 1991). Adherence has been shown to be treatment specific in CF (Abbott et al 1994) and adherence with one treatment does not guarantee adherence with all self-care. Treatments that are complex, requiring time and effort with no immediate benefit, e.g. chest clearance and nebulized antibiotics, have lower adherence rates than other treatments which are quick and give immediate relief of symptoms (Dodd & Webb 1999). Over the years, studies have reported only 50% of patients to have 'good' adherence with chest clearance (Abbott et al 1994, Conway et al 1996, Passero et al 1981). Large sputum production, feeling better following treatment and help with treatment were significant factors influencing adherence with chest clearance (Abbott et al 1994).

Exercise is perceived differently; adherence is higher and should be encouraged for all its therapeutic benefits. Self-management and self-efficacy should be encouraged to improve adherence but support and praise are essential to avoid the feeling of loneliness and isolation (McIllwaine & Davidson 1996). Knowledge is considered an important precursor to adherence and it is important to appraise knowledge of treatments and correct any misunderstandings (Conway et al 1996). Assessing patients' understanding of specific treatments and providing individualized specific teaching has been shown to improve knowledge and reported adherence in the short term (Unsworth et al 1998).

The reasons for non-adherence are complex. Psychological influences, patients' perceptions and health beliefs (Abbott et al 1996) and coping styles (Abbott et al 2001) influence adherence. It is important to recognize that non-adherence is normal and encourage openness with self-reporting by adopting a non-judgemental approach. Treatment plans and decisions that are tailored to daily lifestyle should be agreed and compromise accepted by the medical team.

Continuity of care

Continuous assessment and reassessment of patients with cystic fibrosis is essential for effective management. The patient's needs will change as he progresses from infancy through school, higher education, work and parenting. The emphasis is on leading as normal a life as possible while making time to include the many aspects of treatment. Visits to schools to support individual patients and to increase the awareness and knowledge of the teachers are beneficial (Dyer & Morais 1996). Children should be encouraged to attend normal schools.

Although the majority of parents and patients can take the responsibility for physiotherapy treatments, it is essential that there is a regular review of the techniques by a physiotherapist. This also provides an opportunity to update the techniques and to discuss any problems. There are times when the parents or patient are unable to cope effectively on their own and the need for assistance during these periods should be recognized and help should be arranged.

If the patient is treated at both a local hospital and a specialist cystic fibrosis unit, communication between physiotherapists is essential to avoid confusion about treatment.

The physiotherapist must remember that she is a part of a multidisciplinary team and must be aware of the roles of the other members. Good communication within the team is essential. Members of the team may experience considerable stress from long-term involvement with patients with a chronic progressive illness. Coping with this stress can be helped by the team members recognizing each other's needs and providing the necessary support.

In caring for the patient with cystic fibrosis, the physical care is important but the psychological effects on both the family and the patient must also be considered. Many countries have cystic fibrosis associations which offer encouragement and support for patients and their families. In spite of the frequently high demands of treat-ment, most patients with cystic fibrosis are leading fulfilling lives and many adults are in full-time employment, home owners and parents (Walters et al 1993).

Acknowledgement

The authors would like to thank Barbara Webber and Jennifer Pryor for the sections taken from 'Bronchiectasis, primary ciliary dyskinesia and cystic fibrosis' in the second edition of *Physiotherapy for respiratory and cardiac problems* and wish to acknowledge material which reflects the *Clinical guidelines for the physiotherapy management of cystic fibrosis* of the Association of Chartered Physiotherapists in Cystic Fibrosis (2002 Cystic Fibrosis Trust, Bromley, Kent).

REFERENCES

Abbott J, Bilton D, Dodd M, Webb AK 1994 Treatment compliance in adults with cystic fibrosis. Thorax 59: 115–120

Abbott J, Dodd M, Webb AK 1996 Health perceptions and treatment adherence in adults with cystic fibrosis. Thorax 51: 1233–1238

Abbott J, Dodd M, Gee L, Webb AK 2001 Ways of coping with cystic fibrosis: implications for treatment adherence. Disability and Rehabilitation 23: 315–324

Alfaham M, Goodchild M 1996 Aspergillus lung disease In: Dodge JA, Brock DJH, Widdicombe JH, (eds) Cystic fibrosis – current topics. John Wiley, Chichester, pp. 273–275

Alton E, Caplen N, Geddes D, Williamson R 1992 New treatments for cystic fibrosis. British Medical Bulletin 48: 785–804

Anderson DH 1938 Cystic fibrosis of the pancreas and its relation to celiac disease: clinical and pathological study. American Journal of Disease in Childhood 56: 344–399

Andreasson B, Jonson B, Kornfalt R et al 1987 Long-term effects of physical exercise on working capacity and pulmonary function in cystic fibrosis. Acta Paediatrica Scandinavica 76: 70–75

App EM, Kieselman R, Reinhardt D et al 1998 Sputum rheology changes in cystic fibrosis lung disease following two different types of physiotherapy – VRP1 (flutter) versus autogenic drainage. Chest 114: 171–177

Armstrong DS, Grimwood K, Carzino R et al 1995 Lower respiratory tract infection and inflammation in infants with newly diagnosed cystic fibrosis. British Medical Journal 310: 1571–1572

Asher MI, Pardy RL, Coates AL 1982 The effects of inspiratory muscle training in patients with cystic fibrosis. American Review of Respiratory Disease 126: 855–859

Astrand PO, Rodahl K 1977 Text book of work physiology. McGraw-Hill, London.

Bachrach LK, Loutit CW, Moss RB 1994 Osteopenia in adults with cystic fibrosis. American Journal of Medicine 96: 27–34

Baldwin DR, Hill AL, Peckham KG et al 1994 Effect of addition of exercise to chest physiotherapy on sputum expectoration and lung function in adults with cystic fibrosis. Respiratory Medicine 88: 49–53

Balfour-Lynn IM, Klein NH, Dinwiddie R 1997 Randomised controlled trial of inhaled corticosteroids (fluticasone proprionate) in cystic fibrosis. Archives of Disease in Childhood 77: 124–130

Balfour-Lynn IM, Prasad SA, Laverty A 1998 A step in the right direction: assessing exercise tolerance in cystic fibrosis. Pediatric Pulmonology 25: 78–84

Bargon J, Viel K, Dauletbaev N et al 1997 Short-term effects of regular salmeterol treatment on adult cystic fibrosis patients. European Respiratory Journal 10: 2307–2311

Barker AF, Couch L, Fiel SB et al 2000 Tobramycin solution for inhalation reduces sputum Pseudomonas aeruginosa density in bronchiectasis. American Journal of Respiratory and Critical Care Medicine 162: 481–485

Bar-Or O, Blimkie CJ, Hay JA et al 1992 Voluntary dehydration and heat intolerance in cystic fibrosis. Lancet 339: 696–699

Bhudmkanok GS, Lim J, Marcus R et al 1996 Correlates of osteopenia in patients with cystic fibrosis. Journal of Pediatrics 97: 103–111

Bilton D, Webb AK, Foster H et al 1990 Life threatening haemoptysis in cystic fibrosis: an alternative therapeutic approach. Thorax 45: 523–524

Bilton D, Dodd ME, Abbot J et al 1992 The benefits of exercise combined with physiotherapy in the treatment of adults with cystic fibrosis. Respiratory Medicine 86: 507–511

Birrer P, McElvaney N G, Rüdeberg A et al 1994 Protease–antiprotease imbalance in the lungs of children with cystic fibrosis. American Journal of Respiratory and Critical Care Medicine 150: 207–213

Bisgaard H, Pederson SS, Nielsen KG et al 1997 Controlled trial of inhaled budesomide in patients with cystic fibrosis and chronic pseudomonas aeruginosa infection. American Journal of Respiratory and Critical Care Medicine 156: 1190–1196

Boas SR, Danduran MJ, McColley SA 1999 Parental attitudes about exercise regarding their children with cystic fibrosis. International Journal of Sports Medicine 20: 334–338

Bourke S, Rooney M, Fitzgerald M et al 1987 Episodic arthropathy in adult cystic fibrosis. Quarterly Journal of Medicine 64: 651–659

Bradley J, Howard J, Wallace E et al 1999 The validity of a modified shuttle test in adult cystic fibrosis. Thorax 54: 437–439

Bramwell EC, Halpin DMG, Duncan-Skingle F et al 1995 Home treatment of patients with cystic fibrosis using the 'Intermate': the first year's experience. Journal of Advanced Nursing 22: 1063–1067

British Thoracic Society 2000 Recommendations. Managing patients with lung disease planning air travel. British Thoracic Society, London

Britto MT, Garrett JM, Konrad TR et al 2000 Comparison of physical activity in adolescents with cystic fibrosis versus age matched controls. Pediatric Pulmonology 30: 86–91

Brueton MJ, Ormerod LP, Shah KJ et al 1980 Allergic bronchopulmonary aspergillosis complicating cystic fibrosis in childhood. Archives of Disease in Childhood 55: 348–353

Bureau MA, Lupien L, Begin R 1981 Neural drive and ventilatory strategy of breathing in normal children and in patients with cystic fibrosis and asthma. Pediatrics 68: 187–194

Bush A, Cole P, Hariri M et al 1998 Primary ciliary dyskinesia: diagnosis and standards of care. European Respiratory Journal 12: 982–988

Button BM, Heine RG, Catto-Smith AG et al 1997 Postural drainage and gastro-oesophageal reflux in infants with cystic fibrosis. Archives of Disease in Childhood 76: 148–150

Carr L, Smith RE, Pryor JA et al 1996 Cystic fibrosis patients' views and beliefs about chest clearance and exercise – a pilot study. Physiotherapy 82: 621–627

Cecins NM, Jenkins SC, Pengelly J et al 1999 The active cycle of breathing techniques – to tip or not to tip? Respiratory Medicine 93: 660–665

Chartered Society of Physiotherapy 1999 Physiotherapy guidelines for the management of osteoporosis. Chartered Society of Physiotherapy, London

Chen HC, Liu CY, Cheng HF et al 1998 Chest physiotherapy does not exacerbate gastroesophageal reflux in patients with chronic bronchitis and bronchiectasis. Respiratory Medicine 21: 409–414

Cheng K, Smyth RL, Motley J et al 2000 Randomised controlled trials in cystic fibrosis (1966–1997) categorised by time, design and intervention. Pediatric Pulmonology 29: 1–7

Chua HL, Collis GG, Le-Souef PN 1990 Bronchial response to nebulised antibiotics in children with cystic fibrosis. European Respiratory Journal 3: 1114–1116

Cohen AM 1992 Hemoptysis: role of angiography and embolization. Pediatric Pulmonology (suppl) 8: 85–86

Cole P 1995 Bronchiectasis. In: Brewis RAL, Corrin B, Geddes DM, Gibson GJ (eds) Respiratory medicine, 2nd edn. WB Saunders, London ch 39

Congleton J, Hodson M, Duncan-Skingle F 1997 Quality of life in adults with cystic fibrosis. Thorax 52: 397–400

Conway JH, Fleming JS, Perring S et al 1992 Humidification as an adjunct to chest physiotherapy in aiding tracheo-bronchial clearance in patients with bronchiectasis. Respiratory Medicine 86: 109–11

Conway SP, Watson A 1997 Nebulised bronchodilators, corticosteroids and rhdnase in adult patients with cystic fibrosis. Thorax 52 (suppl 2): S64–68

Conway SP, Pond MN, Watson A et al 1996 Knowledge of adult patients with cystic fibrosis about their illness. Thorax 51: 34–38

Corless JA, Warburton CJ 2000 Surgery vs non-surgical treatment for bronchiectasis. Cochrane Database Systematic Review 4: CD002180

Cornaccia M, Zenorini A, Braagion C et al 2001 Prevalence of urinary incontinence in women with cystic fibrosis. British Journal of Urology International 88: 44–48

Cropp GJA, Pullano TP, Cerny FJ et al 1982 Exercise tolerance and cardiorespiratory adjustments at peak work capacity in cystic fibrosis. American Review of Respiratory Disease 126: 211–216

Currie DC 1997 Nebulisers for bronchiectasis. Thorax 52 (suppl 2): S72–74

Currie DC, Munro C, Gaskell D et al 1986 Practice, problems and compliance with postural drainage: a survey of chronic sputum producers. British Journal of Diseases of the Chest 80: 249–253

Currie DC, Cooke JC, Morgan AD et al. 1987 Interpretation of bronchograms and chest radiographs in patients with chronic sputum production. Thorax 42: 278–284

Cystic Fibrosis Trust 1999 Burkholderia cepacia. Cystic Fibrosis Trust, Bromley

Cystic Fibrosis Trust 2000 Antibiotic treatment for cystic fibrosis. Cystic Fibrosis Trust, Bromley

Cystic Fibrosis Trust 2001 Pseudomonas aeruginosa infection in people with cystic fibrosis. Cystic Fibrosis Trust, Bromley

Davidson AGF 2000 Gastrointestinal and pancreatic disease in cystic fibrosis. In: Hodson ME, Geddes DM (eds) Cystic fibrosis. Arnold, London, pp 261–289

Davis PB, Drumm M, Konstan MW 1996 Cystic fibrosis: state of the art. American Journal of Respiratory and Critical Care Medicine 154: 1229–1256

de Boeck K 2000 Improving standards of clinical care in cystic fibrosis. European Respiratory Journal 16: 585–587

de Jong W, Kaptein AA, Van Der Schans CP et al 1997 Quality of life in patients with cystic fibrosis. Pediatric Pulmonology 23: 95–100

Desai M, Weller PH, Spencer DA 1995 Clinical benefit from nebulised human recombinant DNase in Kartagener's syndrome. Pediatric Pulmonology 20: 307–308

Di Sant'Agnese PA, Davis PB 1979 Cystic fibrosis in adults. American Journal of Medicine 66: 121–132

Dodd ME, Webb AK 1999 Understanding non-compliance with treatment in adults with cystic fibrosis. Journal of the Royal Society of Medicine 93 (suppl 38): 2–8

Dodd ME, Abbott J, Maddison J et al 1997 The effect of the tonicity of nebulised colistin on chest tightness and lung function in adults with cystic fibrosis. Thorax 52: 656–658

Dodd ME, Haworth CS, Webb AK 1998 Practical application of oxygen therapy in cystic fibrosis. Journal of the Royal Society of Medicine 91 (suppl 34): 30–39

Dodge JA, Morison S, Lewis PA et al 1993 Cystic fibrosis in the United Kingdom, 1968–1988: incidence, population and survival. Paediatric and Perinatal Epidemiology 7: 157–166

Doring G, Conway SP, Heijerman HGM et al 2000 Antibiotic therapy against *Pseudomonas aeruginosa* in cystic fibrosis. European Respiratory Journal 16: 749–767

Du Bois R M 1995 Respiratory medicine – recent advances. British Medical Journal 310: 1594–1597

Dyer J, Morais JA 1996 Supporting children with cystic fibrosis in school. Professional Nurse 11: 518–520

Edenborough FP, Stableforth DE, Webb AK et al 1995 Outcome of pregnancy in women with cystic fibrosis. Thorax 50: 170–174

Edlund LD, French RW, Herbst JJ et al 1986 Effects of a swimming program on children with cystic fibrosis. American Journal of Diseases of Childhood 140: 80–83

Elborn JS, Shale DJ, Britton JR 1991 Cystic fibrosis: current survival and population estimates to year 2000. Thorax 46: 881–885

Elborn JS, Prescott RJ, Stack BH et al 2000 Elective versus symptomatic antibiotic treatment in cystic fibrosis patients with chronic *Pseudomonas* infection of the lungs. Thorax 55: 355–358

Elkus R, Popovich J 1992 Respiratory physiology in pregnancy. Clinics in Chest Medicine 13: 555–565

Eng PA, Morton J, Douglass JA et al 1996 Short term efficacy of ultrasonically nebulized hypertonic saline in cystic fibrosis. Pediatric Pulmonology 21: 77–83

Evans SA, Turner SM, Bosch BJ, Hardy MA, Woodhead MA 1996 Lung function in bronchiectasis: the influence of *Pseudomonas aeruginosa*. European Respiratory Journal 9: 1601–1604

Fairfax AJ, Ball J, Batten JC et al 1980 A pathological study following bronchial artery embolization for haemoptysis in cystic fibrosis. British Journal of Diseases of the Chest 74: 345–352

Finnegan MJ, Hughes DV, Hodson ME 1992 Comparison of nebulised and intravenous terbutaline during acute exacerbations of pulmonary infection in patients with cystic fibrosis. European Respiratory Journal 5: 1089–1091

FitzSimmons SC 1993 The changing epidemiology of cystic fibrosis. Journal of Pediatrics 122: 1–9

Freeman W, Stableforth DE, Cayton R et al 1993 Endurance exercise capacity in adults with cystic fibrosis. Respiratory Medicine 87: 252–257

Freitag L, Bremme J, Schroer M 1989 High frequency oscillation for respiratory physiotherapy. British Journal of Anaesthesia 63: 44S–46S

Fuchs HJ, Borowitz DS, Christiansen DH et al 1994 Effect of aerolized recombinant human DNase on exacerbations of respiratory symptoms and on pulmonary function in patients with cystic fibrosis. New England Journal of Medicine 331: 637–642

Gee L, Abbott J, Conway SP et al 2000 Development of a disease specific health related quality of life measure for adults and adolescents with cystic fibrosis. Thorax 55: 946–954

Godfrey S, Mearns M 1971 Pulmonary function and response to exercise in cystic fibrosis. Archives of Disease in Childhood 46: 144–151

Govan J, Brown PH, Maddison J et al, 1993 Evidence for transmission of *Pseudomonas cepacia* by social contact in cystic fibrosis. Lancet 342: 15–18

Gozal D 1997 Nocturnal ventilatory support in patients with cystic fibrosis: comparison with supplemental oxygen. European Respiratory Journal 10: 1999–2003

Greenstone M, Rutman A, Dewar I et al 1988 Primary ciliary dyskinesia: cytological and clinical features. Quarterly Journal of Medicine 67(253): 405–430

Gremmo ML, Guenza MC 1999 Positive expiratory pressure in the physiotherapeutic management of primary ciliary dyskinesia in paediatric age. Monaldi Archives of Chest Disease 54: 255–257

Gudas LJ, Koocher GP, Wypij D 1991 Perceptions of medical compliance in children and adolescents with cystic fibrosis. Journal of Behaviour in Pediatrics 12: 236–42

Hasani A, Pavia D, Agnew JE, Clarke SW 1994 Regional lung clearance during cough and forced expiration technique (FET): effects of flow and viscoelasticity. Thorax 49: 557–561

Hassan JA, Saadiah S, Roslan H et al 1999 Bronchodilator response to inhaled beta-2 – agonist and anticholinergic drugs in patients with bronchiectasis. Respirology 4: 423–426

Hathaway T, Higenbottam T, Lowry R, Wallwork J 1991 Pulmonary reflexes after human heart-lung transplantation. Respiratory Medicine 85 (suppl A0: 17–21

Haworth CS, Selby PL, Webb AK et al 1999. Low bone mineral density in adults with cystic fibrosis. Thorax 54: 961–967

Haworth CS, Dodd ME, Atkins M et al 2000 Pneumothorax in adults with cystic fibrosis dependent on nasal intermittent positive pressure ventilation (NIPPV): a management dilemma. Thorax 55: 620–662

Heijerman HG, Bakker W, Sterk PJ et al 1992 Long term effects of exercise training and hyperalimentation in adult cystic fibrosis patients with severe pulmonary dysfunction. International Journal of Rehabilitation and Respiration 15: 252–257

Hilal EHE, Stockton P, Meaden B et al 1999 The prevalence of urinary stress incontinence in adult CF patients. Thorax 54 (suppl 3): A67

Hill AT, Edenborough FP, Cayton RM et al 1998 Long-term nasal intermittent positive pressure ventilation in patients with cystic fibrosis and hypercapnic respiratory failure (1991–1996). Respiratory Medicine 92: 523–526

Hill LS, Slater AL 1998 A comparison of the performance of two modern multidose dry powder asthma inhalers. Respiratory Medicine 92: 105–110

Hodson ME, Madden BP, Steven MH et al 1991 Non-invasive mechanical ventilation for cystic fibrosis patients – a potential bridge to transplantation. European Respiratory Journal 4: 524–527

Hodson ME 1994 Adults. In: Hodson ME, Geddes DM (eds) Cystic fibrosis. Chapman and Hall, London, pp 237–253

Hodson ME 1996 Principles of antibiotic management. In: Issues in cystic fibrosis: antibiotic therapy. Report of a meeting held at Royal College of Pathologists, November (Zeneca), pp. 6–14

Hodson ME 2000 The respiratory system: adults. In: Hodson ME, Geddes DM (eds) Cystic fibrosis. Arnold, London, pp. 218–242

Hodson ME, Shah PL 1995 DNase trials in cystic fibrosis. European Respiratory Journal 8: 1786–1791

Hodson ME, Madden BP, Steven MH et al 1991 Non-invasive mechanical ventilation for cystic fibrosis patients – a potential bridge to transplantation. European Respiratory Journal 4: 524–552

Høiby N, Koch C 1990 *Pseudomonas aeruginosa* infection in cystic fibrosis and its management. Thorax 45: 881–884

Houtmeyers E, Gosselink R, Gayan-Ramirez G et al 1999 Effects of drugs on mucus clearance. European Respiratory Journal 14: 452–467

Hutchinson GR, Parker S, Pryor JA et al 1996 Home-nebulizers: a potential primary source of *Burkholderia cepacia* and other colistin-resistant, gram-negative bacteria in patients with cystic fibrosis. Journal of Clinical Microbiology 34: 584–587

Johnson S, Knox AJ 1994 Arthropathy in cystic fibrosis. Respiratory Medicine 88: 567–570

Jones DK, Davis RJ 1990 Massive haemoptysis. British Medical Journal 300: 889–890

Jones NL 1988 Clinical exercise testing, 3rd edn. WB Saunders, Philadelphia, pp. 306–307

Karadag B, Gultekin E, Wilson N et al 1997 Exhaled nitric oxide (NO) in children with primary ciliary dyskinesia (abstact). European Respiratory Journal 10 (suppl 25): 339s

Kartagener M 1933 Zur Pathogenese der Bronchiektasien. Beitrage zur Klinik der Tuberkulose 83: 489–501 B

Keens TG, Krastins IRB, Wannamaker EM et al 1977 Ventilatory muscle endurance training in normal subjects and patients with cystic fibrosis. American Review of Respiratory Disease 116: 853–860

Kerem E, Reisman J, Corey M et al 1992 Prediction of mortality in patients with cystic fibrosis. New England Journal of Medicine 326: 1187–1191

Khan TZ, Wagener JS, Bost T et al 1995 Early pulmonary inflammation in infants with cystic fibrosis. American Journal of Respiratory and Critical Care Medicine 151: 1075–1082

King AD, Cumberland DC, Brennan SR 1989 Management of severe haemoptysis by bronchial artery embolisation in a patient with cystic fibrosis. Thorax 44: 523–524

Koch C, Lanng S 2000 Other organ systems In: Hodson ME, Geddes DM(eds) Cystic fibrosis. Arnold, London. pp 314–328

Koh YY, Park Y, Jeong JH et al 2000 The effect of regular salbutamol on lung function and bronchial responsiveness in patients with primary ciliary dyskinesia. Chest 117: 427–433

Kolbe J, Wells A 2000 Inhaled steroids for bronchiectasis. Cochrane Database Systematic Review 2: CD000996

Konstan MW, Hilliard KA, Norvell TM et al 1994 Bronchoalveolar lavage findings in cystic fibrosis patients with stable, clinically mild lung disease suggest ongoing infection and inflammation. American Journal of Respiratory and Critical Care Medicine 150: 448–454

Kotloff RM, Fitzsimmons SC, Fiel SB 1992 Fertility and pregnancy in patients with cystic fibrosis. Clinics in Chest Medicine 13: 623–635

Kuhn RJ, Nahata MC 1985 Therapeutic management of cystic fibrosis. Clinical Pharmacology 4: 555–565

Kuo C, Lin S, Wang J 1991 Aerosol, humidity and oxygenation. Chest 99: 1352–1356

Langlands J 1967 The dynamics of cough in health and in chronic bronchitis. Thorax 22: 88–96

Lanng S, Thorsteinsson B, Nerup J et al 1992 Influence of the development of diabetes mellitus on clinical status in patients with cystic fibrosis. European Journal of Paediatrics 151: 684–687

Lapin CD 2000 Mixing and matching airway clearance techniques to patients. Pediatric Pulmonology Supplement 20: S12.3

LiPuma JJ, Dasen SE, Nielson DW et al 1990 Person-to-person transmission of *Pseudomonas cepacia* between patients with cystic fibrosis. Lancet 336: 1094–1096

Madden BP, Hodson ME 1995 Rehabilitation considerations for the lung transplant patient. In: Bach JR (ed) Pulmonary rehabilitation. Hanley and Belfus, Philadelphia, pp 193–202

Maddison J, Dodd M, Webb AK 1994 Nebulised colistin causes chest tightness in adults with cystic fibrosis. Respiratory Medicine 88: 145–147

Mahadeva R, Webb AK, Westerbeek RC et al 1998 Clinical outcome in relation to care in centres specialising in cystic fibrosis: cross sectional study. British Medical Journal 316: 1771–1775

Marcotte JE, Grisdale RK, Levison H et al 1986 Multiple factors limit exercise in cystic fibrosis. Pediatric Pulmonology 2: 274–281

Marcus CL, Bader D, Stabile M et al 1992 Supplemental oxygen and exercise performance in patients with cystic fibrosis with severe pulmonary disease. Chest 105: 52–57

McBride G 1990 More progress in cystic fibrosis. British Medical Journal 301: 627

McIlwaine MP, Davidson GF 1996 Airway clearance techniques in the treatment of cystic fibrosis. Current Opinion in Pulmonary Medicine 2: 447–451

Moorcroft AJ, Dodd ME, Webb AK 2000 Individualised home exercise training in cystic fibrosis. Proceedings of the XIIIth International Cystic Fibrosis Congress, Stockholm S259, p 15

Muhdi K, Edenborough FP, Gumery L et al 1996 Outcome for patients colonised with *Burkholderia cepacia* in a Birmingham adult cystic fibrosis clinic and the end of an epidemic. Thorax 51: 374–377

Mukhopadhyay S, Singh M, Cater JI et al 1996 Nebulised antipseudomonal antibiotic therapy in cystic fibrosis: a meta-analysis of benefits and risks. Thorax 51: 364–368

Nelson LA, Callerame ML, Schwartz RH 1979 Aspergillosis and atopy in cystic fibrosis. American Review of Respiratory Disease 120: 863–873

Nikolaizik WH, Jenni-Galovie V, Schoni MH 1996 Bronchial constriction after nebulised tobramycin preparations and saline in patients with cystic fibrosis. European Journal of Pediatrics 155: 608–611

Noone PG, Bennett WD, Regnis JA et al 1999 Effect of aerolised uridine-5'-triphosphate on airway clearance with cough in patients with primary ciliary dyskinesia. American Journal of Critical Care Medicine 160: 144–149

O'Neill PA, Dodd M, Phillips B et al 1987 Regular exercise and reduction of breathlessness in cystic fibrosis. British Journal of Diseases of the Chest 81: 62–66

Orenstein DM, Franklin BA, Doershuk CFet al 1981 Exercise conditioning and cardiopulmonary fitness in cystic fibrosis. Chest 80: 392–398

Orenstein DM, Nixon PA, Ross EA et al 1989 The quality of well-being in cystic fibrosis. Chest 95: 344–347

Oriols R, Roig J, Ferrer J et al 1999 Inhaled antibiotic therapy in non-cystic fibrosis patients with bronchiectasis and chronic bronchial infection by Pseudomonas aeruginosa. Respiratory Medicine 93: 476–480

Orr A, McVean R, Webb AK et al 2001 A questionnaire survey of the prevalence of urinary incontinence in females with cystic fibrosis: a marginalised and undertreated problem. British Medical Journal 322: 1521

Park RW, Grand RJ 1981 Gastrointestinal manifestations of cystic fibrosis: a review. Gastroenterology 81: 1143–116

Passero MA, Remor B, Salomon J 1981 Patient-reported compliance with cystic fibrosis therapy. Clinical Pediatrics 20: 264–268

Pasteur MC, Heliwell SM, Houghton SJ et al 2000 An investigation into the causative factors in patients with bronchiectasis. American Journal of Respiratory and Critical Care Medicine 162: 1277–1284

Penketh ARL, Knight RK, Hodson M et al 1982 Management of pneumothorax in adults with cystic fibrosis. Thorax 37: 850–853

Phillips G 1996 To tip or not to tip? Physiotherapy Research International 1: 1–6

Phillips GE, Thomas S, Heather S, Bush A 1996 Airway responsiveness in primary ciliary dyskinesia: intrasubject variability and the effects of exercise and bronchodilator therapy (abstract). European Respiratory Journal 9 (Suppl 23): 36s

Phillipson GTM, Petrucco OM, Mathews CD 2000 Congenital absence of the vas deferens, cystic fibrosis mutational analysis and intracytoplasmic sperm injection. Human Reproduction 15: 431–435

Piper AJ, Parker S, Torzillo PJ et al 1992 Nocturnal nasal IPPV stabilizes patients with cystic fibrosis and hypercapnic respiratory failure. Chest 102: 846–850

Poole S 1995 Dietary treatment of cystic fibrosis. In: Hodson ME, Geddes DM (eds) Cystic fibrosis. Chapman and Hall, London, pp 383–395

Prasad A, Main E 1998 Finding evidence to support airway clearance techniques in cystic fibrosis. Disability and Rehabilitation 20: 235–246

Prasad A, Randall SD, Balfour-Lynn I 2000 Fifteen-count breathlessness score: an objective measure for children. Pediatric Pulmonology 30: 56–62

Pringle MB 1992 Swimming and grommets. British Medical Journal 304: 198

Ramsey BW, Dorkin HL 1994 Consensus conference: practical applications of Pulmozyme. Pediatric Pulmonology 17: 404–408

Range SP, Knox AJ 1995 rhDNase in cystic fibrosis. Thorax 50: 321–322

Ranieri E, Lewis BD, Gerace RL et al 1994 Neonatal screening for cystic fibrosis using immunoreactive trypsinogen and direct gene analysis: four years' experience. British Medical Journal 308: 1469–1472

Reid L, De Haller R 1967 The bronchial mucous glands – their hypertrophy and changes in intracellular mucus. Bibliotheca Pediatrica 86: 195–200

Robinson M, Regnis JA, Bailey DL et al 1996 Effect of hypertonic saline, amiloride, and cough on mucociliary clearance in patients with cystic fibrosis. American Journal of Respiratory and Critical Care Medicine 153: 1503–1509

Rodwell LT, Anderson SD 1996 Airway responsiveness to hyperosmolar saline challenge in cystic fibrosis: a pilot study. Pediatric Pulmonology 21: 282–289

Rogers D, Goodchild MC 1996 Role of a domiciliary physiotherapist in the treatment of children with cystic fibrosis. Physiotherapy 82: 396–402

Rommens JM, Iannuzzi MC, Kerem B et al 1989 Identification of the cystic fibrosis gene: chromosome walking and jumping. Science 245: 1059–1065

Rubin BK 1988 Immotile cilia syndrome (primary ciliary dyskinesia) and inflammatory lung disease. Clinics of Chest Medicine 9: 657–668

Rubin K 1998. Emerging therapies for cystic fibrosis lung disease. Chest 115: 1120–1126

Rush PJ, Shore A, Coblentz C et al. 1986 The musculoskeletal manifestations of C.F. Seminars in Arthritis and Rheumatism 15: (3) 213–225

Rutland J, Cole PJ 1980 Non-invasive sampling of nasal cilia for measurement of beat frequency and study of ultrastructure. Lancet ii: 564–565

Sahl W, Bilton D, Dodd M, Webb AK 1989 Effect of exercise and physiotherapy in aiding sputum expectoration in adults with cystic fibrosis. Thorax 44: 1006–1008

Sawyer E, Clayton TL 1993 Improved pulmonary function and exercise tolerance with inspiratory muscle conditioning in children with cystic fibrosis. Chest 104: 1490–1497

Scherer TA, Barandum J, Martinez E et al 1998 Effect of high-frequency oral airway and chest wall oscillation and conventional chest physical therapy on expectoration in patients with stable cystic fibrosis. Chest 113: 1019–1027

Schneiderman-Walker J, Pollack SL, Corey M et al 2000 A randomised controlled trial of a 3-year home exercise program in cystic fibrosis. Journal of Pediatrics 136: 304–310

Schöni MH 1989 Autogenic drainage – a modern approach to chest physiotherapy in cystic fibrosis. Journal of the Royal Society of Medicine 82(suppl 16): 32–37

Shah PL, Scott SF, Knight RA et al 1996 In vivo effects of recombinant human DNase I on sputum in patients with cystic fibrosis. Thorax 51: 119–125

Shah PL, Scott SF, Geddes DM et al 1997 An evaluation of two aerosol delivery systems for rhDNase. European Respiratory Journal 10: 1261–1267

Shale DJ 1997a Predicting survival in cystic fibrosis. (Editorial) Thorax 52: 309

Shale DJ 1997b Commentary. Thorax 52: 95–96

Sharp JT, Drutz WS, Moisan T, Forster J, Machnach W 1980 Postural relief of dyspnea in severe chronic obstructive pulmonary disease. American Review of Respiratory Disease 122: 201–211

Shepherd SL, Hovell MF, Slymen DJ et al 1992 Functional status as an overall measure of health in adults with cystic fibrosis: a further validation of a generic health measure. Journal of Clinical Epidemiology 45: 117–125

Simmonds EJ, Littlewood JM, Evans EGV 1990 Cystic fibrosis and allergic bronchopulmonary aspergillosis. Archives of Disease in Childhood 65: 507–511

Sindel BD, Maisels MJ, Ballantine TVN 1989 Gastroesophageal reflux to the proximal esophagus in infants with bronchopulmonary dysplasia. American Journal of Disease in Childhood 143: 1103–1106

Smith IE, Flower CDR 1996 Review article: imaging in bronchiectasis. British Journal of Radiology 69: 589–593

Speechley-Dick ME, Rimmer SJ, Hodson ME 1992 Exacerbation of cystic fibrosis after holidays at high altitude: a cautionary tale. Respiratory Medicine 86: 55–56

Spier S, Rivlin J, Hughes D et al 1984 The effect of oxygen on sleep, blood gases and ventilation in cystic fibrosis. American Review of Respiratory Disease 129: 712–718

Stanley P, MacWilliam L, Greenstone M et al 1984 Efficacy of a saccharin test for screening to detect abnormal mucociliary clearance. British Journal of Diseases of the Chest 78: 62–65

Stead RJ, Davidson TI, Duncan FR et al 1987 Use of a totally implantable system for venous access in cystic fibrosis. Thorax 42: 149–150

Stern M, Geddes D 1994 Gene therapy for cystic fibrosis. Respiratory Disease in Practice Winter: 18–23

Strauss GD, Osher A, Wang C et al 1987 Variable weight training in cystic fibrosis. Chest 92: 273–276

Super M, Schwarz MJ, Malone G et al 1994 Active cascade testing for carriers of cystic fibrosis gene. British Medical Journal 308: 1462–1468

Suri R, Wallis C, Bush A 2000a Tolerability of nebulised hypertonic saline in children with cystic fibrosis. Pediatric Pulmonology 30 (suppl 20): 306

Suri R, Wallis C, Bush A 2000b In vivo use of hypertonic saline in CF. Pediatric Pulmonology 30 (suppl 20): 125–126

Tattersall R, Callaghan H, Groves D, Walshaw MJ 2000 Assessment of posture by Quantec scanning in adult cystic fibrosis (CF) patients. Proceedings of the XIIIth International Cystic Fibrosis Congress, Stockholm S237, p 148

Taylor CJ, Threlfall D 1997 Postural drainage techniques and gastro-oesophageal reflux in cystic fibrosis. Lancet 349: 1567–1568

ten Berge M, Brinkhorst G, Kroon AA et al 1999 DNase treatment in primary ciliary dyskinesia – assessment by nocturnal pulse oximetry. Pediatric Pulmonology 27: 59–61

Thomas J, Cook DJ, Brooks D 1995 Chest physical therapy management of patients with cystic fibrosis: a meta-analysis. American Journal of Respiratory and Critical Care Medicine 151: 846–885

Tomashefski JF, Bruce M, Goldberg HI et al 1986 Regional distribution of macroscopic lung disease in cystic fibrosis. American Review of Respiratory Disease 133: 535–540

Touw DJ, Brimicombe RW, Hodson ME et al 1995 Inhalation of antibiotics in cystic fibrosis. European Respiratory Journal 8: 1594–1604

Turner JA, Corkey CW, Lee JY et al 1981 Clinical expression of immotile cilia syndrome. Pediatrics 67: 805–810

Turner M, Baildam E, Patel L et al 1997 Joint disorders in C.F. Journal of the Royal Society of Medicine 90 (suppl 31): 13–20

Unsworth R, Davis A, Dodd ME et al 1998 Does education improve patient understanding and adherence with airway clearance techniques? Proceedings of 22nd European Cystic Fibrosis Conference

Valerius NH, Koch C, Høiby N 1991 Prevention of chronic *Pseudomonas aeruginosa* colonisation in cystic fibrosis by early treatment. Lancet 338: 725–772

van der Schans CP 1997 Forced expiratory manoeuvres to increase transport of bronchial mucus: a mechanistic approach. Monaldi Archives of Chest Disease 52: 367–370

van der Schans C, Prasad SA, Main E 2000 Chest physiotherapy compared to no chest physiotherapy in cystic fibrosis. In: The Cochrane Library, Issue 2. Update Software, Oxford

Vibekk P 1991 Chest mobilization and respiratory function. In: Pryor JA (ed) Respiratory Care. Churchill Livingstone, Edinburgh, pp. 103–119

Vizza CD, Yusen RD, Jynch JP et al 2000 Outcome of patients with cystic fibrosis awaiting lung transplantation. American Journal of Respiratory and Critical Care Medicine 162: 819–825

Walters S, Britton J, Hodson ME 1993 Demographic and social characteristics of adults with cystic fibrosis in the United Kingdom. British Medical Journal 306: 549–552

Wanner A, Rao A 1980 Clinical implications and effects of bland, mucolytic and antibiotic aerosols. American Review of Respiratory Diseases 122: 79–87

Webb AK, Dodd ME 1997 Nebulised antibiotics for adults with cystic fibrosis. Thorax 52 (suppl 2): S69–71

Webb AK, Dodd ME 1999 Exercise and sport in cystic fibrosis: benefits and risks. British Journal of Sports Medicine 33: 77–78

Webb AK, Dodd ME 2000 Exercise and training for adults with cystic fibrosis. In: Hodson ME, Geddes DM (eds) Cystic fibrosis. Arnold, London, pp 433–444

Webb AK, Egan J, Dodd ME 1996 Clinical management of cystic fibrosis patients awaiting and immediately following lung transplantation. In Dodge A, Brock DJH, Widdecombe JH (eds) Cystic fibrosis: current topics, vol 3. John Wiley, Chichester, pp 311–337

Weeks AM, Buckland MR 1995 Anaesthesia for adults with cystic fibrosis. Anaesthesia and Intensive Care Journal 23: 332–338

Weinberger JBL, Weiss ST, Cohen WR et al 1980 Pregnancy and the lung. American Review of Respiratory Disease 121: 559–581

Westaby D 2000 Liver and biliary disease. In: Hodson ME, Geddes DM(eds) Cystic fibrosis. Arnold, London, pp. 289–300

Wills PJ, Wodehouse T, Corkery K, Mallon K, Wilson R, Cole PJ 1996 Short-term recombinant human DNase in bronchiectasis. American Journal of Respiratory and Critical Care Medicine 154: 413–417

Wilson R, Sykes DA, Chan KL et al 1987 Effect of head position on the efficacy of topical treatment of chronic mucopurulent rhinosinusitis. Thorax 42: 631–663

Wood RE, Wanner A, Hirsch J et al 1975 Tracheal muco-ciliary transport in cystic fibrosis and its stimulation by terbutaline. American Review of Respiratory Disease 111: 733–738

Zach MS, Oberwaldner B, Forche G et al 1985 Bronchodilators increase airway instability in cystic fibrosis. American Review of Respiratory Disease 131: 537–543

FURTHER READING

Bluebond-Langner M, Lask B, Angst D2001 Psychosocial aspects of cystis fibrosis. Arnold, London

Brewis RAL, Corrin B, Geddes DM, Gibson GJ (eds) 1995 Respiratory medicine, 2nd edn. WB Saunders, London, vols 1, 2

Cystic Fibrosis Trust 2001 Clinical guidelines for the physiotherapy management of cystic fibrosis (ACPCF).

Cystic Fibrosis Trust, Bromley (In Press)

Dinwiddie R 1997 The diagnosis and management of paediatric respiratory disease, 2nd edn. Churchill Livingstone, Edinburgh

Hodson ME, Geddes DM (eds) 2000 Cystic fibrosis. Arnold, London

Normal values and abbreviations

NORMAL VALUES

Age group	Heart rate Mean (range) (beats/min)	Respiratory rate range (breaths/min)	Blood pressure systolic/ diastolic (mmHg)
Preterm	150 (100–200)	40–60	39–59 / 16–36
Newborn	140 (80–200)	30–50	50–70 / 25–45
< 2 years	130 (100–190)	20–40	87–105 / 53–66
> 2 years	80 (60–140)	20–40	95–105 / 53–66
> 6 years	75 (60–90)	15–30	97–112 / 57–71
Adults	70 (50–100)	12–16	95–140 / 60–90

Conversion tables

0.133 kPa = 1.0 mmHg		$pH = 9 - \log [H^+]$ where $[H^+]$ is in nmol/l	
kPa	mmHg	pH	$[H^+]$
1	7.5	7.52	30
2	15.0	7.45	35
4	30	7.40	40
6	45	7.35	45
8	60	7.30	50
10	75	7.26	55
12	90	7.22	60
14	105	7.19	65

Arterial blood

pH	7.35–7.45 $[H^+]$ 45–35 nmol/l
PaO_2	10.7–13.3 kPa (80–100 mmHg)
$PaCO_2$	4.7–6.0 kPa (35–45 mmHg)
HCO_3^-	22–26 mmol/l
Base excess	–2 to +2

Venous blood

pH	7.31 – 7.41 [H^+] 46 – 38 nmol/l
PO_2	5.0–5.6 kPa (37–42 mmHg)
PCO_2	5.6–6.7 kPa (42–50 mmHg)

Ventilation/perfusion

Alveolar–arterial oxygen gradient A–aPO_2:
Breathing air   0.7–2.7 kPa (5–20 mmHg)
Breathing 100%   3.3–8.6 kPa (25–65 mmHg)
  oxygen

Pressures

		mmHg	kPa
Right atrial (RA) pressure	Mean	−1 to +7	−0.13 to 0.93
Right ventricular (RV) pressure	Systolic	15–25	2.0–3.3
	Diastolic	0–8	0–1.0
Pulmonary artery (PA) pressure	Systolic	15–25	2.0–3.3
	Diastolic	8–15	1.0–2.0
	Mean	10–20	1.3–2.7
Pulmonary capillary wedge pressure (PCWP)	Mean	6–15	0.8–2.0
Central venous pressure (CVP)		3–15 cmH$_2$O	
Intracranial pressure (ICP)		< 10 mmHg (< 1.3 kPa)	
Peak inspiratory mouth pressure (PiMax)	Male	103–124 cmH$_2$O (age dependent)	
	Female	65–87 cmH$_2$O (age dependent)	
Peak expiratory mouth pressure (PeMax)	Male	185–233 cmH$_2$O (age dependent)	
	Female	128–152 cmH$_2$O (age dependent)	

Blood chemistry

Albumin	37–53 g/l
Calcium (Ca^{2+})	2.25–2.65 mmol/l
Creatinine	60–120 μmol/l
Glucose	4–6 mmol/l
Potassium (K^+)	3.4–5.0 mmol/l
Sodium (Na^+)	134–140 mmol/l
Urea	2.5–6.5 mmol/l
Haemoglobin (Hb)	14.0–18.0 g/100 ml (men)
	11.5–15.5 g/100 ml (women)

Platelets	$150–400 \times 10^9/l$
White blood cell count (WBC)	$4–11 \times 10^9/l$
Urine output	1 ml/kg/h

ABBREVIATIONS

AAA	abdominal aortic aneurysm
A–aDO_2	alveolar–arterial oxygen gradient
A–aPO_2	alveolar–arterial oxygen gradient
ABPA	allergic bronchopulmonary aspergillosis
ACBT	active cycle of breathing techniques
ACT	airway clearance technique
AD	autogenic drainage
ADH	antidiuretic hormone
ADL	activities of daily living
AF	atrial fibrillation
AHRF	acute hypoxaemic respiratory failure
AIDS	acquired immune deficiency syndrome
ALI	acute lung injury
AMBER	advanced multiple beam equalization radiography
AP	anteroposterior
APACHE	acute physiology and chronic health evaluation
ARDS	acute respiratory distress syndrome
ARF	acute renal failure
ASD	atrial septal defect
ATN	acute tubular necrosis
ATPS	ambient temperature and pressure saturated
AVAS	absolute visual analogue scale
AVSD	atrioventricular septal defect
BDI	baseline and transition dyspnoea index
BiPAP	bilevel positive airway pressure
BIPAP	bilevel positive airway pressure
BIVAD	biventricular device
BM	blood glucose monitoring
BMI	body mass index
BP	blood pressure
BPD	bronchopulmonary dysplasia
BPF	bronchopleural fistula
bpm	beats per minute

BSA	body surface area		DIOS	distal intestinal obstruction syndrome
BTPS	body temperature and pressure saturated		dl	decilitre
			DLCO	diffusing capacity for carbon monoxide
Ca^{2+}	calcium		DMD	Duchenne muscular dystrophy
CABG	coronary artery bypass graft		DNA	deoxyribonucleic acid
CABGS	coronary artery bypass graft surgery		DO_2	oxygen delivery
CAD	coronary artery disease		DVT	deep vein thrombosis
CAL	chronic airflow limitation			
CAVG	coronary artery vein graft		EBV	Epstein–Barr virus
CBF	cerebral blood flow		$ECCO_2R$	extracorporeal carbon dioxide removal
Ccw	chest wall compliance		ECG	electrocardiograph
CF	cystic fibrosis		ECMO	extracorporeal membrane oxygenation
CFA	cryptogenic fibrosing alveolitis		EECP	enhanced external counter-pulsation
CFTR	cystic fibrosis transmembrane conductance regulator		EEG	electroencephalogram
CHD	coronary heart disease		EIA	exercise-induced asthma
CHF	chronic heart failure		EMG	electromyogram
CK	creatine kinase		EOG	electrooculogram
C_L	lung compliance		EPAP	expiratory positive airway pressure
CLD	chronic lung disease		EPP	equal pressure point
cm	centimetre		ERV	expiratory reserve volume
CMV	controlled mandatory ventilation		$ETCO_2$	end-tidal carbon dioxide
CMV	cytomegalovirus		ETT	endotracheal tube
CO	cardiac output		ETT	exercise tolerance test
CO_2	carbon dioxide			
COAD	chronic obstructive airways disease		FDP	fibrin degradation product
COPD	chronic obstructive pulmonary disease		FEF_{50}	forced expiratory flow at 50% of forced vital capacity
CPAP	continuous positive airway pressure		FEF_{75}	forced expiratory flow at 75% of forced vital capacity
CPP	cerebral perfusion pressure		FET	forced expiration technique
CRF	chronic renal failure		FEV_1	forced expiratory volume in 1 second
CRP	conditioning rehabilitation programme		FG	French gauge
CRQ	chronic respiratory disease questionnaire		FGF	fibroblast growth factor
CSF	cerebrospinal fluid		FH	family history
CT	computed tomography		FHF	fulminant hepatic failure
CV	cardiovascular		FiO_2	fractional inspired oxygen concentration
CV	closing volume		FRC	functional residual capacity
CVP	central venous pressure		ft	feet
			FVC	forced vital capacity
DH	drug history			
DIC	disseminated intravascular coagulopathy		g	gram

GA	general anaesthetic	IPAP	inspiratory positive airway pressure
g/dl	gram per decilitre	IPPB	intermittent positive pressure breathing
GCS	Glasgow coma scale		
GOR	gastro-oesophageal reflux		
GPB	glossopharyngeal breathing	IPPV	intermittent positive pressure ventilation
GTN	glyceryl trinitrate		
h	hour	IPS	inspiratory pressure support
H^+	hydrogen ion	IS	incentive spirometry
$[H^+]$	hydrogen ion concentration	IV	intravenous
H_2O	water	IVH	intraventricular haemorrhage
Hb	haemoglobin	IVOX	intravenacaval oxygenation
HCO_3^-	bicarbonate	IVUS	intravascular ultrasound
Hct	haematocrit		
HD	haemodialysis	JVP	jugular venous pressure
HDU	high dependency unit		
HFCWO	high-frequency chest wall oscillation	K^+	potassium
		Kcal	kilocalories
HFJV	high-frequency jet ventilation	KCO	coefficient of gas transfer
HFO	high-frequency oscillation	kg	kilogram
HFOV	high-frequency oscillatory ventilation	kJ	kilojoule
		kPa	kilopascal
HFPPV	high-frequency positive pressure ventilation	kVp	kilovoltage
		l	litre
HIV	human immunodeficiency virus	LAP	left atrial pressure
HLA	human leucocyte antigen	LED	light-emitting diode
HLT	heart-lung transplantation	LRTD	lower respiratory tract disease
HME	heat and moisture exchanger	LTOT	long-term oxygen therapy
HPC	history of presenting condition	LVAD	left ventricular assist device
HPOA	hypertrophic pulmonary osteoarthropathy	LVEF	left ventricular ejection fraction
		LVF	left ventricular failure
HR	heart rate	LVRS	lung volume reduction surgery
HRQol	health-related quality of life		
HRR	heart rate reserve	m	metre
Hz	hertz	μm	micrometre (10^{-6} m)
		μs	microsecond
IABP	intra-aortic balloon pump	MAP	mean airway pressure
ICC	intercostal catheter	MAP	mean arterial pressure
ICP	intracranial pressure	MAS	minimal access surgery
ICU	intensive care unit	MCH	mean corpuscular haemoglobin
Ig	immunoglobulin	MCV	mean corpuscular volume
IHD	ischaemic heart disease	MDI	metered dose inhaler
ILD	interstitial lung disease	MEF_{50}	maximal expiratory flow at 50% of forced vital capacity
IMA	internal mammary artery		
IMT	inspiratory muscle training	MEF_{75}	maximal expiratory flow at 75% of forced vital capacity
IMV	intermittent mandatory ventilation		
in	inches	METs	metabolic equivalents
INR	international normalized ratio	MHz	megahertz

MI	myocardial infarction	PAWP	pulmonary artery wedge pressure
MIE	meconium ileus equivalent	PCA	patient-controlled analgesia
min	minute	PCD	primary ciliary dyskinesia
ml	millilitre	PCIRV	pressure-controlled inverse ratio ventilation
mm	millimetre		
MMAD	mass median aerodynamic diameter	PCP	*Pneumocystis carinii* pneumonia
mmHg	millimetres of mercury	PCPAP	periodic continuous positive airway pressure
mmol	millimole		
mph	miles per hour	PCV	packed cell volume
MRI	magnetic resonance imaging	PCWP	pulmonary capillary wedge pressure
MRSA	methicillin-resistant *Staphylococcus aureus*		
		PD	peritoneal dialysis
ms	millisecond	PD	postural drainage
MVO_2	myocardial oxygen consumption	PDA	patent ductus arteriosus
MVV	maximum voluntary ventilation	Pdi	transdiaphragmatic pressure
		PE	pulmonary embolus
n	number	PEEP	positive end-expiratory presssure
Na^+	sodium	PEF	peak expiratory flow
NEPV	negative extrathoracic pressure ventilation	PEFR	peak expiratory flow rate
		$PeMax$	peak expiratory mouth pressure
NICU	neonatal intensive care unit	PEP	positive expiratory pressure
NIPPV	non-invasive intermittent positive pressure ventilation	pH	hydrogen ion concentration
		PIE	pulmonary interstitial emphysema
nm	nanometre		
nmol	nanomole	PIF	peak inspiratory flow
NO	nitric oxide	PIFR	peak inspiratory flow rate
NPV	negative pressure ventilation	$PiMax$	peak inspiratory mouth pressure
NREM	non-rapid eye movement	PIP	peak inspiratory pressure
NSAID	non-steroidal anti-inflammatory drug	PMH	previous medical history
		PMR	percutaneous myocardial revascularization
O_2	oxygen		
OB	obliterative bronchiolitis	PN	percussion note
OHFO	oral high-frequency oscillation	PND	paroxysmal nocturnal dyspnoea
OI	oxygen index	POMR	problem oriented medical record
OLT	orthotopic liver transplantation	PTB	pulmonary tuberculosis
		PTCA	percutaneous transluminal coronary angioplasty
PA	posteroanterior		
PA	pulmonary artery	$P_{TC}CO_2$	transcutaneous carbon dioxide tension
$PaCO_2$	partial pressure of carbon dioxide in alveolar gas		
		PTFE	polytetrafluoroethylene
$PaCO_2$	partial pressure of carbon dioxide in arterial blood	PTT	partial thromboplastin time
		PVC	polyvinyl chloride
PaO_2	partial pressure of oxygen in alveolar gas	PVH	periventricular haemorrhage
		PVL	periventricular leucomalacia
PaO_2	partial pressure of oxygen in arterial blood	PVR	pulmonary vascular resistance
		PWC	peak work capacity
PAP	pulmonary artery pressure	$\dot{Q}$	blood flow

QOL	quality of life
RAP	right atrial pressure
R_{AW}	airway resistance
RBC	red blood cell
RDS	respiratory distress syndrome
REM	rapid eye movement
RMT	respiratory muscle training
ROP	retinopathy of prematurity
RPE	rating of perceived exertion
RPP	rate pressure product
RSV	respiratory syncytial virus
RTA	road traffic accident
RV	residual volume
RVF	right ventricular failure
s	second
SA	sinoatrial
SaO_2	arterial oxygen saturation
SG_{AW}	specific airway conductance
SGRQ	St George's Respiratory Questionnaire
SH	social history
SIMV	synchronized intermittent mandatory ventilation
SOB	shortness of breath
SpO_2	pulse oximetry arterial oxygen saturation
SVC	superior vena cava
SV	saphenous vein
SVO_2	mixed venous oxygen saturation
SVR	systemic vascular resistance
SWT	shuttle walk test
TAA	thoracic aortic aneurysm
$TcCO_2$	transcutaneous carbon dioxide
TcO_2	transcutaneous oxygen
TED	thromboembolic deterrent

TEE	thoracic expansion exercises
TENS	transcutaneous electrical nerve stimulation
TGA	transposition of the great arteries
TLC	total lung capacity
TLCO	transfer factor in lung of carbon monoxide
TMR	transmyocardial revascularization
TV	tidal volume
UAS	upper abdominal surgery
$\dot{V}$	ventilation
$\dot{V}_A$	alveolar ventilation/alveolar volume
VAD	ventricular assist device
VAS	visual analogue scale
VATS	video assisted thoracoscopy surgery
VC	vital capacity
V_D	dead-space ventilation
$\dot{V}_E$	minute ventilation
VEGF	vascular endothelial growth factor
VF	ventricular fibrillation
VF	vocal fremitus
$\dot{V}O_2$	oxygen consumption
$\dot{V}O_2$max	maximum oxygen uptake
$\dot{V}/\dot{Q}$	ventilation/perfusion ratio
VR	vocal resonance
VRE	vancomycin-resistant enterococcus
VSD	ventricular septal defect
V_T	tidal volume
W	watt
WBC	white blood count
WCC	white cell count
WOB	work of breathing

Index

625

Piers Anthony was born in Oxford in 1934, moved with his family to Spain in 1939 and then to the USA in 1940, after his father was expelled from Spain by the Franco regime. He became a citizen of the US in 1958 and, before devoting himself to full-time writing, worked as a technical writer for a communications company and taught English. He started publishing short stories with *Possible to Rue* for *Fantastic* in 1963, and published in SF magazines for the next decade. He has, however, concentrated more and more on writing novels.

Author of the brilliant, widely acclaimed *Cluster* series, and the superb *Tarot*, he has made a name for himself as a writer of original, inventive stories whose imaginative, mind-twisting style is full of extraordinary, often poetic images and flights of cosmic fancy.

VIRTUAL
MODE

Piers Anthony

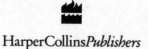

HarperCollins*Publishers*

HarperCollins*Publishers*
77–85 Fulham Palace Road
Hammersmith, London W6 8JB

Published by HarperCollins*Publishers* 1991
9 8 7 6 5 4 3 2 1

A catalogue record for this book
is available from the British Library

ISBN 0–246–13860–2
ISBN 0–246–13887–4 (Pbk)

Set in Palatino

Printed in Great Britain by
HarperCollinsManufacturing Glasgow

CONTENTS

1

COLENE

Colene had a study hall during the last period, and as an Honor student she had a regular hall pass. RHIP, she thought: Rank Hath Its Privileges. She smiled marginally, remembering a cartoon she had seen: two gravestones, one plain, one quite fancy. The plain one was lettered RIP, the fancy one RHIP. She liked the notion. No one challenged her as she got up and walked out of the room and down the hall to the bathroom.

She was in luck: it was empty at the moment. She went into the farthest stall, closed and latched the swinging door, lifted her skirt, took down her panties, and sat on the seat. But she did not actually use the toilet. Instead she held up her left arm, and used her right hand to unwrap the winding around her left wrist. It was a style only a few girls affected: bright red cloth on both wrists, complementing her blue skirt and yellow blouse. It was attractive, of course, and Colene preferred to be esthetic, but it was more than that.

For as the band came loose, her wrist showed, horribly scarred. There were welts all across the inner side, some old and white, others fresh and raw. She gazed at it with mixed awe and loathing. She was artistic and creative as well as smart, but this was none of these things. This was closer to her real nature, ugly and dull and tragic, that had to be hidden from others.

Then she reached down to fetch her compass from her purse. A knife would have been better, but might also have

7

brought suspicion on her. She lifted the point, set it against her wrist, and made a sudden, sharp slice across. 'Oh!' she exclaimed as the pain came. She hated the pain, but it was the only way. Maybe she could get a small, sharp knife, seemingly decorative and harmless, that would cut almost painlessly, and deeper. If she had the nerve. The nerve was not in the cutting, but in the acquisition; if anyone saw her with the blade out, and asked . . .

The scratch was stinging, but only a bit of blood was showing. She clenched her teeth and made another pass, in the same track, harder. This time the surge of pain was rewarded by some real blood. It welled out and flowed slowly across her wrist. It was beautiful, like a rich red river wending across a desolate terrain.

She spread her legs and nudged back on the toilet, so that she had more space in front. She angled her wrist so that the blood could drip directly into the water below. The first drop gathered itself, bunched, and finally let go. It struck the water and spread out, losing its identity as the water diluted it. It was dying.

Dying. There was the thought that counted. Oh to fall like that drop into the water, and dissolve, and dissipate, and be no more. Just to fade away, forgotten.

Drop by drop, coloring the water, turning it slowly pinkish. Like menstrual flow, only more vital. Menstrual flow was associated with life, or potential life. This was associated with death, and that was infinitely more important.

Another drop fell to the water, but this one was not red. It was a tear. That seemed fitting: blood and tears. For a man it would be blood, sweat and tears, but it wasn't feminine to sweat, so just the blood and tears would do. Her life, gone into the water, flushed down the toilet, cleanly. Part of the problem with death was the sheer messiness of it. She didn't like mess. She liked things neat and clean and in order. If only she could find a way –

The bathroom door opened. Instantly Colene snapped out of it. She put her wrist to her mouth, licking off the salty blood. She dropped the compass into her purse. She rebound her wrist with a practiced motion, and tucked in the end so it was tight. Then she slid forward on the toilet and used it as was its custom, taking care to make a splash so that the sound advertised the fact of her urination. There were levels and levels of concealment, and she had learned not to assume that others would get the message she intended. It had to be too obvious to miss. Nothing but pissing going on here, ma'am.

The other girl chose another stall and settled down. She was not suspicious. Still, it was nervous business. If anyone were to catch on, Colene would just die of embarrassment. That was not the way she wanted to die!

She stood, reassembled herself, and flushed the toilet. No blood showed; the drops had fallen cleanly into the water, leaving no giveaway stains. Yet somehow she feared that the traces were there, a guilty ambience, so that the next person who used this toilet would somehow know that a person had flirted with suicide here.

But maybe not. A girl could have changed her tampon, and that was where the blood had come from. Not a pad, because that couldn't be flushed. A tampon would leave no evidence. Some girls used pads so as to maintain the pretense that they were virginal, but most preferred convenience, as did Colene herself. So she was covered.

She went to a sink and washed her hands, carefully. No blood showed on her wrist, thanks in part to the wrapping: red covered red. The inner layer was absorbent, and would take up the blood and help it thicken and clot. She would have to wash out the cloth at home, but she was used to that.

Back in the study hall she brought out her compass and wiped the point on a tissue, just to be sure. Then she brought out her geometry homework, so that no one would wonder about the compass. Geometry was a snap; in fact it was boring, because it was two dimensional. It would have been more of a challenge in three dimensions, or four. If only they had a class in cubic geometry, or multi-dimensional constructions. Or fractals: now there would be one she could truly sink her teeth into. *Class, today we shall take our little pencil and graph paper and define the complete Mandelbrot Set.*

Colene stifled a smile. The Mandelbrot Set was said to be the most complicated object in mathematics. Even mainframe computers could not fathom the whole of it. Yet it was simply an exercise in algebra, plotted on paper. How she would love to explore that beautiful picture! To lose herself in its phenomenal and diminishing convolutions, for ever and ever Amen.

But this was mundane school, where brains were routinely pickled in trivia. No hope here.

As the final bell approached, Julie came to sit beside her. It was Friday, and the teacher in charge knew better than to try to keep things totally quiet in the closing minutes. As long as they didn't make a scene, they were all right.

Julie had long yellow hair, which she liked to swirl about her face and shoulders. It was a nice complement to Colene's similar brown tresses. But in other respects they differed more widely. Julie wore glasses and braces, which made her by definition unattractive; Colene, with neither, was far more popular. That was a barrier between them, and their friendship was only nominal, because it was mutually convenient to walk home from the bus stop together.

Actually, Colene had no friends, by her definition, though many others called her friend. It was as if she had an invisible barrier around herself that kept all others at a certain distance. No one touched her heart, and her heart was lonely. She wished it could be otherwise, but the truth was that no one she knew at school was the type she cared to sincerely like and trust. Maybe she was just an intellectual snob, and she felt slightly guilty for that, but only slightly. If she ever encountered someone with really solid intelligence and integrity, someone she could truly admire for maintaining standards she herself could not, then maybe –

'Did you hear?' Julie inquired in a breathless whisper. 'The Principal canceled the rally tomorrow!'

Colene had planned on skipping the rally anyway, but she acted properly outraged. 'The nerve of the nerd! Why?'

'Too many Bumper Stinkers in the parking lot.'

Colene remembered: there had been a rash of bad-taste stickers, using four letter words and concepts. Principal Brown had laid down the law: no more of them on the school grounds. Evidently some of the stupid high school boys had tried it anyway. The Principal wasn't satisfied to

10

punish the errant boys; he had to punish the whole school too. Actually there was reason for this: those stickers would keep reappearing until there was a climate of rejection among the students, and that would come only if all of them paid the penalty. Colene understood, but it would be traitorous to argue the case.

'What will we do with Brown?' Julie demanded rhetorically. It was a matter of definition: no matter what happened, the Principal was always wrong. That was one of the unifying principles of the student body.

Colene glanced around, saw that the teacher in charge was not paying attention while nearby students were, and launched into one of her clever little stories. She was good at this sort of thing, and she enjoyed it in her fashion.

'Why, we should hold a benefit for him,' she said brightly.

'A benefit?' Julie asked blankly, playing the straight man to Colene's act.

'Yes. When he drives up in his Datsun with the tags saying OBITCH –' She paused, giving them time to put that together: DATSUN OBITCH. An expanding circle of sniggers indicated that the joke had registered. 'Then we should stage a gala fund-raising extravaganza, a dunk-the-idiot benefit, with Principal Brown as the main event. Three balls for a dollar, and whoever scores on the target makes Brown fall on the biggest, loudest, smelliest whoopee cushion ever put out by the Ack-Mee Novelty Company!' She put the back of a hand to her mouth and blew the whoopee noise.

It came out too loud. The teacher glanced quickly over at them, and they all had to stifle their laughter. Then the bell rang, saving them. That reminded Colene of a recording she had once heard at a party she wasn't supposed to attend: a 'crepitation' championship match, in which the contestants broke wind in novel ways, each effort appropriately named, such as the sonorous 'Follow-up Blooper' and cute little 'Freeps', and the end of the round was signaled not by a bell but a flatulent horn. The school buzzer was actually more like that than a church bell.

Julie and Colene got off the bus and walked home. It was a

11

pleasant neighborhood, with neat lawns, trees, and even some overgrown lots that were almost like little jungles. Drainage ditches were forming into the beginning of a stream that wound on out of the city. Colene had explored the recesses of that nascent river many times, on the assumption that there had to be something interesting there, like buried treasure or a vampire's coffin. Maybe even, O Rapturous Joy, a lost horse looking for someone to love it. But all she had ever found were weeds and mud.

'Groan, I have to go in for X-rays tomorrow,' Julie was saying. 'Those damned hard ridges on the pictures always slice up my gums. I don't know why they can't make them softer.'

'Easy to fix,' Colene said brightly. 'Just bring the president of Code-Ack in for X-rays, and have *his* gums and roof-of-mouth cut up by those corners. Make him really have to chew down on them for retakes, and tell him "Don't be a difficult child now; those things don't hurt!" I guarantee: next day those edges would be soft as sponges.'

'Yes!' Julie agreed, heartened. 'If only we could!'

But they both knew that nothing that sensible would ever be done, and that sharp edges would continue to find their helpless victims. That was just the way of it. The people who manufactured things never actually used them themselves.

As they approached Colene's house, her wandering glance spied something in the ditch. It was probably just a pile of cloth, or garbage tossed from a car; there were creeps who routinely did such things. But she felt a chill, and surge of excitement. Suppose it was something else?

She said nothing to Julie. She wanted to check this by herself. Just in case.

They walked on. Julie's house was beyond Colene's house, so Colene turned off. Her parents weren't home at this hour, of course; they both worked. Not that it mattered. She had ways in her imagination to glorify the empty home. She liked to pretend that the drainage ditch behind was a great river that wended its way past the most illustrious regions: The Charles. Her simple residence became a gloomy mansion on the bank of this river, where death was a familiar presence. Thus it was the Charles Mansion, a takeoff on a grim killer

12

in a text on legal cases. Her folks wouldn't have thought that funny, and her schoolmates wouldn't have caught the allusion. That seemed to be typical of her life: she couldn't relate well to either parents or peers. But she was the only one who realized this.

She unlocked the door and entered. She set her books on the table and walked straight on through to the back door. She unlocked that and went out, glancing back over her shoulder to make sure that there was no one to see her. It was fun being secretive, despite the fact that her whole life was pretty much an act, papering over her secret reality. She fancied that she was a princess going out to discover a fallen prince from a far land. What she would find would most likely be garbage, but for thirty seconds she could dream, and that was worth something. Even garbage might be better than tackling her stupid homework early.

She came to the cloth, and froze. It was a man! A grown man, lying face down on the weedy bank. His clothing was strange, but it was definitely a man. Was it a corpse, thrown here by some drug gang? Such things did happen, though not in this neighborhood. Of course the neighborhood wasn't what it represented itself to be, either; a lot was covered up for the sake of appearances.

Thrilling to this morbid adventure, she approached. Death fascinated her, though she hated it. This was as good as watching her blood flow. Would the body be riddled with bullet holes?

She remembered one of her favorite lines, from a song she could not otherwise remember. It was about some great Irish or Scottish battle, and a sore wounded soldier had staggered back from the front line. But he had not given up. 'I'll lay me down and bleed a while, then up to fight again!' he declared. She knew she would have liked him. Maybe this was such a man, who had laid him down to bleed and had forgotten to get up again before overdoing it.

Then it moved. Colene stifled her scream, for all that could do was alert the neighbors and bring a crowd, and her little adventure would be over. Cautiously, she approached.

The man lifted his head, spying her. He moved his right

arm, reaching toward her. He groaned. Then he sank back, evidently too weak to do more.

But if she stepped within reach, he might suddenly come to full life, and grab her ankle, pull her down, and rape her. It could be just a ruse to get her close. After he had his way with her, he might kill her and roll her body under the brush near the trickle of water that was the river. After several days she would be found, covered by flies, and he would be long gone.

It was as good a way to die as any. When it came right down to it, it hardly mattered whether death was pretty or ugly; what counted was that the escape had finally been made. A certain amount of messiness could be tolerated for the sake of the novelty. She stepped deliberately within reach.

But the man did not respond. He just lay there, breathing in shudders. Maybe he was sick with some deathly malady, and she would catch it, and die in horrible agony of a disease unknown to science.

She squatted. 'Who are you?' she asked.

The man reacted to her voice. He lifted his head again, and uttered something alien, and sank down once more.

He really did seem to be too tired to do more. He hadn't even tried to grab her ankle or to look up her skirt. He didn't look diseased, just worn out.

That clothing was definitely strange. His language, too, was unlike anything she had heard before. Could he be a diplomat from some faraway little kingdom who somehow got off at the wrong stop and was hopelessly lost? Unable to speak the local language, perhaps with no local money, he might simply be starving.

Or he might be hideously dangerous in a way she couldn't fathom. As an innocent fourteen year old girl, she definitely ought to get quickly away from him and phone the police. They could handle it, whether he was a diplomat or a criminal. That was the only proper course.

Colene felt the thrill of danger, and knew she was about to do something monumentally stupid.

She leaned close to his ear. 'You must come with me. I will help you. I will help. Help. Do you understand?'

14

His hand slid across the ground, toward the sound of her voice, the fingers twitching.

Maybe he was dehydrated. The day had been hot, though the night would be cold; that was the way fall was in Oklahoma.

'I'll be right back,' she said.

She straightened up, paused as dizziness took her because of the sudden change of position, then walked quickly back to her house. She went to the messy kitchen and fetched a plastic glass. She filled it with water from the tap, and carried it out.

The man had not moved. She sat down beside his head, set the water down in a snug depression, and reached for him. 'I'm back,' she said. 'I brought you water. Can you drink it?'

He tried to raise his head again. She put her hands on it and lifted; then she scooted on her bottom so that she could set his head in her lap. She held it tilted up, then reached for the glass. It was a stretch, and she had to lean over his head. Her bosom actually touched his hair. He did not seem to notice, but the contact sent new waves of speculation through her. Wasn't this the way the Little Mermaid had rescued the drowning prince? Holding him close, helping him survive – until he recovered and married somebody else, never realizing what he owed to the mermaid. The tragedy of not even knowing!

She got the glass and brought it to his face, which was now propped against her front. 'Water,' she murmured. 'Water. Drink. Water.' She touched his mouth and tilted the glass.

Suddenly he realized what it was. Eagerly he sipped. She tilted further, spilling some, but he managed to drink most of it. She had been right!

'More?' she asked, still holding his head and feeling very maternal. 'More water?'

His hand came up, questing for something. He seemed to have more strength than before, but that wasn't saying much.

She set aside the empty glass and caught his hand with her free one. His fingers were cold. She squeezed them with her warm ones. His squeezed back.

She was thrilled again. Communication!

Then she decided that she had better get away from him

before he recovered too much. She had already taken a phenomenal chance; it was time to stop pushing her luck to the brink. 'More water,' she said firmly, and pulled herself away. She set his head back on the ground, scrambled up, got the glass and hurried back to the house.

When she returned with the next glassful of water, the man was struggling to his hands and knees. He was definitely gaining strength. It would be absolutely crazy to get near him again. Anything could happen.

She brought the glass to him. But he had now recovered to the point where he might walk, and he was trying to get to his feet. He was a good deal larger than she was, and surely stronger, which meant yet again that it was time for her to get away from him. So she dropped the glass and stepped in and helped him stand.

She put her arms around his body and heaved, and he lurched to his feet. They staggered toward her house.

At which point Colene thought things through just a bit further. It didn't matter whether she was being sensible or foolish – as if there were any question! – because once the man got to her house, and her parents came home, the game would be over. They would call the police, and the police would take the man away, and both parents would bawl her out for her stupidity before settling into their usual pursuits for the evening. Her father would head off for his date with his current liaison, and her mother would settle down to serious drinking. Things would be back to normal.

'No!' she gasped. 'Not there – there!' She shoved him away from the house and toward her shed. This was a solid structure, larger than a dollhouse but considerably smaller than a real house, perhaps originally intended for storage, but she had taken it over and made it her own private place. Her parents had learned not to bother her there. It was often enough her main link with sanity. Sometimes she spent the full night there, rather than watching her mother drink. She called it Dogwood Bumshed, because a small dogwood tree grew beside it. It wasn't a great tree, and it wouldn't survive at all if she didn't water it, but it did flower nicely in the spring, its moment of glory.

16

The man moved in that direction, yielding to her shove. She wrenched the door open and he stumbled in. He collapsed on her pile of cushions; his brief strength had been exhausted. Perhaps that was just as well. 'More water,' she told him, and shut the door on him. Now he would not be discovered, by her parents or anyone else.

She fetched the glass, which had fallen and spilled when she helped the man walk. She took it to the house, filled it again, then checked the supplies of food. There was a loaf of bread; she took it whole. That would do for a start.

She brought the things to the shed. The man lay where he had settled, but revived when she entered. Now he was able to drink by himself; he accepted the glass from her.

He did not seem to know what the bread was. She opened the package and took out a slice. He gazed at it blankly. She took a bite of it. Then his face lighted; he finally understood. He took a slice and bit into it with considerably less delicacy than she had. Oh yes, he was hungry!

Standing there, watching him eat, Colene finally had time to reflect on what all this might be leading to. She had rescued a man; now what was she going to do with him? He did not seem to be aggressive, but of course he was weak from hunger and thirst. What would he be like when he had his strength back? She really should report him, now; she had taken much more risk than she should have, and gotten away with it, but there were limits. She knew nothing about him except that he was a man, and that was warning enough.

She returned to the house and fetched two blankets from her closet. She knew already that she was not going to turn him in. He might turn on her and kill her, but that risk intrigued her more than it frightened her. She would see this through to wherever it led, no matter what. If she could only keep anybody else from finding out about him.

Did that mean she was going to try to keep him captive? After all, how could she stop him from simply walking out? She didn't know, but until he did depart, she would take care of him.

The man finished the loaf of bread, and Colene returned to the house to get more food. She couldn't take anything

17

else that would be missed; it would be difficult enough explaining the bread. She found some old cookies, and some leftover casserole in the back of the refrigerator; she could say it was getting moldy so she threw it out. It *was* getting moldy, but she trimmed off the mold and took it anyway. She was an old hand at trimming mold, because her mother constantly forgot things; she knew it wasn't anything to freak out about.

The man was glad to have the additional food. But he remained weak, and she knew she couldn't send him back out into the world. He would just collapse again.

But there was something she had to make clear to him. How could she establish communication, so as to tell him what she needed to? For the fact was that her parents would be getting home soon, and if the man showed himself, the game would be up. He had to remain hidden.

Well, all she could do was try. First maybe they could exchange names. She tapped herself on the breastbone: 'Colene. Colene.' Then she pointed to him.

He looked at her, then tapped himself similarly. 'Colene.'

Oops. She cast about for something else. She picked up a notepad and pencil, and quickly drew two figures, one small and female, the other larger and male. She pointed to herself, then to the female. 'Me. Colene.' Then to the male. 'You.' She paused expectantly.

He took the paper. 'Me. Colene,' he said, pointing to the female. 'You. Darius.'

Well, it was progress. 'Me Colene, girl,' she said, tapping herself again. 'You Darius, man.'

He nodded, pointing to her. 'Me –'

'No, *you*.'

He looked perplexed, but managed to get it. 'You Colene girl. Me Darius man.'

She smiled. 'Yes.' It was a beginning. He did not know her language, but he could learn. She drilled him on Yes and No until she was sure he understood them, and tested him on the picture of the horse on the wall, titled 'For Whom Was That Neigh?' 'Man?' she asked, pointing to it. No. 'Girl?' No. 'Horse?' Yes. He had it straight. Then she gave her message.

18

She opened the door and pointed to the house beyond. 'House. Colene. Yes. House. Darius. No.'

After some back and forth, he seemed to understand. But he seemed uneasy, even uncomfortable.

'What's the matter?' she asked.

Finally he made what might have been taken as an obscene gesture, but he did it in such an apologetic manner that she knew he wasn't trying to insult her. He touched and halfway squeezed his groin.

'The bathroom!' she exclaimed, catching on. 'You have to use the –' But she couldn't bring him to the house for that!

'Wait,' she told him, and dashed back to the house. She dug out a big old rusty pot and brought it to the shed. 'This.' She pantomimed sitting on it. She even made the whoopee noise.

He looked extremely doubtful. 'No, I won't watch you!' she said, knowing he couldn't understand the words, but hoping the sense of it came through. 'I have to go to the house, there.' She pointed to it. 'So my folks won't know anything's up. I'll try to check back on you, when I can. You just stay here.' Then she stepped out, and closed the door on him.

She was just in time: her father's car was pulling into the drive. She hurried to the back door and in. She checked the kitchen to make sure that nothing there would give her away, then went to the front room to pick up her school books. But no, this was Friday, and she never did homework on Friday. She didn't want to arouse suspicion. She had to be perfectly normal. So she turned on the TV too loud and plumped down on the couch.

Her father came in. 'Turn that thing down!' he snapped.

She grabbed the remote control and diminished the volume just enough to accede without quite ceasing to annoy him. He went on to his bedroom.

One down. One to go.

An hour later her father, clean, shaved and neatly dressed, went out again. Colene stared at the TV, pretending not to notice. She didn't care about his date with his mistress, as long as he was discreet. Well, maybe deep-down she did care, but that was worse than pointless: it only cut her up further.

There was nothing she could do about it anyway. So it was safer not to care.

Fifteen minutes after that, her mother's car arrived. Colene remained before the TV. Actually her mind was on the man in the shed; she wasn't paying any attention to the program. But she had to play her role, more so today than usual.

Her mother went straight to the kitchen, and Colene heard the first drink being poured. Good; there would be no trouble from that quarter this evening.

She got up, leaving the TV on, and went to the kitchen. 'I'll just take a snack out to the shed, okay?' she said, picking up some candy bars and raisins. She put tap water into a plastic bottle. Her mother, intent on hiding what could not be hidden, offered no objection.

Colene carried her things out. It was strictly live and let live, in her family; none of them wanted the hassle that a challenge to any of them would have brought. If someone insisted on visiting, all three of them shaped up to put on a good act for the required time. What was to be gained by letting the truth be known? A philanderer, an alcoholic, a suicidal child. Family love? It was a laugh. Ha. Ha. Ha. Maybe there had once been love. Now it was merely strained tolerance. Typical American family, for sure!

She knocked on the shed door, just to warn Darius. Then she opened it.

He had used the pot. She could tell by the smell. She should have brought a cover for it. Without a word she walked across, set down the candy bars, picked up the pot, and carried it outside and around to the back of the shed. There was an old rusty spade there with a broken handle. She used that to dig a hole, and she dumped the pot and covered up the stuff. She had had some experience with this sort of thing, and knew that it wasn't worth even wrinkling her nose. It wasn't as bad as cleaning up her mother's vomit, after all.

She found a battered piece of plywood, banged it against the ground to get the dirt and mold off, and set it on the pot. She brought the set back into the shed. She put them down in a corner.

Then at last she faced Darius. 'I can't stay long,' she said.

He nodded as if he understood. He smiled.

She smiled back. Then she picked up the candy and raisins. 'More food for you.'

He insisted this time on sharing it with her, so she ate one bar while he ate the rest. He was much more alert than he had been, which was a relief. He was also halfway handsome under his dirt. There was nothing wrong with him that food and a washcloth wouldn't cure.

Well, that she could handle. She found a tatter of colored cloth she had pretended was the flag of her imaginary kingdom in the Land of Horses and poured some of her cup of water on it. 'Clean,' she told him, and proceeded to rub it across his face. He did not protest; in fact he seemed used to having such a thing done for him. Finally she fetched her comb and combed his hair back. Oh, yes, he was handsome, when allowance was made for his stubble beard. But that kind of beard was considered macho, because of all the undercover criminal-playing cops on TV.

They drilled on vocabulary. Darius was a quick study – a very quick study – and so was she. Soon they had the words for the parts of the body and items of clothing, and were working on other parts of speech. For the first time Colene appreciated basic grammar, now that she was teaching it. It was convenient to say 'noun' or 'verb' in some cases when clarifying the use of a word. When Darius indicated the door and said 'verb' she knew he was zeroing in on things like 'open' and 'close' and 'walk through'.

One bit was fun in its own fashion. She had a little box of wooden matches in the shed, which she used for lighting her canned heat so she could do a tiny bit of cooking. An electric hotplate would have been better, but she didn't have one. This was good enough.

Darius saw the box, and inquired. 'Matches,' she explained. Then she demonstrated by striking one. He gaped as it burst into flame. Then he wanted to try it himself. She let him – and he burned his fingers on it. But he was really intrigued by the phenomenon, like a little child. 'Keep them,' she told him generously. 'I can get more.'

He put the box away in a pocket, smiling. It was as if he had found a charm.

She tried to learn his words for things, but they were melodious and extremely strange, with nuances she was sure she was missing. She was apt at language, but knew that there was nothing like this on this side of the world. So she concentrated for now on teaching him. When he could talk well enough to tell her where he was from, she would look it up and learn a whole lot more about him. Somewhere in the Orient, maybe, though he did not look Oriental.

She realized in the course of this session that she had lost her fear of Darius. He was unusual and mysterious, but not dangerous. He was also fascinating.

It grew dark in the shed, for though there was a line here, Colene had used it only to listen to tapes in the day, and had never brought out a light. Now a light would be disastrous, because it would show that Darius was there.

'I have to go,' she said abruptly. 'Mom will wonder if I stay out here too long. But you stay here, and I'll bring you more food in the morning.'

'Yes,' he said. She hoped that he really did understand. She slipped out the door, not opening it wide, just in case her mother were looking this way, and closed it quickly behind her. Actually there would be nothing visible inside except darkness, now, but it made sense to practice safe management. She returned to the house.

Her mother was pretty much out of it by this time. Good. Colene scrounged in the refrigerator for more to eat, and gobbled it down without bothering to sit. Then she went to her room. There was her bed, neatly made, and her desk where she normally did her homework, and her dresser and mirror, and the guitar she hoped someday to learn to play decently. All very conventional. She kept it that way deliberately, so that no one could garner any secrets about her by analyzing her living space. There was even a set of standard dolls on the dresser, Ken and Barbie. What a visitor would not know was that she had renamed the male: he was really Klaus. Thus the pair was Klaus Barbie. There had been a notorious Nazi criminal by that name. She flossed her teeth, brushed her hair, changed into her pajamas, and lay down on her bed. She stared at the ceiling.

Sleep didn't come. All she could do was think about Darius, out there in the Bumshed, and her heart was beating at a running place. She had to slow it to a walking pace before she could nod off. She knew from experience with bad nights.

After a time she got up, went to the closet, and changed into her silky nightgown. She loved the feel of it against her skin. It was long enough so that she wore nothing under it, which gave her a deliciously wicked feeling. It was a good outfit in which to dream. Very good.

In fact, too good.

Now her heart slowed, but her thoughts turned darker. She remembered the time a few months ago when her beloved grandmother, one of the mainstays of her young life after the default of her parents, had sickened with cancer and then died. It was as if the last leg had been knocked out from under Colene's will to live. Without Grandma, what was the point? She had not exactly told Grandma about the horrors she had experienced, or how her life had been falling apart, but she suspected that Grandma knew. It was better to go where Grandma was, and have her reassurance again. Colene had taken her mother's pills from the cabinet, one sniff of which, as an *Arabian Nights* tale put it with suitable hyperbole, could make an elephant sleep from night to night. She swallowed three, then another, pondered, and finally two more. Six was a good number. Six-six-six was the devil's own number. Sick-sick-sick was what these pills would make her. Sick unto death. Then she lay down in her sexy nightie – the one she was wearing now. She wanted to expire in maidenly style.

The elephant pills did not exactly kill her. They put her into a trancelike state in which she had a vision. In the vision she was exactly as she was, in her naughty nightgown, and gloriously dying; the church bells were warming up for the somber death toll, and there would be mourning until the funeral. How sweet she would look in the casket, a red-red rose on her cold-cold bosom. Other girls would envy her the beauty of that nightgown, knowing that they would not have the nerve to be shown dead in such an outfit.

23

Three figures entered the room, coming through the wall, so it was obvious that they were of the spiritual persuasion. Two were her grandparents, now reunited in the afterlife. Grandma approached. 'Dear, you may not yet die, because there is something you have yet to do with your life. We love you and will always be with you.'

Then the third figure, the stranger, approached. He was clothed in a dark robe and wore a cowl over his head, and his face was shaded by mist. Who he was she dared not guess, but there was an inherent glow about him that bespoke his authority. 'Colene,' he said, his voice full of compassion and knowledge. 'You have to go on. You will not be able to quit. Your life will get better.'

Buoyed by that message, she had roused herself from the vision, stumbled to the bathroom, poked her finger down her throat, and gagged out the remaining contents of her stomach. 'Just call me bulimic,' she had gasped with gallant gallows humor as her heaves expired. She had changed her mind about dying. For a while.

No one had known. Her mother hadn't even missed the six pills.

Had she done the right thing? Colene could not be sure. Yet now, with the appearance of Darius, it seemed that there was indeed something for her to do with her life. Maybe her vision was coming true.

After more time she got up again, slipped her feet into her slippers, turned out the light, and cracked open the door. She made her way through the house. If her mother asked, she was just going for another snack. But her mother didn't notice her passage.

Colene got the spare house key, stepped quickly out the back door, and locked herself out. That way her mother would assume that she had locked them in for the night, and would not check her room. Colene would use the key to let herself in again later.

It was chill outside, and she shivered as she made her way across the dark back yard to the shed. Her heart was pounding, but not because of the temperature. She was embarking on another suicidally foolish risk.

She knocked on the door, then opened it. She couldn't see anything inside, but knew he was there.

Indeed he was, hunched under the blankets. They really weren't enough, considering his weakened state. He needed more warmth.

'I should have brought another blanket,' she murmured. 'But I would have had to take it from my own bed, and that would be chancy. I'll see what I can do.'

She sat down beside him, and pulled at the blankets, rearranging them. Then she lay down, full length beside him, and drew the blankets over them both. 'It's warmer, this way,' she explained.

He rolled over to face her, and she stiffened with fear. 'Please don't rape me,' she whispered. 'I really don't like it.' Yet she had come out here in her provocative nightgown. He couldn't see it, of course, but he could feel it. She had gotten under the blankets with him, in the dark. No jury would convict him.

'Rape?' he asked, not knowing the word.

Now she had to define it! How could she do that? If she managed to get the concept across, without the use of her pad and pencil, it would have to be by touch, and he might think she was asking for it. But she had used the word, and she had to explain it.

She pondered, her heart beating so wildly she almost thought her mother in the house could hear it, let alone Darius. Then she found his right hand under the blanket. She brought it across his body and up to touch her head. 'Yes,' she said. Then she took it down to touch her right breast through the nightgown, as she lay on her back. 'Maybe.' Finally she put it against her thigh. 'No.'

He considered that, while she lay breathing rapidly, her body stiff. Then he reached across her, not to embrace her, but to find her left arm. He brought it across her body and up to his head. Her fingers touched his mouth. 'Yes,' he said. Then he took it down to his clothed crotch. 'No.'

He understood! 'That's right,' she said, squeezing his fingers with hers. 'I'm here to warm you, and that's about it.'

'Thank you.' He brought her hand to his lips again, and kissed it.

25

Colene experienced a wild thrill. She knew she should just lie where she was, having made her point. But it was her nature to risk disaster. Suicide was merely the most extreme extension of a syndrome that permeated her existence. Whatever she did, she had to push the limit, courting trouble. This was folly, but it was her way. Had she been a man, she would have been a daredevil cyclist, hurdling lines of cars soaked in gasoline, daring the flames to get her. But she was only a teenage girl, so had to settle for lesser dares.

She rolled over toward him, scooted up a bit, found his head, and lifted hers to kiss him on the mouth. Then she lay against him, her body touching his full length. Of course he was clothed, but she wasn't; all she had was the flimsy nightgown. With her wickedly bare torso within it, her breasts nudging him with each breath she took.

He put his right arm around her and drew her close. His hand did not wander. She put her left arm around him. They were embraced.

She had intended only to remain for half an hour or so, but this was such dangerous delight that she couldn't bring herself to break it off. Slowly her heart eased its horrendous pace, and she relaxed.

She woke, and realized that she had been asleep for some time, nestled against Darius. He was warm and she was warm. As far as she knew, he had not touched her even in the 'maybe' region. She was almost disappointed. She fell back into sleep.

She became aware of the creeping light. 'Ohmigod!' she squeaked. 'Morning!'

She scrambled out from under the blanket, startling Darius awake. 'My parents!' she said. 'I have to get back to my room, so they don't know where I was!'

He nodded, seeming to understand. She found her slippers, slipped out the door and almost flew, wraith-like, across the yard to the door.

The door was locked. 'The key!' she breathed in anguish. She turned about and flew back to the shed.

A hand reached out. It held her key.

'Thanks!' She snatched it and ran back. The door seemed

to make a thunderous noise as it unlocked and opened. She went in, then turned to lock it again. She put the key away.

Then she forced herself to walk slowly through the house to her room. No one was up. She was unobserved.

She entered her room, went to the bed, and threw herself into it. She had made it!

Now she remembered how Darius had given her the key. He knew what it was for and where it was. He could have kept it from her. He could have raped her. He could have taken the contact of his hand on her breast last night as a pretext to go wild. It wasn't the kind of breast found in macho male magazines, but it didn't exactly require padding for a formal gown, either. She had given him every opportunity.

He was either a decent man or he just wasn't interested.

She cursed herself for her total, absolute, unmitigated folly – and knew she would try to find out exactly which it was. Decency or disinterest. If it killed her. And it just might. Which was perhaps the point.

2

DARIUS

Darius woke as the maiden jumped out of bed in the wan light of dawn. For a moment he was disoriented, but it quickly came back: she was Colene, and she had come back to spend a chaste night with him, warming him with her company. He appreciated that very much.

She hurried out. She did not speak his language, unsurprisingly, but had taught him some of hers. She had made it plain that she shared her domicile with her parents, who would not understand Darius' presence here. That too was understandable. Certainly he did not want her to be distressed before he could get to know her well enough.

He felt something cold against his ankle. It was her key. She would need that to enter her locked house. He picked it up and moved to the door.

In a moment she appeared, shivering in her pretty nightdress, her breath fogging in the chill morning air. He saw her small high breasts heaving enticingly. He extended the key. She took it and ran back the way she had come. He shut the door.

Colene. She was young, but by the same token fresh and pretty. She had courage, too, and intelligence. She seemed eminently suitable. But would she want to do it? It was too soon to tell.

He had time to find out. Unless there was trouble before he did. If there was trouble, he would have to –

28

Then he remembered that aspect. He couldn't! He had lost the signal key!

What was he to do? Without that key he couldn't return. He would be locked in this reality, and he had already discovered that he was not equipped to survive here.

Well, did it really make a difference?

It was pointless, but the knowledge of his likely demise here caused him to set a higher value on his life than hitherto. With renewed interest, he reviewed the events of the last few days.

The post of Cyng of Hlahtar was an enviable one, but it had its desperate drawback. A castle was provided, fully staffed and supplied. The Cyng's magic was virtually limitless. As long as he performed.

It was impossible to endure alone for long; every Cyng soon was depleted. The only practical way to survive was to marry a strong, abundantly happy woman, and draw on her resources until she was depleted, and then cast her aside in favor of a new one. Because the post was prominent and the perquisites excellent, many women were willing to endure this, and it was feasible to maintain a chain of marriages indefinitely. But Darius, new to the post, had rebelled after divorcing his second wife. She was not a bad person, and they got along well, but she was depleted. He did not want to marry a series of women for their life forces, daring to love none. He wanted to marry one for love, and to remain with her for the full tenure.

The wiser heads had nodded. It was often thus with newlings; they just had to learn from experience. Once a Cyng came to proper terms with the inevitable, he generally settled down and performed adequately.

Darius went to the Cyng of Pwer. 'What are my options?' he inquired.

'If you will not heed the wisdom of experience, you must learn in your own fashion,' the old man said. 'You may marry for love, but you can not keep her long. She will die if you do not let her go in time. I think you will find it better to marry for other than love.'

'The Modes,' Darius said. 'What are my options there?'

'The Modes are dangerous,' the man reminded him. 'Of every ten folk who risk them, three do not return. Of those who do return, half do not achieve their desire. This leaves about one in three who are successful. I do not recommend this course.'

'You would have me suck the joy from endless innocent women instead?'

The Pwer shook his head. 'No one forces them. They do it to escape poverty, nonentity or pointlessness. It is a good bargain for them. They do not die, and they recover slowly after you turn them loose. It is a feasible system.'

'Not as I see it!' Darius retorted. 'I see love and marriage as ennobling.'

'You are young.'

'Tell me more about the Modes. What can I expect?'

'You can expect the unexpected. Do you understand the theory of it?'

'I understand only that when I appealed to the Cyng of Mngemnt, to provide me some better way, he sent me to you for the Modes. I never heard of them before.'

'Then I will tell you in capsule what we know of them. As you surely do know, I handle the broadcasting of the magic power that enables all other magic to operate. That power must have a source. The first Cyng of Pwer found the source in the Modes. We have a number of what he termed Chips which enable us to relate to the realms beyond our own, and one of these has limitless raw power. He constructed mechanisms to harness this power and convert it to a form we can use. It is my special ability to channel it, and to keep the mechanisms operative. The Chips still relate to what seems to be an infinite number of other Modes. But we explore these others at our considerable risk. We conjecture that they are alternate realities, and that each Chip attunes to the spot where it would be in that other Mode. In many modes that spot is empty, without even earth, water or air, and whoever goes there immediately dies. In other modes there is something there, but not what we like. We have brought back the bodies of those we have sent through, and they have been burned or dehydrated or mauled, as by some monster. But in some Modes there are worlds like ours, only different. By that I mean they may have a comfortable environment, and people, but those people have drastically different customs from ours. In fact, it seems that even the fundamental laws of magic differ in them, so that much of what is truth here is falsity there.'

He looked hard at Darius. 'We have located a region of fairly safe Modes. But even there, the risk is as I described. Also, there seems to be imprecision in the tuning of the Chip; no person seems to go to the same other Mode that any other person has been to. Thus we can not get to know any one of them well, and it is always a serious gamble. I suggest to you that it is unwise in the extreme for you to take this gamble, because not only do you risk your own life, you risk the welfare of our society, which truly needs your ability as Cyng of Hlahtar.'

'Another can assume the post,' Darius said.

'But not one as talented as you. That is why it came to you, after the retirement of the prior Cyng of Hlahtar. You can be the best, and if we lose you, we will have only the next best, and that will hurt us all to some degree.'

He spoke truth. Darius felt guilt. But it was not enough to sway him from his purpose. 'What I may gain must be worth the risk,' he said.

'Exactly what do you hope to gain?' Pwer asked sharply.

'A woman who will not be depleted by close association with me. A woman I can love and not lose. A woman I can marry and never divorce.'

'There is no such woman.'

'Not in this reality,' Darius agreed. 'But elsewhere, where other fundamental rules obtain, there may be women of another nature, who can not be depleted. If I can find one of them, and bring her back here –' He broke off, alarmed. '*Can* I bring her back?'

'Oh, yes. If you are in contact with her when you signal for the return, she will come with you. Your problem will be finding her – and if you do, convincing her to come with you. There are several problems in that connection.'

'This has been done before?'

'Yes. Not by a Cyng of Hlahtar, but by others. They have

31

brought back people or things. Some women have brought back babies or odd animals. But if you want to marry and love her, you must explain to her what this entails; you must not abduct her, for then she will hate you and be no true wife to you.'

'Well, of course I wouldn't abduct her!' Darius exclaimed. 'If I were inclined to treat women in that manner, I would be better off simply marrying a chain of wives here and casting them aside!'

'Precisely.'

'If that is the only problem, then certainly I will –'

'No. There is worse. We have ascertained through some-times bitter experience that not all people or things can be taken. It seems that any person who plays a significant role in his or her or its Mode –'

'Its?'

'Some Mode-folk are sexless, and some are mechanical.'

Darius shuddered. 'Go on.'

'No person of significance can be taken. Apparently there is a certain stability; a Mode will not let go of what it needs to make it what it is. This has a peculiar effect.'

'Go on,' Darius said, experiencing a chill.

'In general, only those folk who are destined to have minimal impact on their realities can be taken. It may be that their Modes know that these folk are soon to be lost anyway, and do not try to hold them.'

'Do you mean they are about to be accidentally killed?'

'Not necessarily. They may have some terminal malady. You could bring such a one here, but she would soon die anyway. Or possibly she merely is of little account, so will live but will have no significant impact. You might find that she has similarly little effect here.'

Darius was still struggling with another aspect of this. 'You said their Modes know, and hold those they want. The Modes are conscious? The Modes are like people?'

'We don't think so. It seems more like a stone that does not readily give up any of its substance. But if part of it has been cracked, a chip may be flaked off with less effort. So you will have to find a loose flake.'

32

Darius pondered this. A diseased woman? It would be better to take one who was about to be killed. But what kind would that be? A criminal? He did not want to marry that kind either. The prospects were dimming.

'I anticipate your next question,' Pwer said.

That was good, because Darius didn't know what to ask next. 'Yes.'

'How do you locate such a woman?' the man said. 'The answer is that we can help you there. There are settings on the Chips. Not many, but enough. We can put you through to a reality that is livable, with human beings much like us, and where one is suitable. We can make that one female. We can not guarantee that she is not already married, but of course if she dies that will not matter. We can not guarantee her age or health or personality. But we can put you close to her. Not completely close, for our command of this alien device is imperfect, but in her Mode and in her vicinity. Then you can inspect her, and bring her back here with you if that seems appropriate. Which brings up your final question.'

'Yes,' Darius agreed, as before.

'How do you return? And the answer is that you will have a signal device, an aspect of the Chip. When you activate that, I will receive the signal, and will revert you and whatever you hold to this reality. If you do not signal within a month, I will assume you are not going to. Because you are dead or unable to signal. Without that signal we can not bring you back, because the Chip is unable to fix on you.'

So now Darius had all the information, and was not reassured. He understood perfectly how three of ten could fail to return, and three or four others would not attain their desire. But at least some did succeed. That left him hope.

'Suppose I go, and return without a woman,' he said. 'Could I then go again, and perhaps that time find one?'

Pwer stared at him. 'Go again? Few have been interested in that! Each time a person goes, he has about one chance in three of not returning. If you went twice, you would double your chance of that.'

'But I would also double my chance of finding what I need,' Darius pointed out.

'Perhaps. But you could not return to the same other Mode. There are too many of them, and our way is imprecise. Some few have tried to go again to the same one, but none we know of has succeeded.'

None we know of. Because some did not return. 'Could that mean that they liked it there, and stayed voluntarily?'

Pwer shrugged. 'It could. But it does seem doubtful. It seems more likely that they found a wholly new situation, and could not survive it. Those who did return the second time reported that their experience was just as difficult as the first time.'

'I want to do it,' Darius said. 'If I lose once, I may try again. If I lose twice, I may decide to do it the conventional way, and marry the chain of women.'

Pwer sighed. 'We are a free society. Your position and your need entitle you to take this foolish risk if you choose. Return tomorrow, and I will have the Chip prepared.'

'My thanks to you,' Darius said gratefully.

Darius got up, for he needed to urinate. The maiden had brought a pot and indicated that he should use it for such purpose. Her method of communication in this respect had been quaint: she had made a vulgar poop noise. He was not easy about this matter, but realized that it was best to oblige her desires. Surely she had reason to keep him out of sight; his limited experience here had suggested the merit of her case. So he remained confined, and did what was necessary. He used the pot and covered it.

He was hungry again, and hoped she would bring more of her strange food. He knew that she could not act with complete freedom, because she was young and had to maintain the semblance of her normal life-style. She seemed to be resourceful, and she was certainly healthy. How could it be that she would either have minimal impact in her Mode, or soon die?

He thought of the night just past. He had expected to be alone. Evidently she had sneaked out to join him for a while, then stayed longer than intended. He was grateful for that; he had been cold, and her warm little body had been a great comfort.

34

More than that. It was clear that she knew the effect such a body could have on a man, and she had addressed the matter forthrightly, considering their lack of a common vocabulary. She had set his hand on her head, breast and hip, identifying what was a permissible touch and what was not. Then she had slept against him, trusting him. He liked that.

Of course he had not touched even that part of her where the proscription was vague. It was not that her breasts were inadequate; they were extremely nice, being neither insignificant nor ponderous. They had the filling perkiness of youth. It was that he could tell by her nervousness and tightness that she was afraid. She had offered him somewhat, hoping that he would be satisfied with that, but even that much was not her desire.

Why, then, had she come at all? Because he was cold, and she wanted to warm him. She was generous despite her fear. He liked that too; in fact he was quite impressed.

But that was not quite all. She had come dressed in only the sheerest of garments, no protection against the cold. No protection against any inclination he might have had. She had made sure he knew it, by causing his hand to touch it. Her pulsing breast might as well have been bare. Was it to tease him? No, for she had not labeled that breast 'No.'

Why had she placed herself at what she surely believed was serious risk, when she could have avoided it by wearing more substantial clothing?

Perhaps she had come out on a whim, and not thought to dress more appropriately. She had intended to sleep in her warm house, but stepped out to check on him; then, finding him cold, she had warmed him. Yes, that would explain it. She was young, and therefore somewhat foolish, not thinking things through. If he remained here another night, and if she came again, she would be better clothed.

She was obviously the one he had come for, and he liked her very well. He had maintained a mental blank in lieu of a picture of the kind of woman he sought, but Colene was far superior to whatever he might have envisioned. As soon as he knew enough of her language to make his mission clear, he would ask her whether she would like to return with him

35

to his reality and be his wife. He would of course have to make clear the nature of the relationship, which was no ordinary marriage. She would have to understand that if she turned out to be unable to withstand depletion, he would have to divorce her despite still loving her. He could appreciate how that might annoy her.

Then the brutal realization struck him. How could he even risk taking this sweet maiden to be depleted? She was evidently no special type who would be immune to the effect. And even if that were not the case, how could he bring her back – when he could not return himself? *He had lost the key!*

Dispirited, he returned to the blankets and buried himself under them. The cold was not merely of the body, now.

He returned to his review of recent events. What else was there to do?

So Darius went to the alien Mode, armed with the signal chiplet and a pack with supplies of food and water, because he had no certainty of finding either quickly in the other reality.

The actual process was simple enough, from his perspective. Just a matter of standing in the circle that marked the focal point of the Chip. Pwer did something – and Darius found himself standing at the edge of a level place, surrounded by what were evidently domiciles. But what oddities they were! Each had many crystalline windows, and peaked roofs, and bits of vegetation around. The level place sent out squared-off offshoots which reached right to the edges of the structures, and sometimes right into them, as if feeding on them.

He stepped out onto the level region. It was completely hard, as if fashioned of stone. But it was not stone, and not packed dirt. He squatted, touching it with his finger. Less hard than stone, actually, but still impressive.

There was the blaring of a horn. Darius looked up and saw some kind of creature charging him. It was not a dragon, for the smoke puffed from its tail, and it seemed to have no mouth. But it was definitely aggressive.

He scrambled erect and stepped back. The creature charged

on by him. There was the sound of a human shout. A human arm projected from the side of the creature and made a gesture with one lifted finger. Apparently there was a person inside who remained alive.

Uncertain how to respond, Darius emulated the gesture. He signaled the creature with one finger.

The creature squealed as it turned and slewed back toward him. Darius retreated farther. It halted, and mouths on its sides abruptly opened. Human men emerged, in unfamiliar apparel. They converged on Darius, shouting incomprehensibly. They looked angry.

He tried to withdraw, as he did not want trouble, but the men attacked him. He was so surprised at this uncivilized behavior that he invoked an elementary pacification spell – and it had no effect.

Then he knew: this was one of the realities in which magic was not operative. At least not the type he knew. He was defenseless.

He tried to explain that he sought no quarrel, but his words seemed only to enrage the young men further. They struck at him with their fists, knocked him down, and kicked him. One of them grabbed at his pack and wrenched it away. Then they sent him rolling down the incline toward what might have been a stream.

His head collided glancingly with a rock. His consciousness faded.

After a period, the maiden came again, bearing food. This time she was somewhat better prepared: she had a box and a jug and a bowl and a curious spoon. She opened the box and poured some bits of something into the bowl, then opened the jug and poured something he recognized – milk – into the bowl with it. She gave him the bowl and spoon, and made gestures as of using the spoon to eat the peculiar mixture.

He tried it. He dipped out both milk and food-bits and put the spoon in his mouth. The bits were crunchy, and the milk not sufficient to slake his thirst, but of course this was only one spoonful.

Colene smiled. Evidently this was the proper way to do it.

She was now attired in a completely different outfit: a heavy shirt, solid cloth shoes, and some kind of tight blue trousers. No woman in his reality would allow herself to be seen in such clothing, for it was disturbingly similar to nakedness from the waist down. The muscles of her posterior flexed visibly as she walked, and there was no looseness at all in the region of her groin. The contrast between her decorous upper section and indecorous nether section was startling.

She sat on the floor to watch him eat, folding her legs so that her feet were crossed and her thighs were wide apart. He tried to avoid looking at this embarrassing display, but he could not do so without turning his face completely to the side. The worst of it was that the maiden seemed to be completely oblivious to her erotic display. Her manner suggested that her concern was only with his consumption of the milk-and-bits concoction.

He tried to be similarly oblivious, but her spread crotch was directly in the line of sight of his bowl and spoon, and his gaze could not help but center on it. There was no doubt: she wore no diaper beneath those alarming trousers. He was getting a reaction. He felt a flush coming to his face.

'Trouble?' she inquired, becoming aware of his distress. 'Food bad?'

How could he explain, without similarly embarrassing her? But she insisted on knowing. Finally he set down bowl and spoon, put his two hands on her projecting knees, and pushed them together.

For a moment she was confused, then startled. Then she burst out laughing. She laughed so hard that she fell over backwards, drawing her legs up against her body and kicking her feet from the knees. This was no improvement; not only was her indecorous region in view, it was flexing. His face was now burning.

Finally she exhausted her mirth. Then she kneeled beside him, kissed him on the cheek, and gave him another lesson in clothing and culture. 'Blue jeans,' she said, touching the tights. 'Okay. No show bad.'

Maybe so, by her definition, but the suggestion was nevertheless overpowering.

She pointed to his crotch. 'You. Sit. Same.'

That was true, but he was a man. Also, his clothing was considerably looser in that region, revealing no private contours.

Colene was unconvinced. 'Oh, Darius – you me laugh.'

True, he had made her laugh – and he had experienced no depletion. But he realized that was because magic was not operative in this reality. Here, it seemed, the transfer of emotion did not cost the source. Indeed, he had not even been trying to make her laugh; she had done it on her own.

That gave him something to think about. Was it possible that she was a self-generating joy person? If so, she was perfect! But he could not presume too much; her ready laughter might merely be because her level was high, and could be as readily depleted as that of any other person.

At least he had learned something: in this reality, the mere fact of physical material covering a region was considered sufficient discretion. Her entire genital region had been exposed in outline, but because there was opaque material between her flesh and his vision, she had no concern. That explained her action of the night, too: her breast had been quite tangible to his touch, soft and warm, yet because there had been a thin barrier of material, she considered it no exposure. Apparently she believed that he could have no sexual excitement if he saw or touched the outline, rather than the direct flesh. Perhaps that was the way of men here, being unmoved by views that would have maddened men of his own reality. He would school himself to react accordingly, difficult as it would be.

Now he was glad he had been cautious during the night! Had a woman of his own reality come to him in the manner Colene had, lightly garbed, sharing his bed, and placing his hand on parts of her body, it could only have been because she wished very much to fornicate with him. Her Yes and No would have been merely indications of the approach he was to make: first kissing, then fondling, and finally copulation if she did not change her mind. It would have indicated phenomenal trust in him, for men were not known for diffidence once embarked on the exploration of female flesh. He had assumed that her actions were not identical in significance to those of women of his own reality, and made no attempt at all to pursue a sexual experience. This, as it had turned out, had been the correct course.

But how would it have been, if he had not been greatly depleted from exposure, thirst and hunger? At that time, the thing he needed most had been warmth. She had brought him that, and it had enabled him to sleep in comfort and to recover more of his well being. A sexual effort might have been beyond his means. So he had taken her warmth, and nothing else, gambling that her ways differed from those of women in his own reality. Had he been robust, he surely would have interpreted her actions as an invitation. In that he would have been gravely mistaken, as he now understood, after seeing her way with clothing.

He had, he knew, been lucky.

'You. Think.' She tapped her head as she spoke, watching him.

'Yes. I. Think.' He tapped his own head. That was a new word, but clear in this context.

'Think. What?'

'What' was a general query term he had learned to use. When he pointed to an object and said 'What?' she would name the object. Now she was inquiring what he was thinking.

How could he tell her? It was complicated, and he lacked the vocabulary, and perhaps the information would affront her. 'No,' he said, smiling to show that this was intended as a positive negation rather than bad feeling.

'Yes,' she said insistently. He was beginning to realize that she did not respond well to 'No' when she wanted something. 'Tell. Me.'

He was obliged to try. He cast about for some way, and saw a small inert figure in the corner, in the likeness of a very young girl. There was something common to both realities! Like all who were serious about magic, she had effigies.

Serious about magic? But there was no magic here, as far as he had been able to ascertain! He had been making another potentially dangerous assumption.

'Try,' he agreed. He pointed to the effigy. 'What?'

Colene looked. 'Doll,' she said, picking it up. She cradled it as if it were a baby. 'Play.'

Play? Was that what they called sympathetic magic? No, probably it meant something quite different. He would have to be extremely careful about that term, until he was sure of its nature. 'Doll. Me.'

She gave him the effigy. He held it with his left hand, and extended his right hand. 'Doll. Me.'

Colene considered momentarily, then went to the corner. There, in a box, was another figure. This one was male. Good.

She gave him the second doll. He held up the male. 'Me.' Then the female. 'You.'

She nodded. She was paying close attention.

He put the male down and covered it with a corner of a blanket. Then he brought the female, as if she were walking. She came to lie beside the male.

'Last Night,' Colene said.

'Night,' he agreed; that seemed to be the time of darkness. But he made sure. He waved his hand, indicating their surroundings. 'What?'

'Day. Light.'

'Night – Light,' he said, pairing the opposites.

'No. Night. Day. Dark. Light. Night–Dark. Day–Light.'

After a moment they got it straight. This was Day, and the time of sleeping was Night.

He indicated the dolls. 'Day. No. Night. Yes.'

She nodded again. 'You. Me. Night.' There was no doubt of her interest.

Now he needed to convey the concept of his home reality. That might be impossible. 'You. Me. Things. Here.' He gestured, trying to show themselves and their surroundings. 'Day. Night. Day. Night. There.' He tried to indicate something far away.

Colene said something, seeming to understand. He hoped that was the case. 'Here.' He touched the two dolls. He moved the arm of the male to touch the female's head section. 'Yes.' Then her chest region. 'Maybe.' Finally her leg. 'No.' After that he put them close together without motion.

Colene nodded. 'Us. Last Night.'

Us. Evidently the two of them. 'Yes.' Then he made the

41

faraway gesture. 'There.' He moved the dolls to another place. Then he repeated the action between them. But this time the male doll did not sleep. Instead it became more active, covering the female.

She still seemed to understand, but was not concerned. 'You. Me. Here,' she said firmly. 'No. There.'

Clear enough. She understood that in his Mode, she could not expect to be left alone at night. But in her Mode, the local customs prevailed.

Days passed. Each night Colene came to share her warmth with him, though she brought another blanket that sufficed against the cold. He held her and did no more, though his strength was returning and he did desire her. She was young, he reminded himself, probably not more than five years into nubility, but enticing.

They continued to talk, and he learned enough of her language so that in due course they could cover more sophisticated topics. Now he could tell her where he had come from, and what his mission had been – and what had happened. Their dialogue was extended and fraught with misunderstandings and missing terms, but in essence it was this:

'So you came all the way here from your fantasy world to marry me?' she asked. 'Only you got mugged and lost your ticket home?'

'This is too simple,' he protested. 'I came here to discover whether you were right to marry. But this is uncertain. Now it does not matter, since I can not return.'

'And am I?'

She cut so quickly to her aspects that he often had to pause to follow them. 'Are you right to marry? I am not sure, but I am hopeful.'

'What would make you sure?'

'That is complicated to tell. But there is no need, since I will die here.'

'Why will you die?'

'Because I cannot endure without magic. I have no way here to support myself, and soon you will tire of bringing me food.

Already I feel the depletion of my separation from my reality. When it becomes too great, I will seek as easy a death as I can manage.'

'You hurt, and you will die?'

'Yes. I am not like you. But I thank you for the great comfort you have given me.'

She looked at him intently. 'You are not joking, are you?'

'The King of Laughter does not joke.' This was hardly a precise translation of his role in his own Mode, but it was what she best related to.

'If you were going back, would you take me with you?'

'If I could return, I would want to do that. But only if I knew that it was right, and that you wished to. Marriage to Hlahtar is no easy matter.'

'Even though I am only fourteen?'

Darius was startled. 'I thought you were older! Unless our years differ.'

'I don't think they do. Everything you have told me suggests that your world is the same as mine, except for the way you live. So does it matter?'

'In my reality it does not. Every person does what he chooses, if he can do it well enough. If you truly understood the requirements of the marriage, it would be honored.'

'Like having sex with you?'

'No, marriage is not necessary for that. It is a more important commitment.'

'Because of the mergence of life forces?'

'Yes.'

She shook her head. 'You know I don't believe you.'

'Yes. I think you would believe only if you could be in my reality. What you have done for me has been most generous, since you can gain nothing in return.'

'Do you really live in a castle with many servants, and do magic?'

'My servants usually do the magic for me. My ability is joy, not conjuring.'

'Tell me again about what you do.'

'Colene, I will not be doing it any more, because –'

'Tell me!'

43

He did not understand her intensity. 'I bring joy to the multitudes. I make them laugh.'

'Then you are a comedian.'

'No. I do not tell funny stories or do funny things. I infuse joy directly, so that they can laugh at what merits it.'

'That's what I don't understand! How can you – I mean, that's not the way it works!'

'How does it work here?'

'Each person's pleasure and pain come from inside him. If he sees or hears something funny, he laughs and feels good. If he sees something bad, he is unhappy. If something hurts his body, he feels pain, but the pain is from his nervous system, not the other thing. If he loves or hates, the emotion is all in himself. He can't receive it like an electric current from anyone else.'

'Physically that is true for us too. But emotionally we can transfer. It is my post to transfer joy to others.'

'But if you can do that, that doesn't mean you lose it yourself!'

'Indeed it does! It is my emotional substance being shared.'

'But then you would be miserable after making one person happy.'

'No. I have a special qualification for the post. I can magnify my joy as I transfer, making a thousand people happy, while I suffer only a little depletion. Most people can exchange only on an even basis, as you say, but some can multiply, and I can multiply better than any other. That is why I am Cyng.'

'Then what's your problem?'

'There are many thousands who need joy. So many that I cannot serve them all without eventually being depleted. But I can not stop, because then everyone would become unhappy.'

'What does a wife have to do with it?'

'My wife shares her joy with me. I can then share it with others, multiplied. Were she able to share on an even basis, that would double my ability to serve. But normally women are found who can multiply somewhat themselves, so that I may receive what two or three others might provide. That can enable me to carry on for a year or more, before we are both depleted.'

'What happens then?'

'I must divorce her before she dies, so that she can recover. Then I must marry another, so that I can continue my work.'

'How could you do that to one you loved?'

Darius spread his hands. 'I can not. That is why I elected to search in other realities.'

'So you could find me, and take me back, and deplete me, and cast me aside after a year?'

'Oh, no, Colene! I am looking for a woman who can multiply the way I do, so that I can love her and never cast her aside. There are none in my reality.'

'And you think I might be one like that?'

'I hope you are. The Chip oriented on women who might be like that. But the Chip is fallible. It may be that it is a misreading.'

'How can you tell?'

'There is no sure way except to bring you back with me.'

'And if I am not right?'

'Then I could not marry you. You would be provided for; I could make you one of my servants.'

'One of your servants!'

'The Chip can not focus on precisely the same reality twice. You could not return to your own realm. But you could have a good life with me. Just not as my wife.'

'Thanks a lot!'

She was evidently angry. 'I do not understand.'

'That's for sure!' She lurched to her feet and charged out of the shed.

But later she returned, with more food. 'I am sorry I blew up at you, Darius,' she said. 'I know your culture is way different from mine, and you didn't think you were insulting me.'

'That is true. I am sorry I insulted you. Please tell me in what manner I did that, so that I can avoid doing it again.'

'With us, a wife is different from a servant. A wife you love; a servant you maybe don't care much about. If you see me as a potential servant –'

Darius was stricken. 'No! It is this way in my land too! It is that at least I could be with you, if I couldn't marry you.'

She stepped close to him. 'How do you really feel about me, Darius?'

'It is my hope that you are suitable, and that you will be willing too –'

'Forget suitability! What about *me*?'

'I *can't* forget suitability, because marriage to me would kill you if –'

'But you can't go back, so that doesn't matter! All there is is you and me. So how do you feel?'

That made him pause. She was right; he could not go back. All he could do was remain here until he died. 'I can not marry you here either, because –'

'Nobody asked you to!' she flared. '*Will* you answer the question!'

He looked at her with an altered appreciation. He had been so girt about by the problems of his isolation and his dependence on her for food and information that he had not allowed himself to think of her as a feeling creature.

She was small, the top of her head reaching just above his shoulder. Her hair was brown, with slight curving, just touching her shoulders. Her face, framed by it, was rounded, except for a slightly pointed chin. Her eyes were large and round and brown. She wore a dress, perhaps in deference to his problem with the blue jeans, and she never sat in that particular position when wearing it. But now she was standing, nicely proportioned, small of chin, breast, waist and hip but well balanced and extremely feminine.

But appearance was only one aspect of a person. Colene had shown great patience, teaching him her language, and good judgment in the food and clothing she had brought for him, and had been responsible about things like emptying the privy-pot. She had wanted him kept out of sight, and though it made him a virtual prisoner here, he felt she was correct in her judgment about this. She had made it as comfortable for him as was feasible. Her personality was nice; she laughed often, and was direct in her dealings with him. She was generous, going to the trouble and discomfort of sharing her warmth with him at night despite the risk of discovery.

Yet still he could not answer, for there was more than all of this in the question. Feelings were bidirectional things, and if hers were not there, his could not be either. There was one more thing he had to know.

'May I handle you?' he inquired.

'You want to have sex with me?' Now she was guarded.

'I must give that a qualified answer. I do find you desirable, but that is not my intent at the moment.'

'You may handle me,' she said, understanding that this was not a casual thing. He had to do this in order to determine the answer to her question. How he felt about her depended in considerable part how she felt about him.

He put his arms around her back, drawing her in close. Her body yielded to him, and she lifted her face. He knew that magic did not work here, but perhaps just a bit of his peculiar power could be invoked. His power to relate to the emotions of others: to receive and return their joy. Perhaps, with the closest and most evocative contact, he could know.

He kissed her: just a touching of his lips to hers.

3

KEY

She knew it had not been long, externally, but internally it was
as if she had stepped across realities, or Modes as Darius put
it. Then she was sobbing against his shoulder, and it wasn't
disappointment but relief: now she knew how he really felt
about her – and he knew how she felt about him. She had
not really believed in electricity between people, or in instant
knowing. Not until now.

Soon enough she pulled herself together. She had learned to
make quick recoveries. She drew him down, and they sat side
by side, leaning against the back wall of the shed, her right
fingers interlaced with his left fingers.

'So it's love,' she said matter-of-factly. She had to tackle it
this way, as if it were something she had observed from afar,
that didn't concern her, because that was the only way she
could handle it at the moment. 'We have to talk.'

'We have talked,' he said.

'Not this way. You can't marry me here, because I'm underage and you'll die soon anyway. But you can –'

'No. Your love suffices.'

She laughed. She did that often with him, and now she knew
why. 'I wouldn't tell, Darius. I'm good at keeping secrets, honest. You've been a real gentleman, and I like that a lot. But that's
not it. You can tell me exactly how to get to your reality.'

'But even if I could return, and take you there, there would
be no certainty –'

'I know. If we went there, and you couldn't marry me, I'd be your servant. The forms don't matter. Now I know how you feel. I want to go with you, Darius. Just tell me how.'

He seemed surprised. He thought this kind of discussion was useless. He might be right, but she had a notion. 'I must have the key. That, in my hand, becomes the signal. Then Pwer will revert me to my reality, together with what I hold.'

'So if you are holding me, I'm there too.'

'Yes.'

'How do you activate the key? Is there a button on it?'

'No. My mind does it. I touch it to my forehead and make my desire.'

'You make a wish!' she exclaimed. 'That makes sense!'

'Yes. No one else can activate it. It is attuned to me. It amplifies my wish to return, and that signal crosses the realities, and the Chip responds. I need it, and it needs me. Separate, we both are useless.'

She squeezed his fingers reassuringly. 'So if you could recover that key –'

'I could return. But it is lost.'

'But if I found it for you –'

His fingers stiffened against hers. 'If you could do that –'

'I can't promise, Darius, but I'll try.'

'You give me hope! If I had that key, I would take you with me.'

'That's the idea, you know.'

His face turned to her. 'But you don't believe.'

'I believe you love.'

'That is enough, I think.' They leaned together and kissed. Again she felt the magic tingle of passion, intimacy and commitment. All that she lacked in her own poor life she had found in Darius. She *knew*.

She spent the afternoon stocking supplies. She had some money of her own, and she used it to buy groceries at the only store within walking distance that was open on Sunday. She piled them into the shed. 'These are canned goods,' she explained. 'You open them with this can opener. They may not taste good, cold, but they'll feed you.'

'But why are you doing this?' he asked.

She faced him seriously. 'This is Sunday. Tomorrow I go back to school. I think I know how to find your key. But getting it may be tricky. If I don't come back, I don't want you to starve. Stay here as long as you can, and when you can't, well, you'll just have to go out. But I'll try to get back here okay. This is just in case.'

'Just in case what?' he demanded, alarmed.

She shook her head. 'Darius, it's been beautiful here with you. You have made me believe in human decency again. But out there's the real world. It's not all that nice. Please don't ask me to tell you any more.'

'If I ask, you will tell?'

'Yes. But please don't.'

'Then I ask you only to be careful.'

'Thank you.' She kissed him. She liked doing that. Not only did it make her feel good, it made her feel good about it. He was a good man, and he welcomed her kisses, and he asked no more than that. It was love fulfilled. For now. Until she had the chance to prove her love, in a way he might not understand if he knew.

Monday, school-day, Colene headed out to the bus with her books. Her attendance the past two weeks had been spotty; she had pleaded illness, then sneaked out to be with Darius. But she had done her homework, because she didn't want to bring any unnecessary suspicion on herself. She had done it with Darius, teaching him words and explaining things as she went along, and it had actually been pleasant.

The thing about Darius was this: he might be crazy, or he might be lying, making up a story about a magic land so he wouldn't have to say where he really was from. But she liked his story, and the meticulous detail of it, and she liked him, with his archaic ways and respect for her body. It was fun having a man to herself. Since she had found him, she had not sliced her wrists. Her skin was healing over; she could probably take off her wrist wraps now, and the scars would not be fresh enough to attract attention.

In fact, all the time she had known him, she had been very like a normal girl. She had laughed, meaning it, liking his

50

confusions, liking his company, liking him. When at last he had kissed her, she had become a normal woman. A woman in love.

Love. At first she had held it at arm's length, uncertain what to do with this weird emotion. Was it real, or just something she imagined? She had heard that girls her age only thought they could love, and were actually in love with the idea of love. Maybe that was true for some. Maybe for most. But not for her. What she felt swept all other considerations aside. It was like a magic fire, burning away all her prior supports, making ashes of other interests. Now there was only Darius. Everything she did was with his welfare in mind. Even what she would do today.

'Tell Biff I want to deal,' she said to a boy she knew had a connection.

He was startled. 'You?'

'Not his way. But if he has what I want, I'll deal.'

She went to classes, and she shone. That extra homework time was paying off. Normally she skimped on schoolwork, and was bright enough to get by with high grades anyway; now she was prepared with research done for the joy of doing it with Darius, who was unfailingly interested in all the things of her world. What had been dull became interesting with him, and by the time she got it all explained to him, she knew it better than she had thought possible. But her performance was incidental; it was only to reassure everyone that Bright Little Colene had everything to live for, and nothing on her mind except classwork.

At lunch she was about to sit down with her tray when she saw a young man of about eighteen standing in the doorway to the rear exit. That was Biff. He was theoretically a student, but somehow he never attended classes. Students carefully ignored him unless they wanted something illegal. Then they dealt, making what deals they could. If the school administration knew about it, it pretended ignorance, knowing that Biff could quickly be replaced by something worse.

She set her tray on a table, picked up the half-pint carton of milk, opened it, and walked to that door. Biff faded back out of sight. She came to stand between the doorway and the large

51

trash container, drinking her milk. She faced back toward the main chamber.

'Yeah?' It was Biff's voice from the other side of the doorway.

'I want something.'

'What?'

'It's a sort of gray metal button, like a slug, only thicker and brighter. It was on a bum who got rolled two weeks ago. He wore funny clothes. He gave some punks the finger, and they pounded him.'

'What's it to you?'

'It's a memento. I heard it's a luck charm.'

'I don't mess with luck charms.'

'I want it bad. This one, no other.'

'How bad?'

'I'll game for it.'

He laughed, harshly. 'You want it, you bring money.'

'I have no money. Make another offer.'

'Stand out where I can see you.'

She finished her milk, dumped the balled carton into the container, and stepped into the center of the doorway. She was wearing a light white sweater and black skirt, both too tight. She inhaled, turning. She hated this part, but it was all she had to bargain with. Biff could get girls, but they were either his type, which was no novelty, or under duress, which was no fun. What he wanted was a high class young one who would pretend she liked it. Colene had acted high class for years, and she knew how to pretend.

'Okay. One week.'

Now she laughed. 'I'm a clean girl! One night.'

'You ain't clean! Four guys had you.'

'Not lately. I'll put four guys in jail, they come near me again. I never ate or sniffed. I'm clean.'

'But you drank.'

'Never again!'

'No jail, if you deal. None of that.' He meant no charges against him.

'None of that,' she agreed. 'Two nights.'

'You don't want it bad enough.'

52

'You don't even have it.' Then, signaling the approach of someone dumping a tray in the trash, 'Pause.'

When the person moved on, she said 'Resume.' Part of the deal, when anyone talked with Biff, was to keep it quiet.

'I can get it.'

Her heart leaped. 'You know of it? It has to be only that one.'

'They couldn't fence a slug. No value. I can get it. Tomorrow.'

'I said I'd game. I win, what I want. You win, what you want.'

'That slug against one week, smiling.' Not only would she have to do anything he wanted, short of drugs – there were reasons to keep a clean girl clean – she would have to take his side if they were caught, swearing she was his girlfriend and that there had been no coertion. She gagged at the notion, but had to accept. There was a screwball honor in this sort of dealing, enforced by those who had no conscience, just business sense.

'Yes.'

'What game?'

'I'll decide.'

'Before my friends.'

'Before your friends. But I deal only with you.'

'For sure! Tomorrow, after school. Come to my car.'

'Only if you have what I want.'

'I'll have it.'

She walked away. The preliminary deal had been struck. He would bring the key and she would bring her body. The outcome of the game was uncertain, but if she had to, she would game again for the key after paying off the first game. The important thing was that he knew what it was and would get it. Darius could have it back.

This was the part Darius might not understand. He had odd notions about honor and chastity. If she had to give her body to a lout like Biff to win back the key – well, she had a ploy she hoped would avoid that.

In the afternoon she was in a daze. She went through classes mechanically. She would get the key – but would that really solve anything? For she simply did not believe in that alternate universe of his. If she gave him the key, what could he do except prove that it didn't work? Then his fantasy would be exposed, and a major part of his appeal for her would be diminished. As long as he lacked that key, he was the King of Laughter from an alien reality. With it, he might be only a deluded refugee from some mental hospital.

Why was she risking so much, for such likely disappointment?

Maybe she had been fooling herself. She remained as suicidal as ever. She had merely found a new way to flirt with death. Because if she lost the game, and Biff had his way with her for a week, she might as well die. Maybe the key was just a pretext. Maybe her love for Darius was just a pretext.

No!

The teacher paused. 'A problem, Colene?'

Her pain had shown on her face. 'I'm better, Miss Grumman, honest! Maybe I ate too fast.'

The teacher let it pass. Colene suppressed her thoughts and paid better attention in class. It was a fair deal.

But on the way home that question resumed. She hardly responded to Julie's chatter. Was she making a mistake? Was she about to torpedo her dream? For even if the illusion didn't end for Darius, it would for her.

Back home, she hurried to the shed. 'Oh, Colene, I am so glad to see you!' Darius exclaimed, embracing her. 'I feared I would not.'

'I have made a deal to recover your key,' she said. 'Tomorrow.'

He stared at her. 'You really can recover it?'

'The punks who mugged you couldn't fence it. They thought it was just a fancy slug. I can get it.'

'You can buy it?' He had had trouble with the concept of money, but understood it reasonably well now.

'I asked you not to ask.'

He was silent. She kissed him, and it was good.

But that night she broached the matter herself. She had discovered that an aspect of love was an extreme reluctance to deceive the object of that love. That was awkward, but there was nothing for it but to play it through. 'Darius, there are two ways to do this. I am going to gamble, and if I win, I will have the key for you. If I lose, I will have to be away from you for a week, at night, anyway. I – you said you desire me. I think maybe tonight –'

'No. I want to marry you, unsullied according to your code.'

'But I –' She could not continue. How could she tell him she might be bound for a week of disgusting sex with a criminal lout, pretending she liked it, when she had told Darius no? He thought she was pure. 'All the same, I think –'

'No.'

If she won the game, and got the key without having to pay, and he used it and it didn't work, then the dream would be gone and it would be foolish to have sex with him. If she lost, she would have no pretense of being the kind of girl he wanted. Now was the only time.

'Darius, I told you no, before, but now I tell you yes. Please –'

'No. I will not have you sully yourself by your code for me. I will marry you in honor.'

She had never expected this. It wasn't that she was eager for sex; that was far from the case. It was fraught with liabilities the sex-ed teachers hardly imagined. But if she had it with anyone, she wanted it to be him. If she had to have it with someone else, she wanted it first with Darius. But he, with his incomplete understanding of the situation, would not hear of it. If she told him the full truth, he would probably forbid her to recover the key that way.

They were, in their fashion, having a lover's quarrel. It was not nearly as delightful as she had thought such a thing would be.

She thought of trying to seduce him, of sleeping naked with him. But she realized that this would only demean her in his eyes, and she didn't want that.

How she wished she could believe in his reality!

Tuesday after school, modestly garbed, she sought Biff's car in the parking lot. Students she knew were runners stood casually here and there, making sure there were no authorities. That protected her as well as him, because both wanted to deal in private.

'You have it?'

He lifted a gray disk that exactly fitted the description Darius had given.

'May I see it?'

He handed it to her. She turned it over. There, in tiny etching, was the coding Darius had described. She had not told anyone of this. It was genuine.

She handed it back. 'This is it.'

'In,' he said. 'Down.'

She walked around the car and got in. She ducked down so that she was not visible from outside. He drove cautiously out, and around the block, checking for pursuit. Satisfied there was none, he drove to his club house across town.

'Up,' he said, and she sat normally in the front seat. 'How come a clean chic like you wants a damn slug so much?'

She was prepared. 'There's a man. He said I could have what I wanted if I got it for him. He doesn't really want it; he just thought I couldn't get it. So I'm getting it.'

Biff did not seem to believe her, but was satisfied that she did want it. Few people in his business cared to give their real reasons.

They arrived at the club house. They entered. Inside were four men. She had expected disreputable types, but these were clean-cut. They were also older, in their thirties and forties. No juvenile thugs, these; they were the real thing.

'Before we deal,' Biff said. 'This never happened. No one was here.'

'Yes. You too. No one talks. You win, no one knows how I paid. Not like those four rapists.'

Biff nodded. 'No one talks. It's private.' There was, as she had reflected before, a certain honor in such transactions. No one wanted the police to get wind of either drug operations or juvenile sex. The police wouldn't get rid of either, they would only complicate things for all parties.

'And no welshing,' she said. 'I win, you give me the slug and take me back near where I live. No rape.'

56

Biff smiled. 'If you win to the satisfaction of my friends, no problem. I settle my deals.'

'You win, you have me smiling for a week,' she said, making sure they were agreed. 'Nights only; I can't skip more school. No drugs, no bondage, no hurting. No marking.'

'Kid, I like you,' Biff said. 'Agreed. Now what's your game?'

Colene nerved herself. Then she began removing her clothes. 'You, me, naked. Endurance. The one who fills most cups without falling wins.'

Biff smiled. 'Naked endurance? Chick, I know you ain't thinking what I'm thinking!'

'For sure,' she agreed, removing her shoes and socks. 'Naked to prove there's no cheating. No hidden tubes or things. We stand separate. Each has a bucket, or whatever. Several cups, maybe. No one touches either of us. We get no help.'

'We got buckets,' Biff said. He gestured, and one of the men left the room, returning in a moment with two plastic buckets. He set one before each of them.

Colene continued to strip. She had her shirt off, and removed her bra. She was doing something she had dreamed of: a strip tease before strange men who were honor-bound not to touch her or to tell. She could see that all of them were now fascinated, and not just because of her increasing nudity; they wondered just what she was up to.

'I can do that,' Biff said. He removed his own shirt.

Colene started on her lower half, pulling down her skirt. 'Knives. Good ones. Sharp and clean.'

'I got a blade,' Biff said. A handle appeared in his hand, and from it suddenly snapped a wicked narrow four inch blade. It was obvious that he knew how to use it.

'I need one too,' Colene said. She turned to one of the spectators. 'May I borrow yours?'

The man was surely a killer, but he looked startled. Then he reached into his jacket and brought out an old fashioned barber's shaving knife. He unfolded it. The blade was a good inch longer than Biff's, but it wasn't the same kind of weapon. It was a slicer, not a stabber. The kind used to slit throats. She felt a chill, now realizing the nature of his business. He was an enforcer, a contract man. He extended it to her, holding it by the blade.

Colene smiled most sweetly, though there was a layer of the ice of fear coating her heart. 'Thank you sir,' she said, taking the handle. 'I will return it to you soon.'

Now they were twice as curious as before. 'Kid, I got to tell you, if you figure to knife-fight Biff –' the owner of the razor started.

'Not exactly,' Colene said. Holding the razor carefully so as not to cut herself, she tucked her fingers into her panties and slid them down. Now she was all the way naked, and the eyes of all five men were locked onto her body. What a fantasy she was playing out, for real! She turned in place, all the way around, so that they could see everything. She was really pleased that they liked it; this did wonders for her self esteem, in its macabre fashion.

Biff had meanwhile stripped to his jock, but here he hesitated. She knew why: her little show was giving him an erection, and he didn't want to bare it unless sex really was part of the game.

'You can wear that,' she told him. 'I'm satisfied there's nothing in there.'

Biff scowled, but one of the men chuckled.

'All right, what's your game?' Biff demanded.

Then she dropped her bombshell. 'Just this: who can bleed the most before falling. You know, like a knockout, count to ten, you're out. The one left standing wins.'

'Bleed?' Biff asked, dismayed.

'I'll cut my arm, you cut yours. We bleed into our buckets. The men measure the blood. If I faint at two pints and you're still standing, and you've bled two and a half pints, you win.'

'That's no game!' Biff protested.

'It's *my* game,' she said evenly. 'It's as good a game as knife-fighting, only we bleed ourselves. Isn't it fair?' She looked at the other men.

They looked at each other. Then the one who had lent her the razor shrugged. 'It's fair, Biff,' he said. 'We knew she wasn't coming here to play posies. She said endurance. She didn't say what kind.'

Biff swallowed. He was now in the position of put up or shut up. 'Okay. You start.'

He thought she was bluffing. He didn't know she was suicidal. 'Gladly.' She extended her left arm over her bucket, lifted the razor, and made one fast pass across her forearm. No bluffing here!

The edge was, by no coincidence, razor sharp. It cut much deeper than she had expected, almost painless in the first seconds. Blood welled out immediately, flowed across her arm, and dripped into the bucket. There was so much of it that it threatened to spill onto the floor. She had to lower her hand, so that the blood flowed down and off her fingers. Now the pain was coming, but it really wasn't bad. It was masked by excitement. She had done it! With aplomb, even. She had never cut herself like this before! What a sight it was!

She looked up. Biff was standing there, staring. So were the others.

'What's the matter?' she inquired sweetly. 'Never seen blood before?'

This time two of them chuckled.

She addressed Biff. 'You're a lot bigger than I am,' she said. 'You must have twice as much blood in you as I have in me. You can beat me easy, if you care to.'

'She's right,' the razor man said.

Still Biff stood, not moving.

'But you have to play the game,' Colene said. 'It's not fair to let me bleed myself out if you don't even start.'

The men nodded. 'Do it, Biff,' one said.

'But what good's a bled-out chic to me?' Biff demanded somewhat plaintively. 'Me weakened, and her unconscious –'

'There's no time limit on the payoff,' Colene said. 'I thought you'd want it right away, but you can take a rain check. Make it six months from now. I'll be there. You know where I live.' She looked down again at the blood dripping from her hand, so bright and beautiful. She felt dizzy, and knew it wasn't from the blood loss; it was exhilaration.

Still Biff hesitated.

'Biff, she's got you,' the razor man said. 'Cut or yield.'

Biff considered a moment more. At last he smiled. 'Okay, kid, you beat me. You win.'

'Thank you,' she said. But she didn't move.

'Here's your slug,' he said, handing it to her. She took it with her knife-hand, carefully.

'Thank you,' she repeated. She had the victory, if she didn't lose her nerve now and do something monumentally stupid. So she did nothing. That seemed safest.

Biff took his clothes and walked from the room. One of the other men fetched some bandage material. Trust them to have such supplies; they probably had to doctor their own bullet wounds. 'You won, kid; we won't touch you. But you gotta let us help you before you bleed to death.'

'Thank you,' she said a third time, smiling.

They did a competent job of closing and bandaging her wound, and helped her get dressed. Not one tried to handle her body even 'accidentally', but they seemed to like handing her the panties, bra and skirt. It was as if each wanted to have a personal part in what had turned out to be a most unusual game. 'I'll take you home, if that's okay with you,' the razor man said. 'I don't think Biff feels like it.'

'Just remember, no –'

'Kid, you *won*. No one touches you. Not now, not ever. Not until you say so. We're – you know what we are. But you got our respect. Just keep your mouth shut, and it's done.'

'Thank you,' she said once again. 'You may take me home.' She completed her dressing, donning her shoes.

The razor man extended his elbow. Startled by this bit of chivalry, Colene put her hand on it, and walked with him out of the building.

He drove her home. 'Kid, you're as gutsy as I've ever seen,' he said. 'If you're ever in bad trouble, ask for Slick. We'll make a deal.'

'Thank you.' It seemed to be the only thing she was able to say, now. She was riding on a high like none before. She had played her scene flawlessly, every part of it, and it had worked exactly as she had hoped. What a dream come true! It wasn't just that she had won the key, it was that she had made one of her weird fantasies come true, and gotten away with it.

She had *liked* stripping before those tough men, having them admire her body. Rape she did not like at all, but this had been showmanship. See, no Touch. There was all the difference in the world.

He drew to a stop a block from her home. 'You can walk from here. I'll watch, then go.'

'Thank you.' She slid out.

'You got a nice little body,' he said as she closed the door. 'Damn nice. Keep it clean, kid. Don't mess with our kind if you don't have to.'

'Thank you,' she said yet again, experiencing another thrill of pleasure. Then she walked away, knowing he was watching that body in motion. His name was Slick, as in slick-as-a-razor. She would remember.

Things were normal at home: Dad was out and Mom was drunk. Colene fixed herself a generous meal and bundled it up and took it out to the shed. If she was spending more time there now than she used to, nobody noticed. As long as she kept her grades up and stayed out of trouble, nobody cared. There had been a time when that bothered her.

She knocked, then entered. Darius had been snoozing; there really wasn't much for him to do, as he had not made much progress learning to read her books.

She brought out the key and held it up.

He seemed almost afraid to touch it. But when he turned it over and saw the coding, he knew.

'Colene, I didn't think you could do it!' he said, hugging her. 'But you have! You have recovered the key! We can go to my reality!'

Now she was descending from her euphoria. She had not actually lost that much blood, but she had taken a phenomenal risk, and knew it. It had been her luck that Biff had been squeamish about letting his own blood, and that his criminal friends had had a sense of honor about a game played by their rules. In the letting of her own blood she had shown guts, not quite literally, and they had respected that. She knew that some killers had very conservative family lives and were kind to children. But some were otherwise. She had gambled that not only could she beat Biff, but that his friends would side with her. She had won, but she wouldn't care to try it again.

Now she faced another gamble: that Darius wasn't crazy or a con-man. Because either that key would work or it wouldn't. And she knew it wouldn't. Which meant that the lovely bubble would burst, and things would be back as they had been before.

She set down her bundle of food. 'I think we'd better talk,' she said. She spread out the makings, and they began to eat.

'Yes, of course.' His actual speech was much more limited, but she liked to think of it as educated and courtly, and her fancy filled in the nuances. 'I realize that it is a daunting decision, to leave your family and your entire Mode, without any guarantee that –'

''Snot that, Darius. I want to go. I love what you have described. I have nothing much to hold me here. And if you can't marry me, but all the rest is real, well, I'll be your lover instead. You've been up-front about that aspect. But there's a problem.'

'You don't believe me,' he said.

'I wish I could! But I just don't.'

'When I take you there, you will believe. I will take you there now, if you wish. With the key –'

'Here's the thing: suppose you take that key, and hold it to your head, and make your wish – and nothing happens? What then?'

'Colene, it will work. The same Chip that sent me here will bring me back. But as I said, you do not need to believe, because this is not a matter of faith. I will take you there, and then we shall discover whether you can multiply your joy, and – oh, I want so much to marry you!'

'You have faith, but I don't, and these things don't necessarily work unless you believe in them.'

He smiled. 'If it doesn't work, I will be amazed!'

'If it doesn't work,' she said doggedly, 'you will be crazy.' There: she had said it.

He glanced more intently at her. 'You believe I am not sane?'

How she hated this. 'Darius, I think I love you, but I'm

a realist. I think you are deluded. I think you have a dream that's a wonderful thing, and you've spent years perfecting it, but somehow you got out of the institution and I found you, and now it's my dream too, but I know that's all it is. When you try to use that key, the dream will be over. Because I'm not crazy, and I'm not going to be. So what do we do, after you try that thing and nothing happens?'

'You do not wish to try it, and discover the truth of it directly?'

'Discovering the truth directly can be a whole lot of trouble,' she said, pushing down memories that were trying to rise, like bodies buried in muck. 'I'd rather know what I'm getting into first.'

'What would persuade you to try it?'

'If there were some way it could be believed. I mean, I don't believe in ghosts either, but if one came in here and said "Boo!" to me, I'd sure check it out and maybe change my mind. Same thing for a flying saucer, a UFO.' Here it took some time for her to get the concept across, and they finally settled on Ship Containing Alien Creatures. 'But if one landed beside my house, I'd consider it. Can you show me anything to make me believe you?'

'I fear I can not. But perhaps I can clarify the rationale.'

'How about this: if you try it, and it works, we're both there and we see about getting married or whatever. If you try it and it doesn't work, you turn yourself in for mental treatment.'

He laughed. 'If they provide food and shelter, I will not mind if they think I am deluded! If I can not return, my life will not be long in any event.'

'Because if they cure you, I'll still marry you,' she said. And there was another crazy thing she was doing! Seriously talking of marriage to a man she believed to be crazy! But crazy or not, he was a lot better for her than death.

'Let me clarify the rationale,' he said. 'Because then I can use the key, and it will be done. There are an infinite number of Modes, in which different people live and different fundamental laws obtain. The Chips enable us to establish contact with the others. In mine, magic —'

'Like computer chips,' she said.

'You know of the Chips?'

'A chip is a sort of section of a computer that enables it to do what it does,' she said. 'To address a lot of memory, for example. The fancier the chip, the more sophisticated the computer. Take the 86 series, for example.'

'There are eighty-six of these "computers"?'

She laughed. 'No, silly, that's what they're called! The 8086, 80286, 80386 and so on. There was an 80186 but I think it was the same as the 8086. Anyway, they may seem similar, but the amount of RAM they can manage is –'

'Ram? A male sheep?'

She laughed so hard she let herself fall over backwards, which was fun. She tended to be happy when she was with him, which was an exhilarating experience. Then she remembered that she wasn't in her blue jeans now; she didn't want to freak him out. Not right at this moment, anyway; better to save it for when she needed it. He had endearingly quaint notions of propriety. She drew herself up and forced herself into sobriety. 'No, RAM stands for Random Access Memory. Memory you can change about, any which way you want. So you can do a lot with it. But that's irrelevant. The point is that when you said you had chips to make contact with other realities, well, I thought of the way our computer chips make contact with a lot of memory, among other things. It's just an analogy.'

'Perhaps,' he said seriously. 'But it sounds so much like an aspect of what I was discussing that I think I had better learn more of it. Exactly what is a computer, and how does the chip relate to it? The chip is an integral part?'

'You really don't know?'

'I really don't know, Colene, and it may be important.'

'Okay. We use computers in school for homework papers and math problems and things. Oh, we still use books, but the computers make it easier. We can set up our problems and push a few buttons, and it's much faster. We can write papers on the screen, and edit them, and print them out when they're all done.'

'Where do you get these devices?'

'We make them. There are companies in California and Japan and all over. Where do you get your chips?'

'They are ancient relics apparently deriving from some other Mode. We do not know their origin, only their power, and we understand only a little of that.'

'Gee – mysterious ancient otherworld science! I like it!'

'You like everything. You are wonderful.'

She felt a warm thrill. When she was with him, that was the way she felt. If she could be with him forever, would she become normal? It was an intriguing notion.

But there was business to handle. She had to go into some detail about exactly what problems and papers were, and how they were done with computers. Then they got down to the essence:

'So the 186 chip addressed one megabyte RAM,' she said. 'One million bytes. Maybe 165,000 words if you used up all the space in writing a novel: one pretty solid book. But the software only addressed about two thirds of that, six hundred and forty kilobytes. Then the 286 chip addressed sixteen megabytes RAM, but the software was still limited to six forty K. So what was the point? They had to develop a new operating system to catch up with the hardware. The way I see it, the 186 was like a line: it did a lot, but was sort of limited. The 286 was like a square, adding a whole dimension to computing. Then the 386 was like a cube, because it addressed four thousand megabytes RAM and could do stuff the other chips only dreamed of. So it's the 86 series, with the numbers telling how many dimensions: one, two or three. And then four, for the 486, and so on. But each one is based on just that key chip.'

'Dimensions,' Darius said. 'How many points does it take to establish a dimension?'

'Huh? We were talking about computers!'

'We were talking about an analogy. Chips, computers and dimensions. In my reality, when we deal with a line, it requires two points to establish the orientation of that line. Is it the same here?'

'Oh, sure. You can measure a line with two points, marking it off.'

'And three points for a plane? Defining it in space?'

'You mean like balancing a tray on three fingers? Sure.'

'And four points for a three dimensional object.'

'Sure, I'm with you. Length, width, thickness and time, 'cause if it doesn't exist for some time, it's not there at all. What's your point?'

'Five points for a four dimensional Mode,' he continued. 'To fix it in space and time. The Cyng of Pwer mentioned that. The infinite number of Modes are each fixed in their own places, like planes in a cube, and one of these is mine and another is yours.'

'Oh, you mean like – like mica. That rock that you can just peel apart?'

'Mica,' he agreed, after she had clarified the nature of the stone for him. 'Each layer infinitely thin, but a universe to those who are of it. The Chip enabled me to cross vertically, from my layer to yours. Because it addresses many megabytes. But my finding you was essentially random, because there are only a few parameters we could specify, and infinity to choose from.'

'Gee, I wonder if it could set up a Virtual Mode?' she said musingly.

'What is that?'

'Well, I told you how each new chip addressed a whole lot more memory. But that's not the half of it. The 386 can extend that way beyond by making it seem that there's a lot more memory. There's not, really, but you can use it same as if it's real. Fake memory, I call it.'

'Pretend memory? But surely that would be a fantasy!'

'No. Like when you have the disk drive, and it's too small for what you want to do, but you have a whole lot of memory, so you make up a virtual drive out of memory, and it acts just like a real disk. Or the other way around, making memory out of extra storage on your hard disk. When you turn off the computer, it's gone, but as long as you're running it, it works. Virtual memory is real, it just isn't quite what it seems. The 386 can make your memory act like sixty-four million megabytes, which is a lot. And it can set up a Virtual Mode, too.'

'Tell me of Modes.'

Colene had been privately convinced that he was crazy, but he now seemed more like an ignorant but smart person.

Like someone who was from another reality. She began to doubt, and to believe, as she talked. 'I don't remember all the computer modes; it's been a while since I had that class. I think there's Native Mode, that's sort of whatever the 386 chip would do if left to itself. Then there's Real Mode, used to run the regular AT software; it's limited, just sort of choking down the chip's potential to make it seem like a simpler one.'

'Like one slice of mica,' he said.

'Yes. And Protected Mode, used for the Operating System Two multitasking. That's like a three dimensional chunk of mica. And Virtual Mode, that will take the chip as far as it will go; it can be set up any which way, and however it's set up, it acts just as if it's real.'

'With that we could institute a reality that included you with your science, and me with my magic, yet we would be together, neither giving up anything.'

'So it wouldn't have to be one or the other!' she agreed. 'I'd like that, Darius! Then I could just walk across to you, and if I couldn't marry you, I'd just walk back to here.'

'A reality that consisted of a slanting place across the block of mica, permanently linking us,' he agreed. 'Unfortunately, that is not what brought me here. I am a mere intruder into your reality, with no permanence. When I take you with me, you will be an intruder into my reality.'

She shrugged. 'So I guess there's no way you can show me your reality, without my actually going there and not being able to return.' A journey into madness?

'I see I have not convinced you.'

'Right. That computer analogy is nice, but I never fooled myself that I can step into the picture on the screen. My reality is a lot uglier.'

'Ugly? But you are beautiful and cheerful!'

She sighed. 'Something you better know about me, Darius, before you marry me. I'm not happy. I'm suicidal.'

He was astonished. 'You seek to destroy yourself? I can not believe –'

'Believe it!' She began unwinding the bandage on her arm. 'I slice my wrists and watch the blood. Some day I'll get up the courage to go all the way, and then I'll be free.' She showed the inner padding, soaked in blood. 'See this? This is how I got your key back for you. I challenged the punk who had it to a bleeding contest. He thought I was bluffing, but I wasn't. Freaked him out. So I won. If I had lost, I'd either be dead or as good as dead, paying off my bet.'

'You are depressed!' he exclaimed, horrified.

'You bet! I think the only time I've been happy this year is when I've been with you. So I guess I'm crazy too. It's been fun dreaming of being in your world with its magic, and loving you, and I guess I do love you, but I don't believe you. It's my misfortune to be too firmly grounded in reality, and I don't mean your kind.'

'Oh, Colene, this is terrible!' he cried.

'Why?'

'Because it means I can't marry you.'

'Well, if you get treatment and get cured –'

'Not so. If I take you to my reality, where joy can be transferred, you would have no joy to give me. You have the opposite. That makes it impossible.'

'You're changing your mind?' she asked. Her feelings were horribly mixed. She wanted to love him and have him love her, but she knew that marriage between them had always been an impossible dream. Now that he had his key, and his fantasy would soon be dashed, it was time to end it. But how she wished this sweet interlude could have been forever!

'Colene, I love you, and I want nothing more than to bring you home and marry you! But that would destroy us both! I was willing to take you as long as there was a reasonable chance of it being right, but now I know there is not. I blinded my mind to one of the major possibilities for your availability, and that was my folly. My mission has failed. The kindest thing I can do for you is to leave you behind.'

So he knew the key wouldn't work, and was calling it off. That did make sense. It also meant he didn't have to make the deal, and go to a mental hospital when he failed to go where he thought he was going. He was defaulting, just as Biff had. Getting set up to walk out of her life when his bubble of illusion was popped.

She felt the tears starting down her cheeks. 'I guess you're

68

right. I guess you'd better use your key now. You know where I am, if you ever change your mind.' For now she did not have to disparage the fantasy; she could let him depart in his own way. It hurt terribly, but it was for the best.

'If there were any way –'

'If there were any way,' she agreed.

He came to her and kissed her, and it was excruciatingly sweet. It was like an old movie, with them parting at the train station, knowing they might never see each other again. Maybe that analogy wasn't so far off.

'I can't even leave you anything, to repay you for your great kindness to me,' he said. 'It has been for nothing.'

'For nothing,' she agreed. 'But I really liked being with you, Darius. I'm sorry I can't believe in you. If I did, I'd go with you, even if you had to marry someone else.'

'I would not care to do that to you.' He lifted the key to his forehead. 'Farewell, Colene.'

'Goodbye, Darius.'

He closed his eyes, seeming to concentrate.

Then he disappeared.

Colene blinked her tears out of the way. She stepped forward and swept her hand through the space where he had stood. There was nothing except the faint smell of him; he had not been able to wash up well, here.

The door was closed. He had not walked out. He had just – gone. Exactly as he had said he would.

Now she knew that she should have believed. She should have gone with him to his magic reality. Her disbelief had cost her everything.

4

VIRTUAL MODE

Darius looked around him. The familiar landscape of his home reality was newly unfamiliar, after his acclimation to the alternate reality. He gazed at it with a new appreciation.

He stood on a dais, the one addressed by the Chip. One hop distant – or about twenty meters, in Colene's system – was the larger dais of the Cyng of Pwer. Between was the serrate wilderness: a land surface so jagged that it was not possible to walk on it. Only by pounding a temporary path through the crystals could it be made passable by foot, and that was pointless, because in days the crystals would regenerate, and their new, smaller spikes would be sharper than the old ones had been. Also, who would want to damage such prettiness? The original crystals were all the natural colors and some generated ones, shifting iridescently in the changing light of the sun.

He glanced up. There were good cloud formations, pink above green and yellow. A heavy purple cloud was slowly descending, and below it the trees on their common dais were extending their black leaves, ready to draw nourishment. The light of the sun was refracting through a colorless cloud, its beams reradiating out to be intercepted by other clouds, each of which took its color from the color of the light it received.

It was good to be home!

A figure appeared on the main dais. The man spied Darius.

70

He made a gesture, and a bridge appeared, spanning the ragged gap between them.

Darius stepped onto the bridge, and felt his weight diminishing. It was what Colene would have called a virtual bridge: it acted like a real one, but it was mock. He was able to use it because his weight was being reduced almost to nothing. Pwer had simply invoked a miniature bridge with a figurine, and was marching the latter across the former. Darius had allowed him to make the figurine because it was essential to the process of traveling to another reality. Otherwise the magic would not have had effect.

He completed his crossing and stood before the Cyng of Pwer. 'You return alone,' the man said.

'I found her,' Darius said. 'I love her. But I misjudged her. She was depressive.'

Pwer was startled. 'How could you make an error like that?'

'There is no transfer in her reality. I judged by appearances, not direct mental contact, and she laughed much. But it was because she liked me. Her contacts with me were limited, and her joy was limited to her time with me. Her underlying nature was suicidal.'

'Your power did not work there?'

'Not at all. I thought it did when I kissed her and felt love, and she felt love, but it seems we were each generating our own in the company of the other. I was entirely dependent on verbal language. Much of my time was spent learning it, so that we could communicate. It was in that period of close association that we came to love each other.'

'You should have brought her.'

'I could not marry her! It would have killed her.'

'And what will she do, alone?'

That made Darius pause. 'She – she could kill herself.'

'Could? You fool! She surely will!'

'We can't know that! Maybe her experience with me will change her outlook, and she will become less suicidal.'

'Unlikely, since she is slated to die anyway.'

'What?'

'Don't you remember? Only those who are destined to have

71

little effect on their realities can be removed from them. That is why the Chip oriented on her.'

'I know. Yet in her case, it seemed to me –' Darius shook his head. 'I blinded myself.'

'The Chip was set to orient only on those whose impact is minimal. Some may have more impact by dying than by living. But in most cases, an early death best accounts for it. This may usually be by accident or disease, but it is evident that your young woman will soon kill herself.'

'I left her there, to do what she would, alone!' Darius cried, stricken. 'I lost track entirely. I forgot the larger picture.'

'Whereas here she could have been with you, and at least died happy.'

'But she did not believe. She fetched me the key, but thought it was my fantasy. She did not want to commit to one she thought crazy.'

'She surely believes now.'

'Surely now,' Darius agreed, crushed. 'I should have insisted – but when I knew I could not marry her –'

'Cyngs of Hlahtar do not remain functional indefinitely. You might have married her when you gave up the post.'

'I was a fool,' Darius said.

'Will you now settle to the normal course?'

Darius thought of marrying a woman he did not love, instead of Colene. 'I can not.'

'Or try the Chip again?'

He thought of searching for another woman of a suitable nature to love and marry. 'I can not.'

'Then it appears we have a problem.'

'There must be another way!' Darius exclaimed. 'I must go to her again! She would come with me, now that she believes.'

'There is a way. But it is fraught with complication and danger.'

Darius grasped at it. 'What way?'

'Before, we set up the simplest connection between realities, as it were a line. It is possible to set up a more complicated connection, if more than one point is established, as it were a plane. The line could be flung out and recalled only once, but the plane would be more durable.'

'A Virtual Mode!' Darius breathed.

'A what?'

'A temporary Mode that crosses other Modes, like a block of mica sliced crosswise. It would be possible to walk from one part to another, from this Mode to her Mode.'

'I had not pictured it that way, but it is true. However you picture it, it may be the way to do what you desire. However, the complications –'

Darius was abruptly certain. 'Describe them.'

'Because it would entail some time away from this Mode, you can not go without finding another Cyng of Hlahtar to serve in your stead, at least temporarily. One as competent as you.'

'There is none!'

'Not among those who have not yet served.'

Now Darius understood his reference. 'A retired Hlahtar? But none of them would serve again!'

'Not unless the inducement were considerable.'

'What possible inducement could there be? They have wealth and power and respect already; they need nothing. None would wish to suffer the agonies of depletion and wife discarding again.'

'You might inquire.'

'And if I can get one to serve, you will set up the Virtual Mode?'

'After this warning: no person who has gone this route has returned. We do not know whether each has found what he sought and been satisfied, or has died. We know nothing, except that we shall wait with no expectation for your return.'

That was why another Hlahtar had to serve in his stead.

Darius was at the moment poorly acclimated to his native Mode, having been so long unable to do any magic, but he did not wait. He did not know how long Colene would linger before letting the rest of her blood drain away.

He walked into the forest and found several twigs and bits of vine. He bound these together into a crude man-figure. Then he pulled out five hairs from his head and tucked them into the two legs, two arms, and one head of the figurine. Now he had made an icon of himself. It was crude, but it should do.

He touched his tongue to it, anointing it with his saliva. Now it was twice tuned to him, to his solid and his liquid. All it required was his air.

He breathed on it. 'You are the icon of the Cyng of Hlahtar,' he murmured, activating it and tuning it in. Then he set it on the ground and marked a circle around it. He also marked several irregular shapes, and a wavy line. 'You are here, among these trees, and near this river.' He marked a square a short distance away, with several points beside it. 'The Castle of Hlahtar is there, beside the mountains.' Then he jumped the figure from the circle to the edge of the square.

The world around him wrenched. He caught his balance, almost falling. Yes, he was clumsy after the layoff! But he was here before his castle, having conjured himself here by the use of sympathetic magic. It was good to be able to travel normally again!

He lifted the icon to his mouth. 'You are inert,' he breathed on it. It wouldn't do to carry an active personal icon around with him, its feedback from his motions interfering with his activities! He put it in his pocket – and realized that he was not in his normal attire, but in the odd clothing of Colene's Mode. It was a good thing he had decided to come home before visiting the former Hlahtars!

A maid spied him and shrieked. 'A strange man-form!' she cried.

'No, a familiar one, in strange attire,' he called. 'You know me, Ella!'

She shrieked again. 'It's the Cyng!' She ran out to come to him, her breasts bobbing, and flung herself into his arms. 'Did you find a wife?'

'Not exactly.'

'Oh, too bad! Then you must settle for me in your bed a while longer.'

'That is no chore,' he said, patting her shapely derriere.

Indeed, it was late, and he needed to rest. He would have to wait until tomorrow to visit the retired Cyngs.

*　　*　　*

74

That night, after celebrating his return with a minor feast, he came to his bed. Ella was there, moving over so he could have the spot she had warmed for him. She had always been thoughtful in such little ways, and often forgetful in big ways. She was cheerful, buxom and pretty, but not phenomenally smart, and she had not the slightest ability to multiply joy. Therefore she would never be other than a servant and in due course a servant's wife. She could be very pleasant as a nocturnal companion.

But tonight he found himself unmoved. 'Please, do not expect more of me than sleep,' he said.

'You are annoyed with me?' she asked, hurt.

'No, Ella, merely indisposed.'

'Why?' This was not a proper question, but part of her delight was her social naivete.

'I have another woman on my mind.'

'Who?'

'The one I wished to marry. But I could not.'

'Oh. Why not?'

'Because she is depressive.'

'But you could have her in bed as a servant, same as me.'

'Somehow I forgot that. I wanted to marry her.'

'Well, you could, if you weren't Cyng.'

It was a foolish statement, readily dismissed. But somehow it struck home. *If he were not Cyng of Hlahtar.*

But he could not just step down. He was the only one who could serve the post with the necessary expertise. Except for the former Cyngs, who would not resume the post any longer than absolutely necessary. If he could step down, without having completed his term, he would be no better than a servant himself, and Colene might not have liked that. No, the only way was to complete his term and retire; then he could have the blessing of marriage for love and permanence.

But if he could use the Virtual Mode to find Colene, and bring her back, and keep her here in servant status until he retired, then he could marry her, and their love would never have been sacrificed. Colene had said she would be willing to endure something of the kind; he just hadn't quite listened.

It was feasible. He just had to get her back.

'Thank you, Ella,' he said, and kissed her.

'Oooo,' she exclaimed, thrilled to have pleased him. She clasped him to her, and didn't mind that all he did was fall asleep.

In the morning he used one of his established icons to travel to the castle of the Cyng of Hlahtar who had preceded him. This was Kublai, a huge red-bearded man. The man's dais was extremely high, so that the trees on it could feed from the higher level, before other plants depleted the nutrients. As a result, the trees were impressive, their trunks brilliant green and their foliage extensive.

Darius stood at the edge of the dais, in the region reserved for visitors. 'I am Darius,' he said. 'Cyng of Hlahtar, come for a dealing.' Again he remembered Colene, who had spoken of dealing for the Mode key. She had done so much for him, considering her unbelief – and he had done nothing for her.

Kublai appeared. 'Welcome, Darius! Come into my house!'

With that invitation, Darius stepped out of the visitors' area and walked the path to the castle. Had he tried to do it uninvited, he would have invoked the dais defenses, which could be of any nature. He would not have attempted to breach courtesy even if prepared for the defenses; a man's castle was his home.

Kublai's young and pretty wife served them condensed cloudfruit while they talked. Her name was Koren. She was evidently happy; there had been no depletion of her joy. That was the delight of retirement. Gazing at her, Darius knew his mission here was lost; Kublai would not give up his love-marriage to resume the post.

'News has spread of your concern,' Kublai said. 'Not widely, but I believe I know how you feel.'

'Surely you do!' Darius agreed. 'I have divorced my second wife, and she was a good woman, and loyal. I could have loved her, but never dared.'

'I divorced ten,' Kublai said. 'Each one was painful. Some I did love. But it was a great relief when you came of age and displaced me.'

'I did not truly appreciate the onus, until I saw my first wife depleted,' Darius said. 'We had known it would happen from the start, and there was no blame, no rancor. But her joy was gone, and I think even now she can not take pleasure in the good life she has as a retired wife.'

'She will recover her joy in time,' Kublai said. 'She may remarry a normal man, and have offspring. Several of mine did.'

'But the flower of her youth will be gone in depression.'

'It is an unkind price,' Kublai agreed.

'I think this is hopeless, but I must ask,' Darius said. 'I can not allow any person to take my place who can not perform as well as I would. Only former Cyngs of Hlahtar can do that.'

'Tell me of the need that brings you to this pass.'

Darius described his visit to the other Mode, and his encounter with Colene. 'I hoped she would be a multiplier,' he said. 'The Chip was tuned to such. But she was depressive. She would have multiplied a negative balance.'

'But you love her,' Kublai said.

'I love her. I thought it was just my expectation, and would fade when I realized that I was mistaken about her. But I hadn't realized that she was doomed to die. Here, at least, perhaps she could live. If not, at least we could try for some happiness before it happened. Pwer says he can institute a Virtual Mode that will enable me to seek her. Perhaps I can bring her here, and if it is suicide she contemplates, she may postpone it while we love. But –'

'But you need a substitute for the post.'

'That is the case. So I come to inquire whether there is anything I can offer you that would incline you to do this for me, and I fear there is not.'

Kublai nodded. 'I am in a position to know exactly how much you are asking of me. Not only would I have to resume the burden of Hlahtar, I would have to divorce my lovely love-wife Koren and marry another for other than love. That is not a thing I would do lightly.'

'You would risk much, while I would have no guarantee of accomplishing my mission.'

'You would have no guarantee of surviving yourself!' Kublai

77

said. 'I well might be stuck with a full term, until some other prospect matured. That might be a decade!'

'And even if I succeed, and find her, and bring her back here safely, I will not be able to marry her – unless there is someone else to assume the post,' Darius said. 'So I can not even promise that your loss would be my gain; probably I would gain less than you lost, even with full success.'

'You are candid.'

'I am desperate. I made a terrible mistake. I will do whatever I must to ameliorate it to the extent I can. Is there a price that will tempt you?'

Kublai was silent. He gazed at Koren. She had of course overheard their conversation, and now stood with tears flowing down her cheeks.

Suddenly Darius understood the significance of those tears. *There was a price!*

'There is a price,' Kublai agreed gravely.

'Tell me.' He did not want to evince unseemly eagerness, but that was what he felt. At the same time he felt guilty, seeing the dawning misery of Kublai's wife. This was the classic Hlahtar trade-off: joy for many at the expense of a few. But in this case it was joy for one at the expense of one: not a suitable ratio.

Kublai glanced at Koren. 'Come here, my love; this is not the disaster you envision; I am not about to cast you aside. This is something it is best that you also know.'

She went to him and cast herself into his arms, burying her face in his shoulder. He looked at Darius over her shoulder, holding her, stroking her lustrous black hair as he talked.

'When I was young, I encountered a woman. She called herself Prima. I was attracted to her not for her beauty or personality, for she was not remarkable in these respects, but for her ability to multiply. Her power was on a par with my own –'

'With yours?' Darius asked, startled. 'But no woman –'

Kublai smiled. 'In general, women are not as capable as men in this respect, so that while a man may multiply by a factor of a thousand, a woman may do it by a factor of three. But there is no absolute limitation. It may be that women would be as capable as men, were this encouraged in our culture. Certainly Prima was in this respect. She was fiercely independent and assertive, which of course did not endear her to others. She wanted to be the Cyng of Hlahtar, but of course this was not allowed. When I appeared, she asked me why I should assume the post simply because I was male, my talent being no greater than hers. I had not before considered the matter, but I was persuaded by her, and agreed that it was not right. Indeed, I came to love her, and she loved me, for we were one in our ability.

'We went to the council of Cyngs and asked that she be allowed to assume the post. I agreed to marry her and support her in that post, for my talent feeding into hers would make us the most effective and enduring Hlahtar our Mode has known. But they would not allow a woman to be dominant.

'Then we asked whether we could assume the post as co-equals, taking turns being the lead, one supporting the other. But they would not allow this either. They would allow only my own assumption of the post. I could marry her, but she would be only my wife, supporting me. She would never be Cyng herself.

'Neither of us was willing to do that, at this point. We discussed the matter at length, and finally she decided to explore the realms of the Chips. So the Cyng of Pwer set up what you have termed a Virtual Mode, and she went there to seek some suitable situation. Perhaps there was a realm in which women were equal to men, and she could assume the post there without quarrel, and they would appreciate what she was able to do for them.

'So Prima departed, and I became Hlahtar. We agreed that if she did not find her situation, and returned, she would marry me and accept secondary status. I hoped privately that this would be the case, for I could ask no better support than hers. But she had to do it of her own will.' Kublai paused.

'And she never returned,' Darius said.

'She never returned,' Kublai agreed. 'I married ten wives in succession, depleting each, and retired when you appeared. Now I have love, and it is sweet.' He patted Koren's shoulder. 'But always I have wondered what became of Prima. Did she find her situation, or did she die, or is she still searching? My curiosity has become overwhelming. But I lack the incentive to explore the alternate realms myself, now that I have a good life here. So I would ask two things of you: first, that you seek Prima, or news of her, so that I may finally know the truth. If you should find her, and she is ready to return, bring her back. If you did that, I would be happy to maintain the post indefinitely, for with her support it would represent no burden.'

'If you enabled me to search for my love, and bring her back, I would be glad to search also for yours, and bring her back too,' Darius said. 'Once I know the way, any who are with me can come along.'

'But you will cast me aside!' Kublai's wife protested, her voice buried in his shoulder.

'No, my love,' he said reassuringly. 'I would have to divorce you and keep you as my love companion, but that would be little other than a matter of legality. You would remain my love, as you are now. What I felt for Prima has faded in twenty years, and certainly she is no longer young, and never was she winsome. It would be a business relationship, based on my respect for her talent, and the enormous power that talent would provide me. You would remain my love, and you would not be depleted.'

'I still would rather be your wife,' she said.

'The chances are that Darius will return without her,' Kublai said. 'Then he will resume the post, and I will remarry you. I think this is a fair gamble.'

'But you mentioned two things you would ask of me,' Darius said. The second was likely to be the crusher.

'The second is both larger and perhaps easier,' Kublai said. 'I have developed a curiosity not only about Prima's situation, but about the alternate realms themselves. I wish to know the nature of ultimate reality. I would ask you to explore these alternate realms, seeking to understand them, and to formulate and test an explanation for the way things are. Who made the Chips and left them here? Who made it possible for Modes to be crossed? Why? I would like, before I die, to have that explanation.'

'But my mind may not be good enough to compass such

knowledge,' Darius protested. 'I hardly understand the one other Mode I have seen, and I did not understand the nature of the young woman I came to love there.'

'Yet you would make the effort, and tell me all you learn. It might be considerable, and certainly it would be far more than I know now – discovered at no risk to me.'

'But no one has returned!' Darius pointed out. 'I may be unable to honor any part of such an agreement.'

'That is why I ask for two favors: the news on Prima, and the nature of the Modes. If I win, I win all that I have wanted to know. If I lose, I am Cyng until another suitable prospect appears. I am experienced; it is not the worst of fates. In fact, I find myself bored with retirement. Oh, not with you, my dear,' he added quickly as his wife lifted her head. 'You are my perpetual delight! But the rest of it – there is only so much ease and luxury a man can tolerate. I think I am ready to resume useful activity – and keep my love with me.'

She settled back, mollified.

'I can only agree,' Darius said. 'If you will take my place, I will seek what you wish.'

In this manner it was agreed. Darius and Kublai had merged their hopes, and it would be done.

It took time to set up the Virtual Mode and to arrange for the temporary resumption of the post by Kublai. Darius had to do a tour, for the need was growing. The public had to be served.

But he lacked a wife. He did not want to marry for just one tour, but it would not be wise to deplete himself immediately before embarking on the treacherous journey that was the Virtual Mode. What was he to do?

Kublai came up with the answer. 'Borrow Koren.'

'What?'

'My wife Koren. She has it in her pretty head that she wants to remain married to me, even as I resume the post. This is foolish.'

'Of course it is! But –'

'I need to persuade her to step down, and to allow me to marry a woman suitable for that office. But I do not wish to hurt or offend her. However, if she went with you on the tour, she would quickly learn the cost, and I think that would be more persuasive than anything I could say.'

'Surely it would!' Darius agreed. 'But the intimacy of the borrowing –'

'I would rather have you do it, than do it to her myself. I prefer to convince her without instituting that barrier between us.'

'But she is your wife!' Darius said, at a loss.

'Who has never felt my power. Let her feel yours. By the time the tour is done, she will have had enough.'

The man did know what he was suggesting. Reluctantly, Darius agreed.

So it was that Koren came to his castle as ad-hoc wife. She made it quite plain that there was no private aspect to the relationship. She was here because Kublai had asked her to be, and she was certain that her mind would be changed not one iota by this experience. She expected to prove herself to her husband.

'I understand your reticence,' Darius said. 'I will honor your privacy in all things, but when the time of multiplication comes, I shall have to embrace you closely and publicly. You will find it a unique experience.'

'I doubt it,' she said coldly. 'If you touch me anywhere else, I will slap you.'

Yes, she did not understand. She would learn a great deal in the next day.

Sexual energy was part of what enabled multiplication, and it was customary for the Cyng to indulge in it with his wife the night before a tour. This was out of the question with Koren, but he did need to do it with someone. If only Colene had returned with him! If only he had understood all of what was at stake, and had insisted that she come here!

So that night he used a device that he feared would shame him if he thought about it: he closed his eyes and visualized Ella as Colene. Then he was most passionate with her. She was quite pleased.

In the morning they set out on the tour. Darius, Koren, a comedian, a props man and the castle's regular conjurer stepped onto a large disk, and the conjurer lifted a small disk containing a hair from each of them and activated it. They moved upward as the miniature disk did, floating from the castle court until they were high above the dais. Then the conjurer moved the little disk south toward the Model of a castle, and the big disk zoomed in that direction.

It was routine, but Darius' awareness of the other Mode remained, and he continued to appreciate how novel this would seem to Colene. She had told him that her people had huge flying machines, but she didn't believe in magic, so this flying disk would surprise her. Also, the landscape below was beautiful. The rugged crevices of the land formed patterns of ridges, their crystals scintillating, so that it was possible to see circles, triangles, squares, pentagons and hexagons forming and dissipating as they moved across. Some crystals sent up beams of reflected light that formed three-dimensional figures, the green beams intersecting the red beams and yellow beams, the whole being bathed by diffused light from other crystals. It might be impossible to walk across such terrain, but it was lovely to float across.

The sky, too, was a continuing pleasure. They floated around, above and below the colored clouds, swerving as necessary, and these too were beautiful. Some had patterns on their surfaces, projected from the crystals, and the patterns changed as the perspective did. Yes, Colene would love this, and he would do his best to bring her here and show it to her. If only he had thought it properly through before, and brought her with him despite her nature and her doubt!

Then they came into sight of a village dais, much larger than those for the castles or solitary trees. Here there were thousands of villagers, and around it were the lesser platforms where gardens flourished. At such enclaves the fundamental supplies of the realm were grown and made. A potato, for example, did not just appear when conjured; it was grown and saved, and so was ready for conjuration at need. The children of Cyngs sometimes believed that food came into existence when summoned, but the children of peasants well understood the labors of production.

At locations like these the animals were also raised: cows

to produce milk, chickens to produce eggs, and so on. There were grazing dais, and sections where the crystals of the nether terrain were less prominent, so that vegetation could grow and creatures could forage. But people had to watch over these animals, and keep them safe from predators. There were also artisans of many types: woodworkers, metalworkers, stoneworkers, clothworkers and on. All laboring patiently for their sustenance. No, nothing was free; at every stage there had to be the hands of dedicated men and women. Without such workers, the fine society of mankind would not be possible.

These were the folk who needed joy, for their lives did not provide great amounts of it naturally. Each Cyng was granted a good life, but each Cyng repaid it with the unique service which was the speciality of his post. Thus the society was interactive, but the lives of Cyngs were better than most.

Their disk landed. Immediately the group stepped off and proceeded to the setting up. Soon there was a little stage, and the villagers were seated around it in concentric circular rows. The whole village assembled; every member of it was eager for joy.

The comedian took a prop and went into his act. He pranced, he twirled, he made grotesque faces. The villagers watched passively. They were not much entertained. This was exactly according to expectation; had they reacted positively, it would have been an indication that their need was not sufficient to warrant this presentation.

Then Darius stepped to the center of the stage. There was a hush of expectation. He turned and gestured to Koren.

The woman came up on the stage. No one introduced her; the villagers were allowed to assume that she was his wife. The wives of Cyngs of Hlahtar changed often, so her newness here did not excite suspicion. She was young, she was beautiful, and she came when called: that was evidence enough.

Koren came to stand immediately before Darius. She was in a glossy black dress that matched her hair, so that it was hard to tell where one left off and the other began. The upper portion flared so as to conceal the shape of her bosom, and the nether portion spread out similarly to hide her legs, in the

84

decorous manner, but it was not possible to completely mask her beauty.

Darius embraced her. He drew her in very close, so that the full length of her body was tight against his own. She was stiff, not liking this, thinking that he was being too familiar. She averted her face, and kept her arms immobile at her sides. But only with close contact could he exert his power efficiently; the effect diminished with distance, causing needless waste.

Then he drew from her. Her vitality came into his body, measure by measure in its measureless fashion, strengthening him while depleting her. It was not a large transfer, but it was significant.

She stood without moving, evidently uncertain what she was experiencing. Then she tried to struggle, but her determination was weak, being the first thing tapped. Her head snapped around; her eyes came to stare into his with the wonder and horror of a captive animal. She would have felt better giving a quantity of the blood of her body. She sank into herself, her vitality waning. She was helpless. Left to her own devices at this moment, she would soon lie down and die, having no further joy of life. She was depleted.

Darius let her go, and turned. He was flush with Koren's joy, taken from her. Then he fed it out to the multitude. It magnified enormously as it extended from him and bathed every seated peasant. Every man, woman and child received almost as much joy as Koren had lost.

Koren herself received a similar amount, for she was now among the recipients. But her joy was less than it had been, by that small margin, for the multiplying was like the level of water: it might spread to many, but would never exceed the level of its source. She had lost most of her joy, and had most of that loss restored, but that remaining level was lower. Only time would make up that small loss, and she would lose more before she could get that time.

The comedian stepped out again, capering, and now the peasants laughed. Their joy had been lifted to a height not recently experienced. Now they were well satisfied with their lot, and ready to enjoy the festivities.

Darius waved to them, and they cheered him lustily. Then

he took Koren by the hand and led her to the traveling disk. She came without resistance, shaken by her recent experience. Her level of joy was now the same as that of the peasants, but to her it seemed inadequate. She had known better; they had not. She had also suffered the shock of sudden depletion, as they had not; their depletion was gradual, as they went about their dull business. She had perspective.

The party gathered on the disk, and the conjurer lifted it, using his small icon-disk. The power for this came from the Cyng of Pwer, who drew it from the Modes and sent it out to be used as needed. The magic was used only to control it; the power itself was physical, like the things grown and made by the peasants.

They floated to the next village, where they repeated the process. This time Koren was not stiff but was afraid when he embraced her, and familiarity did not seem to make her more comfortable with the process. She looked less beautiful than before, even when most of her joy had been restored. Something new and awful had been introduced to her experience. She was coming to understand why her husband believed that love and marriage were incompatible, with a Cyng of Hlahtar.

They served ten villages on this tour, catching up on those that most needed joy. In a few days there would be another tour, to other villages. The process was continuous, for by the time every village had been served, the first village needed to be served again. The break Darius had taken had allowed many villages to get behind, and a faster schedule would be necessary to restore them.

At last they floated home. Now Darius spoke to Koren. 'This is what your husband seeks to spare you. You have lost only about a tenth of your joy this day, but before you can recover that, there will be another tour, and another. In two years, perhaps less, you will be depleted to the extent that it is no longer safe to draw from you, and you will have to be set aside for a fresher woman. Of course I hope to return long before that time, and resume the post. But your love will be better if you become his love-servant instead, for that period.'

She stared back at him with hopeless hate. Yes, now she

understood. How much better for her to hate Darius, than to hate her husband!

His thoughts turned to Colene. She, too, did not understand. She thought love could conquer all. She had been angry when he saw the impossibility of marrying her. Had the transfer of joy been possible in her Mode, he could have demonstrated; then she would have known. As Koren now knew.

The Chip was ready. It would institute the Virtual Mode. 'Now you must understand the deviousness of this process,' the Cyng of Pwer said. 'It seems that we are sending out several lines of force, and that those lines will anchor in several other Modes, and fix in place the Virtual Mode. One anchor is here, and another should be at the site of the girl you encountered – but only if she catches on to it. If she does not, some other person may do so, fixing the Mode, but your girl will not be in that Mode.'

'Colene may not be there?' Darius asked, appalled.

'We can send the line past her, but we can not make her take it. You can judge better than I how likely she is to take it.'

'She has to take it!' But there was a troubling doubt there.

'And if she does take it, that anchors only two points. Three more are required, because –'

'Because it takes five points to fix a four dimensional Mode,' Darius said.

'Ah, I see you understand! But we have no control at all over those remaining three. They can be anywhere, and the Virtual Mode may be strange indeed.'

'At least they will all be human.'

Pwer frowned. 'Not necessarily. I have made the setting sapience rather than humanity. Humanity can include anything from our level to complete primitives. With sapience, at least there will in all cases be minds to which you can relate. We hope they will be human.'

Darius hoped so too! 'I am ready,' he said. He had a new pack of supplies, and this time he had something he had not thought to take before: a weapon. It was a primitive sword, which did not require any spell for its effect. It had a sharp point and a sharp edge. He was not proficient in its use, but was satisfied that it would be effective against either animals or unarmed attackers, such as the young men who had attacked him without provocation in Colene's Mode. He also had primitive tools for cutting wood, breaking stone or making fire. In fact he had the little box of 'matches' Colene had given him. One thing he had learned: not to depend on magic in that realm!

'I hope to return soon,' he said. 'But if I do not, I thank you for enabling me to make this quest.'

'This time I can not bring you back by orienting on a signal key,' Pwer reminded him grimly. 'You must return by yourself. If you do not return soon, you will gradually lose contact, until finally you will be unable. Do not leave any of your things behind; only you can carry them across the boundaries of the Modes. The Virtual Mode will remain anchored until you come here and touch the anchor-place and will it to let go. The Mode exists on its own; we are merely catching an aspect of it and fixing it in place for a time.'

'Fix it now,' Darius said, stepping into the marked circle. Pwer was full of cautions, but not all of what he said was believable.

The Cyng of Pwer nodded. He lifted his hand, invoking the necessary spell.

Something changed.

5

SEQIRO

Colene remained in a daze. *He had been right!* Darius really *was* from a far Kingdom of Laughter where magic worked. She had not believed, and so had thrown away her chance for happiness.

Yet he had changed his mind, too. He had thought she was full of joy, and had recoiled when she told him the truth. He had wanted only one thing from her, and that had been not her body but her happiness. She had been happy with him; without him she was the same old suicidal shell.

Now she was paging through her Journal, which she kept under lock and key here in Dogwood Bumshed, trying to distract her mind from her present distress by contemplating her past distress. She called it a Journal and not a diary, because 'diary' sounded like 'diarrhea' and she was not about to put her sanitary thoughts in an unsanitary place like that. She made her entries in the form of letters to her friend Maresy, who was actually an imaginary horse. Colene had never had a horse, but always wanted one, not just to ride, but to be her understanding companion. People were not necessarily fit to understand, but Maresy had more than human fathoming. Maresy was a most unusual animal.

Dear Maresy,

My friend Eney Locke did the craziest thing last night! She was at this party, and she wandered out on a balcony and gazed down into the concrete alley one floor down, thinking her usual dark thoughts. A boy came out, someone she knew mostly casually, a decent type. He said 'Oh, are you looking for the way out?' and she said 'Yes, but it's not far enough.' Then she realized that she had spoken aloud, and he realized that she was neither lost nor joking. He was appalled. 'Eney – you mean you're –?' he asked. And she, faced with this excellent chance to confess her secret and perhaps have some sympathy, blew it. 'I was joking!' she snapped, and pushed on past him, back into the party where everyone was drunk and happy.

The key to this was that Colene spelled backward was Eneloc, broken in two with letters added for camouflage: Eney Locke. She was talking about herself, but not directly, in case someone should get at her Journal before she had a chance to destroy it. She had the need to talk to someone, a desperate need, but obviously her parents were out, and she couldn't afford to trust anyone she knew at school. Once she had made the mistake of trusting a friend at camp. Never again! But Maresy was the epitome of equine discretion, partly because she could not speak in any human language. That did not mean that Maresy could not communicate, just that it required special comprehension to know what was on her mind. A horse could say a lot just in the orientation of her ears.

Actually, the address was fake. Maresy lived only in her mind. So she had made up a place for the horse to live, and used her own zip code rounded off to the nearest even hundred. As far as she knew, there was no such number, which was fine. She was never actually going to mail any of those letters. For one thing, Maresy didn't live where she seemed; that OK in her address stood for Okay. She was always Okay.

There were boxes in the margins of the Journal. They weren't exactly code; it was just that she drew them when she was disturbed, and the more disturbed she was, the more numerous and elaborate those little boxes became. She didn't need to read the actual entries to know how she had felt when making them; the boxes told. Sometimes there were only one or two plain cubes; sometimes there was an elaborate network of boxes that completely surrounded the text. Sometimes they resembled stalls for Maresy, though the truth was that Maresy was a free horse, unbridled, unsaddled, and unstalled. Maresy was as free as Colene was bound.

She turned to the last entry she had made. It was the day before she had found Darius in the ditch. It was a box done in the shape of an optical illusion, with three projections that weren't actually there when traced back to their sources; one was really the space between the other two. Variations on the figure were common; many people were intrigued by it. She thought the original was like a tuning fork, but it didn't matter. The point was, this was her. She looked just exactly like a girl, but when the lines were traced, there was nothing; she was a girl-shaped space between others, and if the others went away, she would cease to appear to exist. She had really been twisted up, then. The day before her adventure had begun.

But from the moment she spied Darius, she had neither written to Maresy nor scratched her wrists. Not till she freaked out Biff with a wholesale slash. No boxes, either. Her inner life had changed completely.

Now she was back in her own reality, as it were. She started to draw a box, and watched it take form as if of its own volition. It looked like a cross between a prison cell and an execution platform.

'Oh, Maresy, I need you now!' she breathed. 'What am I to do? I didn't trust the man I loved, and now I am alone.'

But that wasn't quite true. She had trusted Darius; she just hadn't believed him. She had been willing to sleep practically naked in his arms, but not to stand with him when he tried to go home. Maybe he had seen that, and made it easier for her by pretending she was unsuitable for him.

Pretending? Why should he pretend? He hadn't pretended about anything else. He had told her where he came from though he knew she didn't believe him. He had made her cover her crotch, because blue jeans didn't do the job to his satisfaction. He had learned enough of her language to talk with her, and had shown how well he understood what she told him. He had been his own man throughout, despite the indignities of being confined to the shed and having to use the pot. He had embraced her nightly without even trying to take any advantage of her. In fact, he had refused sex with her when she offered it. Pretend? He had never pretended! He had said she was unsuitable because that was exactly what she was. She was fourteen years old and suicidal. How could she ever have thought he would want to marry her?

Because he had told her he did. He had always told her the truth, and now she knew that even the least believable part of it had been valid. So he had been willing to marry her, until he learned that she was depressive. He had to have joy, to take and magnify and spread about. That was her most awful liability. She could make others laugh by her cutting humor, but if they had been able to read her inner nature, they would have been appalled. Darius would have read it, in his realm. So he had done what he had to do, and had been kind to her, he thought, letting her go.

'Oh Darius!' she cried, grief-smitten. 'I would have been satisfied to go with you, as your servant or your slave, just to be near you. If only I had believed! Now I have gotten what I deserved. I hope you find a woman you can marry.' But that last was insincere. Colene had wanted to be his wife. Deep-down, she didn't want him to be satisfied with any other woman. Oh, she wanted him to be happy, but not as happy as he might have been with her. And to know it.

She closed her Journal and locked it away. She knew what she had to do. There was a good knife in the kitchen, maybe not as sharp as Slick's razor, but it would do the job. No more fooling around with compass points.

She went to the house. But her mother was in the kitchen and she couldn't get the knife. Anyway, she hadn't figured out the right place to do it. She didn't want to splash blood all over Bumshed, for it didn't deserve to be soiled that way. It wouldn't be safe in her room in the house; her parents hardly

92

ever went there, except those few times when she especially didn't want them to. They had some kind of parental radar that made them home in at the exact worst times. Outside wasn't good; someone would be sure to see her. So she would have to figure out a place first; then she could take the knife there and do it quickly.

There was nothing to do except wrap up her homework, so that no one would be suspicious. She would go to school as usual Monday, and keep her eye out for a suitable place. She would certainly find it, and then she would act.

Monday she found herself in the bathroom, contemplating her scarred wrist. But she didn't touch it. She had been playing with suicide, before; this time she would do it right. That meant the right place and the right knife. She had seen how easy it was with the sharp razor; she could bleed herself out quickly by slashing both arms similarly. Once she decided on the place that was right. Where she could do it cleanly, and not be discovered until long after she was dead. She had to guarantee that she would not wake up in a hospital, to the shame of failure. Boys had it easy; they used guns, which were easy, quick and sure. But she didn't know a thing about guns; they frightened her. It had to be by a knife, so the blood could flow gently and prettily.

No place seemed right. Finally, Tuesday night, she did something foolish: she sneaked out to Bumshed in her nightie. She made a mound of books and a pillow, pretending it was Darius, and lay next to him in the darkness. 'Take me now,' she breathed to the quiet form, spreading her legs and breathing heavily. 'Do anything you want to do.' Of course he did not, but that did not interfere with the fancy; Darius would not have done it anyway.

By morning she had come to three conclusions. First, she wasn't fooling herself; she knew there was no man there. So this was pointless. Second, it was too darned cold out here alone, and lonely too. Third, *this* was the place she had been looking for. Here where she had known him, and brief happiness. She could make it sanitary by having plenty of basins to catch the blood, and she could empty them out as long as she was able. She could make a small hole beside Dogwood and pour it carefully in and cover it up; not only would it be practically untraceable, it would fertilize the tree. She liked the idea of her decorative little tree being nourished by her blood. When she was unable to take out the basin, there might not be enough blood left in her to overflow, so it would be all right. They would find her pale cold body, and a neat brimming basin of blood. That would be nice.

She went to school again Wednesday, concentrating on being absolutely normal. She did not give any of her things away to friends, because that was a recognized tipoff for suicidal intention. She did not mope. She laughed and paid attention in class. As far as she knew, no one had a clue to her plan.

That evening she fetched her favorite belongings and arranged them in a circle in Bumshed. Her ancient Teddy bear, Raggedy Ann doll, her book on odd mating customs of the world, one on exotic computer viruses (for 'safe' computing), her guitar, the picture of Maresy grazing, and the artificial carnation she had worn to the Prom last year. The dance itself had not been great, her date had been gawky, she had been gawky too, being thirteen, but it had become her first significant dance, and now would be her last, so this symbol of it deserved respect. Maybe she would float it in the final basin of blood, her last deliberate act. A white flower on a red background, the opposite of a red rose on a white gown.

Then she fetched the knife.

But as she set up for it, she realized that she had forgotten the most critical thing: the basin. It was too late to fetch it; she would be risking the curiosity of her parents. Dad happened to be home this night, so naturally the two were arguing: 'What's the matter, dear – your paramour have a snit?' 'What do you care, you tipsy lady?' That sort of thing. As it progressed, the language would get less polite, and finally they would come to physical contact and have sex on the floor. They fought verbally, not physically, but the sex was in lieu of hitting, and could get pretty violent. Her mother got bonus points for bitchiness if she made him cheat on his mistress. That made him angry, but the woman was sexiest when bitchiest, and he couldn't resist. Colene hated that scene, but also was morbidly fascinated by it. Maybe if she had taunted Darius as impotent, the way her mother did her father, he would have gotten mad and put it to her hard. That tempted her now, in retrospect, but also repelled her. She did not like anything even hinting of rape. Yet at least she would have *had* him! Maybe then she would have felt obliged to believe him, and would have gone with him to his fabulous land of laughter. So what if she was a stranger there, unable to marry him? It couldn't be worse than what she faced here.

So she had no basin, and was not about to go back to the house for it. What else would serve? She was definitely not going to spill her precious clean blood on the floor!

Her eye fell on the privy pot. Oh, ugh! Yet what else was there? And it had the remnants of *his* substance. That was about as close as any part of her could get to any part of him, now. So it would have to do. What an image for a romantic song: Blood and Feces. A sure hit with the anti-establishment crowd.

She brought the pot and removed the cover. The stink smote her nose. Quickly she covered it again. Maybe she could put a clothespin on her nose, if she had a clothespin. Anything else? She leaned on the board over the pot, and set the knife down on it while she considered.

She concluded that it didn't really matter. She would get used to the smell soon enough. So she sat cross-legged, in her nightie without panties, in a position that would have freaked Darius all the way out to the moon, dear man, drew the pot in to her, nestled it inside her crossed ankles, held her breath, lifted the knife, removed the cover board, leaned over, and paused.

Should she do the left arm first, or the right one? She was right handed, so maybe she should do the right one first, so if her left handed slash was clumsy she could do it again, and again until she had a proper blood flow into the pot. Then she could transfer the knife and do the left one with one excellent slice. Then she could grasp the far rim of the pot, keeping her arms locked in place, and watch the twin blood flows. It would be glorious!

95

So why was she hesitating? She was sure there was a reason. There always was.

She explored her motives, and found the relevant one. 'Oh, Darius, I don't want to die away from you!' she said. 'I'd so much rather die *with* you!'

She pondered some more, then decided to sleep on it. She could slice herself as well in the morning as at night. Maybe she would have a chance to sneak into the house and get a better basin, after her parents had sex-sotted themselves out and turned in. It was worth a try.

She lay down, shivering in the cold. She wrapped the blankets around and around her, and curled up into an almost fetal ball. She knew she would not sleep, but at least she wouldn't freeze.

She woke shivering, after an interminably restless night. The floor was hard, the air was chill, and the blankets seemed to have holes that exactly matched the path of the draft coming in under the door.

But it was her troubled thoughts that caused the greatest disruption of sleep. She was reviewing her life, trying to total up the credits and the debits, to justify her decision to end it. In snatches of dreams she talked to Maresy:

'Dear Maresy, today I decided to end it. Well actually I decided several days ago, but today was the day to do it. Only I didn't want to use a filthy potty for my blood.'

'You lost your nerve,' Maresy replied.

'No! I just want to do it right!'

'You really don't want to die. You never did.'

'That so, smarty? Then what do I really want to do?'

'You want to love and be loved.'

Maresy was right. She always was. She knew Colene better than Colene knew herself, because she was more objective. Death was merely the most convenient escape from a life without love. That was why she had not been suicidal in the time she had known Darius. She had had love.

Now she had lost that love. Oh, she still had it, in a sense: she definitely still loved him. But he was gone, and he had explained how he couldn't come back, because it had been

96

a random setting. So even if he loved her – and she thought he did – it was no good. They were apart forever.

'Why do you think he loves you?' Maresy asked.

'Because he told me he did.'

'But men lie about that.'

'To get sex from women,' she agreed. 'But he never had sex with me, even when I offered it. So he wasn't saying it for sex. Oh, yes, he did want something from me! He wanted my joy. And I would have given him that, if I had had any to give. So he loved me, but couldn't marry me without destroying me, and he wouldn't do that. I believe him. I believe him. I believe him.'

'So you do love, and you are loved,' Maresy said. 'So why do you want to die?'

That made her ponder for some time. She did have love; why wasn't it enough? 'Because it's apart,' she said at last. 'I want to love and be loved and have it close – like hugging close. Like kissing close. Like sex close. I want to be part of him, and have him be part of me, forever and ever. I want eternal romance.'

'You have foolish juvenile notions. It isn't that way.'

'How do you know?' Colene shot back.

'I know from what you've read. The half-life of romantic love is one and a half years.'

'What do you mean, half-life of love?'

'Remember your physics? Radioactive materials keep losing their radiation, getting less dangerous but never entirely finishing. So you can't say how long they last. But you can say how long it takes for their level of radioactivity to drop to half of what it was. That's their half-life, which may be a fraction of a second, or millions of years. So when it comes to the declining excitement of love, the half-life is eighteen months, on average.'

'I don't believe that! True love is forever!'

'Look at your parents.'

Accurate counterthrust! Where was the romance in her parents' marriage? As far as she knew, there had never been any. There had just been absence and alcohol and occasional bouts of hostile sex. Yet there must once have been love, or else why had they married?

So apply the half-life law. Suppose they had fallen in love, and in six months gotten married. She had been born the following year. Presto: their love had halved by the time she appeared on the scene, and halved again in the next year and a half. How many times had it halved by now? Take her age, fourteen, and add that first year and a half before her birth: fifteen and a half years since their first love. Enough for ten halvings. Plus maybe a quartering, or whatever. So if their love had started at a hundred per cent, it had gone to fifty per cent, then twenty five per cent, then – brother! How low had it sunk by this time?

Her thoughts fuzzed out, but her agile brain kept mulling it over, and in due course she concluded that it was just under one per cent. So what she was seeing now was only a hundredth of what they had started with. So now it was just a shared house, some ugly sex, and a messed-up daughter. Their love-child, as it were. More like a tough-love-child.

'You desire that with Darius?' Maresy inquired alertly.

'It wouldn't be that way with Darius!' she protested. But uncertainty was closing in, like dark fog at dusk. If she could be with Darius, and go to his wonderful Kingdom of Laughter, and everything was just perfect, would the romance be down to one per cent in fifteen years? Would she be an alcoholic and he be having affairs with other women? Would they have a suicidal daughter?

Maresy faded out, for Colene was now absolutely, totally wide awake. Now she knew: it was time to end it. There was no hope for romance, even if it were possible for her to join Darius. So she had lost nothing, really; there had never been anything to make her life worth continuing.

The dirty pot would do. It wasn't as if her life were clean. She was the offspring of a garbage marriage, and faced more garbage if she tried to grow up and get married herself. The whole thing was pointless.

She sat with the pot, uncovered it, bared her arms, and picked up the knife. Now was the time. Two swift, deep slices, then hang on. 'I'll lay me down and bleed a while,' she murmured. 'Then ne'er up again.'

Yet somehow she didn't make the first cut. She shivered

from the cold and the anticipation, and her arms were goosepimply, but she just sat there not doing it. She couldn't quite take that final step. She knew she had been playing at suicide, before; she couldn't bleed to death from the scratch of a compass point. She could have done it from the slash of Slick's razor, but that had been in company; she had known they wouldn't actually let her die. But now it was real, and she just couldn't.

'What a hypocrite I am!' she exclaimed. 'I know what to do, and I'm too cowardly to do it!'

The knife dropped from her hand. She sat there and sobbed. She had come to the final test of her life, and flunked it.

Yet she could not quite give up the death, either. She sat there, congealing with cold, breathing the miasma of the pot. Everything was hopeless! Maybe she would die of the cold, or at least catch pneumonia and expire. Or would that be cheating?

Colene! Wait for me!

She snapped out of her drift. Time had passed, maybe a little, maybe a lot. She must have nodded off, and dreamed.

Yet something had changed. She felt a certain imperative, or potential, or something.

Take hold!

It was Darius! It was no dream. Maybe she was crazy, but she was ready to go for it. If it was to be a one per cent romance fifteen years down the line, so be it, but it was a hundred per cent now, and now was what counted. She would give him everything immediately, before the joy of it could fade.

She reached out with her mind and took hold. She felt something settle into place. That was all.

But she knew reality had changed. It was a Virtual Mode: a ramp spanning the realities from his to hers. Darius was coming for her! If he was crazy, she would be crazy too. Gloriously crazy in love!

What now, of the futility of romance? She didn't care; she was going for it. Because while she was orienting on love, she wasn't orienting on death.

She got up and looked around. Nothing had changed, physically. But this was here, in her reality. It would be different in Darius' reality.

But how was she to get from here to there? Well, if this was a true Virtual Mode, all she had to do was walk there. She would be at one end, he at the other. It should be easy enough to cross the ramp and join him.

Why wait for him to come for her? She had wanted to depart this life. Now she could do it – without killing herself. She would meet him half way.

Still, it might be a fair distance. She should travel prepared. She wasn't sure how far it might seem in miles. If there were an infinite number of realities, was that an infinite number of miles? No, it had to be fewer than that. But she should use her bicycle, just in case.

She gathered up her scattered things, such as the canned food she had bought for Darius to eat. He had used some, but she had continued to bring in more as she scrounged it. Now she would eat it herself, if she had to. She also dressed and packed a change of clothing, though what she had here in Bumshed wasn't exactly clean.

Her bike was leaning against the wall of the shed, under the overhang. It wasn't in top condition, but it was functional. She hadn't ridden it much in the past year, because a bike was really kid stuff, and a teenager was not a kid. But a bicycle was the most efficient mode of transport known to man; a person on a bike used less energy than any walking animal or any traveling machine. So she would be a kid again to travel – so that she could be a woman when she got there.

Hastily assembled, she walked the bike out to the road. It wasn't nearly as late as it had seemed in the shed; actually her watch said eight o'clock. Things were hardly stirring outside. She could get cleanly away before her parents caught on.

That made her pause. How would they react to her disappearance? For she knew she wasn't coming back.

She walked back to the shed. There she dug out a pad of paper and a pencil. DEAR FOLKS: DON'T WORRY; I AM FINE. I JUST HAVE SOMEWHERE TO GO. COLENE

She tore off the sheet and set it on top of the board covering

100

the pot. Eventually someone would look in here, and then the note would be seen. That should be enough. They might put out an alert for her, but she was going where their alert could not reach. As she understood it, the ramp intersected her reality only at this spot; everything else was in other realities, no matter how similar to hers it seemed.

She walked her bike back out to the street, got on it, and started pedaling. Immediately her sense of 'whereto' went wrong. This wasn't the way.

She looped the bike and went the other way. Now it was better. It felt like going uphill, only it wasn't physical and it wasn't hard. It was like orienting on a distant light.

Actually the light was a little to the side; the street wasn't going in quite the right direction. But neither were the intersecting streets. She had to turn and go down one, then turn again.

Then she reached a region where there weren't cross streets, and had to keep going straight. Gradually her awareness of the proper direction faded. This was no good; it seemed that she had to stay pretty close to the center of the ramp, or she lost it.

Finally there was an intersection, and she turned and rode at right angles. Before long she felt it: the attuning. Good; that meant that she didn't have to stay on it all the time; she could detour and pick it up later. She might have to do S shaped figures, crossing and recrossing the ramp, but it did give her more freedom.

But was she getting anywhere? Everything looked ordinary, not magical. She had now biked more than a mile. That wasn't far, but how far would it be before something changed? She just didn't know.

Well, she would give it a real try regardless. After all, she was skipping school, and that would get her in trouble if they caught her. She had to get far enough to be sure they couldn't.

She came to a red light, and stopped. She knew that the rules of the road applied to cyclists the same as cars, and she obeyed them scrupulously. To do otherwise was dangerous. It was ironic that people who wanted to live were suicidally

101

careless about such rules, while she who was suicidal was careful. But she knew how close death was. She didn't want her blood splatted across the busy highway; she wanted it handled neatly.

She saw a car going through the intersection. It was a limousine. At the wheel was a seedy looking man; in back was a well manicured dog, sitting up high as if the car belonged to it. That made her smile.

Then the light changed to blue, and she pedaled across. She was entering a parklike section, with trees growing fairly near the pavement. She liked that. She didn't remember any park, here; in fact she didn't remember this neighborhood at all, now that she actually looked at something other than the road in front of her, but that was all right, since she wouldn't be back.

Blue?

She skewed to a stop. Then she turned and stared back, expecting to correct the glitch in her memory.

No, the green light was blue.

She resumed travel. She had never seen a blue GO light before, but that didn't mean they didn't exist. Maybe it was a faulty lens, or maybe somebody had sprayed blue paint on it.

But all the lights thereafter were blue too. Soon the red lenses turned to orange. The color scheme was definitely different!

Move over, human!

Startled, Colene veered off the road. A car zoomed by, with another dog sitting up in the rear. It was as if the dog had yelled at her!

But the yell had been in her mind.

Colene stopped under a tree near another intersection and pondered. Blue traffic lights. Dogs being chauffeured. Telepathy. Was she imagining things, or was reality changing?

A car slowed and stopped near her. The black and white head of a Dalmatian dog poked out of the rear window. *Are you lost, human girl?*

'No, thank you,' she said before she could think. 'Just resting.'

Best get on to your obedience school, the thought came. Then

102

the dog's head withdrew, the window closed, and the car nudged back onto the road and accelerated.

There was no doubt now! Telepathic dogs! 'I don't think we're in Oklahoma any more, Tonto,' she murmured, taking brief pleasure in mixing her references.

Heartened but also nervous, she resumed travel. If this was a region where dogs governed people, it wasn't what she was looking for. Evidently Darius lived somewhere beyond this. She had somehow thought the ramp would proceed straight from her place to his, but of course that wasn't necessarily so. There could be any number of different realities between, and one with telepathic dogs was evidently among them.

The dog had stopped to check on her, as a person might when seeing a lost puppy. The dogs were evidently in charge here, using human beings as drivers. And people were sent to obedience schools? She had better move on through!

But it was good to have this assurance that the Virtual Mode was in place. She had wanted to die, then had loved Darius, then had lost him and wanted to die again, and now was on her way to find him again. Girl meets man, girl loses man, girl regains man: standard story, happy ending. And if she ran afoul of that one per cent factor, fifteen years down the line, well, at least she'd have the pleasure of wearing out the romance the hard way: by loving him to pieces.

The surface of the road changed. Now it was rougher, and the cars had wheels that were more like caterpillar treads. And the animals riding in them were no longer dogs, but cats – big ones.

She paused at another intersection, waiting for the traffic to clear. Almost all of the vehicles were traveling at right angles to her route, which was maybe just as well. She had heard a couple coming up behind her, but they seemed to have turned off before reaching her.

A car came toward her, slowing. A tiger bounded out. *You will make a fine meal, tender girl!*

Terrified, Colene pedaled desperately, bumping her bike over the road-ground. The tiger leaped – and disappeared before reaching her.

What had happened? Had someone vaporized it? No, there

had seemed to be no violence, other than that being practiced by the tiger. It had just phased out.

She had ridden into another reality, where the tiger wasn't after her! It looked much the same, but was different. Her ramp evidently made the terrain of the realities merge smoothly, so she could travel along it, but the inhabitants were not continuous in the same way. That was probably just as well; otherwise there might have been an endless chain of Colenes setting out on their bicycles, all heading for the same set of Dariuses. One of each was enough!

Now she knew two more things: there was direct danger to herself in these realities, and she could get out of it by moving quickly forward. But the farther she moved, the stranger things were becoming. She could get into trouble before she knew it, and be stuck. If that tiger had caught her –

She delved into her pack and brought out the kitchen knife. Now it was not to cut her arms, but to protect her! But she doubted she would be very effective against a telepathic tiger. Surely worse lay ahead.

She realized now why so few cars had been traveling her way. She was going in the 'steep' climb through realities, and the cars were remaining in their own realities, so never reached her. But the streets going at right angles were all in whatever reality she was passing at the moment, like long rungs on a ladder.

Should she turn back? She would be safer in more familiar territory. But that would not get her to Darius. So she would have to go on, and hope she found him before she got into an inextricable predicament, as Principal Brown would put it. Or an inedible picklement, as the kids would translate it.

She rode forward. But this just wasn't cycling terrain. It was more work to ride than to walk. So with regret she walked her bike, hoping to find a better road in another reality.

Suddenly a huge bear was in front of her. It wore a woodsman's hat and held an axe. *A wild human!* it thought. *Exterminate it!*

Colene wanted to run forward into the next reality, but the bear blocked the way. She would have to retreat, and hope it would go away soon. She stepped back, and the bear vanished.

But suppose it didn't go away? Suppose it brought in its henchbears and waited for her return? She could be caught before she could move! Suddenly her life, so worthless a few hours ago, was excruciatingly precious.

She couldn't wait here long, anyway; before long something similar to a bear or a cat would come along the road, and nab her. Maybe she could hide in the forest to the side, but there were two problems with that. One was that she didn't know what monsters were in there, or what bugs. The other was that she didn't want to drift any farther than she had to from the direct ramp, because she might not be able to find it again. Then she would really be in trouble, lost in shifting realities!

Even if she managed to handle those problems, what about night? When that came, and she got tired, and had to sleep, she would be vulnerable. She had to get somewhere safe before night – and how could she find such a place, in these strange worlds? How could she trust even the safest-looking place?

I'm in trouble! she thought, fearing that she was vastly understating the case. She really should have waited for Darius to come for her!

But was he any better equipped to handle these realities? His realm was magic, not telepathy, not animal dominance. He had almost died in her reality, because he couldn't cope without magic. She feared he wouldn't do any better than she, and might do worse – which would mean that he would not survive the journey. So maybe she had better meet him half way, or three quarters of the way, to be sure they both were alive to love when they met.

Are you from afar?

There was another thought, faint but clear. Was it a tiger or a bear? It felt friendly, but that could be deceptive. Should she answer?

Why not? She was in trouble anyway. Maybe this represented some kind of help.

Yes! she thought as hard as she could.

Are you in distress?

Yes.

Are you human?

Yes. I am Colene, a human girl.

Come to me. I need a companion.

So did she! But if this was a tiger trying to lure her in, she would be a fool to go.

Also a fool to pass up a potential friend. *Who are you?*

I am Seqiro. Please come quickly; this mental contact across realities represents a strain.

Across realities? That didn't sound like a tiger! She would risk it. *How can I find you?*

I am on your path. I have felt your approach. Come to my reality, and follow my mind to my stall.

But there was the bear lurking for her. She considered briefly, then walked several feet to the side, faced forward again, and started running.

Her strategy worked. She saw a bear to the side, but by the time it turned to spot her, she was beyond its plane and the way was clear.

She forged on, trusting to blind luck to keep her out of serious trouble. The road deteriorated further, becoming a beaten path. But maybe this was ridable. She got on her bike, set her gears to the lowest ratio, and pedaled hard. Yes, she was moving well.

Here! You are passing my reality!

Oops! She turned and rode back, until the thought agreed that she was on the right plane. Then she turned to the side and followed it, walking the bike over forest floor.

Follow my thought, Seqiro sent. His signal was much stronger now. *There is some danger for you, but my thought will avoid it.*

She hoped so. She followed his thought out of the forest and to a rustic village. There were many oddly dressed people, and horses, dogs, and cats, each going about his business. She did her best to look as if she were one of them, going about her business, but wasn't sure she wasn't ludicrously obvious as a foreigner. At least this didn't look like a bear or tiger camp.

In the course of this travel, she wandered across the reality lines several times, but his mental contact remained. Sometimes she stepped across the boundary deliberately, to avoid being spotted, then back in farther along. She was getting better at using the Virtual Mode.

Seqiro led her through a back alley that passed several stalls where horses were stabled. He had used the term stall; evidently he had meant it literally. But what kind of man would live in a stall? A stable hand?

The presence of horses reminded her of her imaginary friend Maresy. Colene had always liked horses, not in the sense of riding them but in the sense of just liking them. She knew they were not considered very intelligent as animals went; cows did twice as well on maze tests. But there was a basic niceness about horses that other animals lacked. Oh there were those who swore by cats because they were cuddly and purring and quiet, but cats were actually pretty selfish creatures who made friends only with those who fed them well. Some folk swore by dogs, supposedly man's best friend, but there were thousands of dog bites every year, suggesting how thin that veneer of friendship was. There were pet birds, locked in cages or in houses; hardly any of them would remain if given a chance to fly into the wild. But horses – there was just something *about* horses. Oh, some could be mean and some could be lazy, of course. But, taken as a whole, they were better than people. That was why she wrote to Maresy Doats in her Journal. Maresy was a whole lot more serious than her name suggested.

But of course a family living in a suburb, scraping along in the middle class two-incomes-one-child mode, could not even think of having a horse. This had never been an issue; Colene had seen from the outset that it was impossible. Even had it been possible, she would have hesitated to bring a horse into such a situation, because at any moment her mother could lose her job – when her alcoholism began manifesting at her job – or her father could lose his, when he had a fight with a mistress and she made a scene that embarrassed his company. Even without one of those events, there was no love in the family, not even that one per cent romance. The family was a bomb waiting to be detonated. A horse wouldn't like associating with that. So Maresy would always be a mere dream.

Still, it was nice passing through this region, for a reason irrelevant to what she was actually doing. By the look of it, this was an ordinary primitive hamlet where horses were the main animals, instead of a reality in which telepathy was practiced. She wouldn't mind living here, near the stalls, and maybe sneaking treats to the horses when their masters weren't looking. That was the nature of girls and horses.

But she certainly hoped that her telepathic friend really was a friend, because she was getting physically tired and needed a safe place to rest. If it turned out to be another bear or tiger —

Finally she stopped at a particular stall. There was a large brown stallion in it, gazing out.

Where next, Seqiro? she thought.

Duck down and enter my stall, the thought came back. *We must explore motives.*

Enter the stall? Colene stared at the horse with dawning wonder. Could it be?

There had been telepathic dogs, cats and bears. Why not a horse? *You?*

Slowly, the horse nodded.

Something very like instant love blossomed in her heart. A tiger or bear she would not have trusted, but a horse! Of course!

She ducked down under the heavy gate that closed the stall, and came up inside. She stood next to Seqiro. He was about eighteen hands tall at the shoulder, or about six feet in human terms. Almost a foot higher than the top of her head. He smelled wonderfully horsy.

It was all so suddenly ecstatic. A mind-reading horse! What more could any girl ask?

May I pat you? she thought.

Yes.

She reached up and patted his massive neck on the left side. His mane fell to the right side, so didn't get in the way. His hide was sleek and warm. What a beautiful creature!

May I hug you?

Yes.

She reached up with both arms and clasped his neck as well as she could. She put her face against his hide and just sort of

108

breathed his ambience. He was just such a totally magnificent animal!

May I adore you?

Yes.

She felt her emotion surging into overload.

May I cry on you?

Yes.

She stood there and wept, her tears squeezing down between her face and his hide. It was a great relief.

Finally she lifted her face. *I like horses,* she thought belatedly.

I like girls.

That seemed to cover the situation.

6

PRIMA

The world seemed unchanged. He stood on the dais, within the marked circle beside the castle. But the Cyng of Pwer was gone.

He stepped out of the circle, in the direction that seemed proper. A plume-bird took wing, startled. Darius was startled too; that bird had appeared from nowhere.

No, not nowhere. Darius was the one who had stepped into its reality. The geography might be so similar as to be identical, and the animal life too – but men and creatures did not follow the same schedules here as in his own reality. So a bird had been roosting here. He had better move on before the local Cyng of Pwer spied him and asked what he was doing here. He didn't know how many others there might be like him, in these very similar Modes.

He walked on toward the rim of the disk. He hesitated, then brought out his personal icon. He squatted and drew the crude likeness of the dais of the Castle of Hlahtar. He activated the icon and jumped it to that likeness.

He made it, but it was a gut-wrenching experience. Evidently his sympathetic magic was not well attuned to this Mode.

He gazed at the castle. It looked the same, but now he doubted that it had the same personnel. If it did, could he meet himself? That promised only complication! So he decided not to approach it; he would get well away from anything similar

110

to what he knew. In fact, he should get away from the dais region, too, because if his magic stopped working, he would be stranded on a dais.

He knew where there was a lowland region that was almost level. It was almost uninhabited, too; an assortment of wild animals roamed there, and that was about all. His sword should protect him from any predators, if he remained alert.

He stepped his icon there, and immediately arrived, his gut further wrenched. But now he had another problem: he did not know where to go. Pwer had told him that there should be a feel to the right direction, and he had felt it at first. Now he did not. He had gone off the path.

But he should be able to pick it up again. He turned slowly around, concentrating, and felt a faint tingle in one direction. That should be the way to go.

He stepped in that direction. Nothing seemed to change. He continued, and saw an animal: a big reptile, one of the dragons that roamed this region. Some of them could do enough magic to blow fire, but they were no threat to a man who could do magic to douse fire, or simply conjure the creatures elsewhere.

He continued walking, and the feeling of rightness grew stronger. Good enough; he could reach the proper path without having to struggle with the impassable terrain in the vicinity of the daises.

Could he conjure himself along the path across Modes? A moment's thought made him decide not to try. Probably he had done that when he conjured himself before, which was why he had the gut wrenches. The Modes were close together; Pwer had indicated that about three paces should take him from one to another. He had conjured himself many leagues, so must have crossed hundreds of Modes. In so doing, he had almost lost the path. As he progressed on the path, his magic would fade, so it was best not to depend on it.

Were it otherwise, he might have conjured himself all the way to Colene's Mode, and fetched her back immediately. But he knew he could do no magic there. He needed to forge a path by foot, so he could bring her back the same way.

He continued until he reached the strongest sense of the

path. As he did, the terrain changed around him. The plain became a ragged slope, but not as rough as in his home Mode. He could manage.

He had been traveling, as it were, slantwise across Modes. Now he crossed them directly, following the path, and Pwer was right: about three paces took him across. He could tell because though the terrain did not change much if at all, the vegetation changed somewhat and the animal life could shift abruptly, as the first plume-bird had shown.

He passed a pair of ridges between which nestled a small clear lake. He approached it cautiously, alert for danger, because such water was apt to be a drinking hole for animals. Indeed, odd creatures did appear and disappear as he crossed Modes, while the lake remained constant. This brought home to him the fact that though for him each Mode was only three paces wide, he saw the whole of it while he was in it. The lake was in each Mode, so appeared constant, but every three paces it was actually a different lake he saw. He was not approaching the lake he saw, but the lake that would be in the Mode he would stand in when he got there.

He did get there, and there were no animals. There were fish in the water, however, so it was probably clean. He lay down and drank deeply, then filled his water bag. Water was precious!

He stepped into the next Mode. There was a wrenching in his stomach and a lightening of his water bag. What had happened?

He stepped back. There were two wet places on the ground beside the lake, where water had evidently been recently spilled. And his bag was low, and he was thirsty.

Then he remembered Pwer's warning: he could not assimilate the stuff of other Modes. Not rapidly. He could not carry anything with him across Modes except what was of his own Mode or the Mode of one of the other anchors. He could eat or drink the substance of another Mode, but it would not remain with him when he departed it, unless he gave it time to be assimilated by his body. It seemed that it was the isolation of the molecules amidst many more of his own molecules that caused them to become detached from their Mode and

112

to join his. This could happen fairly rapidly with water, and more slowly with food.

He drank again, more moderately, and waited an hour. Then he resumed his journey, and the water did not disappear from his stomach. It had already done that, to be distributed elsewhere in his body, and was captive.

Suppose he ran out of water? Then he would have to remain in a single Mode long enough to drink a lot of it, urinate it out, and filter it through sand to make it pure. That pure water would be of his system, and could travel with him in his bag. It was not the most pleasant mechanism, but necessary. Food was harder; he would not have time to excrete it and grow new plants from it, so he carried what he needed with him. He could mix it with water, expanding its mass, and it would last a good length of time.

He moved on, and now the lake was left behind him, as constant as before, while plants and animals flickered in and out of sight with each change of Modes. The animals he understood, but why the variation in plants? Probably because the animals grazed on them, so changes in animal life meant changes in plant life. Since adjacent Modes tended to be similar, if he saw a dramatic shift in plant life, he would have to be extremely cautious about the animal life, even if he didn't see it. Because it was probably nearby and the next Mode might put him abruptly face to face with it.

The glimpses he got of animals were not reassuring. There seemed to be an increasing number of dragons, and they were getting larger. They seemed to be squeezing other animals out, almost as if –

Suddenly he was caught in a net. He struggled to get free of it, but it hauled him into the air and held him. It was an animal trap, triggered by touching. He hadn't seen it because it had not existed until he stepped into its Mode, moving swiftly.

He drew his sword and started cutting the threads of it. Who could have set up this trap, and why? The second question was readily answered: it was to snare wildlife alive, probably for domestication or later slaughter. The setters of the snare had not figured on a Mode traveler passing through.

113

He completed his cuts, sheathed the sword, and let himself down through the hole he had made. He landed on the ground – and discovered himself facing a dragon. A big one. A maneater.

The creature had evidently come up while Darius was cutting himself free. He decided to risk a conjuration, because this one was big enough to eat him. He activated his icon and moved it back away.

There was a bit of wrenching in the gut, but his body did not move. He had passed beyond the range of magic already.

Well, he could escape the monster simply by stepping into the next Mode; that was what he should have done first. He started to move – and the dragon leaped.

Darius found himself on his back, with the dragon's snoot at his face. The monster could bite off his head in a moment!

Then a monkey appeared. The creature had another net, a smaller one. It put this net over Darius' head, then yanked it up as the dragon backed off. Darius had to sit up, then stand, with the net covering him from head to knees. The monkeys were in charge of this Mode?

The monkey held a cord connected to the net and walked to the side. When Darius tried to step toward the next Mode, the dragon growled and breathed down the back of his neck. That monster could snap him up in an instant; dragons had hunting reflexes. He had to walk exactly where the monkey indicated.

The path veered to the side, but the monkey guided him in a straight though not level line up a bank and into a forest of giant ferns. The dragon followed closely. The way was marked by dabs of colour on the ferns or ground.

They knew! They knew he was crossing Modes, and they were keeping him in this one!

He figured it out as he was required to scramble across the irregular terrain, hewing to the line that was this Mode's intersection with his route. They had set out nets to snare wild creatures, but also to catch Mode travelers. They could recognize the latter by their odd clothing or alien nature. Then they brought the captives in, confining them to the narrow channel. As long as they were alert, they could do it.

And what did they do with their special captives? He was surely about to find out! He doubted he was the first one; the marked special path showed that. It wasn't regularly used. Probably there were many such, so that they could bring in captives from whatever nets they were found in. With ordinary captures, they used the ordinary paths. So this was't a common occurrence, but neither was it unknown.

In due course they traveled down a sloping field and to a collection of artificial structures. They weren't exactly houses, but they weren't exactly anything else. They had sloping upper surfaces, and walls made of bars.

Most of them were empty, but some did contain creatures. It was hard to see well, because one structure tended to obscure his view of another, but there seemed to be a wide variety of animals and birds. One animal had eight legs and long antennae, but also a cowlike udder, which suggested that it was a mammal, not a huge insect. One bird had four wings, translucent and extended like those of a dragonfly, but it also had a beak and feathers.

This divergence of animal creatures intrigued him despite his present peril. As far as he knew, the animals of Colene's Mode were similar to those of his own, so he had assumed that they differed no more than did the people. He had evidently been mistaken, because he was only part of the way between their two Modes, and had seen no people and a wide divergence of animals.

Certainly it smelled of animals! The odor thickened as they approached the structures, becoming stifling. But he had no way to escape it. He did his best to tune it out. After all, it had not smelled nice in Colene's shed, because of the presence of the fecal pot, but that had not bothered him or apparently her when they were together.

Colene: how he hoped he would reach her! Whether he lived or died was less important to him than whether he was reunited with her. If only he had brought her with him! But he had been put off by the realization of her youth and her depressive nature, and had blundered terribly.

He was brought along his straight line until it intersected one of the structures. Now he saw that the thing was fairly large. Indeed, large enough for him to step inside. The monkey put him in, took his pack, sword, and all his clothing, and carried them out to the dragon. The bars slammed down, sealing him in. This was a cage!

Dragon and monkey departed. Darius looked around. He was now naked, but the air was warm and he wasn't in physical discomfort. There was straw or the equivalent on the floor, and a pot whose function he recognized from recent experience. That was all.

He checked the bars of his cage. They were set close enough together so that he could not get past them, and were firmly anchored in the floor. They seemed to be of wood or something similarly hard, perhaps cut from the stems of the big ferns. The floor under the hay was of the same substance, seamless. So was the roof. Whatever it was, it was too strong for him to bend or break. His sword might have chopped through it, but they had been smart enough to deprive him of that, as well as his food.

He tried to peer beyond his cage, but all he could see was other cages, all empty. Evidently recent trapping in this particular slice of the Mode had not been good.

But *he* had been caught! What was he to do? If he didn't get out of here soon, not being able to complete his mission might be the least of his problems. The monkeys could be building the fires for a roast.

He sat on the straw. If he got any chance, he would dive out of the cage and into the next Mode. Better to be naked and free, than risk recapture by trying to recover his clothes. But he doubted that he would get the chance.

At least now he had a notion why so few ever returned from the Modes! It wasn't that they got lost, but that they were caught and dispatched. It had not occurred to him that there could be predators among the Modes, but it was all too clear in retrospect.

There was a stir beyond the cages. He peered out, and saw a figure approaching, followed by a dragon. It was a human being!

Indeed, it turned out to be a woman. She seemed to be about forty and not unhandsome, but there were deep lines of sadness or weariness on her face. She wore what might once have been a good conventional shirt, its buttons crossing from left shoulder to right hip in the style for the unmarried, but its color had long since faded to gray and it had been patched many times. Her skirt was evidently homemade from native material, puffing out from her hips and extending to the calves; her original one must have worn out. Her feet were in sandals, and were filthy, the toenails growing down and around in a manner that might be practical in a wilderness for protection against abrasions, but was detestable aesthetically. Her hair was long and somewhat unkempt, as if maintaining appearance were pointless here. Surely that was true!

She carried his clothing, which was in a tangle. She came to stand outside his cell, staring at him. Darius would have been uneasy about this at the best of times; he was even less at ease now.

'Ung,' she said, and passed the wad of clothing through the bars. She set his pack on the ground beside her. 'Ung, ung!' She made motions as of dressing.

Human but not of his culture, obviously. Darius said nothing, because it seemed pointless. He untangled his clothing and quickly put it on.

'Ung,' she said. 'Ung pretend ung you ung ung don't ung understand.'

It was his turn to stare. Words came through clearly amidst the nonsense syllables. There was no doubt: she spoke his language, and wanted to conceal that fact from the captors. That probably meant she was on his side!

'Ung?' he asked, scratching his head.

The woman turned to the dragon and said something. The dragon exhaled steamy breath and settled down for a snooze.

'Play dumb,' the women said. 'Look blank. I am testing you for responses to see whether we can learn to communicate. The dragon doesn't understand the words, but he is watching you. If you give me away, we both are dead.'

Darius shook his head in feigned bafflement. 'Ung?'

'You are from my Mode, or close to it,' she said. 'I can tell by your clothing and supplies. Look to my right if you mean yes, and to my left to indicate no. Make no other responses,

117

except obvious ones.' She twitched her right and left hands as she spoke, clarifying the signals. 'Do you understand?'

'Ung?' he said, looking to her right.

'That is agreement. Now indicate disagreement.'

He did not move his body, but he glanced to her left.

'Good.' She stood straight and made a grand gesture of pointing to herself. 'Me Prima.'

Darius had to grab onto the bars for support. Prima! The would-be female Cyng of Hlahtar he had promised to look for! Just like this he had found her!

Actually it made sense. She would have been trapped the same way he had been, and probably many others. She must have proved useful to her captors, so they had kept her alive.

'Me Prima,' she repeated, touching herself again.

This time he responded more appropriately. 'Me Darius,' he said, touching himself. Establishing names was elementary; he had done it with Colene. But he realized that it was important not to let the captors know that he was from the same Mode as she, and that he knew of her.

'Listen closely. The dragons govern this Mode. They have hunted most other species to extinction and are desperate for new creatures to prey upon, because that is their nature. They know about the Modes, but can not travel between them. They are hoping to capture a Mode traveler who can give them the secret. Failing that, they will do what they can to restock this Mode with prey. We must work together to escape. If we do not, they will breed you to me to produce prey they hope will be more of a challenge to hunt. Will you cooperate with me?'

Darius looked firmly to the right.

'They will not let you have your sword. They will let you have your food. Magic is not operative here. Do you have anything that might be used as a weapon that is not obvious as such?'

Darius had to think about that. Then he got a bright notion. He glanced right.

She squatted and began drawing things out from his pack. 'Identify the things in your language,' she told him. 'I have to appear to be making progress. Let your eyes tell me what your weapon is.'

118

She held up a package of beans. 'Beans,' he said.

'Beans,' she repeated, and set the package down. She brought out a loaf of bread.

'Bread.' He remembered how he had been confused by what had turned out to be white (not brown) sliced (not whole) bread in Colene's Mode.

'Bread,' she repeated. So it went, item after item. Then, near the bottom, there was a tiny box with slivers of wood inside.

'Matches,' he said, looking to the right. This was the box he had gotten from Colene and brought back with him. Matches were much like magic, but were actually science, and they fascinated him.

'Matches,' she repeated, this time truly unfamiliar with the term. 'What are they?'

'Ung,' he said, holding out his hand. The watching dragon made a warning puff of steam.

She handed him one match.

Darius held it by the business end and poked into his mouth with the bare wood end. He was using it to pick his teeth!

Both the woman and the dragon looked disgusted. Evidently they had anticipated something more significant.

He reached, signaling for another. The woman gave him one more match. He stuck this in the other side of his mouth.

'This is a weapon?' she asked as she rummaged in his pack for what remained.

He glanced again to the right. Then he put the matches in a pocket.

After the woman completed the pack inventory, Darius risked telling her. 'Ung. Kublai. Ung ung.'

Now she was the one who reeled. Oh yes she knew that name! She had loved Kublai, twenty years ago.

She recovered. 'When can you use your weapon?' she asked. 'At any time?'

He looked to the right.

'Can it kill dragons?'

He looked left.

'Better in privacy?'

He looked right.

'I will come to you at night, to feed you. I can not open the cage; only a dragon can do that. But they will put me in with you if I ask, because they are aware that breeding is not instantaneous with strangers. Can you use your weapon then?'

He looked right.

She verified some words, holding up things they had identified from the pack. Then she departed. The dragon glanced at him, then settled back to sleep.

Darius lay on the straw and closed his own eyes. He had a lot to assimilate!

Dusk came, and then darkness. Prima came, carrying not only his pack with its food, but a bottle of water. She said something to the dragon, and the barred gate swung open. She stepped inside, and the gate closed. How it worked Darius couldn't fathom, except that it was under the control of the dragon. If magic didn't work here, there must be some other type of force. The dragons must have used it to establish dominance in their Mode, just as humans had used magic to achieve power in his own Mode.

'Now you must eat and drink,' she told him, making broad gestures of food-to-mouth so that the dragon could see that she was doing her job. 'And after that, if I am to remain here with you, I must make obvious attempts to seduce you, so that the dragon will know that we are potentially breedable. I realize that this will be distasteful to you because I am too old and unattractive, but our lives are at stake, so I ask you to behave in a manner the dragon will find reasonable.'

'Ung,' he said, taking bread from her. He certainly was hungry!

'As I interpret it, all you need to do to escape this Mode is to step into the next, which is just beyond this cage. If I am in direct contact with you at that time, I should be able to accompany you. This is because it is my home Mode too; were it not, I would be unable to join you regardless of our contact. We shall have to maintain contact continuously thereafter, because I fear I will slip away when we lose it, and be lost in infinity.'

'Ung,' he said around his mouthful. He saw how this could

get complicated, but if the alternative was to be trapped here, it was necessary.

'I believe that once I emerge at the anchor site, I will be secure,' she continued. 'So I will ask you to conduct me there. I realize that this will delay whatever mission you are on, but perhaps I can provide you with information that will facilitate your mission, and in this manner make up for it. I think, for example, I can enable you to avoid similar capture in the future.'

He looked to her right, indicating his interest. It had become obvious that he had entered the Virtual Mode woefully unprepared.

'Now how do you propose to use your weapon?' she inquired. 'I confess to being baffled how those two toothpicks can hurt anything.'

'They make fire,' he murmured. 'I will burn the straw, and burn through the wooden bars. It will also distract the dragons.'

'Fire!' she repeated, surprised. 'But a pyro spell won't work here.'

'This is not magic.' He spoke into his bread, so that the dragon could not see him or hear him. He hoped. 'All I'm concerned about is how long it will take to burn through the bars. If the fire is too big, I'll be burned too; if too small, the dragons will put it out too soon.'

'Correct. Here is a better way: start the fire and feign sleep. I will scream to be released. When the gate opens, you must launch yourself out, and sweep me with you across the boundary.'

Darius was impressed. That did seem to be a better way to do it. Risky, of course, but probably less so than his imperfect notion. 'Then let's do it,' he murmured. 'Say when.'

'Finish eating. Eliminate. Settle down to sleep. I will join you, but you will not yet be responsive. I will tell you when to make the fire.'

He glanced significantly to her right. Then he proceeded to stuff himself, for if their escape was effective, it might be some time before they had another chance to eat. She ate some with him, evidently trying to spark his interest in her.

121

His experience with Colene assisted him with the next stage. He did have to defecate. Prima turned her back, and he did it on the pot. The dragon seemed to be snoozing, but he knew better than to trust that.

He formed a bed of straw and lay down on it. Prima brought some more straw and joined him. Now he smelled her body odor over that of the environment. She must not have washed in years! But probably that was not her fault; the captors seemed to have little concern for the hygiene of their captives.

She made as if to take off his clothing, and he demurred with a curt gesture even the dragon could not mistake. Then she removed her worn shirt, showing her haltered bosom. It was a good one, considering her age. She took his hand and brought it to her halter, and he drew his hand back, but with less force than before. Thus the dragon could see that she was making some progress.

However, he was evidently tired, and dropped into his feigned sleep without being seduced. Prima dug in his pack and brought out his blanket-pac, unfolding it and spreading it over him. He had feared that its magic would be inoperative here, so that its thinness would offer no protection against the cooling night, but it remained effective. Then she rested quietly beside him, seeming a bit frustrated but patient.

He had almost fallen asleep for real when she murmured 'Now.'

He had the two matches in his hand. He brought one slowly out, his arm motion screened by his body and hers, and struck it against the hard wood under the straw. First it sputtered, then it caught. He moved it under more straw, setting fire to it. He nudged the straw away from him so that he would not be burned. He was in luck; there was a slight breeze, and it not only fanned the nascent flame, it moved it away from him.

Prima waited until the fire was well established. Then she screamed. It was a truly piercing sound; it was all he could do to maintain his pretense of sleep. Would the dragon believe that the scream hadn't jolted him awake?

Prima ran for the other end, shouting in what seemed to be the dragon language and pointing back at the fire. The dragon's head snapped up, the big eyes blinked, and the gate swung open to let her out.

Darius scrambled up and caught the strap of his pack as he launched himself after her. The gate began to swing closed, but Prima wasn't clear of it, and it couldn't complete the motion. Then he came through, sweeping his free arm around her waist, and rammed on to the side.

The dragon had been caught by surprise, and had made the mistake they had hoped for, but now its hunter reflexes came into play. It leaped forward, intercepting the two of them and shoving them back and down with its nose. But Darius clambered over its nose, lifting Prima with him, and they tumbled to the other side. The dragon turned to snap at them, its jaws opening – and they rolled into the next Mode. It looked the same as the other, but there was no fire and no dragon. Only the light of the moon and stars. It was as if those two things had ceased to exist. Actually they had never existed, in this Mode.

'Don't let go of me!' Prima gasped.

He had been about to. Instead he tightened his grip around her waist. 'Are you sure we have to maintain contact, if we're not actually crossing Modes?'

'No, but it's a strong likelihood. I've been trapped for twenty years; I don't want to be trapped for the next twenty.'

'But I have pulled you into my Virtual Mode,' he argued. 'You should stay on it now.'

'We must talk,' she said. 'Until then, do not let go of me. Let's get away from here; there are surely other dragons, because this is an adjacent Mode, almost identical to the one we left.'

Sure enough, he saw the outline of a dragon approaching. It looked just like the one they had escaped, but it was beyond several cages. They needed to get away from this entire set of Modes.

Arms around one another's waists, like lovers, they walked into the next Mode. The dragon vanished. They continued to walk, until the cages shrank and finally disappeared. The landscape looked the same, in the dim moonlight, but there was now no sign of artificial structures.

'We had better tie ourselves together,' he said as they paused. 'Otherwise we could lose contact by accident, if we are surprised.' He set down the pack, wondering how to put it on without letting go of her.

'There's no cord in your pack, and I have none,' she said.

'Maybe I can tear off a sleeve of my shirt, and use that,' he suggested. Why hadn't he thought to carry a good length of cord? Its advantage was obvious.

'You may need that to protect your arm from the sun.' She considered a moment. 'I have something. Put your arms around my waist.'

He did so. She turned within his grasp, so that she faced away from him. Then she leaned forward, reached behind her, up inside her shirt, and untied her halter. The front of it, loosened, dropped down against his hands. She reached inside the front and hauled it out, leaving him with her breasts on his hands. He was too startled to react. This woman was of his Mode? 'This.'

They linked arms, his left to her right, hands clasping forearms, the halter bound around the wrists in the middle. It wasn't ideal, and if they fell they could wrench their arms, but they were unlikely to let go by accident.

'As I recall, it requires more than a day to walk to your anchor, and this is night,' she said. 'It will be better to find a secure place to sleep.'

'That may be a problem. I have lost my sword, and have only one match left. A high place may be subject to predator birds, and a low place to predator reptiles. I saw each kind during my journey out.'

'Yes. We had better make weapons. I would also like to bathe.'

That was a relief! Her odor had been bad in the cage; now it was overwhelming. The folk of his Mode were normally scrupulous about cleanliness; he was glad to learn that she remained true to form.

'I passed a mountain lake not far back.'

'Were there trees nearby?'

'Yes. Not any variety I know.'

'Let's go there first. Then perhaps we can hide in a tree, after we talk.'

She seemed to have a better notion how to proceed than he did, so he agreed. He realized that this was good experience; what he was learning now should help him rescue Colene.

They moved on to the lake, proceeding carefully and quietly in the darkness. When they reached it they stripped, but remained linked. More correctly, they remained linked and tried to strip. Their shirts could not pass their linked arms. So they walked into the chill water and washed in tandem, he standing in front with his left arm reaching back, she with her right arm reaching forward. She held his shirt and other clothing while he washed. Then he held the bundle of their clothing while she stepped forward and washed. He felt distinctly awkward putting his hands on her shirt, halter, skirt and diaper, but it was necessary. This reminded him that Colene had not used diapers; she had had almost sheer panties that barely sufficed for concealment. But she normally wore trousers, so that her undergarment could never be seen by accident. The purpose of diapers, of course, was to cushion the secret region from gaze and touch, making it unfeasible to see the shape of it. Now, he was seeing everything, in a manner normally reserved only for one about to undertake sexual contact. But this was a very special situation.

Unable to do much else, he stared mostly into darkness while she washed. After she got the caked grime loose, she rinsed her hair, and though it remained tangled, it assumed better color. It was not proper of him, but linked as he was to her, it was difficult for him not to glimpse her body in the moonlight. He saw that she was lean rather than plump, but her posterior was well rounded and her breasts were of adequate mass. Kublai had said she was not a pretty woman – no, he had said she was not remarkable in appearance or personality, which wasn't quite the same – and that was true. But she had evidently had the stamina to survive twenty years of captivity and retain her ability to speak her native language, and to act promptly to escape when the opportunity presented itself. That spoke well for her personality, and in the appropriate apparel her body would be attractive enough. Perhaps he

125

had been comparing her to a young beauty, such as Colene, which was unfair.

In moments they were both shivering. They came out and shook themselves. Their clothing was dry, but they wanted to keep it that way. 'We must hug for warmth until we dry,' she said.

He was constrained to agree. They embraced face to face, their linked arms somewhat awkward to the side. He was too cold to be sexually stimulated; he was just glad for her warmth.

When they were dry enough, they put their dirty clothes back on. They scrounged for some sticks, but not for a fire; these were makeshift weapons. Then they sought a suitable tree with branches both big enough and high enough to enable them to settle comfortably above the ground. That should protect them from nocturnal ground animals, and the foliage might shield them from great birds.

It was awkward climbing with their arms linked, and awkward getting comfortably settled. Finally they sat facing each other, with their backs braced against the large forking branches of the tree, his feet wedged against knots to the side of the opposite branch, her legs lifted and spread so that her knees embraced his waist while she sat partly on his thighs. His inadequate blanket covered their shoulders.

'I could wish that I were younger,' she murmured, 'for this position would surely drive you mad.'

He remembered how Colene's naivete about the spread of her clothed legs had nearly done so. 'You are not old enough to avoid that risk. Fortunately it is too dark to see.'

'I thank you for that courtesy. However, you have seen my body. Please answer with candor: do I retain sexual appeal?'

'Yes, but –'

'I mean, allowing for my age, of course.'

'That was not the nature of my qualification. I am a man of honor.'

'I thank you again, Darius. You are very much a man of my culture.'

He tried to tilt his head back, so as to rest it against the branch behind him, but that was awkward. 'Please do not misunderstand. I think I must put my head forward, on your shoulder, to sleep.'

'Understood. We shall embrace as necessary to be comfortable.' She put her head on his left shoulder, and he put his on her left shoulder. They linked their free arms to complete the solidity of the position. Thus braced, it would be possible to sleep safely, and their closeness helped shield them from the cold. It was far from ideal, in several respects, but feasible.

'We shall sleep soon, but now we must talk,' Prima said, as if they had not been doing so all along. 'You have been most patient and accommodating. Please, if you will, tell me of your mission here. You surely have most pressing reason to risk the Modes.'

'I made a spot trip to a far Mode, searching for a woman I could both love and marry,' he said. 'I am the current Cyng of Hlahtar. I think you know the problem.'

'Indeed I do! I think you know mine, too.'

'Yes. Kublai wanted most sincerely to learn of your fate. He agreed to take my place if I would search for you as I went.'

She was silent for a moment. Then she asked: 'What is Kublai's present feeling for me?'

'I think it is not love. He has had to marry many times, and discard all his wives, until he retired. Now he has married for love, at last. But he loved you once, and remains sorry it could not be worked out. I think he holds his emotion in abeyance, expecting either to learn nothing of you, or of your death. Now of course, while he takes my place, he has had to divorce his love-wife and make her his love-mistress. She is not pleased with that.'

'I know the feeling.'

'Yes, of course.' Not only had she not been able to marry for love, she had not been able to assume the post for which she was plainly qualified.

'If I return, would he marry me?'

'But the Cyngs of Hlahtar don't marry for love!'

She merely lifted her head and looked at him in the darkness.

Embarrassed, he gave her the answer. 'Yes, I believe he

127

would. Your power would make no other wife necessary. But I understood that this was not a role you sought.'

'It was not. But I had time to think, in twenty years, and I realized that such a marriage was a better use for me than what I had with the dragons.'

'What did they make you do?'

'Very little. They were saving me for the chance arrival of another of my kind. Then I was either to discover his secret of Mode travel, or to breed with him.'

'But there is no secret!' he protested. 'The Chip must be set from the anchor point.'

'So I tried to tell them. They were not sure they could believe me. So I helped feed the captives, until their Modes expired and they could be freed.'

'Freed?'

'There is no sport in hunting a caged creature. But one that has fled the cages and gone out into the wilds can be a pleasant challenge. I was smart enough never to do that, so I survived.'

'I am glad you did. I think I would not have escaped without your help.'

'I did it for myself as much as for you. But now we must ascertain where we stand.'

'I thought we had done that.'

'No. What do you suppose the chances of your encountering me were?'

'Obviously good enough!'

She shook her head. Her hair moved against his own. 'That is not the case. There are an infinite number of Modes. How did we meet in one?'

'I was crossing Modes, until I was trapped in the same way you were. Thus there was no chance involved.'

'Not so. Infinity is broader than that. There are not only an infinite number of types of Modes, there are an infinite number of each type. An infinite number of Cyngs setting out in search of love. An infinite number of dragons trapping travelers. How is it that you encountered me, when there are an infinite number of variations of you and an infinite number of variations of me?'

That had not occurred to him. 'Perhaps it was a fortunate chance.'

'I think not.'

'What are you saying?'

'I am saying that we did not meet.'

He lifted his head, startled. 'This is humor?'

'No. I shall explain. We are from different Modes.'

'But we speak the same language! We have the same conventions! And I know of you, and you know of Kublai! Our Modes match!'

'No. Our Modes are very similar, but they surely do not match. That is why I must remain bound to you until I reach your anchor. Were I identical, I would not need such contact; once you drew me onto your Virtual Mode, I would remain on it, being of the substance of your universe. Were I too far removed, I would not be able to cross with you at all. But I am in between: close enough to cross with your help.'

'But perhaps you *are* identical,' he said.

'No. When I came close to you, and touched you, I did not step on to your Virtual Mode, though I could feel its ambience. I was one of the infinite number of near misses. So you see, there is no great coincidence in our meeting. There are infinitely more mismatches than perfect matches.'

'But then why do you want to return with me?'

'Because your Mode is also infinitely better than the alternative. At least once I am through your anchor point I will be able to remain, for your Mode will surround me far more solidly than does the Virtual Mode. A man very like the one I loved will be there. I hope he will marry me.'

'But surely you would not deceive him!'

'Surely not! I will tell him the truth, and offer him my body and my power for his disposal, as long as he wishes either.'

Darius nodded. 'I think he will accept. But he will be concerned about the fate of his original Prima.'

'She may well be traveling back to the Mode of another Darius, to marry another Kublai.' Her chest heaved with silent laughter. 'We are interchangeable.'

He did not laugh. 'But when I return, he will vacate the post, and need no Cyng wife.'

129

Her face lifted again and turned to his. 'If you return with your love, would you marry me then? I can do for you what I can do for him, and I would be discreet about your love mistress.'

Darius was startled. A power of multiplication rivaling his own! 'Why yes, I believe I would! You understand the nature of the marriage.'

'I certainly do. Consider us affianced, in that unlikely event.'

Darius sank into thought, his mind racing. He had visited the other Mode in search of exactly a woman such as this: one who could expand his power so greatly as to make it no burden, without being depleted herself. He had found her. She was not young and lovely and sweet; she was old and smart and cynical. She was not his love. She was Kublai's lost love. What a strange solution!

'You were correct,' he remarked. 'There was something to talk about.'

'Yes. There is more, but I felt it necessary to clarify our relationship as I believe it is, so as not to deceive you.'

'More?'

'I have had twenty years to ponder the nature of the Modes,' she reminded him.

'Kublai will be most interested in what you have to say.' He might be interested himself, but right now he was tired, and wanted to sleep.

'Delicately put. Let me mention just one other question, whose answer I believe I know.'

'One other thing,' he agreed.

'We are in a provocative position, physically. If this causes you to desire –'

'No. No offense.'

'That is the answer I anticipated, and prefer. We are of different generations, and thrown together only by the chance of our Mode involvement. Now we must share warmth and sleep.'

Darius was glad to agree. He relaxed, adjusting his head on her shoulder, cushioned from her shoulder bone by her shirt and hair and the thin blanket, and closed his eyes. She relaxed similarly against him, and drew him in closer for that warmth.

Her bosom touched his chest, and he became conscious of her breasts as she breathed.

His imagination shaped her body into that of Colene. He did desire a woman, and Colene was that woman. But the two of them had been hedged by imperfect understandings, and it had not been right. Were they traveling the Virtual Mode, together like this, then – well, if it had been Colene who had made that offer, this time, he would have accepted.

'You are thinking of your loved one,' Prima murmured.

'We are sharing minds?' he asked, surprised.

'Some. Bear in mind that I have similar power to multiply as you do; that is a kind of emotional interaction. It is stifled now because I am isolated from your Mode and your special Chip connection, but our minds will interact increasingly as we associate and are in close contact.'

'Surely true,' he agreed. His power had been stifled in the alternate Modes, but she derived from his own Mode, or one very similar. He had no experience with such interaction, because he had never before encountered a woman of her level of power.

'But mainly I felt the tenderness of your touching, and knew it was not for me.'

She was embarrassingly perceptive. 'It is true.'

'If I marry Kublai, I will try to pretend he still loves me. I hope that at least he desires me.'

'He has a young and beautiful and attentive wife,' he said. 'She is Koren. I impressed on her the need to be unmarried from the Cyng of Hlahtar, and she hates me. She will hate you, if you evoke his desire.'

Her body stiffened, then relaxed. 'True. I thank you for that reminder. I have no right.'

Evidently she had been quite lonely, trapped in the dragon's Mode. She had loved Kublai, and perhaps still loved him, having had neither satisfaction nor any other man to dream of. She could represent disaster for Kublai's love life. Yet she had a power that would be invaluable to any Cyng of Hlahtar, himself included.

'If I may make a suggestion –'

'By all means.'

131

'Marry Kublai, but take a lover. Make it obvious. Then it will be seen that the marriage is purely convenience.'

'That is good advice,' she said sadly. Then she was silent, and they drifted to sleep.

In the morning they were both quite stiff and uncomfortable. It occurred to him that this was indeed a provocative position, but that even had it been Colene here, it would have become relatively unexciting in this situation.

They unkinked their legs, and Prima got her skirt decorously down so that her diapers no longer showed, which was a relief. They worked their way down to the ground and stretched and exercised, jumping together to get warm.

'I must undertake natural functions,' she said. 'But we can not untie our arms.'

'What exactly would happen if we did?' he asked. 'I mean, if we are careful to remain right here in this Mode – or if I stepped across, I could return for you.'

'It might be all right,' she said. 'But my fear is that because I am now a creature of the dragon's Mode, and have no alternate Mode anchored in that, I would fall through the Modes and return there. That is a risk I prefer not to take.'

'Fall through? But if you do not walk across the borders –'

'If you will humor me while I relieve myself, I will explain in more detail.'

'As you wish.' He was sure she had good reason.

He stood facing away while she squatted to do her business and bury it in the dirt. Then she faced away for his turn. This was another firm reminder that there was little actual romance in being bound to a woman; instead the details he would have preferred to ignore were made uncomfortably evident.

Then they made a meal from his supplies, and she explained while they waited for the water they had drunk to be assimilated. 'You understand that a traveler's tenure is limited on the Chip Mode, because he gradually loses contact. If he does not return fairly soon, he never will.'

'Yes. I call it the Virtual Mode, because it is analogous to a state of functioning by that name in the Mode where I met my love. It is presumed that a traveler has been killed or lost or trapped as you were. Now that I have learned what happened to you, I consider this presumption confirmed.'

'Virtual Mode,' she repeated musingly. 'As if it is something not quite real, yet seems real. A useful concept.' She paused, evidently assimilating the notion. 'However, the presumption of the reason a traveler through the Modes does not return is not confirmed. He may indeed be killed, lost or trapped, but the mechanism is more basic than that. You are aware how you must eat and drink cautiously in foreign Modes, because you can not immediately assimilate the food.'

'Yes. I was warned, but forgot. I drank at this lake, and lost the water from my stomach. I had to do it again, and wait.'

'Precisely. Your body isolates the foreign molecules and separates them from their Mode; they must join yours. But the corollary is more dangerous: the more foreign matter you incorporate in your body, the less remains of your original substance. Eventually your body is more foreign than native, and you are unable to remain on the Virtual Mode. Then you are trapped, regardless of the rest of your situation. This happened to me.'

'But the dragons caged you!'

'Yes. They caged me and fed me, and in due course I became too much of their Mode, and could not escape. I had little choice: had I refused to eat, I would have died of starvation. They knew that. They would have done that with you. They allowed me to feed you your own food because they wished me to ingratiate myself with you. They knew that in time your food would be exhausted, and the process of assimilation into their Mode would accelerate. The very process of breathing was already beginning that.'

'Breathing!' he exclaimed.

'When you breathe, you exchange molecules of your substance with those of the air. The longer you breathe, the greater amount of foreign matter you incorporate.'

'I never thought of that! Of course you are right.'

'I have had a long time to ponder the aspects of my failure,' she said with a wan smile. 'It is not surprising that some of my realizations are new to you. I would have told you this had we remained trapped, and the dragons would have noted your reaction and seen that I was impressing you.'

'And if you succeeded in winning my confidence, you might learn from me how to cross the Modes,' he said. 'I see their logic. But you succeeded too well.'

'That was my desire. I think now that I could have addressed you directly without trying to mask it with nonsense syllables; the dragons are not highly vocal and do not really understand the versatility of it. But I was determined not to squander my only chance for escape.'

'So your body is mostly of the dragon Mode,' he said. 'But I am aware of no actual attraction of a Mode. I do not find myself sliding back to my anchor Mode when I relax. Why should it pull you back?'

'It may not,' she admitted. 'But it could work in this way: if I became separated from you, I would be unable to cross Modes toward your anchor. But I might be able to cross them toward the dragon realm, because it is as it were downhill for my present substance. Since the Virtual Mode intersects only a narrow segment of each Mode, I would inevitably stumble across and be moved back. Certainly I would not reach your anchor. My fear is that even a brief separation would prevent you from finding me, for you would not know in which Mode to search, or where within it.'

'Needle in a haystack,' he agreed.

'I do not follow your reference.'

'It is a saying I learned from Colene. They use fine needles for stitchwork, as I understand it, and should such a needle fall into a pile of hay, it would be exceedingly difficult to find.'

'That is apt. So I prefer to take no risk, being sensitized by my long captivity. I shall do my best to repay this inconvenience for you. For example, I may be able to show you how to cross Modes more safely, so that you run no further risk of being trapped.'

'That would be a great help!'

'When we reach your anchor, and I am safe there, I will fetch you mirrors. It should be easy to make a structure to hold a set of them, one reflecting to the other. When the forward mirror is poked across the border of Modes, its light could be reflected through a closed tube to the backward mirror. I think you could then see in the backward mirror the image from the forward one, not overwhelmed by the images of the Mode in which you stood.'

Darius was intrigued by the concept. 'If light can be reflected across the border, why can't we just look across?'

'I think we could, if we were not attuned to the Mode in which we stand. We need to isolate our sight from that, just as we need to isolate our flesh from it if we wish to depart it. Perhaps I am mistaken. It is a concept I played with, and I would like to discover whether it works.'

'I will certainly try it!' he said. 'If it protects me from walking into a net, this delay will have been worth it.' Then he reconsidered. 'I do not mean to imply that it is not worthwhile to rescue you.'

She laughed. 'I understand perfectly!'

She surely did. She was older than he, and not beautiful (though not ugly), but she had a good mind to go with her excellent power. He was adjusting to the notion of marrying her, when he returned with Colene. That would indeed give him love and advantage in his post, though not in the same woman. It would make his foray onto the Virtual Mode a success.

Having assimilated the water, they moved on across the Modes. Darius was now conscious of a resistance in his body, as if the foreign molecules were dragging behind. But it was so slight as perhaps to be his imagination. After all, Prima, who had twenty years' accumulation of foreign substance in her body, was having no apparent difficulty crossing. Unless it was the resistance of her substance, in contact with his, which caused the drag.

He expected their return to be slower than his original journey, but it was faster. His familiarity with the route and her eagerness to reach the anchor made for excellent progress. They did encounter a large predator at one point, but a quick dodge back across the Mode border solved that. Prima also insisted on leading the way, so that she rather than he would catch the brunt of danger. She seemed almost fearless in her cooperation.

135

When they reached the point at which he had diverged from the direct route, he explained, and she agreed as to the wisdom of that course. They retraced his route across the plain. When he judged they were close to his Mode, he conjured them to the dais of the Cyng of Pwer.

Then sudden doubt assailed him. 'How can I be sure it's *my* anchor?' he asked. 'If there are an infinite number of Darius's entering an infinite number of Virtual Modes –'

'Each should relate to his own anchor,' she said. 'Your Virtual Mode slants across Modes at such an angle that three paces separate them. When you take the final three paces, you should be at the correct anchor. My case differs; I lost my Mode, so have no such orientation and must depend on yours.'

'I hope you are right,' he said.

'And if it is a different anchor, but so similar that it accepts you, and no one can tell the difference, does it matter?'

'Of course it matters! Those awaiting my return would wait in vain, for I would be in the wrong Mode!'

'But that wrong Mode would stand in the same need of your return as your own, and your return would be as beneficial to it.'

He did not feel equipped to answer that. He just hoped it was the right one.

They reached the anchor and stepped onto the marked circle.

7

UNDERSTANDING

But why were you calling me? Colene inquired after recovering control of herself.

I need help to escape, Seqiro replied. *I felt the invitation of the Virtual Mode, and accepted it. But I must step out of my stall to utilize it, and can not without breaking it down.*

I can open it for you, she said. *The latch looks simple enough.*

The horse twitched an ear. *For your human fingers, yes. For my hoof, no.*

She stepped toward it. *I will do it now.*

He brought his nose about to intercept her. *Not yet. I will need feed and some supplies before I travel, for grazing has disadvantages on the Virtual Mode.*

But I thought horses liked to graze!

We do. But the food of other realities is difficult to assimilate, and best avoided until the journey is complete.

She was surprised. *What's wrong with it?*

When you cross realities, what you have recently eaten remains behind, for it is not of your reality.

She had packed supplies because she had been uncertain what she would find along the way. Now she was very glad she had done so!

I'm going to find my lost love, Darius, she thought. *Where are you going?*

With you.

But you may not like it in his reality!

I will like it with you.

He wasn't just saying it, he was thinking it, and the sincerity of his thought was not to be doubted. *Oh, Seqiro, you are so much more than I ever dreamed of!*

I know. I felt you coming from afar, and hoped you were human. It is a strain to think across realities, but with the Virtual Mode it is possible, and I had to find you and bring you to me.

This was sudden, but right. Colene knew her life had changed, in a way she had never expected. She had loved Darius quickly; she loved Seqiro instantly, but in a different way. Instant love was supposed to be foolish, as it was based on infatuation rather than knowledge, but with direct mind contact, that rule was irrelevant.

Soon she learned his situation, because he made a comprehensive explanatory mental picture: this was a reality in which the horses governed, just as the dogs, cats and bears governed some of the realities she had passed. They did it by telepathy, imposing their will on human beings. To an outside observer, this was much like a human reality, but here the humans acted at the behest of the horses, feeding them, exercising them and guarding them.

But Seqiro had too much of a mind for leisure. He wanted to explore new frontiers and gain new understandings. He also tended to be generous to his handlers. This had made other horses look bad, and finally they had acted by removing his handlers, effectively confining him to his stall. He was being pressured to change his ways. He had resisted – and then felt the questing of the Virtual Mode.

There had been such questings before, but he had not cared to risk them. Now he had to, for it was his only likely escape, physically and mentally. It was no coincidence that this connection had come; only those in great need established Virtual Modes, and only those in similar need attuned to them. They were like calls across the realities: I NEED YOUR HELP. SHARE MY ADVENTURE. But such adventure could be extremely strange. Thus only specially receptive minds felt the questings, and only the most strongly motivated folk accepted them.

But there was serious risk entailed, for though he knew he could escape via the Virtual Mode, he did not know who had instituted it, or for what purpose. He did know that other animals had mental powers, and that many of these were predator species. If this happened to be a tiger mode, he would have difficulty relating and would probably perish. If, on the other hoof, it was a compatible species, he might do very well, and gain intellectual satisfaction.

When he had tuned in to her approach, he had perceived what seemed to be a human personality. Could it be a human mode? That possibility had not occurred to him before, but of course any species could institute a Virtual Mode if it knew how. He had never noted any telepathic power in the human kind, but it was certainly possible that it existed in variants of that species in distant realities. Certainly a human animal could be compatible; human animals were a horse's best friend, here.

Then it turned out that the approaching human was only potentially telepathic. This was very promising, because such a human would need a horse for mental contacts, just as a horse needed a human for physical chores. Would the human be amenable to such cooperation? It was female, and females tended to like horses for themselves, apart from their power; that was another positive sign.

By the time Colene reached his stall, he had the answer. The sheer chance of the Virtual Mode had brought him the ideal companion. Their two realities might be different in most cultural and practical respects, but they aligned in what counted most for this purpose: the affinity of horses and girls. It was a bond that needed no further justification.

Yes, Colene agreed.

Now you must get my things, for I can not do it, and bring them to me, so I can travel with you.

But I am limited to a ten-foot swath, she protested. *If I step out of it, I will leave this reality and lose you.*

Not once you pass through the anchor, as you did when you entered my stall. Now you are in my reality, until you approach it from the other side.

She found that hard to believe, but it turned out to be true: she could now leave the stall and cross the aisle without losing track of him. She was now in his reality, all the way.

They got it organized: she would hide her bicycle in his stall, then fetch his feed and supplies, then open his gate and they would depart his anchor, as he called it, and resume progress toward her destination. Seqiro had no destination for himself; he merely wished to be free to explore and learn, without suffering undue hardship.

He made a mental picture for her, how she should dress and deport herself so as to pass unnoticed among the local attendants. Any human folk she should ignore, but she would have to respond to any equine queries. She should indicate that she was on private business for her steed, and move on.

The uniform was simple: a loincloth, cape and sandals. There was a supply shed near the stall; she went and changed, under his mental guidance. She removed her own clothing, then put on the loincloth. It circled her waist once, looped into two ends in front, and one end passed down between her legs and up and over in back. It rather resembled the cloth worn by the American Indians, being supremely simple and functional. When she had that properly wrapped, she donned the cloak, which was a circle with a hole in the center; it came down to about her waist. Then sandals, each one fashioned of two slabs of wood linked by cord, for heel and toe, and a loop of cord for the ankle. Again: about as simple and functional as clothing could be. Obviously the human folk of this reality did not rate fancy outfits.

Then she donned the hat. This was what identified her status and affiliation. It was like a beanie with a hanging tassel, and the manner the tassel fell indicated her degree of autonomy. Some humans had more responsibility than others, and could act without constant direction from their horses.

Now she walked to the granary for the feed. She passed other humans, who were similarly garbed. They ignored her. She knew they would not have, had she appeared publicly in her own clothing. Had Seqiro not been guiding her as she first came onto these premises, she would have run afoul of others.

The granary was stocked with bags of grain. *Take two, if you can carry them*, Seqiro thought. *Each represents approximately one day's feed, and I will need eight.*

She picked up two, putting their straps over her shoulders. She walked back with them and set them in Seqiro's stall. She made another trip, bringing two more. She was surprised how easy it was; others seemed not to see her at all. She could take the whole granary, load by load, and no one would care. She tossed her head, feeling carefree for the moment; this was fun in its way. Her cap almost fell off, and she had to jam it back.

Then someone did notice. It was a young man. He glanced passingly at her, did a doubletake, and approached her. He stared at her hat.

Seqiro — something's wrong, she thought, hoping he was tuning in. She could not broadcast her thoughts; it only seemed like it. He was able to think to her alone, so that others of his kind did not know he was breaking confinement, but he might not do that continuously now that she knew what she was doing.

I am here.

She pictured the situation, hoping she didn't have to put it into words, because that would take too much time.

Give me your eyes.

Eyes? could he see through her eyes? She relaxed, trying to let her mind go blank. She hoped that was enough.

Her eyes moved on their own. They cast about, then focused on the man. *He is looking at your tassel. It must have changed position.*

Oops! I did that without thinking.

He is sexually interested. Your tassel must be in the position of urgent invitation.

She had done that when she so blithely tossed her head? Sexual invitation? *I didn't know it could say that!*

There is no spoken language among humans of this reality. Signs of several types suffice. We allow humans to choose their own times and partners for procreation, provided they are proper workers. You signaled him that you find him desirable and wish to conceive by him.

What disastrous luck! *I don't want sex with him! How can I get out of it?*

That will be difficult without causing a commotion. Human males are unsubtle creatures.

What else was new! *I don't care how! Just do it!*

Seqiro considered, while the man attempted to embrace her. Her two bags of grain got accidentally-on-purpose in the way. But that dodge would not last long. He was starting to untie his loincloth. *Hurry!* she thought.

Smile and make a fist. Move it slowly down, then open your hand.

She did as bid. The man watched intently, then did the same. Then he got out of her way.

She walked on toward the stall. *What did I tell him?*

That you would meet him here at sundown with your loincloth off.

But I don't want to do that!

We shall be gone by then.

Oh. *But I didn't mean to lie to him either! That's not right.* Actually there were qualifications; sometimes a lie was necessary. It depended on the situation.

I will mind-touch another female and suggest to her that one who finds her desirable will be there at that time.

So she would go to meet the man. That might do it. Obviously he had no great prior relationship with Colene! *But I thought you couldn't telepath to other humans.*

I can do so. But my own servitors have been confined, and it is bad form to mind touch others. However, a subtle touch of the mind of a female not otherwise occupied should pass unnoticed. It is any effort to gain freedom for myself that the authorities are guarding against.

But I'm helping you do that!

He made a mental suggestion of unconcern. *You are not of this reality. They do not know of you.*

And that made all the difference for them both! She needed help, he needed help, and they both needed to have nobody else know what they were doing. *I guess it's all right. I hope she gives him a good time. I never meant to be a tease.*

When he sees her without her loincloth, he will not care about any other matter. This is the nature of humans.

These were primitive humans, she realized, stultified by having no real power over their own affairs, no pun. But perhaps not much different from those of her reality. She knew boys who would grab any girl they could, and girls who would tease unmercifully. She had done her share, when she got that key for Darius. In fact she had done more than her share of teasing when she had come to sleep with him in her bottomless nightie and told him no sex.

Straighten your tassel.

She paused to do it. She didn't need any more hot encounters!

She finished hauling the grain and got to work on the other things. There were small tools, and bags of water, and a kind of harness so that he could carry the things on either side of his body. She followed his mental guidance and got the harness put on correctly and the things set in it, working with far greater facility than she ever could have by figuring everything out for herself. This mental contact was like riding the bicycle: it tripled efficiency in a fun way.

She went for other things, and brought them back and put them in their loops in the harness. The horses were mental creatures, here, but obviously they could handle physical work too. It was probably easier than making the relatively puny humans do it. The humans were for minor chores.

She loaded her bicycle on top of his other things, because he thought she would be unable to use it in this vicinity. She was amazed at how much of a load he could bear, but he was unconcerned.

But as she was fetching one of the last items, a block of salt, there was a different mind touch. *What are you doing?*

That wasn't Seqiro! Which meant it was another horse. Which meant trouble. What was she to do? She shouldn't answer, but if she didn't there might be trouble too.

She kept her mind quiet. As far as she knew, a thought had to be conscious to be read. The ordinary mind was such a jumble of this and that and reactions and temporary concerns that it was hopeless as far as any outside perception went. But when she made something conscious, she formulated it, and that was what Seqiro read. So if she formulated no response, the other horse should find her mind a muddy slate. She hoped.

Identify yourself, the thought came imperiously.

Could she risk a thought directed to Seqiro? She doubted it,

143

because she wasn't sending, he was reading, and the other horse could do the same. Maybe Seqiro was able to read the other thought, so already knew. In that case he probably couldn't send to her, because the other horse would pick it up. The other horses might not even know it was Seqiro she was working for; that was why they had to inquire. So she maintained her mental silence, or at least her mental mud. In fact, she should stop thinking of his name, in case they picked that up. It was best if they thought she was just a simple human intruder stealing things.

Pain lanced through her. It felt like what she thought a heart attack would be, hurting from shoulder to gut. The other horse was whipping her with its mind!

The block of salt fell from her twitching hands. She staggered and almost fell. These horses did have ways to enforce their demands!

Identify!

Instead she focused on her legs, and broke into as much of a run as she could manage. She had to get to Seqiro's stall before that creature knocked her unconscious or worse. The boss-horses must have caught on that something was happening, and were investigating.

Now she heard rapid human footsteps. They were summoning the minions! She had to reach Seqiro before the others intercepted her.

But as she rounded a corner, she saw that she had not made it. Three young men were between her and Seqiro's stall. How was she to get past them, even if the other horse didn't blast her mind?

A notion percolated up through her mud-mind, and she put it into effect before a horse could read it. *Humans! They are catching me!* she thought loudly. That should satisfy the horse that he didn't need to stun her; the situation was in hand. One threat sidetracked, maybe.

Meanwhile she reversed her course and broke into a run, away from the men. It was also away from Seqiro's stall, but that was part of the point: if they didn't know about Seqiro, this would keep the secret. Maybe she would be able to lead them astray, then duck back to the stall unobserved.

She whipped around the corner she had just rounded from the other direction. There was a supply nook here; she knew because she had recently fetched things from it. She swung herself into it, ducked down, and held her breath.

The men rounded the corner and pounded down the aisle. They ran right by the nook. It had worked! She had given them the slip by acting fast – by stopping here immediately after turning the corner, when they expected her to keep running. They couldn't read minds; they depended on the horses for that, and meanwhile the horses thought the humans had the situation in hand. She was slipping through a crack.

She resumed breathing, cautiously. She listened, and heard only the receding footsteps. Good enough.

She stepped out of the nook, and walked around the corner. The way was clear. She approached Seqiro's stall. She knew that at any moment things would heat up again, so she wasted no time. She reached into the supply shed near his stall and fetched her clothing and pack.

She came to stand before his stall. Was it safe to think a clear thought yet? She doubted it. Better just to get on with the escape without further mind talk.

She reached for the bar which only human hands could remove, not hoofs. It came up, releasing the gate.

The grain and supplies would have to be enough; she couldn't chance going back for the salt. She got her pack on her back, stuffing her original clothing into it; there was no time to change now, either. She pointed to the aisle before the stall, indicating her eagerness to go before anyone returned. She hoped Seqiro agreed.

Then she heard something. She looked back.

There were two more men, barring the way. They held pitchforks in a manner that made them look exactly like weapons.

Now we know whom you serve, the hostile thought came. *We gave you the chance to show us.*

Go, Seqiro! she thought desperately. She realized that their mental silence had been for nothing; the boss-horses had out-tricked them. *Before they can attack you!*

Seqiro started to move out. The men moved to bar his way,

the tines of the pitchforks orienting on his head. They were the servants of horses, but not of Seqiro.

Colene ran out ahead. 'Get away! Get away!' she cried, hoping to startle them into retreat just long enough to let Seqiro out of the stall.

Instead one man dropped his fork and grabbed her, while the other continued to hold his tines at Seqiro's eye level. They were under expert control, all right. They had neither startled nor panicked.

She struggled, but all she did was get her cape jammed up against her neck; the man was strong. So she tried another tactic: she twisted some more, deliberately causing her cape to ride up farther, exposing her breasts. 'See how nice I am,' she said. 'Watch me, not the horse.'

The man holding her looked down, interested. He evidently did not understand her words, but he could see her body well enough. The other one was looking too, now, his fork dropping low. Colene both loved and hated herself for doing this; it was akin to the way she made others laugh while she thought of the blood flowing from her wrists. She delighted in the power of her body to make men stare, while knowing that she was cheapening herself in the process.

Then, suddenly, the second man forgot her and turned back to Seqiro. The other horse had taken control of his mind! The horses got no sexual thrill from seeing her torso. The fork lifted again. But the man holding her did not let go. Instead he started to drag her back, away from the horse.

Go, Seqiro! she thought again. At least he would get free.

Then the man with the fork doubled over, the weapon clattering to the floor. The one holding her dropped similarly. *Go, Colene!* Seqiro thought back at her.

She realized that Seqiro had used his own power of stunning on the men, now that there was no point in further mind silence. She caught her balance and ran for the stall. She had to go into it, and then out of it on the Virtual Mode. Like passing the other way through a tunnel to another valley.

But before she got there, the other horse stunned her too. It was like a hammer blow to the head; she felt her consciousness fleeting. Just as the other horse had not been able to protect

146

its minions from Seqiro's blows, Seqiro could not protect her from the blow of the other horse.

But it wasn't quite complete. The other horse was farther away, so some force was lost. She fought to hang on to what she could before it overwhelmed her. If she could make it through before losing consciousness –

She found herself falling into the stall. She had made it! But now that she was down, she could not get up. Her body would not respond. She could only lie here, at the anchor but not through it. So close, so far!

Go, Seqiro! she thought again.

Something brushed her face. It was the end of his tail. She grabbed onto it and clung with what she hoped was a death grip.

She felt herself being dragged forward, out of the stall. She was unable to fight any more.

She found herself face down in the aisle. *Rise, Colene,* Seqiro's thought came urgently. *Get on me.*

She lifted her head. Only a few seconds had passed, she thought, but the men were gone. What had happened?

Up! Up!

She responded sluggishly to his thought. She dragged herself to her hands and knees, then caught hold of part of Seqiro's harness and hauled herself up that.

A horse appeared down the aisle. It looked surprised.

Hold on. Seqiro stepped forward, dragging her with him. In a few steps the other horse disappeared.

At last she caught on to what was happening. They were crossing realities! Seqiro had dragged her from the anchor into another reality on the Virtual Mode, leaving the men and horses of his own reality behind. Perhaps that change had eased the pressure on her mind, allowing her to recover a bit. But the adjacent reality was very similar, with more telepathic horses, who would surely interfere if they realized what was happening, so they had stepped into a third one.

Buoyed by that realization, she clung to the harness and made her legs move. She started to walk beside Seqiro. The motion helped restore circulation and clear her mind.

147

They turned and walked down the aisle, then turned again at the corner and resumed crossing realities. The stalls began to change appearance. They were on their way!

Colene's head cleared. Apparently the other horse's stun-thought had done no physical damage.

They left the village, or maybe the village just faded away in the new realities. They were now in open countryside, with some trails going who-knew-where. It was nice. She realized that the details of her own anchor reality must have been constantly changing similarly, when she started out. She had been focusing only on the road ahead, and had been embroiled in her own confused thoughts, so had paid almost no attention to her surroundings. Also, it had been morning, in the suburbs, with little traffic, so she had not seen cars popping in and out of existence at first. From the first ten feet, she had been in a far weirder environment than she had realized!

'Say, maybe we can find a salt block out here, to replace the one I dropped,' Colene said brightly.

That will not be effective, Seqiro replied. She realized that she had spoken rather than thought, but it seemed to make no difference: he tuned in to her focused thoughts, and she had to focus them to talk. In fact, that was easier.

'Why not? Salt is salt, isn't it? It won't hurt you just because it's from another reality?'

It will not hurt me. But we can not carry such a block across realities.

'Now wait a minute! You explained about not being able to eat anything in other realities, but you're carrying a whole big load of supplies across realities right now, just as I am.'

These are from our anchor realities. You may carry substance from your own reality with you, or from my reality, and I may carry from either reality, but not from the intervening realities.

'Are you sure? These realities seem pretty solid to me.'

It is easy to demonstrate. Pick up an object.

Colene stooped to pick up a pretty stone. She had always liked stones, and not just the pretty ones; she knew that each stone was a fragment of something that had once been much larger, and had formed by dint of terrific pressures or unimaginably long time or both. How was it described in class?

Metamorphic, which meant being squished; sedimentary, which meant settling in the bottom of the sea; and igneous, which meant being squeezed out like toothpaste around a volcano. But that was really one of the other two kinds, because it had to have started somewhere else before getting cooked under the mountain. So each stone had its history, and every stone was interesting in its own way. She wished she could collect them all. This particular one looked like mica, which was about as appropriate as it could be.

Carry it across realities.

They stepped forward. The scenery barely changed, but the stone vanished.

Startled, Colene looked back. There was the stone on the ground, where she had picked it up. But she knew that what she saw was not the stone she had picked up; it was the one of this reality. She could not see across realities, as she had discovered when the bear appeared before her. If she stepped back, she would then see the rock she had picked up.

So she stepped back. The rock was on the ground, but not where it had been. It was in the path where she had dropped it. Except that she *hadn't* dropped it.

'So I crossed, but it didn't,' she said, turning back to face Seqiro.

That is correct. We are on the Virtual Mode, and we can transport only substance from our own realities, because the Mode is tied in to them. Other realities have only partial effect on us, and we on them.

Colene stared. She was receiving his thoughts, but he was not there! The countryside was empty.

Then she caught on. She stepped toward him, and as she crossed into the next reality he reappeared.

She went to him and hugged him again. 'Point made, Seqiro,' she said. 'I guess I just hadn't thought it through. I hadn't tried to pick up anything, or eat anything – brother! I guess food would vanish the same way, wouldn't it!'

Yes, it should. My understanding is that it may be possible to retain the substance of intervening realities if it is digested, but that there is danger in doing that.

149

'Let's not risk it! Oh, I'm glad I met you! I would have been in trouble pretty soon, just from ignorance.'

It is no shame to be ignorant, when you lack a source of information.

They resumed their walk, angling toward the route she had been following before she detoured to meet the horse. 'How is it that you know all this, when you haven't done this before?'

I learned it from reading the minds of other Virtual Mode travelers.

'But other horses don't seem to read minds across realities. How can you?'

It is quite limited. I could read your mind because we share this particular Virtual Mode. I can read the minds of other creatures only when we intersect their particular realities. The other horses of my reality can not perceive the Virtual Mode, because only I am its anchor in my reality.

'Just as only I am the anchor in my reality,' she said. 'And Darius is the anchor in his reality. Only it's the place too, isn't it? Because otherwise when we left our realities, the anchors would fade away.'

Correct. The anchor place becomes inoperative when the anchor person departs; only when the two are together can the connection be invoked or abolished.

'Abolished? You mean it won't last?'

It will remain until you return and renounce it, just as you accepted it at the start. Or until the Chip that is the source of the full Virtual Mode is changed.

'That would be at Darius' end.' She considered as they entered a forest and climbed a slope. When the way became difficult, she explored ahead a little to find a better passage for Seqiro's bulk, because he weighed about a ton, literally, and could not squeeze through places she could, especially with his load making his body wider. 'You read the minds of folk on other Virtual Modes before this one, though you were not part of those Modes?'

This seems to be my special ability. I have always sought to explore the unknown, and when I became aware of a trace mental current I could not identify, I sought it avidly. Perhaps others of my kind could do the same, but they have had no interest. In time I was able to fathom enough of the occasional Virtual Modes to understand their nature. I learned that I could join one, if I wished, if I exerted my will at the time it was being formed. I decided that I would do so, when the time was right – and this was that time.

'I'm glad you did,' she said sincerely.

I am glad it was you who was on it.

She turned and hugged him again. 'I hope you don't mind all this physical contact, Seqiro. I – I guess I have this need, and you're so wonderful –'

I have not before been loved by a human girl. I feel your emotion, and I revel in it.

'I revel too,' she said. 'I never knew I'd meet you, and I never want to lose you.'

I see no immediate need for us to separate. We shall find Darius, and then I will remain with you if you desire. There is no conflict between me and your human contacts.

'No conflict,' she agreed. 'But suppose it is dull for you, in Darius' reality? You want to learn new things, and magic might not be to your taste.'

Then I can embark on another Virtual Mode.

'But then we would have to separate, because I'll want to stay with Darius forever and ever!' she protested.

Unless he too wished to explore farther on a Virtual Mode.

She hadn't thought of that. 'Well, first we have to get there. From what I've seen so far, that's not necessarily a cinch.'

True. We are entering the region of telepathic carnivores. I can feel their thoughts as we progress.

'Oh! Can they hurt you?'

That depends on their size. I would prefer not to get bitten or scratched.

'And you can't read their minds until you're in their reality,' she said. 'So a tiger could pounce on you by surprise. But not if I go ahead.'

So it can pounce on you? We had better go together.

'Maybe I can get a weapon to fend off – oops, but I can't carry it across realities!'

My hoof knife may serve.

She dug out the knife. It was a solid, ugly thing. 'I don't

know. Most of my experience with knives has been cutting myself, not others. I don't know whether I could use it effectively against a tiger or bear.'

With my direction you could.

'You mean you could tell me in my mind? But still I might miss, or drop it, or something. Girls really aren't much for physical combat.'

Allow me to demonstrate. Pretend that tree is a tiger.

Colene took the knife and stepped to the side, toward the tree, remaining in the same reality. 'Okay, it's a tiger. Suddenly I see it, and it sees me, and it gets ready to spring and I panic and –'

She ducked down, then straightened like an uncoiling spring. Her hand snapped violently forward. The knife plunged into a knot on the trunk of the tree.

Colene fell back, letting go of the knife, shaking her hand, for it had taken a jolt. The knife remained in the tree. She had thrust with more speed and force than she had known she possessed. 'What –?'

I guided your body. We are experienced in controlling humans.

'And that tiger has the knife through his snoot!' she exclaimed, amazed. 'I didn't hurt the tree much, but that tiger would have had one hell of a surprise!'

I believe the knife will be an effective weapon for you.

That was the understatement of the day! Colene went to the tree and tugged at the knife. It wouldn't come. She pushed up and pulled down on it, trying to wiggle it free, but the wood clung to it. Then Seqiro sent a thought, and she wrenched and twisted with special force and skill, and it came out. She had physical ability beyond what she had thought were her limits. Seqiro seemed to bypass her restraints and draw on her full potential.

Holding the knife, she proceeded with more confidence. Actually the chances of encountering a bear or tiger right up close by surprise were small; her episode with the bear might have been the only one that would happen.

You thought of cutting yourself, Seqiro thought. *I do not understand this.*

She laughed self-consciously. 'I'm suicidal. It's a secret, but

152

I think I'll have no secrets from you. I think about death a lot, and blood. Or I did, before I met Darius. Before I got on the Virtual Mode.'

I still do not understand. Why should you wish to die? You are a comely and intelligent young woman.

'Well, that gets complicated, and maybe I don't know the whole answer myself. I don't think you'd like me as well if you saw what's down inside me.'

I read a wellspring of pain. This does not surprise me. You would not have undertaken the Virtual Mode if you had been satisfied with your situation. Think through your pain while we travel. Perhaps I will be able to help.

She laughed bitterly. 'Only if you could make me forget!'

This I could do.

Startled, she realized that it was probably true. He could read her mind, and could make her body perform in a way it never had before. Why not block off a bad memory?

'Okay, Seqiro. But stop me if you get disgusted, because I don't want to make you hate me. When I told Darius how I was suicidal, he –' The pain of that misunderstanding and separation cut her off. At least Darius had changed his mind, and set up the Virtual Mode so they could be together again. She knew there were still problems, because he had to marry a woman with a whole lot of joy, but if she could just be with him, things would work out somehow.

She turned her mind back to the times of special pain. There were several, and she didn't know what related most directly to what or how they tied in with how she felt later. Maybe they really didn't mean much; maybe she had reacted the wrong way, or maybe they shouldn't have bothered her. *Would* they have bothered her, if her folks' marriage hadn't become a shell, forcing her to seek elsewhere for emotional support – which she hadn't found? Maybe the whole business was too dull to review, and she should have forgotten it long ago. Maybe worse had happened to others and they had shrugged it off, and Colene was peculiar to have failed to have done that.

'I don't know. Maybe this is a bad idea. I would feel foolish just speaking some of this stuff, and –'

153

Then feel it. I am attuning to you and learning to read your nuances. I can read your memories, if you allow me.

He could do that? He could reach deep into her and see her most secret things, if she did not resist? That was scary! Yet she remembered lying with Darius, telling him he could touch her breasts but not her genital region, and he had done neither. Then later she had offered it all to him, and he had not taken it. She had respected him for that, yet also been annoyed. It might have been better if he had been unable to control himself. That would have given the control to her, odd as that seemed considering that he would be having his will of her. He had not, and so she had not had her will of him, which wasn't quite the same.

Spreading her legs for Darius. Spreading her mind for Seqiro. What was the difference? One was a secret of the body, the other a secret of the mind. Of the two, the mind was more private. Yet it was something she wanted to do, wanton as it might reveal her to be. She wanted to tell *someone*, just as she had wanted to show her body to someone. To lay the guilt bare, just because it was there.

'Okay.'

She laid open her mind. It traveled back two years.

She was twelve years old, and visiting Catholic relatives in Panama, in the Canal Zone. One parent was Catholic, so maybe that made her one too, but she wasn't sure whether it did or whether she wanted it to. She went to Mass on Sunday, undecided and really not caring a whole lot. She just loved visiting here, where everything was so much nicer than back at home. If church was part of it, well, it was worth it.

And it did make her feel very close to God. God loved the sparrow as He loved His Son. Surely He loved this whole region, and that was why it was so nice. The American enclave was beautiful, very like paradise, with lovely gardens and ultimate contemporary luxury. After a distance it faded to the natural landscape, which was not manicured but which remained interesting in its tropicality. Every palm tree was a novelty, to one raised in Oklahoma.

She walked to the nearby native village, curious how the

154

Panamanians lived. Was it the same as the Americans, or different in some intriguing way? They must be very happy, living in a place like this.

Nothing in her life had prepared her for what she saw in that village. The houses were huts with thatched roofs and dirt floors. The people were filthy, their clothing odd. Naked children of both sexes ran wildly in the streets. Young mothers held soiled babies to their bare breasts, nursing them in public. There were sores on the children's legs, scabbed over, with flies clinging to the crust. Insects gathered around their mouths, and no one even bothered to brush them away. It was horrible.

She rushed back to the enclave, back to the church. 'A priest, a priest!' she cried. A priest came to her; perhaps this was confession.

Tearfully, she expressed her feelings of shock and grievance. Suddenly she had seen the real world, right next to paradise. It wasn't better than what she had known, it was worse! It had been hidden from her. Hurt and outraged, she wept bitterly. She felt betrayed. She blamed the church, she blamed the priest, she blamed herself, and she blamed God. Everything was wrong, and she wanted this wrong to be corrected.

The good father was patient. When she wound down, he spoke softly and kindly to her. 'My child, you have seen reality, and it is as uncomfortable for you as it is for all of us. You now have a decision to make. Whatever you have or will get in the future, you may give equally to each poor Panamanian. It is possible to give each one a good meal for one day. Then you will be just as poor as they are. You are allowed to do this, but you are not required to give up your birthright.'

It was her first real lesson in logic, and a giant one. She had thought herself a fast learner, but now she saw how slowly she was learning about reality. Even then, she did not appreciate how much more she had to learn.

She remained shaken when she returned home to the States. She had not been satisfied with her life, and was less satisfied now that the crevices in her parents' marriage had opened into significant faults. Yet she had material things and good health, which was much more than what she had observed in the villagers. What good would it have been to have a unified family, if she had to run naked and hungry in the streets, the flies eating at her open sores? She had too much, and she felt guilty for being dissatisfied.

She went again to a priest. He advised her to donate some of her spare time to work at a charitable institution. She did so, helping out as a junior candy-striper, bringing mail, newspapers, drinks and phone messages to the patients. She had a pretty little uniform and the patients liked her. She was, some said, a breath of fresh air in hell.

For these were not people in for pleasant recuperation following hangnail surgery. This was the accident ward, and some patients were bandaged all over, in casts, or with amputated limbs. Some could not move at all, yet their minds were whole. She read to them from the newspapers, and they appreciated it. She was doing good; she was giving back to the world some of what she owed it.

She was moved to the Sunday morning shift. The wee hours: midnight to six AM. This wasn't properly candy-striper business, it was more like Gray Lady business, but few cared to take those hours, and she volunteered. The doctors knew she was underage, but she was a good worker and mature for her age of just thirteen, so they did not make an issue of it. The nurses needed the help, and it wasn't as if she was alone. So when patients were restless, the nurses did not force sleeping pills on them, they had Colene come in and read the paper. As often as not, that did put them to sleep, and it was always appreciated.

One man was recovering from abdominal surgery. He had fallen on a spike and punctured his gut; they had had to cut out the affected intestine and sew the ends together. He had lost a lot of blood, and they didn't have enough of his type. Infection had set in. But he was tiding through, though too weak as yet to lift his arms. When the nurses were busy at the far end of the ward, he spoke to Colene: 'Not that dull stuff. There's a novel under my mattress. Read me that.'

She felt under the mattress and found it. A visitor must have left it for him, or read it to him during the day. There was a marker in it. She opened it at the marker and started reading.

156

It was an erotic novel. Colene was fascinated. She had never read anything like this, and knew she wasn't supposed to. The four letter words were there, and not as expletives. The man didn't know how young she was, probably. She did not let on. Instead she read the text as it was, about steamy hot women who approached virile men with indecent offers, and amply fulfilled those offers. Colene learned more about raw sex in one hour (with pauses; she had the wit to switch to the newspaper when a nurse came within hearing range) than in all her prior life. She learned exactly what men did with women behind closed doors, squeeze by squeeze and inch by inch. She was doing the man a favor, but he had done her a much greater one, inadvertently: he had completed her education in a forbidden subject. She was grateful.

A week later, wee Sunday morning, she read to him again. The marker was well forward of the place she had left it, but that didn't matter; plot was the least of this story. This time she read about man, woman, and animal, and it was a further education. It was as if God were rewarding her for her good work by sneaking in this secret information she so valued.

The third week the man was gone; he had recovered enough to be moved to another ward, along with his book. A new patient was in the bed: a perfect young man with a bandaged head. He had shot himself, trying to commit suicide. This, too, fascinated her. She offered to read for him, but the nurse told her not to bother. 'He's in a coma. He'll die soon. He's a vegetable. We are waiting for him to die.'

'But he's so handsome!' Colene protested, as if that counted for anything in this ward.

The nurse laughed. She was old, with decades of grim experience; she had seen death hundreds of times, and was callused. She lifted one of the man's legs and let it drop with a thud onto the bed. 'Look, he is as good as dead. He can't feel, see, or hear. Don't waste your time.' She went on about her business.

But Colene lingered, unwilling to believe that such perfection of body could simply die. Why had he shot himself? What reason could someone this handsome have to want to die? It was a mystery that lured her moth-like to a candle flame.

She bent over him. 'Don't die, elegant man,' she whispered. 'God loves you – and I love you too. You are too beautiful to die!'

Suddenly his eyes opened, focusing on her. Colene was startled and frightened, for it was the first motion he had made on his own. She ran from the room and told the nurse. 'He's conscious! He looked at me!'

The nurse returned with her. She checked the man's pulse and eyes. There was no reaction. 'You are mistaken,' she said gruffly. 'There is no change in him.'

Colene couldn't believe it. She *knew* the man had looked at her. She went to the bed and took the patient's hand. 'Please open your eyes,' she pleaded.

His eyes opened. But when he saw the nurse, his eyes closed. Tears trickled down his cheeks.

The nurse was staring. In all her decades of experience, it seemed she had never before seen this happen.

Next week the man remained, undead. It seemed he had not moved a limb or an eyelash in the intervening time. But when Colene took his hand and spoke to him, his eyes opened, and his mouth tried to smile.

He began to recover after that. Week by week he improved, most dramatically when Colene was present, until he was well enough to be taken home. He could not speak or walk without help, but perhaps that would come.

Two weeks later came the news: the beautiful man had gotten his hands on another gun. This time his shot had been all the way true, and he was dead.

What had she accomplished, by interfering with the natural course? She had thought she was doing so much good; instead she had hastened the man's death. She should never have done it. She should have had the humility to know that she could not change another person's destined course.

Suicide. What was its attraction?

She continued with the wee hours Sunday shift, but the heart was gone from it. What was right and what was wrong? She had no sure answers.

Then there was an emergency. A bus had been involved in an accident, and there were horrendous injuries. The call went out: all available personnel report to assist in the emergency room.

Colene went down. In the throes of it, no one challenged her. She carried bandages and ran errands for the harried doctors. There were so many bodies to deal with all at once, they were doing triage.

A teenager not much older than Colene herself was hauled in on a stretcher, his legs crushed. Colene passed the bandages as the doctor tried to stanch the flow of blood; as he said, succinctly, the legs would have to wait, because they would do the kid no good if he bled to death. A woman was almost unmarked on the body, but she had been struck across the face and her eyes gouged out. Colene held her hand while the doctor gave her a shot to abate her screaming. A man was sitting, waiting his turn, coughing up blood, helpless, bewildered and in despair. Colene went to him and put her arm around his shoulders. 'The doctor will be with you in a moment,' she whispered in his ear. He turned his face to her, started to smile, and slumped. Now at last the doctor came, performing a hasty check. 'He's dead.' And he was; they could not revive him.

Now a nurse recognized Colene. 'Child, you don't belong here!' she exclaimed, horrified.

'Yes I do,' Colene said. But she left, knowing the nurse would not report her if she got out before anyone else caught on. Most of the injured had been classified by this time, anyway.

But it was enough. She asked to be relieved of her job, saying the night hours were interfering with her sleep and her homework. The hospital administration, covertly aware of what had happened, gave her a fancy Certificate of Merit and let her go. It was their secret. Colene was learning about secrets, learning well.

Now Colene's interest in death, a sometime thing before, became dominant. The last man had smiled as he died. Death had been a relief. The way those people had been suffering, death would have been a relief for all of them. What right did she, an undistinguished girl, have to be healthy and happy?

But she told no one of her experiences, and indeed she wasn't sure what significance they had. Was death the proper destiny of man? If not, what was? Until she knew the answer, she hid her feelings and acted normal.

She started dating. Her mother thought she was too young, at mid thirteen, but her mother didn't want to quarrel about it. A quarrel could lead to a discussion of her mother's drinking habit. Secrets – Colene was learning how to borrow against their power, how to finesse them, to get her way. So she went to the movies with a boy she hardly cared for, and let him kiss her, while in her mind ran the scenes from the dirty novel of twining bare bodies. What would it be like, actually?

An older boy asked her out. He had a car, but he didn't drive her to the movie. He said it would be more fun at the party his friends were having. There would be great entertainment. Colene didn't care about the movie either, so she didn't object.

There were three other boys there at an apartment, and no other girls. They were drinking. They gave her a drink, and she tried it, curious. This, too, was new experience. Soon she was pleasantly dizzy. She had another drink, and another, reveling in the feeling.

Then she was in the bedroom with her date, and he had his trousers off. Suddenly the descriptions in the dirty novel registered, and she knew what he was after. She started to protest, but he pushed her down on the bed and got her dress up and her panties off and rammed into her with a whole lot less art than the novel had described. By the time she realized that it was rape, it was done, and he was getting off.

Rape? Even tipsy as she was, she realized that no one would believe her. So she played it cool, and pretended she had liked it. That way maybe she would get home safely.

But the other boys came in, and she had either to continue the pretense or make a scene, and if she made the scene she feared she would not only get raped, she would get beaten up and maybe killed. That wasn't the way she wanted to die! So she smiled and said it was all right, and one by one they pressed her down and jammed in, and it was so slick and messy now that it didn't hurt the way the first time had.

She did make it home safely, and her mother was so drunk she couldn't smell the liquor on Colene or see her condition.

160

Colene went to the bathroom and washed and washed, but she couldn't get the awful feel of those men out of her. The novel had been wrong; it was no fun for the woman.

She never told, and neither did the boys. Not where it counted. They knew the trouble they would be in if news got to the authorities, considering her age. So the secret was kept, to a degree. But Colene stopped dating. Her reputation in certain circles was shot. Her mother, ignorant and relieved, did not question that decision.

Time showed that she was neither pregnant nor infected with VD. She had gotten away with it, such as it was. But she was saddled with a deep, abiding disgust. The worst of it was that she couldn't really condemn the men; they were what they were, opportunists. It was herself she condemned, for being such a fool. She had indeed asked for it, by her naiveté. How could she have read all about it in the dirty novel, and not caught on that to such men a girl was nothing more than a walking vagina waiting to be unwrapped and plunged? Fool! Fool!

Why was life such a grubby mess? She hated every aspect of this, but still didn't know what to do about it. There seemed to be no justice, only opportunity and coping. Opportunity for the men and coping for the women.

After that her double life had come upon her. She was bright and cheery in public, suicidal in private.

Did you share your feeling with anyone?

She had forgotten that Seqiro was tuning in. Well, not really; she had gone through it all for his benefit, buoyed somewhat in the fashion of her nude display before criminals at the time of the bleeding contest. In that she had in a devious manner made up for her disastrous date: instead of getting raped by four men and having to pretend to like it, she had tempted them and beaten them in sheer nerve, and they had had to pretend to like it. They weren't the same men and it wasn't the same situation, but it aligned in her perception. This wasn't the same situation either, but it also aligned: instead of baring her fascinating body (it had to be fascinating, or there was no point) she was baring her fascinating mind, and there was a dubious glory in it, a thrill of release, almost of expiation.

161

No, this was not parallel to the physical business, she realized as she reviewed it. It was parallel to mental business. She *had* shared her feeling with a friend, once before. And that had been another bad mistake.

It was this past summer, at camp. Naturally her folks got her out of the house when they could, not because they disliked her but because they were more concerned with their own problems than with hers. Camp wasn't bad, actually. There was swimming and hiking and dancing and woodwork and nature. She liked all the events, yet her depression remained. It was as if she were a mere shell going through the motions. What was real was the blood on her wrist.

But her roommate Mitzi spied the scars. Things could be hidden from parents, teachers, friends, psychologists, and the man on the street, but roommates were deadly. Rather than try to bluff through, which was a bad risk, she was frank, telling how she secretly wanted to die but didn't quite have the courage to do it. So she flirted with it, and the flowing blood relieved something in her, a little, and one day she would get up the nerve to go all the way and truly be dead.

Mitzi expressed sympathy and promised to keep her secret. She watched out for Colene after that, as if afraid she would keep her head under water too long or eat poison instead of dessert or throw herself off the precipice instead of admiring the view from it. It was fun for a while, having this constant attention. But soon it became annoying, and then oppressive. For one thing, the roommate was alert at night too, and the toilet wasn't sufficiently private. Colene just couldn't cut herself, and was getting restive.

She tried to distance herself a bit, to go on events without the roommate, so she could get the necessary privacy to do what she hated to do. Otherwise she was afraid she really *would* hurl herself over a cliff, having been unable to alleviate her need in a lesser and more controlled manner. The problem with the cliff was that she knew she would be unable to change her mind in mid air, and that the job might not be complete; she might survive, broken and ashamed. But mainly it would be messy. Instead of lying pale and beautiful in her coffin, she would be bruised and

162

battered, with her nose broken and teeth stoved in. That was no way to die.

It came to arguments, not about anything in particular, but about what wasn't said: Colene's need to do her own thing, even if that was self destructive. First they were private, then they spilled over into public. Finally, in the last week of camp, the roommate blew up: 'I'm sorry I ever tried to stop you from killing yourself!' she cried.

There was an abrupt silence in the mess hall. Then, studiously, the other kids resumed eating and talking, not looking at Colene. Colene got up and dumped the rest of her meal in the trash and left. She went to her room and bared her arm, but couldn't do it; she was too humiliated and angry to focus even on this.

That night the roommate came, but they did not speak to each other. Camp life went on as usual. But something had changed. Colene realized that people were speaking to her, about nothing in particular and everything in the ellipses – and they weren't speaking to Mitzi.

A girl approached her, seemingly by coincidence. The girl was younger and seemed perky. But she showed Colene her arm, and it was scarred where the sleeve normally covered it. 'I thought I was the only one,' she murmured, and moved on.

A boy approached at another time. He was handsome, and Colene liked his look, but had had no personal interaction with him. 'I, ah, she shouldn't have done that,' he said. 'I didn't know. I didn't ask you before, but now, ah, maybe there isn't much time. The last-night dance, will you, ah –?'

'Because you're sorry for me?' Colene asked, witheringly.

'Ah, yeah, I guess. I guess I'd be mad too, if –'

'Okay.'

'What?'

'I will go to the dance with you.'

He seemed stunned. 'Ah, okay, then.'

They did go. He gave her a small corsage of wild flowers he had made himself. Her held her very close as they danced, and suddenly she realized something. She halted on the floor. 'Was that the truth?'

163

He knew what she meant. 'Ah, no. I lied. I just didn't have the nerve to tell you I liked you. Are you mad?'

'Furious,' she said, and pulled his head down and kissed him firmly on the mouth.

There was applause from the other couples and those along the sidelines. A counselor forged her way to them. 'Go to your rooms,' she said severely. 'You know that's not permitted.'

'See, I got you in trouble already,' Colene told him as they separated.

'Yeah. Thanks,' he replied, looking stunned again.

Mitzi was there in the room. Colene looked at her, surprised.

'No one asked me,' the girl said. 'No one would dance with me.' She was near tears.

She was not suicidal, but she was suffering worse than Colene was, now. 'Maybe I can fix that,' Colene said.

'No! I don't deserve anything from you. I'm sorry I – I said what I did. I knew it was wrong the moment I – Colene, I'm *sorry*!' She buried her face in her handkerchief.

'I know. But I guess you did me a favor.'

The head counselor arrived. 'Colene, whatever possessed you to let him kiss you like that?' she demanded. 'You know I shall have to report both of you to your families as well as apply demerits for discipline.'

'You kissed him?' the roommate asked, astonished.

The counselor glanced at her, startled. 'Why aren't you at the dance?'

Colene spoke before Mitzi could answer. 'We had a quarrel. I got back at her. I got her date to take me instead, at the last minute, so she was frozen out. He didn't kiss me; *I* kissed *him*. Ask anyone; they all saw it, except the chaperon, who only looked when she heard the applause. So I fixed them both good.'

The counselor stared at the roommate. 'Is this true?'

'Why do you think she's been crying?' Colene demanded.

The counselor was at a loss for only a moment. Then she acted in the decisive fashion of her kind. 'Colene, I am appalled at you. I will deal with you later.' She turned to Mitzi. 'You come with me. You *will* attend the dance with your date.'

164

In moments they were gone. Colene lay on her bunk bed, gazing at the ceiling. She was proud of herself. She knew her date would play along. Not only would it get him out of trouble with the counselors, it would make him a celebrity for the night. Two girls had fought to date him!

Next day the buses came and the kids went home. They were from all over the country and had no contact with each other apart from the camp. The counselors were busy keeping things moving, and there wasn't much chance for any talking. But every time a camper caught Colene's eye, he or she smiled and made a little gesture of a finger across the throat. It was a temporary camp convention, signifying credit for getting punished for doing something daring or decent. It had special meaning in Colene's case. They all knew, and all were pleased. Naturally no one told the counselors. Secrets – secrets were the stuff of life.

That was it. When Colene's mother received the discipline report, she was perplexed. 'What did you do?'

'I kissed a boy in public.'

Her father burst out laughing. 'About time!'

Colene wondered what he would have said if he had known about the rape. Her world was such a schizoid place, where a gang rape went unnoticed while an innocent kiss got a girl in trouble. For all that, the last week of camp, betrayal and all, had been a high point in her life.

Why did she want to die, anyway? Now she felt far more positive. It was because of Darius, she knew: even the hope of him made her want to live, for she had to live to love, and she did love. Even the notion of sex, which had pretty much turned her off, now turned her on. With *him* it would be beautiful, she knew.

But it was also Seqiro. She had loved horses from afar. Now she loved one from up close. Very close. Right-inside-her-mind close. She could tell him her secrets, and he would not betray them. That made her feel much better about living.

'Seqiro!' she exclaimed. 'Are you helping me? I mean, messing with my mind, making me forget the pain or whatever?'

I could do this, but have not, because I see that it was that pain

165

that caused you to embark on the Virtual Mode. Without it you might give up your quest.

'You mean you're selfish, Seqiro? You want my company?'

That is true. He sent a non-specific companion thought of agreement that was so complete it had to be believed.

She was thrilled in much the way she had been when she learned that the boy at camp had really wanted to dance with her. It meant he was not just putting up with her. 'Don't worry. I want to get together with Darius, and I want to stay with you. I'm glad you didn't mess with my mind. That means I really *am* feeling better. Just going through those memories with you makes me feel better.'

What is your desire of life?

Colene thought for a moment, and then it poured out of her. 'I like to consider myself apart from the whole earth. There is no dignity left. I would like to be able to float away with my books and music and my guitar. It just seems to me that there are few people left with any integrity, and two of them happen to be my favorite writer and my favorite musician. I do too much thinking for my own good. I compose poetry in my head, but it won't come out right on paper. It's depressing. I dream too much, also. I have so many ambitions, and I am crushed when I realize how very few will ever be achieved. I want to be an author, a musician, a veterinarian, a researcher working with dolphins and other marine life, a friend of those I admire. I want to be someone who would die for her cause. I want to be creative. I want to be a starving artist. I want always to be traveling, never in one place for long. I want to be defending everyone's rights, especially animals and women. I want to be free, inspiring, compassionate. I want to be everything. I want to live under a night sky with someone I love intensely, and never have to move. To sit and gaze at the heavens with someone. I want never to be tied down or held back as I am now. Above all, I want to be free. I want it to be nighttime forever.'

I share your feeling. But what you have thought is not all. His thought was sympathetic.

She laughed. 'No, that's not all! It's not even consistent. I want never to have to stay in one place and never to have to move. I want total freedom and total irresponsibility and total dedication. I want everything and nothing, all at the same time. I know it doesn't make any sense, but this isn't sense, this is desire. So does it make any sense to you, or would it, if you were a girl?

I am a stallion, neither human nor female, and I have similar desires. You express them better than I could formulate them.

She felt another surge of the continuing thrill of being with him, of telling him her secret heart and being understood. She was talking, but her mind was carrying harmonics that made her whole feeling come across, so much greater than mere words could ever convey. His mind was sending back background washes and waves of understanding and support, so she knew he meant it. Telepathy: it was like being in a hot tub together, their bodies dissolved away and their minds sharing the essence.

'Do you have religion, Seqiro?'

There was a quick exploration of the concept she lifted to the surface. *No.*

'Maybe that's better. I don't know whether I have religion either. I feel that it's better for me to take my own decisions about religion than to have my beliefs dictated to me. I hate people who go to church just so they can feel better about doing other things that they know are bad. I think I believe more in nature than in God. I can see nature, and feel and be a part of it. God is more of a closed case. I like to feel a little different from other people and have a different view of things. That's part of the reason I'm not too wild about school. Everyone is expected to be the same. It leaves no room for freedom of thought. If you're not like everyone else, you stand out and are not tolerated. I want to break away from this everybody-must-be-the-same type of society. Routine is awful. To do the same thing every day, every week, is torture. I hope, someday, to do something that allows for a lot of freedom and creativity. To live in a small house with natural wooden floors that creak beneath my feet. My home will be on the coast where it stays dark for a long time. I will go outside at night and be inspired by the storm clouds over the ocean. There will be a rocky cliff that I can sit on while I think.'

Yes.

Colene opened her eyes. 'So you see, I dream wonderful things, but in the back of my mind I have always known that I will just end up in some stupid job and live like everyone else. I couldn't even speak of my dreams before, because people would just laugh. They think the dull world is all there is.'

Now you know about the other realities, and are on the Virtual Mode. Your life will after all be different.

'That's right! Say, Seqiro, if everything else doesn't work out, let's you and me just keep traveling à la Mode!'

We do not know how far we shall have to travel as it is, or what dangers we shall face. The day is late; we had better seek sanctuary for the night.

'Yes, that's right. I didn't realize how tired I've gotten, with all this walking.' Which made her realize that it had never occurred to her to ride the horse. Seqiro just wasn't that kind of horse.

They came into a series of realities in which there were thickly forested mountains. Colene knew that there was nothing like this within a day's walking distance of Oklahoma, which meant that the geography changed in nearby realities as well as the creatures and the underlying rules of nature.

'You were right, Seqiro,' she said. 'I can't ride my bike here! But if we come to a region where it's flat or paved, I'll be able to.'

I shall be interested to see how this device operates. I have seen nothing like it before.

They found a clear stream. 'That sure looks nice!' she exclaimed. 'I'd like to have a deep drink and wash up, but if the water won't stay with me –'

There is no problem about washing, for you do not need to have the water stay. As for drinking – perhaps it should be done, as we can remain the night in this reality and assimilate the water. We are sweating, so may excrete some of the alien water in the normal course, without being bound to its reality.

Colene, suddenly desperately thirsty, focused on one thing. 'You mean it's all right to use this water?'

Provided we remain here for some time.

'That's good enough for me!' She threw herself down and

drank deeply. All that water on top of all that exertion made her feel giddy, but it was worth it.

Seqiro drank more cautiously. Then they both washed. Colene got out of her loincloth and cape and splashed naked, screaming with pained pleasure at the shock of the cold water. Then she took a sponge they had packed and sponged off the horse's hide where the bags of supplies weren't in the way. Seqiro did not let her remove his burdens; wary of possible danger, he preferred to keep everything on him, so as to be able to step quickly into another reality without leaving important things behind. Colene had to admit that made sense. She was able to clean him pretty well by pushing away one bag at a time and sponging under it. His hide was steaming hot, but the chill water helped cool him.

It is a delight to have this attention from you without coercion.

'You don't get washed off at home?'

Our humans act only under our imperative. We direct them in all things, and punish them when they do not perform.

'Where I live, girls do these things for horses because they love horses.'

It would seem that the activities are similar, but the motives dissimilar.

'It would seem,' she agreed.

Colene bent twigs and scuffed the forest floor to mark the borders of the other realities on either side, so they would not cross unawares. They had a channel ten feet wide and endlessly long to remain in. It was hard to believe, because the forest and stream were uninterrupted, but she had now had enough experience to treat the boundary with extreme respect.

I have quested through this vicinity of this reality, and found no hostile or dangerous creatures, Seqiro thought. *There may be danger in the adjacent realities, but we need not be concerned about those until we resume our travel.*

'That's nice,' Colene said, relieved. 'Are you going to lie down to sleep?'

That is not necessary. I can rest and sleep on my feet.

'The reason I asked is if you lie down, I can lie down with you, and be warm.'

That is true. As it is safe, I shall lie.

So it was that they lay down in their narrow channel beside the stream. Colene took a heavy blanket from Seqiro's supplies and spread it over him, then settled down against his side, between two bags of feed. It was really quite comfortable, all things considered. She slept, feeling about as happy as she could remember since losing Darius.

8

PROVOS

Darius resumed his quest alone, having delivered Prima to his anchor Mode. His feelings were mixed. He was not glad for the delay occasioned by this encounter, yet it had enabled him to satisfy about three quarters of his commitment to Kublai: he had found Prima, and she had a lot of information about the nature of the Modes that Kublai would find most interesting. He was now about two days behind wherever he would have been, but it was possible that he would have been captive or dead by now if it had not been for her. Probably he was ahead, overall. For one thing, he was now the first in a long time to enter a Virtual Mode and return.

Prima had fashioned for him the mirror tube she had promised. It did seem to work. He experimented by setting a package of food on the ground, stepping across the boundary, looking back to see nothing, then poking the tube cautiously across. He did see the package in the mirror, when it wasn't visible directly. So it seemed that the way the tube excluded the light of the Mode in which he stood did enable it to carry the light of the Mode beyond. Or perhaps it was just that the device was fashioned of the substance of his anchor Mode, so was able to transmit the light along the Virtual Mode.

But it was not feasible to stop to check every Mode boundary as he went. He would take ten times as long to get anywhere if he did that. So he would have to use it judiciously, when there

171

seemed to be danger. Such as in the region of the dominant dragons.

He moved much faster this time, using magic to take himself as far along the route as it would. Magic seemed to have no difficulty taking him across Modes, in the region of the Virtual Mode where magic was operative. Beyond that he walked rapidly, with the confidence of his prior experience in two directions.

Soon he reached the lake. He had learned a lot here, from Prima. Now he became more cautious. He needed to get safely past the region of the dragons. But he didn't depend on the tube alone. He had another sword, and also a heavy pair of shears which could cut through cord. For this he had more confidence in the shears than the sword, because they would be faster. He also had a fair coil of cord of his own, strong enough to sustain several times his weight without breaking. Experience counted.

He came to the geographic region of the dragons, which on the Virtual Mode was the same as the Mode of the dragons. This time he intended to keep the two separate! He paused to use his mirror tube before crossing each boundary. He could even see his footprints in the soft dirt, in places. To a creature watching, he would seem to appear, walk three paces, and disappear, leaving the prints.

Now he was almost at the place where he had been netted; he recognized the tree ahead from which the net had been suspended. There was no net visible, of course, because it didn't exist in this Mode. But the dragons, or their monkey servitors, had surely restored the damaged one, ready to trap the next unwary Mode traveler.

He moved to the side, then slowly poked his forward mirror across. He turned it, so that the image in the near mirror swept across the region.

There was the net, cunningly set so that a creature who plowed into it would cause it to close and rise, completing the trap. There was no dragon in sight, but he knew how quickly one could come when a trap was sprung.

He pondered a moment. Suppose he threw something across into the net, then crossed behind the dragon when it approached the net? No, he could not move anything from one Mode to another except his own belongings, which he had no intention of risking. It would be better to avoid the issue. He knew how dangerous those dragons were, because they understood about the Modes.

He surveyed the section carefully, turning the mirror around. There seemed to be nothing to the side of the net. Yet how could the dragons be so sure of catching something at that particular place?

He became aware of an itching on one leg. He looked down. He was standing in a bed of nettles. Their spikes seemed to be actually clinging to his trousers and seeking to stab through. That was why: the path he had been following was the only place clear of the nettles. Animals in several Modes must have found the best place through, and it made sense for him too. He had followed it before without even being conscious of the nettles.

He looked beyond. The nettles extended as far as he could see. The mystery of the net's placement was becoming less. There really was no other way through.

He could step cautiously, and cut the anchor line, disabling the trap, and go on quickly. But adjacent Modes tended to be similar. There could be another net in the following Mode, or a pit, or something worse. He did not like this region at all.

He decided to avoid the whole thing. He retreated through the Modes until he found a way through the nettles, then proceeded down the slope toward what had been the dragon's camp in its own Mode. He came to the field, then turned and proceeded across Modes again. There had been no trap in this vicinity, so it was probably a safe crossing. Still, he slowed and tested each Mode as he came to that vicinity.

When he passed the one showing the cages in the valley, he was relieved. There were several Modes with cages; then they faded and the countryside resumed.

He considered whether to find a way back to his original path, which proceeded most directly through Modes toward wherever he was going. But there could be other traps along it, so he continued through the field, and then through the forest, until the slope changed and the hill became a plain. Only then did he return to his direct path, slowly.

Time had passed, and nightfall was approaching. He had come a long way, and his legs were tired, but he was surprised at how fast the day had passed. He had not even paused for lunch, and was only now getting hungry. Was it possible that the length of the day changed along with other things, in other Modes? Yes, that did seem possible. Too bad he did not have a time piece of the type Colene had. It was a little device she wore on her left wrist, which helped to cover the scars there. Tiny pointers moved in it, indicating the hour of the day. Superfluous in Darius' Mode, of course, where things happened when they happened. But now that time might be changing, such a device might have enabled him to verify just how much difference there was.

Colene. She kept returning to his thoughts. On one level he recognized this quest as foolish, because he had already found his answer. He could go home and marry Prima and have an excellent career as Cyng of Hlahtar. She was older than he, but that was irrelevant; Hlahtar's wife was neither for love nor offspring, but for a ready source of joy to spread. Prima was the best possible source. But he was intent on Colene, who offered him none of that. All she offered him was private love.

Well, that was what he wanted. He would fetch Colene, then see about Prima. It might be foolish, but it was what he wanted. At least he knew that Kublai had a good situation during his absence.

He came to a lake at dusk, or perhaps the shore of a sea. There was no such body of water within walking distance in his Mode, but he had long since recognized that though geography changed gradually, it also changed significantly, and it resembled that of his home only in the immediate vicinity of his anchor. Were he to become trapped in the Mode in which he stood at this moment, and walk back through it the way he would come until he reached the spot where his anchor was supposed to be, he would probably find a completely different geography. The Modes changed vertically as well as horizontally, as if each sliver of mica had a different pattern that matched that of its neighbor slivers only when they were close. It was possible that when he had made the first foray into Colene's Mode, it had been to the same geographic spot in her Mode as the one he had left in his.

He searched out a tree whose larger branches spread from one Mode to another. That was ideal. Prima had shown him that a tree was a good place to spend the night, removed from nocturnal creatures of the ground. But attack could come, and the best way to deal with it was to avoid it – by stepping into the next Mode. If he could do so without leaving the tree, so much the better.

He drank from the lake, washed, and ate from his pack. He realized that this must be a lake, because the water was not salty. But he could not see across it. Then he drew out his light blanket, climbed into the tree, braced himself, wrapped himself, and settled down for sleep. He thought of Prima, who had slept in his embrace, sharing warmth. At the time he had wished it could have been Colene, but now he realized that Prima herself had been good company. She had been intelligent and practical and not finicky about niceties, an easy person to travel with despite the awkwardness of their arms being constantly bound together. She was not at all the kind of woman he had been looking for, consciously, but very much the kind he actually needed. Colene, in contrast, was young and pretty and devoted, matching his desire, but quite unsuitable for marriage to the Cyng of Hlahtar. So said his logic. So much for logic. He wanted Colene.

As he was nodding off, something occurred to him that woke him up again. If Colene was at the same spot on the globe as he, one Mode directly over the other, so that his first foray with the Chip had plunged him straight up or down – how could he reach her by traveling on the slant? He was walking horizontally, stepping down into each new infinitely-thin Mode in the course of three paces. It wasn't a physically vertical thing, or the slopes of hills would have put him into new Modes at a great rate. But he was definitely moving across the terrain. By the time he reached Colene's Mode, he should be far from the spot on the globe he had started at, and therefore far from her. How would he be able to find her?

No, he had to be near her when he reached her Mode, because she had an anchor there. So that should be no problem. But how was it possible to travel horizontally and arrive vertically?

Then he remembered another part of the explanation the Cyng of Pwer had given, whose significance had bypassed him at the time. The Virtual Mode was like a plane cutting through the Modes at an angle, but it was not infinite. It was really a plane segment bounded by the five anchors. Like a pentagon, or roughly circular in outline. He could be walking around the edge of it. When he got half way around, there would be Colene.

The image helped reassure him, but it did not do the whole job. This Virtual Mode was really not a simple thing, and some of its incidental aspects, such as the business of drinking the water of foreign Modes along the way, were tricky. His image might be all wrong.

At any rate, he slept.

In the morning Darius resumed his travel. He traveled around the lake. At one point he encountered a family of otter-like animals who spooked at his appearance and swam rapidly away. At another he came across a small dragon or large lizard, similarly shy. But he became wary, because where there were small dragons there could also be large ones.

Beyond the lake was a settled region. At first it was just a planted field, but as he passed by it, successive Modes brought it to more intense cultivation and a road appeared. This looked human, but his wariness increased. Human beings would not necessarily be friendly. In fact he felt far more at ease among the animals of the wilderness, for very few of them represented any danger to him, and those few could be fairly readily avoided. But human beings were potentially worse than the dragons. Certainly he would not walk into the center of a village and announce himself!

He walked clear of the fields and found a forested section. The trees were unlike those he knew, being yellow of trunk and blue of leaf, but a tree of any color remained reassuring and protective. This was no jungle, and there was little undergrowth, but it did provide some privacy for his passage.

Then he spied a woman. She was standing in the center of a glade as if expecting him. She wore a small hat with two very long projections like the antennae of insects, a gray woolen sweater, an ankle-length brown knit dress, and high black boots laced up the front. She had what was evidently a traveling bag beside her. She was old, perhaps sixty. What was on her mind?

He approached her cautiously, following the sideways channel of this Mode. He could have stepped into the next Mode and avoided the contact, but she had seen him and he preferred to be polite as long as it was safe to be so. 'A greeting,' he said, speaking in his own language.

She said something indecipherable. Her language was not only different, it was weirdly different; he could not tell whether she had uttered a greeting, curse or gibberish. She picked up her bag. It had straps, and he realized that it was actually a kind of backpack, which she now donned. She was certainly prepared!

He tried again in Colene's language. 'Hi.'

She smiled and put her hand on his arm. She stepped forward, drawing him along with her.

She was evidently harmless, and of course she could not go any distance with him. Having tried to communicate, and failed, he decided simply to walk along with her, and step through to the next Mode when he reached the boundary. He would fade from her sight and touch, and she would think she had had a supernatural experience. An unkind trick to play on her, perhaps, but kinder than rejecting her gesture outright. It was evident that she expected to go somewhere with him.

They walked back to the point where he had been when he had first seen her, then turned to resume his original route. They stepped through the invisible boundary together.

Darius did a doubletake. *She was still there!* Still walking beside him, her hand on his arm.

But Prima had been able to cross Modes with him, as long as she touched him. He had understood that this was because she was of his Mode, or very close to it, despite not being an anchor person. This woman was not close at all. Had his notion been wrong? Could a person of another Mode cross simply by maintaining contact with an anchor person on the Virtual Mode? So it seemed to be.

But that would mean that she would be stranded in a Mode that was foreign to her. It would be wrong to leave her like that.

He turned and stepped back into the woman's Mode, bringing her along with him. 'I must go where you can not,' he told her firmly, withdrawing his arm from her hand. 'I am sorry. I am unable to explain, but I must leave you here.' He stepped across, alone.

He looked back. The woman was gone, of course; she did not exist in this Mode. The glade remained, and there was a small creature in a tree that he thought had not been there in the other glade. It must have watched him appear, disappear, and reappear, with an understandable perplexity.

Then the woman reappeared. She had stepped through after him.

Darius just stared. She had done it on her own! No physical contact! But that was impossible, unless –

Then he realized what the answer had to be. She was an anchor person! There were five of them, and he did not know the identity of three. It had not occurred to him that he would meet any of them, but if he truly was walking around the edge of a figurative plate, he would indeed encounter other anchor folk.

Somehow he had not expected an old woman, despite expecting nothing. What was he to do with her? He couldn't take her with him!

She took his arm again and urged him forward. She did want to go with him, and seemed to know the situation. It was hard for him to say no, because he couldn't speak her language and couldn't stop her from following him. That did not make the situation any less awkward.

He sighed inwardly and resumed walking. What was to be, was to be.

'Yes,' she said.

178

He was startled again. He stopped in place. 'You speak my language?'

'No.'

'But you are speaking it now! You –'

She uttered a mellifluous stream of unintelligibility. Evidently she knew only a few of his words.

'How did you learn "yes" and "no"?'

'Yes, future,' she said. 'No, past.'

Now he understood the words, but could not fathom the meaning. She might not mean the same thing by those words that he did. But in case she did, it could mean that she expected to travel with him from now on, and had not done so in the past.

They resumed walking. The forest disappeared, but the cultivated fields were gone; they had gone beyond the group of Modes in which these folk operated.

'Provos,' she said.

He glanced at her. She removed her hand from his arm and tapped herself above her slight bosom.

Oh. He tapped himself. 'Darius,' he said.

They stepped into another Mode. Abruptly her hand tightened on his arm. 'No!' she said, trying to hold him back.

He stopped. 'What's the matter?'

She merely shook her head, unable to clarify the matter.

He looked around. There was nothing threatening in view. 'I have somewhere to go,' he said. He started to step forward again.

'No!' She hauled him back again.

Could there be something in the next Mode that she knew about and he could not see? He brought out his mirror tube and extended it forward. But as he started to take a cautious step, she stopped him a third time.

He almost lost his balance. The end of the tube dipped to touch the ground.

A pointed stake shot up from the ground, right beside the end of the tube. The end of the stake was discolored.

'A poison trap!' Darius exclaimed. 'If I had stepped there, it would have stabbed my leg!' Or worse.

He put away the tube, found a stick, and poked beside the

stake. In a moment another stake shot up, and then another. There was a row of them slanting across this Mode segment.

'I think you just saved my health or life,' he told Provos, shaken. 'How did you know?'

But she now seemed to be ignoring the situation, as if it were of no further concern.

He walked to the side, beyond the stakes, and poked some more. There was no further reaction from the ground, and Provos did not balk him. The danger seemed to be limited to that one segment.

All the same, he used the tube to check the next Mode carefully before crossing. This escape had been quite too narrow!

Nothing was in view. They crossed, cautiously. He fetched a stick in this Mode and poked ahead. There was nothing. The stakes seemed to be an artifact of a single Mode, in much the way the net of the dragons had been.

They continued until the afternoon grew late. Darius didn't know how to ask Provos about camping arrangements, so he simply went ahead and trusted her to protest if she chose.

And protest she did, after he had located a suitable tree to use for the night. At first he thought it was because she was prudish about climbing or sharing warmth, but it seemed that she was becoming increasingly nervous about this whole region. He saw no reason for it, but after the experience with the stakes he took it seriously.

He offered to make the same camp in the Mode they had just crossed. To that she agreed. She opened her bag and produced what seemed to be homemade bread and a sweet spread, which she shared with him. He wasn't sure whether he could eat it, because of the problem retaining foreign food when crossing Modes, but realized that if it had traveled with her through all the prior Modes, it was safely on the Virtual Mode and should remain with them. The substance of her Mode was as real for him as the substance of his own or of Colene's. That was the thing about the anchors; they really were firm.

'Thank you,' he said. She did not acknowledge.

They performed their separate natural functions in different

180

nooks of the Mode, then mounted the tree and shared his blanket. Provos seemed to be entirely at ease with the closeness, which surprised him. He was considerably more at ease than he would have been before the experience with Prima.

Prima. Provos. There was a certain similarity of names. Did it mean anything? He decided that it didn't. It was a minor coincidence until proven otherwise.

In the morning they got down and unkinked their bodies. Provos was old but spry; she must have had camping experience. Indeed she produced a set of stones which struck a spark that started a fire, and they were able to have a hot meal of some kind of tasty tubers she brought from her bag. She was certainly doing her part.

Then they doused the fire, got organized, and stepped back across the boundary.

Darius stared. There were foot prints where there had been none before; something had come here in the night. Huge claws had dug into the ground, as if a giant bird had landed here. The bark of the tree they would have slept in was torn away in patches.

'Something came here and smelled our traces,' he said, awed. 'It scratched the ground where we stood, and scratched at the tree where I had started to set up for the night. By the marks, it was huge and predatory: a dragon or carnivorous bird. I think we would have been dead.'

But Provos seemed unconcerned, hardly noticing the marks. She was just interested in going on.

He refused to settle for that. 'What is it with you?' he demanded. 'Twice you may have saved my life, yet you act as if it is nothing.' He pointed to the marks, making her look. 'How did you know?'

'Yes, future,' she said. 'No, past.'

'You said that before, but I don't know what it means!'

She tried to explain. 'I yes future. You yes past. I no past. You no future.'

He tried to make sense of this, in the context of what he had seen. She was yes future and no past. He was no future and yes past. He had no future and she did? He couldn't accept that!

And that couldn't be it, because the corollary would be that she had no past while he did. The only thing that made remote sense was that he could not foresee the future, while she –

She could see the future? She had precognition? That did seem to be the case! And the barrier of language prevented her from telling him exactly what it was that she saw, so she was able to warn him only by crude gestures. But that could not be the whole of it. What did she mean about no past? She could not see the past?

He walked on with her, his mind laboring. How was it possible for her not to know the past? She would have no memory! She would be completely unconcerned with yesterday.

Which was exactly the attitude she showed. Concern for the future, none for the past. It seemed unbelievable, but she *was* from an alien Mode, and its ordinariness in the physical aspect might mask a truly amazing difference in the mental aspect.

He reviewed specifics as they went. She had balked at one place, and there had been a deadly trap there. She had surely not been there before; she was as new to the Virtual Mode as he, and had been waiting for someone to come along it, so she would not have to go alone. She had probably been waiting for days, and acted the moment she saw him. Why had she not been afraid of the stranger? Because she had foreseen his arrival! She might not be concerned about what was past, but she knew she would be traveling with him, so she had made sure to be there at the right time.

Yet she had not seemed to foresee the poisoned stakes, exactly. She had just been very nervous. It was the same with the monster of the night. She had not been concerned about that immediately; only after camping preparations were well along had she insisted on leaving the area. It didn't seem to be straight anticipation of future events.

She had likened her situation to his. 'I yes future, you yes past.' He did not foresee the past, he remembered it, and the farther in the past it was, the foggier his memory tended to become, unless it was something important. Could she *remember* the future? 'I no past, you no future.' She could not remember the past, though she might have a notion of it by judging from the present. If she was here with him, and remembered what they would be doing in the future, she could safely assume that they had met in the past and had some kind of understanding. Just as he could assume that he would be traveling with her for a while.

But that monster of the night – that was not a threat to be forgotten quickly! Why had it taken her a while to catch on to it?

Because it happened in a foreign Mode! He could not remember the past of Modes he had not been in; she could not remember the future of Modes she would not be in. But if he stayed in a Mode for a while, and got some experience in it, he could remember that much of it. She must have become acclimatized to it, gradually, and then realized that something terrible was about to happen there. So she had warned him. When they moved into the adjacent Mode that feeling did not come on her, so she relaxed.

It did seem to make sense. But if so, there would always be some problems. How could they relate, if she remembered only what they would be doing, and he remembered only what they had been doing?

He saw Provos nodding as if she had just come to understand something. Yet there was nothing unusual about the landscape of the Modes they were passing through, and they had not spoken.

But maybe they were about to speak, and she was remembering that! He was concerned with the problem of relating to a woman who could not remember their dialogue after it happened – but could remember it coming.

So maybe there was a way. 'Provos,' he said – and realized that she had started turning to him before he spoke. Yes, she was remembering that he was about to say something to her! 'Night, monster,' he said, making clawing motions with a hand.

She looked concerned. 'Monster,' she repeated.

'You saved me,' he said. He took her hand, put it on his own arm, and acted as if he were being pulled back. 'Escaped monster.'

'Monster no?' she asked.

'Monster yes,' he said. He repeated the gesture. 'Then monster no. You warned me.'

'Day monster no,' she said.

Which should mean that no monster was in their immediate future. Except that her perception might be limited to the Mode they were now in. So there could be a monster in the next one. If something threatened in the next step, she might pick it up, as she had with the stakes; but if it threatened in several hours, she might take a while to attune to it.

Did that make sense? Suppose something awful had happened several hours ago in one Mode; would he forget about it in the last half hour before they left that Mode? He didn't think so. Also, if she remembered something bad that was about to happen, and told him, and he changed it, then it wouldn't happen. So how could she remember it? It seemed like paradox.

But maybe not. If something she remembered didn't happen, her memory should change to what *would* happen. But it might be foggy, because of the change. So it could be a while before it clarified for her. The future was not a simple reversal of the past; it was mutable, so her memories could be changed or confused at times. The more distant something was, the longer it might take her to orient on it. Thus a danger in the next step she could catch immediately, but one several hours away would not clarify until she had more experience with the Mode in which it was to occur. Not just because it took her time to attune, but because the more time passed, the more chances there were for it to be changed, fogging her memory. She had to get closer to the event to be sure of it.

At any rate, he hoped he had a workable system. He had just informed her of what had recently happened, and she had informed him of what was about to happen. She had remembered what he was going to tell her, so knew something of the prior adventures despite not being able to remember them directly. She had remembered his telling her. Tomorrow he would tell her again, so she could always have a notion what had been going on. Meanwhile she had told him that nothing bad was about to happen, and he would remember that. When she told him that there would be danger, he would be suitably warned by his memory of her words. It seem like a feasible way to relate. If he had it straight. His mind tended to stretch out of shape as he reviewed the matter.

But if he were correct about the way the new Modes cut off her awareness of the future, she would not do him much good while they were actually traveling. Only when they camped for a time. But that was when they most needed warning of danger, so they could sleep.

His thoughts mostly settled, he resumed his awareness of the terrain. They were out of the forest and were climbing a gentle slope overgrown with waist-high plants whose leaves were pale blue. They made a faint jingling noise as the progress of the two human beings pushed them aside. At irregular intervals there were outcroppings of the underlying rock, which was red. It was a pretty enough scene.

They crested the hill and started down the other side. The plants shifted from blue to purple, and the outcrops to pink, as the Modes shifted. The sky was turning deep green.

Suddenly the two of them were falling. Darius felt a moment of panic. Then his feet struck steeply sloping pink sand. He tried to stand, but could not, so he tried to sit, and it made little difference; he continued sliding down. Provos was beside him, doing her best to maintain a decorous attitude despite being out of control. They were rapidly descending into a huge pit.

Another drop, and another rescue by a steep slope. Then they landed in a pile of pink sand. They climbed out of it and surveyed their situation.

This was evidently an artificial excavation of enormous scope. On three sides it rose so steeply that climbing it was out of the question; they had been fortunate that it had even slowed their fall. The fourth side was flat: a terrace, narrowing into a level road leading out between the towering pink sides.

So why hadn't Provos warned him of this? Because they had stepped into it in a new Mode. Because it was artificial, there was no natural warning, nothing they could see ahead. This ground had once been whole, and now it was hollow, and they had stepped from the ground of

185

one Mode into the emptiness of the next. He had known that she could not anticipate such a thing, yet had somehow depended on it, thinking their periodic descriptions of past and future events would suffice. Only when they remained for a time in a single Mode would that system work well.

Who had dug this monstrous hole? Probably some civilization similar to the one Colene shared. She had told him how they mined deep in the ground, sometimes leaving just such pits as this. So maybe he was getting close to her Mode. That was encouraging.

But not identical, because this was not her village with its paved streets and angular houses. So it was best to get on by this pit before those who dug it arrived. Trying to go back was hopeless; they couldn't even stand on that slope, and could never climb to the top.

Provos evidently agreed. They dusted themselves off and started walking across the level base.

Suddenly there was a giant thing bearing down on them. It resembled one of the traveling machines Colene had described, but was much larger and fiercer.

Both of them stepped hastily back across the boundary. The machine vanished. It least it was easy to avoid, with the Modes.

Darius got out his mirror tube and poked it across the boundary. The machine had passed beyond them, and was now stopping beside another machine, one with a giant set of jaws on the end of a long neck.

They stepped across again. Now he saw that the jawed machine was gouging great mouthfuls of orange sand from the base of the pit, and spitting them into the back of the traveling machine. So that was how the pit was made. The machines must have been working at it for a long time, evidently wanting the pretty sand.

They crossed another boundary. The sand brightened a trace, now possessing more of a yellow component. The pit seemed larger, and there were several dark blue machines eating at the edge of it. All the machines of this section of the Virtual Mode were hungry for this sand!

It seemed that all they needed to do was keep walking across the pit until they reached the far side. Then –

Then what? The far side looked as forbidding as the near side. They would not be able to climb out of it either.

They would have to walk down the road, which surely led out. It was not going in the direction Darius wanted, but once they were free of the pit they could recover their course.

Darius turned to follow the road, and Provos went with him. Now they were remaining longer in one Mode, because the road slanted slowly across it.

A green machine came charging out of the pit. They stepped hastily into the next Mode, and the vehicle vanished. But there was a gray machine coming from the opposite direction. If they ducked back, they could get run over by the first. So they ran on across and jumped into the next Mode before the gray machine reached them.

Here there were yellow machines. These were smaller, though still formidable, and looked like huge insects with antennae. The antennae rotated, seeming to orient on the two living folk. Then two machines started toward them.

They ran on across, to the edge of the road where the next boundary would take them away. But something alarming happened.

They bounced off the boundary.

Darius stared at Provos. She seemed as dismayed as he. This had never happened before.

The machines were closing in on them. As one, they turned and ran back the way they had come, barely crossing the prior boundary before the machines arrived.

Another gray machine was coming. This one slowed, seeming to see them. It too had antennae.

'I don't like this,' Darius muttered. 'These things are aware of us!'

Provos agreed. But it wasn't safe to cross this Mode in front of the machine; it was too big and fast. They had to duck back into the Mode they had just left.

The two yellow machines were waiting. As soon as the two living folk reappeared in this Mode, the machines resumed motion, closing in.

Provos was becoming increasingly agitated. Darius knew that meant that she was starting to tune into future trouble here. They had to get away!

Their best chance seemed to be to cross rapidly through the Mode of the gray machines, so as to be out of this squeeze. He grabbed Provos' arm and pointed. But she demurred. She pointed down this Mode, at right angles.

If she was tuning in, she knew what she was doing. He nodded agreement, and they ran in that direction.

The yellow machines accelerated, quickly overtaking them. But they ran straight ahead, while the road curved, and the mechanical devices couldn't follow well. There was a ditch which was treacherous for wheels on frames to navigate. They had to swerve aside, and the two living folk got clear.

But other machines were now approaching from the opposite direction. One of them had large wheels that could handle the terrain.

Provos ran on, though she was now breathing hard and holding her side. She was an old woman, and evidently not in condition for such activity. But she must remember something to make this effort worthwhile.

Darius drew close to her, matched her steps, and put his right arm around her mid section. He drew her in close and lifted, taking some of her weight off her feet. This might have seemed unduly familiar, but she would remember that he had done this without familiar intent.

So it seemed. She put her left arm around him and leaned into him. Now they ran as one, with his legs assuming much of the burden. He was used to walking and running, and could handle this for a short distance.

A building came into sight. It was large, with several metal lacework towers rising from its top. It crossed their path, and they were headed straight for it.

But if the machines were chasing them now, what would happen when they reached that building? Surely there were many more machines in there!

The machines cut them off. Now Provos urged him to the left, across the boundary. The yellow machines vanished.

The ground was now flat, without the ditches that limited

the machines, and the gray machines were lurking. They were clustered in the vicinity the two living folk had left, but quickly reoriented and renewed the pursuit.

Provos kept running. As the gray machines caught up, she drew the two of them back to the Mode of the yellow machines.

They were now beyond the machines that had cut them off, and close to the building. This was not the kind of structure that creatures of flesh lived in; it was formed of a metal lattice, with spaced supports. He could see through the gaps into its center, where machines and parts of machines seemed to be clustered. Perhaps this was where the machines were bred, birthed and trained.

Provos drew free of him, squatted, and picked up a handful of orange sand. She stuffed it in whatever pockets she possessed. Darius, bemused, did the same. He had to trust her memory of the immediate future, as she had to trust his memory of the past. Then she put her hands on the edges of the lattice, and started climbing. Darius did the same, moving to her right to climb, though the point of this exercise baffled him. The machines would only trap them on the building.

Indeed, yellow machines were moving inside the building, on a platform that was rising by itself. The machines would reach the top before the people did.

Darius tried to find better climbing by moving to his right, but his shoulder banged into the impenetrable wall that was the next Mode. He didn't know what to make of that; surely the machines had not found a way to block it off to travelers!

Provos lost a handhold on her left and hung for a moment in doubt. He quickly steadied her with his left arm. Then she gestured with her left hand, and he saw it pass right through the metal of the wall. No wonder she had missed her hold! The building did not exist in the next Mode, though they could see it clearly from this one. On the ground it didn't matter if they strayed across a boundary, but here it could be fatal.

This minor misadventure had cost them time, and the platform with the machines was passing them. They would surely be made captive or worse when they reached the roof.

Provos held on firmly with one hand, and with the other

dug into a pocket. She brought out some sand and hurled it at the side of the platform, where toothed wheels turned. So Darius did the same. Was this a form of magic, a ritual throwing of sand? If so, it was useless, for this was obviously a nonmagical Mode. But he reminded himself again that she could remember the future, so should know what she was doing to make it memorable. He heaved another handful of sand into the works.

There was an unkind sound. The platform shuddered and slowed. Sparks flew out.

Now it was making sense. The gears did not like sand.

They climbed on to the top of the building, and walked across the metal roof. They remained carefully in their three-paces-wide channel, because the Mode on one side was an impenetrable wall, and on the other was a drop-off. It was a big building, and a fall from it would be devastating.

Provos went to the tower that was in their channel. But it was near the boundary. In fact, half of it was across the boundary; they had to pass it to the right, lest they fall.

But she did not try to pass it. Instead she started climbing it, though she was evidently tired. Her backpack surely weighed her down, with all the running and climbing. Yet the tower went nowhere except up. What was her urgency?

'This thing is only half anchored!' he warned. 'It will fall over with your weight!' But then he realized that this was not the case. The tower was quite firmly anchored, in this Mode. The fact that they could not touch its other side did not mean that it lacked that support. They could climb it, until it narrowed into nothing. Then what?

The yellow machines were getting their platform unjammed. Soon they would be here.

Darius shrugged and started up the tower after her. He hoped she was remembering something that he was unable to foresee, because otherwise they were doomed.

They climbed high on the narrowing tower. Now there was scarcely room for them, even in tandem, because of the half that didn't exist for them. A stiffening breeze tugged at them, making Darius even less comfortable about the height. What could possibly be the point of this?

Meanwhile the machines reached the roof and clustered around the base of the tower. It seemed that they could not climb it, but surely they had ways to get at those who did. Probably the only thing that had saved the two living folk so far had been the machines' desire to capture them alive. Maybe the machines, like the dragons, were interested in learning how to cross Modes, and thought that firm persuasion would elicit the secret from the travelers.

Provos stopped. He looked up and saw that she was struggling to get something from her pack. But she was now so tired that she couldn't twist around without being in danger of falling.

'I'll do it!' he said. 'What do you want?'

She made a gesture of throwing.

'Sand,' he said. He dug into a pocket and threw some sand down on the machines.

She shook her head no.

'Throw something else? But all we have is our supplies, and we need those.'

She nodded yes.

Darius gazed down at the machines. Now they were bringing something with a portable platform. They would be getting up here soon.

He sighed. He drew out a package of bread. He opened it and tore off one chunk with his teeth. He wanted to eat it, but this mouthful was for another purpose. What a waste! He threw it in the direction the woman had indicated.

The chunk flew out and down. It bounced against the invisible wall of the next Mode.

Provos signaled for him to throw again, higher.

He tore off another chunk, and threw it in a higher arc.

It disappeared.

'Yes!' Provos cried.

It took Darius a moment to realize the significance of what had happened. That last chunk had passed above the blank wall and entered the next Mode!

The woman made another gesture of throwing.

He worked it out. They had been unable to enter that Mode because there was no deep pit there. They could not step into

191

solid rock. But if they got above the level of the ground, they could jump onto it!

Provided they knew the exact level. Too low, and they would strike the barrier and drop way down. Too high, and they would make it, but hurt themselves landing.

He ripped off more bread and began throwing in earnest. He found the level, about a body length below him. But it was also a body length away from him. How could they reach it?

The rope! If they could tie it to the tower above, they might be able to swing across on it. He could push Provos so that she would go far enough, and then she could let go on the other Mode.

He reached over his shoulder and plunged his hand into his pack. He found the rope and brought it out. It was fine thin cord, light but strong, with plenty of length. But how was he to tie it to the tower above them? There really wasn't room for him to climb up past Provos, and if he did, it would take time, and the machines' capture-platform was now in place and rising toward them. There wasn't enough time!

He gazed up. At the top, the tower had a crosspiece with hooked ends. That should be ideal to tie the rope to, had he the time and position to do it.

Provos looked down. She extended one hand. She wanted the rope?

He passed up one end. She worked the rope around her upper body and through part of the tower, tying herself to it. Then she leaned back, freeing both hands while her body was held by the rope. She formed a double loop in the cord, with an intricate knot. She fished a solid little package out of her pack and tightened the loops around it. Then she untied herself and passed the end of the rope down to him.

Darius realized that she had effectively weighted the end of the rope. Now he knew what to do. He held on firmly to the tower with his left hand, leaned out, and hurled the end straight up as hard as he could. He let the cord play out, holding tightly on to the other end.

It sailed up beyond the crosspiece, and down again, missing. He borrowed from Provos' technique, tying himself to the tower so as to free both hands. Then he hauled up the rope, leaned way out, and threw it with a more looping motion. This time his aim was good, but not his power; it passed just under the crosspiece.

He tried a third time, and a fourth, while the machine platform slowly came up at him. The fourth time did it: the rope passed over and swung down beyond. The weighted end came down and he caught it. He drew on the two ends, working the rope out to the edge of the crosspiece, where it was caught by the hook. Now they were ready to swing, and none too soon, because the machine platform was uncomfortably close.

Provos took the rope again. She removed the package and returned it to her pack. Then she formed a harness with the two ends, and put her legs through it. She certainly knew how to do things with that rope! In a moment she was dangling free of the tower, seated in the harness.

Darius climbed up, glad to get his feet farther away from the machines. He gave her a push to start her swinging. She swung out toward the invisible wall, then back past the tower, and disappeared.

Darius stared, then realized that this was not disaster. She had passed into the Mode of the gray machines. There was no building or tower there, but she was anchored by the rope to this yellow machine Mode. He could see the rope above, angling down and disappearing about halfway down.

Sure enough, in a moment she reappeared. First her bent knees and feet showed, then the rest of her. She swung past him, and he put out his hand and shoved her farther in the direction she was going. She went farther toward the wall Mode, but did not disappear.

In a moment she was passing him again, the other way. He gave her knees a shove, but it wasn't straight, and it started her turning. That couldn't be helped.

He looked down. The machines had stopped advancing. Their platform was still. Their feelers seemed to be focused on the vanished woman. They didn't know what was happening. Well, he would be surprised too, if a machine came through his home region, climbed a tower, dangled from it, and started swinging in and out of existence.

Provos reappeared. He gave her another good shove. She

swung far out – and half of her disappeared. Her feet remained in view, evidently snagging on the wall.

Then she was coming back. 'I gone!' she exclaimed. She remembered what was about to happen.

Pleased, he gave her another shove back, and another forward when she reappeared. This time she lifted her legs and disappeared entirely, and the rope went slack without returning. She must have put her feet down on the ground, stopping her swing.

Then the rope swung back to him, the harness empty. He caught it and worked his way into the harness.

Now the machines resumed activity, evidently catching on that the prey was escaping. The platform rose again.

Darius shoved off from the tower. He did not swing out far enough. He swiped at the tower, trying to increase his motion, and set himself spinning.

He swung into emptiness. There a dizzying distance below him was the pit, with the gray machines waiting. Then he was back passing the tower. He shoved at it again as well as he could, slowing his spinning but not gaining much on his swinging.

Then he was back over the gray machines. One was aiming what seemed to be a metal tube at him. From the tube came a rope which narrowly missed him. They were trying to catch him in the air and haul him down to them!

He swung back into the yellow-machine Mode. The platform was almost up to the level of his feet, and a machine with big pincers was reaching up. The pincers appeared to be padded so as not to do damage; they wanted to catch him, not kill him, as he had suspected. They were coming close to succeeding, because he simply could not get himself swinging enough.

Swinging. Something clicked. The children's game with swings – they could pump themselves up higher without touching anything else.

He started pumping, extending his feet and moving his body. Why hadn't he thought of this before? He gained momentum.

A pincer reached up to catch his passing leg. He kicked it

194

away. That started him spinning, and he was unable to pump. Trouble! He reached out and banged a hand into the tower as he passed, trying desperately to get straightened out. He succeeded, but at the expense of momentum.

He resumed pumping – and saw the yellow pincers directly in front of him. He could not avoid them this time!

He held his breath, tucked his feet under him, then swung them out in a two-legged kick. He smashed into the pincer machine, shoving it back. The platform moved, its support tower beginning to fall.

As Darius pumped himself up, he saw the gray machines taking aim again, and the platform falling, in alternate Modes. Then he broke through and caught a glimpse of a new green world, its surface barely under him. He could not quite stop at it; he needed one more good swing. But those swings were dangerous!

Then hands caught his feet. Provos had tackled his legs, trying to hold him there. But if he dragged her back with him –

She managed to hold him long enough so that he could pitch his upper body forward and brace against the ground. He struggled out of the harness.

Provos caught the harness, quickly undid it, and let go of one rope. She pulled, and the other rope disappeared. Soon the length of it had been hauled in. They had made it, with their equipment.

Later, several more Modes away from the pit and at a suitable camping site, they talked. Provos no longer remembered the business with the tower and rope, but he told her of it, and she told him that nothing dangerous was to occur during their stay in this particular Mode.

'Provos come why?' he asked her. Now he was sure that she was an asset to his journey, and wanted to know what she was getting from it. Was she along for the duration, or would she be deserting him when she found what she wanted?

She tried to convey a confusing concept, and it seemed that she had forgotten part of it, because it was in the past. But his memory of their meeting, and her memory of what he was to tell her in the future, enabled him finally to put it together.

195

Her memory of future events was hazy or null, but she did have memories of him, because he was to be a constant part of her next few days.

Provos suffered from amnesia. She had been able to remember her future perfectly, in as much detail as she desired, right up until a mysterious blank. As it approached, she viewed it with increasing trepidation, until she realized that it was not necessarily the end. Perhaps it was better viewed as a great new adventure occurring after some mishap such as a blow to the head. Since she could not avoid it, she decided to approach it positively. So she had packed her things, as for a long journey, and told her friends she was going to another region. That way they were not concerned about the future absence of her presence in their lives.

Now she was in that adventure, and enjoying it. She still suffered amnesia of the future, but not as badly. She understood the reason: because she had no future experience in most of the Modes they were crossing.

She had no plans for the future. She would know the future when she remembered it, and she was content to wait for that memory. It was actually rather exciting, being unable to tell what she was doing tomorrow, in contrast to the deadly dull existence she suspected she had been having in the past. She was not concerned about Darius' convenience, as she did not remember him telling her he disliked her company. When he preferred to move on alone, she would know it before the time came, and they would part.

Indeed, Darius realized that he did not object to her company. He was not looking for any personal complications along the way, and she presented few, which were more than compensated for by her brief insights of mischief forthcoming. She was a good companion for this treacherous journey.

'But how do you feel about your own death?' he asked. 'Will you see it coming?'

She certainly hoped so! She was not at all disturbed by his question. It turned out that she feared her death no more than he feared his birth. It was merely one end of a person's existence. But that part of her life she could not remember, which was in the past, she preferred not to think about, for it was filled with unkind mystery and foreboding, as well as with hopeful speculation. Exactly as was his future for him.

'But now you have a taste of what my perspective is like,' he told her. 'Because you can not anticipate most of your future either.'

She agreed that was frightening, but she would bear up under the challenge of it, knowing that it was bound to be alleviated one way or another before too long. She put her hand on his, with pity and comfort for his misfortune to be locked always in the past.

'Thank you,' he said, moved in mixed manner. But she had already lost the dialogue, and proceeded in a businesslike manner to the settling in for the night.

9

DDWNG

There were more realities than Colene had dreamed of. Some were inhabited by what were probably human beings or the equivalent; most were not. They passed quickly through the inhabited ones, which tended to cluster, and lingered in the wilderness ones. Wild creatures, as a general class, were not as dangerous as civilized ones. Seqiro was able to stun any creature who threatened, or simply to change its mind. In fact, she discovered, he could generate a mental field around them that discouraged insects, so that mosquitoes and biting flies did not come close. The first time she had slapped at a mosquito he had inquired, and then sent out the no-insect thought. Just like that, no problem. He had been satisfied to use his tail to flick away pests, until then.

She had liked him from the start. Each new thing she learned about him enhanced the feeling.

They walked for another day and slept another night. She kept no count of the number of realities they crossed, but judged that such a day's travel should represent about five thousand of them. The calculation was simple enough: ten feet per reality, if they crossed it at right angles as they usually did. Ten miles in the day, because they walked maybe ten hours at maybe three miles an hour, taking time for eating and rest. The tens canceled out, and the number of feet in a mile – about five thousand – was the number of realities. But it didn't matter. What counted was that they were making progress

198

toward Darius. She knew they were; she felt the strengthening rightness of the route.

Most realities were overgrown with vegetation, but they did encounter a series of them with rocky sections, and she was able to ride her bicycle through these. Otherwise she would have been dead tired, because this was a whole lot more walking than she had done in a long time. She was lucky that her camping experience had prepared her somewhat; she knew how to conserve her strength and not push her limits.

Seqiro, in contrast, seemed indefatigable. He had evidently made it a point to maintain his health and stamina, and it showed.

I could carry you, he thought. *It would not represent a burden to me, as you weigh little.*

'I just don't think of you as a riding horse,' she said. 'You're my companion.'

Granted. But a companion may walk or be carried.

She smiled briefly. 'If it comes to the point where we really need to get somewhere, and I'm really holding us back, then you carry me. Until then, I feel more equal afoot.'

Because in your home reality horses are beasts of burden.

'Never to me!' she protested.

But your mind indicates that the association is there. You are concerned with what others will think, though none are here to see.

'Never argue cases with a mind reader!' she said ruefully. 'Or with someone smarter than you.'

I am quite stupid compared to you.

'No way! Everything I tell you, you understand right away, better than I do. So you're smarter or older or both, or just plain have more experience.'

None of these. I am your age in years: fourteen. That is mature for my kind, but my experience of my reality is less than yours of yours. I depend on your mind.

'Do you, Seqiro? Maybe you needed me to fetch your supplies and load them on you, and to open your gate. But once you got out of your reality, I became superfluous. You have just remained with me out of sympathy.'

By no means. I remain with you because I need you, and because we are compatible.

199

'A girl needs a horse,' she argued. 'But does a horse need a girl? Wouldn't you be happier out grazing, if the grass would stay with you?'

I would be satisfied grazing, he agreed. *But I am also satisfied to be traveling with you. Since I can not safely graze, and can comfortably travel with you, this is the preferable course.*

'But you could travel just as well without me! I'm really holding you back.'

Not so. I would be unable to travel without you. This is the major reason I did not break out of my confinement and enter the Virtual Mode alone.

'I don't believe that!' She was feeling that self-destructive urge, trying to persuade him to do without her. She didn't want to be alone; in retrospect she found her prior travel frightening. But to be a drag on this beautiful horse – that just wasn't right. 'Give me one good reason why you can't travel without me.'

My intelligence would revert to its normal level, and I would be unable to fix on a specific distant destination. I would soon be captured by any creatures who saw me as a beast of burden.

'But you're smart! I couldn't be talking with you like this if you weren't!'

I draw on your intelligence, which is excellent. In your absence I would retain only the memory of you, not the power of your mind. If other creatures captured me, and none shared minds with me, I would remain dull. I was dull until I made contact with your mind from afar; then I became more intelligent than any of my kind.

Colene was amazed. 'You mean – it's all me? I'm really talking to myself?'

You are talking to me, and I am as intelligent as you – because you share your mind with me. If you withheld your mind, I would indeed be just a stupid horse.

'But your kind controls my kind, in your reality! I saw it, I felt it. Your minds make hash of our minds.'

Our leaders retain intelligent humans who provide them with good power of the mind, much as your leaders retain strong horses who provide them with rapid transportation. In your reality your riders control your horses despite the inferior strength of the humans. In mine, the horses control the humans despite the inferior intelligence of the horses. It is a matter of who is in charge, and how power is wielded.

She was coming to accept it, reluctantly. 'So you needed a smart companion, so you would understand where you were going and how to get there. And I'm that companion.'

Yes.

'And if I'd turned out to be a bad human man, you'd still have had to go with me, because it would have been either that or stay under stall arrest.'

Yes.

'But I turned out to be a sweet human girl, and you like that better.'

Yes.

She turned to him. 'I was joking, Seqiro.'

No.

'I mean, about being sweet. I'm not sweet, I'm suicidal.'

Yes, you were suicidal once, and sweet. Now you are only sweet.

'You believe that?' she demanded

Yes. So do you. This is why I believe it.

She stepped into him and hugged his neck as well as she could. 'I love you, Seqiro.'

Yes. I also love you.

'But would you love me if you weren't picking it up from my mind?'

No. That is not an emotion I would understand alone. But it is pleasant now.

'I think I like you even better this way. You are my ideal companion.'

Yes.

'Yes,' she echoed. 'We are ideal for each other. Seqiro, we must stay together!'

Yes.

'You keep agreeing with me, and I love it!' she exclaimed.

Yes.

'Yet how is it you know so much, when I don't know it?'

A horse has good memory. I have learned much in my life, and when I am with you I am able to apply it relevantly.

She walked on with restored attitude. Seqiro did need her,

201

perhaps more than she needed him, and this was an enormous comfort. She had made it possible for him to escape his fate, and he would remain with her until he found what he was looking for – which he could best find only while he was with her, sharing her mind. That might be forever. That was long enough.

They stepped across a boundary, and suddenly there was barrenness. As far as they could see, the forested slopes had been abruptly denuded. The air was cold and dry.

They retreated, and the friendly trees reappeared. 'What happened?' Colene asked, baffled.

Nothing in my reality explains this. But you have thoughts of nuclear war in yours.

'I don't think it's that,' she said with a shiver. 'No slag. No green glass. No deadly radiation – I hope.' She glanced at him. 'I don't suppose you can detect radiation with your mind?'

Focus on it, and I will try.

She concentrated on deadly rays, uncertain of their names or how they would feel, but sure that they would cut up the tender cells of her body and mess up her genetics. Invisible shafts of destruction, like X-rays only worse. Would this be enough for him to fathom? She doubted it, yet she hoped, because otherwise they were at an impasse. How could they risk that barren waste, without being sure it wouldn't kill them just because they were there? They couldn't go around it, because it was evident that it extended everywhere on that planet. There had not even been any clouds. It was just so utter and final!

I can detect such radiation, Seqiro thought. *My telepathic mind is very sensitive to intrusion, and such rays would intrude. There are none.*

'Are you sure?' she asked eagerly, but knew it was a foolish question. Seqiro knew what he knew.

Yes, I am sure. But this may be immaterial. If that waste extends across many realities, we shall not be able to cross it.

'It can't extend forever!' she exclaimed. 'My sense says that where I'm going is somewhere beyond it. Darius didn't say anything about a desert.' But she realized that Darius hadn't said anything about the intervening realities, because the first time he had simply cut through directly. Only with the Virtual Mode did every reality between them become significant.

Then we must cross.

'But suppose it *does* cross many?' she asked, flipping across to the other case, as was her fashion when in doubt. 'Do we have supplies to make it? I don't want to be stuck in Death Valley without water!'

I see the bones of horses in your vision of that valley.

'Yes! It's awful! I've never been there, but I've seen it in movies. Oh, Seqiro, what shall we do?'

You love my company, but you would not be satisfied with it indefinitely. You must rejoin your human man. Therefore we must cross, because the alternative is not suitable.

'Yes, we must cross,' she agreed. She wished she could say it with more confidence. Where was the hero-istic, die-for-her-beliefs girl she longed to be? Not here, unfortunately.

They camped for the night, so as to be able to start early in the day. They agreed that the desert might get hot in the day, and cold at night. They might do best to cross it rapidly and get back into comfortable realities. But if it turned out to be more than a one day trek, they would be better off to maintain a measured pace, resting in the heat of noon and in the cold of night, preserving their strength. They could make a three day crossing, but not if they exhausted themselves on the first day.

Colene fetched dry sticks of wood, and bunches of dry grass, and used one of her precious matches to light a fire. Seqiro had checked and ascertained that there were no high powered minds in this reality, so that the fire would be safe. She was very pleased to have it, for psychological as well as physical reasons.

While she stared into the blaze, she reviewed plans with Seqiro. He would quest ahead for minds. He could tune in to both animals and plants, but the distance depended on circumstances. A strong telepathic mind similar to his own could be contacted across a continent, while dialogue with a nontelepathic mind was limited to about half that. The Virtual Mode was similar, making the different realities seem like one;

without it he would be confined to one reality. The less similar a mind was to his own, the more limited the range. Thus plants had to be fairly close for him to receive.

'Plants have minds?' Colene asked, startled.

Indeed they do. But not similar to yours. We find the best grazing by tuning in to the healthiest grass.

'But doesn't the grass hurt when you bite it off? Why would it tell you where it is?'

It does not suffer in the way you would. It is philosophical about being eaten. It accepts what is. Since grazing promotes the growth of more grass at the expense of weeds, there is a certain compatibility between us.

Colene shook her head. 'I hope so! I'd hate to have my head chewed off every week or so!'

A plant would hate to have to eat through its head, or to pull its roots from the ground and walk about.

She considered. 'I see your point, maybe.'

Everything was normal, for a single reality. But Colene was unable to relax, let alone sleep, for a time. The barrenness ahead of them worried her.

'Can we talk, Seqiro?' she asked after a bit as the darkness closed in.

We may talk, he agreed.

'Say, I just realized: you never argue with me. Not really. You point out things, you clarify what I don't know, but you always go along with what I'm thinking about.'

It is true. I reflect your interests, as mine are not of great moment.

'How can you think that? You're the most wonderful person I've met, next to Darius!'

True. But I am not wonderful without you.

'You're a horse! A horse is wonderful by definition.'

As is a girl.

'Let me tell you what a horse is to me. I'm going to introduce you to Maresy Doats.' She summoned her mental picture of her imaginary friend.

She is a winsome mare.

'Well, I never thought of her as having sex appeal!'

I would have to smell her to determine that.

She laughed. 'So you're just like any man!'

No. Human males are always interested in reproduction. Horses are interested only when the mare is ready. We do not waste energy. We regard this as more sensible.

'Well, Maresy is sensible. She always knows what to do. The trouble is, others aren't always sensible, and they don't listen. It's all recorded in my book, *For Whom Was That Neigh?* It's based on a picture I have of Maresy Doats. Do you want an example?'

Yes.

'Now why did I know you would say that? Okay, here it is. Maresy and another mare were grazing in this pasture. It was the only pasture they had, and there was no other source of food. Just the grass. A tough variety that hung on through the winter. Now Maresy is smarter than the average horse, and she did some figuring, and realized that at the rate they were grazing, they would run out of grass before spring, and then starve in the winter. But if they slowed down their grazing, and ate less grass, they could stretch it out so that it would last until spring, when it would start growing again, and they would survive. They might be lean, but okay. So it made sense to do that.

'So she told the other mare. But the other mare just went right on grazing, paying no attention. She wasn't smart like Maresy, and didn't understand anything except eating until she was full. She ate like a horse.

'So what was Maresy to do? If she stopped grazing, then there would be enough for the other mare, but Maresy would starve now. If she didn't stop, they would both starve later. So should she give up her life so that at least one of them would survive, even though it was the undeserving one? Or should she prolong her own life for a while by continuing to graze?'

She should kill the other mare, and have enough for herself.

'But Maresy wouldn't do that!' Colene protested. 'She believes in life, not death!'

But if there is life only for one –

'Yes. So she's in trouble. I call it the pacifist's dilemma.'

'How does the story end?

'I don't know. We'll just have to wait and see.'

How long?

'I don't know.'

I do not see the point of this story.

'It has no solution, but it does have a point. You see, Maresy stands for me, and for people like me, who are smart enough to see that the world – I mean, in my reality – can't go on this way. It is using up all its resources, and when they are gone, it will be impossible to feed everyone, and most or all of us will die. It doesn't have to be that way, but everyone else, like the other mare, refuses to see the problem, and just goes on grazing at top speed. So we will all suffer, when we don't have to, because of the shortsightedly selfish ones. We won't know exactly what happens until it happens, and then it will be too late. I think that's part of what makes me suicidal. I mean, what's the point in hanging onto life, when it's all going to end anyway, too soon?'

But you are free of that, now, with the Virtual Mode.

'Yes. So I'm not suicidal now, maybe. But I feel guilty for bugging out on my world.'

With the situation as you present it, that is your only choice. You are freeing your world of your presence, so that someone else can survive.

'Say, yes! That's a good way to look at it.' Somewhat cheered, she relaxed, and soon was asleep.

They did start early, as soon as they could see their way. Immediately the barrens, as Colene thought of this region, were all around them, before and behind. It was as if life had never existed anywhere.

At first the land was reasonably level, but this changed with realities, and it became so ragged as to be an unkind challenge. Bare stone rose up in twisted contours, and sank into rubble. Tors gave way to pits, forcing them to wind around their edges, slowing progress. Meanwhile the sun rose in the bleak sky and the bright light beat down on them. Colene fashioned a hat from cloth to protect her face and arms, and covered Seqiro's head and neck similarly, fearing damage from the intensity of the rays. They were a strange looking pair, swathed in coverings fashioned of loose clothing, but there was no one to see.

Then the land descended. It was a great cavity, so large that it featured its own mountains and pits and convolutions, as if it were a continent in reverse. It extended ahead until the rim of the horizon cut it off.

Colene gazed at it with dismay. Then she had a revelation. 'It's a sea!' she exclaimed. 'An ocean! We've come to the end of a continent! A sea without water!'

All water is gone from these realities, Seqiro agreed.

There was nothing to do except descend into it, because her sense told her that Darius was somewhere across this region. 'I hope we don't have to cross the whole Atlantic or Pacific!' Because that would be doom; they could not walk that far.

That brought another concern. 'How will we know if it's too far? I mean, if it is, we should turn back, so at least we don't die of hunger or exposure. But if we turn back, when we could have made it across –'

If we reach what we deem to be half our ability to travel without new supplies, and I still can not detect life ahead, then we should turn back.

'You can detect life behind us?' she asked. 'I mean, you're not just thinking that to reassure me?'

It is fading, but I can feel that life behind.

'Okay. If you get so you can't feel it behind, and you still can't feel it ahead, we'd better turn back. That's not the same as giving up; it just means we'll have to find a better way.'

Agreed.

Yet privately she wondered what better way there could be. They would not be able to go around the barrens the way she had around the hostile bear, because these were entire realities, each one a universe in itself. If there were a million of them, they just had to be crossed, because there didn't seem to be any way to skip over parts of the Virtual Mode.

Well, if they had to retreat, maybe Darius would be able to find a way from the other side. She was sure that he was looking for her, too; he wouldn't have set up the Virtual Mode and then just twiddled his thumbs. They could meet in the middle. So maybe he was coming to the other side of this, now, and was thinking about how to cross, and all she had to do was go back and wait.

But she was more independent than that. She wanted to make it on her own. So she hoped they made it across.

I echo your sentiment.

'Oh, was I thinking too close to the surface? I didn't mean to bother you with this!'

I am becoming increasingly attuned to your mind, so can read more deeply with less effort. I did not mean to intrude.

'Oh, no, that's all right, Seqiro! You understand me, the way Maresy did. I don't mind you in my mind. I just didn't want to burden you with my worries.'

You are concerned about survival now, rather than death.

She laughed, somewhat self-consciously. 'For sure, I'm not being suicidal, now that I'm up against possible death! I'm reacting in a disgustingly normal way. I guess that's an improvement.'

You have reason to live, now.

'Yes. Because of Darius – and you, Seqiro.'

But if you lacked these folk, your self destructiveness would return.

'I guess it would. I'm no bargain, emotionally.'

If you had not had those bad experiences, you would not have become self destructive.

'Well, I don't know about that. Those experiences weren't necessarily bad, just different or shocking. I hadn't known how the people lived in Panama; plenty of other people do know, and they aren't suicidal. I did a lot of good at that hospital, and the doctors and nurses aren't suicidal. The rape scene – that I could have done without. But I didn't get beaten up or anything, and it sure taught me to be wary of liquor and of men! That camp episode really worked out okay, and word never got back to my folks what had really happened. It taught me not to trust anyone, not with my true secrets, and that was a good lesson.'

But you trust me.

'Now why did I know you were going to come up with that? I guess I am breaking my rule. But I also guess I meant not to trust anyone *human*. I trusted Maresy, because she's a horse, and horses can be trusted. You're a horse. Trust just sort of comes with your territory.'

I like Maresy. But there are many horses in my reality who can not be trusted. You are as foolish to trust an animal blindly as to trust a human being blindly.

Colene sighed. 'I guess I am. Okay, I won't trust any other animals either. But is it okay to trust *you*, Seqiro?'

Me alone, he agreed. *Yet do you not also trust Darius, who is human?*

That set her back. 'I don't think I do trust him, exactly. I love him, but that's another matter. When he told me of his wonderful magic land, I didn't believe it. I wish I had! So I guess there is danger in not trusting people, too. I hope he forgives me!'

He must have forgiven you, because he set up the Virtual Mode, so that he could rejoin you.

'Yes, he did that.' Then she paused in her descent of a slope. 'Seqiro! Is it possible that it wasn't Darius who set it up? But someone else? I mean, how would I know, for sure?'

If it was Darius, you will know when you meet him.

'Unless it's someone just pretending to be him, because he wanted an innocent girl or something. Lots of men want young sex-slaves. I really don't know Darius that well.'

I will be with you. I will know his mind.

'Yes! You will know his mind, Seqiro! You must let me know whether it's really him, and how he truly feels about me. I'm not going to marry him, I know that, but I'm willing to be his mistress and helper if I just know he loves me.'

I will inform you of his feeling for you, if you don't object to my intrusion into your private matters. Understand that I will be partial to his sexual sentiment as well as his emotion.

'I understand! I want him to want me, every which way from Sunday! Just so long as he loves me!'

It shall be known.

They continued into the waterless ocean, which seemed even more barren than the continent, because of what should have been there. A continent could be a natural desert, but an ocean could only be an unnatural desert.

That brought another horrible realization. 'Seqiro! Suppose we reach the next living reality – and we're at the bottom of the sea? We could drown!'

209

She felt a wash of panic, and knew that her thought had struck through to his natural mind. It was a horse's nature to spook and run from danger. *So it seems. But your intellect suggests that we might simply retreat through the boundary between realities and be dry again.*

'Well, at least we wouldn't be thirsty!' she exclaimed too cheerily. The notion of being suddenly under a mile or so of water terrified her. She realized increasingly that though she had been suicidal, she was quite choosy about the way she might die. Water would be too suffocating, and she didn't like that.

It would also be crushing. Suppose they were crushed to death before they could retreat? 'I think we had better be pretty careful how we cross boundaries,' she said, shaken.

I will detect the ocean life, which will give us warning.

'Not if it's a sterile sea!' For now she realized that the presence of water was no guarantee of life.

I will flick my tail across them, Seqiro suggested.

'But you would have to travel backwards! No, let me take something of ours – here, this kerchief of mine will do – and I'll flick it ahead of me, and when it gets wet, we'll know.'

Agreed.

They moved on, with Colene ahead, constantly flicking her kerchief as she approached each boundary. It became automatic: one, two, three steps, flick, step, flick and step across, and start over. It was about five of her steps between boundaries, about two feet per step, but she wanted no accident. It would have looked strange to an outsider, but it was a sensible precaution.

Now she was not sure whether she did or did not want to encounter such an ocean. If they found no water, they might have to walk thousands of miles through this dread desert, and would die of dehydration; already their water supply was diminishing at an alarming rate. But if they did find it, how would they get through?

Suddenly there was something. Colene clapped her hand to her mouth to stifle a possible scream. A light was blinking to the south!

I see it, Seqiro thought, responding to her thought. *A beacon. It seems that we are not alone.*

'But can you detect life?'

No. But life must have placed it there.

'Then maybe it's safe to check it,' she said. 'Unless it's got killer machines or something.'

What would be the point of that?

'I don't know. But whatever sterilized all these realities may intend to keep them that way. If that beacon picks up a sign of life, it may trigger another sterilization treatment.'

I suspect it can spot us as readily as we have spotted it. I am aware of no harmful radiation associated with it. Is it possible that it simply marks a path through the barrens?

'Maybe so!' she agreed, encouraged. 'There has to be a way through, so maybe someone left markers. If we have to gamble, let's gamble on the positive interpretation.'

Nevertheless, they were diffident as they approached the beacon. It disappeared when they crossed realities; it existed only in one. But it was easy to approach, because of its constant flashing.

It turned out to be a simple machine: a ball mounted on a thin metal pole stuck into a porous section of the sea floor, which blinked. At its base was an arrow painted in bright red, pointing east.

'A direction marker!' Colene exclaimed. 'Pointing the way!'

Could it be your friend Darius?

'You mean, to show where he's been? Or to find his way back?' She focused seriously on that for a moment. 'No, I don't think so. He's from the reality of magic, and this is plainly science. Super-science, I think; that ball's opaque, yet it flashes. It must be someone else. Maybe there's a regular caravan through here, with markers to steer it straight.'

I doubt it. This Virtual Mode has existed only a week in your terms.

She nodded. 'Well, one person, maybe, but not Darius. But it will do for us, certainly; this should be much faster, because now we know where we're going, sort of.'

I agree.

Heartened, they resumed travel.

211

Meanwhile the contours of the bottom of the ocean were a revelation to her. Instead of being flat and sandy, as she had somehow fancied, they were phenomenally more varied than those of the continental land. There were mountains and valleys and rifts and lattices of twisted stone. There were holes so deep they filled her with dread, and slopes so sharp that they resembled walls. One section was like a monstrous banyan tree, with thousands of pillars reaching down to lower platforms, from which more pillars extended on down. Another was like an upside-down mountain with mounds supporting its edges. Elsewhere there were what seemed to be worm holes in myriads, ranging from pinhead to handspan diameter, disappearing into darkness. And the opposite: pencil-thin towers of packed sand, their sedimentary origins showing in streaks crossing the formation. There had surely been water here once; what had happened to it?

In fact, how could this region have been rendered so dry, without disturbing these natural formations? She was able to knock over the pencil towers with her hands; they were not made for sidewise pressure. Any heat great enough to vaporize all the water should have generated savage storms. If some cosmic drain had opened in the bottom and let it all flow out, there should have been some pools remaining and some gouging as the drainage rivers formed. Instead it was as if the water had simply vanished, without even making any currents.

Then her bandanna snagged on something. She jerked it back, startled, for to her eye she was merely flicking it in air before a sea of air. She checked it.

The tip was dry, but looked as if it had recently been wet. Because the water couldn't cross the boundary.

'Oopsy, Seqiro! We've struck water!'

The horse stepped up and turned broadside. He flicked his tail. It struck something.

I felt the liquid, he agreed.

Colene put up her hands, carefully, and felt the air before her. The boundary was icy cold and slick. 'Like ice,' she announced. 'I guess we didn't have to worry about drowning; it's under such pressure we can't get into it anyway.'

212

I sense no life.

So it was lifeless water. Some realities had been dried, some frozen, or at least sterilized. The two of them could not continue crossing boundaries.

This was not exactly a relief. 'What do we do, Seqiro? Do we turn back? We can make it from here, at least.'

But if we find a way to enter the next reality, we will have water, greatly extending our range.

'I don't think so. We can't take it with us.'

'We can if we drink it carefully, saving our own water for emergency use.'

'But it must be salt water! We can't drink that!'

It is my understanding that we can. In my reality we have a technique for filtering impure water through sand to make it pure. We can do that.

'Or we can evaporate some, and condense the vapor!' she agreed, turning more positive. 'But we still have to get up to the top of it, and then what will we do – sail across it?'

Seqiro sorted through the picture in her mind, of a girl and horse standing precariously on a raft. *I prefer not.*

She laughed, humorlessly. 'I guess not! So unless there's a big change coming beyond the water-reality, we're sunk anyway, no pun.'

I fear that is the case. But we should try to explore it if we can. If we can find land, and cross more realities, I can quest farther for life.

'I guess you're right. This is about midday now; let's see if there is any rise to the level of the surface north or south.' She meant to the left or right, because their progress was generally eastward. 'Maybe an island, at least. But which direction do we go? It would be a shame if there is a perfect island north, and we go south and fail to find it and have to give up and go back.' She tried to make it sound cheery, but knew that her dark forebodings were coming through clearly to the horse.

Perhaps we could explore both directions, one going north, the other south, and double our chances. We may discover another beacon.

'Seqiro, you're a genius!' she exclaimed. 'And we can stay in mental contact, so the other will have the news first thing.'

They did it. Colene went north. She tried to suppress her belief that they were wasting time and energy, because even if they found an island and were able to cross the boundary, they would still have virtually impassable water to cross. These barren realities were an awful barrier!

She came to a rise, but it was followed by a depression. She saw a mountain in the distance, which should be an island, but it was to the northeast, in the territory of another reality, impossible to reach from here.

'How about you?' she asked, thinking at Seqiro.

I may have found an island. But I can not find an ascent.

'Keep looking!' she exclaimed. 'I have nothing here; I'll come join you.'

She hurried south, now trying to suppress unreasonable hope. 'Have you found a path up yet, Seqiro?'

No. I fear I am lost. I am caught in an endless trench.

'I'll watch out for it!' Suddenly she thought how much worse it would be if her companion got trapped, and she had to choose between staying with him or saving herself. Even if she had no choice, if something happened to him, how could she go on alone? His marvelous mind had become her main emotional support.

Thank you. But away from you I am just a horse.

'You're so much more than a horse!' she protested. 'But a horse is good enough.'

In due course she reached the mountain. It did seem to rise high enough to be an island, depending on how high the surface of the water in the other reality was. But between her and it was a deep channel, as if the mountain had sunk down in the semi-molten floor eons ago, making a depression. This must be Seqiro's endless trench.

She found a place where she could safely drop down into it, the drop not so far that she couldn't scramble back. 'I'm in the channel, Seqiro. Where are you?'

Not far from you. I shall wait.

Soon she caught up with him. He was standing, breathing

214

hard, the sweat rolling off his hide. 'Why Seqiro! What happened to you? You're steaming hot!'

I'm afraid I panicked. I galloped, but found no end to the channel. I recognized landmarks I had passed before, and realized that I was trapped.

'You ran all the way around the mountain!' she exclaimed. 'Oh, Seqiro, you wasted valuable energy and are losing water in your sweat. Didn't you know better?'

I did not.

'But you're so smart!'

No. Away from you I am not. I maintained contact with you, but only your thoughts came through, not your underlying power of mind.

She realized that he had meant it literally when he warned her about that before. So, alone, he had reverted to his underlying nature, and spooked when unable to figure out how to escape the channel.

Then she realized something else. 'You couldn't have run around the mountain! Half of it's in the other reality, under the water!'

True. I realize that now. The loop evidently is completed on this side.

'Well, let's get you out of this and climb that mountain,' she said. 'Now that you're smart again, did you see a good way for you to do that?'

Yes. There is a navigable slope to a dead-end path.

They walked back to it. Sure enough, it was possible for a horse to climb up on the mountain side, but then the path ended as it seemed about to cross over the top of the channel, which was deep and narrow here. It was as if there had once been a bridge here.

And there, in an adjacent reality beyond the trench, was another stick-ball beacon. This was certainly the right place!

But I will do better with your help.

'Sure! What do you need from me?'

Tell me when my front feet are about to land just before the bridge. I am unable to see them when my head is up.

'Okay.'

Seqiro got up speed and galloped toward the brink. 'Now!'

she cried as his front feet came down. He brought his hind feet up close to them, then heaved up his forefeet and leaped over the gap. He recovered his balance and slowed to a stop. He was out.

'I guess maybe we should stay together after this,' she said. 'I really didn't like being apart from you anyway, Seqiro. I worried –'

I understand. And of course he did, for he could read the complex of her emotions as she spoke.

They explored the mountain from outside the channel, and found a likely ascent. But it was a narrow ledge in places. 'Um, will you be able to turn around, there? I mean, if –?'

Perhaps you should explore ahead, and I will rejoin you when you come across a turning place.

'Okay. But let's just not separate any farther than we absolutely have to, okay?'

Agreed.

So she ran and hurdled the trench and mounted the twisty steep path, catching handholds on the carved stone abutments to help haul herself up. She found a kind of landing, and thought its description to Seqiro, who then followed her up. They continued similarly, by stages, their progress complicated by the wall of cold water. When the best path crossed that boundary, they had to back off and find an alternate path. Thus it was evening by the time they reached the top, and they were tired. They had seen no other beacons or signs of life.

'You know, if this doesn't give us some way to move on rapidly, we're sunk,' she said. 'It will be all we can do to get down the mountain and back to the last habitable reality.'

I shall be disappointed for you in that event. But perhaps Darius will find a way to cross from the other side, and you will still be unified.

'Gee, I hope so! It's not that I'm not satisfied with your company, Seqiro, but –'

You need a human male like Darius, just as I need a mare like Maresy, to complete your life.

'Yeah.' She led the way along the leveling summit, looking for a good place to camp for the night. But the only good one was on the east side of the mountain, beyond the boundary.

She knew exactly where that boundary was, now, after bumping into it so many times on the way up.

Then she did a mental doubletake: this was the top. They should be able to cross that boundary now – if they ever could. So she stepped gingerly into it – and passed through.

It was indeed an island. Ahead it sloped to a rocky shore just a few feet below the level she stood. The waves washed against the barren stone, making froth.

'Seqiro! We're across!'

I saw it with you. The horse appeared behind her as she looked back, seeming to materialize from nothing. *But I fear that this too is impassable.*

'Yeah.' Her elation of the moment faded quickly. The surface of the ocean extended to the horizon, featureless. Then she had another thought. 'But the beacons pointed this way, so there must be something.'

At least we can wash.

She forced her mind away from the disappointment. She really hadn't expected any more than this. 'Yes, we can both take a good dip, and I can wash my clothes.'

This time Seqiro let her remove his load and harness, and she stripped. Nakedness didn't matter with an animal, and if it did, it wouldn't have mattered with this one. He could see her naked mind.

They stepped cautiously toward the limited shore, passing through another boundary just at the verge of the water – and stopped short.

There was a pontoon wharf projecting into the sea. It cut off abruptly about ten feet out, and seemed of recent vintage, with bright paint and gleaming metal chains connecting the floats.

But what was the point of a wharf, here? Was it waiting for a ship?

It is a bridge. We can see only what is in this reality.

Suddenly it made sense. The path hadn't ended; it continued on across the water. But only part of it was in this reality, because it was on the Virtual Mode. 'So the beacons did know what they were doing,' she breathed. 'Well, let's wash, and – maybe we had better spend the night here, and eat and rest, before we start across. We don't know exactly what we may encounter out there.'

True.

They washed up, finding the water chill but refreshing. Colene felt a special freedom, being naked in the open. Somehow it seemed that if she could be naked all the time, she would never be suicidal.

She walked out along the bridge, crossing the next boundary. The pontoons continued unbroken. But the appearance was of a ten foot segment ending before and behind her. It looked far more precarious than it was. There was no doubt now: the bridge was part of the Virtual Mode. Someone from an anchor reality must have set it up. But who?

We shall discover that when we follow it to its source.

'But how do we know that source is friendly?' she asked as she toweled herself off, using a dry shirt. She would have preferred to let herself dry naturally, but she was shivering and had to get clothed before she did herself harm.

I will be able to tell, if I am let into the mind of the anchor person.

'You can't just peek?'

I can enter only a willing mind. Once I do, I can communicate freely, regardless of the language of the person, and can control that mind, and therefore the body. But I can not penetrate a hostile mind, or even an indifferent one.

'But you controlled the minds of those human servants in your reality, so we could escape.'

Not exactly. Our humans have been tamed, in the manner of your horses and other animals, so are receptive. Wild humans would not be receptive, any more than wild horses in your reality allow themselves to be ridden. They had discussed the differences between their two societies as they walked; Seqiro now understood her framework well enough. *Even so, particular humans associate with particular horses, and do not allow unfamiliar horses to govern them if their own horses forbid it. In the stress of the moment I was able to strike through, but that was a limited opportunity.*

'But you and I made immediate connection!'

Because you are highly receptive.

'Well, I'm not tame!' she said indignantly.

218

But you desired compatible company. You were extremely lonely and nervous. That enabled me not only to join you, but to reach you from a distance, and across realities.

She nodded, now chewing on cold bread from his supplies, because there was nothing here from which she could make a fire. He was eating a ration of mixed grains. 'I was that, for sure! I still am. I need you, Seqiro, I really do! Back when I started getting depressed I did some research, and decided I fit the profile of BPD: Borderline Personality Disorder. I mean, alienation from my parents, sexual betrayal by a date, inability to cope with what I was learning about the evils of the world, and I was sort of on a roller-coaster of mood swings with nowhere to go. I really didn't know who I was, yet I hurt something awful with rejection even when maybe it wasn't real. I would get so damn depressed, even when there didn't seem to be any good reason. I didn't dare trust anyone, especially not after that business with Mitzi, even though that worked out okay, in a way. But I couldn't stand being alone, either. Even when I was in the middle of people who seemed like friends, I knew it wasn't true, and I just kept cutting my wrists and hiding them. I kept sort of wanting to tempt men, make them get hot, make them really want my body, but I didn't want sex with them. I knew that was crazy but I couldn't stop. Little Miss Self Destructive, that was me – until I loved Darius. Then I lost him. Then came the Virtual Mode – and you.'

I understand you and need you as you do me, but I have no sexual desire for you.

'Yeah. I can parade around naked with you, and it doesn't matter. I thought I just wanted to tease men, but now I think it's something else. I just want my freedom, freedom from what's bugging me, and throwing away my clothes in public makes it seem as if I'm doing that, but it doesn't mean anything with other girls, that happens in the showers anyway, so it has to be men, and when they get hot it sort of proves I'm getting there, I mean I want to be attractive, but it's sort of dangerous too. Like – you know, once I was eating cereal, and it wasn't sweet enough, so I put sugar on it, and it still wasn't sweet enough, so I put more, but no matter how much I put it wasn't there.

219

Then someone said "Try salt," so I put a little salt on it, and suddenly that stuff was so sickly awful sweet I couldn't stand it. I'd been putting on the wrong stuff, not knowing, because it hadn't tasted sweet enough. So with the nakedness and me – I'm looking for salt, but sugar is all I have, so I keep trying but it keeps not quite working. Does that make sense?'

Yes.

'And then when I found the salt – Darius – everything sort of came together. But I didn't quite believe him, and –'

Suddenly she was sobbing. She leaned her forehead against his warm side and the tears flowed down.

You were afraid of intimacy, both physical and emotional.

'I guess so,' she said into his hide. 'Did I ever blow that one!'

Yet you did what any practical person would have. Magic is not believable in your reality.

'If I had loved him enough, I would have believed him!'

Love is not precisely what horses experience, but we have learned something of it from our association with humans. In our judgment, the best love is based on practical considerations. Trust should not follow love; love should follow trust. You condemn yourself because you were unable to do it backwards. You should not.

She lifted her head. 'I never thought of that!'

Because you had no compatible and objective mind to explore it with. You do need me – and with me, you are whole.

'With you I am whole,' she echoed. 'But Seqiro, are you whole with me?'

Yes. My need for you is primarily physical and mental, for I have neither hands nor intelligence alone, but I had those things in my normal existence. You provide also the emotional factor I need, the quest for new things and new meanings. In this you are my completion, as I am yours.

'Yes,' she breathed. 'Yes! We are whole!'

Then they settled down for sleep, Colene curled against his warm side with a blanket over them both.

Naturally her own thoughts interrupted it. 'Seqiro! If you have to be let into a mind, if it's a wild mind, how come you could handle those mosquitoes?'

Their minds are comparatively simple. The complex human minds

220

*are another matter. Mosquitoes could bar my penetration, had
they the wit. But they don't realize that, and I would not advise
them of it.*

'So it does make sense, after all.'

Yes. He seemed amused. She snuggled against him and
drifted off.

In the morning they set out on the pontoon bridge. It was
solid enough to support Seqiro's weight, though it did sink
somewhat where he stood. Now it was Colene's turn to shore
up his confidence. 'These things are strong. See, the platform
part of it consists of long metallic planks, so even if the pontoon you're over sinks, the others take up the slack, and you'd
have to weigh a lot more than you do to make them all sink.
In my reality they drive trucks across these things. So it may
feel insecure, and look insecure because all we can see is one
little segment at a time, but believe me, you're safe.'

Now I have confidence. For he had seen her mental picture of
the heavy trucks driving safely across such bridges, and her
trust had become his.

However, she led the way, with a hand lightly touching his
nose. This was so that her light body would encounter any
possible weakening in the bridge first, and to guide him,
because his eyes were not well placed to see the bridge. Her
mind and hand became his guidance. Only the lack of a halter
on his head would have showed an outsider that this was not
a girl leading her horse. It *was* a girl leading her horse, but the
relation between them was different.

The surface of the sea continued, but the color of the
water shifted as they crossed realities. *Life!* Seqiro thought.
*I sense faint life ahead – perhaps very primitive, in the depths of
the ocean.*

'Then we're getting somewhere!'

The signs became stronger. It was as if they were stepping
through a paleontological exhibit, tracing the world from its
sterile inception through the first suggestions of life and to
the first multi-celled organisms. Things started showing in
the water, living froth, then tiny jellylike creatures, then
swimming crustaceans, and then actual fish.

And another island. This one had shrubbery on it, or primitive trees. The bridge went right to it, each short segment appearing as they proceeded until one touched the island, and for the first time in hours they set foot on land.

It was a relief to have the shade of fernlike trees, but they decided not to linger, because the pontoon bridge seemed endlessly long on the Virtual Mode despite its shortness in any one reality, and they were limited to the supplies they carried. They could more readily rest after they got safely past this region.

So with regret they moved out on the bridge again, trusting it to extend itself on through the Virtual Mode, and soon found themselves back in the middle of the placid sea.

Until Colene stepped through a boundary and found herself in a wind-screaming storm. Big waves rocked the bridge so hard it seemed about to be torn away.

She ducked back, and the storm cut off abruptly. Her hair was matted across her face and her blouse and jeans were wrinkled. 'We've got a problem.'

So I saw. Seqiro had not yet crossed, but his mind had been with her. *If it is confined to one reality, we can cross quickly.*

'Maybe so. But suppose it isn't?'

We can wait for it to subside.

'We don't know how long these storms last. Maybe it's always stormy in that reality.'

They discussed it, and decided to let Colene cross to the following reality, tied with a rope to Seqiro. The rope was part of his supplies, so would remain firm across the boundaries. If she got washed off the bridge, he would back away and haul her to this calm section. If she found that the following reality was calm, he would move across and rejoin her. They would remain in constant mental touch.

She knotted the rope firmly around her middle, and passed a loop down between her legs and up around her shoulders, so that there was no way for her to slip out of it. She was afraid of that terrible storm, but knew this was the best way to tackle it.

She ventured across the boundary again, wishing there were handholds. But there was only the level planking, which she now realized was vibrating with the force of the storm beyond. That had not been evident while Seqiro was walking, but now he was still and they both saw that part of the motion was not from his hoofs.

The storm caught her again. This time a wave was washing over the bridge, making the pontoons tip at what seemed like a precarious angle. She lost her balance and fell, and the water carried her into the sea. She inhaled to scream, involuntarily, and took in a mouthful and some of a lungful of froth.

Then she was in the calm water, having been carried across the boundary by the wave. Seqiro was backing away, hauling her in. She managed to catch hold of the edge of a pontoon and cling there, choking.

Calm. Cough. Calm. Inhale. Cough.

It was Seqiro, assuming control of her breathing, getting her to clear her lungs without panicking. She let him do it; it was much easier to ride along with his procedure.

Sooner than otherwise, she was back on the bridge and on her feet. 'Thanks, Seqiro,' she gasped. 'I needed that.'

Then she gathered her strength and charged back through the boundary.

This time a wave had just passed. She forged through the knee-deep water, able to keep her footing, and by the time the next wave loomed, she plunged across.

Into bright sunlight. The storm was only one reality wide! 'Come on, Seqiro!' Then, immediately, she reconsidered. 'Wait – let me spy the waves. It's much easier to cross between them.'

She sat at the edge of the boundary, clung to a pontoon, and cautiously poked her head across. She got a faceful of salt water. She drew back, blinking the salt out of her eyes. Then she tried it again, and found a lull. 'Now!'

The bridge vibrated with extra force. Suddenly the horse appeared, almost galloping along the bridge. The water splashed up from his legs.

Colene threw herself to the side, into the water, lest she be inadvertently trampled. How big Seqiro looked from this vantage! He was a massive horse, and splendid in his motion. She had forgotten that, in her constant communion with his mind.

He entered her current reality, and she had to scramble up before he overshot her position too far and yanked her along by the rope. They were across, but she hoped they did not have to do that again soon.

The nature of the ocean changed faster than any individual reality suggested, and land came into view by jumps with each crossed boundary. Adjacent realities tended to be similar, but sometimes differed by significant stages within that similarity. Now they seemed to be headed for a reality whose far shoreline was considerably west of the one they had started with. Perhaps this world was turning slightly faster, so that it had gained on the others. No, it would be the other way: if it turned more slowly, a given spot on the globe would be west of the others. It hardly mattered; what counted was that they were getting across the ocean much faster than they might have.

By nightfall they set foot on what in her reality might have been Europe. Now she remembered how quickly they had reached what seemed to be the Atlantic Ocean; she had not walked any twelve hundred miles to the coast! So this effect must have existed all along; she just hadn't paused to realize its significance. Now she was glad they weren't traveling in the other direction!

Life had continued to progress, and now there were modern fish and animals and birds, though she did not recognize the individual species.

The pontoon bridge stopped at the shore, but here there was a well marked path leading east. Someone certainly had set this up – but who traveled it? They had encountered no one, and seen no footprints or other signs of use. It had to have been done recently – within the past week – because before then this Virtual Mode hadn't been in place. What did it mean?

We are approaching superior minds, Seqiro thought. *Not many realities away. They are closed to me; I can fathom only their power.*

'Not Darius' reality? Magic?'

No. I suspect science, like yours, because if they set up the bridge –

'High-tech,' she agreed.

224

They seem to be human. They may be friendly. However –

'Um, Seqiro,' she murmured, really not speaking at all, more or less subvocalizing so as to focus her thoughts. 'We don't know what we're headed into, but I think maybe they're expecting us. Maybe we should, you know, not let them know too much about us. Until we know more about them.'

This was my thought.

They considered, then decided to do something neither of them really liked. Colene made a loop of rope and tied it about Seqiro's nose, and held the other end like a rein. She climbed up on his back with the supplies and rode. Now it seemed that he was a plain unintelligent horse – she could not bring herself to think 'stupid' – under the control of a human. It seemed to be a necessary charade – just in case.

They advanced through more realities, the path broadening as if to signal that they were close to their destination. Other paths intersected it at acute angles to their route, evidently going the same way. Were there paths reaching as far out as theirs, in other directions? All constructed in the past week? What an effort that must have been! And why? Colene still didn't trust this.

'You know,' she subvocalized, 'if this turns out as suspicious as it seems so far, and you have to keep on acting like a dumb animal, you'll be put in a stall and I won't be able to be with you without giving you away.'

True. But a stall is no discomfort for me, and we can remain in mind contact throughout. I believe I can now reach you across a continent, so we will not truly be separated.

'I hope not! But I have an ill feeling about this. Someone has gone to an awful lot of trouble to show us in.'

We must continue as we have, until we are able to proceed through this reality and resume our journey. Obviously they know someone will be coming on the Virtual Mode, but not who or from what direction, or they would not have fashioned so many paths.

'That's what bothers me. This is obviously another anchor. Why didn't the anchor person just come on out to meet us? If he wants to escape his reality, why take all this trouble to bring us *in* to it?'

I think we shall find out. I doubt we can avoid the encounter which threatens, so it is better to proceed into it as if innocent.

'We *are* innocent,' she muttered bleakly.

They crossed several more realities – and were abruptly in a huge building. This was evidently the anchor place.

A man stood before them. He was in what was evidently a uniform: a princely robe of what looked like silk or fine artificial material. A metallic band circled his head at forehead level. His hair was reddish and receding, and his eyes were black and piercing. He looked to be in his fifties, running to density rather than fat.

Seqiro stopped immediately. Colene, uncertain what to do, decided to remain mounted. That way she could go with Seqiro if he bolted. 'Hello,' she said tentatively, her throat feeling somewhat constrained.

'Hello,' a ball hanging near them said, mimicking her voice and intonation precisely.

I can not get into his mind, Seqiro thought. *But I think that device is trying to communicate.*

A translator! That made sense. She faced the ball. 'Hello. I am Colene, and this is my horse Seqiro. We are from a far reality, and only passing through this one. We would like to stay the night and go on in the morning.'

'Hello. I am –' the ball said.

Colene tapped her collarbone with a thumb. 'I am Colene.' She glanced down. 'This is my horse, Seqiro.' She indicated him. 'Who are you?' She pointed to the ball, and then to the man.

'Hello. I am –' the ball said. Then the man lifted one hand and tapped himself. 'Ddwng.' The ball spoke again. 'You are Colene. This is my horse Seqiro.'

She smiled. 'My horse, not your horse. This is your palace.' She gestured around the chamber.

'Seqiro is your horse. This is my palace. You are from a far reality.'

That machine was fast! 'A far reality,' Colene agreed. 'On the Virtual Mode.' She gestured back the way they had come. Then she oriented on the man. 'You are Deedwing.'

226

'Ddwng,' he corrected her. There seemed to be a stutter at the beginning and no vowels in the middle.

'D-dwng,' she agreed, almost getting it. 'Who are your people?'

The translator ball took some dialogue to get that straight, but in due course answered: 'My people are the –'

'DoOon,' Ddwng finished.

'Do-Oh!-on,' she repeated, noting the three different 'o' sounds. 'Ddwng of the DoOon. I am Colene of the Americans.'

The introductions completed, Ddwng stepped forward. He smiled, offering his arm for Colene to brace against so she could dismount without tumbling. She put both hands on it, finding it very strong, and jumped down.

Other people appeared. Except that they weren't exactly people. Colene tried not to stare, sure that it would be bad form. They had the heads of sheep!

'These are nulls of the Ovine persuasion,' Ddwng said through the ball, noting her surprise. The actual words were less precise, but that was the essence. 'Palace servants. They are of human intelligence and perception.'

'Oh. Thank you.'

First the Ovines saw to her horse. Colene made clear that she wanted her mount well treated, and Ddwng led them to a chamber that would do for a stall. They were now in the anchor reality, and things did not shift every ten feet. She arranged with Ram, the male Ovine, to get good hay and grain and water for the horse, for Seqiro could eat the food of an anchor reality and retain it. Plus a block of salt! Then, with regret, she left him, for it would not do to show too great an attachment to a mere beast of burden. Seqiro advised her in this mentally, while playing the part of animal perfectly. They still did not know whether they could trust the folk of this reality. At least the DoOon seemed to have no notion of telepathy; their sophisticated ball indicated that they depended on computerized data banks for translation.

Then they saw to Colene. Ewe, the female sheep, approached bearing silken robes. Colene realized that she must look pretty ratty, after the day's hike and the soaking down in the storm.

Her clothing had dried on her and must look that way. She nodded affirmatively.

The sheep-woman led her to an elegant private chamber. Ddwng did not follow; evidently he honored basic human protocol with regard to males and females. But she still didn't trust him. She remembered how her date had behaved well enough, until he got her alone with his friends and their liquor. This could be a fancier version of something similar.

There was another hanging ball here, and it continued to respond to all her remarks. Evidently it was all part of a network, and they wanted to get as much of her language as possible, quickly. That was fine with her. She gave it all the words that came up, and instructed it in basic syntax, correcting it when it made an incorrect assumption. This was the easy way to establish communication!

Meanwhile she suffered herself to be undressed, bathed, and redressed by the quiet female. She was very good at her profession, evidently born to be a servant to nobility. For Colene was being treated like a princess, and garbed like one. Whenever she spoke to Ewe, that creature nodded her head forward in a set motion, evidently both bow and acknowledgment, and did her best as quietly and efficiently as possible.

Soon enough Colene was not only clean and clothed, her hair was flowing and lustrous, and she wore a diadem that scintillated iridescently. Her fingernails matched the diadem, and her toenails too, in comfortable yet elegant sandal-slippers. The fatigue of the day was fading; the sheer luxury of her apparel was banishing it.

She looked at herself in a mirror. She was stunning! As lovely as she had ever imagined herself to be in her most foolish flights of fancy. She showed no private flesh, yet somehow the gown made her look utterly feminine.

Then they guided her to another ornate chamber. This was evidently a dining room, and suddenly she realized how hungry she was. She and Seqiro had been so busy following the pontoon bridge that they hadn't stopped to eat since breakfast.

Seqiro: the horse was doing fine. His thoughts told her of his best meal in days, and the attention of servants who had the heads of horses, who scrubbed off his hide and brushed out tangles in his mane. He could not read their minds, but their attitude indicated that they had not seen a genuine horse before, but understood hoofed animals, so had a general notion how to treat him.

Ddwng was waiting for her. He showed her to a seat at a table for two, and sat opposite her. 'You are comfortable?' the ball of this room inquired.

'Yes, thank you,' Colene replied. Indeed she was, physically. But what was this leading up to? She tried not to show her continuing tension.

'You are beautiful,' the ball said.

'Thank you.' Then, aware that it spoke at the direction of Ddwng, she made the servant nod-bow to him.

Evidently pleased, he returned the nod. If he had had doubt about whether she was civilized, it was being resolved.

Ovines brought in platters. Each had an array of odd but interesting-smelling substances. But she hesitated to choose, not wanting to make some gauche error. 'Please – you choose,' she said to Ddwng.

He nodded again. In a moment she had a plate of things, similar to his own. She watched him lift a utensil resembling a single chopstick. When he touched it to a morsel, a bite-sized segment of that morsel adhered to it. Good enough.

They ate in silence. The food, strange as it was, was excellent; she could get used to this in a hurry. There was a beverage too, tasting like a cross between beer and chocolate milk; she hoped it wasn't alcoholic, and it didn't seem to be. Ddwng evidently wasn't trying to get her drunk. Why should he bother? She was in his power. That was the fly in this lovely ointment: soon enough Ddwng would get down to business.

They completed the meal, and the servants brought mouthwash that left her mouth feeling absolutely clean after one rinse. That was certainly easier than brushing her teeth!

Then they adjourned to a chamber containing a fountain whose fluid changed colors as it moved. Around it were exotic plants – perhaps ordinary here, but alien to her.

'Now we shall formulate our understanding,' the ball said.

'Of course,' Colene agreed, hoping that her suddenly

renewed tension did not show. 'What is your interest in me?'

'You are traveling the Virtual Mode with your animal. I have an interest in the Virtual Mode. I would like to know where its Device of origin is located.'

'I don't really know about that,' she admitted honestly enough. 'It must have been set up by Darius. I am traveling along it to reach his home reality, or to meet him along the way, I hope.'

'Darius is your promised man?' The ball was doing the talking, but the expressions were on the face of Ddwng, and soon it was as if he were talking. He evidently had some kind of ongoing translation, so that he understood what she said.

'Yes. I love him.' She wanted no misunderstandings: she was taken.

'He is a fortunate man.'

She tried to suppress her girlish delight in being flattered. 'I would like to get moving again tomorrow, with my horse. We had to cross quite a number of realities that were, well, empty. Do you know whether the ones in the other direction are okay?'

'We have not had occasion to explore far, but they seem to be similar to those through which you passed.'

'You went to a lot of effort, setting up those paths. Why did you bother?'

'When the Virtual Mode was established, we could not know its origin or mission,' the ball said. 'We knew that those on it would have difficulty with this region, and perhaps suffer harm. So we constructed paths as far as feasible, and set markers beyond them. This seems to have been effective, as you arrived on one of these paths.'

'Well, I'm sorry I can't help you. Why do you want the Chip?'

'A Virtual Mode is normally a temporary thing. With the Chip, we could establish Virtual Modes at our discretion. This would be an excellent thing for our society.'

'The Chip can do that? Can set up a Virtual Mode from anywhere, anytime?'

Ddwng smiled. 'Indeed it can, Colene,' the ball said. 'So you can see that a Chip is one of the most valuable things in all the realities.'

'I sure do, now! I thought it was just some routine thing they could do in Darius's reality.'

'That may be the case. But I gather it is not routine in your reality, as it is not in mine.'

'In my reality, we don't even know there's more than one reality!'

'How did you discover that?'

He seemed interested, and nice, so she told him. In fact she was acting just a bit more naive than she was, because deep down she definitely did not trust him. Stupidity and ignorance could be significant assets for a girl, when they weren't actual. 'Darius was looking for a wife, and he didn't like the ones where he was, so he made a spot trip to my reality. Somehow he knew that I wanted out of my situation and might go with him. But I didn't quite trust it, and didn't go. Then he set up the Virtual Mode, and now I'm trying to get back to him. But it's one hell of a trip!'

'Evidently so. But have you considered that if you are traveling toward his reality, and he is traveling toward yours, you may pass each other without meeting?'

'Se –' she started, then caught herself. She didn't want him to know that the horse could pick up Darius' mind when he came within several realities. 'Seems I didn't think of that! Gee, I hope I haven't already missed him!'

Ddwng smiled again, evidently becoming satisfied about her naiveté. The ball spoke again. 'I am sure you have not, because he has not passed through this reality, which seems to be between his and yours.'

'But maybe he went through a corner of it and you didn't see him.'

'That is unlikely. The void realities are extensive, and difficult to pass. He should have intercepted one of our paths and followed it here, as you did.'

That did make sense. She now saw where Ddwng was leading, so she set it up for him. 'But how will I know which path he's coming in on? I mean, if I go out tomorrow –'

'Readily solved. You will simply wait here for him, and be

reunited here. This will surely be best in any event, because we have excellent facilities, and he may be tired from the struggle with the void realities.'

'Gee, that's nice of you!' she exclaimed happily. But inside she was not at all sanguine. This person had gone to an extraordinary amount of trouble to make long paths, and she doubted that he was doing it from sheer niceness. He wanted the Chip, as he said, and that meant he needed Darius to lead him to the reality where the Chip was.

But that Chip was evidently the potential source of almost unimaginable power. What would Ddwng do once he had it?

She wished she could think of a way to see that Ddwng didn't get it. But if she made any suspicious move, she was now afraid that she would proceed from the status of Guest to that of Prisoner.

She would have to wait until Darius came, and then warn him not to tell where his reality was. Maybe they could head back to hers, until they got free of Ddwng, then cross this region somewhere else. Or start toward his reality, and turn aside. There were surely ways and ways, if she could just warn him without alerting Ddwng.

'It sure is lucky that you're here, with a good reality in the middle of the bad ones,' she said brightly. 'I'm afraid we would have been in real trouble otherwise.'

'It is fortunate,' the ball agreed.

It was a disaster, she feared.

10

CAPTAIN

Suddenly they were in a barren region. There seemed to be no life at all in this Mode, though the prior Mode was lush.

Darius looked at Provos. 'Do you have any memory of this?'

'I have no memory of this,' she said, not answering so much as anticipating his coming response. 'We do not remain here long.'

'Let's move on, then,' he agreed.

They crossed into the next, and the next, but the barrenness continued. This seemed to be an entire segment of lifeless Modes, unlike any they had passed before. The ground was nothing but rock and sand; there was no water.

She could not remember their future as long as they kept crossing to new Modes. But suppose there was no resumption of living Modes within their walking range? Her memory of the future would do them no good; they would be dead.

'Provos, you may not remember the terrain,' he said carefully. 'But can you remember your association with me? Do you know me from more than a few days in the future?'

'I remember you from a fortnight in the future,' she said. 'Then it becomes confused.'

Two weeks. That suggested that it was safe to plow ahead, because they would not die in that time. Heartened, he did just that.

But the barren Modes continued for the course of half a

day's travel. The naked sun beat down, making an oven of the landscape. Darius became doubtful. Yet Provos seemed unconcerned, so he said nothing.

Then they spied a flash of a light to the side. It turned out to be a little signaler stuck in the sterile sand. Near it was an arrow pointing onward.

Evidently someone had been here before them. Since the Virtual Mode had not existed for a long time, this had to be recent. Could Colene have passed this way? No, her arrow should have been pointing back the way he had come.

They moved on. Now the sun was descending, so that they had to shield their faces from it as they proceeded westward. Several hours later they found another flashing signal, with its arrow. Then they found a path. It was just a thin layer of silvery material laid on the rock, disappearing as it crossed to the next Mode. But it wound on through the bleak crevices and dunes, going somewhere. It was dusk now, and they decided to camp, then follow the path in the morning.

Provos remembered no problems in the coming hours. With neither weather nor animals to contend with, this seemed reasonable. But there was also no shield against the chill of night. The stone had been burning hot, and it retained much of its heat, but the air was turning frigid. There was no wood from which to make a fire. His thin blanket was not enough to shield them from the intensity of the chill that was developing.

Provos looked around. Then she stooped to lift the end of the path. The material came up readily. She walked with it, bunching up a length. Of this she made a blanket. She signaled him to join her.

The path material turned out to have a good insulating property. Whether as tent or blanket, it held in the radiating heat of the stone and kept them warm.

By morning, even so, it was very cold, and the two of them were closely embraced, huddled under the path. Darius wished it could have been Colene with him, with her lovely little body and innocently seductive manner. But with the dawn came the heat of the sun, and soon the air was warming.

The reflective path remained cooler than the surrounding

stone. They walked on it and were more comfortable than they had been the day before. Now they were obviously going somewhere. But who had set this up, and why?

The path was leading in the direction of the steepest change of Modes, which meant it was going toward an anchor. But probably not the right one. Darius had found his way first to Provos' anchor Mode. Now they must be going to a third one, and they could not know what to expect of it.

Suddenly there was water. The land had been desert-dry, but now there were lakes to the sides and vapors rising from the stone. Farther along there was life: thin, tenacious lichen coloring the rocks. But as they proceeded, this became more ambitious, until there was a general covering of primitive vegetation, and the appearance of insect life.

Then there was animal life. At first it was not far removed from the lakes, and was small, but it progressed rapidly. When man-sized reptiles appeared, Darius got nervous. But it was easy to avoid a predator by stepping across a Mode boundary. They just had to be careful not to walk directly into one, as there was no way to spot them ahead. They learned to count their paces, pause, and use his mirror-tube before moving on. This slowed them, but seemed necessary.

The path became bolder, and the scenery more recent. There seemed to be no large predators in this section, so they put away the mirror tube and moved more rapidly, because night was coming again.

Suddenly they were in an enormous chamber. There was an extremely elegant young woman, obviously of high social standing. She turned and saw him.

'Darius!' she cried, and flung herself into his arms.

It was Colene! Thus suddenly they had come together.

'Beware,' she whispered into his ear before she kissed him.

But already a man was walking toward them. He had reddish hair and piercing black eyes under a metallic band resembling a crown, and wore a kingly robe.

'You must be Darius,' a voice said in Colene's language. It came not from the man but what appeared to be a hanging ball.

'I am Darius,' he agreed as Colene relaxed enough to let him speak. Her whispered warning: what did it mean? That this was a hostile figure of some sort? Yet what could he do if it was?

'And your companion?' the ball asked.

Provos did not speak Colene's language, and not a great deal of his own language. 'She is Provos,' he said.

'This is not good,' Provos murmured in his language.

What was she beginning to remember? He knew it took a while for her to clarify her memories of a new Mode. Since her warning coincided with Colene's, he knew he had to be very careful.

'I must talk with you,' the ball said. 'Come with me.'

It seemed that it was the man who was really talking, as he was gesturing.

'Go with him,' Colene said. 'I will see to your companion.'

Darius looked at Provos, but she seemed to be willing to go with Colene despite the barrier of speech. He nodded.

In a moment he was in a separate chamber with the man, evidently private. 'I am Ddwng of the DoOon,' the ball said, still in Colene's language. 'I need your Chip.'

'The Chip that set up the Virtual Mode?' Darius asked, surprised. 'It is not mine to give.'

'But you could lead me to it.'

'To my Mode, yes. But the Cyng of Pwer would not give it to you. Chips are valuable.'

'I know. If you lead me to your Mode, I will get it from your official.'

'Why do you want it?'

'We are confined to our Mode. The Chip will enable us to visit other Modes.'

Darius considered. He did not like this situation. Both Colene and Provos had expressed doubt. Why should this evidently powerful man be so eager to go to other Modes? Could he be a human version of the dragons, seeking to invade new territory to the disadvantage of the folk there?

But it might not be wise to turn him down flatly. 'I will think about the matter.'

Ddwng frowned. 'There are things you should know, as you think,' the ball said. 'Colene will be withheld from you during that period.'

'Withheld?' Darius asked, dismayed. 'But I entered the Virtual Mode only to fetch her!'

'Then your decision should be easy. I shall grant you ten days to decide. If you are negative, we shall sterilize Colene and make her a common concubine.'

Suddenly Darius understood how accurate the warnings were. Ddwng was holding Colene hostage to Darius' performance! Surely there was no good motive there.

'In the interim, you shall perform an assignment,' the ball continued. 'The manner in which you acquit yourself will determine your situation after your decision.'

Darius suspected that anything he could say would only complicate his situation. But there was one way he could improve his chances. 'I will need the services of Provos.'

Ddwng hesitated, then evidently concluded that a small concession was in order. What he wanted was Darius' cooperation, not his antagonism. 'She will join you.'

Then a servant appeared. His head was that of a sheep. The creature was evidently waiting for Darius, so Darius got up and accompanied him from the room. They walked to a relatively tiny chamber. 'Stand in there,' a nearby hanging ball said.

Darius stepped into the little chamber. A panel closed him in. The chamber shook. Then the panel opened.

A man stood outside, but not the same one. This one was fully human, and wore a rather handsome deep red uniform. He lifted his right hand, spreading his fingers. 'Welcome aboard, Captain,' a ball said.

Darius shook his head. 'You have mistaken me for someone else. I am here only to do an assignment for Ddwng of the DoOon.'

'This is true, sir,' the ball said, evidently speaking for the man. 'You are to complete a mission as Captain of this ship, the FTL *Flay*. I am your executive officer, Jjle.'

Darius stepped out of the little chamber. 'But I know nothing of ships! I can't even find the sail!'

Jjle smiled. 'This ship has no sail, sir,' the ball said. 'It is a destroyer-class thousand-light-year craft. I am competent to operate it, as I shall do at your command.'

'No sail?' Darius asked blankly.

'Sir, if you will permit the personal remark, I suspect you have come into this command rather suddenly. May I proffer a suggestion?'

'Yes, please, J-jlee! I have no idea what —'

'Allow me to show you to your quarters, where your nulls will acquaint you with the necessary background. When you emerge, no other member of the crew will know that this is new to you.'

This had the sound of good advice. 'Yes, thank you.'

'The appropriate term is "affirmative", sir. When we reach your quarters, tell me to "carry on".'

'Affirmative,' Darius said.

They walked down a short squared-off metal hall to another door panel. 'Your touch will key it open, sir.'

Darius touched the panel. It slid aside to reveal a chamber beyond.

'I look forward to serving with you, sir,' Jjle said.

'Uh, yes. Uh, carry on.'

The man lifted his hand again, fingers splayed. Then he turned smartly and departed.

Darius stepped into the chamber. The panel closed behind him. How he had come from the palace on the ground to this 'space' ship he did not know, but it was actually no stranger than stepping through Mode boundaries.

The chamber was opulent. Lush carpeting covered the floor, and fine murals were on the walls. Three odd statues lined one side. Near the ceiling were ornate cabinets set into the corners. There was a huge picture window overlooking a lovely placid river valley. This was definitely not where he had been! But neither was it on the water.

Then he saw a statue move. It was breathing!

He looked more closely. The bodies of the figures were human, but the heads resembled those of cats. One body was evidently male, for it was of masculine proportions and had a cod piece fitted obviously into his shorts; another was female, with full breasts and hips distending her tight dress; the one between them seemed to be neuter.

'Who are you?' he asked.

The male stepped forward marginally. 'We are your nulls, Captain Darius,' a ball he hadn't noticed before said. 'We are of the Feline persuasion. I am Tom.'

The neuter figure stepped forward. 'I am Cat.' The pitch and intonation differed, though it was still the ball speaking.

Then the female: 'I am Pussy.' This time the tone was sultry.

'Nulls?'

'Nulls are subhuman servants. We exist to serve you in any capacity you desire.'

Darius pondered that, not knowing what to make of it.

'Your attention, sir,' the ball said in a neutral voice. 'A person is beyond the panel.'

'Who?'

'The woman Provos.'

'Let her in,' he said, relieved.

The panel opened. Provos stepped through. She seemed to take this reunion for granted, evidently remembering their future association. 'I presume you interceded to bring me here,' she said.

'I interceded to bring you here,' he repeated, because that was evidently the dialogue she remembered.

She turned to the three feline nulls. 'It is pleasant to commence our association, Tom, Cat and Pussy,' she said.

She spoke in Darius' language, which the folk here did not seem to know. So he translated.

The three were startled. Darius was sympathetic. 'Provos is a woman of special ways,' he said.

'These folk are to be trusted,' Provos advised him. 'You will get to know them while I clean up and retire.' She walked across the room to a panel set in the wall, and tapped on it. It didn't open.

'Uh, obey her touch as you would mine,' Darius said to the panel. It opened, and Provos stepped inside another tiny chamber. The panel closed after her.

Darius addressed the felines. 'I would like to sit down and get to know you.'

239

Immediately Tom walked to another panel. It opened, and from it slid an oblong board. The board puffed out and became a chair. Tom set it down before Darius.

Darius sat in it. 'Make yourselves comfortable,' he said.

The three got down on the floor before him and curled up rather in the manner of cats, their limbs tucked under them, their heads up, watching him. This was all right for Tom and Cat, but it caused Pussy to show such a generous cleavage that it was distracting.

'Pussy, get yourself a chair,' he said. 'I will talk with you.'

She rose and produced a chair. She sat on it in the human manner, crossing her legs somewhat loosely. Her skirt was not long enough for this maneuver, so that the whole of her inner thighs were now visible for his inspection. She wore no diaper. Indeed, she seemed to wear no panties either.

He decided to try to ignore this, lest he seem too fussy. 'Pussy, please clarify for me what it is the three of you are expected to do for me.'

'We exist to serve you in any capacity you desire,' the sultry voice of the ball said. The cat-woman's thighs spread a bit more.

'Yes, so you said before. But what capacities do you expect me to desire of you?'

'Information, body attendance, sex,' she said via the ball, confirming the message her legs had been sending.

'Information is the one I desire now. How did you come to be the way you are?'

'We are androids, manufactured in the factory from reconstituted human genetic material. We have no souls. Our heads are modified to conform to several animal patterns, though we retain the ability to perceive and communicate as humans do. As a class we are the nulls; as a subclass we are the Felines, male, neuter and female. Our only pleasure comes from being of significant service to our human masters, and we must perform at least one such service each day or suffer.'

Evidently this was a set speech for the edification of ignorants like himself. Darius appreciated it. 'You are performing such a service to me by giving me this information?'

'Yes,' she agreed eagerly.

240

'What happens to a null who fails to perform such a service?'

'On the first day we suffer emotional pain. On the second, physical pain. On the third we die.'

The DoOon did not treat their servants gently! 'Suppose I just tell you that I need no services, and to relax?'

'The nature of acceptable services is listed and programmed,' the ball said in her voice. 'We can not deviate. If you wish some service which is not programmed, you must arrange it by having us reprogrammed on a temporary basis.'

'Suppose I do not need a service, but another human being does. May I have you do it, abating your need?'

'No,' she said sadly. The ball seemed to be fading out of awareness.

The neuter null lifted a hand, evidently a signal for attention. 'Speak, Cat,' Darius said.

'Pussy's answer is incomplete. We are differentiated by type as well as by sex. Tom is strong and capable of violence at your behest; he will defend you against attack, even by a human being. Pussy is sympathetic and versed in the arts of gentleness, massage, seduction and sexual peformance. I lack either nature, but am the most objective and intelligent of your Felines. I am capable of interpreting your commands and questions and verifying your actual intent when you misspeak yourself or are vague. Accordingly I advise you that while Pussy's response is technically correct, there are ways to circumvent this restriction.'

'Then I should be talking with you, rather than Pussy,' Darius said, interested.

'We would not presume to say that,' the ball said for Cat.

Darius faced Pussy. 'Should I be talking with Cat instead of you?'

'Yes.'

'Thank you, Pussy. I will talk with him, if this will not hurt your feelings.'

She looked confused. 'He means kindness, Pussy,' Cat said to her. 'He appreciates what you have done so far.'

'Oh, thank you!' she said, relieved. As always, it was the

ball that spoke, but the distinction had become meaningless; it was her voice, and her thought.

Cat faced Darius. 'This was an example. When you said "if" this would not hurt her feelings, she was not sure whether they should be hurt, which would mean she had in some way failed you. I provided the reassurance you intended. If I interpret your intent incorrectly, or if you prefer that I not do this, advise me and I will desist.'

Darius was fascinated by this information. It was apparent that these servants could indeed be useful. 'How may I circumvent the restriction against assigning a service to another person?'

'One way would be to volunteer to do a service yourself for that person, begin it, then have one of us complete it for you. You are free to make commitments in ways we are not.'

Darius nodded. 'You serve me because you serve the Captain?'

'We serve you because we have been assigned to you. An officer of the Navy normally keeps his own nulls to serve him wherever he is employed. If you wish other nulls, we can be exchanged. But for the duration we are loyal to you, not the office, and you may trust us always to serve your interest to the best of our understanding and ability.'

Provos emerged from the cleaning chamber, looking refreshed. She glanced at Darius. 'You need more sleep and rest than you get this night,' she said reprovingly in his language. 'At least have them give you a nourishment pill.'

'I will show you to a bedchamber,' Darius said, rising. He walked toward her, having no idea where it was or whether it existed. He looked back. 'Pussy, please complete this task for me, and see that Provos is as comfortable as I would make her.'

Pussy jumped up, her breasts bouncing. 'It is this way,' she said, almost purring as she led Provos to another panel and through to another chamber.

'Thank you, Darius,' Provos said, familiar with this protocol from her memory.

He settled down with the remaining two Felines. He realized that he was hungry. 'Nourishment pill?'

242

'Immediately,' Tom said, and rose to fetch a tablet.

Darius accepted the pill, and gazed at it. 'This will feed me?'

'Yes. You may order a conventional meal if you prefer.'

'No, I'll try this.' If Provos remembered it as satisfactory, it probably was. He popped the pill in his mouth and swallowed it with saliva.

He was no longer hungry. Evidently this was something like magic. That made it acceptable. He returned to business. 'The executive officer called me sir. Why did he do this, and why don't you?'

'"Sir" is a token of respect given by a human to one of a higher rank in the Navy,' Cat said. 'We are not human, so lack the status to show respect. One must possess sufficient status to have his token of respect be worthy.'

'Pussy has performed a service for me, and you are performing one now. If it is not convenient for me to find a service for Tom to do, how can I avoid causing him distress?'

'His distress has no force against your convenience. You may ignore it.'

'It would cause me distress to cause any of you needless distress.'

'Then I can suggest tasks which would not cause you inconvenience.'

'Yes.'

'Is there anything you desire which would be awkward or inconvenient for you to achieve at present by your own action?'

'I'd like to be with Colene!' Darius said before he thought.

'This is a human person?'

'This is the human person I came to be with. But Ddwng has separated us, pending a mission I must complete for him. I don't want to do a mission, I want to take Colene home with me. But I think this is beyond your capacity to remedy.'

'It is,' Cat agreed. 'But we can provide you with partial satisfaction with no more effort on your part than you choose to exert.'

'Then do it.'

Tom got up. He touched a section of the wall opposite

Darius, and the mural became a scene of an office so realistic that there seemed to be a window between the two chambers. A null with the head of a dog sat at a desk.

The Canine glanced at them and spoke in an incomprehensible language.

'Speak English, Bitch,' Tom snapped.

'What do you want, Tom?' she inquired. It was probably a ball speaking for her, but since the sound came through the window it made no difference.

'Information, by order of Captain Darius of the *Flay*,' Tom said curtly.

'I will give you Dog.' She touched a button. The picture changed. Now there was another office, with what appeared to be a neuter Canine. 'What information, Tom?' it asked.

'The present location and accessibility of the human Colene, visitor to this Mode.'

Dog touched buttons of his own. He studied what might have been a screen they could not see. 'The human Colene is the present consort of the Emperor Ddwng. As such she is accessible only by his leave.'

Darius was stunned. Consort?

'The Captain requests that leave,' Tom said.

'This may require some delay.'

Cat glanced at Darius. 'We'll wait,' Darius said.

'Proceed,' Cat said.

The picture changed again. Now it showed a woman with the head of a pig. 'Tom, why do you seek this contact?' she asked.

'I speak for Captain Darius, Sow. He does not answer to you.'

Darius appreciated the imperious attitude Tom was showing. That was about the way he felt. It seemed appropriate that the bureaucracy should be represented by swine.

A male pig-head appeared. 'By order of our master Ddwng, Darius will answer to the Swine,' he snorted. His tone was arrogant in the masculine fashion.

'Boar, Darius wishes contact with Colene, with whom he has had prior connection. Screen contact will do on an interim basis.'

244

A third Swine appeared, evidently the neuter. 'This may be granted. But there is information I must impart first.'

Tom glanced at Darius again. Darius nodded.

'Impart it, Pig.'

'Colene's present status is nominal. She is not subject to present sexual use by the Emperor, but is required to present herself and comport herself as his consort. This is a compatible existence, and her status is one to incite the envy of all women. If Darius fails to accommodate Ddwng in the required manner at the deadline, Colene's ovaries will be removed for the genetic bank and she will be given as a full-human concubine to whatever officer is selected. Should she resist, she will be lobotomized to the degree necessary to make her docile. She has not been informed of this.'

Darius felt faint. He had known that pressure would be brought to bear on him, to make him help Ddwng obtain the Chip. Sterilization of Colene had already been threatened. But he had not realized how ruthless the full course would be. Colene was hostage to his cooperation – and he seemed to have no way to fight it.

'And should Darius do the Emperor's will?' Tom inquired.

'Colene will be restored to him whole, and they will be given their freedom, either as ranking persons within the Empire or to travel to another Mode.'

What choice did he have? Yet a person who would make this kind of threat and back it up would probably also break his word. It might be pointless to agree. At least he had ten days to think about it.

'Message received,' Tom said. 'May Darius now see Colene?'

The screen changed again. Suddenly Colene was there, in her ornate gown, sparkling hair and bracelets. She was beautiful in her vibrant youth. No one would know from her appearance that she was suicidal, and she had surely kept the secret.

She saw him. 'Darius!' she exclaimed, stepping toward him.

Unable to help himself, he stepped toward her too. They met at the screen/wall between them, the images of their hands touching the cold surface. They tried to kiss, but again it was only images meeting.

245

'I asked to be with you,' he said.

'We're not even in the same stellar system,' she replied. 'I'm still on Earth, and you're on an FTL ship crossing the galaxy.'

'Ddwng wants me to lead him to the Chip.'

'Don't do it!' she exclaimed. 'He wants to conquer the other Modes too!'

'But if I do not –'

'We won't be allowed together,' she finished. 'I know that, Darius. But we owe something to our realities. We can't let them be despoiled. I love you, and I want to be with you, but not this way.' Her face shone with tears. 'If you find a way to escape, don't wait for me. Just get gone!'

'Colene, I love you too, and I curse the moment I failed to bring you with me. There are other ways – we don't have to marry – I found a woman who can – we can love, if –'

'Prima,' she agreed. 'I understand. It is good. It's not what I first dreamed of, but I love you so, I don't care. But not – you know. Not this way.'

'Not this way,' he agreed.

'They're not cutting us off,' she said, surprised.

'Because the more we see of each other, the more we will be willing to sacrifice for each other,' he said.

'Yes. So I guess we'd better quit, now.' Her tears were streaming down her face. 'But it's been great, Darius!'

'It is not over!' he protested. 'It can't be over! I went to the Virtual Mode only for you!'

'My life is nothing. It's complete. But you – thank you for stepping into my life, Darius, however briefly. You made it all worthwhile.'

She turned away. He did the same. What irony, to seem so close, yet be so far! To exchange vows of love, yet to have to deny the realization of them.

He became aware of the three Felines. Pussy had rejoined the group.

He stepped into her and embraced her. She was completely soft and responsive. He buried his face in her furry hair and let himself hurt.

246

'You may take me in your bedroom, or here, as you wish,' she murmured.

She misunderstood the nature of his emotion. 'Another time,' he said. 'I have much still to learn, here.' Then he disengaged, resumed his chair, and organized his thoughts.

He looked at Tom. 'That was a significant service,' he said. 'Now you may retire; I will not need you until morning.'

Tom walked to a niche, lay on the floor, curled up, and put his head down. In a moment he was asleep.

'You also,' he said to Pussy. She selected another nook and curled up similarly, showing firm upper thigh. Apparently it was simply her nature to display her body.

'From you I need more information,' he said to Cat. 'What does "FTL" mean?'

'It is an acronym for "Faster Than Light,"' it explained. 'This ship, for example, is the FTL *Flay*, capable of traveling a great deal faster than the velocity of light through a vacuum. It is proceeding at that rate to the site of your mission, and will arrive in approximately fifty hours travel time.'

'I am from a culture where the velocity of light does not matter. Translate that into something I can follow.'

'If you walked entirely around the globe of Earth, you would travel about twenty-five thousand miles, as this language has it. If you completed that circuit seven or eight times, you would cover the distance light travels in a single second. The spans between stars are such that we prefer to measure them in multiples of the amount light travels in a year. This ship traverses a thousand light-years each hour, so its destination is fifty thousand light-years from Earth, or about half way across the galaxy.'

Darius found that translated version was not much more intelligible than the original. 'So we are now an enormous distance from Earth, and going farther away.'

'That is correct. But we shall return as readily as we go.'

'What is the mission I am to accomplish?'

'A monster is rampaging on a colony planet, and the natives are unable to dispatch it. You will do that.'

With magic, Darius knew he could set a monster back. But

247

magic had not worked for him in any of the Modes beyond the region of his own.

Still, he should test it. He removed his pack and brought out his golem-figure of himself. 'To the far corner of this chamber,' he murmured, and made the figure jump.

Nothing happened. There was not even a tug in his stomach. Magic was not operative here.

Darius sighed. He was in effect a man without special power. 'I am not skilled in this.'

'It is not necessary that you be so.' The Felines seemed to have no interest in his peculiar action with the figurine; evidently his business was his business, unless he made it theirs. 'You will have merely to give the necessary directives. Nulls will assume the risk and complete the job.'

'So I'm a figurehead,' he said.

'No, nulls have no initiative in such respects,' it reassured him. 'A ranking human being must be in charge of the operation.'

'But any human could do it, even a complete ignoramus.'

'Yes.'

'So why did Ddwng bother to send me? Just to get me out of the way for a while?'

'I can not speak for the motives of the Emperor, but it seems reasonable that he has several reasons. He may wish to give you time and experience so that you can come to the conclusion that it is best to accede to his wishes. He may wish to keep you away from Colene. He may wish to prevent you from departing via your Virtual Mode. He may wish to keep you out of mischief without imprisoning you. And he may wish to discover how competent an officer you have the potential of being, in the event that you are converted to his cause. This mission accomplishes these things.'

The reasoning was formidable. 'I think I had better do as good a job as I can, until I decide what I will do.'

'That seems appropriate,' it agreed.

'What is known about this monster?'

'It seems to be a beast set on wanton destruction. It sets fire to villages, floods pastures, and fouls food supplies. No one has seen it, but its presence is manifest.'

248

'Why don't they lock doors and set guards?'

'They do, but the monster is extremely cunning about locks, and can stun guards.'

Darius pondered that. 'What are the natives like?'

'They are similar in outline and manner to Earthly snails, but larger. They are reasonably intelligent and capable, but slow.'

That surprised Darius. He had assumed that the natives were human, with a culture distinct from that of the colonists. Snails? This was a far land indeed!

He continued to question Cat, learning more about the various aspects of this Mode. It seemed that there were many intelligent creatures in what was called the galaxy, but that the humans had become dominant and now governed and exploited all of it they wished. They had risen to dominance thousands of years before, because of their ability to make ships that traveled faster than light, to nullify the effects of gravity, and to make weapons that could kill individual creatures or destroy entire planets.

But when they had sought to invade other Modes, the dominant cultures of those had taken action. The humans in most Modes were isolated on their home planet, causing trouble only to the creatures there; only in this Mode had they mastered the elusive secrets of super-science that enabled them to spread out and molest the larger galaxy. The creatures of other Modes had an ancient compact which prevented them from committing genocide in any single Mode. So they isolated this Mode by sterilizing the adjacent Modes and barring any contact from beyond. So it had been for a thousand years.

That explained what he and Provos had seen on the way here. 'But then how did this come to be an anchor Mode for our Virtual Mode?'

'We can only conjecture,' Cat said. 'The lives of empires are long, but the lives of individual creatures are short. Some creature must have become careless, and not been watching when your Virtual Mode was instituted. In fact, the possession of a Chip by human beings in any Mode constitutes a violation of the proscription. It seems likely that in due course this error will be corrected, and human beings will be confined again, to either their conquered Mode or their individual world in other Modes.'

'Unless Ddwng succeeds in getting his hands on the Chip in my Mode first,' Darius said. 'Then he will spread his minions across many Modes in a hurry, making it impossible to isolate them without doing enormous damage to innocent creatures.'

'This I suspect is the strategy,' Cat agreed.

'I see why he wants my Chip.' Darius was careful not to mention that it was only one of many in his Mode, evidently a forgotten hoard. 'But why is he giving me ten days to make up my mind? Surely time is of the essence.'

'Ddwng is competent, and comes from a lineage of competent Emperors. He is surely doing what is most advantageous to his purpose, considering all factors. It may be that the risks of forcing the issue rapidly are worse than those of giving you time, despite the danger of having the error discovered. Perhaps it is unlikely that the error will be noted until the Chip begins to be exploited. But it seems that the Emperor is not willing to risk too much time, as he has set the limit.'

That reminded Darius of the threat against Colene. Evidently Ddwng didn't know that she was suicidal, so that he was unlikely to get any long servitude from her if she didn't like it. But the nature of the threat was perplexing. 'Why have her ovaries cut out? There are surely more painful tortures that would not disfigure her.'

'She would not be disfigured,' it said. 'The surgery would be painless. Torture is done not by mutilation, but by infliction of harmless pain.'

'Harmless pain! How can that be?'

Cat got up and went to another panel. It opened, and from it it took a small disk. 'This is a pain control. It is attuned to you, so that it will not affect you. But it will cause discomfort in any other person, whether human or null, within its range, to whatever degree you choose. This dial sets the level.'

'Harmless pain?' Darius repeated.

'You may demonstrate it on me if you wish. However I must caution you that if you do not wish to render me unconscious, do not turn it to the highest range.'

250

'Demonstrate it on you? I have no wish to hurt you, and what would it prove? Demonstrate it on me.'

'This is a thing I may not do, for I think you do not understand what you are asking.'

'Set it at the minimum level, and show me how to turn it on. And how to detune it so that it affects me as well as you.'

'This setting will detune it,' Cat said. 'This is the minimum level.' It moved the dial. 'This activates it.'

Darius touched the detune setting. Then he turned it on.

Abruptly he experienced an ugly feeling. It was as if he were just coming down with a fever: a malaise not yet incapacitating, but a harbinger of worse to come.

He looked at Cat, who seemed unaffected. 'You feel it too?'

'Yes. But I am accustomed to it.'

Darius moved the dial. The discomfort increased. His body began to shake, and sweat appeared on his skin. His breathing became irregular. 'You feel this?'

'Yes.' The Feline did look a bit uncomfortable, but not nearly as much so as Darius felt.

He nudged it up farther. It felt as if he were walking into a furnace which was heating his bones, causing them to swell and split. Yet he was only three notches up, on a scale of ten.

He turned it off. 'It is effective,' he agreed. 'And I do seem to feel no aftereffect. I can see that this would be effective for discipline. But that leaves my question: why do surgery on Colene?'

'That is a prerequisite to demoting her to servant status,' Cat said. 'Humans, unlike nulls, are capable of reproduction. On colony planets they still do it naturally; on the more civilized worlds they do it via the birth banks. Once her valuable human eggs are safe, she can be treated in any manner. This is expected to cause you distress.'

'It does,' Darius said. 'I don't want any part of her removed, and I want to be with her myself. But surely there are many human women in this Mode; why take the eggs from Colene?'

'The human genetic pool has been highly refined and modified,' it said. 'As you can see by the manner that we nulls have

251

been crafted from the leftover parts of it. No human suffers from genetic maladies; none grow fat or weak or are stupid. All live long lives by primitive standards, and enjoy health throughout. But the genetic pool has become inbred, and the rate of population increase is declining. Fewer eggs are viable. It seems that primitive vigor has been sacrificed along with primitive liabilities. New genetic input is needed, to broaden the base and invigorate the pool. Colene represents an excellent source of that input, being young, intelligent, and healthy. It is unfortunate that the other woman, Provos, is beyond the age of similar harvest.'

Darius was horrified anew. 'So they aren't going to let her escape with her ovaries. But then why should I cooperate? Ddwng's word means nothing.'

'That is not true. The Emperor's word is always good. It would be beneath him to make any false statement. There is reason for you to cooperate: if you provide the Chip that enables Ddwng to transcend Modes, he will be able to bring in other women with their genes, and will have no need of Colene's genes. He will release you both as promised, together with Provos and the horse.'

'The what?'

'Colene has a horse. You were not aware?'

'I was not aware,' Darius said, surprised. 'I thought she came alone.'

'No, she preferred to ride, so she brought her horse. He was loaded with supplies for them both.'

Darius did not know what to make of this. Colene had had no horse! How had she gotten one? She wouldn't have stolen it. However, she was welcome to it, as far as he was concerned. A horse could be a useful animal when properly trained, and evidently this one was.

It was coming clear why Ddwng was giving Darius time to think about his decision. The more he learned, the more futile it seemed to try to oppose the Emperor. He still didn't like the notion of letting a conqueror loose among the Modes, but he feared increasingly that if he did not cooperate, Colene would suffer immediately, and then increasing pressure would be brought to bear until he capitulated. Darius did not consider

252

himself to be a brave man; if he were put in pain from the pain dial, he would be in serious trouble. Ddwng had surely known that Darius would discover this. There was probably more to learn, which was not good news.

'I think I had better retire,' he said. 'I seem to have used up half the night already.'

'True. Do you wish for a sleep ray, or for Pussy's company?'

'Neither, thanks. Let me just clean up and turn in.'

'As you wish.' Cat settled to the floor, but did not sleep; it was alert for any other directives.

Darius stepped into the cleaning chamber he had seen Provos use. He got out of his clothes. Light flashed. That seemed to be it; he was clean. He picked up his clothes and discovered that they were clean too. Probably he had not had to remove them. But since he did not intend to sleep in them, it didn't matter. He bundled them up and stepped back out.

'My bedroom?' he inquired.

Cat jumped up. 'Here.' It indicated another panel.

Darius entered, and found a chamber with an excellent bed. He suspected that only the Captain rated such accommodations. That was all right; he was ready for this. He dumped his clothing into a shelf-niche and lay down naked.

But before he slept he remembered his screen contact with Colene. How lovely she had been! He had not chosen her for beauty, if he had chosen her at all; somehow he had just gradually discovered that she was the one he wanted to be with. She had been kind to him in her Mode, but it was more than that.

How had she come by a horse?

And – *how had she known about Prima?*

He remembered now: he had been telling her that he had found a suitable woman to marry, so that that part of his search was over. It freed him to love Colene. Colene had said she understood, and she had named Prima. But he had not mentioned that name this time, and he could not have mentioned it before, because he had not encountered Prima before embarking on the Virtual Mode. Somehow Colene had learned the name and what it signified.

253

It had not been Colene directly with whom he talked, but an image. With magic, images could be false. Surely that was true in this super-science realm. Yet Colene's ways had rung true. She had wept when she told him they must part, and she had reacted in other authentic ways. She was suicidal; she would not have told Ddwng that, because she told no one. Only Darius himself, and then only when she loved him. This time she had said that her life was complete, and he knew too well what that meant. Complete because she intended to end it. When she lost him. That had to be Colene! A false image would have tried to convince him to capitulate; she had done the opposite. Had she begged him to do it, he might have yielded; she had begged him not to. That rang true.

But the name. Colene could not know of Prima. Yet how could a false image know it either? No one should know it, not even Provos. He had not mentioned her to Provos. Or had he? He had used the mirror tube Prima had devised; perhaps he had after all mentioned its origin. Or Provos could have remembered the name from some remark he would make in the future. And Provos had been with Colene for a while.

Yes, it was possible, he realized. Provos must have told her. Colene would naturally have asked about him, and Provos would have told what she remembered of future conversations. So the little mystery was solved.

Relieved, he slept.

He must have slept longer than intended, because he had the impression that too much time had passed. But he woke refreshed.

He got up and looked for his clothes. But they were gone. 'Pussy!' he called.

Immediately she appeared, and he realized that he had in his haste spoken the wrong name. He had wanted Tom, the male. Now he was sitting naked on the bed, and the voluptuous female Feline was gazing at him expectantly. 'May I be of service now?' she asked.

'Yes. Fetch me my clothes.'

She touched a panel, and out came a glittering robe. She proffered it.

'That's not mine,' he protested.

'It is the Captain's robe,' she explained. 'It would be amiss for you to go about the ship out of uniform.'

Darius acquiesced to the inevitable. 'Very well. Carry on.'

He meant for her to depart, so he could dress. Instead she proceeded to dress him. Well, she did know what she was doing, and he did not. She had to perform her daily service, and he hoped this counted.

Did it? He realized that he had better be sure, lest he cause inadvertent mischief by assuming too much. 'Does this acquit you of your daily service, Pussy?'

'No. This is routine. I must do more for you than this.' She smiled, inhaling, and her breasts swelled, making the fabric of her dress turn translucent in that region. The signal was clear enough.

So much for that. 'I think you know that I love the human woman Colene. I do not have sexual interest in others at this time.'

'But I am not a woman!' she protested happily. 'I am a null. There is no conflict with your woman.'

'No conflict? Colene comes from a culture where men and women are supposed to be true to each other during their association. She would not appreciate my doing anything with you.'

'Then you must explain to her. It is quite normal. Married couples use their nulls all the time. It eases the stress of monogamy and provides variety. A null is much more accommodating than a spouse, because a null has no pride and no rights.'

No pride and no rights. Darius had been coming to like the nulls, but now he realized that the culture that fostered them had a brutal disregard of human pride and rights, and had to be condemned. If he cooperated with Ddwng, he would be facilitating the spread of that system to other Modes, like a loathsome disease.

But it would not be expedient to express his doubt to her. She would only take it as rejection, and therefore some defect in the quality of her service. 'Perhaps another time,' he said

255

gently. 'I have much to learn of the ways of the DoOon, and must get to it.'

'Yes,' she said, disappointed.

Provos was in the main chamber, with a meal set up for them both. She remembered the time of his awakening, of course. 'This is an interesting society,' she remarked. 'But I am sorry you are giving them the Chip.'

'I am?' he asked, startled.

'I understand that it is what you must do to be united with your young woman, and I appreciate your desire, but I wish there had been some other way. Or is there some factor in the past which changes the effect of your action?'

'No, there is not,' he said. She remembered that he was going to agree to Ddwng's demand! He had hoped that her knowledge of the future would enable him to do the opposite. Apparently he was to discover no such device.

The meal was catered by Pussy, eager as always to be of any possible service. But how was he going to find daily services for her other than the one she expected?

Provos glanced at the buxom feline woman. 'I also fear that Colene will not understand your sexual use of this creature,' she said. 'I suspect she will be hurt, considering that you will so soon be rejoined. It would seem to be a virtue in a man to be able to wait a few days.'

He was going to do that? Provos was a good woman who spoke her mind plainly, and it was not possible to argue with her. She was not condemning him, merely voicing her disapproval. But in the light of his determination not to use Pussy in this manner, this was a distressing revelation.

Provos was speaking in Darius' language, which he thought the translator balls did not understand. But now Pussy perked up. 'Oh, thank you, Darius!' she exclaimed. Then, to Provos: 'When?'

'Before he kills the monster,' the old woman replied.

So he was going to succeed in his mission, though he knew so little about it. Actually, he would give the order and a minion would dispatch the monster, giving Darius the credit. No genuine accomplishment there!

He made no comment. He realized that the folk of this Mode,

256

however loyal they might seem to Darius, were all minions of Ddwng and would report to him. Darius could afford to say nothing of his true thoughts – especially since it seemed that his course was already plotted.

Darius went out to see to the operation of the ship. It was indeed traveling rapidly through the night sky; the simulation – he found it more comfortable to think of it as a magic picture – showed stars passing by at the rate of one or two close ones each minute. The executive officer Jjle with his Caprine nulls saw to the routine; in fact Buck was seeing to it, with authority delegated by his master, and Doe was keeping track of the internal operations of the ship. Goat was at the communications center, coordinating with the planet of destination and with other FTL ships in the area; it seemed that it was important that no two ships pass too close to each other, because of harmonics of hypershift. Darius made no pretense of understanding the technical details; this was obviously a smoothly functioning system.

'We shall rendezvous with Planet Yils in twenty-three hours, sir,' Jjle informed him. 'Have you any directives?'

'Carry on,' Darius replied.

The exec nodded without trace of a smile. Darius completed the tour of the ship, gradually becoming comfortable with it and his position in it. He was a figurehead, true – but it seemed that all captains were figureheads, normally.

He repaired to the ship's library, which was merely a chamber with screens in contact with a number of planets in the galaxy, and with the help of Cat and the resident Ovine neuter, Sheep, he learned as much as he could assimilate about the colony on Planet Yils. The first human mission had come there approximately a thousand years before – all times were scaled to the Earthly measurements, because this was a human empire – and settlement had proceeded. There had been a lively export of 'escargot' for wealthy cuisine, until someone had noticed that the big snails were intelligent. Technically they qualified for sapient-species recognition and protection. But the Empire had never been much for technicalities, so the export continued on a muted basis. The natives were placid folk who did not hold grudges, so there was no fuss.

Now, however, the marauding was becoming an embarrassment. The actual value of the damage was not great, but the seeming inability of the colonists to stop it reflected adversely on the Empire. There was also the suspicion that the natives might be finally developing notions of objection to human rule, and of course that had to be emphatically squelched. It was necessary not only to stop the monster, but to ascertain exactly how it had come on the scene and what had enabled it to operate so long without being stopped. The suggestion of mind-blasting was especially sensitive. The Empire had overwhelming superiority in conventional weapons of all types, but something that could stun a mind without physical contact was alarming.

Darius retired to his quarters and pondered. This just might prove to be a more difficult mission than had been suggested. Was it possible that Ddwng really was providing him with a challenge that would prove his mettle one way or the other? Mind-stunning, if done by intelligent creatures who were organized, could prove to be a threat to more than just a single colony.

Then why assign the mission to an ignorant outsider? It wasn't to get rid of him, because Ddwng wanted him to survive to show the way to his home Mode and the Chip there. Darius was not a conspirator by nature, but he had a certain notion of the ways in which people of doubtful loyalty could be tested. They could be provided with the opportunity to do some secret wrong. Believing they were unobserved, they usually revealed their basic natures.

Suppose Ddwng hesitated to trust himself to the Virtual Mode with only Darius as a guide? The Emperor would not be able to take any of his loyal minions along unless he remained in constant contact with them, which would be awkward. How well Darius knew! That meant he would have to trust Darius and his companions of the Virtual Mode. After requiring Darius' cooperation by threatening the young woman he loved. That would seem chancy indeed!

But if Darius turned out to be trustworthy, the risk became

feasible. If Darius' nature was honest, then his word, once given, was good. That might well be more important to Ddwng than the outcome of the mission on Planet Yils. That ten day deadline might be as much for Ddwng as for Darius: time to study the visitor to this Mode, to come to a conclusion about him.

Darius was a Cyng, a man of inherent power. He had never had the need to deal in anything other than the truth, and hardly cared to demean himself by doing so now. But he had never before been faced with such a difficult choice. Should he save the woman he loved by pledging to enable a conqueror to ravage other Modes? That would represent a loss of honor. But if the alternative was to lose Colene –

Well, he still had most of nine days to make the decision. Or did he? Could this span of time be another kind of test? A person who waited until the end to make the pledge surely was doing it only as a last resort. One who made it at the outset might simply be saying it as a matter of convenience, without sincerity. The sincere man would take time to study the situation and think it through, then make his decision in timely fashion.

Provos believed he would make the pledge. But she could not know what was in his heart, and neither could Ddwng. A liar and a truth-teller would say the same thing, to get his way. But in a situation of challenge and decision, the reactions of the two would probably differ. Ddwng and his minions had surely had a great deal of experience in judging how the two differed.

But a single episode was not enough. It was necessary to know a person as well as possible, and to judge whether his decision was consistent with the pattern of his personality. Even if a person made a commitment with sincerity, he could not be trusted if it was not in accord with his nature. Men did not always know their own wills.

Darius realized that he had probably been under observation throughout, waking and sleeping, and would be for the duration of this venture. It didn't matter; he had been too busy getting his bearings to act in any way atypical of himself. But now that he realized this, it did matter. He could not form a pattern of action consistent with one decision, then decide the other way.

But he hadn't made his decision! How could he be consistent with an unknown?

Provos had given him the key to that. He would have to comport himself in a manner consistent with a decision to accede to Ddwng's demand. If he then did so, it would be trusted. If he did not, then the pattern would be inconsistent – but that would not matter, because an inconsistent pattern was similar to a negative one, for Ddwng's purpose. Either would mean that it was not safe to enter the Virtual Mode with him.

Was the choice truly between Colene and the welfare of the Modes? He would have to search for some compromise. But meanwhile he would assume that he was going to agree to give Ddwng the Chip. He did love Colene, and this was the only likely way to save her.

He looked up. There were the three Felines, not watching him, but alert for any required service. Cat had been of service today; the other two had not. He had to do something about that.

'Tom, try to enable me to see Colene again,' he said.

Tom jumped to manipulate the screen. This time he quickly got through to the Swine. However far the ship was from Earth, it seemed to entail no delay in communication.

But the bureaucracy would not be rushed. Tom had to go through the litany of requests and clarifications. Finally a man with the seeming head of a horse appeared on the screen. 'The Lady Colene is not accessible at the moment,' Stallion said.

'Why not?' Tom demanded.

'Because she is riding her horse.'

Darius was surprised. A horse had been mentioned, and it had slipped his mind. She was allowed to ride it? But of course they wouldn't let her ride it into the Virtual Mode. She must have ridden it all the way to this Mode, to prevent it from being lost in the intervening Modes.

'Stick with it,' Darius said. 'She won't ride forever, and when she's done she will be available.' He did want to see Colene again, but that was not all of it; he wanted to be sure that Tom

260

had enough of a challenge even if he failed to get Colene so that it counted as a full service.

Meanwhile, what should Darius do? His research and his thinking had fatigued him more than he realized, but it was too early to go for his night's sleep. He wanted to maintain a regular sleeping schedule if he could. He wasn't hungry yet. And he hadn't figured out a service for Pussy.

'What can you do for me?' he asked her with mock exasperation. 'That requires no thought on my part?'

She inhaled.

'What else?' he asked quickly.

'I can give you a relaxing massage.'

He considered that. He liked it. 'Agreed.'

'On your bed,' she purred, guiding him to his bed chamber. He let her do it. She was probably very good at this, and his body did feel tight.

Before he knew it, she had pulled off his robe. But of course it wouldn't be good to crumple the Captain's uniform. He lay face down on the bed.

She was good at it. She kneaded his shoulders, and the tension melted away from the muscles there. She stroked his back, and it relaxed. She massaged his calves, and they felt like new. She worked on his thighs, and they were invigorated.

Then she started in on his buttocks. He had been sitting for much of the time he had been on the ship, and there was tenseness to be released here too. But as her hands reached around and inside, a new kind of tension developed. Embarrassed, he lay still and did not say anything.

Until she turned him over. 'Uh, no,' he said, resisting.

'But I have to do the other side, or my service is not complete,' she explained, sounding hurt.

He was stuck. He turned over, revealing his erection. She had surely seen similar before. He closed his eyes.

'Oh, what a beautiful member!' she exclaimed, delighted.

She did his chest muscles with similar finesse, and his stomach. Then she got on the bed, straddling him, her thighs outside his. He opened his eyes and saw that she was naked; she was evidently able to doff her tight dress in a single fluid motion. She leaned forward, her breasts

261

descending invitingly toward him. She was trying to seduce him.

All he had to do was tell her no. But if he did, what would that indicate about his impending decision to cooperate with Ddwng? And if he refused her offerings, then told Ddwng yes, and Ddwng considered his maladaption to the customs of this culture, and concluded that he could not be trusted, what then of Colene? Pussy was nice, but she was meaningless; she would be exactly as nice in exactly this way to any man she was required to serve. It was Colene who counted. He could not risk anything to imperil Colene's welfare.

The safest thing to do was nothing.

Pussy took that as assent. She lay on him full length, sliding up enough to kiss him with her feline mouth. It was a human mouth; it only looked feline. All of her cat features were more suggestive than actual, as if she had had just enough cosmetic surgery to lend the effect.

His resolve to be passive dissolved. His arms closed around her body. His hands stroked the sleekness of the small of her back, and below. Her posterior was as marvelous to touch as to see. Then they were turning over, his eagerness taking charge. She was intended for this use, and –

The wall became a window screen. Colene stood there, as if right beside the bed, staring down. Everything was visible. She blinked.

Darius froze in place. The call! How could he have forgotten the call! Tom had kept at it, finally completed it, and put it right through to Darius, where he happened to be at the moment. In the middle of a sexual act with another woman.

'I guess you're busy right now,' Colene said, turning away. The screen faded and became the wall.

Pussy looked at him, concerned. 'Have I done wrong?'

'No.' She had been true to her nature.

'She was not supposed to see?'

'I was not supposed to be doing it.' An understatement!

'I will tell her what I did!' Pussy said, tears starting down her face as she sat up. 'You did not tell me yes! I have done you a disservice, my master!'

What could he say? What was the penalty for a disservice?

He feared it was formidable. He was already in critical trouble with Colene, and no apology by a null would make that right. What would be the point in punishing Pussy?

'You were not at fault,' he said. 'I let you do what I wanted you to do. I did not know Colene would see, but if I had done it without her seeing, I would have been deceiving her. The fault was mine, either way.'

'You must not take the blame for me!' she protested. 'I have done you a disservice, and I must pay. I am so sorry to have done this to you. I wanted only –'

'Enough!' He spoke more forcefully than he had intended, startling her. 'You have done me no disservice. I have done myself the disservice. But if you feel you had any share in it, I will require two services of you tomorrow, and thereafter the matter shall be forgotten.'

She had to think about that a moment. 'You want my service tomorrow?'

'Yes, of course. Not necessarily of this type, but a service. Or two. Be ready.'

'Oh, yes, my master! I will be ready! But now –'

'Dress me. Now I shall eat.'

She hastened to oblige. They emerged to the main chamber, and she hurried to fetch food.

Provos was there. She had evidently been walking around the ship, knowing her way by memory, and the members of the crew tolerated her as a guest of the Captain. 'Something happened?' she inquired.

'So to speak.' He knew what she thought he had done, and she was not far off. He came close to her, needing the illusion of privacy. 'Provos, do you remember what the penalty is for a null who does a disservice?'

'Why of course. The null is destroyed immediately. It is unfortunate, because no null ever does such a thing intentionally, but it seems that some mistakes are not allowed. Why do you ask?'

'I had a concern that one might have made such a mistake.'

'No, not that I remember. The nulls of this ship are very competent.'

'I am glad to know that.' He was indeed! Pussy had been offering her death, to try to spare him embarrassment. He had managed to avoid that as much by luck as intent. His luck had been opposite with Colene. He knew it would be useless to try to call her back.

And all because he had allowed his passion to get out of control. He had indeed done himself a disservice.

The following day he had to worry about the two services from Pussy, as well as the single ones from Tom and Cat. So he did the obvious: he asked Cat.

'You do not wish to make sexual use of Pussy?' Cat inquired.

'I do and I don't. She is an attractive and innocent creature. But Colene would not understand.'

'Colene already does not understand.'

'All too true! Still, my feeling for Colene is such that I prefer not to be guilty of what disturbs her, even if it is too late for such restraint. I punish myself by denying myself that which I foolishly desired.' It was, he knew, a pointless gesture, but the hurt he had done Colene was gnawing at him, and this was the only way he could think of to ameliorate it even slightly.

'As you prefer. There is another alternative. On rare occasions, at the master's discretion, services may be postponed, pending greater service at a later time. You are about to undertake a mission with some risk. You can require Pussy to join you on that mission, as a bodyguard.'

'A bodyguard! Is she good at that?'

'No, violence is against her nature. Tom will be with you, of course; he is adapted for violence. It would be a stressful thing for her, worthy of several services.'

'I don't want to put her under stress!'

'She is already under stress.'

As with Colene, he was damned either way. 'I'll do it.'

Darius did some more thinking about the possible nature of the monster. It seemed unlikely to him that even the most intelligent snail could do the type of mischief described. That suggested that the monster was human. That in turn suggested that something more than incidental vandalism was involved. Perhaps Ddwng knew it.

He discussed it with Jjle, without speaking of his suspicion. 'What is the standard way to deal with a problem like this?' He had learned the answer from Cat, but he had a reason to clear this with the exec.

'Locate the troublemaker with a fair degree of certainty and bomb the region,' Jjle replied.

'But doesn't that kill many innocent folk along with the guilty one?'

'It does. But since the normal trouble is terrorism or incipient rebellion against the Empire, and the penalty is known, this is an effective mechanism. Few loyal creatures would seek to shield a guilty one.'

'I will do it in another manner. I will not bomb the region; I will enter it myself and try to nullify the monster. I intend to kill no innocent folk, either human or native.'

'I do not recommend this,' the exec said, alarmed.

'Neither do my Felines,' Darius said with a smile. 'They are unanimous against it. But I believe it is my authority to handle this mission as I choose.'

Jjle gazed at him with a certain wary appreciation. 'That is correct, Captain. But I must insist that you be appropriately protected.'

'I will take Tom and Pussy as bodyguards, carrying weapons.'

'A female null? This is irregular.'

'But my prerogative.'

'True, sir.' There was a slight emphasis on the 'sir', a nuance of disapproval. 'But two nulls is not sufficient protection. You will require shielding.'

'Armor?'

'It could be called that. It will shield you from both physical and environmental threats.'

'Agreed. The three of us will be so protected.'

He returned to his chambers, knowing that a message would be sent to Ddwng, and that the Emperor would confirm Darius' authority, because Ddwng wanted to learn more about him. None of the members of this ship owed allegiance to Darius, only to the Emperor. All thought him foolish and perhaps crazy, but they had to go along with him as long as Ddwng did. They feared he might only get himself killed.

But Provos had remembered him killing the monster, so the success of his mission was not in doubt, merely the manner of its accomplishment. Of course Provos had been in error about him having sex with Pussy, but only because she had made the reasonable assumption about his session in the bedroom. Provos did not know the literal future, only that part of it she was to learn. Darius had been caught in compromise. Anyone would have drawn a similar conclusion. Especially Colene. And he was in effect guilty. But however Colene now felt about him, he still loved her, and the thought of her being sterilized and lobotomized was intolerable. He *had* to save her.

So if Ddwng wanted to discover Darius' nature, this would provide a clear indication. He would accomplish this mission in his own style. But he still had not decided whether to accede to Ddwng's demand for the Chip. If he could find a way to save Colene without giving up the Chip, he would do so. Just as he hoped to find a way to nullify the monster without hurting anyone.

'Tell me about shielding,' he said to Cat.

'It is an electronic armament which prevents any fast-moving missiles from touching the wearer,' Cat replied. 'It also intercepts any radiation or sonics which would be harmful. Only officers of the Empire are allowed to utilize it.'

'Or those designated by such officers.' Darius was catching on to the rules of Empire.

'True.'

'Do you think it will intercept the mind-stunning attack of the monster?'

'It should, as there surely is some physical aspect of this. True mental transmission between minds is unknown; all claims of such have been investigated and debunked. But it seems indiscreet to expose yourself to it.'

'It seems indiscreet to me not to,' Darius said. 'Tom and Pussy and I will go after the monster protected in this manner.'

266

Cat was silent. That was his indication of disagreement so strong as to be a possible disservice if voiced. No null could afford to call its master a fool.

The *Flay* arrived at Planet Yils on schedule. There was no fanfare; it simply took up what Jjle described as an orbit, and Darius stepped into the transfer chamber with his two Feline bodyguards. Tom was confident; Pussy was nervous. Tom carried what was called a laser rifle, and Pussy the pain dial. She had to bear a weapon for this type of service to count, though she seemed afraid of it.

The shields they wore were invisible. They were generated by small boxes carried in pockets. Darius knew the power of magic, but distrusted the power of super science, so tested the shields by having his Felines make mock attacks against each other and himself. They could make contact with each other, but the moment any motion became swift enough to harm a person, the shields cushioned it and slowed it down to safe range. The faster the motion, the greater the cushioning effect, until it became quite un-cushionlike. When Darius, emboldened by slower maneuvers, attempted to strike Tom with a stick, the stick seemed to smack into a wall, and it broke in half. Thrown stones bounced off harmlessly. A direct charge at Pussy resulted in both of them bouncing back, cushioned by their shields so that neither was hurt.

This did seem to be about as good as magic. But would it really be effective against the monster? Darius had a nagging doubt.

They met the commandant of the colony, an old human man in an Empire robe. 'It struck again six hours ago,' he announced. His language was unfamiliar, but Darius now carried a translation ball which worked both ways. 'We have set up a cordon, and believe we have it isolated. Unfortunately a number of colonists reside in that sector.'

'We are not going to bomb the sector,' Darius said.

'You have a way to point-spot the monster?' the commandant asked, relieved.

'We are going to search for it ourselves.'

'But it can stun human minds!'

267

'We are shielded.'

The commandant looked doubtful. 'I would not wish to seem critical of Navy equipment, but unless your shields are more potent than ours, they will not be effective. This seems almost to be a case of – something unknown.'

So maybe it *was* direct mind contact! The commandant didn't want to name it as such, fearing ridicule for believing what was supposedly supernatural, but he was hinting. 'I have had some experience of this type,' Darius said, understating the case. Receiving and amplifying and broadcasting mental power was his specialty of magic. If by any chance the monster's power related, Darius might be uniquely equipped to handle it. He had tested sympathetic magic here and found it to be inoperative, but perhaps mental magic would work. Certainly the two were different, because even in his own Mode, few folk possessed the power of multiplying feeling, while anyone could do ordinary magic.

Could this be coincidence? Colene had arrived at this Mode before him, perhaps because of his delay when he returned Prima to his own Mode. Ddwng had surely questioned her. She could have told him what she knew of Darius' power of magic, which the Emperor well might have interpreted as supernatural mental power. By the definitions of this culture, that was what it was. Darius had not been aware of any mental interactions with the folk of this Mode, but it was possible that though most were deaf to the transfer of joy, some few might be receptive.

Ddwng was evidently no ignorant functionary. He had given Darius a mission that might exploit his particular talent, if it were operative here. Ddwng might be extremely interested in knowing the status of that talent.

Darius decided to assume that this was a good connection and that he could be effective in dealing with the monster. He let his peculiar awareness extend, seeking a mind that was in some fashion similar to his own. A mind that could transfer joy – or other emotion. Or simply the deadly absence of emotion that was unconsciousness.

In a moment he found it. To his perception it was a nucleus of malignancy. Something was hating.

Darius had not had occasion to magnify or broadcast hate. There just was no market for it. But the principle was the same as for joy. He could transfer it without affecting himself. If there were no suitable recipients, the emotion would be lost – but that was a suitable way to deal with hate.

All this happened in a moment. Meanwhile, he was answering: 'It shall be known soon enough.' Then he set forth with his Felines into the cordoned region.

Most of it was native. The Yils came out to meet them. They were indeed like snails with the body mass of men or greater, slow moving. One had positioned itself to be in the main aisle they were following. Did it want a dialogue?

Darius stopped before it. 'What is your concern?' he inquired.

The snail wiggled feelers. 'You are the Empire Captain come to abolish the menace?' the translator ball inquired.

'I am.'

'This mischief is not of our doing.'

'But is it of your toleration?' Darius inquired sharply.

'It is known that we have no power to inhibit human beings from doing what they choose.'

'Such as exporting your citizens as cuisine?'

'This is a concern.'

'I will ask the Emperor that this be stopped. But the power is his, not mine.'

'We thank you, Captain.' The snail withdrew into its shell, clearing the aisle ahead.

Pussy lifted a hand. Darius nodded, giving her leave to speak. 'Why should you do anything for the natives?'

'Because they are feeling creatures, and deserve sympathetic treatment.'

'This is an odd concept.'

'You deserve it too.'

'That is odder yet.'

Darius smiled, not arguing the case. He tuned in on the bolus of hate, walking that way. 'I suspect your weapons will not be effective,' he told them both. 'But have them ready. Should I fall unconscious, kill whatever creature is before us. It may be a human being.'

They nodded. They were responsive to his will.

The snails did not use houses; their shells were sufficient. They had many slick paths through their cultivated sections; the paths branched and rebranched, becoming smaller, like the structure of trees. It was evident that there was no centralized feeding system; each snail had its own patch to graze. It seemed to be a live and let live society. Unfortunately the human conquerors did not have a similar philosophy. Now they wanted to break into other Modes, so as to get new genes to revivify their stock, so they could maintain and expand their empire. His sympathy was with whatever power had decided to confine this empire to this one Mode.

But if he told Ddwng no, what then? Destruction for Colene, if torture of her did not make him yield. Then probably torture of him. And in the end, if he died without yielding, Ddwng would still be able to set out on the Virtual Mode and perhaps find Darius' Mode and the Chip. He was an anchor person; he should be able to sense the right direction the same way Darius and Provos did, and as Colene surely had. He merely wanted to avoid the serious risks of traveling alone into unknown territory. But he could take them if he chose. What would defiance accomplish, in the end?

They were coming close to the source of the hate. But there seemed only to be a snail snoozing at the end of its pathlet, having grazed its fill. It was withdrawn into its shell.

But hiding behind that shell was a human child. 'I see you,' Darius said.

The child stood, and the nucleus of hate shifted with his body. This was the monster: a boy of perhaps seven years. No wonder he had escaped detection! He was just an ordinary gamin, a neglected urchin, probably stealing food to survive. But his mind was an absolute horror.

'In the name of the Empire, I am come to bring you to justice,' Darius said, observing the ritual. 'Yield, and you will not be killed.'

Both Felines looked at Darius, evidently suspecting that he had gotten severely confused. A little human boy? Hardly a monster!

For answer, the boy unleashed his fury. It struck Darius –

and was rebroadcast outward. He was unaffected. But he had learned something: the boy could direct his power. He did not strike at every mind within his range. Harnessed, this could probably be useful to the Empire.

'Yield, and perhaps you will be granted a good life in return for the use of your power on behalf of the Empire,' Darius said.

He sensed the lad's understanding. But there was no trust there. The boy hated his own kind. He must have been rejected, cast out, orphaned. There was something strange and vulnerable about his mind, as if it had been weakened, not strengthened, and in its distress had channeled most of its force to this incubus of hate. So great was that destructive force that it could overwhelm even a 'deaf' mind, such as those of this Mode. But the hammer that could shatter a stone could not do the same with a sponge or a rubber ball. The boy could not prevail against Darius.

The lad seemed shaken by the failure of his attack on Darius. But his little face was set in a grimace of hate which echoed that of his mind. He had no intention of yielding to the Empire. But Darius tried again. 'I have the means to destroy you. I ask you to yield and save yourself.'

Apparently it was a lost cause. The mind-monster would not or could not be reasonable. He would have to be stunned and taken in; perhaps the empire super-scientists could do something with him, or at least confine him so that he could not do physical damage, such as torching granaries.

'Dial him, Pussy,' Darius said.

The Feline lifted the dial and turned it on. Level Three discomfort struck Darius. He had never reset the device! It was tuned to him as well as to others. The Felines expected to be affected, and were prepared to endure it in order to accomplish the mission. It would surely be far more potent against the boy than against them.

Indeed, the boy felt it. He staggered as if physically struck. Then he sent a jolt of hate directly at Pussy.

Pussy collapsed with a little meow of pain. She could not ward off the power.

The boy staggered forward and snatched the dial from her

hand. He touched the detune switch, then turned the dial up to maximum.

He had not understood the dial well enough. All he had done was to restore Darius' exemption – and hit himself with the maximum degree of pain. He collapsed.

Darius stepped forward and took the dial from the boy's flaccid hand. He turned the dial down to zero.

But it was too late. Pussy, already unconscious, was unaffected. Tom, caught by the dial, was now sprawled on the ground. And the boy was dead.

Darius had after all killed the monster. And, in his own judgment, bungled the mission.

Back on the *Flay* with his staggering minions, Darius was the object of covert stares of awe. 'The monster took out your bodyguards, sir – and you killed it alone?' Jjle inquired. 'Without a weapon?'

'Not exactly. It was the pain dial that killed him. His mind was more vulnerable to it than others. But my success was chance as much as design.'

'As you say, sir.' But the awe remained.

When he reached his chambers, the wall-screen was on. There was Colene, in her preternatural beauty. 'Oh Darius – you're all right!' she cried.

He was taken aback. 'You are speaking to me?'

'Of course I'm speaking to you! I love you!'

She couldn't have forgiven him! 'And I love you. But –'

'I know your culture's different. You can't be expected to – I understand that – and anyway, you're a man. Oh, Darius, please give Ddwng the Chip! It's the only way we can be together!'

'Colene, I want to be with you more than anything. But if I –'

'It'll be all right! Honest it will! He'll let us go, if – please, Darius!'

Why had she turned about so completely? She should be furious with him, yet she was urging him to betray their Modes so that she could be with him. He would have to think about this.

'I will consider,' he told her.

'Please,' she repeated, and faded out.

Darius sat in the chair and considered. He thought of the monster-boy, so recently dead. He thought of Provos, who had said he would kill the monster, and who had also said he would agree to commit to Ddwng. He though of Colene.

He had offered the boy the chance for a kind of amnesty: fair treatment and a chance to serve the Empire, if he turned his talent to the welfare of the Empire. He knew Ddwng would have honored that, because it made sense. Instead the boy had attacked him – and destroyed himself in the process. Utter folly.

There was no doubt that Ddwng had power over Darius and Colene. He could make them happy together, or keep them apart, or torture them or kill them or let them go. He was no fool. If Darius tried to cross him, Darius would be destroyed. But if he cooperated, he would be rewarded. He was to the Emperor as the monster/boy was to Darius himself. What was his choice?

Provos said he would accede. Colene had begged him to. He didn't like it, but it did seem to be his only practical choice.

'Get me the Emperor,' he told Cat. The two other Felines were recuperating from their ordeal.

In a moment Ddwng was on the screen. He must have been waiting for this.

'I have destroyed the monster,' Darius said to the Emperor. 'I promised the natives I would seek to end the exploitation of their kind as food. I am requesting –'

'The word of a minion of the Empire is good. That exploitation shall cease forthwith.'

That was certainly swift! Darius had promised only to ask, and here he had succeeded in changing empire policy. But that was the minor issue. He braced himself for the major one.

'Today I am in your Mode, sir, in your power,' Darius said. 'In my Mode the power will be ours. I will guide you there, but the Chip is not mine to give. I will introduce you to the Cyng of Pwer, who may elect instead to kill you. You must

273

let Colene and her horse and Provos and me into the Virtual Mode, and we shall do you no harm there. This is the deal I proffer.'

'Agreed.'

Darius stared at the man. 'No bargaining? You will risk yourself this way?'

'You are a man of honor. You will advise me of the appropriate manner to approach your official. It is enough.'

'A man of honor? How can you know that?'

'It is not only your words and actions we have watched. We know the physical and brain-wave patterns of deceit. You have at times withheld information, but you have not given false information. You are to be trusted, and after I possess the Chip you will be given a ranking position in the Empire, if you wish it.'

'You can not trust a person whose cooperation has been obtained under duress.'

'That depends on the man. Now relax, Captain Darius; your mission has been accomplished, and you will return to Earth.' Ddwng faded out.

So it was done. Darius did not feel uplifted. He had done it to save Colene.

Colene. What were her feelings toward him, now? She had seen him with Pussy, then called him back to plead his acquiescence to the demand of the Emperor. She did not know the threat against herself. What could account for the change?

Was there a threat against him, too, which she knew about? But if she was angry with him, she could simply let it happen. Instead she had said she loved him and wanted to be with him.

Maybe she really did understand. But maybe she was doing what was expedient now, and there would be a reckoning later. After they were free of the DoOon. If they got free.

11

CONSORT

Colene looked at her wrist. The scars had faded. She had not cut herself since meeting Darius. But now she was getting that feeling again.

When she had come here and realized that she and Seqiro were prisoners, she had hoped they would be able to escape soon after Darius arrived. But he had been whisked away almost immediately to a distant stellar system. That prevented her from even trying to flee. She knew she would have to wait until he returned to Earth.

Oh, Ddwng was treating her well enough. He dined with her often, and was always exceedingly polite. One might have supposed that an Emperor of a Galaxy would have better things to do, but apparently his staff was more than competent, and he seldom had crisis decisions to make. She had feared that his interest in her was that of a man for some wild primitive strange woman, but he seemed genuinely curious about her ways and feelings. What she would do if another type of interest manifested she didn't know. She didn't want to make him mad – not while Darius was far away – but she didn't want any more to do with him than absolutely necessary.

She had three nulls of the Equine persuasion to tend to her every need and want. Indeed, they were compelled to do one or more services for her each day. Had she been a man, she would have had no trouble finding something for Mare each day; she was as luscious a piece of woman-flesh as could be imagined, from the neck down. But Colene was a girl, and though Stallion would have been glad to do for her what a man did, hired sex was not her interest. So she was kept busy keeping them busy.

She was allowed information on Darius' progress, and she followed it compulsively. Unfortunately that meant being aware of the time he spent with *his* nulls, particularly Pussy. What an apt name for that juicy Feline!

He called her, to her surprise; she had assumed that direct dialogue between them would be forbidden. So she tested it farther by urging him not to agree to give Ddwng the Chip. Then she waited somewhat apprehensively for the Emperor's reaction.

There was none. She did not trust that one bit.

She was allowed access to Seqiro, too. Actually she was in constant mental contact with him, but she wanted more than that. So they played the game of riding, because both agreed that his mental powers should be hidden. The people of this reality had no awareness of telepathy, treating it as a supernatural notion. Seqiro reported that their minds seemed opaque to it, not because of being guarded but because they just did not seem to be organized that way. The animals could be touched, but Seqiro did not even send the mosquitoes away, lest an attendant notice. He was being the complete dumb animal.

She returned to the palace interior to learn from Horse that Darius had tried to call her again. 'Well call him back!' she said, her heart leaping. 'Immediately!'

It placed the call. Tom received it. 'Darius is busy at the moment,' the cat-head said.

'Oh, he'll talk to *me*!' she said confidently.

'As you wish.' The picture changed.

There was Darius, naked, in the process of having sex with Pussy. She was so surprised and dismayed that she couldn't think of any appropriate reaction. 'I guess you're busy right now,' she said lamely, and faded out. That description was appropriate: she thought she was going to faint.

'You seem surprised at his activity,' Horse said. 'I should clarify that it is normal to –'

'Oh, shut up!' she snapped. She charged to her bedroom and flung herself down among the plush pillows, sobbing.

Your mind is in turmoil, Seqiro remarked.

She let him have her feeling in an inchoate blast. Then, aware of his distress, she apologized. *I'm sorry, Seqiro! It's just that – oh, what will I do?*

The horse pondered, using her intelligence and his objectivity. *You are being polite to Ddwng, because you fear what he might otherwise do. Those watching you are under the impression that you like him. Perhaps Darius finds it similarly expedient to give others the impression that he likes his situation.*

By screwing the pussy? she demanded, her image savage.

Yes. It would suggest that he was not acclimatizing, were he to spurn her.

Colene struggled with that. She did know the nature of men; they were always interested in sex, and took it when they got the chance. That night with the boys – she had represented Opportunity. She had had no illusions after that. Darius was a man, and he had treated her decently, and he said he loved her. But how was he with other women? He had not tried to hide that from her: he expected to marry some other woman, and have sex with her if she wanted it, and in his castle he had mistresses. In fact, as Seqiro had read in Darius' mind in that brief time he was in the palace, he had found the perfect woman to marry, named Prima, who could greatly extend his ability to radiate joy to others. Prima was no love-match; she was twice Darius' age. The only thing distinguishing Colene from those other women was the fact that he loved her.

Yes.

With a woman, sex and love were aspects of the same thing. That was why the abuse of sex was so horrible; it soiled love. But with a man they were in different ball-parks. A man could love one woman and have sex with another. It was part of the basic misunderstanding between the sexes. She had learned the hard way. So Darius could love Colene and have sex with Pussy. She understood that with her mind.

Yes.

Why, then, couldn't she understand it with her emotion?

You do understand it with your emotion, Seqiro thought.

It merely requires time for the pain of that understanding to subside.

She did understand it. Her problem was in accepting it. When she walked carelessly and stubbed her toe and it hurt, she understood what had happened, but the pain remained. After a while the pain faded, and she made sure not to stub her toe there again.

Darius might not even want to dally with the cat-woman. But as Seqiro suggested, if he did not give the impression of going along with the system, he would not be trusted, and would never be given any real freedom.

In fact, she realized something else: if the very walls of Darius' bedroom could become video screens when he didn't want it, they must have that capacity any time. Was it possible that they were always tuning in on him, wherever he was? The four of them – Darius, the old woman Provos, Seqiro and herself – were strangers here, and there was something Ddwng wanted from them. Why wouldn't he watch them closely? If he had thrown them in dark prison cells he wouldn't have had to watch. But not only did he keep them in excellent style, he had given Darius a significant mission to perform.

Because Darius can show him where the Chip is.

Yes. In order to get that Chip, Ddwng would have to trust himself to the Virtual Mode, where Darius could dump him in a deep hole in some barren reality and let him die. If Ddwng had to trust Darius, he wanted to know him well. So it figured that Darius would be watched closely, and all his actions judged. If Darius had caught on to that, he would play the role, because the alternative might be much worse than being a ship captain.

You are forgiving him.

She was forgiving him. Or at least finding reason not to blame him, which wasn't exactly the same thing. There was a hard core of rancor that remained, but she was good at burying such things. She was capable of accepting what had to be accepted, and moving on.

Meanwhile she had a date with Ddwng for another meal. It was time for Mare to get her ready for it.

Ddwng was the root of her problem. He was the one who

278

kept her apart from Darius, and put him in the position of having to hold women other than Colene in his arms. If her core of anger needed a focus, that was where it should orient.

Seqiro, link with me when I'm with the Emperor. I want to know what's truly on his mind.

The horse was doubtful. *I have not been able to penetrate any mind in this reality.*

But Seqiro couldn't get into any un-tame mind in his own reality without that person's permission. This might merely be a more extreme case of that. *I will try to open his mind.*

Then she summoned Mare. 'Let's see what you can do when you go all out,' she told the Equine. 'Make me into a princess. That is your service today.'

Mare smiled. This was a challenge she was ready to tackle. She swung into a program that demonstrated more competence than Colene had realized existed.

Soon she was clean and garbed in a scintillating pale green dress which made her look twice as good as she could ever be. She had never thought of herself as voluptuous, but in this outfit she was long-legged, sleek-hipped, narrow-waisted, and with a decolletage that could have come from a classic painting. Her face and hair were angelic; special reflective pins even gave the impression of a halo.

Colene stared at herself in the mirror. She would not have believed that she could be this adorable! It was said that clothes made the man, but men were pretty dull physically, regardless. It was the woman that clothes made. She was the living proof of it.

Too bad she had to waste this on Ddwng. She would much rather have wowed Darius. But it was in her mind that the Emperor did have some reason for this frequent interaction with her, and it probably wasn't sexual, so it was suspicious. If she could manage to dazzle him just a little, to get him closely focused while Seqiro was tuning in, maybe, just maybe there would be an avenue to get Seqiro into his mind. It was certainly worth a good try.

Stallion guided her to the shuttle. Here in the palace the windows to other cities or ships or worlds weren't used;

it was more physical. Maybe because such windows represented accesses to the palace, and it was supposed to be
secure from intrusion. The shuttle was nice enough; it was
like an enclosed amusement park ride, gently wafting to its
destination. Stallion maneuvered it to Ddwng's dining hall,
let her out, and took it back; private personal nulls were not
welcome in the hall itself. Only the palace nulls.

Ddwng was there, resplendent in a purple robe which
complemented her dress perfectly. A little alarm sounded
somewhere in her head: coincidence? No, probably he had
known what she was wearing – because probably those walls
had eyes here, just as on the FTL *Flay*, and he had access to
those eyes. This could be confirmation of her prior suspicion
that they were all being watched.

But no one here could see what was in their minds. Seqiro
had ascertained that. So if she never voiced her true feelings,
they could be known only through her actions – and she was
pretty good at masking feelings.

She took the Emperor's elbow and walked with him to the
table. The Ovine nulls were there. Ram placed Ddwng's chair,
Ewe placed Colene's, and Sheep stood by for their order.

Colene hardly noticed the excellent exotic food. She was
genuinely interested in Ddwng this time, but not in as flattering
a way as he might suppose. She wanted to tune his mind to
things which Seqiro might read. She hoped that if the subject
were narrow enough, and the interest strong enough, and
she were close enough, serving as a focusing point, it just
might work. It *had* to work, because it just wasn't safe to be
ignorant.

She started obliquely. 'You know, in my reality, things like
anti-gravity and faster-than-light travel are impossible. They
just can't be done. Are you sure that –?'

'The fundamental laws of physics differ from reality to
reality,' Ddwng said. 'We have known that, and understand
that there are realities in which our science is inoperative, but where magic is operative, or psionic powers.
Darius comes from a reality with magic, and his companion Provos appears to remember the future. That, to us, is
paradoxical.'

'She knows the future?' Despite herself, Colene got distracted. 'I was with her only briefly, before she was mattermitted to the ship to rejoin Darius, but it was my impression that even if we had spoken a common language, we wouldn't have gotten far. She seemed to know what we were about to do, but not what had just happened.'

'We are studying her. We find it interesting that her ability does appear to operate in this reality. That suggests that the fundamental laws may not be what they seem.'

Was there a chance that Darius could do magic here? That he could conjure them both away? That seemed too wonderful to be believed!

If she knows the future here, she knows what is to become of us, Seqiro thought.

But Colene was determined not to just let the future happen. She wanted to do whatever was in her power to make it the right future.

She smiled most innocently at Ddwng. 'Maybe you should ask her about your own future. I mean, about getting the Chip.'

'You do not want me to have it?'

'I didn't say that!'

I am getting a bit, Seqiro thought. *He knows you are trying to deceive him.*

'You do wish me to have it?' Ddwng asked, amused.

'I didn't say that either,' she said ruefully.

I am finding an avenue. It is very narrow, but I am attuning. He is fascinated by you, but not as a woman. He is intrigued by the challenge of fathoming your motives.

'Perhaps it would be best if you were open with me,' Ddwng said.

'I'm afraid you're going to rape me,' she said, her deathwish causing her to tread the brink.

He guffawed. For that the sound was direct rather than through the translation ball. 'I have no interest in taking any woman involuntarily. I have any I want, either null or human. Set aside your fear.'

'Rape can be more than physical. What do you want with my mind?'

He studied her for a long moment before responding.

There is something horrible, Seqiro thought. *Maintain the dialogue, if you can.*

'There are three things I want of you,' Ddwng said. 'I want the information you possess about the neighboring realities, so that at such time as I enter them, I am aware of their assets and their pitfalls.'

True.

'That's okay by me,' she said.

'I want you to persuade Darius to guide me to the Chip.'

True.

'I guess that's up to him,' she said guardedly. 'I don't see why I should try to influence him.'

'Perhaps you will change your mind when you know more of my rationale.'

There is something devious here.

'What's the third thing you want of me?' Trying to be nonchalant, she took a sip of her alien fizz-drink. It wasn't alcoholic; she would have gotten sick if it was. Ever since the rape scene, she had detested alcohol.

'I want you to be my consort.'

Colene choked, dribbling liquid on her gown. Immediately Ewe was there, with sponges, efficiently cleaning her up. But at least the delay gave her a chance to commune with Seqiro before replying.

This is not an evil thing. It is innocent. Something else is evil.

Innocent? That's marriage!

No, this is form only. You can agree without compromise.

You had better be right, Seqiro! Darius is the only man I – But that remained a complex emotional mess, too.

Her seizure had concluded. 'I thought you had no such interest.'

'I see you misunderstand. I have many consorts. All are attractive women. Most are mistresses. Their proximity to me gives them unique authority, for it is known that I do not like to embarrass them. I sometimes use them as emissaries. I would like to have you with me as I make a business trip this coming period, and the proper format for this is as consort.'

282

True. But there is something else. You have his attention; question him.

Colene leaned forward, evincing the appropriate amount of suspicion as well as presenting a bit more of the flesh of her bosom for inspection. 'You mean I should go traveling with you, and everyone will think I'm having sex with you, but it won't be true?'

'Correct, if that is the way you wish it.'

True.

'And maybe I'll have to do some public task for you, the way Darius is with that far flung mission?'

'Correct. You should find it interesting.'

True.

'And this is the way things are done in the Empire, so it's okay and won't sully my reputation?'

'Correct.'

True.

'And somewhere along the way I should talk Darius into giving you the Chip?'

'Correct. I believe your word will influence him.'

True.

'Though he thinks I'm having sex with you?' she asked sweetly.

He is receiving information. I think you are under constant surveillance, and he knows your heart rate and muscle tension. He knows you are hiding something, and wants to know what it is, but he can not read minds so must persuade you to cooperate. He is enjoying the challenge.

'I see that this would be disruptive,' Ddwng said. 'But there is no problem. Darius will be informed of the nature of the relationship, if you wish.'

Now Colene took a long moment, gazing at him. She was not considering her answer; she was focusing on Seqiro's thoughts.

All that he has told you is true. But there is something he knows would distress you greatly, that he hides. It ties in with Darius. That is what you must ascertain.

'Ddwng, I don't know what's going on in your mind,' she said in what she judged was a three-quarter truth. 'And you

283

don't know what's going on in mine.' Another three-quarter truth. 'You're playing these little games with me, wasting your time, when all you have to do is drug me and make me do anything. It doesn't make sense.'

'You are perceptive. But it does make sense.'

He is playing with you as a cat does with a mouse.

'I'll make you this deal, Ddwng: I'll do all those things you are asking me to do, if you will tell me exactly what your real game is.'

Ddwng smiled. 'Then the game would be over.'

Now he is thinking of it. I have it! Agree to everything. I will cover this with you later.

Colene trusted Seqiro. But she didn't like to capitulate readily, as a matter of obscure principle. 'Then maybe I'll just do none of those things. What do you say to that?'

'I would not recommend such a course.'

There is something else. He is grim.

'So what would you do about it?' she demanded, treading the brink again.

'I would have your horse vivisected.'

True.

She stared at him. 'You aren't kidding, are you!'

'I do not joke. But I would hope that such inducement would not be necessary.'

She sighed. 'Okay, you win. I agree to do the three things you say you want of me.'

'Excellent.'

He is surprised. To him your moods and decisions are strange. He can not be sure when you are telling the truth.

They finished the meal. Then Stallion came to escort her back to her suite.

Colene had Horse tune the wall-screen to an entertainment program. She did not relate well to the sort of television the Empire had, but it gave her a cover for her contact with Seqiro. That business about vivisecting him had her seething. But she knew that was only part of what was wrong. *Now tell me what gives? What's Ddwng's big secret?*

He told Darius that if he does not cooperate, you will be lobotomized and the reproductive cells of your body taken surgically for use by the people of this reality, to replenish their stock. They are too conformist, genetically; they must introduce variety, or suffer slow degeneration.

Colene was stunned. Now she knew why Darius was playing the game! *She* was the cause of it.

She tried to keep her face straight and her body relaxed, so that the hidden sensors could not read her reactions well. Whoever was watching her would know that something was bothering her, but might assume it was the stupid wall-program. Or the threat to her horse, which wasn't far wrong.

The more she dwelt on this news, the firmer her reaction became. It was utter fury. The Emperor was keeping her close to him and treating her like a great lady, while threatening her horse and herself with dire consequences. Rape? He was expert at it!

So what was she going to do about it? Ddwng seemed to hold most of the cards. He was holding them hostage against each other, and was unscrupulous enough to make good on all his threats. But if they all went along, and the Emperor got that Chip, he could ravage the other realities too. Was their welfare worth it?

If they didn't cooperate, it might not stop Ddwng. He would kill them and head into the Virtual Mode on his own, and maybe he would find the Chip anyway. His chances of getting it would be greatly reduced, and his chances of getting lost or killed increased, but he was obviously one tough nut and he well might get through. It which case they would have sacrificed themselves for nothing.

No, the only sure way was to be rid of Ddwng. To agree to do his will, get him into the Virtual Mode, away from his minions, and destroy him. Feed him to a telepathic bear or something.

But right away she saw several problems with that. First, Ddwng wouldn't fall for it; he would know not to trust them. Second, Darius wouldn't give his word unless he meant it, so Ddwng *could* trust him, and for Ddwng's purpose Darius was the only one who mattered. The rest of them were just to make sure Darius didn't change his mind; they had to keep encouraging him to give Ddwng that Chip. How could Colene do anything else, when Seqiro would be hurt? There was probably some sort of threat against Provos, too, so she kept her mouth shut. She might know what was going to happen, but not be able to prevent it.

That gave her a passing notion. *Seqiro – did you tune in on Provos when she was here? Did she know our future?*

Her mind is permeable but strange. She was just beginning to know it. She takes time to remember, in a new reality. She seemed to see us being here for ten days, then going back into the Virtual Mode with Ddwng. She could not see beyond that.

Well, that's enough. So we are going to do it.

Yes, as she sees it.

Colene felt a surge of despair. It was already decided! They were locked in to the Emperor's fell plot. Whatever they did, Ddwng would win, because he was what he was and they were what they were. If only Darius weren't so honest! If he agreed, even under duress, he would carry through. Colene herself would have no such compunction; a pledge made under duress was not binding. Knowing what she now knew of Ddwng, she would have no compunction about lying to him. She would not let the DoOon exploit the other realities as they had this one! But she had no power. Darius didn't want to see her hurt, so he would agree, and that would be that. Should she condemn him because he really did love her?

Damn, damn, damn! Ddwng could tell when others were lying, because his instruments read their body signals. Colene was different; he couldn't quite keep track of her, because she was wildly mixed up inside. The DoOon were pretty much all of a kind, their genetics inbred; that was why they needed new blood, and her ovaries represented that. So Ddwng was trying to understand her, not because he cared about her but because he didn't want to introduce truly crazy blood into the DoOon strain. He was surveying her as he might a new breed of animal, making sure of the quality. Once he was sure that her mind did not represent a genetic danger to the stock –

Could she pretend she was truly crazy, and scare him off? No, because it was Darius he really needed. He could throw her away if he decided she was worthless. She would do better to satisfy him that she was actually a pretty genetically solid creature, and then do something wild in the Virtual Mode, like pushing him off a mile-high cliff into a mile-wide bed of carnivorous oysters who hadn't been fed for two years. But he would surely be well armed, and have electronic armor and an antigravity suit and other super science that would make him invulnerable to any betrayal she might attempt. In fact, he would probably have one of those little pain dials Horse had shown her, tuned to all of them, so that it would go off if anything happened to him and they'd all fry. She would have no way to do him harm, for sure.

But she absolutely refused to let him get away with it. She had faced down Biff in that bleeding contest; there must be some way she could beat Ddwng. Some nasty little plot she could hide in her nutty little mind, that he couldn't fathom. Some little poison needle he wouldn't even feel until it was too late. She had read once about a woman who put slow-acting poison in her vagina, and killed her false lover because after sex with her he just went to sleep, while she got up and quickly washed herself out before she got too bad a dose. If Colene had something like that, and Ddwng did rape her, what revenge! Yet even if she had something like that, and managed to kill him – what would his death do to the Virtual Mode? He was an anchor person. A dead anchor – that just might blow up the whole thing, like a rock in a fan, and kill them all. Could she afford to gamble on that, even if she had the poison, which she didn't? She was ready to die, but she didn't want to do it to Darius or Seqiro.

The anchor – there was the problem. It wasn't safe to touch an anchor person. Ddwng surely realized that, so he wouldn't kill any of them as long as he had any chance to travel their Virtual Mode, and he wouldn't do anything to them while they were on it. So he was muscling them into shape in other ways, taming them, bending them to his will. If only he weren't the anchor for this reality!

Then the answer flashed through her consciousness like a lovely meteor. *Seqiro! We can do it!*

287

Seqiro considered, using her intelligence and his objectivity. *Yes, it is possible, if he does not suspect.*

I'll lull him right to sleep! I'm good at fooling people. Trust me. I do.

Colene had to laugh. Seqiro was the only one who had ever truly understood her. He trusted her because he knew her for exactly what she was: a conniving little wench. *Horse-face, I love you!*

True.

After Darius killed the monster in properly heroic fashion, according to the news release, she called him. 'Oh Darius,' she pleaded in distraught maidenly fashion, 'please give Ddwng the Chip! It's the only way we can be together!'

He seemed taken aback, as well he might be. But she was serious. She did want him to agree. 'It'll be all right! Honest it will! Please, Darius!' She even managed to put a quaver of earnestness into her voice, which would have been excellent acting except that it was real. She was absolutely sincere in this, and she wanted this entire reality to know it. Darius *had* to make the pledge!

He promised to consider. Evidently he did, because soon he did call Ddwng and agreed to guide him to the Chip, with certain manly honorable reservations. It was done.

Colene was the dishonorable one. She dreaded to think of the reckoning she would have with Darius when she did what she hoped to do. But it was better than the choice between lobotomy and loosing the DoOon on the realities. Sometimes deceit was the only way.

Ddwng took her to a far planet elsewhere in the galaxy. She had given up trying to wrestle with the concept of faster-than-light travel; it was contrary to the physics of her reality, but evidently just fine here. The same went for instant communication across the galaxy, antigravity, and all the rest. Super-science, another name for fantasy, in her home town.

They would attend an elegant ball in their honor at the chief city of Planet Kyvrn. Mare got Colene garbed for it in a rehearsal, and Horse drilled her on spot protocol. She was the Emperor's newest and youngest consort, and as such the object of much interest. She would be rather quiet in the Emperor's presence, and rather haughty when alone, for her status on this planet was second only to his. She would dance with him once, and thereafter with any man she chose. Stallion went through the steps with her, making sure she would not misstep.

'But what's my mission here?' she asked.

'This is a rebellious planet,' Horse explained. 'You will need to restore it to harmony with the Empire.'

Colene was aghast. 'A rebel world? And Ddwng is setting foot on it? And I'm supposed to tame it? Why doesn't he just stick his head in a running meat-grinder while he's at it, and I'll just pick up a section of the galaxy and shake some stars loose!'

All three Equines laughed. They had learned early that she made jokes, and accommodated themselves to it. She liked them very well. They were nominally subhuman, but actually they were intelligent enough, with Horse perhaps being smarter than she, and they were perfectly comfortable to be around. She wished there were some way to have such companions with her always, without the degradation of such permanent servitude. She had always liked horses, but would have thought that horse-headed human beings would be disgusting. That was not the case at all; they seemed quite natural now.

'This is not that kind of rebellion,' Horse said. 'This is a retirement colony. Most of the residents are former Empire officials. Here they are out of power, with no requirements, and discover that they are restive. They would never actually rebel, but their discomfort would be an embarrassment were it known, as this is supposedly an ideal world. It will be your task, in the course of the next three days, to make them comfortable with their situation.'

'It's still preposterous!' she exclaimed. 'Does Ddwng expect me to perform magic? I don't know anything about this! and if I did, what could I do? And if I could do anything – three days? I mean, Rome wasn't built in a day, and –'

'Rome?'

'Famous ancient city in my reality. Forget it. The point is, this is like – like – impossible!'

'Evidently the Emperor has much confidence in you,' Horse said dryly, twitching his furry ears.

Colene only wished that Seqiro were here. He might have been able to read the minds of the people, and get a notion how to satisfy them. But he was thousands of light years away, reverted to his dumb animal stage, awaiting her return. She was on her own, and she didn't like it one bit.

Or was she? If telepathy existed, and faster-than-light travel existed, and Provos could remember the future here, showing that it was her talent, not restricted to her reality – why couldn't telepathy and FTL merge, and enable her to commune with her friend regardless? Where was it written that the powers of one reality were nullified in another? Maybe some were and some weren't. Maybe Darius couldn't do magic here, but Seqiro could project his thoughts instantly across interstellar reaches. She had a receptive mind for him, for sure! If anybody could receive him here, she was the one!

She lay down, theoretically resting the hour before the ball, and closed her eyes. But she didn't relax, and she didn't care what the monitors thought; they could assume that she was all twisted up by the enormity of her mission. She opened her mind to her true friend.

Seqiro! Seqiro! Do you read me?

At first there was nothing. Then there was the faintest response. She focused on that, willing it to become stronger. It had to be him!

Seqiro! Read me! I need you!

Faintly, faintly, she felt his mind.

I have to find a way to make these folk feel better about being retired and useless. You must read their minds for me, if you can, to get a glimpse of what will do it. That's my only chance not to blow this mission out of space!

The faint reassurance came. He would do what he could.

It was a pretty planet. The terraforming had evidently made it into one big garden, with neatly laid out cities set up like parkland, so that the houses hardly showed through the trees.

Small lakes were everywhere, set between hills, with paths between them. There seemed to be no motorized vehicles; if there was mass traffic, it was out of sight. This was the sort of place she would like to retire to with Darius, if that ever came.

Of course that was just the image in the screen. She was sure there were slums and garbage and all the rest of the seamy side of civilization. She knew how it was; she remembered Panama. But the illusion was nice, even so.

Then it was time to get ready. All three Equines pitched in, without regard for modesty; Stallion was drawing something like support stockings up her legs while Horse was fitting her invisible bra for proper uplift and Mare was doing her hair. It was all right; there were no secrets from a person's nulls. In a surprisingly short time they transformed her from ordinary messed-up teenager to a vision of unbelievable loveliness. Each time they garbed her, they seemed to exceed prior records for success. Then Stallion took her to the matterport and via it to landfall.

She went in a daze through the halls of the receiving complex, feeling the slightly diminished gravity and breathing the slightly strange air. This was a foreign planet, all right; her body knew it. Ddwng was waiting for her at the entrance, resplendent in his own uniform robe of the day. He was actually rather handsome in his brute fashion. She pictured his Swine doing him as the Equines had done her: support stockings, transparent bra, and hair. She had to bite her tongue lest she let slip an indiscreet titter.

The ball was every bit as opulent as Colene had feared. In her wildest dreams of the distant past – circa one month ago – she had pictured occasions at which she would be the cynosure of all, impressing the ladies with her courtly presence and the men with her sex appeal. Now it had come true, and it wasn't nearly as delightful as her fancy.

The problem was that she had to watch her manners. She couldn't pick her nose or scratch her bottom or say an uncouth word. Maybe full grown ladies never even thought of doing such things, but she was fourteen, which was sort of on the verge. There were a number of pleasures of childhood that she wasn't sure she wanted to give up just yet, like computer games, and multi-decker ice cream cones with nuts and fudge on top, and putting whoopee cushions under the padding of seats in houses of worship. Every time she remembered that joke about the man breaking wind in church and having to sit in his own pew, she broke up. In short, she just wasn't quite ready for ladyhood.

But here she was, ready or not, on the arm of the Emperor of the Milky Way Galaxy (only they called it the DoOon Galaxy here), resplendent as only Mare could make her. Oh, she was breathtakingly lovely all right; every mirror pillar reflected this phenomenal creature virtually floating along in her glow. She wore a brown gown that exactly matched the hue of her hair, and both had been somehow enhanced to make them seem more livingly lustrous than any ordinary woman deserved. Opalescent sequins glittered as she moved. She could have done without the mirror-polished floor, however; she was afraid her dainty hard-soled slippers would slip, putting her into an inglorious spin. She also wondered just what the men were looking at when they bowed their heads to her and gazed into that reflective surface. Most of all she was afraid that the butterflies in her stomach would erupt in a grotesque burp, making her die of shame three times before her blush reached full definition. In sum, fun was not the operative term at the moment.

Be calm. You are making a good impression.

Her nerves lost their ragged edges. What would she do without Seqiro! She reminded herself that every lady faced the same problems, and most of them survived satisfactorily. Anyway, this wasn't forever. After the first dance things would start getting normal.

Ddwng brought her to the center of that stage. He made the little nod to the assemblage, and as one those hundreds returned it. Colene remained frozen, as she had been told to do; her turn was not quite yet.

'I am glad to revisit Planet Kyvrn,' the Emperor said. The miniature translation ball Colene wore at her throat, just above the nascent cleavage of her seemingly-too-low but actually-promising-more-than-could-be-delivered decolletage, murmured his words to her. She was surprised to see that many of the attending men and women wore similar balls. Apparently they could not understand Ddwng's language any more than she could. That gave her another shot of confidence. A dozen more like it, and she might even begin to think about being at ease. But it would help if someone else made a slip first.

'I am sure any questions will soon be resolved,' Ddwng continued. 'To that end I bring you my consort of the moment, Colene, who will be among you three days.' He made an eighth turn toward her, and Colene made the requisite head-nod to him, then did a slow pirouette and bowed more deeply to the audience, so that her upper gown line promised even more of her bosom than before. The material was adhesive, so there was no danger of even a tenth of an inch more exposure than Mare had decreed, which was a relief. She could stand on her head and nothing would pop out. But she might have a problem with her skirt. For a delicious instant she was tempted to do a cartwheel and really wow the audience. But that was her deathwish manifesting, and she had enough to occupy her attention already.

Then Ddwng took her in his arms and danced with her. He was smooth, evidently coached by his own null of the Porcine persuasion. Colene wondered whether he had sex with Sow. But the image wasn't as insulting as intended, because that female swine was both beautiful and sweet-natured. No Miss Piggie there!

She followed his steps, and it was exactly as Stallion had shown her. It was a set format, hardly more challenging than the box step, and she could probably do it in her sleep. The weird thing was that moving in unison with Ddwng this way, being lovely in his arms, she could almost fool herself into thinking that he was a decent character. There was just something about dressing up, and about dancing, that made everything seem better than it was. But deep down she would never be fooled. *Will you dance with me after my lobotomy, dear?* She had to stifle a wry smile; it was her kind of humor. She had been afraid of physical rape, not realizing how much worse it could be. Her reproductive organs cut out of her and put into a cold sere laboratory . . .

Suddenly the dance was done. Ddwng made the little bow to her, then spun about and walked away. She was on her own.

The tableau was frozen. They were waiting for her. She looked at the circle of men, and spied the oldest and by his clothing the most important. Old men were hardly safe, but tended to be less dangerous than young ones. She walked slowly to him.

'I will dance first with the handsomest,' she said. She heard his ball translating as she spoke.

He stepped forward. 'Governor Rrllo,' her ball said. 'I thank you for this significant privilege.'

They danced in exactly the same fashion as before; the set routine was handy this way. His hands did not stray. Around them other couples now danced also. The ball was underway.

Engage him in dialogue.

Yes, so that Seqiro could tune in on Rrllo's focused thoughts. Colene had a mission to perform, and her one in a million chance of succeeding would become even less if she didn't take advantage of every opportunity to try to understand these folk.

'I didn't really choose you for your handsomeness,' Colene said to Rrllo. 'I wanted to talk with you.'

'I am shocked to hear that,' he replied with a chuckle. Their two translation balls were close together and seemed to be talking to each other. 'You thought I would know what's going on behind the scenes?' The translations had become so facile that his idiom was rendered without hesitation into her idiom.

'Yes. I –' She brought a faintly woebegone look to her face, with little effort required. 'I have almost no chance to figure out the problem, let alone solve it, but if there's anything I can do, I'll at least try. I thought perhaps you would help get me started.'

You aren't fooling him, but he is intrigued. You have honored him by selecting him to dance, and he would like to help you. But he is wary.

'You have a better chance than most,' he said. 'You have the ear of the Emperor, for the moment.'

'But what is it that the people here want?'

He shook his head. 'That is no mystery. But the solution – that is the mystery.'

'It is all a mystery to me! This seems like a nice planet.'

'It is very nice,' he agreed.

He knows. But he doesn't want to tell.

'Please, Rrllo! After the ball – may I see you? I mean, visit your house, get to know your family, talk with you off the record?'

He seemed taken aback. 'Nothing is forbidden to a Consort. But our private lives are of little interest.'

He remains wary. You may be trying to trick him into saying something treasonous.

So it was like that. Colene felt that old familiar deathwish gamble urge coming on. It wasn't that she truly needed to solve this riddle; she expected to fail regardless. It was that when she got into something, anything, the underlying nature of her started taking over, and the decorous rules started suffering.

'Do you know what Ddwng does to those who displease him?' she inquired.

The man stiffened. 'I know.'

'Then you know that I face lobotomy if I mess up.' She wasn't sure how true this was; it probably depended more on whether Darius messed up. But it was certainly a threat against her. And perhaps against any of the residents of the planet who contributed to that failure.

'That, no,' he said. 'Surely not merely for failing an impossible mission.'

'Would you gamble on that?'

He considered, now realizing that his own hide could be on the line too. 'I will meet you after the ball. Tomorrow morning?'

She smiled bittersweetly. 'Thank you, Rrllo.' She was learning how to handle the reins of power.

After that, she came close to enjoying the dance, though she kept thinking of the Sword of Damocles. That was the case of the courtier who was given a fine meal to eat, with a heavy sword hanging by a thread over his head; distracted by that threat, he hardly enjoyed the meal. Thus the King showed him the liability of power. Colene now had an excellent notion how the poor man had felt.

Next morning, more appropriately dressed for going places, she went with Rrllo. 'Now show me Panama,' she said.

'I beg your pardon?'

The translator ball hadn't caught up with that one yet. She felt a small morsel of satisfaction. 'I would like to see how the other half lives. The folk who don't get to go to fancy balls. Who don't hobnob with the Emperor.' For it was in her mind that it would be from this class that a revolution would most likely brew.

'The servant class,' he said. 'We can't afford three nulls for each person, but there is a cadre of nulls that passes from house to house to catch up on business.'

Nulls. Her expectation deflated. There would be no revolution there. 'I changed my mind. Let's just go to your place and talk.'

'As you wish.'

His place turned out to be an elegant futuristic (to her perception) cottage on the edge of a lakelet, with pleasantly exotic trees and shrubs surrounding it. His wife was exactly the kind she expected, and the neighbors were too. Rebellion? This just didn't seem to be the place for it.

He remains intrigued by you. There is a certain naive sincerity you evince which is normally lacking in consorts. He may cooperate.

'Look,' she said forthrightly. 'You folk used to have a lot of power in the Empire, and now you've been put out to pasture. I guess that's a comedown. But why would Ddwng think there's a rebellion brewing?'

'There is no rebellion brewing!' Rrllo protested. 'We are satisfied retired citizens.'

'But he has spy-eyes to check every nuance of every reaction of every person. He has to know you're up to something. Why he figures it's anything I can do anything about is beyond me.'

'You are speaking with unusual candor.'

He's getting interested.

'I'm from another reality. I was on my way to meet my – the man I love, and this reality was between, so I passed through here, and he came from the other side, and now we're both in Ddwng's power and if we don't do what he wants we're in trouble. So I'm doing what he wants. He wants me to fix things here. So if there's anything I *can* do, I'm damn well going to do it, so I can get on out of this reality. Now if you'll just tell me what you want, maybe just maybe I can do you and me some good. I admit it's unlikely, but why not give it a try?'

Rrllo was amazed. 'You are from another reality? There has not been a connection between realities in a thousand years!'

'There is now. Ddwng wants to get our Chip so he can go into other realities. We'd rather not give it to him, but we don't have a lot of choice, so we'll do it. It's better than lobotomy.'

Then she realized that she had made a terrible mistake. She should never have mentioned her knowledge of the lobotomy, because now Ddwng would know she knew, and he hadn't told her. He could have the hint that she had a source of information he didn't know about, and that could expose Seqiro and ruin everything.

'You are inadvertently speaking treason,' Rrllo said.

She nodded grimly. 'Yes, I guess the news is already at Ddwng's HQ. But what does he expect when he abducts travelers and threatens them to make them do his bidding?'

He thinks you are trying to trap him into treasonous dialogue.

'There are no recorders here. It would be too expensive to mount and maintain them in an unimportant site like Kyvrn. This conversation is private. But you are mistaken if you suppose we have any animosity toward the Emperor.'

'No cameras?' she asked, hope flaring. 'You mean no one will know what I just said, if you don't tell them?'

'I would not presume to report on the private words of a Consort. Surely you have excellent reason for your utterances.'

She smiled. 'I guess you couldn't tell him anything he doesn't already know.' Apparently the man did not realize the significance of the lobotomy reference. What a relief!

'But I'm really not trying to trick you. I'm just telling you that I have a different perspective. I'm really not the Emperor's mistress; it's just a title he put on me so he has a pretext to put me here.'

'But he introduced you as –'

'Yes. But it's not real. I guess he wanted you to think you rated higher than you do. But Rrllo, I'd sure like to make good even though it's hardly possible. If you'd just help me a little bit, maybe we can both come out ahead.'

He is impressed by your directness. He is inclined to trust you.

'Let me tell you then what I assumed you knew,' Rrllo said. 'This planet is a retirement community for officers of the Empire. As such, it is elite, and we receive excellent care. There is no poverty or crime. But some of us feel that we were retired too soon, and that we could have given further years of service to the Empire, and maintained the associated perquisites. Instead we have been displaced by younger, relatively inexperienced officers. Are you surprised that we feel a certain dissatisfaction?'

Colene shook her head, perplexed. 'Why retire you if you're still doing well?'

'This is our question. We feel the policy is misguided, particularly since genetic deficiencies are appearing more frequently in following generations. In all candor, we feel that those who replace us lack, as a whole, the ability we have, even after allowing for the difference in experience.'

'And I guess it wouldn't do much good just to say that to Ddwng.'

'It has been said to him already.'

'And he responded by sending me.'

'This is the case.'

True.

Colene pondered for about forty seconds. 'Maybe it's his way of changing his mind. If I suggest something he's ready to do anyway, then he can say he's doing it for me, and no one will think he's wishy-washy.'

'Oh, he does not wish to wash anything himself!'

Colene paused, realizing that she had slipped another collo-quialism past the translator. 'I mean that he's given to changing his mind readily.'

Rrllo smiled. 'He is not given to that.'

'See, I'm about as unusual a Consort as he could have, when you get right down to it. I might come up with something pretty wacky, because I'm from out of town. Rather than make it seem that he sent an unqualified Consort, he might just agree to what I suggest. So maybe what you need to do is to tell me what to suggest, and maybe it'll happen.'

Rrllo stared at her. 'You are a most unusual young woman.'

'I guess I am. But why don't we try it? Because suddenly this makes sense of things. That he knows what he's doing, and he thinks you have a case. So my chances and yours aren't nearly as remote as we figured – if we play it right.'

You have surprised him. He has decided to go along with you.

'As it happens, we do have a proposal, if the Emperor does not find it insulting.'

'I have a feeling he knows what it is, and that he's ready to do it.' She was coming to a better appreciation of Ddwng's subtlety. The man was a cunning and unscrupulous customer, but what he did made sense. She only hoped that he had underestimated her more than she had underestimated him. It was an excruciatingly dangerous game she was playing.

'It is this: we would like to bring our expertise back into play. We would like to be designated advisers in our specialities – which cover the gamut of those necessary to the operation of the Empire – and consulted when there are problems which the younger officers might have difficulty with.'

'To pull things out when they bungle.'

'I would not have put it that way.'

'You're not an alien teenage pseudo-Consort.'

He smiled. 'Indeed I am not.'

'Let's try it! Set me up with the detail and the arguments I'll need, and make sure I have it straight, and I'll tell him as if it's my own idea. If we're right, he'll choose to believe that. We have today and tomorrow. Is that enough time?'

'It should be, as our desire is straightforward.'

They got to it, with a growing conviction that this was

indeed what she had been sent here to do. Colene met a number of the other officers in person and by wall video, and rehearsed the arguments as carefully as she had done the protocol of the ball. When the time came, she would be ready.

It happened as expected. It had obviously been choreographed as precisely as the ritual of the dance. Planet Kyvrn was officially designated as an Advisory Resource, and the residents were presumably encouraged and would feel more positive henceforth.

'You did so well!' Mare said enthusiastically as she gave Colene a massage. Her hands were so gentle and proficient that the lingering tension just faded away. She could appreciate how Darius, subjected to such treatment, could – but she shoved that hastily out of mind. She understood, but there was a tight knot of emotions that would have to be picked apart at another time.

She returned to the recent exhilaration of the successful mission. So Ddwng had programmed it to succeed; so it still had been fun. He had used her in a harmless way to justify his change of policy.

But something nagged, and her morbid aspect kept trying to sniff it out. She had never been one to accept things without question, especially when they were nice. She was always alert for the worm in the apple, and she liked to fathom the whole worm. Which reminded her of two things: the question about what it was better to find in an apple one was eating; a whole worm or half a worm? Where was the other half of the worm? She had made a friend sick at lunch with that one, once. The other thing was a bit of verse her grandmother had told her once, and Colene's beady little mental eye for the grotesque had fixed on it instantly. The verse was about a college professor who tended to transpose the first letters of words when he got excited. Once he had the unpleasant task of informing a prominent woman that she had taken the wrong pew in church: 'Mardon me, Padam, but you are spitting in the wrong stew. Please let me sew you to another sheet.' But the one about the worm was what Colene was after now. The

Prof was bawling out a bad student. 'You have hissed three of my mystery lectures. In fact you have tasted the whole worm!' Well, when the worm was some subtle flaw in a person's understanding, it was indeed better to taste the whole thing.

Why had Ddwng used her for this task? Surely he could have used any beautiful, stupid Consort for this purpose. The answer was reasonably plain: he was studying Colene, because if she were crazy underneath, and it was a genetic defect, he didn't want those genes in the DoOon gene-pool. But if he were studying her, did it make sense to turn her loose unsupervised? Surely he would want to have his machines taking her stats all the time, especially when she thought she was unobserved.

So had Rrllo been lying to her when he said he wouldn't report on her indiscretion? No, because Seqiro had found the man true. But why should Rrllo report? He was just another actor in the play. There would be a monitor on Colene, maybe one Rrllo didn't know about, so Seqiro couldn't get it from his mind.

But there couldn't be a camera following her around! So how could it be done?

'Will there be anything else?' Mare inquired, having completed the rubdown. She spoke through the translation ball, as always.

'No thanks,' Colene replied automatically. 'I'll just lie here and sag for a while.'

Mare let her be. Then an almost tangible light bulb flashed. The translation ball! She had worn a special one at the planet. That was the recorder.

So Ddwng knew what she had said, including the bit about lobotomy. He would know that no one had mentioned this to her. So he would have a direct question to ask her, and if she didn't have a direct answer, she might face that lobotomy sooner than she had figured. That would ruin her plan for escape, not to mention her life.

Oh sweet Jesus! she thought. *How am I going to get out of this one?*

You will have to deceive him with a half-truth, Seqiro replied.

She realized it was true. She couldn't tell Ddwng about

301

Seqiro; that would ruin everything and get the horse destroyed. She couldn't claim it was a lucky guess; he would never buy that.

She mulled it over, and finally came to something she hoped would work.

Sure enough, on the way back to Earth Ddwng had dinner with her, and after the amenities he put it to her directly. 'You surprised me, Colene. I may have underestimated you. How did you know about the lobotomy?'

'I'm telepathic,' she replied without hesitation. That was the half-lie, flat out.

He gazed at her. 'We regard such claims as without substance.'

'Yes. That's why you had so much trouble with the monster of Yils. You just couldn't believe it was possible to stun someone by pure mental force.'

'Darius is telepathic too?'

'Not exactly. He can receive and rebroadcast emotion, without being affected. He's more like a catalyst. So the monster couldn't mindblast him. As you suspected.'

'You are evidently well matched to Darius.'

'I evidently am. His mind, my mind – I think it's going to be fun, when we finally get together and explore the interactions.'

'What am I thinking now?'

She shook her head. 'It's not that simple, Ddwng. It's not like watching a program on the wall. Your mind is all guarded and complicated. You have to be unguarded and have a very strong thought, and even then I don't necessarily get it. The lobotomy was so strong, and related to me so directly, that I picked it up. It was when we were eating, and you told me the three things you wanted of me – to be your Consort, and such. I thought it was sex, but it was lobotomy. After that I decided to agree to your three things. You didn't wonder what changed my mind?'

'I did wonder.'

He is concluding that it is true.

'Well, now you know. The only other thing I got was about

302

genetics, but that wasn't clear. What do genetics have to do with me?'

Now he believes he knows what you have been hiding from him. Your knowledge of some of his plans.

'Our gene pool is too limited. We have achieved perfect health and uniformity, but along with the liabilities of genetic diversity, we eliminated some of the strengths. You may have genes we can use.'

'So you're going to breed me like an animal –' she broke off, fixing him with a carefully rehearsed stare. 'Surgery! *You intend to take my ovaries!*'

'So you did receive that thought.'

'How could I miss it! You monster! You told me that you would let us go if we got you the Chip!'

Ddwng lifted his hands in a gesture of conciliation. 'I will do that. If we achieve the other realities, there will be many gene sources, and you will be superfluous. It is only if we fail that we shall have to take whatever offers.'

'Don't take this personally, Ddwng, but sometimes you remind me of a slimy tapeworm. You don't care whose guts you destroy, so long as you get yours.'

He smiled. 'I see we understand each other.'

And it seemed that her ploy had worked. She had shown the correct amount of perception and outrage, and he believed that she could read his mind – in sometime glimpses. He would probably stay clear of her now. But she would have to watch her step most carefully from here on, if she expected to survive and to save her friends. This was no part-time hood she was facing off; Ddwng was deadly dangerous.

They traveled back to Earth, which was a great relief. This super-science stuff was all right, but Colene felt most comfortable with Earth, even in its multiple alternate realities. The five anchors of the Virtual Mode seemed to be on Earth, so that all the anchor folk were human or familiar animal, though the underlying rules of the universe might shift. If Darius made it back, and they set foot on the Virtual Mode, and if her plan worked – but she refused even to think of that, lest she somehow give it away. She could afford to make no more mistakes.

The first thing she did on Earth was hold communion with Seqiro. Now she knew better than to vocalize or subvocalize; pure thought was the only way, and that with circumspection, so that there was no outward hint about where her mind really was. In fact, she made sure to have something doing to account for her emotional reactions, as a cover. In this case another violent entertainment program. DoOon tastes seemed to be similar to lowbrow American, which didn't say much for their improved genetics.

Seqiro! I'm so glad to be close to you again!

It is wonderful, he agreed. His thought came in far more clearly, now that they were close.

It was like a bad connection, there in the region of Kyvrn. I could barely receive you.

Receive me? There was no contact there.

She was startled. *But there was! You gave me key readings on the reactions of others. I needed those.*

We lost contact when you left Earth. I reverted to unintelligent animal level. I am restored only now, with your contact.

Something was wrong. *But I read you!*

There was no contact between us. The conviction was absolute.

All that key support from him – had been only her imagination? Then how had she picked up the attitudes of Rrllo? *You mean – I really did read a mind myself?*

This seems to have been the case. You have been learning from me during our contact, gaining some of my mental ability just as I gain some of yours.

So her half-truth had been a three-quarter truth! An awesome new horizon was opening to her.

Colene gazed at the stupid program on the wall, her mind reeling. What a development *this* was!

12

DECISION

Darius watched the constellation which included Earth's sun approach with mixed feelings. He had accomplished his mission and agreed to give the Emperor the Chip. His choice had been between Colene and the welfare of the other realities. He had chosen selfishly. He was not proud. But it was done, and now he would carry through.

It was the ninth day of their residence in this Mode. Tomorrow was Ddwng's deadline, and their probable venture back into the Virtual Mode. Darius knew the way back to his own Mode. What would happen there? He would have to see Ddwng safely there, and ask the Cyng of Pwer to give the man the Chip. Then what? Would Pwer do it?

Darius feared he would. Because Ddwng would bring a pain dial and use it on him. If that did not work in that Mode, something else would. Ddwng was a hard man.

'You are pensive,' Pussy said via the translation ball. 'How may I make you feel better?'

'I fear there is no way.'

This time she did not offer him sex or a massage. Only her unadorned sympathy. That turned out to be about as effective as anything.

All too soon they were there. The FTL *Flay* took up orbit around Earth, and made ready for the exchange of captains. 'It has been a pleasure to serve you, sir,' Jjle said formally.

'You made it easy,' Darius said. 'I hope you have pleasure

305

in the next mission.' Then he bid parting to his Felines, shaking hands with Tom and Cat and kissing Pussy. 'There were aspects of my mission I did not appreciate. But you were a delight. I am sorry to leave you.'

They did not respond, for he had neither questioned them nor given them a directive. He knew that they would serve the next captain as loyally as they had him, if the man did not have his own set of nulls. Sentimentality was wasted here. Nevertheless, he felt it.

Then he saw a tear in Pussy's eye. That heartened him. Her emotion was surely transient, but it was there.

He stepped into the transporter cubicle with Provos, and out again in the Emperor's palace on Earth. An Ovine neuter was there to guide them to their chamber for the night.

But when he got there, he discovered that it was occupied. There were three Equines, looking very much like his Felines but with their heads shaped to suggest those of horses. They evidently came with the suite.

Then he remembered something. Colene was served by Equines. Could it be?

'Whom do you serve?' he asked the neuter, who would be Horse.

'We serve Colene, who has directed us to make you comfortable until she returns.'

This seemed too good to be true. Ddwng was allowing them to be together? 'Where is she now?'

'Dining with the Emperor, as she normally does.'

Was Ddwng taking more of an interest in Colene than business? Darius felt a tinge of jealousy, but a larger tinge of satisfaction. Colene knew her own mind, once she made it up, and she wouldn't hesitate to use any influence she had. She would have more influence on Ddwng than the Emperor realized, if he wasn't careful, and she would use it to make him do what she wanted. She wanted to return to the Virtual Mode and travel with him, Darius. He was sure of this.

Maybe she had even used that influence to prevail on Ddwng to let the two of them be together this night. She could have hinted that she would make sure that Darius did not change his mind about giving Ddwng the Chip. Ddwng also might suppose that there would be key dialogue between them, which his sensors would pick up, which would reveal any potential treachery.

Well, there would be no treachery. Darius had given his word, and he would honor it. Maybe Colene expected him to do something foolish or deceitful, but he would not. He was betraying the realities, but not his nature. He hoped Colene would never know why.

What, then, was he to do this night? He did not want to be close to her before they could discuss things and come to some understanding, and he had no intention of discussing anything with her in this Mode.

'Please show us to our separate chambers,' Provos said to the nulls. 'We shall eat after we are established.'

There was the answer. Provos remembered what was to happen.

Mare showed Provos to one chamber, and Stallion showed Darius to another. He saw that a bed had been set up; they were ready for the guests. He used the toilet chamber, checked himself in the mirror, and returned to the main chamber.

Horse had already set up the table with the meal of the day. Provos reappeared, and they sat down opposite each other, as they had regularly while on the ship. Darius hardly noticed what he ate, being preoccupied by his thoughts.

They were, oddly, not of Colene at the moment, but of Provos. He had traveled for some time with this odd woman, and still hardly knew her. She had seldom spoken to him recently, maintaining her disapproval of his decision. He hardly faulted her for that; he did not like it himself. But would she have let Colene be destroyed?

Well, her memory of the future was surely short, now, because she could not remember across realities, and tomorrow they would resume those crossings. He could only hope that some agency other than his own prevented Ddwng from getting what he wanted.

Stallion departed. 'He is going to fetch Colene; it is time,' Horse explained. Like Cat, the neuter was the intelligent one. Darius nodded.

Colene returned. She was an absolute vision of beauty, in a

pale blue gown and diadem. Darius caught his breath, unable to speak. He had never seen her like this!

Her gaze fixed immediately on him. Of course she was not surprised; she had known he was coming. 'What, no Pussy?' she inquired with mock wonder. He noted with odd surprise that her words came from her rather than from the translation ball. 'Take Mare for the night.'

'I would be with her as I was with you,' he said with hurt dignity. 'But without the love.'

She looked at him for a moment more. Then her face crumpled. 'Oh, Darius, I'm sorry!' she cried, and flung herself at him. He barely had time to rise from his chair before she collided, bearing him back against the wall. 'I love you, I love you, I love you!' she wailed through her tears, into his shoulder, destroying the careful makeup Mare must have applied.

He wrestled her around until her head came up. Then he kissed her. 'I love you,' he said.

'I would do anything just to be with you!'

'Yes.' That was what they had done, betraying the realities.

'Please – be with me tonight.'

He tried to say no, and could not. His separate chamber would not be used.

But when they were together, he remembered how young she was. In his culture a woman was old enough when her body indicated she was ready, and by that token Colene was legitimate. But in hers there was a set age of consent, and she was below it. They were not in her Mode now, but her values were of it, and it would be wrong to presume on her innocence. What could she know of the reality of sexual indulgence, however pleasurable it might be?

Also, he knew that everything they did was being watched and recorded; the walls were eyes. He had no shame in sexual expression, but with Colene, with love, the first time, there should be privacy. He could not explain this to her, because she did not know the true ways of the DoOon.

Meanwhile she stripped naked for him. He demurred. 'Not yet,' he said. He also refused to take her as a gift from Ddwng.

When this terrible business was done, and they were safely in his Mode, then it would be all right.

'And what of Pussy?' she demanded with mercurial temper.

'I will be with you as I was with her.' He embraced her, and did nothing more, though his desire was manifest.

'Damn you!' she whispered.

'I will not say it would not have been otherwise, had you not appeared when you did,' he confessed. 'After that, I thought only of you.'

She lifted her head. 'Really? You really didn't do it? Because of me?'

'Yes.'

She paused a moment, as if listening to a distant voice. 'Yes, it really was that way, wasn't it! I am so sorry I doubted. Well, it's me now.'

'Yes. That is enough.'

'It's enough,' she agreed. 'Well, almost; you were naked with her. So get naked with me.'

Darius sighed, not annoyed, and removed his own clothing. His body was aroused, and he did not try to conceal this from her. She wanted to know whether he desired her, and this was answer enough. But his desire was matched by his discipline.

Colene gazed at him with evident satisfaction. Then she planted herself against him, her breasts and thighs pressing close.

He knew what she was doing. The little vixen was tempting him, as she had before, but more directly. Well, she could excite him, but she could not make him forget his resolve. He closed his arms around her and stroked her sleek back, and did no more. He was perversely glad she was doing this, because it was her way.

So it was that they slept, embraced, remaining chaste in their fashion, as they had when in her Mode. The odd thing was that she seemed pleased rather than rejected. Why would she offer her body to a man and be happy when he seemed to lack the gumption to use it?

*   *   *

Next day they gathered in the chamber of the palace where the anchor was. Colene stood beside her huge stallion, whom she had named Seqiro, her hand on his nose to guide him. Darius was becoming increasingly curious about that animal, who seemed to be more than ordinary, but he would not inquire where Ddwng could listen, which meant anywhere in this Mode. Provos was as usual impassive.

Ddwng was something else. The man was solidly garbed in an all-terrain suit with many full pockets and assorted devices whose purposes were obscure. He used a personal shield, which didn't show but made him impossible to touch with any velocity, and carried a special pain dial. 'So that we may best understand each other,' he said, 'I shall make a small demonstration.' He touched the dial, and the pain coursed through Darius, at about the second level. He saw Colene stiffen, and Provos, and even the horse twitched his skin as if flies were stinging it. It was tuned to them all.

Ddwng touched the dial again, and the pain abated. 'I believe this will operate throughout the Virtual Mode, as will my shield. I trust Darius, but I do not trust the rest of you, or the horse who is responsive to Colene. Should anything happen to me, the dial will automatically lock on maximum. It will respond only to me.'

'You made your point,' Colene said. 'You don't trust us, but you have promised to let us go once you have the Chip.'

Ddwng nodded. 'Once I have the Chip.'

Darius doubted that the pain dial would be effective across the boundaries, but that didn't matter. It was his word which bound him, not any threat to his body.

'You understand,' Darius said, 'that you and the anchor are linked. You will be able to consume only food you carry with you from the anchor Mode; other food will do you no good. You will not be able to transport any object or substance that is part of a foreign Mode across the boundaries of the Modes, and anything from your Mode that you leave behind will remain in the Mode where you set it. So you must have all the supplies you will require for a journey of several days.'

'I discovered these things when I laid out the paths,' Ddwng said. 'I used machines to facilitate my work, but I had to be in contact with those machines at all times or they would not cross the boundaries. I could not assign the work to any other person, or to a robot.'

'Robot?'

'Computerized machine,' Colene put in. 'Golem, to you.'

'Yes, I thought you understood,' Darius said to Ddwng. 'But I have undertaken to guide you safely to my Mode, and I need to be sure you understand the nature of the inherent threats to you. You must also be cautious about stepping across the boundaries in some sections; there may be rough terrain, or predators, or traps set. We shall have to proceed extremely cautiously when approaching the pit, the region of several realities that has been mined. We can not cross it safely, but we should be able to go around it. So if I tell you to do something, do not take offense; it may be an emergency.'

'I am a realist,' Ddwng said. 'You are the leader for this excursion.'

'One other thing you need to know, in case we become separated: how to tune in on the most direct path. Since anyone who gets isolated from the group will have no way but this to rejoin the group, by converging on a common destiny, we all must be able to do it.' Darius glanced at Colene, realizing something. 'The horse – he is from another anchor? He can cross boundaries without having to be in contact with you? You will nevertheless have to guide him, and not let him get lost.'

'Yes, I won't let Seqiro get lost,' Colene agreed. 'And warn me long before we step into any pit! I don't want to have to haul him out!'

Even Ddwng smiled briefly. 'I wondered whether you would raise this matter. It was evident that none of you were traveling randomly. How do I tune in? I was aware of no path before; I laid out my paths only geometrically, to intercept those who crossed the blank realities. This is not a physical thing?'

'It is a mental thing,' Darius said. 'In your Mode you do not employ magical or mental mechanisms. Magic simply does not operate; I experimented and verified this. I assumed that the same applied to the mental component, but discovered that it did not. The monster was simply a human child with a

311

freak mental talent. It may be that your people have had this ability bred out of them, but that they can recover it with effort and training.'

'We shall try to broaden our gene pool with this in mind,' Ddwng said.

Darius knew how serious that was. Had it not been for that reproductive threat against Colene, his decision might have been different. 'So for your own security, you need to be able to use your mind this way. You need to be able to feel the route. I'm not sure how you can do this, except by trying to blank your mind to other things, until you develop a subtle awareness of direction.'

Ddwng considered. 'And if I can not?'

Darius shrugged. 'You will be dependent on the rest of us to guide you. Should I suffer an accident, Provos or Colene can continue.'

Ddwng glanced at the other two. Provos seemed uninterested; her future was blank at the moment. Colene was leaning against her horse, also seeming unconcerned, which probably meant the opposite. 'I prefer to master this now.'

'That could take forever!' Colene protested. 'Why don't you practice it on the way?'

That only set Ddwng more firmly. 'We shall wait here until I succeed.'

Colene made a face. 'Suit yourself, Emperor.'

Ddwng stood at the anchor and closed his eyes. 'Nothing,' he reported after a moment.

'You are used to making demands which others must receive,' Darius said. 'For this you need to be receptive. I am not sure how to guide you in this. Perhaps it would be better to wait –'

'I may be getting it,' Ddwng said. 'Something very faint, a distant thought – a strong thought. I –'

He looked surprised. Then the universe turned.

Not quite literally. The land seemed to tilt, yet it was level. But the palace chamber tilted, sinking down, and Ddwng with it, while the rest of them remained as they were. The Emperor looked surprised but helpless to stop it.

Provos lurched into Darius, bearing him back toward Colene and the horse. *Hold on!*

He grabbed on to the harness on the horse's body. The horse was a comfortingly stable object right now, while the rest of everything slowly went skew. Ddwng and his chamber sank all the way out of sight, and another floor or ground level descended. This level was a tree-filled landscape. Its trees tilted with it, seeming unaffected.

Darius stared, his eyes unfocused. The forest was passing through the plane the three of them and the horse stood on, but there was no physical contact. Above it came a setting of lesser plants and shrubs, no trees. That entire setting swung through undisturbed.

Another scene swung down. This was a barren desert similar to the one they had crossed coming to this anchor. What was happening?

Ddwng freed his anchor.

It was not a voice but a thought. It felt like Colene.

The desert swung down, gaining velocity. Another desert replaced it, and another.

He tried to speak, but somehow could not. There was no air, but he was not gasping. He seemed to be in suspended animation, though he could move. Anchor? Ddwng wouldn't do that!

Seqiro took over his mind and made him decide to free the anchor.

The horse? Darius stared at the more rapidly moving scenes, which were now sliding through at a blurring rate.

Seqiro is telepathic. He has linked us. I didn't tell you before, because we had to fool Ddwng. We caught him by surprise when he opened his mind, and before he knew it he had freed the anchor, and he's gone. Now we have to find another, so he can't connect up again.

A telepathic horse? Darius had never suspected such a thing! A thought from outside had made the Emperor do what only he could do, and release his anchor, cutting his Mode free of the Virtual Mode? Darius had honestly intended to deliver on his commitment to Ddwng, despite his detestation of the necessity. But now, astonishingly –

313

Yes. It was the only way. I planned it, but I couldn't tell you or anyone. Seqiro tuned in on your mind, so I know how you love me. He says you have a marvelously straightforward and honest mind, no trouble at all to relate to. It was wonderful sleeping in your love last night. But I couldn't tell you, because –

Because he would not have broken his word to Ddwng. Colene had intended all along to do this. Yet she had pleaded with him to cooperate with Ddwng!

I lied. To fool Ddwng.

She had lied – to them all.

I had to do it! It was the only way!

She had practiced deliberate deception. She had broken her given word. In the process she had rendered his pledge void.

Oh-oh.

How could he love a dishonest woman?

The chaos turning around them shifted its nature. There was sound, now, as if the Modes themselves were humming. It was music, but neither pleasant nor innocent.

The passing Modes were forming a new pattern in their larger perspective. Instead of resembling some changing Earthly landscape, with mountains lifting and sinking like ragged waves, they became geometrical. Three dimensional crystalline outlines formed, changing their configurations in odd ways. Lines and balls passed through, strung in endless spirals. Light flared in divergent colors, each color inconstant, becoming a nucleus for lesser flares, and lesser yet, and on. Well defined shapes became cloudy, dissolving into other well defined shapes; the cloudiness was only in the inability of the observer to fathom the nuances.

Fractals! It was Colene's amazed realization.

There came a shape like a hairy bug, growing rapidly larger, with fire playing about its fringe. Within that fire loomed expanding curlicues, and within them spiderweb-like structures linked to each other by smaller webs, and within those patterns forming seeming tunnels to infinity.

The change was slowing, as if the final orientation was coming into alignment. The new anchor was being set.

Then the whirling Modes abruptly firmed. They came to a sudden stop, with no physical impact. It was as if the Mode

314

on which the four of them stood had been still, and the rest of all the universes had stopped their motion.

They stood at the verge of a strange stone cliff overlooking a heaving sea. Into the face of the cliff were set two enormous red roses. Before them was a young woman in a red dress. A stiff sea breeze was blowing her thick black hair to the side. Beyond her was a green valley, and beyond that a hill on which perched a stone castle.

The weird music was stronger now, not loud but penetrating to the gray matter of their bones and the marrow of their minds.

The girl seemed as startled to see them as they were to see her. Darius knew that they had just connected with a new anchor Mode, and that she was the anchor person. But the young woman had no prior experience with Virtual Modes. To her, the three of them and the horse had just appeared from nowhere.

She is Nona, Colene's thought came. *Hello, Nona. We are friends.*

Darius hoped that was the case.

AUTHOR'S NOTE

Now don't get mad at me. This is the first novel of the Mode series, and there's no concealing the fact that there is a whole lot more to go. This is a complete episode, introducing the concept of the Virtual Mode and the major characters. The next novel, *Fractal Mode*, will follow in about a year, featuring Colene, Darius, Provos, Seqiro and Nona in a setting that is not exactly our own. Let's face it: Colene and Darius hardly know each other, and it would be unrealistic to think that they could just get together and live happily forever after. There are real problems for them to work out, and their love is really infatuation. She has a score to settle with him about his sexual attitude, and he has one to settle with her about her lack of integrity. Promising relationships have been known to founder on just such issues. This process will not be simplified by the presence of another attractive young woman as an anchor-figure. And what of those who made the Chips, and isolated the DoOon? With each novel, an anchor figure will be lost, and a new one gained, with the new Virtual Mode. If you object to this sort of complication, don't buy the sequels; the series will languish without your support, and shut down in due course. Oh, it hurts to lose your favor!

I had three fantasy series going, and a collaborative fantasy series. Two are being shut down now, and a third in another year. Only Xanth will continue, and Mode will join it, inheriting aspects of the Adept and Incarnations series. It's

316

not that I don't like fantasy, but that each series has its natural cycle, and the cycles of some are longer than others. You may wonder about my reference to fantasy, as there was little fantasy in *Virtual Mode*. Well, this is to be an anything-goes project, and *Fractal Mode* will have a good deal more magic. It all depends on the Mode, you see. So this may be referred to as a fantasy series, though that pinches its definition. It's an imaginative series which does not shy away from realism, as you may have noticed.

It is also an Author's Note series; readers of my Incarnations series will have a notion what to expect: that slice of my life occurring during the writing of this novel, complete with discussions of social issues and unfinished thoughts. Reaction to such Notes has been fairly neatly polarized, with the critics ranging from grudging acceptance to deep disgust, and the readers ranging from interested to enthusiastic. The most common comment is that the Notes make the author real for the reader. As one reader put it, approximately: I make my characters live; the Notes make *me* live.

So what happened in the three months of this writing? A slew of things, professional, personal and in between. I started in mid Dismember and finished in Marsh – and in this period I learned that the 1990 Xanth Calendar from which these months are borrowed sold well enough to leave me with a probable 50% loss of the money I invested in it. Apparently the publisher underprinted, so that many stores never got it, and many sold out and could not get new stock. I even received a letter from a reader with a wonderful idea: why didn't I do a Xanth Calendar? So much for getting the news spread! I did the Calendar for love rather than money, and feel the artists did a fine job, and there will be similar calendars following, but an ongoing losing proposition can not endure indefinitely. Sigh.

We had an extremely mild winter – possibly the warmest Jamboree and FeBlueberry since American records began, which is a bad sign considering the question of the global warming trend. But just before Christmas Florida was hit by one of its worst cold waves. We live in the middle of a tree farm on a peninsula in Lake Tsoda Popka, and our climate

317

is moderate compared to that of the region, which is mild enough. But our thermometer dropped to 16°F, and we had a light snow flurry – the first I've seen personally in thirty years in the state – and most of our decorative plants died. We had been given a set of poinsettias by our American publisher the year before, and we planted them and they grow very nicely and were just starting to turn their top leaves from green to red in the style of that plant, when the freeze destroyed them. Sigh.

And the mail. I answered 166 letters in Dismember, 160 in Jamboree, and 205 in FeBlueberry. I had tried using a secretary for a year and a half, but discovered that I wasn't cut out for dictating letters; I'm a lot less intelligent and literate when I speak than I am when I write, perhaps because I can revise what I write when I see it on the screen. I hated seeing the stupid words I spoke go out. So finally I returned to typing them myself, and my wife did the filing. I found that I could take two days off a week and do up to fifty letters that way, and that sufficed. The other five days I had to write my novels, trying for 3,000 words of novel text a day, in addition to perhaps 2,000 words of related and unrelated notes. I use my 'Bracket' system, you see: whenever the going gets difficult in the novel, which may be every few minutes, I go to my notes file and enter a dialogue with myself, exploring the problem and possible solutions, until I work it out. Many a week I didn't make my target, because there is more to a writer's life than text and correspondence – phone calls to/from agents, business associates, relatives and fans also take time – and sometimes I try to sneak in a little leisure with my family. I feel properly guilty when I do that, but it happens. In this period I received a package of letters from one publisher dating back as far as nine months. I answered them immediately, but some did come back for want of a current address. I hate that.

I see a parallel between Darius' situation as Cyng of Hlahtar and my own with respect to my readers: publishing my books multiplies the joy I bring to others, but fan mail depletes my resources. I can not keep answering indefinitely. One fan pointed out that I won't be able to cut down on letters as long as I keep writing Author's Notes, because the notes make me

318

seem like a person and a person can be written to. But somehow I don't want to feel less like a person. So I struggle along, my responses getting later and briefer, knowing that this, like the Xanth Calendar, is probably doomed to extinction in due course.

There are limits, however. On FeBlueberry 26 I received three separate solicitations for fund-raising auctions. Each wanted me to contribute an autographed book of mine, or some other item they might sell to raise money for their worthy purposes. Now at first glance this seems reasonable, but I have been on the receiving end of so many such solicitations that my perception has shifted. My objection is based on two main factors. First, the cost to me, considering the value of my time expended in preparing, packaging and mailing an item, is probably substantially more than it will sell for at the other end. Thus it is a losing game, overall; if I wanted to contribute, it would be cheaper for me to send a check. Second, while stocking libraries and such is good, I feel the cost ought to be borne by the community that library serves, rather than folk like me, who will never see it. Such solicitations in their essence boil down to transferring the cost to strangers. I once received a letter from a young man who had decided to become a millionaire by soliciting money from every address he could get; the principle is the same. So a library is a more worthy cause than a greedy person; that simply suggests that the end justifies the means. I feel the means is unjustified, and I oppose it on principle. At first I did contribute to such efforts, until I had a request for copies of every one of my titles, plus manuscripts and magazines, to be shipped overseas at my expense. Thereafter I wrote letters explaining why I did not. This day I decided to stop responding to them at all. Call me ungenerous if you will. The line has to be drawn somewhere.

What kind of fan mail do I get? Mostly compliments on my novels (thanks), requests for pictures (I ran out long ago), and suggestions for future writing (but I have plenty of my own ideas). But some are different. One letter in Dismember was from a woman who had not read my books, but she informed me that I was ignorant and sarcastic. Why? Because her friend had asked me how I really felt about fan mail, and I replied that I'd rather be writing my novel. I responded to her politely, inquiring how she would feel if *she* had to answer up to 160 letters a month which squeezed out all her free time and some of her working time at her own expense, and someone asked how she felt about it, and she said candidly that she'd rather have more time to herself, and that person then called her ignorant and sarcastic? I received no response. Well, that's one way to cut down on mail. God preserve us from the self-righteous.

Another was from a woman who had read the rape scene in *Unicorn Point* and declared herself an ex-Anthony reader. I replied that I was sorry to lose her, but that when a person does something another person deems unconscionable, the latter has little choice but to withdraw support. I mentioned that I had just done something similar myself. Oh, you want to hear about that? Well hang on; this is a major discussion.

More than a year back I heard from a prisoner who had murdered his girlfriend. It was a brutal and to my mind pointless crime for which he was condemned to death. He was politically conservative and believed in the death penalty. His quarrel with the system was that his lawyer kept making appeals on his behalf which he didn't want. He had committed the crime and deserved to die for it, and he was frustrated by the continual delays.

Now I am politically liberal, and I don't like the death penalty. That does not mean I like murder. I don't like killing, whether it is done by private enterprise or the state. I don't like killing animals either, which is why I am a vegetarian. No need to belabor my philosophy here; you are welcome to read all about me in my autobiography, *Bio of an Ogre*, and if your local bookstore doesn't carry it, don't kill the proprietor, just reason sweetly with him. As Ferrovius reasoned all night with a pagan, in G. B. Shaw's *Androcles and the Lion*, and in the morning not only was the man a Christian, his hair was as white as snow. The pacifistic approach can work wonders when practiced by ogres. I'm sure your store will agree to stock the book. But I try to answer my mail without regard to the nature of the letter writer (well, junk mail gets checked and thrown away), and so I answered the murderer's letters. I made no bones about my sympathy for the victim of his crime, and agreed that he had a right to insist that he pay the penalty in his fashion. You see, I believe in the right to life, and also in the right to death, so I support legislation to allow patients to say no to heroic measures used to prolong their lives in the face of terminal maladies. Note that I do not say that all killing is wrong, just that I don't like it. Absolutes are hard to come by, for those of liberal persuasion, and truth does generally seem to be a shade of gray.

Well, the murderer wrote again, and I answered, and it continued. Sometimes I will cut off a too-persistent correspondent, because I really do have other things to do than to engage in frivolous dialogue, but this person's letters were serious and well thought out. It turned out that I was the only one who did keep up with him; his friends and family did not. He assumed it was because I cared for him. No, I was simply being true to my standard. But as long as the correspondence continued, I thought I might as well learn something useful, such as why would a man murder a woman who by his own account was true to him and wanted nothing but good for him? Men murder women every day; is it just their way of proving how macho they are, or do they do it to prevent the women from moving on to other men? If we could only fathom a common underlying motive, and discover how to debate the situation before an innocent person gets killed, we might spare the world much grief. In this case there turned out to be no simple answer.

The murderer expressed interest in science fiction and supernatural phenomena, such as flying saucers. That sparked a notion. I suggested that he write to a fanzine: that is, one of the amateur magazines of the genre where pros and fans exchange remarks in the letter columns. I gave him information on the best one I knew, considering its frequency of publication, the variety of interests of its contributors, and its open-forum philosophy. I had been writing to it for years, taking on its hard core conservatives. I had addressed the feminists: 'I am a man. I like looking at women. That does not make me a sexist.' Indeed, I support much of the feminist agenda, and I value the company and input of women. I suspect I receive more fan letters from women than most writers of this genre, and I often have female protagonists who are sympathetically portrayed, as you may have seen in this novel. I also took on reviewers: I believe that a reviewer should indicate how well a book relates to the needs or desires of its readers, rather than pushing a private agenda. Gun control – I favor it, though the case is not clear-cut. Minimum wage – I favor raising it to keep pace with inflation. Affirmative action – I favor it, not as ideal, but the only practical way to redress a long-standing wrong. In fact, if you run your finger down the classic liberal agenda – or, if you are conservative, poke your finger up at it – you will find me there most of the time. One major exception is abortion; I don't like it because of my objection to killing. But I don't like the anti-abortionists either, because they seem to have little regard for the welfare of mother or baby and generally don't seem to support the obvious method of not having babies: contraception. I took on all comers in this fanzine, being one of two blatantly liberal writers to do so, and as I see it, we showed up the conservatives as ignorant and mean-spirited clods. But fairness requires that I admit that the conservatives didn't necessarily see it that way. One had a sense of humor about it: when I chided him for making sense on one issue, when I depended on him to be always wrong, he replied that it wasn't his intent to make sense. It is possible for folk to disagree and still respect each other. So I thought it would be interesting if the murderer stated his case here, and let the cynics and conservatives argue his case with him. Is the death penalty a deterrent to crime, when a murderer wants to be executed and the system won't oblige? Just why does a person commit murder? Maybe such a discussion would elicit truths which would enable society to deal more realistically with crime. Such a dialogue would also give the murderer some social interaction in a limited environment, which could be a positive thing. I'm generally interested in beating swords into plowshares, philosophically.

He was hesitant, but he did write to the fanzine. The fanzine editors were hesitant, but did publish his letter. The dialogue began. He made it a point to respond to all challenges or questions directed at him, and he made no apologies for his crime; he wanted truth, not sympathy. But once he had honestly addressed the matter, he wanted to get into other subjects of mutual interest. He wrote a positive letter – and the editors refused to run it.

They explained that they had gone to a convention, and several unnamed parties had approached them and expressed dismay at the murderer's presence in the fanzine. So they cut him out, not for anything he said, but because of essentially anonymous objections to his presence. They said they did this to be fair to those hidden folk, and that they had a right to choose who would appear in their fanzine.

Well, they did have that right. But I also had the right to withdraw my support from what I deemed to be invidious editing. I sent one letter putting my position on the line, and when they did not change their policy, I did not write again. Naturally that left me open to charges that I was a bad sport, and there were a number of insults directed at me. Another pro writer wrote in my defense, protesting the 'pre-emptive smear' and upholding the principle of free speech. In fact the 'make no sense' conservative also wrote a stirring objection to their censorship. I could almost get to like conservatives like that. But the editors were adamant about their policy and about my supposed bad nature, accusing me of attacking another contributor and of calling names. Their basis for this was my suggestion that needless cruelty to animals is an early sign of sociopathic behavior, in response to the other's seeming pride in squishing spiders. Readers may remember Jumper, the spider character in *Castle Roogna*. You don't see the Disney folk sit on their hands when someone disparages the Mouse; well . . .

I can't say I was happy to go. I had enjoyed slugging it out with those of differing opinion, and the interactions had been by no means predominantly negative. I had trouble sleeping several nights, upset about the business. But the principle of freedom of expression is fundamental, and I simply could not allow so egregious a violation to pass. It is in the extremes that our philosophies are tested, and those of us who are serious do not set aside our ethics merely because in some cases they become inconvenient or distasteful. Does a murderer have rights too? Yes, even the worst among us must be granted their right to speak. Imagine applying the editors' logic to other cases: anonymous folk approach a city councilman, saying they don't like the presence of blacks in their neighborhood, so in fairness to them he sets up apartheid. Anonymous businessmen approach a congressman, saying they don't like foreign competition, so in fairness to them he introduces a bill to ban all imports. Anonymous fundamentalists dislike certain elements of the Catholic Church, so they have the government ban Catholicism in the name of fairness. Does that seem far-fetched? There are regions where exactly such things have happened. But in America most of us disapprove of them. We believe in freedom of expression, even for those we don't like. It is part of our Constitution.

How did the murderer react to this exclusion? He apologized for causing the magazine this trouble and asked that his subscription money be used to purchase some tapes he liked, and the balance donated for useful purposes. To my mind he acquitted himself in a more honorable manner than those editors did. I continued the correspondence with him. I believe I did come to understand the rationale for what he did, though I disagree with it. Because he spoke in confidence, I shall not describe it here, except to say that I believe it vindicates the liberal case for socially responsible activity as a preventive for disaster.

So yes, I do understand the principle of withdrawing support from an endeavor one has previously valued. Since I am as adamant about maintaining my freedom to incorporate any elements I choose in my fiction as those editors were about their prerogatives, I can only tell readers who object to such elements to go their own ways. The woman who objected to the rape scene was not abusive or anonymous; she stated her case politely and gave her address. So she received a polite response. I do not vilify those who stand on principle, and I tend to value those who do stand on an opposing principle more than those who agree with me while lacking principle. But lest there be any question: I do not approve of rape. I

324

merely defend my right to show rape onstage, as one of the evils of society.

So I departed that fanzine, disliking the smell. The editors are probably still wondering why professionals are so touchy. I had supported the publication with money, letters, and recommendations. I gave it one last item: my report on the convention where I had met Jenny, the girl paralyzed by a drunk driver, and that was it. I left not only because of what had been done, but because the editors were unwilling or unable to grasp why they were wrong. It marked the probable end of my active participation in fanzine fandom, because this had been one of the best fanzines. What are the worst like? Don't ask!

Ah yes, that brings up Jenny. She has been discussed more fully in the Xanth series, where she has become a character, and you may have met her as Jenny Elf in the graphic edition of *Isle of View*. For those who haven't, a compressed recap: in FeBlueberry of 1989 I received a letter telling me how a twelve year old girl had been struck by a drunk driver and almost killed, and had remained almost three months in a coma. I wrote to her, and my first letter did bring her out of the coma. I continued to write, though she remained paralyzed and mute and could not respond. Later I attended a convention in her area, so I could meet her. She was treated well there, and I believe she enjoyed herself, though she remained so weak that most of her time was spent lying on her back. That was the report I sent to the fanzine. The significance for this novel is that during this period we passed the anniversary of my first letter to her: one year. I have an artificial rose from her corsage beside my computer screen as I type this, a memento. It resembles the roses on the clifflike structure as the novel ends; there will be more on them in the next novel. In this period Jenny resumed going to school, but not the one she had attended before; this one is for folk like her, whose needs are special. She seems to like it.

And on to Ligeia. Ligeia is the name I gave to the first of a number of suicidal teenage girls I have heard from. All have the same name, to preserve their anonymity, because often their nature is a secret from their parents and I don't feel I have the right to betray their confidence. What have I to do with girls forty years my junior? The same as with prisoners: I answer my mail. But though I will not name them individually, I will do so collectively. This novel has considerable input from them, as you may have guessed. Colene represents a composite of these bright and tormented creatures. If you know a girl exactly like Colene, she is not any of my sources, because none is that close to her overall.

I am no expert on the subject of suicide, and I can't say I ever properly understood even my daughters when they were teenagers. In this day of the revelation of fathers who abuse their daughters, I have been hyper-conscious of the proprieties. When does a father stop playing with his little girl? Some it seems don't stop; they proceed into sexual molestation. But the other direction is not ideal either: isolation from one's children. We have been a close family, but I stopped physically touching my daughters early, and felt the gradual alienation. Would one of them tell me if she had a serious problem or felt suicidal? Maybe, and maybe not. I have always been there, and ready to help if asked, but they tend not to ask. I suffer the perhaps universal inadequacy of fathers. So I have had the nagging suspicion that the feelings expressed by the Ligeias, which they don't tell their parents, could also be felt by my daughters, and they wouldn't tell me. But mine have not been abused or neglected, and have suffered neither poverty nor family breakup. I hope that's enough. They are now going to college, and thence into the larger world. As has been said: a child is someone who passes through your life and disappears into an adult. Am I sublimating the distancing I regret in my own daughters by being more sensitive to these Ligeia girls? I don't know, but it is possible. I prefer to think that I am simply trying to do what is right, whatever the context.

The first Ligeia was deeply disturbed. She believed that there had never been love in her home, and she was isolated and hurting. Cautious, I put in an indirect query via the school system, to see whether she could be helped by private counseling there. The school counselor went straight to her parents, putting her into deeper trouble. So much for the sensitivity of the system; no wonder girls prefer to keep the secret. 'No one can be trusted,' a later Ligeia told me, and I had to agree. You see that attitude in Colene. First Ligeia One wrote to me; then she phoned me. She declared that she loved me, and was upset when I demurred. She wanted to talk for an hour or more at a time, and on subjects I balked at, such as sex. Call me conservative if you will, but I feel it is not the proper business of a man who is not a doctor or counselor to talk to a girl just about young enough to be his granddaughter about the specifics of sex. There is too much potential for abuse. When she started calling on consecutive days I had to put the brakes on, because she was sticking her family with horrendous phone bills and I was losing time from my work that was worth even more. In addition, my daughters were bothered. 'She's trying to take more of your attention than we are!' one protested with some accuracy. I set a limit: one hour cumulative per month; I would hang up on her if she overreached it. This was no easy thing, because this girl wasn't kidding about suicide; once she was cutting her wrists as she talked to me. There was more, but let me digest it down to this: in due course her folks seem to have put her in some kind of institution, and her outside contacts were abruptly cut off. I do not know whether she is alive today. In fact, I do not know whether any of them are alive, other than those now in contact with me, and I hesitate to inquire.

Perhaps my favorite was the first Ligeia Two, who was artistic and sensitive to her individuality. I think she could have made it professionally as an artist, and she wanted to pursue this career, but her folks had other plans for her. Later I saw the movie *Dead Poets' Society*, which hit home to me on several levels. I attended such a school, and later I taught English at such a school. But in this case I'm thinking of the young man portrayed there who wanted to be an actor, and could have made it, but his father refused, and he committed suicide. Parents can do terrible harm to their talented children that way. I tried to help her by putting her in touch with another person – and this went wrong, and she overdosed on pills. They caught her in time and I heard from her in the hospital, and not thereafter. I could have killed her, just by trying to help her. It is foolish to speak of such emotion in such a connection, but there was that in me that could have loved her. She was a sweet and sensitive girl. Had she been my daughter, her art would have been allowed to flourish.

Others wrote once or twice, and not thereafter. 'Why is life so unfair?' one asked. In that case I had confirmation from a relative of a deeply disturbed girl. But what I said to her was limited; I had become too conscious of the danger of doing harm myself, without meaning to. I stopped trying to keep track of them; I don't know how many there have been. Some women have written, and only later revealed their suicidal tendencies. Others have only skirted the notion, for reason: they had been abused, or raped, or otherwise devastated. There is a lot of grief out there, and only a fraction of it ever goes on record. A number told how they made it through to successful marriage and family. As a general rule, based on my observation, if they make it through their teens, they are probably all right. But it is never certain.

You may wonder whether some are just making it up, to get my attention. I don't think so. Some send me pieces they have written, or sketches they have made, and I think I am experienced enough as a writer and as an adult depressive to have a notion whether they are faking it. Some of this material horrifies me. Some is presented as fiction, but I know that a person that young would not write that kind of fiction or poetry if she didn't have a basis. The details are too real, the material rings true. They are not fooling about death. They are obsessed with it. I believe, I believe.

Why does it seem to be exclusively female? This is a matter of natural selection. There are suicidal boys, but a boy is likely to try to kill himself with a gun, while a girl is more apt to try it with pills or wrist slashing. The gun is more effective. I understand that twice as many girls try suicide as do boys, but that twice as many boys succeed as do girls. So the main reason I heard from relatively few suicidal boys may be that those who might have written were already dead. At least my own depression is mild. One might expect the author of funny fantasy to be light-hearted but professional comics may be quite otherwise privately, and my affinity may be closer to Colene and Ligeia than to the happy folk.

Now I have some credits for elements of this novel. All of them relate to the characterization of Colene, but to protect privacy I will not identify the actual items here. Some of the contributors may have felt suicidal at some time; some have not. Some are young; some are not. What they have in common is that they happened to mention things in letters which I asked to use. They can not in any other way be classified. I list them in alphabetical order by first name:

Amanda Wagner
Frances Wagner
Kimberly Adams
Ligeias – anonymous group
Margaret McGinnis
Yvonne Johnston

And a sketch titled 'Someday' sent by Oria Tripp: a young woman walking through shallow water toward distant mountains, her hair and dress blown out by the wind. She reminds me of Colene, and of the one to come in the next novel, Nona: girls with more hope than prospects. Then there's Emily Ivie, with a literary project: 'It is a waste of paper to speak of it.' Colene would have said that too. But not all the women I hear from are related to such things. Let me tell you about another kind.

Some years back I had one or two fan letters from a young woman in America, unremarkable. Then she sent me a newspaper clipping describing her work with raptors, which are birds of prey. She would take care of injured ones and nurse them back to health and set them free. Folk would bring them to her. She did not get paid for this: she just did it to help the birds. Suddenly this young woman came alive for me, and I dubbed her the Bird Maiden. I mentioned her in the Author's Note in the reprint of my Arabian Nights fantasy tale adaptation, *Hasan*. In that novel, the Bird Maiden had a feather suit which she could put on so that she could fly; Hasan captured her by hiding the feather suit. He married her and took her home. But later she recovered the suit and flew away, with

329

her two children. After a fabulous adventure, Hasan won her back. So there's really not much connection between that bird maiden and the one who cared for raptors, but I was satisfied with the designation and so was she, indeed, she flew overseas (today it is done by airplane) and was captured by a modern-day Hasan in Germany, fulfilling the romance.

So did she live happily ever after? Well, it's too soon to tell, but she had a scary moment in this period of my writing this novel. At this time the Bird Maiden has a daughter, Alessandra, eighteen months old, cute as only that age can be. After the Christmas holiday, with her husband back at work, Maiden decided to catch up on some postponed housework. She got a bucket of water, a sponge and a squeegee and started cleaning the windows of their upstairs apartment. She squeezed out past the heavy glass door, onto the balcony, into the just-above-freezing outer air and started scrubbing from outside while Alessandra watched from the warm inside. Maiden pretended to scrub the little girl's face through the glass: fun.

Then Maiden heard a familiar thud. Alessandra was clasping her hands with pride at her accomplishment. She had managed to operate the lever that effectively sealed the door back in place from inside. She was too small to work the lever the other way. Maiden was locked out on the balcony with the temperature in the 30s with no shoes, just a sweater and sweat pants. She had not expected to stay out long. The apartment's front door was locked from the inside with the key still in the lock; no one could enter that way. What was she to do?

She watched the street below, and hailed a little old lady on her bicycle. The lady tried not to laugh as she went to ring the bell of the folk in the apartment immediately below. The downstairs lady came out and threw Maiden a coat and pair of shoes, which she donned. Alessandra noted that, so she dashed to the coat rack and brought her own jacket and boots. Maiden tried to keep her occupied, but the little girl tired of that and ran to the kitchen, out of sight. What was she getting into?

The locksmith arrived and drilled out the lock. Alessandra reappeared and put her fingers into the new giant-sized key hole. The locksmith had to coax her to the side so he could finish. The door opened, and Maiden was rescued. Oh, sweet warmth; she had been sooo cold! She hugged Alessandra – and the little girl was disappointed. She knew that the excitement was over. But what a grand adventure it had been!

The Bird Maiden wondered how many more days like this there would be before her marvelous little girl turned eighteen years. 'So, how was *your* Christmas?!' she inquired.

Meanwhile, the world continued. Panama was invaded, and the Communist Empire crumbled. The United States population reached 250 million. Robert Adams, author of the Horse-clans series and a Florida resident, died. He was just under a year older than I. TV personality Andy Rooney was suspended because someone else claimed he had made a racist remark, though he denied it and has no record of racism. Apparently the TV executives have minds like fanzine editors. Then the program he was on dropped 20% in the ratings, and suddenly the execs had a change of heart and brought him back. I think those execs should have been suspended, not Rooney.

There is worse. At this time the child of Dr Elizabeth Morgan was discovered with grandparents in New Zealand. Dr Morgan had ascertained to her satisfaction that her daughter was being sexually molested by the father, but the court had decreed that unsupervised visits be allowed. Maybe I'm no expert, but too many correspondents have told me how they were molested as children; a man who does this takes any opportunity he can get, and an unsupervised visit is folly. I feel that Dr Morgan's caution was reasonable. So she hid her child rather than accede to this – and spent two years in jail for defying the will of the court. It took, literally, an act of congress to get her out. So much for trying to protect a child: the innocent gets punished instead of the guilty.

What happens when the mother does not try to protect her child? The book *Dark Obsession*, published at this time, showed how Bobby Sessions admitted in court to having sex five hundred times with his teenage stepdaughter. She finally blew the whistle on him, and he spent six months in a luxury hospital and was released. She was shipped to a fundamentalist home for troubled children where girls were regularly beaten.

But sometimes the worm does turn: she sued her stepfather and won $10 million.

Let's return to more positive business. I had mixed news on my ongoing projects. My erotic novel *Pornucopia*, published in America only in expensive hardcover and forbidden to readers under age 21, was selling well, and there was a flurry of interest by foreign publishers. I don't object to sex, you see, just to sexual abuse. My collaboration with a teenage boy who was killed by a reckless driver before completing his novel, *Through the Ice*, was published at the same time, and reports indicate it is also doing well. My 200,000 word historical novel about the American Indians who encountered Hernando de Soto, *Tatham Mound*, was taken by Morrow/Avon. The collaboration with Robert Margroff, *Orc's Opal*, was taken by Tor. I took time off *Virtual Mode* to do a chapter in my collaborative novel with Philip José Farmer, not yet titled, and a segment of 49,000 words was put on the market. The main female character there is Tappy, a blind thirteen year old girl, a bit like Colene in her isolation and the drama of her changing situation. I had started it as a story in 1963; a complicated situation and a quarter century had brought it to this point. The galleys for my provocative mainstream novel *Firefly* arrived, and I broke to proofread them. In that novel I show voluntary underage sex, the girl being five years old. More of this happens than we care to advertise.

I placed two of the last three novels which remained unsold from the days of my blacklisting in the 1970s, and set up to rework the third with a publisher interested. I had built up a total of eight unsold novels while weathering the blacklist – you can read about that too in my autobiography, but the essence is that I got in trouble for being right, somewhat in the manner of a whistleblower – and it was good to eliminate the last tangible vestige of it. This campaign of mine to get all my novels into print is one reason I may seem more prolific than I am; I've been writing novels steadily for twenty-five years, and by the end of 1990 the number of books I have had published may come to 82. That's about three and a quarter a year, average.

I read the finalists for a story contest and decided on the

winner. I reviewed revisions for the novel *Total Recall*, necessary to bring the paperback edition into conformance with late changes in the motion picture.

The ladies of Putnam/Berkley visited and brought me a print of the cover for *Phaze Doubt*: the editors had finally taken one of my suggestions, and got a beautiful cover painting of a little girl playing hopscotch with a BEM (Bug-Eyed Monster). At last we would see whether the author's notion of a good cover works to sell copies. You see at this writing I have made the *New York Times* bestseller list with eighteen different titles, which may be the record for this genre, but all have been in paperback, none in hardcover. Other fantasy writers make the list in hardcover; why can't I? Grumble. But in this period I did crack the *Publishers Weekly* hardcover list with the final Incarnations novel, *And Eternity*. Barely. I always was a slow starter.

I wrote a letter to a parole officer on behalf of a prisoner with AIDS, urging compassionate release, as he will otherwise be dead before he gets to see his folks outside. I had corresponded with him for two years, finding him to be a pleasant and principled person; I doubt he would be a menace to society.

My laser printer broke down shortly after the warranty expired: a counter which could not be reset, evidently defective when delivered. $20 part, $560 repair bill. Par for that course. Which brings me to my present computer setup, for those who are interested: Acer 900 AT-clone, 73M hard disk, 5.25 and 3.5 inch drives, VGA monitor, laser printer; Fansi-Console for my Dvorak keyboard, Sprint for word processing, XTreeGold for file handling. I got that last program in this period, and had a time-wasting ball playing with its nice features, such as the ability to set up parallel windows, with different directories in each, or to show and work with the files of several drives simultaneously. I had changed from Dec Rainbow with reluctance, but it was the readiest way to get Sprint, which looked like the ultimate word processor for me, and now I am quite satisfied with it. I set up the Piers Anthony Interface, which is in effect my own word processor, following my rules, like no others.

I started exploring the literature on computer games, playing with the notion of crafting a Xanth game that would be superior to what else exists. I know nothing about such games; naturally I figure I can do a better job than the experts, just as ignorant reviewers figure they could be better writers than I am. We shall see.

A reader advised me that the main thing at issue in her divorce settlement was custody of the collection of Anthony novels. Well, that seems reasonable to me.

And my daughter's horse, Blue: at this writing she is 32 years old, and still spry though her head is turning gray. When Blue came into our lives, horses galloped into my fiction, as you may have noticed. Unlike Seqiro, Blue can not read minds – I think.

I had a sore tongue during this novel. Finally, on the last day of editing, I figured it out: there was a roughness on a tooth, and my tongue was rubbing against it as I read my text to myself – I do that to hear it as well as see it, because I relate to it with more than one sense – that chafing was awful. So my wife hauled me into see the dentist the same day. Sure enough: a gold onlay (not inlay) had worn through, and there was an edge. Maybe now my tongue will heal.

Meanwhile the problems of the world accelerate and population runs out of control and the environment degrades apace. We are headed pell-mell for end-of-the-world disaster. About the only saving grace I see is the dawning awareness of increasing numbers of people that this has to stop. My daughter Penny brought home a book titled *How to Make the World a Better Place – a Guide for Doing Good,* which tackles questions of the environment, hunger, socially responsible investment and consumerism in a realistic manner. Many other good books are appearing, and I am getting them as I do preliminary research for a major novel relating to this subject. I feel obliged to turn my resources increasingly to the service of the universe rather than merely to my own well-being, and the talent I have for writing is my chief instrument. I try not to proselytize unduly in my fiction, but this is the Author's Note where I do speak my mind.

But let me finish on more personal notes, because these

Notes as I see them relate not to lectures but to feeling. I'm sure my readers differ from me on many things, but I hope that we share the essence of wonder and longing for what we may never quite understand.

I have pictures in my study of my wife at age one and a half or two, phenomenally cute, with her father. I had been looking at them, and then the song 'Scarlet Ribbons' came on and I suffered a certain siege of nostalgia for a situation I had never really known, for my wife was somewhat older when I met her. Our own daughters were like that, and they too have grown up. How precious children are! It is foolish to wish that time could stand still, yet tempting.

There was another episode in this period that touched my heart for inconsequential reason. My mother visited for two days. She is in the neighborhood of eighty and travels by train, and naturally the hours are inconvenient. We had to get up early to get her to the station on time. We used the house speaker system to wake us: at 5 AM the local radio station blared on throughout the house. As I was blindly scrambling into clothing, a popular song played. It was a pretty one, with touching words, in contrast to my bleary mood. It suggested that he close his eyes and let her take his hand so that he could feel the beating of her heart. I have a mental picture of bittersweet young Colene taking Darius' hand and holding it to her bosom, longing for love. Isn't that the way we all are, in the hell of our anonymity?

Marsh 8, 1990: Harpy Reading!